BRIEF CONTENTS

P9-CME-497

UNIT 1   INTRODUCTION TO COMMUNITY HEALTH NURSING

1 Health: A Community View, 1
2 Historical Factors: Community Health Nursing in Context, 18
3 Thinking Upstream: Nursing Theories and Population-Focused Nursing Practice, 36
4 Health Promotion and Risk Reduction, 49

UNIT 2   THE ART AND SCIENCE OF COMMUNITY HEALTH NURSING

5 Epidemiology, 59
6 Community Assessment, 92
7 Community Health Planning, Implementation, and Evaluation, 106
8 Community Health Education, 122
9 Case Management, 154

UNIT 3   FACTORS THAT INFLUENCE THE HEALTH OF THE COMMUNITY

10 Policy, Politics, Legislation, and Community Health Nursing, 165
11 The Health Care System, 186
12 Economics of Health Care, 202
13 Cultural Diversity and Community Health Nursing, 220
14 Environmental Health, 249
15 Health in the Global Community, 272

UNIT 4   AGGREGATES IN THE COMMUNITY

16 Child and Adolescent Health, 286
17 Women's Health, 314
18 Men's Health, 339
19 Senior Health, 355
20 Family Health, 380

UNIT 5   VULNERABLE POPULATIONS

21 Populations Affected by Disabilities, 403
22 Homeless Populations, 429
23 Rural and Migrant Health, 443
24 Populations Affected by Mental Illness, 468

UNIT 6   POPULATION HEALTH PROBLEMS

25 Communicable Disease, 488
26 Substance Abuse, 515
27 Violence, 542
28 Natural and Man-Made Disasters, 558

UNIT 7   COMMUNITY HEALTH SETTINGS

29 School Health, 580
30 Occupational Health, 598
31 Forensic and Correctional Nursing, 616
32 Faith Community Health, 631
33 Home Health and Hospice, 645

UNIT 1 INTRODUCTION TO COMMUNITY HEALTH NURSING

1 Health: A Community View, 1
2 Historical Factors: Community Health Nursing in Context, 13
3 Thinking Upstream: Nursing Theories and Population-Focused Nursing Practice, 36
4 Health Promotion and Risk Reduction, 49

UNIT 2 THE ART AND SCIENCE OF COMMUNITY HEALTH NURSING

5 Epidemiology, 73
6 Community Assessment, 92
7 Community Health Planning, Implementation, and Evaluation, 108
8 Community Health Education, 122
9 Case Management, 134

UNIT 3 FACTORS THAT INFLUENCE THE HEALTH OF THE COMMUNITY

10 Policy, Politics, Legislation, and Community Health Nursing, 165
11 The Health Care System, 186
12 Economics of Health Care, 202
13 Cultural Diversity and Community Health Nursing, 220
14 Environmental Health, 249
15 Health in the Global Community, 272

UNIT 4 AGGREGATES IN THE COMMUNITY

16 Child and Adolescent Health, 286
17 Women's Health, 313
18 Men's Health, 339
19 Senior Health, 355
20 Family Health, 380

UNIT 5 VULNERABLE POPULATIONS

21 Populations Affected by Disabilities, 401
22 Homeless Populations, 429
23 Rural and Migrant Health, 447
24 Populations Affected by Mental Illness, 464

UNIT 6 POPULATION HEALTH PROBLEMS

25 Communicable Disease, 488
26 Substance Abuse, 515
27 Violence, 542
28 Natural and Man-Made Disasters, 558

UNIT 7 COMMUNITY HEALTH SETTINGS

29 School Health, 580
30 Occupational Health, 598
31 Forensic and Correctional Nursing, 616
32 Faith Community Health, 631
33 Home Health and Hospice, 645

Community/ Public Health Nursing

6th Edition

Promoting the Health of Populations

Mary A. Nies, PhD, RN, FAAN, FAAHB
Dean and Professor School of Nursing
Joint Appointment MPH Program
Division of Health Sciences
Idaho State University
Pocatello, Idaho

Melanie McEwen, PhD, RN, CNE, ANEF
Associate Professor
University of Texas Health Science Center at Houston
School of Nursing
Houston, Texas

ELSEVIER

ELSEVIER
SAUNDERS

3251 Riverport Lane
St. Louis, Missouri 63043

COMMUNITY/PUBLIC HEALTH NURSING: PROMOTING
THE HEALTH OF POPULATIONS   ISBN: 978-0-323-18819-7
Copyright © 2015, 2011, 2007, 2001, 1997, 1993 by Saunders, an imprint of Elsevier Inc.

Notices

Knowledge and best practice in this field are constantly changing. As new research and experience broaden our understanding, changes in research methods, professional practices, or medical treatment may become necessary.

Practitioners and researchers must always rely on their own experience and knowledge in evaluating and using any information, methods, compounds, or experiments described herein. In using such information or methods they should be mindful of their own safety and the safety of others, including parties for whom they have a professional responsibility.

With respect to any drug or pharmaceutical products identified, readers are advised to check the most current information provided (i) on procedures featured or (ii) by the manufacturer of each product to be administered, to verify the recommended dose or formula, the method and duration of administration, and contraindications. It is the responsibility of practitioners, relying on their own experience and knowledge of their patients, to make diagnoses, to determine dosages and the best treatment for each individual patient, and to take all appropriate safety precautions.

To the fullest extent of the law, neither the Publisher nor the authors, contributors, or editors, assume any liability for any injury and/or damage to persons or property as a matter of products liability, negligence or otherwise, or from any use or operation of any methods, products, instructions, or ideas contained in the material herein.

Library of Congress Cataloging-in-Publication Data

Community/public health nursing : promoting the health of populations / [edited by] Mary A. Nies, Melanie McEwen. -- Edition 6.
   p. ; cm.
   Includes bibliographical references and index.
   ISBN 978-0-323-18819-7 (pbk. : alk. paper)
   I. Nies, Mary A. (Mary Albrecht), editor. II. McEwen, Melanie, editor.
   [DNLM: 1. Community Health Nursing. 2. Health Promotion. 3. Public Health Nursing. WY 106]
   RT98
   610.73'43--dc23
                                                                        2014023359

Director, Traditional Education: Kristin Geen
Senior Content Strategist: Nancy O'Brien
Content Development Specialist: Jennifer Shropshire
Publishing Services Manager: Deborah L. Vogel
Project Manager: John W. Gabbert
Design Direction: Karen Pauls

Printed in China

Last digit is the print number: 9 8 7 6 5 4 3 2 1

*To Phil Yankovich, my husband, companion, and best friend, whose love,
caring, and true support are always there for me. He provides
me with the energy I need to pursue my dreams.*

*To Kara Nies Yankovich, my daughter, for whom I wish a happy and healthy life.
Her energy, joy, and enthusiasm for life give so much to me.*

*To Earl and Lois Nies, my parents,
for their never-ending encouragement and lifelong support.
They helped me develop a foundation for creative thinking, new ideas,
and spirited debate.*

Mary A. Nies

*To my husband, Scott McEwen, whose love, support, and encouragement have been my
foundation for the past thirty-five years. I can't wait to see what happens next!*

Melanie McEwen

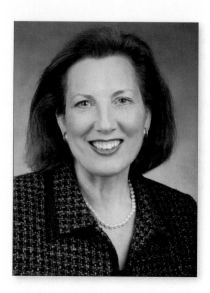

Mary A. Nies

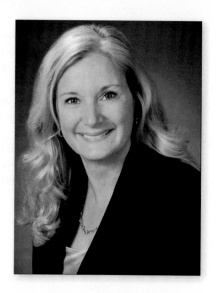

Melanie McEwen

Mary A. Nies, PhD, RN, FAAN, FAAHB is the Dean and Professor School of Nursing, Joint Appointment MPH Program, Division of Health Sciences, Idaho State University. Dr. Nies received her diploma from Bellin School of Nursing in Green Bay, Wisconsin; her BSN from University of Wisconsin, Madison; her MSN from Loyola University, Chicago; and her PhD in Public Health Nursing, Health Services, and Health Promotion Research at the University of Illinois, Chicago. She completed a postdoctoral research fellowship in health promotion and community health at the University of Michigan, Ann Arbor. She is a fellow of the American Academy of Nursing and a fellow of the American Academy of Health Behavior. Dr. Nies co-edited *Community Health Nursing: Promoting the Health of Aggregates,* which received the 1993 Book of the Year award from the *American Journal of Nursing.* Her program of research focuses on the outcomes of health promotion interventions for minority and nonminority populations in the community. Her research is involved with physical activity and obesity prevention for populations, especially women. Her research is involved with physical activity and obesity prevention for vulnerable populations.

Melanie McEwen, PhD, RN, CNE, ANEF is an Associate Professor at the University of Texas Health Science Center at Houston School of Nursing. Dr. McEwen received her BSN from the University of Texas School of Nursing in Austin; her Master's in Community and Public Health Nursing from Louisiana State University Medical Center in New Orleans; and her PhD in Nursing at Texas Woman's University. Dr. McEwen has been a nursing educator for more than 22 years and is also the co-author of *Community–Based Nursing: An Introduction* (Elsevier, 2009) and co-author/editor of *Theoretical Basis for Nursing* (Lippincott, Williams and Wilkins, 2014).

Carrie Buch, PhD, RN
Associate Professor
Oakland University
School of Nursing
Rochester, Michigan
Chapter 13: Cultural Diversity and Community Health Nursing
Chapter 33: Home Health and Hospice

Patricia M. Burbank, DNSc, RN
Professor
College of Nursing
The University of Rhode Island
Kingston, Rhode Island
Chapter 7: Community Health Planning, Implementation, and Evaluation

Holly B. Cassells, PhD, MPH, RN
Professor
School of Nursing and Health Professions
University of the Incarnate Word
San Antonio, Texas
Chapter 5: Epidemiology
Chapter 6: Community Assessment

Stacy A. Drake, MSN, MPH, RN
Instructor
The University of Texas Health Science Center at Houston
School of Nursing
Houston, Texas

Nellie S. Droes, DNSc, RN, CS
Associate Professor, Emerita
School of Nursing
East Carolina University
Rivers Building
Greenville, North Carolina
Chapter 22: Homeless Populations

Anita Finkelman, MSN, RN
Visiting Faculty
School of Nursing
Bouvé College of Health Sciences
Northeastern University
Boston, Massachusetts
Chapter 10: The Health Care System
Chapter 11: The Health Care System
Chapter 12: Economics of Health Care

Susan Givens, RNC-OB, MPH, LCCE
Childbirth Educator
Mount Carmel St. Ann's Hospital
Westerville, Ohio
Chapter 16: Child and Adolescent Health

Lori A. Glenn, DNP, CNM, RN
Assistant Professor
McAuley School of Nursing
University of Detroit Mercy
Detroit, Michigan
Nurse Midwife
Hurley Medical Center
Flint, Michigan
Chapter 17: Women's Health

Deanna E. Grimes, DrPH, RN, FAAN
Professor
University of Texas Health Science Center at Houston
Houston, Texas

Karyn Leavitt Grow, MS, BSN, RN, CCM
Manager, Case Manager
Sierra Surgery Hospital
Carson City, Nevada
Chapter 9: Case Management

Diane C. Hatton, PhD, RN
Consultant
Reno, Nevada
Chapter 22: Homeless Populations

Jené M. Hurlbut, PhD, MSN, RN, CNE
Associate Professor
Roseman University of Health Sciences
Henderson, Nevada
Chapter 18: Men's Health

Kim Jardine-Dickerson, RN, MSN, BC, CADC
Assistant Clinical Professor
Idaho State University
Pocatello, Idaho
Chapter 24: Populations Affected by Mental Illness
Chapter 26: Substance Abuse

Angela Jarrell, PhD, RN
Nurse Consultant
Duquesne University
Pittsburgh, Pennsylvania
Chapter 31: Forensic and Correctional Nursing

Jean Cozad Lyon, PhD, APN
Hospital Surveyor
The Joint Commission
Reno, Nevada
Chapter 9: Case Management

Diane Cocozza Martins, PhD, RN
Associate Professor
College of Nursing
University of Rhode Island
Kingston, Rhode Island
Chapter 3: Thinking Upstream: Nursing Theories and Population-Focused Nursing Practice
Chapter 7: Community Health Planning, Implementation, and Evaluation

Cathy D. Meade, PhD, RN, FAAN
Senior Member and Professor
Population Science
Health Outcomes & Behavior
Moffitt Cancer Center
University of South Florida
Tampa, Florida
Chapter 8: Community Health Education

Julie Cowan Novak, DNSc, RN, CPNP, FAANP
Professor and Vice Dean, Practice and Engagement
Executive Director, UT Nursing Clinical Enterprise, UTHSCSA Student Health Center and Employee Health and Wellness Clinic
UT Health Science Center San Antonio School of Nursing
San Antonio, Texas
Chapter 15: Health in the Global Community

Catherine A. Pourciau, MSN, RN, FNP-C
Family Nurse Practitioner
Internal Medicine and Pediatric Clinic
Baker, Louisiana
Chapter 27: Violence
Chapter 29: School Health

Bridgette Crotwell Pullis, PhD, RN, CHPN
Assistant Professor of Nursing
The University of Texas Health Science Center – Houston School of Nursing
Houston, Texas
Chapter 4: Health Promotion and Risk Reduction

Bonnie Rogers, DrPH, COHN-S, LNCC
Director, NC Occupational Safety and
    Health and Education and Research
Center and OHN Program
University of North Carolina
School of Public Health
Chapel Hill, North Carolina
Chapter 30: Occupational Health

**Mary Ellen Trail Ross, DrPH, MSN,
    RN, GCNS-BC**
Associate Professor of Clinical Nursing
Department of Nursing Systems
University of Texas Health Science Center
Houston, Texas
Chapter 19: Senior Health

**Diane Santa Maria, MSN, RN,
    APHN-BC**
Clinical Faculty
University of Texas School of Nursing
Houston, Texas
Chapter 14: Environmental Health

Beverly Siegrist, EdD, MS, RN, CNE
Professor
Department of Nursing
Western Kentucky University
Bowling Green, Kentucky
Chapter 20: Family Health
Chapter 32: Faith Community Nursing

**Edith B. Summerlin, PhD, MSN, BSN,
    RN, CNS**
Assistant Professor
University of Texas Health Science Center
    at Houston
School of Nursing
Houston, Texas
Chapter 19: Senior Health
*Chapter 28: Natural and Man-made
    Disasters*

Patricia L. Thomas, PhD, RN
Director, Nursing Practice & Research
Trinity Health
Livonia, Michigan
Chapter 23: Rural and Migrant Health

**Meredith Troutman-Jordan, PhD,
    PMHCNS-BC**
Associate Professor
University of North Carolina at Charlotte
College of Health and Human Services,
    School of Nursing
Charlotte, North Carolina
*Chapter 21: Populations Affected by
    Disabilities*

Elaine Vallette, DrPH, RN
Dean, Nursing and Allied Health
Baton Rouge Community College
Baton Rouge, Louisiana
Chapter 27: Violence
Chapter 29: School Health

**Lori Wightman, MSN, DNP, RN,
    NEA-BC**
Chief Nursing Officer
Mercy Hospital Grayling
Grayling, Michigan
Chapter 23: Rural and Migrant Health

ANCILLARY AUTHORS

Joanna E. Cain, BSN, BA, RN
President and Founder
Auctorial Pursuits, Inc.
Atlanta, Georgia
NCLEX Review Questions
TEACH for RN-Case Studies

Penny Leake, PhD, RN
Professor Emerita of Nursing
Luther College
Decorah, Iowa
PowerPoint Slides

Tiffany M. Smith, MSN, RN
PhD student/Graduate Assistant
Roseman University of Health Sciences
University of Nevada
Las Vegas, Nevada
Case Studies

**Anna K. Wehling Weepie, DNP, RN,
    CNE, COI**
Assistant Dean, Undergraduate Nursing
    and Professor
Allen College
Waterloo, Iowa
Test Bank

REVIEWERS

**Edna M. Billingsley, MSN, RN,
    PMHN-C, CLNC, GNP**
Assistant Professor of Nursing
Bethel University
McKenzie, Tennessee

**Barbara Broome, RN, MSN, PhD,
    FAAN**
Associate Dean and Chair Community/
    Mental Health Nursing, Professor
University of South Alabama College of
    Nursing
Mobile, Alabama

**Stephanie Chalupka, EdD, RN,
    PCHCNS-BC, FAAOHN**
Associate Dean for Nursing
Worcester State University
Worcester, Massachusetts

Colleen L. Ciano, MSN, RN, PhD (c)
Instructor of Nursing
The Pennsylvania State University
Middletown, Pennsylvania

Connie Cooper, EdD, RN, CNE
Assistant Professor
Bellarmine University
Louisville, Kentucky

Michelle T. Dang, PhD, RN, APHN-BC
Assistant Professor
California State University, Sacramento
Sacramento, California

Lisa Garsman, MS, FNP-BC
Director BSN Program
Saint Peter's University
Jersey City, New Jersey

**Scharmaine Lawson-Baker, DNP,
    FNP-BC, FAANP**
CEO/Founder
Advanced Clinical Consultants
New Orleans, Louisiana

Lisa M. LeBlanc, RN, BSN
Instructor of Nursing
Wisconsin Lutheran College
Milwaukee, Wisconsin

Patricia S. Martin, RN, MSN
Assistant Professor
University of Louisville
Louisville, Kentucky

**Nancy N. Menzel, PhD, RN, PHCNS-
    BC, CPH**
Associate Professor, Nursing
University of Nevada, Las Vegas
Las Vegas, Nevada

**Lynn M. Miskovich, DNP, ANP-BC,
    APRN**
Associate Professor of Nursing
Purdue University Calumet
Hammond, Indiana

Patti Moss, MSN, RN
Assistant Professor, Nursing
Lamar University
Beaumont, Texas

Jill M. Nocella, MSN, RN
Professor of Nursing
William Paterson University
Wayne, New Jersey

Vicky L. O'Neil, DNP, APRN, FNP-BC
Associate Professor
Dixie State College of Utah
St. George, Utah

Laura Opton, MSN, RN, CNE
Second Degree BSN Program Director
Texas Tech University Health Sciences
    Center
Lubbock, Texas

Susan Palmer, MSN, RN
Lecturer
Fairleigh Dickinson University
Teaneck, New Jersey

Fay Parpart, MS, RN, ANP-BC
Assistant Clinical Professor
Virginia Commonwealth University
Richmond, Virginia

Keevia Porter, DNP, MSN, NP-C, RN
Assistant Professor BSN/MSN Programs
University of Tennessee Health Science
    Center, College of Nursing
Memphis, Tennessee

Cynthia Portman, MSN, RN
Assistant Clinical Professor in Nursing
Department of Nursing and Rehab Sciences
Angelo State University
San Angelo, Texas

Joann Sands, ANP-BC, MSN, RN
Clinical Instructor
The State University of New York – University
    at Buffalo
Buffalo, New York

Charlotte Sortedahl, DNP, MPH, MS, BSN, RN
Assistant Professor
University of Wisconsin – Eau Claire
Eau Claire, Wisconsin

Marnie Lynn Sperling, DMD, MSN, RN, FN-CSA
Assistant Professor, Nursing
Caldwell College
Caldwell, New Jersey

Debbie Sweeney, RN, DNSc
Associate Professor, Nursing
Baptist College of Health Sciences
Memphis, Tennessee

Virginia Teel, DHSc, RN
Assistant Professor, Nursing
College of Coastal Georgia
Brunswick, Georgia

Julie B. Willardson, DNP, FNP-C
Assistant Professor of Nursing
Roseman University of Health Sciences,
    College of Nursing
South Jordan, Utah

PREFACE

More money is spent per capita for health care in the United States than in any other country ($8400 in 2010). However, many countries have far better indices of health, including traditional indicators such as infant mortality rates and longevity for both men and women than does the United States. The United States is one of the few industrialized countries in the world that lacks a program of national health services or national health insurance. Although the United States spent 17.9% of its gross domestic product on health care expenditures in 2010, a record high of $2.6 trillion, before full implementation of the Affordable Care Act, nearly 18.0% of the population had no health care coverage.

The greater the proportion of money put into health care expenditures in the United States, the less money there is to improve education, jobs, housing, and nutrition. Over the years, the greatest improvements in the health of the population have been achieved through advances in public health using organized community efforts, such as improvements in sanitation, immunizations, and food quality and quantity. The greatest determinants of health are still equated with factors in the community, such as education, employment, housing, and nutrition. Although access to health care services and individual behavioral changes are important, they are only components of the larger determinants of health, such as social and physical environments.

UPSTREAM FOCUS

The traditional focus of many health care professionals, known as a downstream focus, has been to deliver health care services to ill people and to encourage needed behavioral change at the individual level. The focus of public/community health nursing has traditionally been on health promotion and illness prevention by working with individuals and families within the community. A shift is needed to an upstream focus, which includes working with aggregates and communities in activities such as organizing and setting health policy. This focus will help aggregates and communities work to create options for healthier environments with essential components of health, including adequate education, housing, employment, and nutrition and provide choices that allow people to make behavioral changes, live and work in safe environments, and access equitable and comprehensive health care.

Grounded in the tenets of public health nursing and the practice of public health nurses such as Lillian Wald, this sixth edition of *Community/Public Health Nursing: Promoting the Health of Populations* builds on the earlier works by highlighting an aggregate focus in addition to the traditional areas of family and community health, and thus promotes upstream thinking. The primary focus is on the promotion of the health of aggregates. This approach includes the family as a population and addresses the needs of other aggregates or population subgroups. It conceptualizes the individual as a member of the family and as a member of other aggregates, including organizations and institutions. Furthermore, individuals and families are viewed as a part of a population within an environment (i.e., within a community).

An aggregate is made up of a collective of individuals, be it family or another group that, with others, make up a community. This text emphasizes the aggregate as a unit of focus and how aggregates that make up communities promote their own health. The aggregate is presented within the social context of the community, and students are given the opportunity to define and analyze environmental, economic, political, and legal constraints to the health of these populations.

Community/public health nursing has been determined to be a synthesis of nursing and public health practice with goals to promote and preserve the health of populations. Diagnosis and treatment of human responses to actual or potential health problems is the nursing component. The ability to prevent disease, prolong life, and promote health through organized community effort is from the public health component. Community/public health nursing practice is responsible to the population as a whole. Nursing efforts to promote health and prevent disease are applied to the public, which includes all units in the community, be they individual or collective (e.g., person, family, other aggregate, community, or population).

PURPOSE OF THE TEXT

In this text, the student is encouraged to become a student of the community, learn from families and other aggregates in the community how they define and promote their own health, and learn how to become an advocate of the community by working with the community to initiate change. The student is exposed to the complexity and rich diversity of the community and is shown evidence of how the community organizes to meet change.

The use of language or terminology by clients and agencies varies in different parts of the United States, and it may vary from that used by government officials. The contributors to this text are a diverse group from various parts of the United States. Their terms vary from chapter to chapter and vary from those in use in local communities. For example, some authors refer to African-Americans, some to blacks, some to European-Americans, and some to whites. The student must be familiar with a range of terms and, most important, know what is used in his or her local community.

Outstanding features of this sixth edition include its provocative nature as it raises consciousness regarding the social inequalities that exist in the United States and how the market-driven health care system contributes to prevention of the realization of health as a right for all. With a focus on social justice, this text emphasizes society's responsibility for the protection of all human life to ensure that all people have their basic needs met, such as adequate health protection and income. Attention to the impact of implementation of the Affordable Care Act as well as the need for further reform of the systems of health reimbursement has enhanced the recognition of the need for population-focused care, or care that covers all people residing within geographic boundaries, rather than only those populations enrolled in insurance plans. Working toward providing health promotion and population-focused care to all requires a dramatic shift in thinking from individual-focused care for the practitioners of the future. The future paradigm for health care is demanding that the focus of nursing move toward population-based interventions if we are to forge toward the goals established in *Healthy People 2020.*

This text is designed to **stimulate critical thinking and challenge students to question and debate issues.** Complex problems demand complex answers; therefore, the student is expected to *synthesize prior biophysical, psychosocial, cultural, and ethical arenas of knowledge.* However, experiential knowledge is also necessary and the student is challenged to *enter new environments within the community* and gain new sensory, cognitive, and affective experiences. The authors of this text have integrated the concept of **upstream thinking**, introduced in the first edition, throughout this sixth edition as an important conceptual basis for nursing practice of aggregates and the community. The student is introduced to the individual and aggregate roles of community health nurses as they are engaged in a collective and interdisciplinary manner, working **upstream**, to facilitate the community's promotion of its own health. Students using this text will be better prepared to work with aggregates and communities in health promotion and with individuals and families in illness. Students using this text will also be better prepared to see the need to take responsibility for participation in organized community action targeting inequalities in arenas such as education, jobs, and housing and to participate in targeting individual health-behavioral change. These are important shifts in thinking for future practitioners who must be prepared to function in a population-focused health care system.

The text is also designed to increase the **cultural awareness and competency** of future community health nurses as they prepare to address the needs of culturally diverse populations. Students must be prepared to work with these growing populations as participation in the nursing workforce by ethnically and racially diverse people continues to lag. Various models are introduced to help students understand the growing link between social problems and health status, experienced disproportionately by diverse populations in the United States, and understand the methods of assessment and intervention used to meet the special needs of these populations.

The goals of the text are to provide the student with the ability to assess the complex factors in the community that affect individual, family, and other aggregate responses to health states and actual or potential health problems; and

to help students use this ability to plan, implement, and evaluate community/public health nursing interventions to increase contributions to the promotion of the health of populations.

MAJOR THEMES RELATED TO PROMOTING THE HEALTH OF POPULATIONS

This text is built on the following major themes:
- A social justice ethic of health care in contrast to a market justice ethic of health care in keeping with the philosophy of public health as "health for all"
- A population-focused model of community/public health nursing as necessary to achieve equity in health for the entire population
- Integration of the concept of *upstream thinking* throughout the text and other appropriate theoretical frameworks related to chapter topics
- The use of population-focused and other community data to develop an assessment, or profile of health, and potential and actual health needs and capabilities of aggregates
- The application of all steps in the nursing process at the individual, family, and aggregate levels
- A focus on identification of needs of the aggregate from common interactions with individuals, families, and communities in traditional environments
- An orientation toward the application of all three levels of prevention at the individual, family, and aggregate levels
- The experience of the underserved aggregate, particularly the economically disenfranchised, including cultural and ethnic groups disproportionately at risk of developing health problems.

Themes are developed and related to promoting the health of populations in the following ways:
- The commitment of community/public health nursing is to an equity model; therefore, community health nurses work toward the provision of the unmet health needs of populations.
- The development of a population-focused model is necessary to close the gap between unmet health care needs and health resources on a geographic basis to the entire population. The contributions of intervention at the aggregate level work toward the realization of such a model.
- Contemporary theories provide frameworks for holistic community health nursing practice that help the students conceptualize the reciprocal influence of various components within the community on the health of aggregates and the population.
- The ability to gather population-focused and other community data in developing an assessment of health is a crucial initial step that precedes the identification of nursing diagnoses and plans to meet aggregate responses to potential and actual health problems.
- The nursing process includes, in each step, a focus on the aggregate, assessment of the aggregate, nursing diagnosis of the aggregate, planning for the aggregate, and intervention and evaluation at the aggregate level.

- The text discusses development of the ability to gather clues about the needs of aggregates from complex environments, such as during a home visit, with parents in a waiting room of a well-baby clinic, or with elders receiving hypertension screening, and to promote individual, collective, and political action that addresses the health of aggregates.
- Primary, secondary, and tertiary prevention strategies include a major focus at the population level.
- In addition to offering a chapter on cultural influences in the community, the text includes data on and the experience of underserved aggregates at high risk of developing health problems and who are most often in need of community health nursing services (i.e., low and marginal income, cultural, and ethnic groups) throughout.

ORGANIZATION

The text is divided into seven units. *Unit 1, Introduction to Community Health Nursing*, presents an overview of the concept of health, a perspective of health as evolving and as defined by the community, and the concept of community health nursing as the nursing of aggregates from both historical and contemporary mandates. Health is viewed as an individual and collective right, brought about through individual and collective/political action. The definitions of public health and community health nursing and their foci are presented. Current crises in public health and the health care system and consequences for the health of the public frame implications for community health nursing. The historical evolution of public health, the health care system, and community health nursing is presented. The evolution of humans from wanderers and food gatherers to those who live in larger groups is presented. The text also discusses the influence of the group on health, which contrasts with the evolution of a health care system built around the individual person, increasingly fractured into many parts. Community health nurses bring to their practice awareness of the social context; economic, political, and legal constraints from the larger community; and knowledge of the current health care system and its structural constraints and limitations on the care of populations. The theoretical foundations for the text, with a focus on the concept of upstream thinking, and the rationale for a population approach to community health nursing are presented. Recognizing the importance of health promotion and risk reduction when striving to improve the health of individuals, families, groups, and communities, this unit concludes with a chapter elaborating on those concepts. Strategies for assessment and analysis of risk factors and interventions to improve health are described.

Unit 2, The Art and Science of Community Health Nursing, describes application of the nursing process—assessment, planning, intervention, and evaluation—to aggregates in the community using selected theory bases. The unit addresses the need for a population focus that includes the public health sciences of biostatistics and epidemiology as key in community assessment and the application of the nursing process to aggregates to promote the health of populations. Application of the art and science of community health nursing to meeting the needs of aggregates is evident in chapters that focus on community health planning and evaluation, community health education, and case management.

Unit 3, Factors That Influence the Health of the Community, examines factors and issues that can both positively and negatively affect health. Beginning with an overview of health policy and legislation, the opening chapter in this unit focuses on how policy is developed and the effect of past and future legislative changes on how health care is delivered in the United States. This unit examines the health care delivery system and the importance of economics and health care financing on the health of individuals, families, and populations. Cultural diversity and associated issues are described in detail, showing the importance of consideration of culture when developing health interventions in the community. The influence of the environment on the health of populations is considered, and the reader is led to recognize the multitude of external factors that influence health. This unit concludes with an examination of various aspects of global health and describes features of the health care systems and patterns of health and illness in developing and developed countries.

Unit 4, Aggregates in the Community, presents the application of the nursing process to address potential health problems identified in large groups, including children and adolescents, women, men, families, and seniors. The focus is on the major indicators of health (e.g., longevity, mortality, and morbidity), types of common health problems, use of health services, pertinent legislation, health services and resources, selected applications of the community health nursing process to a case study, application of the levels of prevention, selected roles of the community health nurse, and relevant research.

Unit 5, Vulnerable Populations, focuses on those aggregates in the community considered vulnerable: persons with disabilities, the homeless, those living in rural areas including migrant workers, and persons with mental illness. Chapters address the application of the community health nursing process to the special service needs in each of these areas. Basic community health nursing strategies are applied to promoting the health of these vulnerable high-risk aggregates.

Unit 6, Population Health Problems, focuses on health problems that affect large aggregates and their service needs as applied in community health nursing. These problems include communicable disease, violence and associated issues, substance abuse, and a chapter describing nursing care during disasters.

Unit 7, Community Health Settings, focuses on selected sites or specialties for community health: school health, occupational health, faith community health, and home health and hospice. Finally, forensic nursing, one of the more recently added sub-specialty areas of community health nursing, is presented in this unit, combined with correctional nursing content.

SPECIAL FEATURES

The following features are presented to enhance student learning:

- **Learning objectives.** Learning objectives set the framework for the content of each chapter.
- **Key terms.** A list of key terms for each chapter is provided at the beginning of the chapter. The terms are highlighted in blue within the chapter. The definitions of these terms are found in the Glossary located on the book's Evolve website.
- **Chapter outline.** The major headings of each chapter are provided at the beginning of each chapter to help locate important content.
- **Theoretical frameworks.** The use of theoretical frameworks common to nursing and public health will aid the student in application of familiar and new theory bases to problems and challenges in the community.
- *Healthy People 2020.* Goals and objectives of *Healthy People 2020* are presented in a special box throughout the text. (The updated *Healthy People 2020* information is new to this edition and based on the proposed objectives.)
- **Upstream thinking.** This theoretical construct is integrated into chapters throughout the text.
- **Case studies and application of the nursing process at individual, family, and aggregate levels.** The use of case studies and **clinical examples** throughout the text is designed to ground the theory, concepts, and application of the nursing process in practical and manageable examples for the student.
- **Research highlights.** The introduction of students to the growing bodies of community health nursing and public health research literature are enhanced by special boxes devoted to specific research studies.
- **Boxed information.** Summaries of content by section, clinical examples, and other pertinent information are presented in colored text to aid the students' learning by focusing on major points, illustrating concepts, and breaking up sections of "heavy" content.
- **Learning activities.** Selected learning activities are listed at the end of each chapter to enable students to enhance learning about the community and cognitive experiences.
- **Photo novellas.** Numerous stories in photograph form depicting public health care in a variety of settings and with different population groups.
- **Ethical insights boxes.** These boxes present situations of ethical dilemmas or considerations pertinent to particular chapters.
- **Veterans' Health boxes.** New to this edition, these boxes present situations and considerations pertinent to the care of veterans.

NEW CONTENT IN THIS EDITION

- New and timely information on **emerging infections** (e.g., H1N1, SARS, West Nile virus) and changing recommendations (e.g., pediatric immunization schedule) are given in the Communicable Disease chapter.

- Reflecting the need for enhanced education and information related to the specific needs and issues for our country's veterans, most chapters include at least one box highlighting veteran's health care in relation to the chapter's topic.
- Most chapters contain new or updated **Research Highlights boxes** highlighting timely, relevant examples of the topics from recent nursing literature and **Ethical Insights boxes** that emphasize specific ethical issues.

TEACHING AND LEARNING PACKAGE

Evolve website: The website at http://evolve.elsevier.com/nies/ is devoted exclusively to this text. It provides materials for both instructors and students.

- **For Instructors:** PowerPoint lecture slides, image collection, and more than 900 test bank questions with alternative item questions as well as the new TEACH for Nurses, which contains detailed chapter Lesson Plans including references to curriculum standards such as QSEN, BSN Essentials and Concepts, BSN Essentials for Public Health, and new and unique Case Studies.
- **For Students:** Quiz with multiple-choice questions with answers and correct answer rationales, Case Studies with questions and answers, a Glossary, and Resource Tools (supplemental material).

ACKNOWLEDGMENTS

Community/Public Health Nursing: Promoting the Health of Populations could not have been written without sharing the experiences, thoughtful critique, and support of many people: individuals, families, groups, and communities. We give special thanks to everyone who made significant contributions to this book.

We are indebted to our contributing authors whose inspiration, untiring hours of work, and persistence have continued to build a new era of community health nursing practice with a focus on the population level. We thank the community health nursing faculty and students who welcomed the previous editions of the text and responded to our inquiries with comments and suggestions for the sixth edition. These people have challenged us to stretch, adapt, and continue to learn throughout our years of work. We also thank our colleagues in our respective work settings for their understanding and support during the writing and editing of this edition.

Finally, an enormous "thank you" to Elsevier editors Jennifer Shropshire, Nancy O'Brien, and Johnny Gabbert. Their energy, enthusiasm, encouragement, direction, and patience were essential to this project.

Mary A. Nies
Melanie McEwen

CONTENTS

UNIT 1 INTRODUCTION TO COMMUNITY HEALTH NURSING

1 Health: A Community View, 1
   Melanie McEwen and Mary A. Nies
      Definitions of Health and Community, 3
         Health, 3
         Community, 3
      Determinants of Health and Disease, 4
      Indicators of Health and Illness, 5
      Definition and Focus of Public Health and
         Community Health, 6
      Preventive Approach to Health, 7
         *Health Promotion and Levels of
            Prevention, 7*
         Prevention versus Cure, 8
         Healthy People 2020, 9
      Definition and Focus of Public Health
         Nursing, Community Health Nursing,
         and Community-Based Nursing, 10
         Public and Community Health Nursing, 10
         Community-Based Nursing, 11
         *Community and Public Health Nursing
            Practice, 11*
      Population-Focused Practice and
         Community/Public Health Nursing
         Interventions, 11
         Community Health Interventions, 13
         The Public Health Intervention Wheel, 14
      Community Health Nursing, Managed Care,
         and Health Reform, 15

2 Historical Factors: Community Health Nursing
   in Context, 18
   Melanie McEwen
      Evolution of Health in Western
         Populations, 19
         Aggregate Impact on Health, 19
         Evolution of Early Public Health Efforts, 20
      Advent of Modern Health Care, 23
         Evolution of Modern Nursing, 23
         *Establishment of Modern Medical Care
            and Public Health Practice, 24*
         Community Caregiver, 27
         Establishment of Public Health Nursing, 28

         Consequences for the Health of
            Aggregates, 30
         Twenty-First Century, 30
      Social Changes and Community Health
         Nursing, 31
      Challenges for Community and Public
         Health Nursing, 32

3 Thinking Upstream: Nursing Theories and
   Population-Focused Nursing Practice, 36
   Diane C. Martins
      Thinking Upstream: Examining the Root
         Causes of Poor Health, 37
      Historical Perspectives on Nursing Theory,
         37
      How Theory Provides Direction to Nursing,
         38
      Microscopic Versus Macroscopic Approaches
         to the Conceptualization of Community
         Health Problems, 38
      Assessing a Theory's Scope in Relation to
         Community Health Nursing, 39
      Review of Theoretical Approaches, 39
         The Individual Is the Focus of Change, 40
         *The Upstream View: Society Is the Focus of
            Change, 41*
         Healthy People 2020, 45

4 Health Promotion and Risk Reduction, 49
   Bridgette Crotwell Pullis and Mary A. Nies
      Health Promotion and Community Health
         Nursing, 49
         Healthy People 2020, 51
      Determinants of Health, 51
      Theories in Health Promotion, 53
         Pender's Health Promotion Model, 53
         The Health Belief Model, 53
         The Transtheoretical Model, 54
         Theory of Reasoned Action, 55
      Risk and Health, 56
      The Relationship of Risk to Health and
         Health Promotion Activities, 57
         Tobacco and Health Risk, 58
         Alcohol Consumption and Health, 60
         Diet and Health, 62
         Physical Activity and Health, 65
         Sleep, 65

UNIT 2   THE ART AND SCIENCE OF COMMUNITY HEALTH NURSING

5 Epidemiology, 69
   Holly B. Cassells
      **Use of Epidemiology in Disease Control
         and Prevention, 70**
      Calculation of Rates, 74
         *Morbidity: Incidence and Prevalence
            Rates, 74*
         Other Rates, 75
      Concept of Risk, 77
      **Use of Epidemiology in Disease
         Prevention, 78**
         Primary Prevention, 78
         Secondary and Tertiary Prevention, 78
         Establishing Causality, 79
         Screening, 79
         Surveillance, 81
      Use of Epidemiology in Health Services, 82
      Epidemiological Methods, 83
         Descriptive Epidemiology, 83
         Analytic Epidemiology, 83
6 Community Assessment, 92
   Holly B. Cassells
      The Nature of Community, 93
         Aggregate of People, 93
         Location in Space and Time, 93
         Social System, 94
      Healthy Communities, 94
      **Assessing the Community: Sources of
         Data, 95**
         Census Data, 97
         Vital Statistics, 98
         Other Sources of Health Data, 99
      Needs Assessment, 99
      Diagnosing Health Problems, 101
7 Community Health Planning, Implementation,
   and Evaluation, 106
   Diane C. Martins and Patricia M. Burbank
      Overview of Health Planning, 107
      Health Planning Model, 108
         Assessment, 109
         Planning, 111
         Intervention, 111
         Evaluation, 112
      Health Planning Projects, 112
         Successful Projects, 112
         Unsuccessful Projects, 113
         Discussion, 114

      Health Planning Federal Legislation, 116
         Hill-Burton Act, 116
         Regional Medical Programs, 116
         Comprehensive Health Planning, 116
         Certificate of Need, 116
         *National Health Planning and Resources
            Development Act, 117*
         Changing Focus of Health Planning, 117
      Nursing Implications, 120
8 Community Health Education, 122
   Cathy D. Meade
      Connecting with Everyday Realities, 122
      Health Education in the Community, 123
      **Learning Theories, Principles and Health
         Education Models, 124**
         Learning Theories, 124
         *Knowles's Assumptions about Adult
            Learners, 126*
         Health Education Models, 126
         Models of Individual Behavior, 126
         *Model of Health Education Empowerment,
            128*
         Community Empowerment, 130
      The Nurse's Role in Health Education, 132
      Enhancing Communication, 132
      **Framework for Developing Health
         Communications, 133**
         *Stage I: Planning and Strategy
            Development, 134*
         *Stage II: Developing and Pretesting
            Concepts, Messages, and Materials, 135*
         Stage III: Implementing the Program, 138
         *Stage IV: Assessing Effectiveness and
            Making Refinements, 138*
      Health Education Resources, 140
         Literacy and Health, 140
         *Assess Materials: Become a Wise Consumer
            and User, 144*
         *Assessing the Relevancy of Health
            Materials, 145*
      Social Media, 148
9 Case Management, 154
   Karyn Leavitt Grow and Jean Cozad Lyon
      Overview of Case Management, 154
         Care Management, 155
         Care Coordination, 156
      Origins of Case Management, 156
         Public Health, 156
         Case Management in Mental Health, 156
         Case Management and the Elderly, 156
         Disease-Specific Case Management, 157
         Patient-Centered Medical Home, 157

Purpose of Case Management, 157
Utilization Review and Managed Care, 157
Trends that Influence Case Management, 158
  Changes in Health Care Reimbursement,
  158
  Access to Health Care for More Americans,
  158
Education and Preparation for Case
  Managers, 158
  Nurse Case Managers, 158
Case Manager Services, 159
Case Manager Roles and Characteristics, 159
Case Identification, 160
The Referral Process, 160
Application of Case Management in
  Community Health, 161
  Community Case Management Models,
  161
  Public Health Clinic Settings, 161
  Occupational Health Settings, 161
  High-Risk Clinic Settings, 161
Research in Case Management, 161
International Case Management, 162

UNIT 3 FACTORS THAT INFLUENCE THE HEALTH OF THE COMMUNITY

10 Policy, Politics, Legislation, and Community
Health Nursing, 165
  Anita W. Finkelman
  Overview: Nurses' Historical and Current
    Activity in Health Care Policy, 166
  Definitions, 166
  A Major Paradigm Shift, 168
  Structure of the Government of the United
    States, 169
  Overview of Health Policy, 171
    Public Health Policy, 171
    Health Policy and the Private Sector, 171
    The Legislative Process: How a Bill
    Becomes a Law, 171
  Major Legislative Actions and the Health
    Care System, 173
    Federal Legislation, 173
    Role of State Legislatures, 176
  Public Policy: Blueprint for Governance, 176
    Policy Formulation: The Ideal, 177
    Policy Formulation: The Reality, 177
    Steps in Policy Formulation and Analysis,
    177

The Effective Use of Nurses: A Policy Issue,
  178
Nurses' Roles in Political Activities, 178
  The Power of One and Many, 178
  Nurses as Change Agents, 179
  Nurses and Coalitions, 179
  Nurses as Lobbyists, 180
  Nurses and Political Action Committees,
  180
  Nurses and Campaigning, 181
  Nurses and Voting Strength, 181
  Nurses in Public Office, 181
Health Care Reform and Restructuring of the
  Health Care Industry, 182
Nurses and Leadership in Health Policy
  Development, 183

11 The Health Care System, 186
  Anita W. Finkelman
  Overview: The Health Care System, 187
  Components of the Health Care System, 187
    Private Health Care Subsystem, 187
    Public Health Subsystem, 188
    Health Care Providers, 192
  Quality Care, 194
    The Institute of Medicine Reports Examine
    Health Care Quality, 194
    Accreditation, 197
    Current Status of Health Care Quality, 197
  Critical Issues in Health Care Delivery, 197
    Managed Care, 197
    Information Technology, 197
    Consumerism, Advocacy, and Client
    Rights, 198
    Coordination and Access to Health Care,
    198
    Disparity in Health Care Delivery, 199
    Globalization and International Health,
    199
    Health Care Reform: Impact on the Health
    Care System, 199
  Future of Public Health and the Health Care
    System, 199

12 Economics of Health Care, 202
  Anita W. Finkelman
  Factors Influencing Health Care Costs, 203
    Historical Perspective, 203
    Use of Health Care, 205
    Lack of Preventive Care, 205
    Lifestyle and Health Behaviors, 205
    Societal Beliefs, 206
    Technological Advances, 206
    Aging of Society, 206

Pharmaceuticals, 206
Shift to For-Profit Health Care, 207
Health Care Fraud and Abuse, 207
Public Financing of Health Care, 207
Medicare, 207
Medicaid, 208
Governmental Grants, 209
Philanthropic Financing of Health Care, 209
Health Care Insurance Plans, 209
Historical Perspective, 209
Types of Health Care Plans, 210
Reimbursement Mechanisms of Insurance
Plans, 210
Prospective Reimbursement, 211
Covered Services, 212
Cost Containment, 212
Historical Perspective of Cost
Containment, 212
Current Trends in Cost Containment, 213
Trends in Health Financing, 214
Cost Sharing, 214
Health Care Alliances, 215
Self-Insurance, 215
Flexible Spending Accounts, 215
Health Promotion and Disease Prevention:
Impact on Health Care Costs, 215
Health Care Financing Reform, 215
Access to Health Care, 216
Historical Perspective, 216
Societal Perceptions, 216
Health Care Reform—2010, 217
Roles Of the Community Health Nurse in the
Economics of Health Care, 217
Researcher, 217
Educator, 217
Provider of Care, 217
Advocate, 218
Best Care at Lower Cost, 218

13 Cultural Diversity and Community Health
Nursing, 220
Carrie L. Buch
Cultural Diversity, 221
Transcultural Perspectives on Community
Health Nursing, 221
Population Trends, 221
Cultural Perspectives and Healthy People
2020, 222
Addressing Racial and Ethnic Disparities
in Health Care, 223
Transcultural Nursing, 223
Overview of Culture, 224
Culture and the Formation of Values, 225
Culture and the Family, 227

Culture and Socioeconomic Factors, 228
Distribution of Resources, 229
Education, 229
Culture and Nutrition, 229
Nutrition Assessment of Culturally Diverse
Groups, 229
Dietary Practices of Selected Cultural
Groups, 230
Religion and Diet, 230
Culture and Religion, 230
Religion and Spirituality, 230
Childhood and Spirituality, 231
Culture and Aging, 231
Cross-Cultural Communication, 232
Nurse-Client Relationship, 232
Space, Distance, and Intimacy, 232
Overcoming Communication Barriers, 232
Nonverbal Communication, 233
Language, 233
Touch, 234
Gender, 234
Health-Related Beliefs and Practices, 235
Health and Culture, 235
Cross-Cultural Perspectives on Causes of
Illness, 235
Biomedical Perspective, 235
Folk Healers, 236
Cultural Expressions of Illness, 236
Cultural Expression of Pain, 237
Culture-Bound Syndromes, 237
Management of Health Problems: A Cultural
Perspective, 238
Cultural Negotiation, 238
Management of Health Problems in
Culturally Diverse Populations, 239
Providing Health Information and
Education, 239
Delivering and Financing Health Services,
240
Developing Health Professionals from
Minority Groups, 240
Enhancing Cooperative Efforts with the
Nonfederal Sector, 241
Promoting a Research Agenda on Minority
Health Issues, 241
Role of the Community Health Nurse in
Improving Health for Culturally Diverse
People, 241
Culturological Assessment, 241
Cultural Self-Assessment, 244
Knowledge about Local Cultures, 244
Recognition of Political Issues of Culturally
Diverse Groups, 244

Providing Culturally Competent Care, 244
Recognition of Culturally Based Health
    Practices, 244
Resources for Minority Health, 245
Office of Minority Health, 245
Indian Health Service, 245

14 Environmental Health, 249
Diane Santa Maria
A Critical Theory Approach to
    Environmental Health, 250
Areas of Environmental Health, 252
The Built Environment, 253
Work-Related Exposures, 254
Outdoor Air Quality, 256
Healthy Homes, 258
Water Quality, 258
Food Safety, 259
Waste Management, 261
Effects of Environmental Hazards, 261
Efforts to Control Environmental Health
    Problems, 262
Emerging Issues in Environment Health, 263
Nursing Actions, 263
Approaching Environmental Health at the
    Population Level, 263
Critical Environmental Health Nursing
    Practice, 264
Taking a Stand: Advocating for Change, 264
Asking Critical Questions, 264
Facilitating Community Involvement, 265
Forming Coalitions, 265
Using Collective Strategies, 266

15 Health in the Global Community, 272
Julie Cowan Novak
Population Characteristics, 273
Environmental Factors, 273
Patterns of Health and Disease, 273
International Agencies and Organizations, 275
International Health Care Delivery Systems,
    277
The Role of the Community Health Nurse
    in International Health Care, 279
Research in International Health, 279

UNIT 4   AGGREGATES IN THE COMMUNITY

16 Child and Adolescent Health, 286
Susan Rumsey Givens
Issues of Pregnancy and Infancy, 287
Infant Mortality, 288
Preterm Birth and Low Birth Weight, 290

Preconception Health, 290
Prenatal Care, 291
Prenatal Substance Use, 291
Breastfeeding, 292
Sudden Unexplained Infant Death, 292
Childhood Health Issues, 293
Accidental Injuries, 293
Unhealthy Weight, 296
Immunization, 296
Environmental Concerns, 297
Child Maltreatment, 297
Children with Special Health Care Needs, 298
Adolescent Health Issues, 298
Sexual Risk Behavior, 298
Violence, 300
Tobacco, Alcohol, and Drug Use, 300
Factors Affecting Child and Adolescent
    Health, 301
Poverty, 301
Racial and Ethnic Disparities, 301
Health Care Use, 301
Strategies to Improve Child and Adolescent
    Health, 302
Monitoring and Tracking, 303
Healthy People, 2020: Child and
    Adolescent Health, 303
Health Promotion and Disease Prevention,
    303
Public Health Programs Targeted to Children
    and Adolescents, 304
Health Care Coverage Programs, 304
Direct Health Care Delivery Programs, 305
Sharing Responsibility for Improving Child
    and Adolescent Health, 306
Parents' Role, 306
Community's Role, 307
Employer's Role, 307
Government's Role, 307
Community Health Nurse's Role, 307
Legal and Ethical Issues in Child and
    Adolescent Health, 308
Ethical Issues, 308

17 Women's Health, 314
Lori Glenn
Major Indicators of Health, 315
Life Expectancy, 316
Mortality Rate, 316
Morbidity Rate, 320
Social Factors Affecting Women's Health, 321
Health Care Access, 321
Education and Work, 321
Employment and Wages, 321

Working Women and Home Life, 321
Family Configuration and Marital Status, 322
Health Promotion Strategies for Women, 322
Chronic Illness, 323
Reproductive Health, 327
Other Issues in Women's Health, 329
Major Legislation Affecting Women's Health, 329
Public Health Service Act, 330
Civil Rights Act, 330
Social Security Act, 330
Occupational Safety and Health Act, 330
Family and Medical Leave Act, 330
Health and Social Services to Promote the Health of Women, 331
Women's Health Services, 331
Other Community Voluntary Services, 332
Levels of Prevention and Women's Health, 332
Primary Prevention, 332
Secondary Prevention, 332
Tertiary Prevention, 332
Roles of the Community Health Nurse, 334
Direct Care, 334
Educator, 334
Counselor, 334
Research in Women's Health, 334

18 Men's Health, 339
Jené Hurlbut
Men's Health Status, 340
Longevity and Mortality, 340
Morbidity, 341
Use of Medical Care, 342
Use of Ambulatory Care, 342
Use of Hospital Care, 342
Use of Preventive Care, 342
Use of Other Health Services, 342
Theories that Explain Men's Health, 342
Biological Factors, 343
Socialization, 343
Orientation Toward Illness and Prevention, 344
Reporting of Health Behavior, 344
Discussion of the Theories of Men's Health, 344
Factors that Impede Men's Health, 346
Medical Care Patterns, 346
Access to Care, 346
Lack of Health Promotion, 346
Men's Health Care Needs, 347
Primary Preventive Measures, 348
Health Education, 348
Interest Groups for Men and Men's Health, 348

Men's Growing Interest in Physical Fitness and Lifestyle, 348
Policy Related to Men's Health, 349
Secondary Preventive Measures, 349
Health Services for Men, 349
Screening Services for Men, 349
Tertiary Preventive Measures, 349
Sex-Role and Lifestyle Rehabilitation, 349
New Concepts of Community Care, 350

19 Senior Health, 355
Mary Ellen Trail Ross and Edith B. Summerlin
Concept of Aging, 356
Theories of Aging, 356
Demographic Characteristics, 357
Population, 357
Racial and Ethnic Composition, 357
Geographic Location, 357
Gender, 357
Marital Status, 357
Education, 357
Living Arrangements, 357
Sources of Income, 358
Poverty and Health Education, 359
Psychosocial Issues, 359
Physiological Changes, 360
Wellness and Health Promotion, 360
Healthy People 2020, 360
Recommended Health Care Screenings and Examinations, 362
Physical Activity and Fitness, 363
Nutrition, 363
Common Health Concerns, 364
Chronic Illness, 364
Medication Use by Elders, 364
Additional Health Concerns, 365
Sensory Impairment, 365
Hearing Loss, 366
Dental Concerns, 366
Incontinence, 366
Elder Safety and Security Needs, 366
Falls, 366
Driver Safety, 367
Residential Fire–Related Injuries, 368
Cold and Heat Stress, 368
Elder Abuse, 368
Crime, 369
Psychosocial Disorders, 370
Anxiety Disorders, 370
Depression, 370
Substance Abuse, 371
Suicide, 372
Alzheimer's Disease, 372
Spirituality, 373

End-of-Life Issues, 374
  Advance Directives, 374
  The Nurse's Role in End-of-Life Issues, 374

20 Family Health, 380
Beverly Cook Siegrist
  Understanding Family Nursing, 382
  The Changing Family, 383
    Definition of Family, 383
    Characteristics of the Changing Family, 383
  Approaches to Meeting the Health Needs of Families, 384
    Moving from Individual to Family, 385
    Moving from Family to Community, 387
  Approaches to Family Health, 388
    Family Theory, 388
    Systems Theory, 388
    Structural-Functional Conceptual Framework, 390
    Developmental Theory, 391
  Assessment Tools, 392
    Genogram, 392
    Family Health Tree, 392
    Ecomap, 393
  Family Health Assessment, 394
    Social and Structural Constraints, 394
  Extending Family Health Intervention to Larger Aggregates and Social Action, 394
    Institutional Context of Family Therapists, 394
    Models of Care for Communities of Families, 396
  Applying the Nursing Process, 397
    Home Visit, 397

UNIT 5   VULNERABLE POPULATIONS

21 Populations Affected by Disabilities, 403
Meredith Troutman-Jordan
  Self-Assessment: Responses to Disability, 404
  Definitions and Models for Disability, 404
    National Agenda for Prevention of Disabilities Model, 405
    Four Models for Disability, 406
    Differentiating Illness from Disability, 407
  A Historical Context for Disability, 407
    Early Attitudes Toward People with Disabilities, 407
    Attitudes Toward People with Disabilities in the Eighteenth and Nineteenth Centuries, 407
    Disability in the Twentieth Century, 408
    Contemporary Conceptualizations of People with Disabilities, 408
  Characteristics of Disability, 409
    Measurement of Disability, 409
    Prevalence of Disability, 409
    Health Status and Causes of Disability, 411
    Culture and Disability, 411
    Aging and Personal Assistance, 412
  Disability and Public Policy, 412
    Legislation Affecting People with Disabilities, 412
    Public Assistance Programs, 414
  Costs Associated with Disability, 414
    Economic Well-Being and Employment, 414
  Healthy People 2020 and The Health Needs of People with Disabilities, 415
    Health Disparities in Quality and Access, 415
    People with Intellectual Disabilities: Undervalued and Disadvantaged, 415
  The Experience of Disability, 416
    Family and Caregiver Responses to a Child with a Disability, 417
    "Knowledgeable Client" and the "Knowledgeable Nurse", 418
  Strategies for the Community Health Nurse in Caring for People with Disabilities, 419
  Ethical Issues for People Affected by Disabilities, 419
    When the Nurse Has a Disability, 423

22 Homeless Populations, 429
Nellie S. Droes and Diane C. Hatton
  Definitions, Prevalence, and Demographic Characteristics of Homelessness, 429
    Definitions of Homelessness, 429
    Prevalence of Homelessness, 431
    Demographic Characteristics, 433
  Factors that Contribute to Homelessness, 433
    Shortage of Affordable Housing, 433
    Income Insufficiency, 434
    Inadequacy and Scarcity of Supportive Services, 434
    Homelessness and Causation, 435
  Health and Homeless Populations, 435
    Federal Health Centers, 435
  Health Status of Homeless Population, 436
    Adults, 436
    Families, 437
    Youth, 437

Chronically Homeless, 438
Community Public Health Nursing: Care of
Homeless Populations, 438
Framework for Community/Public
Health Nursing Care for Homeless
Populations, 438

23 Rural and Migrant Health, 443
Patricia L. Thomas and Lori Wightman
Rural United States, 444
Defining Rural Populations, 445
Describing Rural Health and Populations,
445
Rural, 446
Minority Health and Healthy People 2020,
446
Rural Health Disparities: Context and
Composition, 446
Context: Health Disparities Related to
Place, 446
Composition: Health Disparities Related to
Persons, 449
Perceptions of Health, 454
Specific Rural Aggregates, 455
Agricultural Workers, 455
Migrant and Seasonal Farmworkers, 456
Application of Relevant Theories and
"Thinking Upstream" Concepts to Rural
Health, 457
Attacking Community-Based Problems at
Their Roots, 457
Emphasizing the "Doing" Aspects of
Health, 457
Maximizing the Use of Informal Networks,
457
Rural Health Care delivery System, 457
Health Care Provider Shortages, 457
Managed Care in the Rural Environment,
458
Community-Based Care, 458
Home Health and Hospice Care, 458
Faith Communities and Parish Nursing,
459
Informal Care Systems, 459
Rural Public Health Departments, 459
Rural Mental Health Care, 460
Emergency Services, 460
Legislation and Programs Affecting Rural
Public Health, 460
Programs that Augment Health Care
Facilities and Services, 460
Rural Community Health Nursing, 461
Characteristics of Rural Nursing, 461
Rural Health Research, 462

Capacity of Rural Public Health to Manage
Improvements in Health, 462
Information Technology in Rural
Communities, 462
Performance Standards in Rural Public
Health, 463
Leadership and Workforce Capacity for
Rural Public Health, 463
Interaction and Integration of Community
Health Systems, Managed Care, and
Public Health, 464
New Models of Health Care Delivery for
Rural Areas, 464

24 Populations Affected by Mental Illness, 468
Kim Jardine-Dickerson
Overview and History of Community Mental
Health: 1960 to the Present Day, 469
Deinstitutionalization Cause and Effects,
470
Present-Day Community Mental Health
Reform, 470
Medicalization of Mental Illness, 470
Brain Neuroimaging, Genetics, and Hope
for New Treatments, 470
Healthy People 2020: Mental Health and
Mental Disorders, 471
Factors Influencing Mental Health, 471
Biological Factors, 471
Social Factors, 471
Gender, Racial, and Sexual Orientation
Disparities, 472
Natural and Human-Made Disasters and
Mental Illness, 472
Political Factors, 473
Mental Disorders Encountered in
Community Settings, 474
Overview of Selected Mental Disorders, 474
Depression, 474
Identification and Management of Mental
Disorders, 478
Identification of Mental Disorders, 479
Community-Based Mental Health Care, 481
Role of the Community Mental Health Nurse,
484

UNIT 6   POPULATION HEALTH PROBLEMS

25 Communicable Disease, 488
Deanna E. Grimes
Communicable Disease and Healthy People
2020, 490

Principles of Infection and Infectious Disease Occurrence, 491
  Multicausation, 491
  Spectrum of Infection, 491
  Stages of Infection, 492
  Spectrum of Disease Occurrence, 492
Chain of Transmission, 492
  Infectious Agents, 492
  Reservoirs, 493
  Portals of Exit and Entry, 493
  Modes of Transmission, 493
  Host Susceptibility, 494
Breaking the Chain of Transmission, 494
  Controlling the Agent, 494
  Eradicating the Nonhuman Reservoir, 494
  Controlling the Human Reservoir, 494
  Controlling the Portals of Exit and Entry, 494
  Improving Host Resistance and Immunity, 494
Public Health Control of Infectious Diseases, 495
  Terminology: Control, Elimination, and Eradication, 496
  Defining and Reporting Communicable Diseases, 496
Vaccines and Infectious Disease Prevention, 497
  Vaccines: Word of Caution, 497
  Types of Immunizations, 497
  Vaccine Storage, Transport, and Handling, 498
  Vaccine Administration, 498
  Vaccine Spacing, 498
  Vaccine Hypersensitivity and Contraindications, 498
  Vaccine Documentation, 499
  Vaccine Safety and Reporting Adverse Events and Vaccine-Related Injuries, 499
Vaccine Needs for Special Groups, 499
Healthy People 2020 Focus on Immunization and Infectious Diseases, 499
Healthy People 2020 Focus on Sexually Transmitted Diseases, 506
Healthy People 2020 Focus on HIV/AIDS, 507
Prevention of Communicable Diseases, 510
  Primary Prevention, 510
  Secondary Prevention, 510
  Tertiary Prevention, 510

26 Substance Abuse, 515
Kim Jardine-Dickerson
Etiology of Substance Abuse, 516
Historical Overview of Alcohol and Illicit Drug Use, 517
Prevalence, Incidence, and Trends, 517
  Alcohol, 518
  Illicit Drug Use, 518
  Gender Differences, 519
  Demographics, 520
  Trends in Substance Use, 520
Adolescent Substance Abuse, 521
Conceptualizations of Substance Abuse, 522
  Definitions, 522
Sociocultural and Political Aspects of Substance Abuse, 522
Course of Substance-Related Problems, 524
Legal and Ethical Concerns Related to Substance Abuse, 525
Modes of Intervention, 525
  Prevention, 526
  Treatment, 526
  Pharmacotherapies, 529
  Mutual Help Groups, 530
  Harm Reduction, 531
Social Network Involvement, 531
  Family and Friends, 531
  Effects on the Family, 532
  Professional Enablers, 532
Vulnerable Aggregates, 533
  Preadolescents and Adolescents, 533
  Elderly, 534
  Women, 534
  Ethnocultural Considerations, 535
  Other Aggregates, 535
Nursing Perspective on Substance Abuse, 536
  Nursing Interventions in the Community, 537
  Nursing Care Standards Related to the Patients with Substance Abuse Problems, 538

27 Violence, 542
Cathi A. Pourciau and Elaine C. Vallette
Overview of Violence, 543
History of Violence, 543
Interpersonal Violence, 544
  Homicide and Suicide, 544
  Intimate Partner Violence, 544
  Child Maltreatment, 546
  Elder Abuse, 549
Community Violence, 549
  Workplace Violence, 549

Youth-Related Violence, 550
Gangs, 551
Prison Violence, 551
Human Trafficking, 551
Hate Crimes, 551
Terrorism, 551
Factors Influencing Violence, 551
Firearms, 552
Media, 552
Mental Illness, 552
Violence from a Public Health Perspective, 552
Healthy People 2020 and Violence, 552
Prevention of Violence, 552
Primary Prevention, 553
Secondary Prevention, 553
Tertiary Prevention, 554

28 Natural and Man-Made Disasters, 558
Edith B. Summerlin
Disaster Definitions, 559
Types of Disasters, 560
Characteristics of Disasters, 560
Frequency, 560
Predictability, 561
Preventability/Mitigation, 561
Imminence, 562
Scope and Number of Casualties, 562
Intensity, 562
Disaster Management, 563
Local, State, and Federal Governmental
Responsibilities, 564
Public Health System, 567
American Red Cross, 568
Disaster Management Stages, 569
Prevention Stage, 569
Preparedness and Planning Stage, 570
Response Stage, 571
Recovery Stage, 578

UNIT 7   COMMUNITY HEALTH
SETTINGS

29 School Health, 580
Cathi A. Pourciau and Elaine C. Vallette
History of School Health, 581
School Health Services, 582
Health Education, 583
Physical Education, 586
Health Services, 586
Nutrition, 590
Counseling, Psychological, and Social
Services, 591
Healthy School Environment, 592

Health Promotion for School Staff, 593
Family and Community Involvement, 593
School Nursing Practice, 593
School-Based Health Centers, 594
Future Issues Affecting the School Nurse, 594

30 Occupational Health, 598
Bonnie Rogers
Evolution of Occupational Health Nursing, 599
Demographic Trends and Access Issues
Related to Occupational Health Care, 600
Occupational Health Nursing Practice and
Professionalism, 601
Occupational Health and Prevention
Strategies, 604
Healthy People 2020 and Occupational
Health, 604
Prevention of Exposure to Potential
Hazards, 604
Levels of Prevention and Occupational
Health Nursing, 604
Skills and Competencies of the Occupational
Health Nurse, 607
Competent, 608
Proficient, 608
Expert, 608
Examples of Skills and Competencies for
Occupational Health Nursing, 608
Impact of Federal Legislation on
Occupational Health, 610
Occupational Safety and Health Act, 610
Workers' Compensation Acts, 611
Americans With Disabilities Act, 612
Legal Issues in Occupational Health, 612
Multidisciplinary Teamwork, 612

31 Forensic and Correctional Nursing, 616
Angela Jarrell and Stacy Drake
Subspecialties of Forensic Nursing, 617
Sexual Assault Nurse Examiner, 617
Medicolegal Death Investigation, 618
Legal Nurse Consultants and Nurse
Attorneys, 619
Clinical Forensic Nurse Examiner, 620
Forensic Psychiatric Nurse, 622
Correctional Nursing, 622
Maintenance of a Safe Environment, 622
Health Issues in Prison Populations, 623
Chronic and Communicable Diseases, 623
Women in Prison, 623
Adolescents in Prison, 624
Mental Health Issues in Correctional
Settings, 624
Education and Forensic Nursing, 625

32 Faith Community Nursing, 631
Beverly Cook Siegrist
Faith Communities: Role in Health and Wellness, 632
Foundations of Faith Community Nursing, 633
Roles or Functions of the Faith Community Nurse, 636
Education of the Faith Community Nurse, 637
The Faith Community Nurse and Spirituality, 638
Issues in Faith Community Nurse Practice, 639
Providing Care to Vulnerable Populations, 639
End-of-Life Issues: Grief and Loss, 639
Family Violence Prevention, 639
Confidentiality, 640
Accountability, 641

33 Home Health and Hospice, 645
Carrie L. Buch and Mary A. Nies
Home Health Care, 646
Purpose of Home Health Services, 646
Types of Home Health Agencies, 647
Official Agencies, 647
Nonprofit Agencies, 647
Proprietary Agencies, 647
Hospital-Based Agencies, 647

Certified and Noncertified Agencies, 647
Special Home Health Programs, 647
Reimbursement for Home Care, 648
Oasis, 648
Nursing Standards and Educational Preparation of Home Health Nurses, 649
Conducting a Home Visit, 650
Visit Preparation, 650
The Referral, 650
Initial Telephone Contact, 651
Environment, 651
Improving Communication, 651
Building Trust, 651
Documentation of Home Care, 652
Application of the Nursing Process, 652
Assessment, 652
Diagnosis and Planning, 652
Intervention, 653
Evaluation, 653
Formal and Informal Caregivers, 654
Hospice Home Care, 654
Caring for the Caregiver, 655
Pain Control and Symptom Management, 655
Cultural Differences Related to Death and Dying, 656

Health: A Community View

Melanie McEwen and Mary A. Nies

OBJECTIVES

Upon completion of this chapter, the reader will be able to do the following:

1. Compare and contrast definitions of *health* from a public health nursing perspective.
2. Define and discuss the focus of public health.
3. Discuss determinates of health and indicators of health and illness from a population perspective.
4. List the three levels of prevention, and give examples of each.
5. Explain the difference between public/community health nursing practice and community-based nursing practice.
6. Describe the purpose of *Healthy People 2020*, and give examples of the topic areas that encompass the national health objectives.
7. Discuss community/public health nursing practice in terms of public health's core functions and essential services.
8. Discuss community/public health nursing interventions as explained by the Intervention Wheel.

KEY TERMS

aggregates
community
community health
community health nursing
disease prevention

health
health promotion
population
population-focused nursing
primary prevention

public health
public health nursing
secondary prevention
tertiary prevention

OUTLINE

Definitions of Health and Community
  Health
  Community
Determinants of Health and Disease
Indicators of Health and Illness
Definition and Focus of Public Health and Community Health
Preventive Approach to Health
  Health Promotion and Levels of Prevention
  Prevention versus Cure
  Healthy People 2020

Definition and Focus of Public Health Nursing, Community Health Nursing, and Community-Based Nursing
  Public and Community Health Nursing
  Community-Based Nursing
  Community and Public Health Nursing Practice
Population-Focused Practice and Community/Public Health Nursing Interventions
  Community Health Interventions
  The Public Health Intervention Wheel
Community Health Nursing, Managed Care, and Health Care Reform

As a result of recent and anticipated changes related to health care reform, community/public health nurses are in a position to assist the U.S. health care system in the transition from a disease-oriented system to a health-oriented system. Costs of caring for the sick account for the majority of escalating health care dollars, which increased from 5.7% of the gross domestic product in 1965 to 17.9% in 2010 (National Center for Health Statistics [NCHS], 2013). Alarmingly, national annual health care expenditures reached $2.6 trillion in 2010, or an astonishing $8400 per person.

U.S. health expenditures reflect a focus on the care of the sick. In 2010, $0.31 of each health care dollar supported hospital care, $0.20 supported physician services, and $0.10 was spent on prescription drugs (double the proportion since 1980). The vast majority of these funds were spent providing care for the sick, and only $0.03 of every health care dollar was directed toward preventive public health activities (NCHS, 2013). Despite high hospital and physician expenditures, U.S. health indicators rate considerably below the health indicators of many other countries. This situation reflects a relatively severe disproportion of funding for preventive services and social and economic opportunities. Furthermore, the health status of the population within the United States varies markedly across areas of the country and among groups. For example, the economically disadvantaged and many cultural and ethnic groups have poorer overall health status compared with middle-class Caucasians.

Nurses constitute the largest group of health care workers; therefore, they are instrumental in creating a health care delivery system that will meet the health-oriented needs of the people. According to a survey of registered nurses (RNs) conducted by the Health Resources and Services Administration, about 62% of approximately 2.6 million employed RNs in the United States worked in hospitals during 2008 (down from 66.5% in 1992). This survey also found that about 14.2%, approximately 400,000, of all RNs worked in home, school, or occupational health settings; 10.5% worked in ambulatory care settings; and 5.3% worked in nursing homes or other extended care facilities (U.S. Department of Health and Human Services, Health Resources and Services Administration, Bureau of Health Professions [USDHHS, HRSA, BHP], 2010).

Between 1980 and 2008, the number of nurses employed in community, health, and ambulatory care settings more than doubled (USDHHS, HRSA, BHP, 2010). The decline in the percentage of nurses employed in hospitals and the subsequent increase in nurses employed in community settings indicate a shift in focus from illness and institutional-based care to health promotion and preventive care. This shift will likely continue into the future as alternative delivery systems, such as ambulatory and home care, will employ more nurses (Rosenfeld and Russell, 2012; Way and MacNeil, 2007).

Community/public health nursing is the synthesis of nursing practice and public health practice. The major goal of public health nursing is to preserve the health of the community and surrounding populations by focusing on health promotion and health maintenance of individuals, families, and groups within the community. Thus community/public health nursing is associated with health and the identification of populations at risk rather than with an episodic response to patient demand.

The mission of public health is social justice, which entitles all people to basic necessities such as adequate income and health protection and accepts collective burdens to make it possible. Public health, with its egalitarian tradition and vision, often conflicts with the predominant U.S. model of market justice that largely entitles people to what they have gained through individual efforts. Although market justice respects individual rights, collective action and obligations are minimal. An emphasis on technology and curative medical services within the market justice system has limited the evolution of a health system designed to protect and preserve the health of the population. Public health assumes that it is society's responsibility to meet the basic needs of the people. Thus there is a greater need for public funding of prevention efforts to enhance the health of our population.

Current U.S. health policies advocate changes in personal behaviors that might predispose individuals to chronic disease or accident. These policies promote exercise, healthy eating, tobacco use cessation, and moderate consumption of alcohol. However, simply encouraging the individual to overcome the effects of unhealthy activities lessens focus on collective behaviors necessary to change the determinants of health stemming from such factors as air and water pollution, workplace hazards, and unequal access to health care. Because living arrangements, work/school environment, and other sociocultural constraints affect health and well-being, public policy must address societal and environmental changes, in addition to lifestyle changes, that will positively influence the health of the entire population.

With ongoing and very significant changes in the health care system and increased employment in community settings, there will be greater demands on community and public health nurses to broaden their population health perspective. The Code of Ethics of the American Nurses Association (ANA) (2001) promotes social reform by focusing on health policy and legislation to positively affect accessibility, quality, and cost of health care. Community and public health nurses, therefore, must align themselves with public health programs that promote and preserve the health of populations by influencing sociocultural issues such as human rights, homelessness, violence, disability, and stigma of illness. This principle allows nurses to be positioned to promote the health, welfare, and safety of all individuals.

This chapter examines health from a population-focused, community-based perspective. Therefore it requires understanding of how people identify, define, and describe related concepts. The following section explores six major ideas:
1. Definitions of "health" and "community"
2. Determinants of health and disease
3. Indicators of health and disease
4. Definition and focus of public and community health
5. Description of a preventive approach to health
6. Definition and focus of "public health nursing," "community health nursing," and "community-based nursing"

DEFINITIONS OF HEALTH AND COMMUNITY

Health

The definition of health is evolving. The early, classic definition of health by the World Health Organization (WHO) set a trend toward describing health in social terms rather than in medical terms. Indeed, the WHO (1958, p. 1) defined health as "a state of complete physical, mental, and social well-being and not merely the absence of disease or infirmity."

Social means "of or relating to living together in organized groups or similar close aggregates" (*American Heritage College Dictionary*, 1997, p. 1291) and refers to units of people in communities who interact with one another. "Social health" connotes community vitality and is a result of positive interaction among groups within the community with an emphasis on health promotion and illness prevention. For example, community groups may sponsor food banks in churches and civic organizations to help alleviate problems of hunger and nutrition. Other community groups may form to address problems of violence and lack of opportunity, which can negatively affect social health.

In the mid-1980s, the WHO expanded the definition of health to emphasize recognition of the social implications of health. Thus health is:

> the extent to which an individual or group is able, on the one hand, to realize aspirations and satisfy needs; and, on the other hand, to change or cope with the environment. Health is, therefore, seen as a resource for everyday life, not the objective of living; it is a positive concept emphasizing social and personal resources, and physical capacities. (WHO, 1986, p. 73)

Saylor (2004) pointed out that the WHO definition considers several dimensions of health. These include physical (structure/function), social, role, mental (emotional and intellectual), and general perceptions of health status. It also conceptualizes health from a macro perspective, as a resource to be used rather than a goal in and of itself.

The nursing literature contains many varied definitions of health. For example, health has been defined as "a state of well-being in which the person is able to use purposeful, adaptive responses and processes physically, mentally, emotionally, spiritually, and socially" (Murray, Zentner, and Yakimo, 2009, p. 53); "realization of human potential through goal-directed behavior, competent self-care, and satisfying relationships with others" (Pender, Murdaugh, and Parsons, 2011, p. 22); and a state of a person that is characterized by soundness or wholeness of developed human structures and of bodily and mental functioning (Orem, 2001).

The variety of characterizations of the word illustrates the difficulty in standardizing the conceptualization of health. Commonalities involve description of "goal-directed" or "purposeful" actions, processes, responses, or behaviors and the possession of "soundness," "wholeness," and/or "well-being." Problems can arise when the definition involves a unit of analysis. For example, some writers use the individual or "person" as the unit of analysis and exclude the community. Others may include additional concepts, such as adaptation and environment, in health definitions, and then present the environment as static and requiring human adaptation rather than as changing and enabling human modification.

For many years, community and public health nurses have favored Dunn's (1961) classic concept of wellness, in which family, community, society, and environment are interrelated and have an impact on health. From his viewpoint, illness, health, and peak wellness are on a continuum; health is fluid and changing. Consequently, within a social context or environment, the state of health depends on the goals, potentials, and performance of individuals, families, communities, and societies.

Community

The definitions of *community* are also numerous and variable. Baldwin and colleagues (1998) outlined the evolution of the definition of community by examining community health nursing textbooks. They determined that, before 1996, definitions of community focused on geographic boundaries combined with social attributes of people. Citing several sources from the later part of the decade, the authors observed that geographic location became a secondary characteristic in the discussion of what defines a community.

In recent nursing literature, community has been defined as "a collection of people who interact with one another and whose common interests or characteristics form the basis for a sense of unity or belonging" (Allender, Rector, and Warner, 2013, p. 6); "a group of people who share something in common and interact with one another, who may exhibit a commitment with one another and may share a geographic boundary" (Lundy and Janes, 2009, p. 16); and "a locality-based entity, composed of systems of formal organizations reflecting society's institutions, informal groups and aggregates" (Shuster, 2012, p. 398).

Maurer and Smith (2013) further addressed the concept of community and identified three defining attributes: people, place, and social interaction or common characteristics, interests, or goals. Combining ideas and concepts, in this text, community is seen as a group or collection of individuals interacting in social units and sharing common interests, characteristics, values, and goals.

Maurer and Smith (2013) noted that there are two main types of communities: geopolitical communities and phenomenological communities. Geopolitical communities are those most traditionally recognized or imagined when the term *community* is considered. *Geopolitical communities* are defined or formed by natural and/or man-made boundaries and include cities, counties, states, and nations. Other commonly recognized geopolitical communities are school districts, census tracts, zip codes, and neighborhoods. *Phenomenological communities*, on the other hand, refer to relational, interactive groups. In phenomenological communities, the place or setting is more abstract, and people share a group perspective or identity based on culture, values, history, interests, and goals. Examples of phenomenological communities are schools, colleges, and universities; churches, synagogues, and mosques; and various groups and organizations, such as social networks.

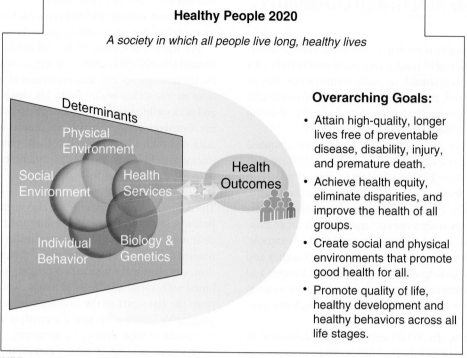

Healthy People 2020

A society in which all people live long, healthy lives

Determinants

Physical Environment

Social Environment

Health Services

Individual Behavior

Biology & Genetics

Health Outcomes

Overarching Goals:

• Attain high-quality, longer lives free of preventable disease, disability, injury, and premature death.

• Achieve health equity, eliminate disparities, and improve the health of all groups.

• Create social and physical environments that promote good health for all.

• Promote quality of life, healthy development and healthy behaviors across all life stages.

FIGURE 1-1 Model: *Healthy People 2020.* (From US Department of Health and Human Services Office of Disease Prevention and Health Promotion. Federal Interagency Workgroup: The Vision, Mission, and Goals of Healthy People 2020. Retrieved July 2013 from http://www.healthypeople.gov/2020/Consortium/HP2020Framework.pdf.)

A community of solution is a type of phenomenological community. A *community of solution* is a collection of people who form a group specifically to address a common need or concern. The Sierra Club, whose members lobby for the preservation of natural resource lands, and a group of disabled people who challenge the owners of an office building to obtain equal access to public buildings, education, jobs, and transportation are examples. These groups or social units work together to promote optimal "health" and to address identified actual and potential health threats and health needs.

Population and *aggregate* are related terms that are often used in public health and community health nursing. **Population** is typically used to denote a group of people having common personal or environmental characteristics. It can also refer to all of the people in a defined community (Maurer and Smith, 2013). **Aggregates** are subgroups or subpopulations that have some common characteristics or concerns (Harkness, 2012). Depending on the situation, needs, and practice parameters, community health nursing interventions may be directed toward a community (e.g., residents of a small town), a population (e.g., all elders in a rural region), or an aggregate (e.g., pregnant teens within a school district).

DETERMINANTS OF HEALTH AND DISEASE

The health status of a community is associated with a number of factors, such as health care access, economic conditions, social and environmental issues, and cultural practices, and it is essential for the community health nurse to understand the determinants of health and recognize the interaction of the factors that lead

to disease, death, and disability. It has been estimated that individual behaviors are responsible for about 50% of all premature deaths in the United States (Orleans and Cassidy, 2011). Indeed, individual biology and behaviors influence health through their interaction with each other and with the individual's social and physical environments. Thus, policies and interventions can improve health by targeting detrimental or harmful factors related to individuals and their environment. Figure 1-1 shows the model of *Healthy People 2020,* which depicts the interaction of these determinants and shows how they influence health.

In a seminal work, McGinnis and Foege (1993) described what they termed "actual causes of death" in the United States, explaining how lifestyle choices contribute markedly to early deaths. Their work was updated a decade later (Mokdad et al, 2004). Leading the list of "actual causes of death" was tobacco, which was implicated in almost 20% of the annual deaths in the United States—approximately 435,000 individuals. Poor diet and physical inactivity were deemed to account for about 16.6% of deaths (about 400,000 per year), and alcohol consumption was implicated in about 85,000 deaths because of its association with accidents, suicides, homicides, and cirrhosis and chronic liver disease. Other leading causes of death were microbial agents (75,000), toxic agents (55,000), motor vehicle crashes (43,000), firearms (29,000), sexual behaviors (20,000) and illicit use of drugs (17,000). Although all of these causes of mortality are related to individual lifestyle choices, they can also be strongly influenced by population-focused policy efforts and education. For example, the prevalence of smoking has fallen dramatically during the past two decades, largely because of legal efforts (e.g., laws prohibiting sale of tobacco to minors and much higher taxes), organizational policy (e.g., smoke-free workplaces), and education. Likewise, later concerns about the widespread increase in incidence of overweight and obesity have led to population-based measures to address the issue (e.g., removal of soft drink and candy machines from schools, regulations prohibiting the use of certain types of fats in processed foods).

Public health experts have observed that health has improved over the past 100 years largely because people become ill less often (Russo, 2011; McKeown, 2003). Indeed, at the population level, better health can be attributed to higher standards of living, good nutrition, a healthier environment, and having fewer children. Furthermore, public health efforts, such as immunization and clean air and water, and medical care, including management of acute episodic illnesses (e.g., pneumonia, tuberculosis) and chronic disease (e.g., cancer, heart disease), have also contributed significantly to the increase in life expectancy.

Community and public health nurses should understand these concepts and appreciate that health and illness are influenced by a web of factors, some that can be changed (e.g., individual behaviors such as tobacco use, diet, physical activity) and some that cannot (e.g., genetics, age, gender). Other factors (e.g., physical and social environment) may require changes that will need to be accomplished from a policy perspective. Community health nurses must work with policy makers and community leaders to identify patterns of disease and death and to advocate for activities and policies that promote health at the individual, family, and population levels.

INDICATORS OF HEALTH AND ILLNESS

A variety of health indicators are used by health providers, policy makers, and community health nurses to measure the health of the community. Local or state health departments, the Centers for Disease Control and Prevention (CDC), and the National Center for Health Statistics (NCHS) provide morbidity, mortality, and other health status–related data. State and local health departments are responsible for collecting morbidity and mortality data and forwarding the information to the appropriate federal-level agency, which is often the CDC. Some of the more commonly reported indicators are life expectancy, infant mortality, age-adjusted death rates, and cancer incidence rates.

Indicators of mortality in particular illustrate the health status of a community and/or population because changes in mortality reflect a number of social, economic, health service, and related trends (Shi and Singh, 2011). These data may be useful in analyzing health patterns over time, comparing communities from different geographic regions, or comparing different aggregates within a community.

When the national health objectives for *Healthy People 2020* were being developed, a total of 12 leading health indicators were identified that reflected the major public health concerns in the United States (See *Healthy People 2020* box). They are individual behaviors (e.g., tobacco use, nutrition,

physical activity, and obesity), physical and social environmental factors (e.g., environmental quality, injury, and violence), and health systems issues (e.g., access to health services). Each of these indicators can affect the health of individuals and communities and can be correlated with leading causes of morbidity and mortality. For example, tobacco use is linked to heart disease, stroke, and cancer; substance abuse is linked to accidents, injuries, and violence; irresponsible sexual behaviors can lead to unwanted pregnancy as well as sexually transmitted diseases, including human immunodeficiency virus/acquired immunodeficiency syndrome (HIV/AIDS); and lack of access to health care can contribute to poor pregnancy outcomes, untreated illness, and disability.

♥ HEALTHY PEOPLE 2020
Leading Health Indicator Topics

- Access to Health Services
- Clinical Preventative Services
- Environmental Quality
- Injury and Violence
- Maternal, Infant and Child Health
- Mental Health
- Nutrition, Physical Activity, and Obesity
- Oral Health
- Reproductive and Sexual Health
- Social Determinants
- Substance Abuse
- Tobacco

From U.S. Department of Health and Human Services: *Healthy People 2020 leading health indicator topics.* Retrieved July 2013 from <http://www.healthy people.gov/2020/LHI/2020indicators.aspx>.

Community health nurses should be aware of health patterns and health indicators within their practice. Each nurse should ask relevant questions, including the following: What are the leading causes of death and disease among various groups served? How do infant mortality rates and teenage pregnancy rates in my community compare with regional, state, and national rates? What are the most serious communicable disease threats in my neighborhood? What are the most common environmental risks in my city?

The community health nurse may identify areas for further investigation and intervention through an understanding of health, disease, and mortality patterns. For example, if a school nurse learns that the teenage pregnancy rate in their community is higher than regional and state averages, the nurse should address the problem with school officials, parents, and students. Likewise, if an occupational health nurse discovers an apparent high rate of chronic lung disease in an industrial facility, the nurse should work with company management, employees, and state and federal officials to identify potential harmful sources. Finally, if a public health nurse works in a state-sponsored AIDS clinic and recognizes an increase in the number of women testing positive for HIV, the nurse should report all findings to the designated agencies. The nurse should then participate in investigative efforts to determine what is precipitating the increase and work to remedy the identified threats or risks.

DEFINITION AND FOCUS OF PUBLIC HEALTH AND COMMUNITY HEALTH

C. E. Winslow is known for the following classic definition of public health:

Public health is the Science and Art of (1) preventing disease, (2) prolonging life, and (3) promoting health and efficiency through organized community effort for:

(a) sanitation of the environment,

(b) control of communicable infections,

(c) education of the individual in personal hygiene,

(d) organization of medical and nursing services for the early diagnosis and preventive treatment of disease, and

(e) development of the social machinery to ensure everyone a standard of living adequate for the maintenance of health, so organizing these benefits as to enable every citizen to realize his birthright of health and longevity. (Hanlon, 1960, p. 23)

A key phrase in this definition of public health is "through organized community effort." The term public health connotes organized, legislated, and tax-supported efforts that serve all people through health departments or related governmental agencies.

The public health nursing tradition, begun in the late 1800s by Lillian Wald and her associates, clearly illustrates this phenomenon (Wald, 1971; see Chapter 2). After moving into the immigrant community in New York City to provide care for individuals and families, these early public health nurses saw that neither administering bedside clinical nursing nor teaching family members to deliver care in the home adequately addressed the true determinants of health and disease. They resolved that collective political activity should focus on advancing the health of aggregates and improving social and environmental conditions by addressing the social and environmental determinants of health, such as child labor, pollution, and poverty. Wald and her colleagues affected the health of the community by organizing the community, establishing school nursing, and taking impoverished mothers to testify in Washington, DC (Wald, 1971).

In a key action, the Institute of Medicine (IOM) (1988) identified the following three primary functions of public health: *assessment, assurance,* and *policy development.* Box 1-1 lists each of the three primary functions and describes them briefly. All nurses working in community settings should develop knowledge and skills related to each of these primary functions.

The term community health extends the realm of public health to include organized health efforts at the community level through both government *and* private efforts. Participants include privately funded agencies such as the American Heart Association and the American Red Cross. A variety of private and public structures serves community health efforts.

Public health efforts focus on prevention and promotion of population health at the federal, state, and local levels. These efforts at the federal and state levels concentrate on providing support and advisory services to public health structures at the local level. The local-level structures provide direct services to communities through two avenues:

BOX 1-1 CORE PUBLIC HEALTH FUNCTIONS

Assessment: Regular collection, analysis, and information sharing about health conditions, risks, and resources in a community.

Policy development: Use of information gathered during assessment to develop local and state health policies and to direct resources toward those policies.

Assurance: Focuses on the availability of necessary health services throughout the community. It includes maintaining the ability of both public health agencies and private providers to manage day-to-day operations and the capacity to respond to critical situations and emergencies.

From Institute of Medicine: *The future of public health,* Washington, DC, 1988, National Academy Press.

BOX 1-2 ESSENTIAL PUBLIC HEALTH SERVICES

- Monitor health status to identify and solve community health problems
- Diagnose and investigate health problems and health hazards in the community
- Inform, educate, and empower people about health issues
- Mobilize community partnerships and actions to identify and solve health problems
- Develop policies and plans that support individual and community health efforts
- Enforce laws and regulations that protect health and ensure safety
- Link people to needed personal health services and assure the provision of health care when otherwise unavailable
- Assure a competent public health and personal health care workforce
- Evaluate effectiveness, accessibility, and quality of personal and population-based health services
- Research for new insights and innovative solutions to health problems

From Centers for Disease Control and Prevention, Office of the Director, Office of the Chief of Public Health Practice, National Public Health Performance Standards Program: *10 essential public health services,* Atlanta, 2012. Retrieved July 2013 from <http://www.cdc.gov/nphpsp/essentialServices.html>.

- Community health services, which protect the public from hazards such as polluted water and air, tainted food, and unsafe housing
- Personal health care services, such as immunization and family planning services, well-infant care, and sexually transmitted disease (STD) treatment

Personal health services may be part of the public health effort and often target the populations most at risk and in need of services. Public health efforts are multidisciplinary because they require people with many different skills. Community health nurses work with a diverse team of public health professionals, including epidemiologists, local health officers, and health educators. Public health science methods that assess biostatistics, epidemiology, and population needs provide a method of measuring characteristics and health indicators and disease patterns within a community. In 1994 the American Public Health Association drafted a list of ten essential public health services, which the U.S. Department of Health and Human Services (USDHHS, 1997) later adopted. This updated list (CDC, 2010) appears in Box 1-2.

PREVENTIVE APPROACH TO HEALTH

Health Promotion and Levels of Prevention

Contrasting with "medical care," which focuses on disease management and "cure," public health efforts focus on health promotion and disease prevention. Health promotion activities enhance resources directed at improving well-being, whereas disease prevention activities protect people from disease and the effects of disease. Leavell and Clark (1958) identified three levels of prevention commonly described in nursing practice: primary prevention, secondary prevention, and tertiary prevention (Figure 1-2 and Table 1-1).

Primary prevention relates to activities directed at preventing a problem before it occurs by altering susceptibility or reducing exposure for susceptible individuals. Primary prevention consists of two elements: general health promotion and specific protection. Health promotion efforts enhance resiliency and protective factors and target essentially well populations. Examples include promotion of good nutrition, provision of adequate shelter, and encouraging regular exercise. Specific protection efforts reduce or eliminate risk factors and include such measures as immunization and water purification (Keller et al, 2004a; McEwen and Pullis, 2009).

Secondary prevention refers to early detection and prompt intervention during the period of early disease pathogenesis. Secondary prevention is implemented after a problem has begun but before signs and symptoms appear and targets those populations that have risk factors (Keller et al, 2004a).

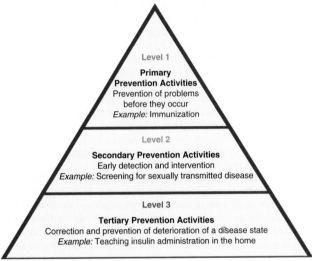

FIGURE 1-2 The three levels of prevention.

TABLE 1-1	EXAMPLES OF LEVELS OF PREVENTION AND CLIENTS SERVED IN THE COMMUNITY		
	LEVEL OF PREVENTION		
DEFINITION OF CLIENT SERVED*	**PRIMARY (HEALTH PROMOTION AND SPECIFIC PREVENTION)**	**SECONDARY (EARLY DIAGNOSIS AND TREATMENT)**	**TERTIARY (LIMITATION OF DISABILITY AND REHABILITATION)**
Individual	Dietary teaching during pregnancy Immunizations	HIV testing Screening for cervical cancer	Teaching new clients with diabetes how to administer insulin Exercise therapy after stroke Skin care for incontinent patients
Family (two or more individuals bound by kinship, law, or living arrangement and with common emotional ties and obligations [see Chapter 20])	Education or counseling regarding smoking, dental care, or nutrition Adequate housing	Dental examinations Tuberculin testing for family at risk	Mental health counseling or referral for family in crisis (e.g., grieving or experiencing a divorce) Dietary instructions and monitoring for family with overweight members
Group or aggregate (interacting people with a common purpose or purposes)	Birthing classes for pregnant teenage mothers AIDS and other STD education for high school students	Vision screening of a first grade class Mammography van for screening of women in a low-income neighborhood Hearing tests at a senior center	Group counseling for grade-school children with asthma Swim therapy for physically disabled elders at a senior center Alcoholics Anonymous and other self-help groups Mental health services for military veterans
Community and populations (aggregate of people sharing space over time within a social system [see Chapter 6]; population groups or aggregates with power relations and common needs or purposes)	Fluoride water supplementation Environmental sanitation Removal of environmental hazards	Organized screening programs for communities (e.g., health fairs) VDRL screening for marriage license applicants in a city Lead screening for children by school district	Shelter and relocation centers for fire or earthquake victims Emergency medical services Community mental health services for chronically mentally ill Home care services for chronically ill

AIDS, Acquired immunodeficiency syndrome; *HIV,* human immunodeficiency virus; *STD,* sexually transmitted disease; *VDRL,* Venereal Disease Research Laboratory.

*Note that terms are used differently in literature of various disciplines. There are not any clear-cut definitions; for example, families may be referred to as an aggregate, and a population and subpopulations may exist within a community.

Mammography, blood pressure screening, scoliosis screening, and Papanicolaou smears are examples of secondary prevention.

Tertiary prevention targets populations that have experienced disease or injury and focuses on limitation of disability and rehabilitation. Aims of tertiary prevention are to keep health problems from getting worse, to reduce the effects of disease and injury, and to restore individuals to their optimal level of functioning (Keller et al, 2004b; McEwen and Pullis, 2009). Examples include teaching how to perform insulin injections and disease management to a patient with diabetes, referral of a patient with spinal cord injury for occupational and physical therapy, and leading a support group for grieving parents.

Much of community health nursing practice is directed toward preventing the progression of disease at the earliest period or phase feasible using the appropriate level(s) of prevention. For example, when applying "levels of prevention" to a client with HIV/AIDS, a nurse might perform the following interventions:

- Educate students on the practice of sexual abstinence or "safer sex" by using barrier methods (primary prevention)
- Encourage testing and counseling for clients with known exposure or who are in high-risk groups; provide referrals for follow-up for clients who test positive for HIV (secondary prevention)
- Provide education on management of HIV infection, advocacy, case management, and other interventions for those who are HIV positive (tertiary prevention) (McEwen and Pullis, 2009).

The concepts of prevention and population-focused care figure prominently in a conceptual orientation to nursing practice referred to as "thinking upstream." This orientation is derived from an analogy of patients falling into a river upstream and being rescued downstream by health providers overwhelmed with the struggle of responding to disease and illness. The river as an analogy for the natural history of illness was first coined by McKinlay (1979), with a charge to health providers to refocus their efforts toward preventive and "upstream" activities. In a description of the daily challenges of providers to address health from a preventive versus curative focus, McKinlay differentiates the consequences of illness (*downstream* endeavors) from its precursors (*upstream* endeavors). The author then charges health providers to critically examine the relative weights of their activities toward illness response versus the prevention of illness.

A population-based perspective on health and health determinants is critical to understanding and formulating nursing actions to prevent disease. By examining the origins of disease, nurses identify social, political, environmental, and economic factors that often lead to poor health options for both individuals and populations. The call to refocus the efforts of nurses "upstream, where the real problems lie" (McKinlay, 1979) has been welcomed by community health nurses in a variety of practice settings. For these nurses, this theme provides affirmation of their daily efforts to prevent disease in populations at risk in schools, work sites, and clinics throughout their local communities and in the larger world.

ETHICAL INSIGHTS

Inequities: Distribution of Resources

In the United States, inequities in the distribution of resources pose a threat to the common good and a challenge for community and public health nurses. Factors that contribute to wide variations in health disparities include education, income, and occupation. Lack of health insurance is a key factor in this issue and a major rationale for passage of the Patient Protection and Affordable Care Act, as about 20% of nonelderly adults and 25% of children in the United States are uninsured. Lack of insurance is damaging to population health, as low-income, uninsured individuals are much less likely than nonpoor insured individuals to receive timely physical examinations and preventive dental care.

Public health nurses are regularly confronted with the consequences of the fragmented health care delivery system. They diligently work to improve the circumstances for populations who have not had adequate access to resources largely because of who they are and where they live.

Ethical questions commonly encountered in community and public health nursing practice include the following: Should resources (e.g., free or low-cost immunizations) be offered to all, even those who have insurance that will pay for the care? Should public health nurses serve anyone who meets financial need guidelines, regardless of medical need? Should the health department provide flu shots to persons of all ages or just those most likely to be severely affected by the disease? Should illegal aliens or persons working on "green cards" receive the same level of health care services that are available to citizens?

Social justice in health care is a goal for all. To this end, community and public health nurses must face the challenges and dilemmas related to these and other questions as they assist individuals, families, and communities dealing with the uneven distribution of health resources.

From Ervin NE, Bell SE: Social justice issues related to uneven distribution of resources, *J N Y State Nurses Assoc* 35:8-13, 2004.

Prevention versus Cure

Spending additional dollars for cure in the form of health care services does little to improve the health of a population, whereas spending money on prevention does a great deal to improve health. Getzen (2010) and others (Shi and Singh, 2011; Russo, 2011) note that there is an absence of convincing evidence that the amount of money expended for health care improves the health of a population. The real determinants of health, as mentioned, are prevention efforts that provide education, housing, food, a decent minimal income, and safe social and physical environments. The United States spends more than one sixth of its wealth on health care or "cure" for individuals, likely diverting money away from the needed resources and services that would make a greater impact on health (Shi and Singh, 2011; NCHS, 2012).

U.S. policy makers must become committed to achieving improved health outcomes for the poor and vulnerable populations. With a limited health workforce and monetary resources, the United States cannot continue to spend vast amounts on health care services when the investment fails to improve health outcomes. In industrialized countries, life expectancy at birth is not related to the level of health care expenditures; in developing countries, longevity is closely related to the level of economic development and the education of the population (Russo, 2011; Shi and Singh, 2012).

A continued overexpansion of the current health care system following passage of the Affordable Care Act (ACA) could actually be detrimental to the health of the population. The focus on obtaining health insurance for more people may defer a large investment of the country's wealth from education and other developmental efforts that would positively affect health. Managed care organizations (MCOs) focus on prevention; therefore, they have determined that the rate of health care cost increases have slowed among employees of large firms (Shi and Singh, 2012). Prevention programs may help reduce costs for those enrolled in MCOs, but it remains unclear who will provide services for those who are required to purchase insurance, those who are currently uninsured and may remain so, the poor, and other vulnerable populations. In addition, still to be determined is who will provide adequate schooling, housing, meals, wages, and a safe environment for the disadvantaged. Increasing health care spending may negatively impact efforts to address economic disparities by reducing investments in sufficient housing, jobs, education, nutrition, and safe environments.

Healthy People 2020

In 1979, the U.S. Department of Health and Human Services published a national prevention initiative titled *Healthy People: The Surgeon General's Report on Health Promotion and Disease Prevention*. The 1979 version established goals that would reduce mortality among infants, children, adolescents and young adults, and adults and increase independence among older adults. In 1990, the mortality of infants, children, and adults declined sufficiently to meet the goal. Adolescent mortality did not reach the 1990 target, and data systems were unable to adequately track the target for older adults (USDHHS, 2000).

Published in 1989, *Healthy People 2000* built on the first Surgeon General's report. *Healthy People 2000* contained the following broad goals (USDHHS, 1989):

1. Increase the span of healthy life for Americans.
2. Reduce health disparities among Americans.
3. Achieve access to preventive services for all Americans.

The purpose of *Healthy People 2000* was to provide direction for individuals wanting to change personal behaviors and to improve health in communities through health promotion policies. The report assimilated the broad approaches of health promotion, health protection, and preventive services and contained more than 300 objectives organized into 22 priority areas. Although many of the objectives fell short, the initiative was extremely successful in raising providers' awareness of health behaviors and health promotional activities. States, local health departments, and private sector health workers used the objectives to determine the relative health of their communities and to set goals for the future.

Healthy People 2010 emerged in January 2000. It expanded on the objectives from *Healthy People 2000* through a broadened prevention science base, an improved surveillance and data system, and a heightened awareness of and demand for preventive health services. This change reflects changes in demographics, science, technology, and disease. *Healthy People 2010* listed two broad goals:

Goal 1: Increase quality and years of healthy life.
Goal 2: Eliminate health disparities.

The first goal moved beyond the idea of increasing life expectancy to incorporate the concept of health-related quality of life (HRQOL). This concept of health includes aspects of physical and mental health and their determinants and measures functional status, participation, and well-being. HRQOL expands the definition of health—beyond simply opposing the negative concepts of disease and death—by integrating mental and physical health concepts (USDHHS, 2000).

The final review and analysis of the *Healthy People 2010* objectives showed decidedly mixed progress for the nation. Some 23% of the objectives were met or exceeded, and another 48% "moved toward target." Conversely, 24% of the objectives "moved away from target" (i.e., the indicators were worse than in the previous decade), and another 5% showed no change. Particularly concerning were the poor responses in two of the Focus Areas: Arthritis, Osteoporosis and Chronic Back conditions (Focus Area 2) and Nutrition and Overweight (Focus Area 19) "moved toward" or "achieved" less than 25% of their targets (USDHHS, 2013).

The fourth version of the Nation's health objectives, *Healthy People 2020*, was published in 2010. *Healthy People 2020* is divided into 42 Topic Areas and contains numerous new objectives and updates for hundreds of objectives from the previous editions. The Topic Areas are listed in the *Healthy People 2020* box. The objectives and related information and materials can help guide health promotion activities and can be used to aid in community-wide initiatives (USDHHS, 2013). All health care practitioners, particularly those working in the community, should review the *Healthy People 2020* objectives and focus on the relevant areas in their practice. Practitioners should incorporate these objectives into programs, events, and publications whenever possible and should use them as a framework to promote healthy cities and communities. Selected relevant objectives are presented throughout this book to acquaint future community health nurses with the scope of the *Healthy People 2020* initiative and to enhance awareness of current health indicators and national goals (see www.healthypeople.gov for more information).

♥ HEALTHY PEOPLE 2020

Topic Areas

- Access to health services
- Adolescent health
- Arthritis, osteoporosis, and chronic back conditions
- Blood disorders and blood safety
- Cancer
- Chronic kidney disease
- Dementias, including Alzheimer's
- Diabetes
- Disability and health
- Early and middle childhood

Continued

- Educational and community-based programs
- Environmental health
- Family planning
- Food safety
- Genomics
- Global health
- Health communication and health information technology
- Healthcare-associated infections
- Health-related quality of life and well-being
- Hearing and other sensory or communication disorders
- Heart disease and stroke
- HIV
- Immunization and infectious diseases
- Injury and violence prevention
- Lesbian, gay, bisexual and transgender health
- Maternal, infant, and child health
- Medical product safety
- Mental health and mental disorders
- Nutrition and weight status
- Occupational safety and health
- Older adults
- Oral health
- Physical activity
- Preparedness
- Public health infrastructure
- Respiratory diseases
- Sexually transmitted diseases
- Social determinants of health
- Substance abuse
- Tobacco use
- Vision

From U.S. Department of Health and Human Services: *Healthy People 2020 topics & objectives—objectives A-Z*. Retrieved July 2013 from <http://www.healthypeople.gov/2020/topicsobjectives2020/default.aspx>.

DEFINITION AND FOCUS OF PUBLIC HEALTH NURSING, COMMUNITY HEALTH NURSING, AND COMMUNITY-BASED NURSING

The terms *community health nursing* and *public health nursing* are often used synonymously or interchangeably. Like the practice of community/public health nursing, the terms are evolving. In past debates and discussions, definitions of "community health nursing" and "public health nursing " have indicated similar yet distinctive ideologies, visions, or philosophies of nursing. These concepts and a third related term—*community-based nursing*—are discussed in this section.

Public and Community Health Nursing

Public health nursing has frequently been described as the synthesis of public health and nursing practice. Freeman (1963) provided a classic definition of public health nursing:

> *Public health nursing may be defined as a field of professional practice in nursing and in public health in which technical nursing, interpersonal, analytical, and organizational skills are applied to problems of health as they affect the community. These skills are applied in concert with those of other persons engaged in health care, through comprehensive nursing care of families and other groups and through measures for evaluation or control of threats to health, for health education of the public, and for mobilization of the public for health action. (p. 34)*

Through the 1980s and 1990s, most nurses were taught that there was a distinction between "community health nursing" and "public health nursing." Indeed, "public health nursing" was seen as a subspecialty nursing practice generally delivered within "official" or governmental agencies. In contrast, "community health nursing" was considered to be a broader and more general specialty area that encompassed many additional sub specialties (e.g., school nursing, occupational health nursing, forensic nursing, home health). In 1980, the ANA defined community health nursing as "the synthesis of nursing practice and public health practice applied to promoting and preserving the health of populations" (ANA, 1980, p. 2). This viewpoint noted that a community health nurse directs care to individuals, families, or groups; this care, in turn, contributes to the health of the total population.

The ANA has revised the standards of practice for this specialty area (ANA, 2013). In the updated standards, the designation was again "public health nursing," and the ANA used the definition presented by the American Public Health Association (APHA) Committee on Public Health Nursing (1996). Thus, public health nursing is defined as "the practice of promoting and protecting the health of populations using knowledge from nursing, social, and public health sciences" (ANA/APHA, 1996, p. 5). The ANA (2013) elaborated by explaining that public health nursing practice "is population-focused, with the goals of promoting health and preventing disease and disability for all people through the creation of conditions in which people can be healthy" (p. 5).

Some nursing writers will continue to use *community health nursing* as a global or umbrella term and *public health nursing* as a component or subset. Others, as stated, use the terms interchangeably. This book uses the terms interchangeably.

RESEARCH HIGHLIGHTS

Public Health Nursing Research Agenda

In 2010, a national conference was held to set a research agenda that would advance the science of public health nursing (PHN). The conference employed a multistage, multimethod, participatory developmental approach, involving many influential PHN leaders. Following numerous meetings and discussions, an agenda was proposed. The agenda was structured around four "High Priority Themes": (1) public health nursing interventions models, (2) quality of population-focused practice, (3) metrics of/for public health nursing, and (4) comparative effectiveness and public health nursing outcomes. The aim of the agenda is to help PHN scholars contribute to an understanding of how to improve health and reduce population health disparities by advancing the evidence base regarding the outcomes of practice and by influencing related health policy. The group encouraged the agenda's use to guide and inform programs of research, to influence funding priorities, and to be incorporated into doctoral PHN education through course and curriculum development. Ultimately, it is anticipated that PHN research will proactively contribute to the effectiveness of the public health system and create healthier communities.

Data from Issel LM, Bekemeier B, Kneipp S: A public health nursing research agenda, *Public Health Nurs* 29:330-342, 2012.

Community-Based Nursing

The term *community-based nursing* has been identified and defined in recent years to differentiate it from what has traditionally been seen as community and public health nursing practice. Community-based nursing practice refers to "application of the nursing process in caring for individuals, families and groups where they live, work or go to school or as they move through the health care system" (McEwen and Pullis, 2009, p. 6). Community-based nursing is setting-specific, and the emphasis is on acute and chronic care and includes such practice areas as home health nursing and nursing in outpatient or ambulatory settings.

Zotti, Brown, and Stotts (1996) compared community-based nursing and community health nursing and explained that the goals of the two are different. Community health nursing emphasizes preservation and protection of health, and community-based nursing emphasizes managing acute or chronic conditions. In community health nursing, the primary client is the community; in community-based nursing, the primary clients are the individual and the family. Finally, services in community-based nursing are largely direct, but in community health nursing, services are both direct and indirect.

Community and Public Health Nursing Practice

Community and public health nurses practice disease prevention and health promotion. It is important to note that community health nursing practice is collaborative and is based in research and theory. It applies the nursing process to the care of individuals, families, aggregates, and the community. Box 1-3

BOX 1-3   THE SCOPE AND STANDARDS OF PRACTICE FOR PUBLIC HEALTH NURSING

The Scope and Standards of Practice for Public Health Nursing is the result of the collaborative effort between the American Nurse Association and the Quad Council of Public Health Nursing Organizations. The Standards were originally developed in 1999 and were updated in 2013. The Scope and Standards of Practice, which are divided into Standards of Practice and Standards of Professional Performance, describe specific competencies relevant to the public health nurse and the public health nurse in advanced practice.

The Standards of Practice include six standards that are based on the critical thinking model of the nursing process, with competencies addressing each nursing process step. The implementation step is further broken down into specific public health areas including coordination of services, health education and health promotion, consultation, and regulatory activities. The Standards of Professional Performance include the leadership competencies necessary in the professional practice of all registered nurses, but with additional standards specific to the public health nurse and advance public health nurse roles. These standards including evidence-based practice and research, collaboration, resource utilization, and advocacy, with competencies specific to public health, such as building coalitions and achieving consensus in public health issues, assessing available health resources within a population, and advocating for equitable access to care and services.

Data from American Nurses Association: *Public health nursing: Scope and standards of practice*, ed 2, Silver Spring, MD, 2013, Author. The Standards can be purchased at <http://www.nursesbooks.org/Homepage/Hot-off-the-Press/Public-Health-Nursing-2nd.aspx>.

---

provides an overview of the Standards for Public Health Nursing (ANA, 2013).

As discussed, the core functions of public health are assessment, policy development, and assurance. In 2003, the Quad Council of Public Health Nursing Organizations (Quad Council) closely examined the core functions and used them to develop a set of public health nursing competencies. These competencies were updated in 2011 and are summarized in Table 1-2 (Quad Council, 2011). Current and future community health nurses should study these competencies to understand the practice parameters and skills required for public health nursing practice.

POPULATION-FOCUSED PRACTICE AND COMMUNITY/PUBLIC HEALTH NURSING INTERVENTIONS

Community/public health nurses must use a population-focused approach to move beyond providing direct care to individuals and families. Population-focused nursing concentrates on specific groups of people and focuses on health promotion and disease prevention, regardless of geographic location (Baldwin et al, 1998). The goal of population-focused nursing is "provision of evidence-based care to targeted groups of people with similar needs in order to improve outcomes" (Curley, 2012, p. 4). In short, population-focused practice (Minnesota Department of Health, 2003):

- Focuses on the entire population
- Is based on assessment of the populations' health status
- Considers the broad determinants of health
- Emphasizes all levels of prevention
- Intervenes with communities, systems, individuals, and families

Whereas community and public health nurses may be responsible for a specific subpopulation in the community (e.g., a school nurse may be responsible for the school's pregnant teenagers), population-focused practice is concerned with many distinct and overlapping community subpopulations. The goal of population-focused nursing is to promote healthy communities.

Population-focused community health nurses would not have exclusive interest in one or two subpopulations, but instead would focus on the many subpopulations that make up the entire community. A population focus involves concern for those who do, and for those who do not, receive health services. A population focus also involves a scientific approach to community health nursing. Thus a thorough, systematic assessment of the community or population is necessary and basic to planning, intervention, and evaluation for the individual, family, aggregate, and population levels.

Community health nursing practice requires the following types of data for scientific approach and population focus: (1) the epidemiology, or body of knowledge, of a particular problem and its solution and (2) information about the community. Each type of knowledge and its source appear in Table 1-3. To determine the overall patterns of health in

TABLE 1-2 SUMMARY OF TIER 1 PUBLIC HEALTH NURSING (PHN) COMPETENCIES (GENERALIST PUBLIC HEALTH NURSES)

DOMAIN	COMMUNITY AND PUBLIC HEALTH NURSING COMPETENCIES
1. Analytic assessment skills	Identifies determinants of health and illness Uses epidemiologic data and ecological perspective to identify health risks, needs, values, beliefs, resources, and relevant environmental factors Identifies variables that measure health and health conditions Uses valid and reliable methods and instruments for collecting data; develops data collection plan Identifies sources of public health data and information; collects, interprets, and documents data in understandable terms Uses valid and reliable data sources for comparisons Identifies gaps and redundancies in data sources Applies ethical, legal, and policy guidelines and principles in data collection, use, and dissemination Practices evidence-based public health nursing to promote the health of individuals, families, and groups
2. Policy development/program planning skills	Identifies policy issues relevant to health; describes the structure of the public health system and its impact on health Identifies the implications of policy options on public health programs Identifies outcomes of health policy relevant to PHN practice Collects information that will inform policy decisions; describes the legislative policy development process; identifies outcomes of current health policy Describes the structure of the public health system; identifies public health laws and regulations relevant to practice Participates as a team member to implement programs and policies Participates in teams to assure compliance with organizational policies Assists in design of evaluation plans
3. Communication skills	Assesses health literacy Communicates effectively in writing, orally, and electronically; communicates in a culturally responsive and relevant manner Solicits input when planning and delivering health care Uses a variety of methods to disseminate public health information Communicates effectively as a member of interprofessional team(s)
4. Cultural competency skills	Utilizes the social and ecological determinants of health to work effectively Uses concepts, knowledge, and evidence of the social determinants of health in the delivery of services Adapts PHN care on the basis of cultural needs and differences Explains factors contributing to cultural diversity Articulates benefits of a diverse public health workforce Demonstrates culturally appropriate public health nursing practice
5. Community dimensions of practice skills	Utilizes an ecological perspective in health assessment, planning, and interventions Identifies research issues at a community level; functions as a member of a participatory research team Identifies community partners for PHN practice Collaborates with community partners to promote health Partners effectively with key stakeholders and groups in care delivery Participates effectively in activities that facilitate community involvement Describes the role of government and the private and nonprofit sectors in the delivery of health services Utilizes community assets and resources to promote health and deliver care Seeks input into plans of care Supports public health policies, programs, and resources
6. Public health sciences skills	Incorporates public health and nursing science in the delivery of care Describes the historical foundation of public health and public health nursing Describes how programs contribute to meeting the core public health functions and the 10 essential services Uses basic descriptive epidemiological methods when conducting a health assessment Interprets research relevant to public health interventions Accesses public health and other sources of information using informatics and information technologies Identifies gaps in research evidence to guide public health nursing practice Complies with requirements of patient confidentiality and human subject protection Participates in research at the community level to build the scientific base of PHN

TABLE 1-2 SUMMARY OF TIER 1 PUBLIC HEALTH NURSING (PHN) COMPETENCIES (GENERALIST PUBLIC HEALTH NURSES)—cont'd

DOMAIN	COMMUNITY AND PUBLIC HEALTH NURSING COMPETENCIES
7. Financial planning and management skills	Describes the interrelationships among local, state, tribal, and federal public health and health care systems
	Describes the structure, function, and jurisdictional authority of organizational units within federal, state, tribal, and local public health agencies
	Adheres to the organization's policies and procedures
	Provides data for inclusion in a programmatic budget
	Describes the impact of budget constraints on the delivery of public health nursing care
	Provides input into budget priorities
	Provides data to evaluate care and services
	Adapts the delivery of PHN care on the basis of evaluation results
	Provides input into proposals for funding from external sources
	Applies basic human relations and conflict management skills in interaction with peers
	Utilizes public health informatics skills
	Provides input into contracts and other agreements for the provision of services
	Delivers PHN care within budgetary guidelines
8. Leadership and systems thinking skills	Incorporates ethical standards of practice as the basis of all interactions
	Applies systems theory to PHN practice
	Participates with stakeholders to identify vision, values, and principles of community action
	Identifies internal and external factors affecting PHN practice and services
	Uses individual, team, and organizational learning opportunities for personal and professional development
	Acts as a mentor, coach, or peer advisor for PHN staff; maintains personal commitment to lifelong learning and professional development
	Participates in quality initiatives
	Adapts the delivery of PHN care in consideration of changes in the health system and the larger social, political, and economic environment; maintains knowledge of current public health laws and policies

Modified from Quad Council of Public Health Nursing Organizations: *Public health nursing competencies,* Washington, DC, 2011, Author.

TABLE 1-3 INFORMATION USEFUL FOR POPULATION FOCUS

TYPE OF INFORMATION	EXAMPLES	SOURCES
Demographic data	Age, gender, race/ethnicity, socioeconomic status, education level	Vital statistic data (national, state, county, local); census
Groups at high risk	Health status and health indicators of various subpopulations in the community (e.g., children, elders, those with disabilities)	Health statistics (morbidity, mortality, natality); disease statistics (incidence and prevalence)
Services/providers available	Official (public) health departments; health care providers for low-income individuals and families; community service agencies and organizations (e.g., Red Cross, Meals on Wheels)	City directories; phone books; local or regional social workers; low-income providers lists; local community health nurses (e.g., school nurses)

a population, data collection for assessment and management decisions within a community should be ongoing, not episodic.

Community Health Interventions

Community health nurses focus on the care of individuals, groups, aggregates, and populations in many settings, including homes, clinics, worksites, and schools. In addition to interviewing clients and assessing individual and family health, community health nurses must be able to assess a population's health needs and resources and identify its values. Community health nurses must also work with the community to identify and implement programs that meet health needs and to evaluate the effectiveness of programs after implementation. For example, school nurses were once responsible only for running first-aid stations and monitoring immunization compliance. Now they are actively involved in assessing the needs of their population and defining programs to meet those needs through activities such as health screening and group health education and promotion. The activities of school nurses may be as varied as designing health curricula with a school and community advisory group, leading support groups for elementary school children with chronic illness, and monitoring the health status of teenage mothers.

Similarly, occupational health nurses are no longer required to simply maintain an office or dispensary. They are involved in many different types of activities. These activities might include maintaining records of workers exposed to physical or chemical risks, monitoring compliance with Occupational Safety and Health Administration (OSHA)

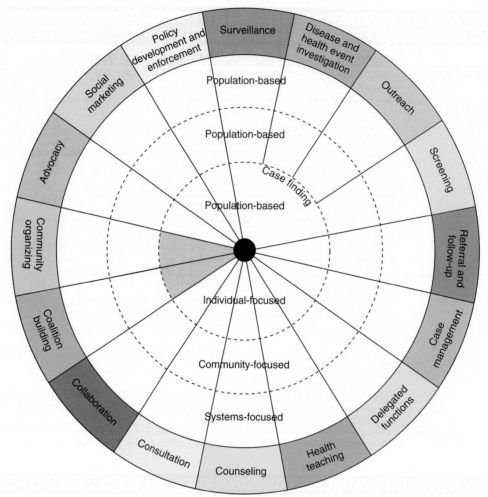

FIGURE 1-3 Public Health Intervention Wheel. (Modified from Section of Public Health Nursing, Minnesota Department of Health: *Public health interventions*, 2001. Retrieved July 2013 from <http://www.health.state. mn.us/divs/cfh/connect/index.cfm?article=phstories.search>.)

standards, teaching classes on health issues, acting as case managers for workers with chronic health conditions, and leading support group discussions for workers with health-related problems.

Private associations, such as the American Diabetes Association, employ community health nurses for their organizational ability and health-related skills. Other community health nurses work with multidisciplinary groups of professionals, serve on boards of voluntary health associations such as the American Heart Association, and are members of health planning agencies and councils.

The Public Health Intervention Wheel

The Public Health Intervention Model was initially proposed in the late 1990s by nurses from the Minnesota Department of Health to describe the breadth and scope of public health nursing practice (Keller et al, 1998). This model was later revised and termed the *Intervention Wheel* (Figure 1-3) (Keller et al, 2004a; Keller et al, 2004b), and it has become increasingly recognized as a framework for community and public health nursing practice.

The Intervention Wheel contains three important elements: (1) it is population-based; (2) it contains three levels of practice (community, systems, and individual/family); and (3) it identifies and defines 17 public health interventions. The levels of practice and interventions are directed at improving population health (Keller et al, 2004a). Within the Intervention Wheel, the 17 health interventions are grouped into five "wedges." These interventions are actions taken on behalf of communities, systems, individuals, and families to improve or protect health status. Table 1-4 provides definitions.

The Intervention Wheel is further dissected into levels of practice, in which the interventions may be directed at an entire population within a community, a system that would affect the health of a population, and/or the individuals and families within the population. Thus each intervention can and should be applied at each level. For example, a systems-level intervention within "disease investigation" might be the community health nurse working with the state health department and federal vaccine program to coordinate a response to an outbreak of measles in a migrant population. An example of a population- or community-level intervention for

TABLE 1-4 PUBLIC HEALTH INTERVENTIONS AND DEFINITIONS

PUBLIC HEALTH INTERVENTION	DEFINITION
Surveillance	Describes and monitors health events through ongoing and systematic collection, analysis, and interpretation of health data for the purpose of planning, implementing, and evaluating public health interventions
Disease and other health event investigation	Systematically gathers and analyzes data regarding threats to the health of populations, ascertains the source of the threat, identifies cases and others at risk, and determines control measures
Outreach	Locates populations of interest or populations at risk and provides information about the nature of the concern, what can be done about it, and how services can be obtained
Screening	Identifies individuals with unrecognized health risk factors or asymptomatic disease conditions
Case finding	Locates individuals and families with identified risk factors and connects them with resources
Referral and follow-up	Assists individuals, families, groups, organizations, and/or communities to identify and access necessary resources to prevent or resolve problems or concerns
Case management	Optimizes self-care capabilities of individuals and families and the capacity of systems and communities to coordinate and provide services
Delegated functions	Carries out direct care tasks under the authority of a health care practitioner as allowed by law
Health teaching	Communicates facts, ideas, and skills that change knowledge, attitudes, values, beliefs, behaviors, and practices of individuals, families, systems, and/or communities
Counseling	Establishes an interpersonal relationship with a community, a system, and a family or individual, with the intention of increasing or enhancing their capacity for self-care and coping
Consultation	Seeks information and generates optional solutions to perceived problems or issues through interactive problem solving with a community system and family or individual
Collaboration	Commits two or more persons or organizations to achieve a common goal through enhancing the capacity of one or more of the members to promote and protect health
Coalition building	Promotes and develops alliances among organizations or constituencies for a common purpose
Community organizing	Helps community groups to identify common problems or goals, mobilize resources, and develop and implement strategies for realizing the goals they collectively have set
Advocacy	Pleads someone's cause or acts on someone's behalf, with a focus on developing the community, system, and individual or family's capacity to plead their own cause or act on their own behalf
Social marketing	Utilizes commercial marketing principles and technologies for programs designed to influence the knowledge, attitudes, values, beliefs, behaviors, and practices of the population of interest
Policy development and enforcement	Places health issues on decision makers' agendas, acquires a plan of resolution, and determines needed resources, resulting in laws, rules, regulations, ordinances, and policies. Policy enforcement compels others to comply with laws, rules, regulations, ordinances, and policies

Modified from Keller LO, Strohschein S, Lia-Hoagberg B, Schaffer MA: *Population-based public health interventions: Practice-based and evidence-supported. Part I*, St. Paul, MN, 2004a, Minnesota Department of Health, Center for Public Health Nursing.

"screening" would be public health nurses working with area high schools to give each student a profile of his or her health to promote nutritional and physical activity lifestyle changes to improve the student's health.

Finally, an individual-level implementation of the intervention "referral and follow-up" would occur when a nurse receives a referral to care for an individual with a diagnosed mental illness who would require regular monitoring of his medication compliance to prevent rehospitalization (Keller et al, 2004b).

COMMUNITY HEALTH NURSING, MANAGED CARE, AND HEALTH REFORM

Shifts in reimbursement, the growth of managed care, and implementation of the Affordable Care Act have revitalized the notion of population-based care. Health insurance companies, governmental financing entities (e.g., Medicare, Medicaid), and MCOs use financial incentives and organizational structures in an attempt to increase efficiency and decrease health care costs. The foundation for managed care is management of health care for an enrolled group of individuals.

This group of enrollees is the population covered by the plan who receive health services from managed care plan providers (Shi and Singh, 2012).

An understanding of enrolled populations and health care patterns is essential for managing health care services and resources effectively. Most MCOs have become sophisticated in identifying key subgroups within the population of enrollees at risk for health problems. Typically, managed care systems target subgroups according to characteristics associated with risk or use of expensive services, such as selected clinical conditions, functional status, and past service use patterns.

In March 2010, President Obama signed the Patient Protection and Affordable Care Act (PPACA) (PL 111-148) into law. Although the law will not be fully implemented until 2017, and challenges to aspects of it are ongoing, it is intended to expand insurance coverage for most of those currently uninsured in the country and to help control health care costs. Expansion of coverage will be accomplished through requiring individuals to purchase health insurance for themselves and their families, implementation of "exchanges" to increase options for individuals to purchase health insurance, and requiring employers of more than 50 people to offer health insurance to employees. Public programs (e.g., Medicaid and State Children's Health Insurance Program [SCHIP]) have been expanded to cover health care for those who cannot afford to buy their own insurance. Cost containment will be accomplished through many activities, including efforts to control waste, fraud, and abuse and simplification of administrative tasks. Finally, the PPACA seeks to improve overall health of the population by encouraging prevention and wellness initiatives (Kaiser Family Foundation, 2011; Kaiser Family Foundation, 2013).

The purpose of public health is to improve the health of the public by promoting healthy lifestyles, preventing disease and injury, and protecting the health of communities. In the past, shrinking public health resources have supported personal health services over community health promotion. In public health practice, the community is the population of interest. With the proposed changes to health care financing, the personal health care system will be under increasing pressure to provide the services that health departments previously provided. Traditionally served by public health, the most vulnerable populations will pose tremendous challenges for private health care providers. Public health agencies and providers will be responsible for partnering with private providers to care for these populations.

Providing population-based care requires a dramatic shift in thinking from individual-based care. Some of the practical demands of population-based care are the following:

1. It must be recognized that populations are not homogeneous; therefore it is necessary to address the needs of special subpopulations within populations.
2. High-risk and vulnerable subpopulations must be identified early in the care delivery cycle.
3. Nonusers of services often become high-cost users; therefore, it is essential to develop outreach strategies.
4. Quality and cost of all health care services are linked together across the health care continuum. (Kaiser Family Foundation, 2013.)

Nurses in community and public health have an opportunity to share their expertise regarding population-based approaches to health care for groups of individuals across health care settings. Today, health care practitioners require additional skills in assessment, policy development, and assurance to provide community public health practice and population-based service. Health care professionals should focus attention toward promoting healthy lifestyles, providing preventive and primary care, expanding and ensuring access to cost-effective and technologically appropriate care, participating in coordinated and interdisciplinary care, and

involving patients and families in the decision-making process. Public health nurses must work in partnership with colleagues in managed care settings to improve community health. Partnerships may address information management, cultural values, health care system improvement, and the physical environment roles in health and may require complex negotiations to share data. The partners may need to develop new community assessment strategies to augment epidemiological methods that often mask the context or meaning of the human experience of vulnerable populations.

SUMMARY

Knowledge and skills enable community health nurses to work in diverse community settings ranging from the isolated rural area to the crowded urban ghetto. To meet the health needs of the population, the community health nurse must work with many individuals and groups within the community. The community health nurse must develop sensitivity to these groups and must respect the community and its established method of problem management. This approach will enable the nurse to become more proficient in helping the community improve overall health.

LEARNING ACTIVITIES

1. Interview several community/public health nurses and several clients regarding their definitions of health. Share the results with your classmates. Do you agree with their definitions? Why or why not?
2. Interview several community/public health nurses regarding their opinions on the focus of community/public health nursing. Do you agree?
3. Ask several neighbors or consumers of health care about their views of the role of public health and community health nursing. Share your results with your classmates.
4. Become familiar with *Healthy People 2020* (www.healthypeople.gov). Review objectives from several of the topic areas covered. How does your community compare with the groups, aggregates, and populations described? What objectives should be targeted for your community?

ⓔ **EVOLVE WEBSITE**

http://evolve.elsevier.com/Nies
- NCLEX Review Questions
- Case Studies
- Glossary

REFERENCES

Allender JA, Rector C, Warner K: *Community health nursing: promoting and protecting the public's health*, ed 8, Philadelphia, 2013, Wolters Kluwer/Lippincott Williams & Wilkins.
American Heritage College Dictionary, ed 3, New York, 1997, Houghton Mifflin.

American Nurses Association: *A conceptual model of community health nursing*, Pub No CH-10, Kansas City, MO, 1980, Author.
American Nurses Association: *Code of ethics*, Kansas City, MO, 2001, Author.

American Nurses Association: *Public health nursing: scope and standards of practice*, Silver Spring, MD, 2013, American Nurses Publishing.

American Public Health Association: *Ad hoc committee on public health nursing: the definition and role of public health nursing practice in the delivery of health care*, Washington, DC, 1996, Author.

Baldwin JH, Conger CO, Abegglen JC, et al: Population-focused and community-based nursing: moving toward clarification of concepts, *Public Health Nurs* 15:12–18, 1998.

Centers for Disease Control and Prevention (CDC): Office of the Director, Office of the Chief of Public Health Practice, National Public Health Performance Standards Program: *10 essential public health services*, 2010. Available from <http://www.cdc.gov/nphpsp/essentialServices.html>.

Curley ALC: Introduction to population-based nursing. In Curley ALC, Vitale PA, editors: *Population-based nursing: concepts and competencies for advanced practice*, New York, 2012, Springer Publishing Co.

Dunn HL: *High level wellness*, Arlington, VA, 1961, RW Beatty.

Freeman RB: *Public health nursing practice*, ed 3, Philadelphia, 1963, WB Saunders.

Getzen T: *Health economics and financing*, ed 4, Hoboken, NJ, 2010, John Wiley & Sons.

Hanlon JJ: *Principles of public health administration*, ed 3, St. Louis, 1960, Mosby.

Harkness GA: Community and public health nursing: present, past and future. In Harkness GA, DeMarco RF, editors: *Community and public health Nursing: evidence for practice*, Philadelphia, PA, 2012, Wolters Kluwer/Lippincott Williams & Wilkins.

Institute of Medicine: *The future of public health*, Washington, DC, 1988, National Academy Press.

Kaiser Family Foundation: *Health reform source*, 2013. Available from <http://healthreform.kff.org/the-basics.aspx>. Accessed March 1, 2013.

Kaiser Family Foundation: *Summary of the new health reform law*, Pub No. 8061. Available from <http://www.kff.org/healthreform/upload/8061.pdf>. Accessed February 5, 2013.

Keller LO, Strohschein S, Lia-Hoagberg B, et al: Population-based public health interventions: a model for practice, *Public Health Nurs* 15:207–215, 1998.

Keller LO, Strohschein S, Lia-Hoagberg B, et al: Population-based public health interventions: practice-based and evidence-supported. Part I, *Public Health Nurs* 21:453–468, 2004a.

Keller LO, Strohschein S, Schaffer MA, et al: Population-based public health interventions: innovations in practice, teaching and management. Part II, *Public Health Nurs* 21:469–487, 2004b.

Leavell HR, Clark EG: *Preventive medicine for the doctor in his community*, New York, 1958, McGraw-Hill.

Lundy KS, Janes S: *Community health nursing: caring for the public's health*, ed 2, Boston, 2009, Jones & Bartlett.

Maurer FA, Smith CM: *Community/public health nursing practice: health for families and populations*, ed 5, St. Louis, 2013, Elsevier.

McEwen M, Pullis B: *Community-based nursing: an introduction*, ed 3, St. Louis, 2009, WB Saunders.

McGinnis MJ, Foege W: Actual causes of death in the United States, *JAMA* 270:2207–2212, 1993.

McKeown T: Determinants of health. In Lee PR, Estes CL, editors: *The nation's health*, ed 7, Boston, 2003, Jones & Bartlett.

McKinlay JB: A case for refocusing upstream: the political economy of illness. In Jaco EG, editor: *Patients, physicians, and illness*, ed 3, New York, 1979, The Free Press.

Minnesota Department of Health: *Definitions of population based practice*, 2003. Available from <http://www.health.state.mn.us/divs/cfh/ophp/resources/docs/population-based-practice_definition.pdf>.

Mokdad AH, Marks JS, Stroup DF, et al: Actual causes of death in the United States, *JAMA* 291:1238–1245, 2004. 2000.

Murray RB, Zentner JP, Yakimo R: *Health promotion strategies through the life span*, ed 8, Upper Saddle River, NJ, 2009, Prentice Hall.

National Center for Health Statistics: *Health, United States*, 2012. Available from <http://www.cdc.gov/nchs/data/hus/hus12.pdf>. Accessed December 27, 2013.

Orem DE: *Nursing: concepts of practice*, ed 6, St. Louis, 2001, Mosby.

Orleans CT, Cassidy EF: Health and behavior. In Kovner AR, Knickman JR, editors: *Health care delivery in the United States*, ed 10, New York, 2011, Springer Publishing.

Pender NJ, Murdaugh CL, Parsons MA: *Health promotion in nursing practice*, ed 6, Upper Saddle River, NJ, 2011, Pearson Education.

Quad Council of Public Health Nursing Organizations: *Competencies for public health nurses*, 2011. Available from <http://www.achne.org/files/Quad%20Council/QuadCouncilCompetenciesforPublicHealthNurses.pdf>.

Rosenfeld P, Russell D: A review of factors influencing utilization of home and community-based long-term care: trends and implications to the nursing workforce, *Policy Polit Nurs Pract* 13:72–80, 2012.

Russo P: Population health. In Kovner AR, Knickman JR, editors: *Health care delivery in the United States*, ed 10, New York, 2011, Springer Publishing.

Saylor C: The circle of health: a health definition model, *J Holist Nurs* 22:98–115, 2004.

Shi L, Singh DA: *Delivering health care in America: a systems approach*, ed 5, Boston, 2012, Jones & Bartlett.

Shi L, Singh DA: *The nation's health*, ed 8, Boston, 2011, Jones & Bartlett.

Shuster GR: Community as client: assessment and analysis. In Stanhope M, Lancaster J, editors: *Public health nursing: population-centered health care in the community*, ed 8, St. Louis, 2012, Elsevier.

U.S. Department of Health and Human Services, Health Resources and Services Administration: *The registered nurse population: Initial findings 2008 national sample survey of registered nurses*, 2010. Available from <http://bhpr.hrsa.gov/healthworkforce/rnsurvey/initialfindings2008.pdf>. Accessed April 6, 2010.

U.S. Department of Health and Human Services, Public Health Service: *The public health workforce: an agenda for the 21st century*, Washington, DC, 1997, Author.

U.S. Department of Health and Human Services: *Healthy People 2000 objectives*, Washington, DC, 1989, Author.

U.S. Department of Health and Human Services: *Healthy People 2010 objectives*, Washington, DC, 2000, Author.

U.S. Department of Health and Human Services: *Healthy People 2010: final review*, 2012. Available from <http://www.cdc.gov/nchs/data/hpdata2010/hp2010_final_review.pdf>.

U.S. Department of Health and Human Services: *Healthy People 2020 objectives*, 2013. Available from <http://www.healthypeople.gov/2020/about/default.aspx>.

Wald LD: *The house on Henry Street*, New York, 1971, Dover Publications.

Way M, MacNeil M: Baccalaureate entry to practice: a systems review, *J Contin Educ Nurs* 38:164–169, 2007.

World Health Organization: A discussion document on the concept and principles of health promotion, *Health Promot* 1:73–78, 1986.

World Health Organization: The first 10 years of the World Health Organization, *Chron WHO* 1:1–2, 1958.

Zotti ME, Brown P, Stotts RC: Community-based nursing versus community health nursing: what does it all mean? *Nurs Outlook* 44:211–217, 1996.

Historical Factors: Community Health Nursing in Context

*Melanie McEwen**

OBJECTIVES

Upon completion of this chapter, the reader will be able to do the following:

1. Describe the impact of aggregate living on population health.
2. Identify approaches to population health promotion from prerecorded historic to present times.
3. Understand historical events that have influenced population health.
4. Compare the application of public health principles to the nation's major health problems at the turn of the twentieth century (i.e., acute disease) with that at the beginning of the twenty-first century (i.e., chronic disease).
5. Describe two leaders in nursing who had a profound impact on addressing aggregate health.
6. Discuss major contemporary issues facing community/public health nursing, and trace the historical roots to the present.

KEY TERMS

district nursing
Edward Jenner
Edwin Chadwick
Elizabethan Poor Law
endemic
epidemic
Flexner Report

Florence Nightingale
health visiting
House on Henry Street
John Snow
Joseph Lister
Lemuel Shattuck
Lillian Wald

Louis Pasteur
pandemic
Robert Koch
Sanitary Revolution
stages in disease history

OUTLINE

Evolution of Health in Western Populations
   Aggregate Impact on Health
   Evolution of Early Public Health Efforts
Advent of Modern Health Care
   Evolution of Modern Nursing
   Establishment of Modern Medical Care and Public
     Health Practice

   Community Caregiver
   Establishment of Public Health Nursing
Consequences for the Health of Aggregates
   Twenty-First Century
Social Changes and Community Health Nursing
**Challenges for Community and Public Health
   Nursing**

* The author would like to acknowledge the contribution of Tom H. Cook, who wrote this chapter for the previous edition.

This chapter presents an overview of some of the historical factors that have influenced the evolution of community health and explains current health challenges. It examines the health of Western populations from prerecorded historic to recent times, the evolution of modern health care, and the role of public health nursing, and addresses the concurrent challenges for public health nursing.

EVOLUTION OF HEALTH IN WESTERN POPULATIONS

The study of humankind's evolution has seldom taken into consideration the interrelationship among an individual's health, an individual's environment, and the nature and size of the individual's aggregate. Medical anthropologists use paleontological records and disease descriptions of primitive societies to speculate on the interrelationship of early humans, probable diseases, and their environment. Historians have also documented the existence of public health activity (i.e., an organized community effort to prevent disease, prolong life, and promote health) since before recorded historic times. The following section describes how aggregate living patterns and early public health efforts have impacted the health of Western populations.

Aggregate Impact on Health

Polgar (1964) defined the following stages in disease history of humankind: hunting and gathering stage, settled villages stage, preindustrial cities stage, industrial cities stage, and present stage (Figure 2-1). In these stages, growing populations, increased population density, and imbalanced human ecology resulted in changes in cultural adaptation. Humans created the ecological imbalance by altering their environment to accommodate group living. This imbalance subsequently had a significant effect on aggregate health.

Although these stages are associated with the evolution of civilization, it is important to note that the information

is limited by cultural bias. For example, the stages depict the evolution of Western civilization from the perspective of the Western world. They consist of overlapping historical time periods, which anthropologists widely debate. However, the stages of human disease can provide a frame of reference to aid in determining the relationship among humans, disease, and environment from prerecorded historic times to the present day. Furthermore, although the stages chronicle the general evolution in the Western world, it is important to realize that each stage still exists in civilization today. For example, Australian aborigines continue to hunt and gather food, and settled villages are common in developing countries.

Public health nurses should be aware that populations from each stage represent a great variety of people with distinct cultural traditions and a broad range of health care practices and beliefs. For example, a nurse currently practicing in an American community may need to plan care for immigrants or refugees from a settled village or a preindustrial city. Community nurses must recognize that the environment, the aggregate's health risks, and the host culture's strengths and contributions affect the health status of each particular aggregate.

Hunting and Gathering Stage

During the Paleolithic period, or Old Stone Age, nomadic and semi-nomadic people engaged in hunting and gathering, with generations of small aggregate groups wandering in search of food. Armelagos and Dewey (1978) reviewed how the size, density, and relationship to the environment of such people probably affected their health. These groups may have avoided many contagious diseases because the scattered aggregates were small, nomadic, and separated from other aggregates. Under these conditions, disease would not spread among the groups. Evidently the disposal of human feces and waste was not a great problem; the nomadic people most likely abandoned the caves they used for shelter once waste accumulated.

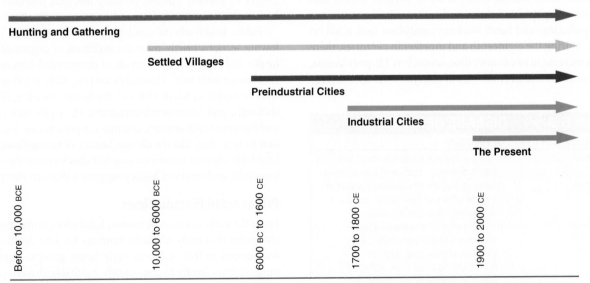

FIGURE 2-1 Stages in the disease history of humankind. Stages overlap and time periods are widely debated in the field of anthropology. Some form of each stage remains evident in the world today.

Settled Village Stage

Small settlements were characteristic of the Mesolithic period, or Middle Stone Age, and the Neolithic period, or New Stone Age. Wandering people became sedentary and formed small encampments and villages. The concentration of people in these small areas caused new health problems. For example, people began to domesticate animals and live close to their herds, a practice that probably transmitted diseases such as salmonella, anthrax, Q fever, and tuberculosis (TB) (Polgar, 1964). These stationary people also domesticated plants, a change that may have reduced the range of consumable nutrients and may have led to deficiency diseases. They had to secure water and remove wastes, often leading to the cross-contamination of the water supply and the spread of waterborne diseases such as dysentery, cholera, typhoid, and hepatitis A.

Preindustrial Cities Stage

In preindustrial times, large urban centers formed to support the expanding population. Populations inhabited smaller areas; therefore preexisting problems expanded. For example, the urban population had to resource increased amounts of food and water and remove increased amounts of waste products. Some cultures developed elaborate water systems. For instance, the Aztec king Ahuitzotl had a stone pipeline built to transport spring water to the inhabitants of Mexico City (Duran, 1964). However, waste removal via the water supply led to diseases such as cholera. With the development of towns, rodent infestation increased and facilitated the spread of plague. People had more frequent close contact with one another; therefore the transmission of diseases spread by direct contact increased, and diseases such as mumps, measles, influenza, and smallpox became endemic (Polgar, 1964). A population must reach a certain size to maintain a disease in endemic proportions (Table 2-1); for example, approximately 1 million people are needed to sustain measles at an endemic level (Cockburn, 1967).

Industrial Cities Stage

Industrialization caused urban areas to become denser and more heavily populated. Increased industrial wastes, air and water pollution, and harsh working conditions took a toll on health. During the eighteenth and nineteenth centuries, there was an increase in respiratory diseases such as TB, pneumonia, and bronchitis and in epidemics of infectious diseases such as diphtheria, smallpox, typhoid fever, typhus, measles, malaria, and yellow fever (Armelagos and Dewey, 1978). Furthermore, imperialism spread epidemics of many diseases to susceptible populations throughout the world because settlers, traders, and soldiers moved from one location to another, introducing communicable diseases into native population groups.

Present Stage

Although infectious diseases no longer account for a majority of deaths in the Western world, they continue to cause many deaths in the non-Western world. They also remain prevalent among low-income populations and some racial and ethnic groups in the West. Western diseases such as cancer, venous disorders, heart disease, obesity, and diabetes are less common among populations from nonindustrial communities. These diseases usually appear, however, when cultures adopt Western customs and transition into urban environments. Epidemiological studies suggest that common risk factors that contribute to chronic health conditions are changes in diet (e.g., increases in refined sugar and fats and lack of fiber), environmental alterations (e.g., use of motorized transportation and climate-controlled living and work sites), and occupational hazards. A rise in population and greater population density also increase mental and behavioral disorders.

In summary, the disease patterns and environmental demands changed when wandering, hunting, and gathering aggregates grew into large populations and became sedentary. Humans had to adapt to more densely populated, largely urban existence with marked consequences for health. As a result, over time, the leading causes of death changed from infectious disease to chronic illness.

Evolution of Early Public Health Efforts

Traditionally, historians believed that organized public health efforts were eighteenth- and nineteenth-century activities associated with the Sanitary Revolution. However, modern historians have shown that organized community health efforts to prevent disease, prolong life, and promote health have existed since early human history.

Public health efforts developed slowly over time. The following sections briefly trace the evolution of organized public health and highlight the periods of prerecorded historic times (i.e., before 5000 BCE), classical times (i.e., 3000 to 200 BCE), the Middle Ages (i.e., 500 to 1500 CE), the Renaissance (i.e., fifteenth, sixteenth, and seventeenth centuries), the eighteenth century, and the nineteenth century, and into the present day. It is important to note that, like the disease history of humankind, public health efforts exist in various stages of development throughout the world, and this brief history suggests a Western viewpoint.

Prerecorded Historic Times

From the early remains of human habitation, anthropologists recognize that early nomadic humans became domesticated and tended to live in increasingly larger groups. Aggregates ranging from family to community inevitably shared episodes of life, health, sickness, and death. Whether based on superstition or sanitation, health practices evolved to ensure the

TABLE 2-1	DISEASE DEFINITIONS
TYPES OF DISEASE	**DEFINITION**
Endemic	Diseases that are always present in a population (e.g., colds and pneumonia)
Epidemic	Diseases that are not always present in a population but flare up on occasion (e.g., diphtheria and measles)
Pandemic	The existence of disease in a large proportion of the population: a global epidemic (e.g., human immunodeficiency virus, acquired immunodeficiency syndrome, and annual outbreaks of influenza type A)

survival of many aggregates. For example, primitive societies used elements of medicine (e.g., voodoo), isolation (e.g., banishment), and fumigation (i.e., use of smoke) to manage disease and thus protect the community for thousands of years (Hanlon and Pickett, 1990).

Classical Times

In the early years of the period 3000 to 1400 BCE, the Minoans devised ways to flush water and construct drainage systems. Circa 1000 BCE, the Egyptians constructed elaborate drainage systems, developed pharmaceutical preparations, and embalmed the dead. Pollution is an ancient problem. The Biblical Book of Exodus reported that "all the waters that were in the river stank," and in the Book of Leviticus (believed to be written around 500 BCE), the Hebrews formulated the first written hygiene code. This hygiene code protected water and food by creating laws that governed personal and community hygiene such as contagion, disinfection, and sanitation.

Greece. Greek literature contains accounts of communicable diseases such as diphtheria, mumps, and malaria. The Hippocratic book *On Airs, Waters and Places,* a treatise on the balance between humans and their environment, may have been the only volume on this topic until the development of bacteriology in the late nineteenth century (Rosen, 1993). Diseases that were always present in a population, such as colds and pneumonia, were called endemic. Diseases such as diphtheria and measles, which were occasionally present and often fairly widespread, were called epidemic. The Greeks emphasized the preservation of health, or good living, which the goddess Hygeia represented, and curative medicine, which the goddess Panacea personified. Human life had to be in balance with environmental demands; therefore the Greeks weighed the importance of exercise, rest, and nutrition according to age, sex, constitution, and climate (Rosen, 1993).

Rome. Although the Romans readily adopted Greek culture, they far surpassed Greek engineering by constructing massive aqueducts, bathhouses, and sewer systems. For example, at the height of the Roman empire, Rome provided its 1 million inhabitants with 40 gallons of water per person per day, which is comparable to modern consumption rates (Rosen, 1993). Inhabitants of the overcrowded Roman slums, however, did not share in public health amenities such as sewer systems and latrines, and their health suffered accordingly.

The Romans also observed and addressed occupational health threats. In particular, they noted the pallor of the miners, the danger of suffocation, and the smell of caustic fumes (Rosen, 1993) (Box 2-1). For protection, miners devised safeguards by using masks made of bags, sacks, membranes, and bladder skins.

In the early years of the Roman Republic, priests were believed to mediate diseases and often dispensed medicine. Public physicians worked in designated towns and earned money to care for the poor. In addition, they were able to charge wealthier patients a service fee. Much as in a modern health maintenance organization (HMO) or group practice, several families paid a set fee for yearly services. Hospitals, surgeries, infirmaries, and nursing homes appeared throughout

BOX 2-1	ROMANS PROVIDED PUBLIC HEALTH SERVICES

The ancient Romans provided public health services that included the following:
- A water board to maintain the aqueducts
- A supervisor of the public baths
- Street cleaners
- Supervision of the sale of food

Data from Rosen G: *A history of public health, expanded edition,* Baltimore, MD, 1993, Johns Hopkins Press.

Rome. In the fourth century, a Christian woman named Fabiola established a hospital for the sick poor. Others repeated this model throughout medieval times (Donahue, 2011).

Middle Ages

The decline of Rome, which occurred circa 500 CE, led to the Middle Ages. Monasteries promoted collective activity to protect public health, and the population adopted protective measures such as building wells and fountains, cleaning streets, and disposing of refuse. The commonly occurring communicable diseases were measles, smallpox, diphtheria, leprosy, and bubonic plague. Physicians had little to offer in the management of diseases such as leprosy. The church took over by enforcing the hygienic codes from Leviticus and establishing isolation and leper houses, or leprosaria (Rosen, 1993).

A pandemic is the existence of disease in a large proportion of the population. One such pandemic, the bubonic plague, ravaged much of the world in the fourteenth century. This plague, or Black Death, claimed close to half the world's population at that time (Hanlon and Pickett, 1990). For centuries, medicine and science did not recognize that fleas, which were attracted to the large number of rodents inhabiting urban areas, were the transmitters of plague. Modern public health practices such as isolation, disinfection, and ship quarantines emerged in response to the bubonic plague (Box 2-2).

During the Middle Ages, clergymen often acted as physicians and treated kings and noblemen. Monks and nuns provided nursing care in small houses designated as structures similar to today's small hospitals. Medieval writings contained information on hygiene and addressed such topics as housing, diet, personal cleanliness, and sleep (Rosen, 1993).

LIFE IN AN ENGLISH HOUSEHOLD IN THE SIXTEENTH CENTURY

In the following account, Erasmus described how life in the sixteenth century must have affected health:

As to floors, they are usually made with clay, covered with rushes that grow in the fens and which are so seldom removed that the lower parts remain sometimes for twenty years and has in it a collection of spittle, vomit, urine of dogs and humans, beer, scraps of fish and other filthiness not to be named.)

Such accounts appeared in literature throughout the nineteenth century.

Quotation from Hanlon JJ, Pickett GE: *Public health administration and practice,* ed 9, St. Louis, 1990, Mosby, p 25.

BOX 2-2   HUMAN PLAGUE CASES IN THE UNITED STATES

Plague is an acute, often fatal bacterial infection spread by the bite of infected fleas, which is endemic and occasionally epidemic in Africa, Asia, and South America. The disease was first introduced into the United States in 1900 through rat-infested steamships that had sailed from affected areas. The last U.S. urban plague epidemic occurred in Los Angeles between 1924 and 1925. Since that time, plague has occurred as scattered cases, largely in rural areas. Sanitary precautions ensure a low frequency of human plague in the United States. The country averages 13 cases of plague each year, and most of these cases occur in New Mexico, California, Texas, and Colorado.

In 2006, 13 cases of human plague were reported and resulted in two fatalities in the United States. This was the largest number of reported cases in the United States since 1994. More recently, in 2010, 2 cases were identified in rural Oregon; both individuals recovered following treatment. Control measures include public education and plague surveillance in rodents and rodent predators. When this surveillance detects plague, local health care providers and the public should receive an alert about possible risks.

Data from Centers for Disease Control and Prevention: Two cases of human plague—Oregon, 2010, *MMWR Morb Mortal Wkly Rep* 60(7):214, 2011; Centers for Disease Control and Prevention: Human plague—four states, 2006, *MMWR Morb Mortal Wkly Rep* 55(34):940-943, 2006; and Centers for Disease Control and Prevention: Plague in the United States, 2012. Available from <http://www.cdc.gov/plague/maps/index.html>. Accessed March 2, 2013.

The Renaissance

Although the cause of infectious disease remained undiscovered, two events important to public health occurred during the Renaissance. In 1546, Girolamo Fracastoro presented a theory that infection was a cause and epidemic a consequence of the "seeds of disease." Then, in 1676, Anton van Leeuwenhoek described microscopic organisms, although he did not associate them with disease (Rosen, 1993).

The Elizabethan Poor Law, enacted in England in 1601, held the church parishes responsible for providing relief for the poor. This law governed health care for the poor for more than two centuries and became a prototype for later U.S. laws.

Eighteenth Century

Great Britain. The eighteenth century was marked by imperialism and industrialization. Sanitary conditions remained a huge problem. During the Industrial Revolution, a gradual change in industrial productivity occurred. The industrial boom sacrificed many lives for profit. In particular, it forced poor children into labor. Under the Elizabethan Poor Law, parishes established workhouses to employ the poor. Orphaned and poor children were wards of the parish; therefore the parish forced these young children to labor in parish workhouses for long hours (George, 1925). At 12 to 14 years of age, a child became a master's apprentice. Those apprenticed to chimney sweeps reportedly suffered the worst fate because their masters forced them into chimneys at the risk of being burned and suffocated.

Vaccination was a major discovery of the times. In 1796, Edward Jenner observed that people who worked around cattle were less likely to have smallpox. He concluded that immunity to smallpox resulted from an inoculation with the cowpox virus. Jenner's contribution was significant because approximately 95% of the population suffered from smallpox and approximately 10% of the population died of smallpox during the eighteenth century. Frequently, the faces of those who survived the disease were scarred with pockmarks.

The Sanitary Revolution's public health reforms were beginning to take place throughout Europe and England. In the eighteenth century, scholars used survey methods to study public health problems (Rosen, 1993). These surveys mapped "medical topographies," which were geographic factors related to regional health and disease. A health education movement provided books and pamphlets on health to the middle and upper classes, but it neglected "economic factors" and was not concerned with the working classes.

Nineteenth Century

Europe. During the nineteenth century, communicable diseases ravaged the population that lived in unsanitary conditions, and many lives were lost. For example, in the mid-1800s, typhus and typhoid fever claimed twice as many lives each year as the Battle of Waterloo (Hanlon and Pickett, 1990).

Edwin Chadwick called attention to the consequences of unsanitary conditions that resulted in health disparities that shortened life spans of the laboring class in particular. Chadwick contended that death rates were high in large industrial cities such as Liverpool, where more than half of all children born of working-class parents died by age 5. Laborers lived an average of 16 years. In contrast, tradesmen lived 22 years, and the upper classes lived 36 years (Richardson, 1887). In 1842, Chadwick published his famous *Report on an Inquiry Into the Sanitary Conditions of the Labouring Population of Great Britain*. The report furthered the establishment of the General Board of Health for England in 1848. Legislation for social reform followed, addressing prevailing concerns such as child welfare, factory management, education, and care for the elderly, sick, and mentally ill. Clean water, sewers, fireplugs, and sidewalks emerged as a result.

In 1849, a German pathologist named Rudolf Virchow argued for social action—bettering the lives of the people by improving economic, social, and environmental conditions—to attack the root social causes of disease. He proposed "a theory of epidemic disease as a manifestation of social and cultural maladjustment" (Rosen, 1993, p. 62). He further argued that the public was responsible for the health of the people; that social and economic conditions heavily affected health and disease; that efforts to promote health and fight disease must be social, economic, and medical; and that the study of social and economic determinants of health and disease would yield knowledge to guide appropriate action.

In 1849, these principles were embodied in a public health law submitted to the Berlin Society of Physicians and Surgeons (Rosen, 1993). According to this document, public health has as its objectives: (1) the healthy mental and physical development of the citizen, (2) the prevention of all dangers to health, and (3) the control of disease. It was pointed out that public health cares for society as a whole by considering the general physical and social conditions that may adversely affect health and protects each individual by considering those conditions that prevent the individual from caring for his or her health. These "conditions" may fit into one of two major categories: conditions that give the individual the right to request assistance from the state (e.g., poverty and infirmity) and conditions that give the state the right and obligation to interfere with the personal liberty of the individual (e.g., transmissible diseases and mental illness).

A very critical event in the development of modern public health occurred in 1854, when an English physician, anesthetist, and epidemiologist named John Snow demonstrated that cholera was transmissible through contaminated water. In a large population afflicted with cholera, he shut down the community's water resource by removing the pump handle from a well and carefully documented changes as the number of cholera cases fell dramatically (Rosen, 1993).

United States. In the United States during the nineteenth century, waves of epidemics continued to spread. Diseases such as yellow fever, smallpox, cholera, typhoid fever, and typhus particularly impacted the poor. These illnesses spread because cities grew and the poor crowded into inadequate housing with unsanitary conditions.

Lemuel Shattuck, a Boston bookseller and publisher with an interest in public health, organized the American Statistical Society in 1839 and issued a *Census of Boston* in 1845. The census showed high overall mortality and very high infant and maternal mortality rates. Living conditions for the poor were inadequate, and communicable diseases were widely prevalent (Rosen, 1993). Shattuck's 1850 *Report of the Sanitary Commission of Massachusetts* outlined the findings and recommended modern public health reforms that included keeping vital statistics and providing environmental, food, drug, and communicable disease control information. Shattuck called for well-infant, well-child, and school-aged–child health care; mental health care; vaccination; and health education. Unfortunately, the report fell on deaf ears, and little was done to improve population health for many years. For example, a state board of health was not formed until 19 years after the report was issued. Around the same time, the National Institute, a Washington, DC, scientific organization, asked the newly formed American Medical Association (AMA) to establish a committee to uniformly collect vital statistics, which the AMA did, beginning in 1848.

ADVENT OF MODERN HEALTH CARE

Early public health efforts evolved further in the mid-nineteenth century. Administrative efforts, initial legislation, and debate regarding the determinants of health and approaches to health management began to appear on a social, economic, and medical level. The advent of "modern" health care occurred around this time, and nursing made a large contribution to the progress of health care. The following sections discuss the evolution of modern nursing, the evolution of modern medical care and public health practice, the evolution of the community caregiver, and the establishment of public health nursing.

Evolution of Modern Nursing

Florence Nightingale, the woman credited with establishing "modern nursing," began her work during the mid-nineteenth century. Historians remember Florence Nightingale for contributing to the health of British soldiers during the Crimean War and establishing nursing education. However, many historians failed to recognize her remarkable use of public health principles and distinguished scientific contributions to health care reform (Cohen, 1984; Grier and Grier, 1978). The following review of Nightingale's work emphasizes her concern for environmental determinants of health; her focus on the aggregate of British soldiers through emphasis on sanitation, community assessment, and analysis; the development of the use of graphically depicted statistics; and the gathering of comparable census data and political advocacy on behalf of the aggregate.

Nightingale was from a wealthy English family, was well educated, and traveled extensively. Her father tutored her in mathematics and many other subjects. Nightingale later studied with Adolphe Quetelet, a Belgian statistician. Quetelet influenced her profoundly and taught her the discipline of social inquiry (Goodnow, 1933). Nightingale also had a passion for hygiene and health. In 1851, at the age of 31 years, she trained in nursing with Pastor Fliedner at Kaiserswerth Hospital in Germany. She later studied the organization and discipline of the Sisters of Charity in Paris. Nightingale wrote extensively and published her analyses of the many nursing systems she studied in France, Austria, Italy, and Germany (Dock and Stewart, 1925).

In 1854, Nightingale responded to distressing accounts of a lack of care for wounded soldiers during the Crimean War. She and 40 other nurses traveled to Scutari, which was part of the Ottoman Empire at the time. Nightingale was accompanied by lay nurses, Roman Catholic sisters, and Anglican sisters. Upon their arrival, the nurses learned that the British army's management method for treating the sick and wounded had created conditions that resulted in extraordinarily high death rates among soldiers. One of Nightingale's greatest achievements was improving the management of ill and wounded soldiers.

Nightingale faced an assignment in The Barrack Hospital, which had been built for 1700 patients. In 4 miles of beds, she found 3000 to 4000 patients separated from each other by only 18 inches of space (Goodnow, 1933).

During the Crimean War, cholera and "contagious fever" were rampant. Equal numbers of men died of disease and battlefield injury (Cohen, 1984). Nightingale found that allocated supplies were bound in bureaucratic red tape; for example, supplies were "sent to the wrong ports or were buried under munitions and could not be got" (Goodnow, 1933, p. 86).

Nightingale encountered problems reforming the army's methods for care of the sick because she had to work through eight military affairs departments related to her assignment. She sent reports of the appalling conditions of the hospitals to London. In response to her actions, governmental and private funds were provided to set up diet kitchens and a laundry and provided food, clothing, dressings, and laboratory equipment (Dock and Stewart, 1925).

Major reforms occurred during the first 2 months of her assignment. Aware that an interest in keeping social statistics was emerging, Nightingale realized that her most forceful argument would be statistical in nature. She reorganized the methods of keeping statistics and was the first to use shaded and colored coxcomb graphs of wedges, circles, and squares to illustrate the preventable deaths of soldiers. Nightingale compared the deaths of soldiers in hospitals during the Crimean War with the average annual mortality in Manchester and with the deaths of soldiers in military hospitals in and near London at the time (Figure 2-2). Through her statistics she also showed that, by the end of the war, the death rate among ill soldiers during the Crimean War was no higher than that among well soldiers in Britain (Cohen, 1984). Indeed, Nightingale's careful statistics revealed that the death rate for treated soldiers decreased from 42% to 2%. Furthermore, she established community services and activities to improve the quality of life for recovering soldiers. These included rest and recreation facilities, study opportunities, a savings fund, and a post office. She also organized care for the families of the soldiers (Dock and Stewart, 1925).

After returning to London at the close of the war in 1856, Nightingale devoted her efforts to sanitary reform. At home, she surmised that if the sanitary neglect of the soldiers existed in the battle area, it probably existed at home in London. She prepared statistical tables to support her suspicions (Table 2-2).

In one study comparing the mortality of men aged 25 to 35 years in the army barracks of England with that of men the same age in civilian life, Nightingale found that the mortality of the soldiers was nearly twice that of the civilians. In one of her reports, she stated that "our soldiers enlist to death in the barracks" (Kopf, 1978, p. 95). Furthermore, she believed that allowing young soldiers to die needlessly of unsanitary conditions was equivalent to taking them out, lining them up, and shooting them. She was very political and did not keep her community assessment and analysis to herself. Nightingale distributed her reports to members of Parliament and to the medical and commanding officers of the army (Kopf, 1978). Prominent male leaders of the time challenged her reports. Undaunted, she rewrote them in greater depth and redistributed them.

In her efforts to compare the hospital systems in European countries, Nightingale discovered that each hospital kept incomparable data and that many hospitals used various names and classifications for diseases. She noted that these differences prevented the collection of similar statistics from larger geographic areas. These statistics would create a regional health-illness profile and allow for comparison with other regions. She printed common statistical forms that some hospitals in London adopted on an experimental basis. A study of the tabulated results revealed the promise of this strategy (Kopf, 1978) (Box 2-3).

Nightingale also stressed the need to use statistics at the administrative and political levels to direct health policy. Noting the ignorance of politicians and those who set policy regarding the interpretation and use of statistics, she emphasized the need to teach national leaders to use statistical facts. Nightingale continued the development and application of statistical procedures, and she won recognition for her efforts. The Royal Statistical Society made her a fellow in 1858, and the American Statistical Association made her an honorary member in 1874 (Kopf, 1978).

In addition to her contributions to nursing and her development of nursing education, Nightingale's credits include the application of statistical information toward an understanding of the total environmental situation (Kopf, 1978). Population-based statistics have marked implications for the development of public health and public health nursing. Grier and Grier (1978, p. 103) recognized Nightingale's contributions to statistics and stated, "Her name occurs in the index of many texts on the history of probability and statistics ... in the history of quantitative graphics ... and in texts on the history of science and mathematics."

It is interesting to note that the paradigm for nursing practice and nursing education that evolved through Nightingale's work did not incorporate her emphasis on statistics and a sound research base. It is also curious that nursing education did not consult her writings and did not stress the importance of determining health's social and environmental determinants until much later.

Establishment of Modern Medical Care and Public Health Practice

To place Nightingale's work in perspective, it is necessary to consider the development of medical care in light of common education and practice during the late nineteenth and early twentieth centuries. Goodnow (1933) called this time a "dark age." Medical sciences were underdeveloped, and bacteriology was unknown. Few medical schools existed at the time, so apprenticeship was the path to medical education. The majority of physicians believed in the "spontaneous generation" theory of disease causation, which stated that disease organisms grew from nothing (Najman, 1990). Typical medical treatment included bloodletting, starving, using leeches, and prescribing large doses of metals such as mercury and antimony (Goodnow, 1933).

Nightingale's uniform classification of hospital statistics noted the need to tabulate the classification of diseases in hospital patients and the need to note the diseases that patients contracted in the hospital. These diseases, such as gangrene and septicemia, were later called *iatrogenic* diseases (Kopf, 1978). Considering the lack of surgical sanitation in hospitals at the time, it is not surprising that iatrogenic infection was rampant. For example, Goodnow (1933) illustrates the following unsanitary operating procedures:

> *Before an operation the surgeon turned up the sleeves of his coat to save the coat, and would often not trouble to wash his hands, knowing how soiled they soon would be! The area of the operation would sometimes be washed with soap and water, but not always, for the inevitability of corruption made it seem useless. The silk or thread used for stitches or ligatures was hung over a button of the surgeon's coat, and during the operation a convenient place for the knife to rest was between his lips. Instruments ... used for ... lancing abscesses were kept in the vest pocket and often only wiped with a piece of rag as the surgeon went from one patient to another. (pp. 471-472)*

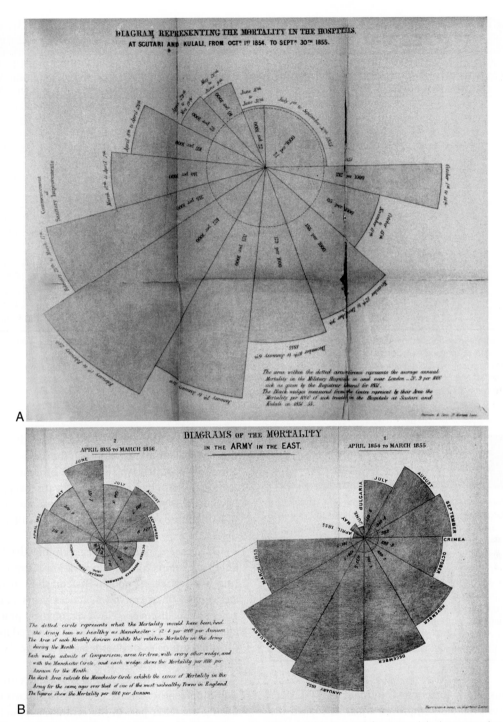

FIGURE 2-2 A, Coxcomb charts by Florence Nightingale. **B,** Photographs of large, foldout charts from an original preserved at the University of Chicago Library. (**A** from Nightingale F: *Notes on matters affecting the health, efficiency and hospitalization of the British army,* London, 1858, Harrison and Sons; **B,** public domain; courtesy University of Chicago Library.)

During the nineteenth century, the following important scientists were born: **Louis Pasteur** in 1822, **Joseph Lister** in 1827, and **Robert Koch** in 1843. Their research also had a profound impact on health care, medicine, and nursing. Pasteur was a chemist, not a physician. While experimenting with wine production in 1854, he proposed the theory of the existence of germs. Although his colleagues ridiculed him at first, Koch applied his theories and developed his methods for handling and studying bacteria. Subsequently, Pasteur's

colleagues gave him acknowledgment for his work (Kalisch and Kalisch, 2004).

Lister, whose father perfected the microscope, observed the healing processes of fractures. He noted that when the bone was broken but the skin was not, recovery was uneventful. However, when both the bone and the skin were broken, fever, infection, and even death were frequent. He found the proposed answer to his observation through Pasteur's work. Something outside the body entered the wound through the

TABLE 2-2 NIGHTINGALE'S CRIMEAN WAR MORTALITY STATISTICS: NURSING RESEARCH THAT MADE A DIFFERENCE*

YEAR	DEATHS THAT WOULD HAVE OCCURRED IN HEALTHY DISTRICTS AMONG MALES OF THE SOLDIERS' AGES†	ACTUAL DEATHS OF NONCOMMISSIONED OFFICERS AND MEN	EXCESS OF DEATHS AMONG NONCOMMISSIONED OFFICERS AND MEN
1839	763	2914	2151
1840	829	3300	2471
1841	857	4167	3310
1842	888	5052	4164
1843	914	5270	4356
1844	920	3867	2947
1845	911	4587	3676
1846	930	5125	4195
1847	981	4232	3251
1848	987	3213	2226
1849	954	4052	3098
1850	919	3119	2200
1851	901	2729	1828
1852	915	3120	2205
1853	920	3392	2472
Total	13,589	58,139	44,550

From Grier B, Grier M: Contributions of the passionate statistician, *Res Nurs Health* 1:103-109, 1978. Copyright ©1978 by John Wiley & Sons, Inc. Reprinted by permission of John Wiley & Sons, Inc.
*Number of deaths of noncommissioned officers and men also shows the number of deaths that would have occurred if the mortality were 7.7 per 1000—such as it was among Englishmen of the soldiers' age in healthy districts, in the years 1849 to 1853—which fairly represent the average mortality.
†The exact mortality in the healthy districts is 0.0077122, with use of the logarithm of 3.8871801.

BOX 2-3 NIGHTINGALE'S USE OF STATISTICAL METHODS IN COMMUNITY ASSESSMENT

London's Southeastern Railway planned to remove St. Thomas' Hospital to enlarge the railway's right-of-way between London Bridge and Charing Cross. Nightingale applied her statistical method to the health needs of the community by conducting a *community assessment*. She plotted the cases served by the hospital, analyzed the proportion by distance, and calculated the probable impact on the community if the hospital were relocated to the proposed site. In her view, hospitals were a part of the wider community that served the needs of humanity. Kopf (1978) noted that this method of health planning and matching resources to the needs of the population was visionary and was not reapplied until the twentieth century.

---

broken skin, causing the infection (Goodnow, 1933). Lister's surgical successes eventually improved when he soaked the dressings and instruments in mixtures of carbolic acid (i.e., phenol) and oil.

In 1882, Koch discovered the causative agent for cholera and the tubercle bacillus. Pasteur discovered immunization in 1881 and the rabies vaccine in 1885. These discoveries were significant to the development of public health and medicine. However, physicians accepted these discoveries slowly (Rosen, 1993). For example, TB was a major cause of death in late nineteenth century America and often plagued its victims with chronic illness and disability. It was a highly stigmatized disease, and most physicians thought it was a hereditary, constitutional disease associated with poor environmental conditions. Hospitalization for TB was rare because the stigma caused families to hide their infected relatives. Without treatment, the communicability of the disease increased. The common treatment was a change of climate (Rosen, 1993). Although Koch had announced the discovery of the tubercle bacillus in 1882, it was 10 years before the emergence of the first organized community campaign to stop the spread of the disease.

The case of puerperal (i.e., childbirth) fever illustrates another example of slow innovation stemming from scientific discoveries. Although Pasteur showed that *Streptococcus* caused puerperal fever, it was years before physicians accepted his discovery. However, medical practice eventually changed, and physicians no longer delivered infants after performing autopsies of puerperal fever cases without washing their hands (Goodnow, 1933).

Debates over the causes of disease occurred throughout the nineteenth century. Scientists discovered organisms during the latter part of the century, supporting the theory that specific contagious entities caused disease. This discovery challenged the earlier, miasmic theory that environment and atmospheric conditions caused disease (Greifinger and Sidel, 1981). The new scientific discoveries had a major impact on the development of public health and medical practice. The emergence of the germ theory of disease focused diagnosis and treatment on the individual organism and the individual disease.

State and local governments felt increasingly responsible for controlling the spread of bacteria and other microorganisms. A community outcry for social reform forced state and local governments to take notice of the deplorable living conditions in the cities. In the New York City riots of 1863, the populace expressed their disgust for overcrowding; filthy streets; lack of provisions for the poor; and lack of adequate food, water, and housing for the people. Local boards of health formed, taking responsibility for safeguarding food and water stores and managing the sewage and quarantine operation for victims of contagious diseases (Greifinger and Sidel, 1981).

The New York Metropolitan Board of Health formed in 1866, and state health departments formed shortly thereafter. States built large public hospitals that treated TB and mental disease with rest, diet, and quarantine. In 1889, the New York City Health Department recommended the surveillance of TB and TB health education, but physicians did not welcome either recommendation (Rosen, 1993). Despite their objections, the New York City Health Department required institutions to report cases of TB in 1894 and required physicians to do the same in 1897.

In 1883, The Johns Hopkins University Medical School in Baltimore, Maryland, formed under the German model that promoted medical education on the principles of scientific discovery. In the United States, the Carnegie Commission appointed Abraham Flexner to evaluate medical schools throughout the country on the basis of the German model. In 1910, the Flexner Report outlined the shortcomings of U.S. medical schools that did not use this model. Within a few years, the report caused philanthropic organizations such as the Rockefeller and Carnegie Foundations to withdraw funding of these schools, ensuring the closure of scientifically "inadequate" medical schools. A "new breed" of physicians emerged who had been taught that germ theory was the "single agent theory" of disease causation (Greifinger and Sidel, 1981, p. 132) (Box 2-4).

Philanthropic foundations continued to influence health care efforts. For example, the Rockefeller Sanitary Commission for the Eradication of Hookworm formed in 1909. Hookworm was an occupational hazard among Southern workers. The discovery of preventive efforts to eradicate hookworm kept the workers healthy and thus proved to be a great industrial benefit. The model was so successful that the Rockefeller Foundation established the first school of public health, The Johns Hopkins School of Hygiene and Public Health, in 1916. The focus of this institution was the preservation and improvement of individual and community health and the prevention of disease through multidisciplinary activities. Foundations made additional efforts, which led to the formation of the International Health Commission, schools of tropical medicine, and medical research institutes in foreign ports.

Community Caregiver

The traditional role of the community caregiver or the traditional healer has nearly vanished. However, medical and nurse anthropologists who have studied primitive and Western cultures are familiar with the community healer and caregiver role (Leininger and McFarland, 2006). The traditional healer (e.g., shaman, midwife, herbalist, or priest) is common in non-Western, ancient, and underdeveloped societies. Although traditional healers have always existed, professionals and many people throughout industrialized societies may

---

BOX 2-4 SCIENTIFIC THEORY/SINGLE AGENT THEORY

The emphasis on the use of scientific theory, or single agent theory, in medical care developed into a focus on disease and symptoms rather than a focus on the prevention of disability and care for the "whole person." The old-fashioned family doctor viewed patients in relation to their families and communities and apparently helped people cope with problems in personal life, family, and society. American medicine adopted science with such vigor that these qualities faded away. Science allowed the physician to deal with tissues and organs, which were much easier to comprehend than the dynamics of human relationships or the complexities of disease prevention. Many physicians made efforts to integrate the various roles, but society was pushing toward academic science.

---

overlook or minimize their role. The role of the healer is often integrated into other institutions of society, including religion, medicine, and morality. The notion that one person acts alone in healing may be foreign to many cultures; healers can be individuals, kin, or entire societies (Hughes, 1978).

Societies retain folk practices because they offer repeated success. Most cultures have a pharmacopoeia and maintain therapeutic and preventive practices, and it is estimated that one fourth to one half of folk medicines are empirically effective. Indeed, many modern drugs are based on the medicines of primitive cultures (e.g., eucalyptus, coca, and opium) (Hughes, 1978).

Since ancient times, folk healers and cultural practices have both positively and negatively affected health. The late nineteenth and early twentieth century practice of midwifery illustrates modern medicine's arguably sometimes negative impact on traditional healing in many Western cultures (Ehrenreich and English, 1973; Smith, 1979). For example, traditional midwifery practices made women rise out of bed within 24 hours of delivery to help "clear" the lochia. Throughout the mid-1900s, in contrast, "modern medicine" recommended keeping women in bed, often for fairly extended periods (Smith, 1979).

HISTORICAL METHODOLOGY FOR NURSING RESEARCH

Historiography is the methodology of historical research. It involves specialized techniques, principles, and theories that pertain to historical matters. *Historical research* involves interpreting history and contributing to understanding through data synthesis. It relies on existing sources or data and requires the researcher to gain access to sources such as libraries, librarians, and databases.

Historical research should be descriptive. It should answer the questions of who, what, when, where, how, and the interpretive why. Historians reconstruct an era using primary sources and interpret the story from that perspective. Historical research in nursing will enhance the understanding of current nursing practice and will help prepare for the future.

Adapted from Lusk B: Historical methodology for nursing research, *Image J Nurs Sch* 29:3555-3560, 1997.

Establishment of Public Health Nursing

Public health nursing as a holistic approach to health care developed in the late nineteenth and early twentieth centuries. Public and community health nursing evolved from home nursing practice, community organizations, and political interventions on behalf of aggregates.

England

Public health nursing developed from providing nursing care to the sick poor and furnishing information and channels of community organization that enable the poor to improve their own health status.

District Nursing. District nursing, which stemmed from public health nursing, developed in England. Between 1854 and 1856, the Epidemiological Society of London developed a plan that trained selected poor women to provide nursing care to the community's sick poor. The society theorized that nurses belonging to their patients' social class would be more effective caregivers and that more nurses would be available to improve the health of community residents (Rosen, 1993).

A similar plan was implemented by William Rathbone in Liverpool in 1859. After experiencing the excellent care a nurse gave his sick wife in his home, Rathbone strongly believed that nurses could offer the same care throughout the community. He developed a plan that divided the community into 18 districts and assigned a nurse and a social worker to each district. This team met the needs of their communities in nursing, social work, and health education. The community widely accepted the plan. To further strengthen it, Rathbone consulted Nightingale about educating the district nurses. She assisted him by providing training for the district nurses, referring to them as "health nurses." The model was successful, and eventually voluntary agencies adopted the plan on the national level (Rosen, 1993).

Health Visiting. Health visiting to provide information for improved health is a parallel service based on the district nursing tradition. The Ladies Section of the Manchester and Salford Sanitary Association originated health visiting in Manchester in 1862. Health pamphlets alone had little effect; therefore this service enlisted home visitors to distribute health information to the poor.

In 1893, Nightingale pointed out that the district nurse should be a health teacher and a nurse for the sick in the home. She believed that teachers should educate "health missioners" for this purpose. The model charged the district nurse with providing care for the sick in the home and the health visitor with providing health information in the home. Eventually, government agencies sponsored health visitors, medical health officers supervised them, and the municipality paid them. Thus a collaborative model developed between government and voluntary agencies.

United States

In the United States, public health nursing also developed from the British traditions of district nursing and home nursing. In 1877, the Women's Board of the New York City Mission sent a graduate nurse named Frances Root into homes to provide care for the sick. The innovation spread, and nursing associations, later called visiting nurse associations, were implemented in Buffalo in 1885 and in Boston and Philadelphia in 1886.

In 1893, nurses Lillian Wald and Mary Brewster established a district nursing service on the Lower East Side of New York City called the House on Henry Street. This was a crowded area teeming with unemployed and homeless immigrants who needed health care. The organization, later called the Visiting Nurse Association of New York City, played an important role in establishing public health nursing in the United States. Box 2-5 contains Wald's compelling account of her early exposure to the community where she identified public health nursing needs.

Wald (1971) described a range of services that evolved from the House on Henry Street. Nurses provided home visits, and patients paid carfare or a cursory fee. Physicians were consultants to Henry Street, and families could arrange a visit by calling the nurse directly or a physician could call the nurse on the family's behalf. The nursing service adopted the philosophy of meeting the health needs of aggregates, which included the many evident social, economic, and environmental determinants of health. By necessity, this effort involved an aggregate approach that empowered people of the community.

Helen Hall, who later directed the House on Henry Street, wrote that the settlement's role was "one of helping people to help themselves" (Wald, 1971) through the development of centers of social action aimed at meeting the needs of the community and the individual. Community organization led to the formation of a great variety of programs, including youth clubs, a juvenile program, sex education for local schoolteachers, and support programs for immigrants.

Additional programs such as school nursing were based on individual observations and interventions. Wald reported the following incident that preceded her successful trial of school nursing (1971):

> I had been downtown only a short time when I met Louis. An open door in a rear tenement revealed a woman standing over a washtub, a fretting baby on her left arm, while with her right she rubbed at the butcher's aprons which she washed for a living.
>
> "Louis," she explained, "was bad." He did not "cure his head of lice and what would become of him, for they would not take him into the school because of it?" Louis said he had been to the dispensary many times. He knew it was awful for a twelve-year-old boy not to know how to read the names of the streets on the lampposts, but "every time I go to school Teacher tells me to go home."
>
> It needed only intelligent application of the dispensary ointments to cure the affected area, and in September, I had the joy of securing the boy's admittance to school for the first time in his life. The next day, at the noon recess, he fairly rushed up our five flights of stairs in the Jefferson Street tenement to spell the elementary words he had acquired that morning. (pp. 46-47)

Overcrowded schools, an uninformed and uninterested public, and an unaware department of health all contributed to this social health neglect. Wald and the nursing staff at the settlement kept anecdotal notes on the sick children teachers excluded from school. One nurse found a boy in school whose

BOX 2-5   LILLIAN WALD: THE HOUSE ON HENRY STREET

The following highlights from *The House on Henry Street*, published in 1915, bring Lillian Wald's experience to life:

A sick woman in a squalid rear tenement, so wretched and so pitiful that, in all the years since, I have not seen anything more appalling, determined me, within half an hour, to live on the East Side.

I had spent two years in a New York training-school for nurses.... After graduation, I supplemented the theoretical instruction, which was casual and inconsequential in the hospital classes twenty-five years ago, by a period of study at a medical college. It was while at the college that a great opportunity came to me.

While there, the long hours "on duty" and the exhausting demands of the ward work scarcely admitted freedom for keeping informed as to what was happening in the world outside. The nurses had no time for general reading; visits to and from friends were brief; we were out of the current and saw little of life saved as it flowed into the hospital wards. It is not strange, therefore, that I should have been ignorant of the various movements which reflected the awakening of the social conscience at the time.

Remembering the families who came to visit patients in the wards, I outlined a course of instruction in home nursing adapted to their needs, and gave it in an old building in Henry Street, then used as a technical school and now part of the settlement. Henry Street then as now was the center of a dense industrial population.

From the schoolroom where I had been giving a lesson in bed-making, a little girl led me one drizzling March morning. She had told me of her sick mother, and gathering from her incoherent account that a child had been born, I caught up the paraphernalia of the bedmaking lesson and carried it with me.

The child led me over broken roadways—there was no asphalt, although its use was well established in other parts of the city—over dirty mattresses and heaps of refuse—it was before Colonel Waring had shown the possibility of clean streets even in that quarter—between tall, reeking houses whose laden fire-escapes, useless for their appointed purpose, bulged with household goods of every description. The rain added to the dismal appearance of the streets and to the discomfort of the crowds which thronged them, intensifying the odors which assailed me from every side. Through Hester and Division Street[s] we went to the end of Ludlow; past odorous fishstands, for the streets were a market-place, unregulated, unsupervised, unclean; past evil-smelling, uncovered garbage-cans; and—perhaps worst of all, where so many little children played—past the trucks brought down from more fastidious quarters and stalled on these already overcrowded streets, lending themselves inevitably to many forms of indecency.

The child led me on through a tenement hallway, across a court where open and unscreened closets were promiscuously used by men and women, up into a rear tenement, by slimy steps whose accumulated dirt was augmented that day by the mud of the streets, and finally into the sickroom.

All the maladjustments of our social and economic relations seemed epitomized in this brief journey and what was found at the end of it. The family to which the child led me was neither criminal nor vicious. Although the husband was a cripple, one of those who stand on street corners exhibiting deformities to enlist compassion, and masking the begging of alms by a pretense at selling; although the family of seven shared their two rooms with boarders—who were literally boarders, since a piece of timber was placed over the floor for them to sleep on—and although the sick woman lay on a wretched, unclean bed, soiled with a hemorrhage two days old, they were not degraded human beings, judged by any measure of moral values.

In fact, it was very plain that they were sensitive to their condition, and when, at the end of my ministrations, they kissed my hands (those who have undergone similar experiences will, I am sure, understand), it would have been some solace if by any conviction of the moral unworthiness of the family I could have defended myself as a part of a society which permitted such conditions to exist. Indeed, my subsequent acquaintance with them revealed the fact that, miserable as their state was, they were not without ideals for the family life, and for society, of which they were so unloved and unlovely a part.

That morning's experience was a baptism of fire. Deserted were the laboratory and the academic work of the college. I never returned to them. On my way from the sickroom to my comfortable student quarters my mind was intent on my own responsibility. To my inexperience it seemed certain that conditions such as these were allowed because people did not know, and for me there was a challenge to know and to tell. When early morning found me still awake, my naive conviction remained that, if people knew things—and "things" meant everything implied in the condition of this family—such horrors would cease to exist, and I rejoiced that I had had a training in the care of the sick that in itself would give me an organic relationship to the neighborhood in which this awakening had come.

To the first sympathetic friend to whom I poured forth my story, I found myself presenting a plan which had been developing almost without conscious mental direction on my part.

Within a day or two a comrade from the training-school, Mary Brewster, agreed to share in the venture. We were to live in the neighborhood as nurses, identify ourselves with it socially, and, in brief, contribute to it our citizenship.

I should like to make it clear that from the beginning we were most profoundly moved by the wretched industrial conditions which were constantly forced upon us.... I hope to tell of the constructive programmes that the people themselves have evolved out of their own hard lives, of the ameliorative measures, ripened out of sympathetic comprehension, and finally, of the social legislation that expresses the new compunction of the community.

From Wald L: *The house on Henry Street*, New York, 1971, Dover Publications (original work published 1915, Henry Holt), pp. 1-9.

---

skin was desquamating from scarlet fever and took him to the president of the Department of Health in an attempt to place physicians in schools. A later program had physicians screen children in school for 1 hour each day.

Twentieth Century. In 1902, Wald persuaded Dr. Ernest J. Lederle, Commissioner of Health in New York City, to try a school nursing experiment. Henry Street lent a public health nurse named Linda Rogers to the New York City Health Department to work in a school (Dock and Stewart, 1925). The experiment was successful, and schools adopted nursing on a widespread basis. School nurses performed physical assessments, treated minor infections, and taught health to pupils and parents.

In 1909, Wald mentioned the efficacy of home nursing to one of the officials of the Metropolitan Life Insurance Company. The company decided to provide home nursing to its industrial policyholders, and soon the United States and Canada used the program successfully (Wald, 1971).

The growing demand for public health nursing was hard to satisfy. In 1910, the Department of Nursing and Health formed at the Teachers College of Columbia University in New York City. A course in visiting nursing placed nurses at the Henry Street settlement for fieldwork. In 1912, the newly formed National Organization for Public Health Nursing elected Lillian Wald its first president. This organization

EXAMPLE OF HISTORICAL NURSING RESEARCH

Thompson and Keeling (2012) presented an historical examination describing how public health nurses contributed to a significant decline in infant mortality in New England between 1884 and 1925. Analyzing archived data and documents from Providence, Rhode Island, they estimated that in the late nineteenth century, the mortality rate of children younger than 2 was between 15% and 20%. Furthermore, they reported that the health officials believed that of those infants and small children who died during those years, 40% to 50% died from digestive-related diseases (e.g., diarrhea).

The germ theory was not widely accepted until the early 1900s. Thus, in the late nineteenth century, nurse were trained to understand "elements of modern hygiene" (e.g., good nutrition, light, cleanliness). But, following acceptance of the germ theory and epidemiological techniques for data analysis in the early 1900s, public health efforts shifted to consideration of factors, including biological, environmental and economic, that contributed to the high infant mortality rate.

To address the problem of infant/child mortality, public health nurses focused on teaching low income mothers how to care for and feed their children. The nurses worked in homes, "milk stations," and other creative settings to meet the identified needs. They set up and participated in "milk dispensaries," which provided pasteurized milk (rather than the widely available unrefrigerated milk— which was frequently days old). They also promoted breastfeeding and provided information on "infant hygiene" along with the milk. These and other efforts, including developing the role of a "children's special nurse," were effective, and the infant mortality rate dropped from 142/1,000 to 102/1,000 between 1907 and 1917.

From Thompson ME, Keeling AA: Nurses' role in the prevention of infant mortality in 1884-1925: health disparities then and now, *J Pediatr Nurs* 27:471-478, 2012.

was open to public health nurses and to those interested in public health nursing. In 1913, the Los Angeles Department of Health formed the first Bureau of Public Health Nursing (Rosen, 1993). That same year, the Public Health Service appointed its first public health nurse.

At first, many public health nursing programs used nurses in specialized areas such as school nursing, TB nursing, maternal-child health nursing, and communicable disease nursing. In later years, more generalized programs have become acceptable. Efforts to contain health care costs include reducing the number of hospital days. With the advent of shortened hospital stays, private home health agencies provide home-based illness care across the United States.

The second half of the century saw a shift in emphasis to cost containment and the provision of health care services through managed care. Traditional models of public health nursing and visiting nursing from home health agencies became increasingly common over the next several decades, but waned toward the end of the century owing to changes in health care financing.

CONSEQUENCES FOR THE HEALTH OF AGGREGATES

An understanding of the consequences of the health care delivery system for aggregate health is necessary to form conclusions about public health nursing from a historical perspective. Implications for the health of aggregates relate to new causes of mortality (i.e., *Hygeia*, or health promotion/care, vs. *Panacea*, or cure) and additional theories of disease causation.

Twenty-First Century
New Causes of Mortality

Since the middle of the twentieth century, the focus of disease in Western societies has changed from mostly infectious diseases to chronic diseases. Increased food production and better nutrition during the nineteenth and early twentieth centuries contributed to the decline in infectious disease–related deaths. Other factors were better sanitation through water purification, sewage disposal, improved food handling, and milk pasteurization. According to McKeown (2001) and Schneider (2011), the components of "modern" medicine, such as antibiotics and immunizations, had little effect on health until well into the twentieth century. Indeed, widespread vaccination programs began in the late 1950s, and antibiotics came into use after 1945.

The advent of chronic disease in Western populations puts selected aggregates at risk, and those aggregates need health education, screening, and programs to ensure occupational and environmental safety. Too often modern medicine focuses on the single cause of disease (i.e., germ theory) and treating the acutely ill. Therefore health providers have treated the chronically ill with an acute care approach even though preventive care, health promotion, and restorative care are necessary and would likely be more effective in combating escalating rates of chronic disease. This expanded approach may develop under new systems of cost containment.

Hygeia versus Panacea

The Grecian Hygeia (i.e., healthful living) versus Panacea (i.e., cure) dichotomy still exists today. Although the change in the nature of health "problems" is certain, the roles of individual and collective activities in the prevention of illness and premature death are slow to evolve.

In 2010, about two thirds of the active physicians in the United States were specialists (U.S. Department of Health and Human Services, Agency for Healthcare Research and Quality [USDHHS/AHRQ], 2011). Medical education is increasingly focused on enhancing the education of primary care physicians (e.g., those specializing in internal medicine, obstetrics-gynecology, family medicine, and pediatrics) to meet the growing need for primary care. This need for primary care providers to address the increase in insured Americans, along with the continued growth of managed care and implementation of the Affordable Care Act, calls for more advanced practice nurses in primary care positions. In addition to primary care, Hygeia (health promotion) requires a coordinated system that addresses health problems holistically with the use of multiple approaches and planning of outcomes for aggregates and populations. A redistribution of interest and resources to address the major determinants of health, such as food, housing, education, and a healthy social and physical environment, is critical (Shi and Singh, 2011).

Additional Theories of Disease Causation

The germ theory of disease causation is a unicausal model that evolved in the late nineteenth century. Najman (1990) reviewed the following theories of disease causation: the multicausal view, which considers the environment multidimensionally, and the general susceptibility view, which considers stress and lifestyle factors. Najman contended that each theory accounts for some disease under some conditions, but no single theory accounts for all disease. Other factors, such as literacy and nutrition, may reduce disease morbidity and mortality to a greater extent than medical interventions alone.

SOCIAL CHANGES AND COMMUNITY HEALTH NURSING

Several social and political changes have occurred in the United States that have affected the development of community health nursing practice. During the twentieth century, the health of the aggregate client, nursing, health, and the environment have been influenced by the development of health insurance and an emphasis on population-based focus.

The advent of and changes in health insurance have dramatically altered health care delivery. The greatest health concerns at the beginning of the twentieth century were lost wages associated with sickness. The cost of health care was so low that there was little understanding of the need for health insurance. Between 1900 and 1920 there was little technology. Treatments available at the time, including surgery, were often performed in private homes.

During the 1920s and 1930s, the costs of health care rose. As the population moved from rural to urban living, the number of large private homes, the delivery points for much of

health care, decreased. Improved technology, the acceptance of medicine as a science, and the closure of several medical schools during the 1920s increased the demand and therefore raised the cost of health care (Rosenberg, 1987).

As hospitals began to organize, they formed the American Hospital Association, whose leaders encouraged the development of health insurance plans. In 1929, the Committee of the Costs of Medical Care, a national group, produced a report that promoted voluntary insurance in the United States. That same year, Baylor Hospital in Dallas, Texas, joined with a local teachers' association to provide health care for those agreeing to pay a small monthly premium. In a short time, this relationship grew to include more employers and evolved into Blue Cross (Getzen, 2010; Sparer, 2011). Improvements in medical technology and the growing practice of employers' offering health insurance in place of employee compensation during and after World War II, further supported the expansion of private health insurance.

During the 1960s, politicians supported the development of federal and state health insurance for the poor and the elderly populations, subsequently enacting Medicare and Medicaid. Currently, most health care is paid for with either public or private insurance plans. Services covered by many insurance plans often do not include community-based health care. Implementation of the Patient Protection and Affordable Care Act (PPACA) should address much of the inequalities that have persisted through the decades. Indeed, considerable attention on current public health initiatives, such as the *Healthy People 2020* campaign and the PPACA, focus on ensuring elimination of disparities in health care. Box 2-6 provides a summary of some of the dramatic effects of public health activities on the health of Americans during the last 100 years.

BOX 2-6   TEN GREAT PUBLIC HEALTH ACHIEVEMENTS—UNITED STATES, 1900-2010

During the twentieth century, the health and life expectancy of persons living in the United States improved dramatically. It is important for nurses to realize that of the 30 years of life expectancy gained during the century, 25 years were attributable to public health efforts. During 1999, the Centers for Disease Control and Prevention published a series of articles outlining ten of the great public health achievements of the twentieth century. In 2011, the agency published an update of highlights from the ensuing decade. Summarized here are the "Public Health Achievements" presented:

Vaccination/vaccine-preventable diseases—Widespread vaccination programs resulted in eradication of smallpox, elimination of polio in the Americas, and control of measles, rubella, tetanus, diphtheria, and a number of other infectious diseases in the United States. In the first decade of the twenty-first century, new vaccines (e.g., rotavirus, herpes zoster, hepatitis A and human papilloma virus) were introduced and are having significant, positive impact on population health.

Motor-vehicle safety—Improvements in motor-vehicle safety contributed to large reductions in traffic deaths. Improvements included efforts to make both vehicles and highways safer and to change personal behaviors (e.g., increase use of seat belts and child safety seats, reduce driving under the influence [DUI] offenses). Between 2000 and 2009, the death rate from motor vehicle accidents continued to decline, largely as a result of safer

vehicles, safer roads, safer road use, and related policies (e.g., graduated driver's licenses).

Safer workplaces—Work-related health problems (e.g., coal worker's pneumoconiosis [black lung] and silicosis) were very significantly reduced during the twentieth century, as were severe injuries and deaths related to mining, manufacturing, construction, and transportation. Following legislation in 1980, safer workplaces resulted in further reduction of 40% in rate of fatal occupational injuries by the end of the century.

Control of infectious diseases—Since the early 1900s, control of infectious diseases has resulted from clean water and better sanitation. Cholera and typhoid were major causes of illness and death in the early twentieth century and have been virtually eliminated today. Additionally, the discovery of antimicrobial therapy has been very successful in helping efforts to control infections such as tuberculosis, sexually transmitted infections, and influenza. Much of the efforts in the last decade of the twentieth century and the first of the twenty-first century focused on prevention and treatment of human immunodeficiency virus/acquired immunodeficiency syndrome (HIV/AIDS). Prevention/education efforts, along with enhanced screening for HIV, early diagnosis, and effective treatment, have resulted in reduction in transmission of the virus, along with enabling access to life-saving treatment and care for those who are HIV positive and their partners.

Continued

BOX 2-6 **TEN GREAT PUBLIC HEALTH ACHIEVEMENTS—UNITED STATES, 1900-2010—cont'd**

Decline in deaths from coronary heart disease (CHD) and stroke—Since 1972, the death rate for CHD has decreased 51%. This improvement is largely the result of risk factor modification (e.g., smoking cessation, blood pressure control) coupled with early detection and better treatment. In the last decade, CHD deaths continued to decline, going from 195/100,000 to 126/100,000. Contributing to the ongoing reduction are better control of hypertension, reduction in elevated cholesterol and smoking, and improvement in treatment and available medications.

Safer and healthier foods—Since 1900, reduction in microbial contamination and increases in nutritional content have led to safer and healthier foods. Food fortification programs and enhanced availability of nutritional options have almost eliminated major nutritional deficiency diseases in the United States.

Healthier mothers and babies—Since 1900, infant mortality in the United States has decreased 90%, and maternal mortality has decreased 99%. These improvements are the result of better hygiene and nutrition, availability of antibiotics, access to better health care, and advances in maternal and neonatal medicine. During the early twenty-first century, there has been a significant reduction in the number of infants born with neural tube defects, a change attributable to mandatory folic acid fortification of cereal grain products.

Family planning—Access to family planning and contraceptives has provided women with better social and economic opportunities and health benefits, including smaller families and longer intervals between children.

Fluoridation of drinking water—Fluoridation of drinking water began in 1945, and by 1999 about half of all Americans had fluoridated water. This achievement positively and inexpensively benefited both children and adults by preventing tooth decay. Indeed, fluoridation has been credited for reducing tooth decay by 40%-70% in children and tooth loss by 40%-60% in adults.

Tobacco control—Recognition in 1964 that tobacco use is a health hazard resulted in behavior and policy changes that eventually led to a dramatic decline in the prevalence of smoking among adults. The rate of smoking peaked in the 1960s, and by 2009 only about 20% of adults and youths were current smokers. Health policy efforts (e.g., prohibition of smoking in worksites, restaurants, and bars), dramatic increases in cigarette taxes, and prohibition of selling to youths have contributed to much of the recent decline.

Data from Centers for Disease Control and Prevention: Ten great public health achievements—United States, 1900-1999. *MMWR Morb Mortal Wkly Rep* 48(12):241-243, 1999; and Centers for Disease Control and Prevention: Ten great public health achievements—United States, 2001-2010, *MMWR Morb Mortal Wkly Rep* 60(19):619-623, 2011.

EXAMPLE OF HISTORICAL NURSING RESEARCH

Fairman's (1996) review of 150 fictional novels from 1850 to 1995 revealed how the image of nursing has changed over the past 140 years. The results showed that the image of nursing improved dramatically from the negative perception of the 1850s. Trained nurses became more common in the early 1900s, and novels began to depict strong, independent, female nurses. The positive image continued until the 1960s and 1970s, when novels presented the negative image of "bed hopping honeys." Popular literature showed the most negative image of nurses, and classics and children's literature showed a more positive image.

Adapted from Fairman PL: *Analysis of the image of nursing and nurses as portrayed in fictional literature from 1850 to 1995*, Dissertation Abstracts, 1996, University of San Francisco.

CHALLENGES FOR COMMUNITY AND PUBLIC HEALTH NURSING

Community health nurses face the challenge of promoting the health of populations. They must accomplish this goal with a broadened understanding of the multiple causes of morbidity and mortality. The specialization of medicine and nursing has affected the delivery of nursing and health care. Well-prepared nurses must be aware of the increased technological advances that specialization has instigated. These advances resulted in an increase in the number and percentage of advanced practice nurses in the past several decades.

The community need for a focus on prevention, health promotion, and home care may become more widespread with the changing patterns of health care cost reimbursement. Holistic care requires multiple dimensions and must have more attention in the future.

The need for education in community health nursing calls for a primary care curriculum that prepares students to meet the needs of aggregates through community strategies that include an understanding of statistical data and epidemiology. Such a curriculum would move the focus from the individual to a broader population approach. Strategies would promote literacy, nutrition programs, prevention of overweight school-aged children, decent housing and income, education, and safe social and physical environments.

Health care services to individuals alone cannot solve today's health problems. All health care workers must learn to work with and on behalf of aggregates and help them build a constituency for the consumer issues they face.

A *population focus* for nursing addresses the health of all in the population through the careful gathering of information and statistics. A population focus will better enable community health nurses to contribute to the ethic of social justice by emphasizing society's responsibility for health (Beauchamp, 1986). Helping aggregates help themselves will empower people and create avenues for addressing their concerns.

EXAMPLE OF HISTORICAL NURSING RESEARCH

In response to public health problems, public health and community health nursing evolved in Louisiana between 1835 and 1927. Yellow fever epidemics in the early 1800s provided the early impetus for nursing growth. A nursing service called the Howard Association began in 1833 and provided food, medicine, and nursing care for yellow fever victims. Natural disasters, such as the Mississippi River flood in 1927, also led to the enhancement of accessible public health efforts.

Maternal and child care was another important area for early community and public health nursing efforts. In 1916, the state board of health employed the first public health nurse to reduce infant and maternal mortality, improve the health of preschool and school-aged children, and decrease the mortality and morbidity of communicable diseases.

Adapted from Hanggi-Myers LJ: *The origins and history of the first public health/community health nurses in Louisiana: 1835-1927*, Dissertation Abstracts, New Orleans, 1996, Louisiana State University Medical Center.

IMAGES OF COMMUNITY HEALTH NURSING IN THE EARLY AND MID-TWENTIETH CENTURY

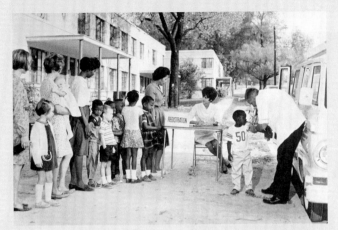

Group Immunization. Multiracial group of women and children in a housing project mobile clinic waiting for and receiving vaccinations. Scene contains a doctor and a nurse. (1972). (Courtesy Centers for Disease Control and Prevention Public Health Image Library [PHIL] Image #1661. Source: CDC/ Reuel Waldrop.)

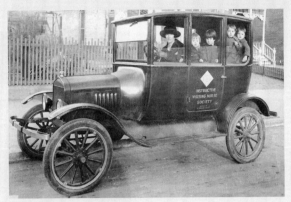

A public health nurse transports children to a clinic. (Courtesy Med-Star Visiting Nurse Association.)

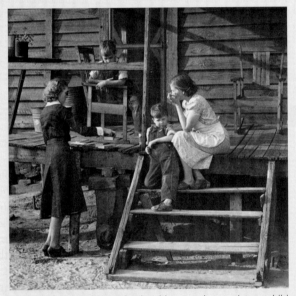

A visiting nurse outside a shack with a mother and two children. (Courtesy of the US National Library of Medicine, History of Medicine Division. Order No. A017986.)

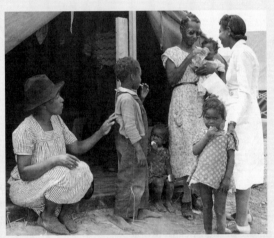

Public Health Nurse performs health teaching. (Courtesy the Library of Congress, Washington, DC.)

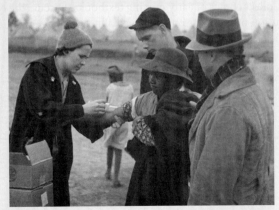

A public health nurse immunizes farm and migrant workers in the 1940s. (Courtesy the Library of Congress, Washington, DC.)

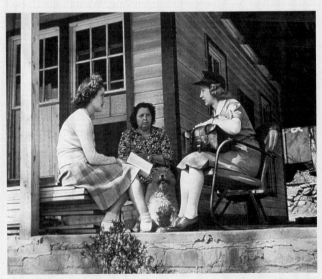

A public health nurse talks to a young woman and her mother about childbirth. (Courtesy the US National Library of Medicine, History of Medicine Division. Order No. A029980.)

Continued

IMAGES OF COMMUNITY HEALTH NURSING IN THE EARLY AND MID-TWENTIETH CENTURY—cont'd

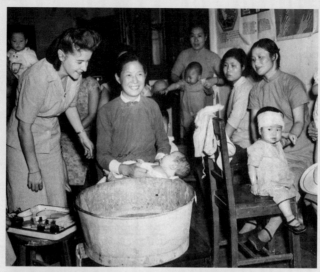

The Shanghai Mother's Club of the Child Welfare and Maternal Health Clinic. United Nations Relief and Rehabilitation Administration (UNRRA) Public Health Nurse Irene Muir instructs Nurse S.U. Zee on child bathing techniques. (Courtesy the US National Library of Medicine, History of Medicine Division. Order No. A016681.)

SUMMARY

Western civilization evolved from the Paleolithic period to the present, and people began to live in increasingly closer proximity to one another; therefore, they experienced a change in the nature of their health problems.

In the mid-nineteenth and early twentieth centuries, public health efforts and the precursors of modern and public health nursing began to improve societal health. Nursing pioneers such as Nightingale in England and Wald in the United States focused on the collection and analysis of statistical data, health care reforms, home health nursing, community empowerment, and nursing education. They established the groundwork for today's public health nurses.

Modern public health nurses must recognize and try to understand the philosophical controversies that influence society and ultimately their practice. These controversies include different opinions about what "intervention" means — specifically in regard to 'cure' vs 'care.' Controversy also surrounds the significance of maintaining a focus on individuals, families, groups, or populations. Finally, public health nurses need to understand social determinants of health and to be part of the solution with regard to coming up with ways to address persistent health problems while addressing the critical problem of escalating health care costs.

LEARNING ACTIVITIES

1. Research the history of the health department or Visiting Nurse Association in a particular city or county.
2. Find two recent articles about Florence Nightingale. After reading the articles, list Nightingale's contributions to public health, public health nursing, and community health nursing.
3. Discuss with peers how Lillian Wald's approach to individual and community health care provides an understanding of how to facilitate the empowerment of aggregates in the community.
4. Obtain copies of early articles from nursing journals (e.g., *American Journal of Nursing* dates from 1900). Discuss the health problems, medical care, and nursing practice these articles illustrated.
5. Collect copies of early nursing textbooks. Discuss the evolution of thoughts on pathology, illness management, and health promotion.

ⓔ EVOLVE WEBSITE

http://evolve.elsevier.com/Nies
- NCLEX Review Questions
- Case Studies
- Glossary

REFERENCES

Armelagos GK, Dewey JR: Evolutionary response to human infectious diseases. In Logan MH, Hunt EE, editors: *Health and the human condition*, North Scituate, MA, 1978, Duxbury Press.

Beauchamp DE: Public health as social justice. In Mappes T, Zembaty J, editors: *Biomedical ethics*, ed 2, New York, 1986, McGraw-Hill.

Centers for Disease Control and Prevention: Two cases of human plague—Oregon, 2010, *MMWR Morb Mortal Wkly Rep* 60:214, 2011.

Centers for Disease Control and Prevention: *Plague in the United States, 2012*. Available from <http://www.cdc.gov/plague/maps/index.html>. Accessed March 2, 2013.

Cockburn TA: The evolution of human infectious diseases. In Cockburn T, editor: *Infectious diseases: their evolution and eradication*, Springfield, IL, 1967, Charles C Thomas.

Cohen IB: Florence Nightingale, *Sci Am* 250:128–137, 1984.

Dock LL, Stewart IM: *A short history of nursing: from the earliest times to the present day*, New York, 1925, Putnam.

Donahue MP: *Nursing: the finest art*, ed 3, St. Louis, MO, 2011, Mosby/Elsevier.

Duffus RL: *Lillian Wald: neighbor and crusader*, New York, 1938, Macmillan.

Duran FD: *The Aztecs: the history of the Indies of New Spain*, New York, 1964, Orion Press (Translated, with notes, by D Heyden and F Horcasitas).

Ehrenreich B, English D: *Witches, midwives, and nurses: a history of women healers*, Old Westbury, NY, 1973, The Feminist Press.

Fairman PL: *Analysis of the image of nursing and nurses as portrayed in fictional literature from 1850 to 1995*, Dissertation Abstracts, University of San Francisco, 1996.

Garn SM: Culture and the direction of human evolution, *Hum Biol* 35:221–236, 1963.

George MD: *London life in the XVIIIth century*, New York, 1925, Knopf.

Getzen T: *Health economics and financing*, ed 4, Hoboken, NJ, 2010, John Wiley & Sons.

Goodnow M: *Outlines of nursing history*, Philadelphia, 1933, WB Saunders.

Greifinger RB, Sidel VW: American medicine: charity begins at home. In Lee P, Brown N, Red I, editors: *The nation's health*, San Francisco, 1981, Boyd and Fraser.

Grier B, Grier M: Contributions of the passionate statistician, *Res Nurs Health* 1:103–109, 1978.

Hanggi-Myers LJ: *The origins and history of the first public health/community health nurses in Louisiana: 1835-1927*, Dissertation Abstracts. New Orleans, 1996, Louisiana State University Medical Center.

Hanlon JJ, Pickett GE: *Public health administration and practice*, ed 9, St. Louis, 1990, Mosby.

Hughes CC: Medical care: ethnomedicine. In Logan MH, Hunt EE, editors: *Health and the human condition*, North Scituate, MA, 1978, Duxbury Press.

Kalisch PA, Kalisch BJ: *American nursing: a history. Lippincott*, ed 4, Philadelphia, PA, 2004, Williams & Wilkins.

Kopf EW: Florence Nightingale as statistician, *Res Nurs Health* 1:93–102, 1978.

Lee PR, Brown N, Red I, editors: *The nation's health*, San Francisco, 1981, Boyd and Fraser.

Leininger M, McFarland MM: *Culture care diversity and universality: a worldwide nursing theory*, ed 2, Sudbury, MA, 2006, Jones & Bartlett.

Logan MH, Hunt EE, editors: *Health and the human condition*, North Scituate, MA, 1978, Duxbury Press.

McKeown T: Determinants of health. In Lee P, Estes CL, editors: *The nation's health*, ed 6, Boston, MA, 2001, Jones & Bartlett.

Najman JM: Theories of disease causation and the concept of a general susceptibility: a review, *Soc Sci Med* 14A:231–237, 1990.

Newbern VB: Women as caregivers in the South: 1900-1945, *Public Health Nurs* 11:247–254, 1994.

Nightingale F: *Notes on matters affecting the health, efficiency and hospitalization of the British army*, London, 1858, Harrison and Sons.

Polgar S: Evolution and the ills of mankind. In Tax S, editor: *Horizons of anthropology*, Chicago, 1964, Aldine.

Richardson BW: *The health of nations: a review of the works of Edwin Chadwick*, vol 2. London, 1887, Longmans. Green.

Rosen G: *A history of public health, expanded edition*, Baltimore, MD, 1993, Johns Hopkins Press.

Rosenberg CE: *The care of strangers*, New York, 1987, Basic Books.

Schneider MJ: *Introduction to public health*, ed 3, Sudbury, MA, 2011, Jones & Bartlett.

Smith FB: *The people's health 1830-1910*, London, 1979, Croom Helm.

Sparer MS: Health policy and health reform. In Kovner AR, Knickman JR, editors: *Health care delivery in the United States*, ed 10, New York, 2011, Springer Publishing Co.

U.S. Department of Health and Human Services, Agency for Healthcare Research and Quality: *The number of practicing primary care physicians in the United States*, 201. Available from <http://www.ahrq.gov/research/findings/factsheets/pcwork1.html>.

Wald L: *The house on Henry Street*, New York, 1971, Dover Publications (original work published 1915, Henry Holt).

Thinking Upstream: Nursing Theories and Population-Focused Nursing Practice

*Diane C. Martins**

*The author would like to acknowledge the contribution of Patricia G. Butterfield, who wrote this chapter for the 4th edition.

OBJECTIVES

Upon completion of this chapter, the reader will be able to do the following:

1. Differentiate between upstream interventions, which are designed to alter the precursors of poor health, and downstream interventions, which are characterized by efforts to modify individuals' perceptions of health.

2. Describe different theories and their application to community/public health nursing.
3. Critique a theory in regard to its relevance to population health issues.
4. Explain how theory-based practice achieves the goals of community/public health nursing by protecting and promoting the public's health.

KEY TERMS

conservative scope of practice
critical interactionism
critical theoretical perspective
health belief model (HBM)

macroscopic focus
microscopic focus
Milio's framework for prevention
self-care deficit theory

theory
upstream thinking

OUTLINE

Thinking Upstream: Examining the Root Causes of Poor Health
Historical Perspectives on Nursing Theory
How Theory Provides Direction to Nursing
Microscopic versus Macroscopic Approaches to the Conceptualization of Community Health Problems
Assessing a Theory's Scope in Relation to Community Health Nursing
Review of Theoretical Approaches
    The Individual Is the Focus of Change
    The Upstream View: Society Is the Focus of Change
Healthy People 2020

It may seem as if many community health problems are so complex, so multifaceted, and so deep that it is impossible for a nurse to make substantial improvements in health. Although nurses see persons in whom cancer, cardiovascular disease, or pulmonary disease has just been diagnosed, we know that their diseases began years or even decades ago. In many cases, genetic risks for diseases are interwoven with social, economic, and environmental risks in ways that are difficult to understand and more difficult to change. In the face of all these challenges, how can nurses hope to affect the health of the public in a significant way? How can the actions nurses take today reduce the current burden of illness and prevent illness in the next generation of citizens?

When nurses work on a complex community health problem they need to think strategically. They need to know where to focus their time, energy, and programmatic resources. Most likely they will be up against health problems that have existed for years, with other layers of foundational problems that may have existed for generations. If nurses use organizational resources in an unfocused manner, they will not solve the problem at hand and may create new problems along the way. If nurses do not build strong relationships with community partners (e.g., parent groups, ministers, local activists), it will be difficult to succeed. If nurses are unable to advocate for their constituencies in a scientifically responsible, logical, and persuasive manner, they may fail. In the face of these challenges and many more, how can nurses succeed in their goal to improve public health?

Fortunately, there are road maps for success. Some of those road maps can be found by reading a nursing history book or an archival work that tells the story of a nurse who succeeded in improving health by leveraging diplomacy skills or neighborhood power, such as Lillian Wald. Other road maps may be found in "success stories" that provide an overview of how a nurse approached a problem, mobilized resources, and moved strategically to promote change. This chapter addresses another road map for success: the ability to think conceptually, almost like a chess player, to formulate a plan to solve complex problems. Thinking conceptually is a subtle skill that requires you to understand the world at an abstract level, seeing the manifestations of power, oppression, justice, and access as they exist within our communities. Most of all, thinking conceptually means that you develop a "critical eye" for the community and understand how change happens at micro and macro levels.

This chapter begins with a brief overview of nursing theory, which is followed by a discussion of the scope of community health nursing in addressing population health concerns. Several theoretical approaches are compared to demonstrate how different conceptualizations can lead to different conclusions about the range of interventions available to the nurse.

THINKING UPSTREAM: EXAMINING THE ROOT CAUSES OF POOR HEALTH

I am standing by the shore of a swiftly flowing river and hear the cry of a drowning man. I jump into the cold waters. I fight against the strong current and force my way to the struggling man. I hold on hard and gradually pull him to shore. I lay him out on the bank and revive him with artificial respiration. Just when he begins to breathe, I hear another cry for help. I jump into the cold waters. I fight against the strong current and swim forcefully to the struggling woman. I grab hold and gradually pull her to shore. I lift her out onto the bank beside the man and work to revive her with artificial respiration. Just when she begins to breathe, I hear another cry for help. I jump into the cold waters. Fighting again against the strong current, I force my way to the struggling man. I am getting tired, so with great effort I eventually pull him to shore. I lay him out on the bank and try to revive him with artificial respiration. Just when he begins to breathe, I hear another cry for help. Near exhaustion, it occurs to me that I'm so busy jumping in, pulling them to shore, applying artificial respiration that I have no time to see who is upstream pushing them all in.... (Adapted from a story told by Irving Zola as cited in McKinlay JB: A case for refocusing upstream: The political economy of illness. In Conrad P, Leiter V, editors: The sociology of health and illness: critical perspectives, ed 9, New York, 2012, Worth, Ch 47.)

In his description of the frustrations in medical practice, McKinlay (1979) used the image of a swiftly flowing river to represent illness. In this analogy, doctors are so busy rescuing victims from the river that they fail to look upstream to see who is pushing patients into the perilous waters. There are many things that could cause a patient to fall (or be pushed) into the waters of illness. Refocusing upstream requires nurses to look beyond individual behavior or characteristics to what McKinlay terms the "manufacturers of illness." McKinlay discusses factors such as tobacco products companies, companies that profit from selling products high in saturated fats, the alcoholic beverage industry, the beauty industry, exposure to environmental toxins, and occupationally induced illnesses. "Manufacturers of illness" are what push clients into the river. Cigarette companies are a good example of manufacturers of illness—their product causes a change for the worse in the health status of their consumers, and they take little to no responsibility for it. McKinlay used this analogy to illustrate the ultimate futility of "downstream endeavors," which are characterized by short-term, individual-based interventions, and challenged health care providers to focus more of their energies "upstream, where the real problems lie" (McKinlay, 1979, p. 9). Downstream health care takes place in our emergency departments, critical care units, and many other health care settings focused on illness care. Upstream thinking actions focus on modifying economic, political, and environmental factors that are the precursors of poor health throughout the world. Although the story cites medical practice, it is equally fitting to the dilemmas of nursing practice. Nursing has a rich history of providing preventive and population-based care, but the current U. S. health system emphasizes episodic and individual-based care. This system has done little to stem the tide of chronic illnesses to which 70% of American deaths can be attributed (Centers for Disease Control and Prevention, 2013).

HISTORICAL PERSPECTIVES ON NURSING THEORY

Many scholars agree that Florence Nightingale was the first nurse to formulate a conceptual foundation for nursing practice. Nightingale believed that clean water, clean linens, access to adequate sanitation, and quiet would improve health outcomes, and she put these beliefs into practice during the Crimean War (Bostidge, 2008). However, in the years after her leadership, nursing practice became less theoretical and was based primarily on reacting to the immediacy of patient situations and the demands of medical staff. Thus hospital and medical personnel defined the boundaries of nursing practice. Once nursing leaders saw that others were defining their profession, they became proactive in advancing the theoretical and scientific foundation of nursing practice. Some of the early nursing theories were extremely narrow and depicted health care situations that involved only one nurse and one patient. Family members and other health professionals were noticeably absent from the context of care. Historically, this characterization may have been an appropriate response to the constraints of nursing practice and the need to emphasize the medically dependent activities of the nursing profession.

Although somewhat valuable, theories that address health from a microscopic, or individual, rather than a macroscopic, or global/social, perspective have limited applicability to community/public health nursing. Such perspectives are inadequate because they do not address social, political, and environmental factors that are central to an understanding of communities. More recent advances in nursing theory development address the dynamic nature of health-sustaining and/or health-damaging environments and address the nature of a collective (e.g., school, worksite) versus an individual client.

HOW THEORY PROVIDES DIRECTION TO NURSING

The goal of theory is to improve nursing practice. Chinn and Kramer (2008) stated that using theories or parts of theoretical frameworks to guide practice best achieves this goal. Students often find theory intellectually burdensome and cannot see the benefits to their practice of something so seemingly obscure. Theory-based practice guides data collection and interpretation in a clear and organized manner; therefore it is easier for the nurse to diagnose and address health problems. Through the process of integrating theory and practice, the student can focus on factors that are critical to understanding the situation. The student also has an opportunity to analyze the realities of nursing practice in relation to a specific theoretical perspective, in a process of ruling in and ruling out the fit of particular concepts (Schwartz-Barcott et al., 2002). Barnum (1998) stated, "A theory is like a map of a territory as opposed to an aerial photograph. The map does not give the full terrain (i.e., the full picture); instead it picks out those parts that are important for its given purpose" (p. 1). Using a theoretical perspective to plan nursing care guides the student in assessing a nursing situation and allows the student "to plan and not get lost in the details or sidetracked in the alleys" (J. M. Swanson, personal communication to P. Butterfield, May 1992).

As with other abstract concepts, different nursing writers have defined and interpreted theory in different ways. Several writers' definitions of theory are listed in Box 3-1. The lack of uniformity among these definitions reflects the evolution of thought and the individual differences in the understanding of relationships among theory, practice, and research. The definitions also reflect the difficult job of describing complex and diverse theories within the constraints of a single definition. Reading several definitions can foster an appreciation for the richness of theory and help the reader identify one or two particularly meaningful definitions. Within the profession, definitions of *theory* typically refer to a set of concepts and relational statements and the purpose of the theory. This chapter presents theoretical perspectives that are congruent with a broad interpretation of theory and correspond with the definitions proposed by Dickoff and James (1968), Torres (1986), and Chinn and Kramer (2008).

MICROSCOPIC VERSUS MACROSCOPIC APPROACHES TO THE CONCEPTUALIZATION OF COMMUNITY HEALTH PROBLEMS

Each nurse must find her or his own way of interpreting the complex forces that shape societies to understand population health. The nurse can best achieve this transformation by integrating population-based practice and theoretical perspectives to conceptualize health from a macroscopic rather than microscopic perspective. Table 3-1 differentiates between these two approaches to conceptualizing health problems.

The individual patient is the microscopic focus whereas society or social economic factors influencing health status are the macroscopic focus. When the individual is the focus,

---

BOX 3-1 DEFINITIONS OF THEORY PROPOSED BY NURSING THEORISTS

- "A systematic vision of reality; a set of interrelated concepts that is useful for prediction and control" (Woods and Catanzaro, 1988, p. 568).
- "A conceptual system or framework invented for some purpose; and as the purpose varies so too must the structure and complexity of the system" (Dickoff and James, 1968, p. 19).
- "A creative and rigorous structuring of ideas that projects a tentative, purposeful, and systematic view of phenomena" (Chinn and Kramer, 1999, p. 51).
- "A set of ideas, hunches, or hypotheses that provides some degree of prediction and/or explanation of the world" (Pryjmachuk, 1996, p. 679).
- "Theory organizes the relationships between the complex events that occur in a nursing situation so that we can assist human beings. Simply stated, theory provides a way of thinking about and looking at the world around us" (Torres, 1986, p. 19).

TABLE 3-1	MICROSCOPIC VERSUS MACROSCOPIC APPROACHES TO THE DELINEATION OF COMMUNITY HEALTH NURSING PROBLEMS	
MICROSCOPIC APPROACH	**MACROSCOPIC APPROACH**
Examines individual, and sometimes family, responses to health and illness	Examines interfamily and intercommunity themes in health and illness
	Delineates factors in the population that perpetuate the development of illness or foster the development of health
Often emphasizes behavioral responses to individual's illness or lifestyle patterns	Emphasizes social, economic, and environmental precursors of illness
Nursing interventions are often aimed at modifying an individual's behavior through changing his or her perceptions or belief system	Nursing interventions may include modifying social or environmental variables (i.e., working to remove care barriers and improving sanitation or living conditions)
	May involve social or political action

the micro focus contains the health problem of interest (e.g., pediatric exposure to lead compounds). In this context, a microscopic approach to assessment would focus exclusively on individual children with lead poisoning. Nursing interventions would focus on the identification and treatment of the child and family. However, the nurse can broaden his or her view of this problem by addressing removal of lead sources in the home and by examining interpersonal and intercommunity factors that perpetuate lead poisoning on a national scale. A macroscopic approach to lead exposure may incorporate the following activities: examining trends in the prevalence of lead poisoning over time, estimating the percentage of older homes in a neighborhood that may contain lead pipes or lead-based paint surfaces, and locating industrial sources of lead emissions. These efforts usually involve the collaborative efforts of nurses from school, occupational, government, and community settings. Doty (1996) noted that macro-level perspectives provide nurses with the conceptual tools that empower clients to make health decisions on the basis of their own interests and the interests of the community at large.

One common dilemma in community health practice is the tension between working on behalf of individuals and working on behalf of a population. For many nurses, this tension is exemplified by the need to reconcile and prioritize multiple daily tasks. Population-directed actions are often more global than the immediate demands of ill people; therefore they may sink to the bottom of the priority list. A community health nurse or nursing administrator may plan to spend the day on a community project directed at preventive efforts, such as screening programs, updating the surveillance program, or meeting with key community members about a specific preventive program. However, the nurse may actually end up spending the time responding to the emergency of the day. This type of reactive rather than proactive nursing practice prevents progress toward "big picture" initiatives and population-based programs. When faced with multiple demands, nurses must be vigilant in devoting a sustained effort toward population-focused projects. Daily pressures can easily distract the nurse from population-based nursing practice. Several nursing organizations focus on this population, and one organization, the Quad Council of Public Health Nursing, is composed of representatives from the following four public health/community health nursing organizations:

- Public Health Nursing Section of the American Public Health Association (PHN-APHA)
- Association of Community Health Nurse Educators (ACHNE)
- Association of Public Health Nurses (APHN)
- American Nurses Association Council on Nursing Practice and Economics (ANA)

The organizations emphasize "systems thinking" in daily practice and the importance of improving health through the design and implementation of population-based interventions (QUAD Council, 2013).

A theoretical focus on the individual can preclude understanding of a larger perspective. Dreher (1982) used the term conservative scope of practice in describing frameworks that focus energy exclusively on intrapatient and nurse-patient factors. She stated that such frameworks often adopt psychological explanations of patient behavior. This mode of thinking attributes low compliance, missed appointments, and reluctant participation to problems in patient motivation or attitude. Nurses are responsible for altering patient attitudes toward health rather than altering the system itself, "even though such negative attitudes may well be a realistic appraisal of health care" (Dreher, 1982, p. 505). This perspective does not entertain the possibility of altering the system or empowering patients to make changes.

ASSESSING A THEORY'S SCOPE IN RELATION TO COMMUNITY HEALTH NURSING

Theoretical scope is especially important to community health nursing because there are many levels of practice within this specialty area. For example, a home health nurse who is caring for ill people after hospitalization has a very different scope of practice from that of a nurse epidemiologist or health planner. Unless a given theory is broad enough in scope to address health and the determinants of health from a population perspective, the theory will not be very useful to community health nurses. Although the past 25 years yielded much advancement in the development of nursing theory, there continues to be a lack of clarity about community health nursing's theoretical foundation (Batra, 1991). Applying the terms *microscopic* and *macroscopic* to health situations may help nurses fill this void and stimulate theory development in community health nursing.

Although the concept of macroscopic is similar to the upstream analogy, the term *macroscopic* refers to a broad scope that incorporates many variables to aid in understanding a health problem. Upstream thinking would fall within this domain. Viewing a problem from this perspective emphasizes the variables that precede or play a role in the development of health problems. Macroscopic is the broad concept, and upstream is a more specific concept. These related concepts and their meanings can help nurses develop a critical eye in evaluating a theory's relevance to population health.

REVIEW OF THEORETICAL APPROACHES

The differences among theoretical approaches demonstrate how a nurse may draw very diverse conclusions about the reasons for client behavior and the range of available interventions. The following section uses two theories to exemplify individual microscopic approaches to community health nursing problems; one originates within nursing and one is based in social psychology. Two other theories demonstrate the examination of nursing problems from a macroscopic perspective; one originates from nursing and another has roots in phenomenology. The format for this review is as follows:

1. The individual is the focus of change (i.e., microscopic).
   a. Orem's self-care deficit theory of nursing.
   b. The health belief model (HBM).

2. Thinking upstream: Society is the focus of change (i.e., macroscopic).
   a. Milio's framework for prevention.
   b. Critical social theory perspective.

The Individual Is the Focus of Change
Orem's Self-Care Deficit Theory of Nursing

In 1958, Dorothea Orem, a staff and private duty nurse who later became a faculty member at Catholic University of America, began to formalize her insights about the purpose of nursing activities and why individuals required nursing care (Eben et al., 1986; Fawcett, 2001). Her theory is based on the assumption that self-care needs and activities are the primary focus of nursing practice. Orem outlined her self-care deficit theory of nursing and stated that this general theory is actually a composite of the following related constructs: the theory of self-care deficits, which provides criteria for identifying those who need nursing; the theory of self-care, which explains self-care and why it is necessary; and the theory of nursing systems, which specifies nursing's role in the delivery of care and how nursing helps people (Orem, 2001).

Application of Self-Care Deficit Theory. During a discussion about theory-based initiatives, a British occupational health nurse lamented over her nursing supervisor's intention to adopt Orem's self-care deficit theory. She was frustrated and argued that much of the model's assumptions seemed incongruous with the realities of her daily practice. Kennedy (1989) maintained that the self-care deficit theory assumes that people are able to exert purposeful control over their environments in the pursuit of health; however, people may have little control over the physical or social aspects of their work environment. On the basis of this thesis, she concluded that the self-care model is incompatible with the practice domain of occupational health nursing.

The Health Belief Model

The second theory that focuses on the individual as the locus of change is the health belief model (HBM). The model evolved from the premise that the world of the perceiver determines action. The model had its inception during the late 1950s, when America was breathing a collective sigh of relief after the development of the polio vaccine. When some people chose not to bring themselves or their children into clinics for immunization, social psychologists and other public health workers recognized the need to develop a more complete understanding of factors that influence preventive health behaviors. Their efforts resulted in the HBM.

Kurt Lewin's work lent itself to the model's core dimensions. He proposed that behavior is based on current dynamics confronting an individual rather than prior experience (Maiman and Becker, 1974). Figure 3-1 outlines the variables and relationships in the HBM. The health belief model is based on the assumption that the major determinant of preventive health behavior is disease avoidance. The concept of disease avoidance includes perceived susceptibility to disease "X," perceived seriousness of disease "X," modifying factors, cues to action, perceived benefits minus perceived barriers to preventive health action, perceived threat of disease "X," and the likelihood of taking a recommended health action. Disease "X" represents a particular disorder that a health action may prevent. It is important to note that actions that relate to breast cancer will be different from those relating to measles. For example, in breast cancer, a cue to action may involve a public service advertisement encouraging women to make an appointment for a mammogram. However, for measles, a cue to action may be news of a measles outbreak in a neighboring town.

Application of the Health Belief Model. Over the years, a number of writers have proposed broadening the scope of the HBM to address health promotion and illness behaviors

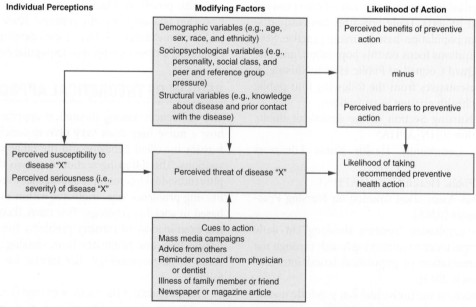

FIGURE 3-1 Variables and relationships in the health belief model (HBM). (Redrawn from Rosenstock IM: Historical origins of the health belief model. In Becker MH, editor: *The health belief model and personal health behavior,* Thorofare, NJ, 1974, Charles B Slack).

(Kirscht, 1974; Pender, 1987) and to merge its concepts with other theories that describe health behavior (Cummings, Becker, and Malie, 1980). The following section contains a brief personal account of the author's perceptions addressing the strengths and limitations of the model.

During my nursing education classes at the undergraduate level, I was exposed to a large number of nursing theories. The HBM was probably my least favorite. Most of the content was interesting, but I found it difficult applying the concepts to patients in the community and home setting. The model's focus on compliance was something that nurses with a critical theoretical perspective would have difficulty applying in their own clinical practice. My perception of the model changed a few years ago when my younger brother had pancreatic cancer diagnosed. This experience allowed me to see how the HBM could offer some insight into an individual's health behaviors. It helped me organize ideas about why people choose to accept or reject the instructions of well-intended nurses and doctors. Concepts such as perceived seriousness, perceived susceptibility, and cue to action afforded new insights into the dynamics of health decision making. I began to apply the model's concepts to guide my work with my family. My brother who became ill had smoked much of his life. Another brother also smoked. My family members believed that you are destined to follow a path of life and death, but this experience clearly modified their health beliefs. Until this point, my family members did not quit smoking because they did not perceive the susceptibility and seriousness of smoking; they belonged to a reference group that disdained most traditional medical practices and favored inaction over action. During the next several weeks, my siblings requested information on strategies that would help them quit smoking and hopefully decrease their chances for the development of cancer.

Over the years, I have become more skilled in assessing and identifying patient needs and issues and have gained a better appreciation for the strengths and limitations that any theoretical framework imposes on a situation.

Limitations of the HBM. The HBM places the burden of action exclusively on the client. It assumes that only those clients who have negative perceptions of the specified disease or recommended health action will fail to act. In practice, this model focuses the nurse's energies on interventions designed to modify the client's distorted perceptions.

The HBM offers an explanation of health behaviors that is similar to a mechanical system. Consulting the HBM, a nurse may induce compliance by using model variables as catalysts to stimulate action. For example, an intervention study based on HBM precepts sought to improve follow-up in clients with hypertension by increasing their perceived susceptibility to and seriousness of the dangers of hypertension (Jones, Jones, and Katz, 1987). The study provided patients with education over the telephone or in the emergency department and resulted in a dramatic increase in compliance. However, the researchers noted that several patient groups, in particular, a group of patients without child care, failed to respond to the intervention. Studies such as these demonstrate the predictive abilities and the limitations of HBM concepts (Lajunen and Rasanen, 2004; Lin et al., 2005; Mirotznik et al., 1998). The Health Belief Model has been used in childhood obesity

prevention research. It was reported that the model accounted for less than 50% of the variance resulting from behavior change interventions (National Heart Lung and Blood Institute, 2007).

The HBM may effectively promote behavioral change by altering patients' perspectives, but it does not acknowledge the health professional's responsibility to reduce or ameliorate health care barriers. The model reflects the type of theoretical perspective that dominated nursing education and behavioral health for many years. The narrow scope of the model is its strength and its limitation: nurses are not challenged to examine the root causes of health opportunities and behaviors in the communities we serve.

The Upstream View: Society Is the Focus of Change
Milio's Framework for Prevention
Nancy Milio conducted extensive research on tobacco policy (1985). Milio's approach to advancing people's health is seen in her seminal book, *Promoting Health through Public Policy*, and through her detailed studies of tobacco policy and Norwegian farm food policy (Draper, 1986). Milio's framework for prevention (1976) provides a complement to the HBM and a mechanism for directing attention upstream and examining opportunities for nursing intervention at the population level. Nancy Milio outlined six propositions that relate an individual's ability to improve healthful behavior to a society's ability to provide accessible and socially affirming options for healthy choices. Milio used these propositions to move the focus of attention upstream by challenging the notion that a main determinant for unhealthful behavior choice is lack of knowledge. She said that government and institutional policies set the range of health options, so community health nursing needs to examine a community's level of health and attempt to influence a community's health through public policy. She noted that the range of available health choices is critical in shaping a society's overall health status. Milio believed that national-level policy making was the best way to favorably impact the health of most Americans rather than concentrating efforts on imparting information in an effort to change individual patterns of behavior.

Milio (1976) proposed that health deficits often result from an imbalance between a population's health needs and its health-sustaining resources. She stated that the diseases associated with excess (e.g., obesity and alcoholism) afflict affluent societies and that the diseases resulting from inadequate or unsafe food, shelter, and water afflict the poor. Within this context, the poor in affluent societies may experience the least desirable combination of factors. Milio (1976) cited the socioeconomic realities that deprive many Americans of a health-sustaining environment despite the fact that "cigarettes, sucrose, pollutants, and tensions are readily available to the poor" (p. 436). Propositions proposed by Milio are listed in Table 3-2.

Personal and societal resources affect the range of health-promoting or health-damaging choices available to individuals. Personal resources include the individual's awareness,

TABLE 3-2   APPLICATION OF MILIO'S FRAMEWORK IN PUBLIC HEALTH NURSING

MILIO'S PROPOSITION SUMMARY	POPULATION HEALTH EXAMPLES
Population health results from deprivation and/or excess of critical health resources.	Individuals and families living in poverty have poorer health status compared with middle- and upper-class individuals and families.
Behaviors of populations result from selection from limited choices; these arise from actual and perceived options available as well as beliefs and expectations resulting from socialization, education and experience.	Positive and negative lifestyle choices (e.g., smoking, alcohol use, safe sex practices, regular exercise, diet/nutrition, seatbelt use) are strongly dependent on culture, socioeconomic status, and educational level.
Organizational decisions and policies (both governmental and nongovernmental) dictate many of the options available to individuals and populations and influence choices.	Health insurance coverage and availability are largely determined and financed by federal and state governments (e.g., Medicare and Medicaid) and employers (e.g., private insurance); the source and funding of insurance very strongly influence health provider choices and services.
Individual choices related to health-promoting or health-damaging behaviors is influenced by efforts to maximize valued resources.	Choices and behaviors of individuals are strongly influenced by desires, values, and beliefs. For example, the use of barrier protection during sex by adolescents is often dependent on peer pressure and the need for acceptance, love, and belonging.
Alteration in patterns of behavior resulting from decision making of a significant number of people in a population can result in social change.	Some behaviors, such as tobacco use, have become difficult to maintain in many settings or situations in response to organizational and public policy mandates. As a result, tobacco use in the United States has dropped dramatically.
Without concurrent availability of alternative health-promoting options for investment of personal resources, health education will be largely ineffective in changing behavior patterns.	Addressing persistent health problems (e.g., overweight/obesity) is hindered because most people are very aware of what causes the problem, but are reluctant to make lifestyle changes to prevent or reverse the condition. Often, "new" information (e.g., a new diet) or resources (e.g., a new medication) can assist in attracting attention and directing positive behavior changes.

Adapted from Milio, N: A framework for prevention: changing health-damaging to health-generating life patterns, *Am J Publ Health*, 66:435-439, 1976.

knowledge, and beliefs and the beliefs of the individual's family and friends. Money, time, and the urgency of other priorities are also personal resources. Community and national locale strongly influence societal resources. These resources include the availability and cost of health services, environmental protection, safe shelter, and the penalties or rewards for failure to select the given options.

Milio (1976) challenged health education's assumption that knowledge of health-generating behaviors implies an act in accordance with that knowledge. She proposed that "most human beings, professional or nonprofessional, provider or consumer, make the easiest choices available to them most of the time" (p. 435). Health-promoting choices must be more readily available and less costly than health-damaging options for individuals to gain health and for society to improve health status. Milio's framework can enable a nurse to reframe this view by understanding the historic play of social forces that have limited the choices available to the parties involved.

Comparison of the HBM and Milio's Conceptualizations of Health. Milio's health resources bear some resemblance to the concepts in the HBM. The purpose of the HBM is to provide the nurse with an understanding of the dynamics of personal health behaviors. The HBM specifies broader contextual variables, such as the constraints of the health care system, and their influence on the individual's decision-making processes. The HBM also assumes that each person has unlimited access to health resources and free will. In contrast, Milio based her framework on an assessment of community resources and their availability to individuals. By assessing such factors up front, the nurse is able to gain a more thorough understanding of the resources people actually have. Milio offered a

different set of insights into the health behavior arena by proposing that many low-income individuals are acting within the constraints of their limited resources. Furthermore, she investigated beyond downstream focus and population health by examining the choices of significant numbers of people within a population.

Compared with the HBM, Milio's framework provides for the inclusion of economic, political, and environmental health determinants; therefore, the nurse is given broader range in the diagnosis and interpretation of health problems. Whereas the HBM allows only two possible outcomes (i.e., "acts" or "fails to act" according to the recommended health action), Milio's framework encourages the nurse to understand health behaviors in the context of their societal milieu.

Implications of Milio's Framework for Current Health Delivery Systems. Through its broader scope, Milio's model provides direction for nursing interventions at many levels. Nurses may use this model to assess the personal and societal resources of individual patients and to analyze social and economic factors that may inhibit healthy choices in populations. Population-based interventions may include such diverse activities as working to improve the nutritional content of school lunches and encouraging political activity on behalf of health care reform (Hobbs et al., 2004; Milio, 1981).

Overall, current health care delivery systems perform best when responding to people with diagnostic-intensive and acute illnesses. Those people who experience chronic debilitation or have less intriguing diagnoses generally fare worse in the health care system despite efforts by community- and home-based care to "fill the gaps." Nurses in both hospital and

TABLE 3-3   COMPARISON OF INDIVIDUAL AND SOCIETAL LEVELS OF CHANGE

INDIVIDUAL LEVEL	SOCIETAL LEVEL
The individual is the focus of change	Society/community is the focus of change
Microscopic	Macroscopic
Downstream activities emphasized	Upstream activities emphasized
Theories:	Theories:
a. Orem's self-care deficit theory of nursing	a. Milio's framework for prevention
b. The health belief model (HBM)	b. Critical social theory perspective

community-based systems often feel constrained by profound financial and service restrictions imposed by third-party payers. These third parties often terminate nursing care after the resolution of the latest immediate health crisis and fail to cover care aimed toward long-term health improvements. Many health systems use nursing standards and reimbursement mechanisms that originate from a narrow, compartmentalized view of health.

Personal behavior patterns are not simply "free" choices about "lifestyle" that are isolated from their personal and economic context. Lifestyles are patterns of choices made from available alternatives according to people's socioeconomic circumstances and how easily they are able to choose some over others (Milio, 1981). It is therefore imperative to practice nursing from a broader understanding of health, illness, and suffering. Public health nurses must often work at both the individual and societal level. As Milio suggested, it is not only individual behaviors but the economic context as well. This can be seen in Table 3-3, which shows that the focus of change can be at the individual or society level.

Critical Theoretical Perspective

Similar to Milio's framework for prevention, critical theoretical perspective uses societal awareness to expose social inequalities that keep people from reaching their full potential. This perspective is devised from the belief that social meanings structure life through social domination. "A critical perspective can be used to understand the linkages between the health care system and the broader political, economic, and social systems of society" (Waitzkin, 1983, p. 5). According to Navarro (1976), in *Medicine Under Capitalism,* the health care system mirrors the class structure of the broader society. According to Conrad (2008), a critical theoretical perspective is one that does not regard the present structure of health care as sacred. A critical theoretical perspective accepts no truth or fact merely because it has been accepted as such in the past. The social aspects of health and illness are too complex to use only one perspective. The critical theoretical perspective assumes that health and illness entail societal and personal values and that these values have to be made explicit if illness and health care problems are to be satisfactorily dealt

with. This perspective is informed by the following values and assumptions:

1. The problems and inequalities of health and health care are connected to the particular historically located social arrangements and the cultural values of society.
2. Health care should be oriented toward the prevention of disease and illness.
3. The priorities of any health care system should be based on the needs of the clients/population and not the health care providers.
4. Ultimately, society itself must be changed for health and medical care to improve (Conrad and Leiter, 2012).

Stevens and Hall (1992) used critical theoretical perspective in nursing to address unsafe neighborhoods as well as economic, political, and social disadvantages of the community we serve. They advocate for emancipator nursing actions for our communities. Proponents of this theoretical approach maintain that social exchanges that are not distorted from power imbalances will stimulate the evolution of a more just society (Allen, Diekelmann, and Benner, 1986). Critical theoretical perspective assumes that truth standards are socially determined and that no form of scientific inquiry is value free. Allen and colleagues (1986) stated, "One cannot separate theory and value, as the empiricist claims. Every theory is penetrated by value interests" (p. 34).

Application of Critical Theoretical Perspective. Application of a critical theoretical perspective can be seen when health care is used as a form of social control. The social control function in health care is used to get patients to adhere to norms of appropriate behavior. This is accomplished through the medicalization of a wide range of psychological and socioeconomic issues. *Medicalization* is identification or categorization of (a condition or behavior) as being a disorder requiring medical treatment or intervention. Examples include medicalization related to sexuality, family life, aging, learning disabilities, and dying (Conrad, 1975, 1992; Zola, 1972). Medicalization can incorporate many facets of health and illness care from childbirth and allergies to hyperactivity and hospitals that have become dominated by the medical profession and its explanation of health and illness. When social problems are medicalized, there is often profit to be made. This can be seen when a patient readily receives a prescription for a medication before the root social cause of the illness is addressed by the health care provider. Using medical treatments for "undesirable behavior" has been implemented throughout history, including lobectomies for mental illness and synthetic stimulants for classroom behavior problems.

In this context, the nurse may examine how the concepts of power and empowerment influence access to quality child care (Kuokkanen and Leino-Kilpi, 2000). The nurse may contrast an organization's policies with interviews from workers who believe the organization is an impediment to achieving quality child care. Data analysis may also include an examination of the interests of workers and administration in promoting social change versus maintaining the status quo.

Wild (1993) used critical social theory to analyze the social, political, and economic conditions associated with the cost of prescription analgesics and the corresponding financial burden of clients who require these medications. Wild compared the trends in pharmaceutical pricing with the inflation rates of other commodities. The study stated that pharmaceutical sales techniques, which market directly to physicians, distance the needs of ill clients from the pharmaceutical industry. Wild's analysis specified nursing actions that a downstream analysis would not consider, such as challenging pricing policies on behalf of client groups.

Challenging Assumptions about Preventive Health Through Critical Theoretical Perspective. The HBM and Milio's prevention model focus on personal health behaviors from a disease avoidance or preventive health perspective; nurses may also analyze this phenomenon using critical social theory. Again, McKinlay's upstream analogy refers to health workers who were so busy fishing sick people out of the river that they did not look upstream to see how they were ending up in the water. Later in the same article, McKinlay (1979) used his upstream analogy to ask the rhetorical question, "How preventive is prevention?" (p. 22). He used this tactic to critically examine different intervention strategies aimed at enhancing preventive behavior. Figure 3-2 illustrates McKinlay's model, which contrasts the different modes of prevention. He linked health professionals' curative and lifestyle modification interventions to a downstream conceptualization of health; the majority of alleged preventive actions fail to alter the process of illness at its origin. Political-economic interventions remain the most effective way to address population determinants of health and to ameliorate illness at its source.

McKinlay (1979) further delineated the activities of the "manufacturers of illness—those individuals, interest groups, and organizations which, in addition to producing material goods and services, also produce, as an inevitable byproduct, widespread morbidity and mortality" (pp. 9, 10). The manufacturers of illness embed desired behaviors in the dominant cultural norm and thus foster the habituation of high-risk behavior in the population. Unhealthy consumption patterns are integrated into everyday lives; for example, the American holiday dinner table offers concrete examples of "the binding of at-riskness to culture" (p. 12). The existing U.S. Health Care System, in a misguided attempt to help, devotes its efforts to changing the products of the illness manufacturers and neglects the processes that create the products. Manufacturers of illness include the tobacco industry, the alcohol industry, and multiple corporations that produce environmental carcinogens.

Waitzkin (1983) continued this theme by asserting that the health care system's emphasis on lifestyle diverts attention from important sources of illness in the capitalist industrial environment and "it also puts the burden of health squarely on the individual rather than seeking collective solutions to health problems" (p. 664). Salmon (1987) supported this position by noting that the basic tenets of Western medicine promote an understanding of individual health and illness factors and obscure the exploration of their social and economic roots. He stated that critical social theory "can aid in uncovering larger dimensions impacting health that are usually unseen or misrepresented by ideological biases. Thus the social reality of health conditions can be both understood and changed" (p. 75).

In the past decade, a critical theoretical perspective has been used with *symbolic interactionism,* a theory that focuses predominantly on the individual and the meaning of situations. **Critical interactionism** brings the two theories together to address some issues of health care reform and thinking both upstream and downstream to make health care system changes (Burbank and Martins, 2010; Martins and Burbank, 2011). Nurses can use both upstream and downstream approaches to address health issues through critical interactionism (Table 3-4).

Nurses in all practice settings face the challenge of understanding and responding to collective health within the context of a health system that allocates resources at the individual level. The Tavistock Group (1999) released a set of ethical principles that summarizes this juxtaposition by noting that "the care of individuals is at the center of health care delivery, but must be viewed and practiced within the overall context of continuing work to generate the greatest possible health gains for groups and populations" (pp. 2, 3). This perspective is an accurate reflection of Western-oriented thought, which generally gives individual health precedence over collective health. Although nurses can appreciate the concept of individual care at the center of health delivery, they should also consider transposing this principle. Doing so allows the nurse to consider a health care system that places the community

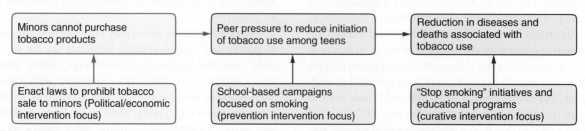

FIGURE 3-2 McKinlay's model of continuum of health behaviors and corresponding interventions foci applied to tobacco use. Data from McKinlay J: A case for refocusing upstream: the political economy of illness. In Gartley J, editor: *Patients, physicians and illness: a sourcebook in behavioral science and health*, New York, 1979, Free Press, pp. 9 -25.

TABLE 3-4 CRITICAL INTERACTIONISM: COMPARISON OF UPSTREAM AND DOWNSTREAM FOCUSES

ISSUE	DOWNSTREAM FOCUS	UPSTREAM FOCUS	CRITICAL INTERACTIONISM: AN UPSTREAM/DOWNSTREAM APPROACH
Clients: Obesity rates	Individual behavior strategies to reduce weight Lifestyle changes Bariatric surgery nursing care	Health policy changes Vending machines in school with healthier choices School lunch program modifications Target corporations that profit from obesity	Individual strategies with weight loss in conjunction with system changes Social marketing at both levels
Client or nurse: Workplace violence	Behavior change at individual level Workplace programs to reduce violence	Address organizational factors that promote workplace violence What organizational structures perpetuate workplace violence?	Change needed in knowledge and skills to address issue of workplace violence at both the downstream and upstream level
Nurse: Workplace errors	Focus on individual: root cause analysis that has individual as focus Change behavior of individual nurse Reeducation of nurse with workplace error	System changes needed What system level factors lead to workplace errors? What organizational structures perpetuate workplace errors?	A dual approach: Providers need changes in knowledge and skills to address root causes of workplace errors that move from individual to system level

Data from Martins DC, Burbank P: Critical interactionism: an upstream-downstream approach to health care reform, *Adv Nurs Sci* 34(4):315-329, 2011.

ETHICAL INSIGHTS

Social Injustice in Community-Based Practice

Chafey (1996) refers to "putting justice to work in community-based practice" and notes that nursing has a rich historic legacy in social justice activities. Although social justice activities are alive and well in nursing practice, many leaders think that the continuing struggle for resources is taking its toll on the scope of social action within community health systems. In addition, the policies of the current federal administration often emphasize market justice values over social justice values. *Market justice* refers to the principle that people are entitled to valued ends (e.g., status, income) when they acquire them through fair rules of entitlement. In contrast, *social justice* refers to the principle that all citizens bear equitably in the benefits and burdens of society (Drevdahl et al., 2001). These are complex concepts that cannot be easily distilled into a clear set of rules or nursing policies. However, in the context of community health nursing, health (and consequently health care) is considered a right rather than a privilege. To the extent that certain citizens, by virtue of their income, race, health needs, or any other attribute, are unable to access health care, our society as a whole suffers. Nurses are well positioned to "stand on the shoulders" of yesterday's nursing leaders and act on behalf of justice in health care access for all citizens.

in the center of health care and holds the goal of generating health gains for individuals. Fortunately, these worldviews of health delivery systems are not mutually exclusive, and nurses can understand the duality of health care needs in individuals and populations.

HEALTHY PEOPLE 2020

Documents from the U.S. program *Healthy People 2020* provide health professionals with a broad mandate to save lives by thinking and acting strategically. The *Healthy People 2020*

documents are classified into 38 "topic areas" that address specific diseases (e.g., diabetes, cancer, chronic kidney disease), care systems (e.g., health care access), and crosscutting issues in public health (e.g., persons with disabilities, family planning). Each of the focal areas specified by the Centers for Disease Control and Prevention and in the *Healthy People 2020* documents encompasses a complex and multifaceted problem, one that can be addressed only by "looking upstream." By thinking about the root causes of health problems, we begin to understand the importance of directing nursing efforts toward the antecedents of poor health and lost opportunities. There is simply no other way to bring positive changes to the more than 290 million U.S. and 6 billion global citizens who inhabit our planet.

The Social Determinants of Health topic area within *Healthy People 2020* is designed to identify ways to create social and physical environments that promote good health for all. All Americans deserve an equal opportunity to make the choices that lead to good health. But to ensure that all Americans have that opportunity, advances are needed not only in health care but also in fields such as education, child care, housing, business, law, media, community planning, transportation, and agriculture. Making these advances would involve working together to: (1) explore how programs, practices, and policies in these areas affect the health of individuals, families, and communities; (2) establish common goals, complementary roles, and ongoing constructive relationships between the health sector and these areas; and (3) maximize opportunities for collaboration among federal-, state-, and local-level partners related to social determinants of health (US Department of Health and Human Services, 2013).

The photos on the following page present environmental health issues and efforts being taken by nurses to address them.

NURSES WORK IN ENVIRONMENTAL HEALTH IN A VARIETY OF WAYS

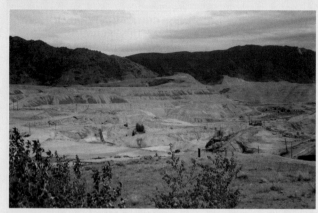

Open mine waste in the rural West can pose a continuing threat to local citizens. Nurses have been involved in advocacy efforts to ensure that citizens receive periodic screening for exposure to lead. Nurses can be active in policy efforts to prevent environmental disasters in the future.

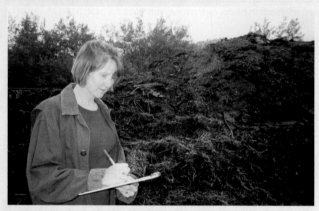

A public health nurse inspects the site of an asphalt spill off a rural railway car. Hazardous materials spills often occur in remote areas away from health care services. Broad conceptual frameworks allow nurses to think upstream and incorporate environmental risks into the consideration of community health issues.

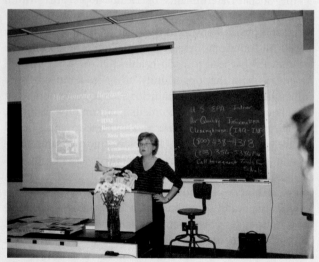

A public health nurse teaches a class on environmental health for local nurses. Environmental health is an important part of community health nursing's expanding practice.

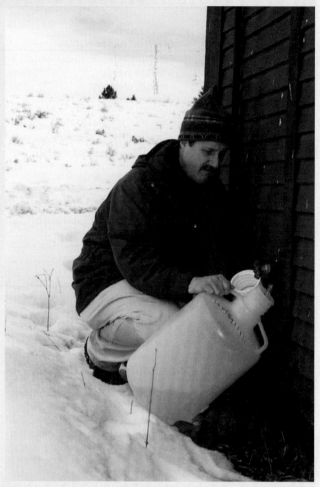

Citizens can be unaware of biological and chemical contaminants in their drinking water. Nurses are playing more active roles in water testing and in communicating the results of such tests to community members. When health is conceptualized broadly, nurses understand and view risk in new ways.

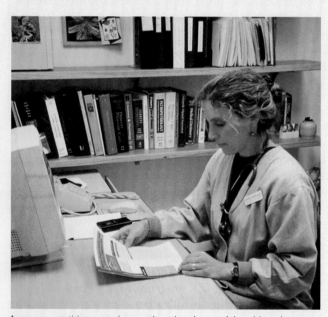

A nurse practitioner reviews educational materials addressing occupational and environmental health risks. By providing guidance for her clients, she is working to reduce risks and empower her clients to reduce their personal and community-based risks.

RESEARCH HIGHLIGHTS

Understanding the Health Experiences of Homeless Populations

How do we understand the health experiences of oppressed populations in the community such as the homeless? Using the lens of the homeless person, a descriptive phenomenological study was conducted. The research question was "What are your experiences with the health care system as a homeless person?" The purposive sample consisted of 15 homeless adults. Four major themes emerged:

1. Living without essential resources compromises health
2. Putting off health care until a crisis arises
3. Encountering barriers to receiving health care to include (a) social triage, (b) feeling labeled and stigmatized, (c) a non-system for health care for the homeless, (d) being treated with disrespect, and (e) feeling invisible to health care providers and
4. Developing underground resourcefulness

Although homeless persons articulated many problems in their health care system encounters, they also described their own resourcefulness and the strategies they employed to manage being marginalized by society and the health care system. Through the use of the critical theoretical perspective, our increased understanding of health care experiences from the homeless persons' view can guide community health nursing emancipatory actions.

Adapted from Martins DC: Experiences of homeless people in the health care delivery system: a descriptive phenomenological study, *Public Health Nurs* 25(5):420-430, 2008.

SUMMARY

Nursing and health service literature often focuses on health care access issues. This topic is interesting because tremendous disparities for access exist between insured and uninsured people in the United States. Access to care is associated with economic, social, and political factors, and, depending on individual and population needs, it can be a primary determinant of health status and survival. Structural variables, such as race-ethnicity, educational status, gender, and income, may be highly predictive of health status. These types of factors, which are also strongly grounded in the sociopolitical and economic milieu, identify risk factors for poor health and opportunities for community-based interventions.

Community health nurses have been instrumental in making many of the lifesaving advances in sanitation, communicable diseases, and environmental conditions that today's society takes for granted. Community health practice helps develop a broad context of nursing practice because community environments are inherently less restrictive than hospital settings. Clarke and Cody (1994) compared the environmental characteristics in community-based settings with those in hospital-based settings. They proposed that the dynamic nature of community settings lends itself best to the education of professional nurses (Clarke and Cody, 1994).

In a discussion addressing the future of community health nursing, Bellack (1998) differentiates between "nursing in the community" and "nursing with the community." This subtle reframing of the nursing role reinforces the notion that the health agenda originates from natural leaders, church members, local officials, parents, children, teens, and other community members. Forming and advancing a shared vision of health can be a formidable challenge for the nurse; as with any other complex issue, multiple viewpoints are the norm. Even "naming" health problems can be difficult, because different constituents are likely to see issues differently and pursue different lines of reasoning. However, allowing the genesis of change to occur from within the community is the essential challenge of nursing with the community. "Nursing with the community" efforts allow the nurse to create agendas that arise from community members rather than those imposed upon community members. Listening, being patient, providing accurate and scientifically sound information, and respecting the experiences of community members are essential to the success of these efforts.

The nursing profession has advanced and with it so has the need to develop nursing theories that formalize the scientific base of community health nursing. The richness of community health nursing comes from the challenge of conceptualizing and implementing strategies that will enhance the health of many people. Likewise, nurses in this practice area must have access to theoretical perspectives that address the social, political, and environmental determinants of population health. The integration of population-based theory with practice gives nurses the means to favorably affect the health of the global community.

LEARNING ACTIVITIES

1. Select a theory or conceptual model. Evaluate its potential for understanding health in individuals, families, a population of 400 children in an elementary school, a community of 50,000 residents, and 2000 workers within a corporate setting.
2. Identify one health problem (e.g., substance abuse, domestic violence, or cardiovascular disease) that is prevalent in the community or city. Analyze the problem using two different theories or conceptual models. One should emphasize individual determinants of health, and another should emphasize population determinants of health. What are some differences in the way these different perspectives inform nursing practice?
3. Review the ANA's definition of community health nursing practice and the APHA's definition of public health nursing practice. What do these definitions indicate about the theoretical basis of community health nursing? How does the theoretical basis of community health nursing practice differ from that of other nursing specialty areas?

⊛EVOLVE WEBSITE

http://evolve.elsevier.com/Nies

- NCLEX Review Questions
- Case Studies
- Glossary

REFERENCES

Allen DG, Diekelmann N, Benner P: Three paradigms for nursing research: methodologic implications. In Chinn P, editor: *Nursing research methodology: issues and implementation*, Rockville, MD, 1986, Aspen Publishers.

Barnum BS: *Nursing theory: analysis, application, evaluation*, ed 5, Philadelphia, PA, 1998, Lippincott.

Batra C: Professional issues: the future of community health nursing. In Cookfair JM, editor: *Nursing process and practice in the community*, St. Louis, 1991, Mosby.

Bellack JP: Community-based nursing practice: necessary but not sufficient, *J Nurs Educe* 37(3):99–100, 1998.

Berwick D, Davidoff F, Hiatt H, et al: Refining and implementing the Tavistock principles for everybody in health care, *British Journal of Medicine*:323, 616–620, 2000.

Bostidge M: *Florence Nightingale: the making of an icon*, New York, 2008, Farrar, Straus and Giroux.

Burbank P, Martins DC: Symbolic interactionism and critical perspective: divergent or synergistic? *Nursing Philosophy* 11(1):25–41, 2010.

Centers for Disease Control and Prevention (2013) National Center for Chronic Disease Prevention and Health Promotion: *Chronic disease prevention*, 2013. Available from <http://www.cdc.gov/chronicdisease/overview/index.htm>. Accessed March 11, 2013.

Chafey K: Caring is not enough: ethical paradigms for community-based care, *N HC Perspect Community* 17(1):10–15, 1996.

Chinn PL, Kramer MK: *Theory and nursing: integrated knowledge development*, ed 7, St. Louis, 2008, Mosby.

Clarke PN, Cody WK: Nursing theory-based practice in the home and community: the crux of professional nursing education, *Adv Nurs Sci* 17(2):41–53, 1994.

Conrad P: The discovery of hyperkinesis: notes on the medicalization of deviant behavior, *Soc Probl* 23:12–21, 1975.

Conrad P: Medicalization and social control, *Annual Review of Sociology* 18:209–232, 1992.

Conrad P: *The sociology of health and illness: critical perspectives*, ed 8, Worth Publisher, 2008.

Conrad P, Leiter V: *The sociology of heath and illness: critical perspectives*, ed 9, New York, 2012, Worth Pub.

Cummings KM, Becker MH, Malie MC: Bringing the models together: an empirical approach to combining variables to explain health actions, *J Behav Med* 3:123–145, 1980.

Dickoff J, James P: A theory of theories: a position paper, *Nurs Res* 17:197–203, 1968.

Doty R: Alternative theoretical perspectives: essential knowledge for the advanced practice nurse in the promotion of rural family health, *Clin Nurs Specialist* 10(5):217–219, 1996.

Draper P: Nancy Milio's work and its importance for the development of health promotion, *Health Promotion International* 1(1):101–106, 1986.

Dreher M: The conflict of conservatism in public health nursing education, *Nurs Outlook* 30(9):504–509, 1982.

Drevdahl D, Kneipp S, Canales M, et al: Reinvesting in social justice: a capital idea for public health nursing? *ANS Adv Nurs Sci* 24(2):19–31, 2001.

Eben J, et al: Self-care deficit theory of nursing. In Marriner A, editor: *Nursing theorists and their work*, St. Louis, 1986, Mosby.

Fawcett J: The nurse theorists: 21st-century updates—Dorothea E. Orem, *Nurs Sci Q* 14(1):34–38, 2001.

Hobbs S, Ricketts T, Dodds J, et al: Analysis of interest group influence on federal school meals regulations 1992 to 1996, *J Nutr Educ Behav* 36(2):90–98, 2004.

Jones PK, Jones SL, Katz J: Improving follow-up among hypertensive patients using a health belief model intervention, *Arch Intern Med* 147:1557–1560, 1987.

Kennedy A: How relevant are nursing models? *Occup Health* 41(12):352–354, 1989.

Kirscht JP: The health belief model and illness behavior. In Becker MH, editor: *The health belief model and personal health behavior*, Thorofare, NJ, 1974, Charles B. Slack.

Kuokkanen L, Leino-Kilpi H: Power and empowerment in nursing: three theoretical approaches, *J Adv Nurs* 31(1):235–241, 2000.

Lajunen T, Rasanen M: Can social psychological models be used to promote bicycle helmet use among teenagers? A comparison of the health belief model, theory of planned behavior and the locus of control, *J Safety Res* 35(1):115–123, 2004.

Lin P, Simoni J, Zemon V: The health belief mode, sexual behaviors, and HIV risk among Taiwanese immigrants, *AIDS Education and Prevention* 17(5):469–483, 2005.

Marmot M: The Marmot Review (2010) Fair Society, healthy lives. Strategic Review of Health Inequities in England. Available at: https://www.google.com/search?q=marmot+priniciples&oq=marmot+&aqs=chrome.1.69i57j69i59j69i61j0l3.3756j0j7&sourceid=chrome&espv=210&es_sm=93&ie=UTF-8

Maiman LA, Becker MH: The health belief model: origins and correlates in psychological theory. In Becker MH, editor: *The health belief model and personal health behavior*, Thorofare, NJ, 1974, Charles B. Slack.

Martins DC, Burbank P: Critical interactionism: an upstream-downstream approach to health care reform, *Advances in Nursing Science* 34(4):315–329, 2011.

McKinlay J: A case for refocusing upstream: the political economy of illness. In Gartley J, editor: *Patients, physicians and illness: a sourcebook in behavioral science and health*, New York, 1979, Free Press, pp 9–25.

McKinlay JB: A case for refocusing upstream: the political economy of illness. In Conrad P, Leiter V, editors: *the sociology of health and illness: critical perspectives*, ed 9, New York, 2012, Worth Pub.

Milio N: A framework for prevention: changing health-damaging to health-generating life patterns, *Am J Public Health* 66:435–439, 1976.

Milio N: *Promoting health through public policy*, Philadelphia, 1981, FA Davis.

Milio N: Health policy and the emerging tobacco reality, *Social Science and Medicine* 21(6):603–613, 1985.

Mirotznik J, Ginzler E, Zagon G, et al: Using the health belief model to explain clinic appointment-keeping for the management of a chronic disease condition, *J Community Health* 23(3):195–210, 1998.

National Heart Lung and Blood Institute: Working Group Report on Future Research: *Directions in childhood obesity prevention and treatment*, 2007. Available from <http://www.nhlbi.nih.gov/meetings/workshops/child-obesity/index.html>. Accessed March 11, 2013.

Navarro V: *Medicine under capitalism*, New York, 1976, Prodist.

Orem DE: *Nursing: concepts of practice*, ed 6, New York, 2001, Mosby.

Pender NJ: *Health promotion in nursing practice*, ed 2, Norwalk, Conn, 1987, Appleton-Century-Crofts.

Pryjmachuk S: A nursing perspective on the interrelationship between theory, research, and practice, *J Adv Nurs* 23:679–684, 1996.

QUAD Council, American Public Health Association: PHN Section, ACHNE, APHN, ANA *Quad council PHN competencies*, 2013. Available at <http://www.achne.org/files/Quad%20Council/QuadCouncilCompetenciesforPublicHealthNurses.pdf>. Accessed November 13, 2013.

Salmon JW: Dilemmas in studying social change versus individual change: considerations from political economy. In Duffy M, Pender NJ, editors: *Conceptual issues in health promotion: a report of proceedings of a Wingspread Conference*, Indianapolis, IN, 1987, Sigma Theta Tau.

Schwartz-Barcott D, Patterson BJ, Lusardi P, et al: From practice to theory: tightening the link via three fieldwork strategies, *J Adv Nurs* 39(3):281–289, 2002.

Stevens PE, Hall JM: Applying critical theories to nursing in communities, *Public Health Nursing* 9(1):2–9, 1992.

Tavistock Group: A shared statement of ethical principles for those who shape and give health care: a working draft from the Tavistock Group, *Image J Nurs Sch* 31:2–3, 1999.

Torres G: *Theoretical foundations of nursing*, Norwalk, CT, 1986, Appleton-Century-Crofts.

U.S. Department of Health and Human Services: *Healthy People 2020: social determinants of health*, 2013. Available from <http://www.healthypeople.gov/2020/topicsobjectives2020/overview.aspx?topicid=39>. Accessed September 4, 2013.

Waitzkin H: A Marxist view of health and health care. In Mechanic D, editor: *Handbook of health, health care, and the health professions*, New York, 1983, Free Press.

Wild LR: Caveat emptor: a critical analysis of the costs of drugs used for pain management, *Adv Nurs Sci* 16:52–61, 1993.

Woods NF, Catanzaro M, editors: *Nursing research: theory and practice*, St. Louis, 1988, Mosby.

Zola I: Medicine as an institution of social control, *Sociol Rev* 20(4):487–504, 1972.

Health Promotion and Risk Reduction

Bridgette Crotwell Pullis and Mary A. Nies

OBJECTIVES

Upon completion of this chapter, the reader will be able to do the following:

1. Discuss various theories of health promotion, including Pender's Health Promotion Model, the Health Belief Model, the Transtheoretical Theory, and the Theory of Reasoned Action.
2. Discuss definitions of health.
3. Demonstrate an understanding of the difference between health promotion and health protection.
4. Define *risk*.
5. Discuss the relationship of risk to health and health promotion activities.
6. Demonstrate an understanding of stratification of risk factors by age, race, and gender.
7. Discuss the influence of various factors on health.
8. List health behaviors for health promotion and disease prevention.
9. Relate the clinical implications of health promotion activities.

KEY TERMS

determinants of health
health
health promotion

health protection
portion distortion
risk

risk communication
risk reduction

OUTLINE

Health Promotion and Community Health Nursing
  Healthy People 2020
Determinants of Health
Theories in Health Promotion
  Pender's Health Promotion Model
  The Health Belief Model
  The Transtheoretical Model
  Theory of Reasoned Action

Risk and Health
The Relationship of Risk to Health and Health Promotion Activities
  Tobacco and Health Risk
  Alcohol Consumption and Health
  Diet and Health
  Physical Activity and Health
  Sleep

HEALTH PROMOTION AND COMMUNITY HEALTH NURSING

Since its inception, nursing has focused on helping individuals, groups, and communities maintain and protect their health. Florence Nightingale and other nursing pioneers recognized the importance of nutrition, rest, and hygiene in maximizing and protecting one's state of health. Though people are responsible for their health and medical care, they often seek advice from nurses in the community regarding health promotion and to help them make sense of the many, often competing, recommendations that appear daily on TV, online, in newspapers and magazines.

Consider the clinical example about Jamie R. on the following page.

Green and Kreuter (1991) define health promotion as "any combination of health education and related organizational, economic, and environmental supports for behavior

Clinical Example

Jamie R. is a lifelong athlete. Married with three grown children, she rises at 4:20 each morning to go to the gym to swim for an hour before going to her job as an executive with a large company. A nonsmoker, Jamie rarely drinks alcohol and eats a diet consisting mostly of vegetables, grains, and fruit. Jamie's body mass index is in the normal range, and, though her cholesterol and triglyceride levels are elevated, she does not require medication for this issue. After work, Jamie and her husband relax by walking their two dogs and reading. An early riser, Jamie is in bed by 9:30 almost every night. At 50 years of age, Jamie is youthful and energetic.

We all have friends like Jamie—people who seem to have an endless amount of energy and self-discipline. The rest of us, however, are typically less successful in achieving our health promotion goals.

---

of individuals, groups, or communities conducive to health" (p. 2). Parse (1990) states that health promotion is that which is motivated by the desire to increase well-being and to reach the best possible health potential. Jamie exemplifies this motivation to stay in her best health, at least at first glance. Let's look further into Jamie's health history.

When it comes to health practices, Jamie is a study in contradictions. Jamie's father had a myocardial infarction (MI) at the age of 48 years and died of an MI at the age of 50 years. Many of Jamie's paternal relatives have died of heart disease. Jamie's mother and one maternal aunt were each diagnosed with breast cancer in their early 50s. Though she has an annual physical examination by her family doctor and

monitors her blood cholesterol and triglycerides, Jamie has never been screened for cardiac disease. Jamie takes the flu vaccine every year but has not had a tetanus-diphtheria vaccine booster in 14 years and has not had the shingles vaccine; though she sees her gynecologist yearly, she has had only one mammogram, 3 years ago.

In skipping annual mammograms and in not pursuing cardiac screening despite her high risk, Jamie is neglecting an important step in maintaining her health—health protection. Health protection consists of those behaviors in which one engages with the specific intent to prevent disease, to detect disease in the early stages, or to maximize health within the constraints of disease (Parse, 1990). Immunizations and cervical cancer screening are examples of health protection activities.

In discussing health promotion, it is helpful to define what is meant by health. One definition states that health is "being sound in body, mind, and spirit: freedom from physical disease or pain" (Merriam-Webster, 2009). As health promotion has become an important strategy to improve health, the way health is defined has shifted from a focus on the curative model to a focus on multidimensional aspects such as the social, cultural, and environmental facets of life and health (Benson, 1996). The well-known definition by the World Health Organization (WHO) states that health is "a state of complete physical, mental and social well-being, and not merely the absence of disease" (WHO, 2009). WHO also states that health is the extent to which an individual or group is able to realize aspirations, to satisfy needs, and to change or to cope with the environment. In this aspect, health is viewed not only as an important goal but as a resource for living (WHO, 1986).

HEALTH PROMOTION IN THE COMMUNITY

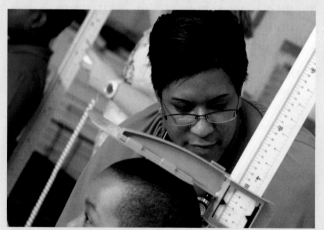

Elementary school screening: A nursing student takes height and weight measurements, which serve as a baseline to measure the growth rate of students.

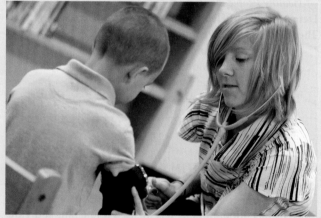

Elementary school screening: A nursing student securely holds the cuff as she takes this little boy's blood pressure.

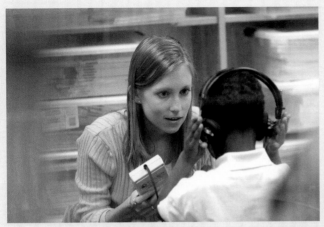

Elementary school screening: A nursing student watches and listens as she gives a hearing test.

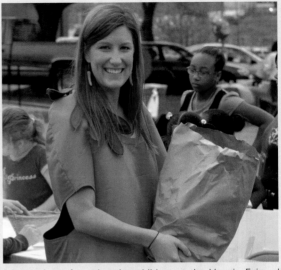

Participants have fun educating children at the Veggie Fair, which will hopefully lead children and their parents to enjoy vegetables as a nutritious part of their daily diet.

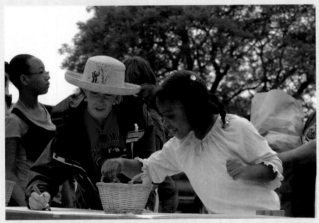

A Veggie Fair in the community teaches children and their parents about the benefits of eating vegetables.

Healthy People 2020

Healthy People 2020 is the health promotion initiative for the nation. Developed through a consortium and managed by the U.S. Department of Health and Human Services (USDHHS), *Healthy People 2020* "challenges individuals, communities, and professionals, to take specific steps to ensure that good health, as well as long life, are enjoyed by all" (USDHHS, 2012).

The broad goals of *Healthy People 2020* are to attain high-quality, longer lives free of preventable disease, disability, injury, and premature death; achieve equity, eliminate disparities, and improve the health of all groups; create social and physical environments that promote good health for all; and promote quality of life, healthy development, and healthy behaviors across all life stages. Objectives toward achieving these goals are organized into 38 topic areas with corresponding priorities for action for each objective. Leading health indicators, or **determinants of health**, in each topic area help track progress toward meeting the goals of *Healthy People 2020*. A list of leading health indicators

common to most of the topic areas is shown in Table 4-1. Figure 4-1 illustrates the relationships among the determinants of health. The home page for *Healthy People 2020* can be accessed at http://www.healthypeople.gov/2020/.

DETERMINANTS OF HEALTH

Biology is an individual's genetic makeup, family history, and any physical and mental health problems developed in the course of life. Aging, diet, physical activity, smoking, stress, alcohol or drug abuse, injury, violence, or a toxic or infectious agent may produce illness or disability, changing an individual's biology.

Behaviors are the individual's responses to internal stimuli and external conditions. Behaviors interact with biology in a common relationship as one may influence the other. If a person chooses behaviors such as alcohol abuse or smoking, his or her biology may be changed as a result (e.g., liver cirrhosis, chronic obstructive pulmonary disease [COPD]). On the other hand, if an individual has a

TABLE 4-1   LEADING HEALTH INDICATORS

FOCUS AREA	PHYSICAL ACTIVITY	OVERWEIGHT AND OBESITY	TOBACCO USE	SUBSTANCE ABUSE	RESPONSIBLE SEXUAL BEHAVIOR	MENTAL HEALTH	INJURY AND VIOLENCE	ENVIRONMENTAL QUALITY	IMMUNIZATION	ACCESS TO HEALTH CARE
Access to quality health services	X	X	X	X	X	X	X		X	X
Arthritis, osteoporosis, and chronic back conditions	X	X					X			
Cancer	X	X	X	X	X				X	X
Chronic kidney disease	X	X	X					X		
Diabetes	X	X	X	X		X			X	X
Disability and secondary conditions	X	X	X	X		X			X	X
Educational and community-based programs	X	X	X	X	X	X	X	X	X	X
Environmental health								X		
Family planning			X		X					X
Food safety				X				X		X
Health communication	X		X	X	X	X	X	X	X	
Heart disease and stroke	X	X	X	X		X	X	X	X	X
Human immunodeficiency virus			X	X	X	X				X
Immunization and infectious diseases										X
Injury and violence prevention	X		X	X	X	X	X	X		
Maternal, infant, and child health		X	X	X	X	X	X		X	X
Medical product safety			X	X	X					
Mental health and mental disorders			X	X	X	X	X			X
Nutrition and overweight	X	X	X	X	X		X			
Occupational safety and health				X			X	X		
Oral health	X	X	X	X	X		X			
Physical activity and fitness	X	X	X	X	X	X	X	X		
Public health infrastructure	X	X	X	X	X	X	X	X	X	
Respiratory diseases	X		X				X	X		X
Sexually transmitted diseases			X	X	X	X	X			
Substance abuse			X	X	X	X	X	X		X
Tobacco use			X	X	X			X		X
Vision and hearing										X

From Office of Disease Prevention and Health Promotion, US Department of Health and Human Services: *Leading health indicators touch everyone, Healthy People 2010*, 2009. Available from <http://www.healthypeople.gov/2020/LHI/default.aspx>. Accessed August 22, 2013.

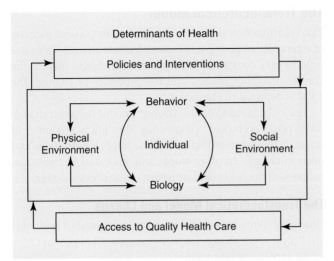

Determinants of Health

FIGURE 4-1 The relationship among the determinants of health. (From U.S. Department of Health and Human Services: *Healthy People 2010: understanding and improving health,* January 30, 2001. Available from <www.healthypeople.gov/Document/tableofcontents. htm#under>. Accessed April 22, 2009.)

history of colon cancer in his or her family, the individual may choose to have regular screenings, thereby preventing advanced cancer and possibly death, and changing his or her biology for the better. One's biology may impact behavior; if a person has hypertension or diabetes, he or she may choose to begin an exercise regimen and to eat more healthfully.

Social environment includes interactions and relationships with family, friends, coworkers, and others in the community. Social institutions, such as law enforcement, faith communities, schools, and government agencies, are also part of the social environment, as well as housing, safety, public transportation, and availability of resources. The social environment has a great impact on the health of individuals, groups, and communities, yet it is complex in nature because of differing cultures and practices.

Physical environment is what is experienced with the senses; what is smelled, seen, touched, heard, and tasted. The physical environment can impact health negatively or positively. If there are toxic or infectious substances in the environment, this is certainly a negative influence on health. If the environment is clean with areas to recreate and play, this is a good influence on health.

Policies and interventions can have a profound effect on the health of individuals, groups, and communities. Positive effects such as policies against smoking in public places, seatbelt and child restraint laws, litter ordinances, and enhanced health care promote health. Policies are implemented at local, state, and national levels by many agencies, such as transportation, health and human services, veterans' affairs, housing, and justice departments.

Expansion of *access to quality health care* is essential to decrease health disparities and to improve the quality of life and the quantity of years of healthy life (USDHHS, 2013).

THEORIES IN HEALTH PROMOTION

Health promotion activities are broad in scope and in setting. Community health nurses and their clients engage in health promotion activities in workplace settings, schools, clinics, and communities. The theories that are used most in health promotion are very diverse to accommodate the variety of settings, clients, and activities in community health. A working knowledge of theory is important in understanding why people act as they do and why they may or may not follow advice given to them by medical professionals, and in helping clients progress from knowledge to behavior change. Some of the most frequently used health promotion theories and models are discussed here.

Pender's Health Promotion Model

Developed in the 1980s and revised in 1996, Pender's Health Promotion Model (HPM) explores the myriad biopsychosocial factors that influence individuals to pursue health promotion activities. The HPM depicts the complex multidimensional factors with which people interact as they work to achieve optimum health. This model contains seven variables related to health behaviors, as well as individual characteristics that may influence a behavioral outcome.

Pender's model does not include threat as a motivator, as threat may not be a motivating factor for clients in all age-groups (Pender et al., 2011). The Health Promotion Model is depicted in Figure 4-2.

Let's relate the Health Promotion Model to Jamie R. in the Clinical Example at the beginning of this chapter. The experience of having relatives who died of heart disease and cancer has probably increased her desire to engage in healthful behavior. Similarly, her busy schedule and lack of communication with her doctor may be reflected in her failure to obtain screenings or immunizations. Jamie has a habit of engaging in exercise and a high self-efficacy related to her success with exercise in the past. Jamie feels better after exercise, and she receives positive comments from significant others regarding her appearance, also increasing her motivation to exercise. Jamie works out in a lovely gym and is very committed to her workout routine. Jamie has found that working out first thing in the morning minimizes the competing demands that may keep her from exercising.

The Health Belief Model

Initially proposed in 1958, the Health Belief Model (HBM) provides the basis for much of the practice of health education and health promotion today. The Health Belief Model was developed by a group of social psychologists to attempt to explain why the public failed to participate in screening for tuberculosis (Hochbaum, 1958). Hochbaum and his associates had the same questions that perplex many health professionals today: Why do people who may have a disease reject health screening? Why do individuals participate in screening if it may lead to the diagnosis of disease? This research documented that information alone is rarely enough to motivate one to act. Individuals must know what to do and how to do it before they can take action. Also, the information must be related in some way to the individual's needs. One of the most widely used conceptual frameworks in health behavior, the Health Belief Model has been used to explain behavior change and maintenance of behavior change and to guide health promotion interventions (Champion and Skinner, 2008).

The Health Belief Model has several constructs: perceived seriousness, perceived susceptibility, perceived benefits of treatment, perceived barriers to treatment, cues to action, and self-efficacy. These components can be found in Table 4-2. All of these constructs relate to the client's perception. How does the client perceive the seriousness of the condition? His susceptibility to the condition? The benefits of prevention or treatment? The barriers to prevention or treatment? The HBM is depicted in Figure 4-3 (McEwen and Pullis, 2009).

Let's apply the HBM to Jamie. She may not perceive that she is susceptible to heart disease or breast cancer, or she may not perceive that there is a benefit of screening, or of treatment for heart disease or cancer—thus, her failure to take up screening for these diseases.

The Transtheoretical Model

The Transtheoretical Model (TTM) combines several theories of intervention, giving it the name *transtheoretical*. Table 4-3 lists the core constructs of the model, which also include the constructs of self-efficacy and the processes of change. The TTM is depicted in Figure 4-4.

The TTM is based on the assumption that behavior change takes place over time, progressing through a sequence of stages. It also assumes that each of the stages is both stable and open to change. In other words, one may stop in one stage, progress to the next stage, or return to the previous stage.

The Transtheoretical Model and Change

Change is difficult, even for the most motivated of individuals. People resist change for many reasons. Change may:

- Be unpleasant (exercising)
- Require giving up pleasure (eating desserts or watching TV)
- Be painful (insulin injections)
- Be stressful (eating new foods)
- Jeopardize social relationships (gatherings with friends and family that involve food)
- Not seem important any more (older individuals or those with the ill effects of lifestyle choices, such as diabetes and hypertension)
- Require change in self-image (from couch potato to athlete) (Westberg and Jason, 1996).

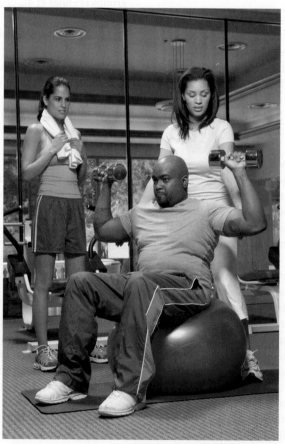

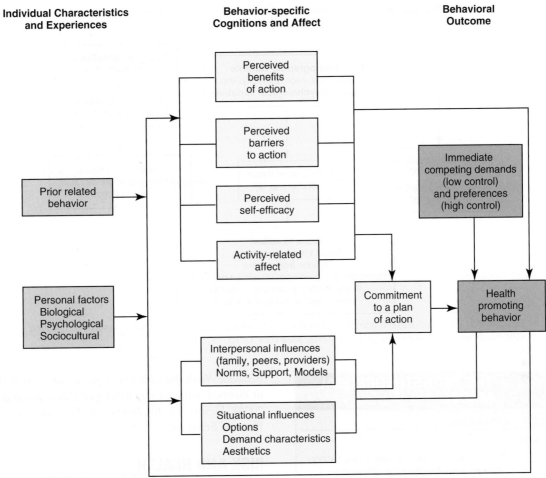

FIGURE 4-2 The Health Promotion Model. (From Pender N: *The Health Promotion Model,* 2009, The University of Michigan School of Nursing. Available from <www.nursing.umich.edu/faculty/pender/chart.gif>. Accessed March 26, 2009.)

TABLE 4-2	KEY CONCEPTS AND DEFINITIONS OF THE HEALTH BELIEF MODEL
CONCEPT	**DEFINITION**
Perceived susceptibility	One's belief regarding the chance of getting a given condition
Perceived severity	One's belief regarding the seriousness of a given condition
Perceived benefits	One's belief in the ability of an advised action to reduce the health risk or seriousness of a given condition
Perceived barriers	One's belief regarding the tangible and psychological costs of an advised action
Cues to action	Strategies or conditions in one's environment that activate readiness to take action
Self-efficacy	One's confidence in one's ability to take action to reduce health risks

From Janz JK, Champion VL, Stretcher VJ: The health belief model. In Glanz K, Rimer BK, Lewis FM, editors: *Health behavior and health education: theory, research, and practice,* San Francisco, 2002, Jossey-Bass.

Theory of Reasoned Action

Developed by Fishbein and Ajzen, the Theory of Reasoned Action (TRA) attempts to predict a person's intention to perform or not to perform a certain behavior (Montano and Kasprzyk, 2008). The Theory of Reasoned Action is based on the assumption that all behavior is determined by one's behavioral intentions. These intentions are determined by one's attitude regarding a behavior and the subjective norms associated with the behavior (Montano and Kasprzyk, 2008). One's attitude is determined by one's beliefs about the outcomes of performing the behavior, weighed by one's assessment of the outcomes. Consider Jamie R. for a moment. Jamie must believe strongly that exercise will have positive results, as she rises early and takes time from her busy schedule to work out daily. Conversely, Jamie may believe strongly that routine immunizations or health screenings will have negative results.

One's subjective norm is determined by one's *normative beliefs,* or whether or not important people in one's life approve or disapprove of the behavior under consideration, weighed by one's motivation to comply with those important persons (Montano and Kasprzyk, 2008). If Jamie believes that her husband or children think that she should get a mammogram, and

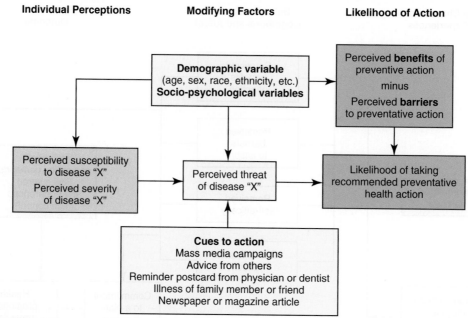

Individual Perceptions   **Modifying Factors**   **Likelihood of Action**

FIGURE 4-3 The Health Belief Model. (From Becker and Maiman: Sociobehavioral determinants of compliance with health and medical care recommendations, *Med Care* 13:10, 1975.)

TABLE 4-3	THE TRANSTHEORETICAL MODEL
CONSTRUCTS	**DESCRIPTION**
Stages of Change	
Precontempla-tion	The individual has no intention to take action toward behavior change in the next 6 months. May be in this phase because of a lack of information about the consequences of the behavior, or failure on previous attempts at change.
Contemplation	The individual has some intention to take action toward behavior change in the next 6 months. Weighing pros and cons to change.
Preparation	The individual intends to take action within the next month, and has taken steps toward behavior change. Has a plan of action.
Action	The individual has changed overt behavior for less than 6 months. Has changed behavior sufficiently to reduce risk of disease.
Maintenance	The individual has changed overt behavior for more than 6 months. Strives to prevent relapse. This phase may last months to years.
Decisional Balance	
Pros	The benefits of behavior change
Cons	The costs of behavior change

Modified from Prochaska JO, Redding CA, Evers KE: The transtheoretical model and stages of change. In Glanz K, Rimer B, Viswanath K, editors, *Health behavior and health education: theory, research, and practice,* San Francisco, 2008, Josey-Bass, pp 97-121.

if she is motivated to comply with their wishes, Jamie will have a positive subject norm regarding getting a mammogram.

Recently, the variable of perceived control has been added to the TRA to account for the amount of control an individual may have over whether or not he or she performs the behavior. With the addition of perceived control, the Theory of Planned Behavior was developed (Montano and Kasprzyk, 2008). Figure 4-5 illustrates the TRA and the Theory of Planned Behavior.

RISK AND HEALTH

Oleckno defines **risk** as "the probability that a specific event will occur in a given time frame" (2002, p. 352). A risk factor is an exposure that is associated with a disease (Friis and Sellers, 2004). Jamie R. has an increased *risk* of heart disease and cancer. Jamie's *risk factors* include a family history of both of these diseases, work stress, her age, environmental exposures, and gender. There are known risk factors for some diseases, such as smoking and its association with lung cancer, and high blood pressure and heart disease. Some risk factors are assumed, such as cell phones and brain tumors. The three criteria for establishing a risk factor, as follows:

1. The frequency of the disease varies by category, or amount of the factor. Lung cancer is more likely to develop in cigarette smokers than in nonsmokers, and in those who smoke heavily than in those who smoke little.
2. The risk factor must precede the onset of the disease. Cigarette smokers have lung cancer after they have been smoking for a while. If smokers had lung cancer before starting to smoke, this fact would cast doubt on smoking as a risk factor for lung cancer.
3. The association of concern must not be due to any source of error. In any research study (especially one involving human behavior), there are many sources of error, such as study design, data collection methods, and data analysis.

Other criteria that have been noted in literature include strength of the association, consistency with repetition, specificity, and plausibility (Friis and Sellers, 2004).

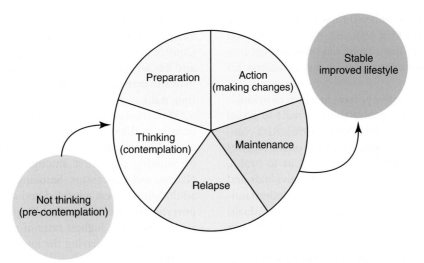

FIGURE 4-4 The Transtheoretical Model. (From Prochaska J, DiClemente C: Transtheoretical therapy: towards a more integrative model of change, *Psychotherapy: Theory, Research & Practice* 19:276-88, 1982.)

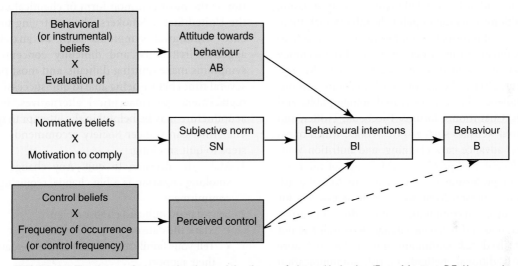

FIGURE 4-5 The theory of reasoned action and the theory of planned behavior. (From Montano DE, Kaspryzyk D: Theory of reasoned action, theory of planned behavior, and the integrated behavioral model. In Glanz K, Rimer BK, Viswanath K, editors: *Health behavior and health education,* San Francisco, 2008, Jossey-Bass, pp 67-96.)

In order to determine the health risks to individuals, groups, and populations, a risk assessment may be conducted. A *risk assessment* is a systematic way of distinguishing the risks posed by potentially harmful exposures. The four main steps of a risk assessment are hazard identification, risk description, exposure assessment, and risk estimation (Savitz, 1998).

THE RELATIONSHIP OF RISK TO HEALTH AND HEALTH PROMOTION ACTIVITIES

Health is directly related to the activities in which we participate, the food we eat, and substances to which we are exposed daily. Where we live and work and our gender, age, and genetic makeup also impact health. In the assessment of risk regarding health and health promotion activities, there are two types of risks: modifiable risks and nonmodifiable risks. *Modifiable risk factors* are those aspects of a person's health

risk over which he or she has control. Examples include smoking, leading a sedentary or active lifestyle, type and amount of food eaten, and the type of activities in which he or she engages (skydiving is riskier than bowling). *Nonmodifiable risk factors* are those aspects of one's health risk over which one has no or little control. Examples include genetic makeup, gender, age, and environmental exposures. A useful tool to help clients assess their family history for possible health risks is available at the U.S. Surgeon General's website at http://www.hhs.gov/familyhistory/. This assessment is easy to use and can create a dialogue between family members to discuss family health history. As the nurse assesses the various aspects of a client's health, it is important to evaluate behaviors that have a positive effect on the client's health, not only those behaviors that are detrimental to health. Healthful behaviors, such as maintaining an exercise regimen and following an eating plan, build self-efficacy and self-esteem. Positive health behaviors also provide a foundation on which a nurse can build to address unhealthful behaviors. If a client has been successful at smoking cessation, the confidence and self-efficacy learned from this change can be drawn upon to help him stick to a low-sodium, low-fat diet to address his hypertension.

Risk reduction is a proactive process in which individuals participate in behaviors that enable them to react to actual or potential threats to their health (Pender, 1996). Risk communication is the process through which the public receives information regarding possible or actual threats to health. Risk communication is affected by the way individuals and communities perceive, process, and act on their understanding of risk (Finnigan and Vinswanath, 2008). Individuals, groups, and communities receive information on health risks from many sources besides health care professionals today. The Internet is a newer source of risk communication for many community members with 60% of Internet users accessing it for health information (Atkinson et al., 2009). Newspapers, periodicals, radio, TV, and billboards are long-standing sources of health information in public health. Though there are many sources of information on health risks available to the public, the quality varies widely in terms of the accuracy of the information presented (Hendrick et al., 2012; Kupferberg and Protus, 2011). The use of social media to communicate with audiences has also increased among public and private entities. Chat rooms, forums, Facebook, Twitter, and many specialized websites such as *Five Wishes*, which offers information on advance care planning, and nutrition websites such as *Eating Well* provide a wide range of information. Health care professionals are endeavoring to make risk communication as personalized and specific as possible for individuals, groups, and communities in an effort to improve uptake of screening and behavior change. Research has not shown personalized risk communication to be any more effective than traditional methods of risk communication (Edwards et al., 2013).

Approximately 50% of annual U.S. deaths occur as a result of modifiable or lifestyle factors (McGinnis and Foege, 1993; Mokdab et al., 2004). Figure 4-6 depicts the leading causes of death and the numbers of deaths related to each. Those causes of death with the highest mortality (heart disease, cancer, stroke, and chronic respiratory disease) are all related to lifestyle factors (McGinnis and Foege, 2004). Table 4-4 details the relationship of the leading causes of death and common risk factors. A 2012 study found that people adopting healthful behaviors such as exercising, eating a healthful diet, not using tobacco, and maintaining a normal weight had a 66% lower risk of death than did those who did not adopt these behaviors (Loef and Walach, 2012).

Tobacco and Health Risk

Smoking cessation is an important step in achieving optimum health. In the United States, smoking is the leading cause of preventable death, accounting for approximately one out of every five deaths or 438,000 deaths per year. Smoking is a causal factor in cancers of the esophagus, bladder, stomach, oral cavity, pharynx, larynx, cervix, and lung, with more

than 90% of lung cancers in men and 80% of lung cancers among women attributable to smoking (Centers for Disease Control and Prevention [CDC], January 2, 2013). Smoking also has an economic impact, costing $97.2 billion annually in health care and lost productivity (American Lung Association, n.d.).

Most smokers are between the ages of 18 and 44 years, and more men than women smoke. In 2010, 21.5% of adult men and 17.3% of adult women were smokers. The prevalence of smoking is highest among American Indians/Alaskan Natives and Caucasians. Smoking is most common among adults who are less educated and adults who live below the poverty level. Kentucky, West Virginia, Oklahoma, and Mississippi have the highest rates of smokers, with Utah, California, and Idaho having the lowest rates (CDC, September 6, 2011).

More than 70% of current smokers report that they would like to quit smoking. (CDC, n.d.). Nicotine addiction is the most common form of chemical dependence in the United States. Smokers who are trying to quit experience withdrawal symptoms such as anxiety, increased appetite, irritability, and difficulty concentrating. These symptoms make quitting difficult, and most people relapse several times before being able to quit successfully. Nicotine replacement, pharmaceutical alternatives, hypnosis, and acupuncture may be helpful in the attempt to quit smoking. The American Cancer Society recommends the following steps to quit smoking:

1. Make the decision to quit. Any change is scary, and smoking cessation is a big change, requiring a long-term commitment.
2. Set a date to quit and choose a plan.
   - Mark the date on your calendar.
   - Tell your family and friends about the date, and ask for their support.
   - Get rid of all tobacco products, ashtrays, and lighters in your environment.
   - Stock up on oral substitutes such as sugarless gum, hard candy, fruit, and carrot sticks.
   - Decide on a plan, and prepare to implement it; register for the stop-smoking class, or see your doctor about nicotine replacement therapy or pharmaceutical alternatives.
   - Practice saying "No thank you, I don't smoke."
   - Think back to your previous attempts to quit, and see what worked and what did not work.
   - If you are taking bupropion or varenicline, take your medication each day of the week leading up to your quit day.
3. Deal with withdrawal through
   - Avoiding temptation
   - Changing your habits. Walk when you are stressed or during breaks. Use hard candy, carrot sticks, or gum to satisfy the need to put something in your mouth. If you feel the urge to light up, tell yourself that you are going to wait 10 minutes before giving in. Usually, the urge will pass within that time.

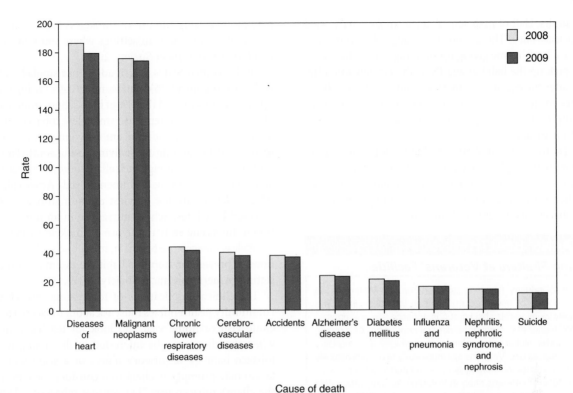

FIGURE 4-6 Leading causes of death, United States, 2008-2009. (From Centers for Disease Control and Prevention, National Center for Chronic Disease: Age-adjusted death rates for the 10 leading causes of death-national vital statistics system, United States, 2008 and 2009. *Morb Mortal Wkly Rep* 60[48]:1656, 2011. Available from <http://www.cdc.gov/mmwr/preview/mmwrhtml/mm6048a7.htm>.)

TABLE 4-4	RELATIONSHIP BETWEEN RISK FACTORS AND TEN LEADING CAUSES OF DEATH							
CAUSE OF DEATH	PERCENT OF TOTAL DEATHS	SMOKING	HIGH-FAT, LOW-FIBER DIET	SEDENTARY LIFESTYLE	HIGH BLOOD PRESSURE	ELEVATED CHOLESTEROL	OBESITY	DIABETES	ALCOHOL ABUSE
Heart disease	25	X	X	X	X	X	X	X	X
Cancer	23	X	X	X			X		X
Stroke	6	X	X		X	X	X		
Chronic obstructive pulmonary disease (COPD)	5	X							
Unintentional injury	5	X							X
Diabetes	3		X	X			X	X	
Alzheimer's	3		X	X					
All other causes	29	X							

From Centers for Disease Control and Prevention: *Health United States 2010.* Available from <http://www.cdc.gov/heartdisease/statistical_reports.htm>. Accessed August 22, 2013.

4. Staying off of tobacco is a lifelong process. Many former smokers state that they experienced strong desires to smoke after weeks, months, even years of smoking cessation. These unexpected cravings can be difficult to deal with.
   - Remind yourself of the reasons why you quit.
   - Wait out the craving. There is no such thing as just one cigarette or just one puff.
   - Avoid alcohol.
   - Begin an exercise program and work on eating a healthy diet to avoid gaining weight (American Cancer Society, 2013).

Information on quitting can be accessed at the CDC website at http://www.cdc.gov/tobacco/quit_smoking/how_to_quit/index.htm. The American Lung Association also has information on smoking cessation at http://www.lung.org/stop-smoking/. The American Cancer Society offers a quit-smoking guide at http://www.cancer.org/healthy/stayawayfromtobacco/guidetoquittingsmoking/guide-to-quitting-smoking-how-to-quit.

Teens are a population of concern regarding smoking. Though the rate of smoking has declined among Americans since the 1990s, more high school juniors and seniors smoke than do adults. Half of high school–aged smokers have tried to quit at least once. Those who start using tobacco in their teens have a harder time giving up smoking later in life. Most smokers pick up the habit at age 18, with very few initiating smoking after the age of 25 (American Cancer Society, 2012). A resource for teens who are trying to quit smoking is available at http://www.lung.org/associations/states/colorado/tobacco/not-on-tobacco/.

Only 4% to 7% of smokers are able to quit smoking on any attempt without pharmaceutical or other interventions to help them, so nurses must provide information and referrals to help clients access resources to help them to get off and to stay off tobacco (see Veterans' Health box).

VETERANS' HEALTH

Smoking Shelters at Veterans' Facilities

The tobacco industry has long targeted the US Military as an important source of new smokers. Among veterans who come from largely working-class backgrounds, tobacco use is estimated to be 40% higher than among the general population. As a result, veterans suffer higher a prevalence of morbidity and mortality related to tobacco use. Veterans are more likely to die prematurely and incur high costs for treating illnesses related to tobacco use.

Almost 70% of veterans seen in Veterans Administration (VA) facilities report that they would like to quit smoking.* (Bastia and Shermann, 2010). Those veterans attempting to quit tobacco face substantial personal and system barriers. Attempts by the military to discourage smoking have been met with great resistance from the tobacco industry, resulting in a federal law requiring that all veteran medical facilities provide an outdoor place for veterans to smoke. Though 60% of civilian hospitals are smoke-free and smoking is prohibited in all federal buildings, VA health facilities must allow smoking on the premises. Veterans are also less likely to receive the optimum treatment for successful smoking cessation of counseling and medication, which are essential given the incidence of depression and post-traumatic stress disorder (PTSD) among veterans (Offen et al., 2013).

As young men and women return from combat and move into the veteran population, it is essential that nurses recognize tobacco use and intervene to help veterans to quit using tobacco. A telephone counseling service is available at 1-800-QUIT NOW. Veterans may receive smoking cessation counseling and treatment without copay and are not required to attend smoking cessation counseling in order to receive medication. Resources and advice on quitting smoking are found on the VA website, at http://www.publichealth.va.gov/smoking/quit_smoking.asp.

Created by Bridgette Crotwell Pullis, PhD, RN, CHPN.

References:

Bastian LA, Sherman SE: Effects of the wars on smoking among veterans, *J Intern Med* 25(2):102–103, 2010.

Offen N, Smith EA, Malone RE: They're going to die anyway: smoking shelters at veterans' facilities, *Am J Public Health* 103(4):604–612, 2013.

Smokeless tobacco also poses a health threat. Commonly called *spit tobacco*, smokeless tobacco is a significant health threat and is not a safe substitute for smoking tobacco. Smokeless tobacco is known to be a cause of cancer and oral health problems. Smokeless tobacco causes nicotine addiction and dependence, and adolescents who use smokeless tobacco are more likely to take up smoking. Smoking bans

may be increasing the use of smokeless tobacco as smokers use smokeless tobacco in settings where smoking is prohibited (American Cancer Society, 2012).

In the United States, 3% of adults use smokeless tobacco, with far more men (6%) than women (0.4%) using smokeless tobacco. It is estimated that 8% of high school students and 3% of middle school students use smokeless tobacco. Smokeless tobacco use is more common among young white males, with its heaviest use among those living in the southern or north central states and among blue collar workers, service workers, and laborers as well as the unemployed. American Indian/Alaska Natives are the heaviest users of smokeless tobacco, followed by whites. School nurses are in an important position to intervene early in the use of smokeless tobacco. Most smokeless tobacco use begins in middle school, and interventions to prevent or stop this habit are essential in the school setting (American Cancer Society, 2012).

The clinical implications of tobacco use are clear. First, community health nurses must ask about tobacco use at every clinic visit or home visit and look for teachable moments, when the client may be interested in discussing his or her tobacco habit (a respiratory illness or a scare with an oral lesion may prompt the client to reconsider the habit). Assess the client's tobacco use: "Do you use tobacco?" "What kind of tobacco (cigarettes, cigars, chewing tobacco, pipe) do you use?" "How much do you smoke (dip, chew)?" "Have you thought about quitting?" Explore with the client why he or she may or may not have considered giving up the tobacco habit, and what options are available to help should he or she desire to quit. Refer the client to smoking cessation websites or other health care professionals for assistance in quitting. Chances are great that the client is very well acquainted with the health risks posed by tobacco but not with the options for helping him or her to quit. Encourage the client to attempt to give up tobacco, and encourage him or her in any attempts to decrease or stop the use of tobacco.

Alcohol Consumption and Health

Alcohol use is very common in our society. In 2010, half of Americans reported being current drinkers, with 5% reporting being heavy drinkers and 17% engaging in binge drinking. Though only 4% of the U.S. population is addicted to alcohol, about 25% of the population drinks excessively. One in five adults reported drinking five or more drinks per day. Men are more likely (63%) than women (55%) to be current drinkers and to binge drink. Men are also more than twice as likely to suffer death or injury related to drinking. Nationally, women are nearly twice as likely as men to be lifetime abstainers, yet one in two women of childbearing age drinks alcohol (CDC, April 2013).

Binge drinking is an unrecognized problem among women and girls. One in five high school–aged girls, and one in eight adult women, reported binge drinking. The intensity and frequency of binge drinking are similar among pregnant and nonpregnant women: about three times per month and six drinks per occasion (Marchetta et al., 2012). It takes less alcohol for females to become impaired than males because of body size and differences in the way alcohol is processed by females. About 7.6% of women use alcohol while pregnant, with about 1 in 20 women using alcohol heavily before discovering that they are pregnant. For both men and women, those aged 25 to 44 years had the highest prevalence of drinking. The drinking prevalence declines at age 44 years and declines steadily with age thereafter. Non-Hispanic white people have the highest drinking prevalence, with non-Hispanic white men being the heaviest drinkers (CDC, April, 2013).

Alcohol use, particularly heavy alcohol use, is responsible for many health problems such as liver disease and for unintentional injuries. *Excessive alcohol use* is drinking more than two drinks per day on average for men or more than one drink per day for women; *binge drinking* is drinking five or more drinks on a single occasion for men or four or more drinks in a single occasion for women. A *drink* is any drink containing 0.6 ounces or 1.2 tablespoons of pure alcohol. A drink is:

- 12 ounces of beer or wine cooler
- 8 ounces of malt liquor
- 5 ounces of wine
- 1.5 ounces of 80-proof distilled spirits or liquor (gin, rum, vodka, whiskey) (CDC, August 6, 2008)

The *Dietary Guidelines for Americans* state that alcohol should be consumed in moderation, no more than one drink per day for women and no more than two drinks per day for men (USDHHS, 2010). People who should not drink are those who:

- Are less than 21 years of age
- Are taking medications that can cause harmful reactions when mixed with alcohol
- Are pregnant or trying to become pregnant
- Are recovering from alcoholism or are unable to control the amount that they drink
- Have a medical condition that may be worsened by alcohol
- Are driving or planning to drive or to perform activities requiring coordination and concentration (CDC, October 1, 2012)

Responsible for 80,000 deaths annually, alcohol use is the third leading lifestyle-related cause of death for the nation. In 2006 there were more than 1.2 million emergency department visits for alcohol-related conditions. The short-term risks of alcohol consumption are usually due to binge drinking or excess drinking and include risky sexual behavior, violence, unintentional injuries from motor vehicle accidents, falls, firearms, and drowning. Miscarriage or stillbirth and alcohol poisoning are also possible immediate effects of excessive alcohol use. The long-term risks of alcohol use are neurological conditions such as dementia and stroke; cardiovascular problems such as MI, hypertension, and cardiomyopathy; psychiatric problems such as depression and anxiety; social problems such as unemployment and family dysfunction; cancer of the mouth, throat, liver, and breast; and liver disease including cirrhosis and hepatitis. Pancreatitis and gastritis are other gastrointestinal consequences of long-term alcohol consumption (CDC, October 1, 2012).

The prevalence of underage drinking declined significantly when states established the minimum legal drinking age as 21 years, and those states with more stringent drinking laws have a lower prevalence of adult and underage binge drinking. Despite age limits for legal consumption of alcohol, alcohol is the number one used and abused drug among U.S. youth. People aged 12 to 20 drink 11% of all alcohol consumed annually in the United States, 80% of it during binge drinking. Alcohol consumption contributes to more than 47,000 deaths among underage youth annually, and 25% of youth aged 12 to 20 reported drinking alcohol in 2011. Initiation to alcohol begins early: a national report found that 33% of eighth graders had tried alcohol and 13% had drunk alcohol in the previous month. Youth who start drinking prior to age 15 are five times more likely to experience alcohol dependence or abuse than those who begin drinking at or after 21 years of age. The prevalence of adult binge drinking behavior is strongly predictive of binge drinking behavior by college students living in the same state (CDC, October 1, 2012; Office of Applied Studies, 2004).

Clinical implications for health promotion related to alcohol consumption emphasize prevention of underage drinking and identifying and assisting groups and individuals at risk for alcohol abuse and dependence. A helpful resource for locating and contacting local agencies for alcohol treatment is the National Drug and Alcohol Treatment Referral Routing Service, available at 1-800-662-HELP. Alcohol Screening and Brief Intervention (SBI) consists of screening for those who are at risk for excessive alcohol consumption and providing brief counseling. In trauma centers and emergency departments where SBI has been implemented, medical costs and readmissions related to alcohol have been reduced (CDC, 2011).

Preventing underage drinking is a public health priority. Enforcement of the legal drinking age, as well as enforcement of bans on sales of alcohol to minors, is an important aspect of prevention. Increased excise tax on alcoholic beverages has also been found to decrease underage drinking. Education of both adults and youth regarding alcohol and the myriad of risks posed by underage alcohol consumption must accompany enforcement efforts. The "Too Smart to Start" program targets parents and caregivers of 9- to 13-year-olds. The goal of the program is to increase the percentage of youth and their caregivers who view underage drinking unfavorably (CDC, April 26, 2013). Preventing excessive alcohol consumption must consider several prominent environmental factors:

- Alcohol is cheap.
- Alcohol is readily available.
- Americans are exposed to 4 billion dollars of alcohol advertising per year.
- New alcohol products cater to youthful tastes and may promote underage drinking (U.S. Department of Justice, 2002).

Decreasing the morbidity and mortality related to over-consumption of alcohol requires a community-wide effort to address the problem on several fronts. Youth tend to model their drinking behavior after adults, and adults are often the source of alcohol for many youth, meaning that interventions must be aimed at the population across the lifespan. Interventions supported by research include:

- Increase taxes on alcohol—a 10% increase in price results in a 7% decrease in alcohol consumption.
- Decrease alcohol outlet density—higher outlet density is associated with greater alcohol consumption and negative impacts of alcohol.
- Hold alcohol retailers responsible for harm caused by inebriated or underage drinkers.

Diet and Health

Diet is one of the most modifiable of risk factors. A healthy diet contributes to the prevention of such chronic diseases as type 2 diabetes, hypertension, heart disease, and some cancers. With 17% of U.S. children 2 to 19 years and 37.5% of U.S. adults being obese (Ogden, Carroll, and Flegal, 2012), diet is an important topic in health promotion. Americans are bombarded with nutrition information, and many are confused and have no idea how to apply the information regarding diet that they have received. As portion sizes get larger, Americans of all ages are spending more time engaged in inactive pursuits such as watching TV and using a computer. Commonly, the terms "portion" and "serving" are misused. A *portion* is the "amount of a single food item served in a single eating occasion." A meal or a snack is a single eating occasion with the amount of green beans or roast beef on your plate being the portion. A *serving* is a "standardized unit of measuring foods" used in dietary guidelines. A cup or an ounce is an example of a serving size (CDC, May 2006).

What does it mean to be overweight or obese? Both of these terms are used to indicate a condition of excess weight for height. Both terms also identify ranges of weight that have been found to be associated with an increased risk of certain diseases or conditions. The body mass index (BMI) is used to determine weight status in adults and children. The body mass index takes both height and weight into account and has been found to correlate well with the amount of body fat present. An adult with a BMI of 25 to 29.9 is considered overweight, and an adult with a BMI of 30 or higher is considered obese. Though there are many contributing factors to overweight and obesity, controlling one's weight is a matter of balancing caloric intake with physical activity. Too many calories in and too few calories out eventually result in overweight. Figure 4-7 illustrates this energy balance. One's body weight is determined by a complex interplay among metabolism, genetics, behavior, environment, culture, and socioeconomic status, making the problem of overweight a difficult one to study and to affect (CDC, August 13, 2012).

The rate of obesity in the United States increased between 1990 and 2010; no state met the *Healthy People 2010* goal to reduce the obesity prevalence to 15%. Mississippi's prevalence of overweight and obesity is the highest in the nation at 34.9%, with Louisiana, Alabama, and Arkansas having the next highest prevalence rates. Colorado has the lowest prevalence of overweight and obesity, at 20.7% (CDC, August 13, 2012). Persons aged 60 and older are most likely to be overweight in the United States, and obesity rates vary among races and ethnicities.

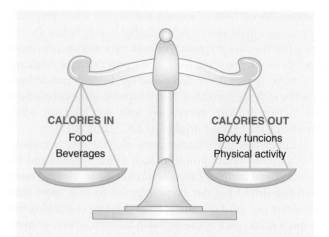

FIGURE 4-7 Caloric balance equation. (From Centers for Disease Control and Prevention: *Overweight and obesity: an overview*, January 28, 2009. Available from <www.cdc.gov/nccdphp/dnpa/obesity/contributing_factors.htm>. Accessed April 20, 2009.)

Non-Hispanic black persons have the highest rates of obesity (49.5%), followed by Mexican Americans (40.4%), all Hispanics (39.1%), and non-Hispanic whites (34.3%) (CDC, August 13, 2012). See Figure 4-8 for specific details on trends in obesity.

Though most obese Americans could not be classified as low income, the prevalence of obesity among women rises as income decreases, with 42% of women whose income is at or below the poverty level being obese. The prevalence of obesity among women also rises as education level decreases. Among men, there is no correlation between obesity prevalence, education, or income level. Rates of obesity have risen among adults at all income levels and all education levels (Ogden, Lamb, Carroll, and Flegal, 2010).

Obesity is also a concern for children. Since 1976 the prevalence of childhood obesity has increased, with 16.9% of children between the ages of 2 and 19 being obese. From 1999 to 2008 there was no trend in obesity prevalence for any age-group among children. There are ethnic disparities in childhood obesity, with Mexican-American adolescent boys having a significantly higher rate of obesity (26.8%) than non-Hispanic white boys (16.7%). Non-Hispanic black girls are more likely to be obese (29.2%) than non-Hispanic white girls (8.9%). From 1988 to 2008 the prevalence of obesity almost doubled among non-Hispanic white girls and non-Hispanic black girls (Ogden and Carroll, 2010). One encouraging development is that the prevalence of extreme obesity among low-income preschool children decreased slightly between 2003 and 2010, from 2.22% to 2.07%. The prevalence of obesity has also declined in this population during the same period, from 15.21% to 14.94% (CDC, April 27, 2012).

As rates of obesity have risen, so has the cost associated with the health comorbidities of obesity. It is well known that obesity is related to the most common causes of death—heart disease, stroke, some cancers, and type 2 diabetes. In 2008, medical costs associated with obesity were estimated to be approximately $147 billion, with obese persons each costing $1429 more in medical expenditures than individuals of

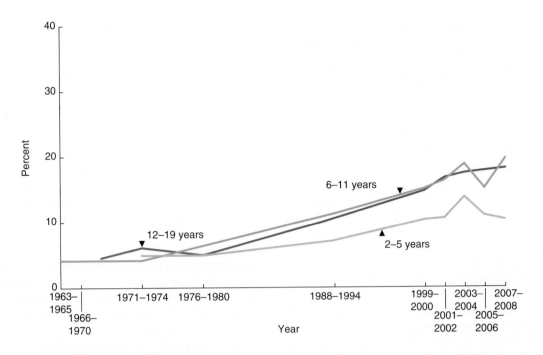

NOTE: Obesity is defined as body mass index (BMI) greater than or equal to sex- and age-specific 95th percentile from the 2000 CDC Growth Charts.
SOURCES: CDC/NCHS, National Health Examination Surveys II (ages 6–11), III (ages 12–17), and National Health and Nutrition Examination Surveys (NHANES) I–III, and NHANES 1999–2000, 2001–2002, 2003–2004, 2005–2006, and 2007-2008.

FIGURE 4-8 Trends in obesity among children and adolescents: United States, 1963-2008. (From Ogden C, Carroll M: Prevalence of obesity among children and adolescents: United States, 1963-1965 through 2007-2008, NCHS Health E-Stat, 2010. Available from <http://www.cdc.gov/nchs/data/hestat/obesity_child_07_08/obesity_child_07_08.htm>. Data from CDC/NCHS, National Health Examination Surveys II (ages 6-11), III (ages 12-17) and National Health and Nutrition Examination Surveys (NHANES) I-III, and NHANES 1999-2000, 2001-2002, 2003-2004, 2005-2006, and 2007-2008.)

normal weight. It is estimated that about 27% of the increase in health care spending between 1987 and 2001 was related to obesity, and about half of this cost was paid for by Medicare and Medicaid. An obese beneficiary costs Medicare more than $600 more annually than a beneficiary of normal weight.

Fats are an essential nutrient for energy and serve many purposes in the body, but too much fat in the diet, especially trans fats, saturated fats, and cholesterol, may increase the risk of heart disease (U.S. Department of Agriculture [USDA]/USDHHS, 2010). In 2009, only about a quarter of persons in the United States reported eating the recommended five or more servings of fruits and vegetables per day. Though the benefits of eating a diet rich in fruits and vegetables is well known, this trend is unchanged since 1996 (USDA/USDHHS, 2010). The CDC has information on incorporating fruits and vegetables into a daily diet at http://www.cdc.gov/nutrition/everyone/fruitsvegetables/index.html.

Although the same eating plan is not appropriate for everyone, USDA does make some key recommendations regarding a healthy diet based on a 2000 calorie per day intake, as follows:

- Select 2 cups of fruit and 2½ cups of vegetables per day. Select a variety of colors and types.
- Consume three or more 1-ounce-equivalent servings per day of whole-grain products.
- Consume 3 cups per day of fat-free or low-fat milk or milk products.
- Keep total fat intake to 20% to 35% of caloric intake.
- When choosing fats, emphasize lean meats, beans, poultry, and fat-free or low-fat milk products.
- Limit intake of trans fatty acids or saturated fats.
- Choose fiber-rich fruits and vegetables often.
- Prepare beverages and foods with little added sugar.
- Consume less than 1 teaspoon of salt per day.
- Consume alcoholic beverages moderately—up to one drink per day for women and two drinks per day for men.

Special populations such as pregnant or lactating women, infants, children, older adults, athletic or very active adults, and adolescents have differing nutritional needs. Specific recommendations for these individuals can be accessed at the website for the *Dietary Guidelines for Americans:* http://www.cnpp.usda.gov/DGAs2010-PolicyDocument.htm (USDHHS, 2010).

The USDA recommends that all Americans go to http://www.choosemyplate.gov/ to develop a personalized eating plan based on individual needs and preferences. *My Plate* (Figure 4-9) was released in 2011, replacing the Food Guide Pyramid. This tool helps users easily translate the USDA guidelines into the kinds and amounts of food to eat each day. *My Plate* is applicable to children as well as adults and is simple and fun enough that children can use it themselves. *My Plate* illustrates a healthful eating plan in a simple and familiar format—a place setting. The key messages of *My Plate* is that half of the plate should be fruit and vegetables; a quarter of the plate should be grains and half of the grains consumed daily should be whole grain; one quarter of the plate should be protein; and a serving of a low-fat or nonfat dairy product should be included in each meal. Oils, a source of essential nutrients, are also included in *My Plate,* with the emphasis on oils low in trans fats. The *Choose My Plate* homepage at http://www.choosemyplate.gov/ contains information on eating on a budget, weight management, and a food and activity tracker to help users balance food intake with activity. Many popular foods, such as pizza and spaghetti, are mixed dishes in that they do not fit into only one food group. The *My Plate* website provides nutrition and calorie information on common mixed dishes (USDA, 2013).

Studies confirm that eating away from home is associated with an increased likelihood of being overweight (Fulkerson et al., 2011; Rafferty et al., 2011). Busy families have more opportunities to eat away from home as the number of eateries has increased in recent years. The latest findings indicate that from 1999 to 2004, American families spent 45% of their food budget on foods eaten away from home (The Keystone Center, 2006). Though parental employment is a benefit to families, the stresses of balancing family and work demands impact nutrition and the kinds of foods consumed. Families with parents who work full time spend less time on food preparation, eat fewer family meals, eat more fast food, and spend less time encouraging healthful eating behaviors (Bauer et al., 2012). Men between ages 40 and 59 years consume the most food prepared away from home (Van der Horst, Brunner, and Siegrist, 2011). (This author can attest to the fact that when her 49-year-old husband is left to fend for himself at mealtime he will most likely eat out). Adolescents also consume a large amount of fast food, with 30% of adolescent males and 27% of adolescent females reporting eating fast food at least three times per week (Bauer et al., 2009). Among adults the percentage of calories consumed from fast food rises as weight status increases, with obese adults consuming the highest percentage of their calories from fast food (Fryar and Ervin, 2013).

Portions served in restaurants are larger than portions served at home, in some cases up to 40% larger. Convenience foods and prepackaged foods contain larger portion sizes than in the 1970s. When presented with a large portion size, individuals often unknowingly eat larger amounts than they would usually eat or than they intend to eat. This phenomenon, called **portion distortion,** occurs frequently when people are dining out (NHLBI, 2013). Portion control is an important aspect of weight management, and distortion of portion sizes makes this difficult task harder. There are several reasons why we tend to overeat when we eat away from home: Foods presented in restaurants are high in energy density (high number of calories for a particular weight of food); restaurant foods are also very palatable, and there is a wide variety of this great-tasting food to choose from; and we want to get more food for our money, so we order the larger entrées (The Keystone Center, 2006).

For many people, eating at home all the time is impossible or impractical, and food is central to many social interactions. In order to consume fewer calories when eating out, one may:

- Patronize establishments that offer a variety of food choices and are willing to make substitutions or changes
- Order lower-fat steamed, broiled, baked, roasted, or poached items, or ask that an item be prepared in a lower-calorie way, such as grilled rather than fried
- Choose lower-calorie sauces or condiments, or do without them altogether
- Substitute colorful vegetables for other side dishes (such as French fries)
- Ask for half of the meal to be boxed to take home before the meal is brought to the table
- Share an entrée with someone
- Order a vegetarian meal
- Select a fruit for dessert

To decrease reliance on away-from-home foods, plan ahead and:

- Pack healthy snacks to avoid the use of vending machines
- Cook a healthful dinner at home, and make extra to pack for lunch the next day
- Purchase healthful foods when grocery shopping to pack for lunch, such as prepackaged salads, fresh fruits, vegetables, and low-calorie soups
- For travel or longer excursions, bring along nutritious foods that will not spoil, such as fresh fruits and vegetables, or pack a cooler with healthy foods

There are various online communities and other support groups available to help individuals manage their weight. Social media is harnessing the power of the Internet to help the public meet fitness goals. Sites such as *Sparkpeople* and *Livestrong* offer interactive and social networking opportunities. Group support is helpful for those who want them, whereas others prefer to have programs that they can implement on their own. The cost to join a weight-management

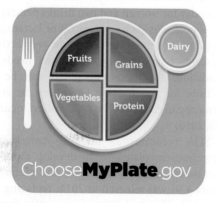

FIGURE 4-9 MyPlate logo. (From the United States Department of Agriculture: *MyPlate 2013,* Retrieved from http://www.choosemyplate.gov/print-materials-ordering/graphic-resources.html.)

community ranges from free to moderate in price. Another popular option for weight control is the large selection of applications for mobile devices. With these applications, it is possible to easily track foods eaten and calories expended throughout the day. Many are free and are available for mobile devices.

Physical Activity and Health

There are many reasons why people engage in physical activity and exercise: for weight management, increased energy, or better appearance; to fit into those favorite jeans; to prevent development or worsening of a chronic health condition; to manage stress; to improve mood and self-esteem; or any combination of these reasons. Despite the many benefits of regular physical activity, less than half (48%) of all U.S. adults meet the U.S. *Physical Activity Guidelines* recommendation to achieve 2.5 hours of physical activity per week (CDC, August 7, 2012).

Several factors acting individually and in concert can affect the likelihood that one is physically active. Men are a little more likely to engage in leisure physical activity and are more likely to engage in strength training than women. The percentage of adults who engage in leisure-time physical activity decreases with age, from its highest among adults aged 18 to 24 years. White adults and Asian adults are more likely to engage in leisure-time physical activity than are black and Hispanic adults. The percentage of adults participating in leisure-time physical activity increases with level of education; adults with advanced degrees are twice as likely to engage in some physical activity than high school graduates. The percentage of adults who engage in regular leisure-time physical activity also increases with income level. Adults whose income is four times the federal poverty level are nearly twice as likely to engage in some form of regular leisure-time physical activity than adults whose income is below the poverty level. Adults living in the southern region of the United States get the least amount of leisure-time physical activity (CDC, August 7, 2012).

As has been previously mentioned, one's surroundings also impact whether one will choose to exercise. The Walk Score has ranked cities across the United States for suitability for walking. So, what makes a city walkable?

- A center: It may be a shopping center, park, or main street
- Mixed use, mixed income: Businesses are located next to homes at all price points
- Pedestrian-centric design: Businesses are close to the street to encourage foot traffic with parking in back
- Density: The city is compact enough to allow businesses to flourish and for public transportation to run frequently
- Parks and public space: There are plenty of public areas in which to gather
- Nearby schools and workplaces: Schools and workplaces are close enough that most people can walk from home (Walk Score, 2013)

Research has found that one's environment is a significant factor in health promotion. Adults and adolescents living in neighborhoods with high walkability engage in significantly more walking and cycling than those living in neighborhoods with low walkability. As a result, the rates of obesity are lower in communities that are walkable than in communities that do not encourage physical activity (Brown et al., 2013; Slater et al., 2013).

How much exercise do I need? What counts as exercise? Nurses in the community hear these questions commonly as they educate the public on the need to increase physical activity. The answers to these questions depend on the age, physical condition, and gender of the client. The CDC website at http://www.cdc.gov/physicalactivity/data/facts.html presents the amount of exercise recommended for adults and children. Videos on the website further explain and illustrate the use of these guidelines. People may feel overwhelmed by the idea that they must add one more demand to an already busy schedule, and some think, "I'm in such bad shape, I'll never be able to exercise." The most important idea is that one must take a first step to try exercise. Walking, biking, taking the stairs, swimming—there is something for everyone, and *any* exercise is better than none. Exercise may also be broken up into smaller blocks of time during the day if it is not possible or convenient to do it all at once. Physical activity can also be a family affair, with the entire family using the time to reconnect and have fun together.

Sleep

Sleep is an essential component of chronic disease prevention and health promotion, yet 74% of adults report having a sleeping problem one or more nights per week. One quarter of the U.S. population reports that they occasionally do not get enough sleep, 39% report getting less than 7 hours of sleep per night, and 37% report being so sleepy during the day that it interferes with daily activities. Insufficient sleep is associated with diabetes, heart disease, obesity, and depression. Insufficient sleep contributes to 100,000 motor vehicle crashes each year and 15,000 deaths. Sleep requirements change as people age (Figure 4-10), and depending on life circumstances, one may require more than the minimum hours listed. If a person is so tired or sleepy that it interferes with his or her daily

How Much Sleep Do You Really Need?	
Age	Sleep needs
Newborns (1-2 months)	10.5-18 hours
Infants (3-11 months)	9-12 hours during night and 30-minute to 2-hour naps, one to 4 times a day
Toddlers (1-3 years)	12-14 hours
Preschoolers (3-5 years)	11-13 hours
School-aged children (5-12 years)	10-11 hours
Teens (11-17)	8.5-9.25 hours
Adults	7-9 hours
Older adults	7-9 hours

FIGURE 4-10 How much sleep do we really need? (Used with permission of the National Sleep Foundation: For further information, please visit www.sleepfoundation.org/how-much-sleep-do-we-really-need.)

activities, that person probably needs more sleep (National Sleep Foundation, n.d.).

As we age, sleep is often interrupted by pain, trips to the bathroom, medications, medical conditions, and sleep disorders. In order to get enough sleep, we must plan to set aside enough time for sleep. Preferably, this means that we can awaken naturally, without an alarm clock, ensuring adequate rest. The need for sleep is regulated by two processes. One is the number of hours we are awake. The longer we are awake, the stronger the desire is to sleep. The other process is the circadian biological clock in the brain, the suprachiasmatic nucleus (SCN), which responds to light. This clock makes us tend to be sleepy at night when it is dark and to be active during the day when it is light. The circadian rhythm is why we are sleepiest between 2:00 and 4:00 AM and 1:00 and 3:00 PM. The circadian rhythm also regulates the 24-hour cycle of the body. While we sleep, important hormones are released, memory is consolidated, blood pressure is decreased, and kidney function changes (National Sleep Foundation, n.d.).

One of the results of lack of sleep is drowsy driving. More than one third of U.S. drivers admit to having fallen asleep while driving, and 4% have had an accident owing to driving while drowsy. An estimated 1550 deaths result from driver fatigue annually. Sleep-related motor vehicle accidents are most common among young people, shift workers, men, and adults with children. Adults between 18 and 29 years of age are the most likely to drive when sleepy. The less people sleep, the greater their risk for being involved in a vehicular crash. People who sleep 6 to 7 hours per night are twice as likely to be involved in a crash as those sleeping 8 hours per night or more. People sleeping 4 to 5 hours have a four to five times higher risk of being involved in a sleep-related accident. Being awake for 18 hours produces the same degree of impairment as being legally intoxicated (National Sleep Foundation, 2013)

Practicing sleep hygiene will help achieve optimum sleep, as follows:

1. Avoid caffeine and nicotine close to bedtime.
2. Avoid alcohol as it can cause sleep disruptions.
3. Retire and get up at the same time every day.
4. Exercise regularly, but finish all exercise and vigorous activity at least 3 hours before bedtime.
5. Establish a regular, relaxing bedtime routine (a warm bath, reading a book).
6. Create a dark, quiet, cool sleep environment.
7. Have a comfortable mattress and bedding.
8. Use the bed for sleep only; do not read, listen to music, or watch TV in bed.
9. Avoid large meals before bedtime (National Sleep Foundation, n.d.).

Sleep assessment is an important nursing function. If a client reports snoring, apnea, restlessness, or insomnia, he or she may have a sleep disorder. Recommend keeping a sleep log that details how many hours are spent in sleep each night and any problems with sleep. If insufficient sleep is causing trouble concentrating or completing daily activities, recommend consulting a doctor, as a sleep disorder may be to blame. A sleep assessment tool and a list of sleep disorders

and descriptions of each may be found at the National Sleep Foundation's website, at http://www.sleepfoundation.org/.

Because of the 24-hour-per-day nature of nursing, nurses are among many workers who must work night shifts. Negative physical effects of working nights include an increased risk for stroke and heart disease, increased development of metabolic syndrome, and irregular menstrual cycles. Sleep deprivation related to shift work can cause practice errors related to a lack of attention to detail, impaired psychomotor skills, and reduced coordination, among others.

An article regarding the effects of shift work and ways to adapt to its rigors, *Help Me Make it Through the Night (Shift)*, is available from Medscape at http://www.medscape.com/viewarticle/757050.

SUMMARY

Health promotion is an essential component to ongoing good health and well-being, yet many Americans have difficulty with one or more of the components of health promotion. Exercise, diet, sleep, and tobacco and alcohol use all affect our health. Nurses, particularly community health nurses, are in a position to assess and counsel clients on their health habits. Community health nurses also possess the unique combination of community familiarity and the knowledge and training to affect health at the policy level. As the environment is made safer and more walkable, or with a lower density of available alcohol or fast food, the community as a whole will benefit.

LEARNING ACTIVITIES

1. How has *Healthy People* changed? Get to know the *Healthy People 2020* proposed objectives at www.healthypeople.gov/hp2020/objectives/TopicAreas.aspx. Read over the new objectives and compare them with the *Healthy People 2010* objectives at www.healthypeople.gov/About/.

2. How did Americans do in meeting *Healthy People 2010* objectives? Choose a focus area from *Healthy People 2010*, and access the periodic reviews for *Healthy People 2010* at www.healthypeople.gov/data/PROGRVW/. Was progress made toward achieving the objectives for this focus area? What are the challenges to meeting the objectives? What are the strategies for meeting the objectives? Did the objective change for *Healthy People 2020*?

3. How is your community doing in comparison with other communities? Prevalence and incidence rates for diseases or health conditions allow us to make comparisons between communities. Rates of activities such as smoking and physical activity allow us to make comparisons between communities regarding other areas of health promotion. Consider a community of which you are a member (e.g., your state, your county, your age-group, or your school). Choose a health promotion topic that is of particular importance to your community of interest, such as sexual health, obesity, communicable disease, or physical activity. How does your community compare with a

similar community in a different area of the state or the country? How does your community compare with a similar community in another part of the world?

4. How do people, groups, and populations meet health-promotion goals? Interview someone who is successful at meeting his or her health promotion goals. For example: How did the person manage to keep his or her weight at a healthy level? How did the person stop smoking? How does he or she make time to exercise daily? Does the individual have a philosophy of health that helps him or her stay on track with health promotion goals? How does the individual incorporate health promotion into daily life? What advice does he or she have for others striving to achieve better health?

5. View the Institute of Medicine series *Weight of the Nation* at http://theweightofthenation.hbo.com/. As you watch the series consider: What is the largest contributing factor to obesity among children? What interventions can you think of that would be effective in preventing or reducing obesity prevalence in your community? What are common barriers to preventing or reducing obesity among people across the lifespan? What negative effects will the US as a whole face due to obesity?

ⓔ EVOLVE WEBSITE

http://evolve.elsevier.com/Nies

- NCLEX Review Questions
- Case Studies
- Glossary

REFERENCES

American Cancer Society: *Child and teen tobacco use*, November 8, 2012. Available from <http://www.cancer.org/cancer/cancercauses/tobaccocancer/childandteentobaccouse/child-and-teen-tobacco-use-child-and-teen-tobacco-use>. Accessed February 27, 2013.

American Cancer Society: *Guide to quitting smoking*, January 17, 2013. Available from <http://www.cancer.org/healthy/stayawayfromtobacco/guidetoquittingsmoking/index>. Accessed February 27, 2013.

American Lung Association: *Quit smoking*, n.d. Available from <http://www.lung.org/stop-smoking/>. Accessed January 9, 2014.

Atkinson LN, Saperstein LS, Pleis J: Using the internet for health-related activities: findings from a national probability sample, *Journal of Medical Internet Research* 11(1):e4, 2009.

Bauer KW, Hearst MO, Escoto K, et al: Parental environments and work-family stress: associations with family food environments, *Social Science and Medicine* 75:496–504, 2012.

Bauer KW, Larson NI, Nelson MC, et al: Fast food intake among adolescents: secular and longitudinal trends from 1999-2004, *Preventive Medicine* 48:284–287, 2009.

Benson H: *Timeless healing: the power and biology of belief*, New York, 1996, Scribner.

Brown BB, Smith KR, Hanson H, et al: Neighborhood design for walking and biking: physical activity and body mass index, *American Journal of Preventive Medicine* 44:23–238, 2013.

Burger KS, Kern M, Coleman KJ: Characteristics of self-selected portion sizes in young adults [electronic version], *J Am Diet Assoc* 107:611–1608, 2007.

Centers for Disease Control and Prevention: *Smoking cessation* (n.d.). Available from <http://www.cdc.gov/tobacco/data_statistics/fact_sheets/cessation/quitting/index.htm>. Accessed August 22, 2013.

Centers for Disease Control and Prevention: *Do increased portion sizes affect how much we eat? Nutrition resources for health professionals*, May 2006. Available from <www.cdc.gov/nccdphp/dnpa/nutrition/pdf/portion_size_research.pdf>. Accessed April 20, 2009.

Centers for Disease Control and Prevention: *Ways to reduce cancer risk*, January 2, 2013. Available from <http://www.cdc.gov/cancer/dcpc/prevention/other.htm>. Accessed February 25, 2013.

Centers for Disease Control and Prevention: *Adult smoking in the United States: current estimates (updated 2011): smoking and tobacco use*, November 11, 2007; updated 2011. Available from <http://www.cdc.gov/VitalSigns/AdultSmoking/index.html#StateInfo>. Accessed February 27, 2013.

Centers for Disease Control and Prevention: *US obesity trends 1985-2007: overweight and obesity*, July 24, 2008a. Available from <www.cdc.gov/nccdphp/dnpa/obesity/trend/maps/index.htm>. Accessed April 19, 2009.

Centers for Disease Control and Prevention: *Excessive alcohol use and risks to women's health*, October 1, 2012. Available from <http://www.cdc.gov/alcohol/fact-sheets/womens-health.htm>. Accessed February 28, 2012.

Centers for Disease Control and Prevention: *Underage drinking*, April 9, 2013. Available from <http://www.cdc.gov/alcohol/fact-sheets/underage-drinking.htm>. Accessed February 28, 2013.

Centers for Disease Control and Prevention: *Alcohol use and health*, April 9, 2013. Available from <http://www.cdc.gov/alcohol/fact-sheets/alcohol-use.htm>. Accessed February 28, 2013.

Centers for Disease Control and Prevention: *Alcohol screening*, April 9, 2013. Available from <http://www.cdc.gov/injuryresponse/alcohol-screening/index.html>. Accessed March, 2013.

Centers for Disease Control and Prevention: *Facts about physical activity*, August 7, 2012c. Available from <http://www.cdc.gov/physicalactivity/data/facts.html>. Accessed March 2013.

Centers for Disease Control and Prevention: *Quick stats: age 21 legal minimum drinking age. alcohol and public health*, September 3, 2008b. Available from <www.cdc.gov/alcohol/quickstats/mlda.htm>. Accessed May 4, 2009.

Centers for Disease Control and Prevention: *Incorporating eaten-away-from-home food into a healthy eating plan: nutrition resources for health professionals*, December 22, 2008a. Available from. <www.cdc.gov/nccdphp/dnpa/nutrition/pdf/r2p_away_from_home_food.pdf>. Accessed April 13, 2009.

Centers for Disease Control and Prevention: *Overweight and obesity*, August 13, 2012d. Available from <http://www.cdc.gov/obesity/data/adult.html>. Accessed March 26, 2013.

Centers for Disease Control and Prevention, National Center for Chronic Disease Prevention and Health Promotion: *Fruit and vegetable consumption per day, nationwide—2007. nutrition information for health professionals*, November 6, 2008. Available from <apps.nccd.cdc.gov/5ADaySurveillance/displayV.asp>. Accessed April 13, 2009.

Centers for Disease Control and Prevention: *Trends in the prevalence of extreme obesity among US preschool-aged children living in low-income families, 1998-2010*, 2012. Available from <http://www.cdc.gov/obesity/data/childhood.html>. Accessed March 2013.

Champion VL, Skinner CS: The health belief model. In Glanz K, Rimer BK, Viswanath K, editors: *Health behavior and health education: theory, research, and practice*, San Francisco, 2008, Jossey-Bass.

De Castro JM, King GA, Duarte-Gardea M, et al: Overweight and obese humans overeat away from home, *Appetite* 59:204–211, 2012.

Edwards A, Naik G, Ahmed H, et al: Personalised risk communication for informed decision making about screening tests (Review) [update], *The Cochrane Library* (2): CD001865, 2013.

Finklestein EA, Trogdon JG, Cohen JW, et al: Annual medical spending attributable to obesity: payer- and service-specific estimates, *Health Affairs* 289(5):w822–w831, 2009.

Finnigan JR, Vinswanath K: Communication theory and health behavior change. In Glanz KR, Rimer BK, Vinswanath K, editors: *Health behavior and health education*, ed 4, San Francisco, 2008, Jossey-Bass, pp 363–384.

Flegal K, Carroll O: Johnson Prevalence and trends among US adults, 1999-2000, *JAMA* 288:1723–1727, 2002.

Frank LS: Linking objectively measured physical activity with objectively measured urban form: findings from SMARTRAQ, *Am J Prev Med*(28)117–125, 2005.

Fryar, CD, & Ervin, RB (2013). Caloric intake from fast food among adults: United States, 2007-2010. NCHS Data Brief No. 114. Available from www.cdc.gov/nchs/data/databriefs/db114.htm Accessed March 2013.

Friis R, Sellers: *Epidemiology for public health practice*, London, 2004, Jones & Bartlett.

Fulkerson JA, Farbakhsh K, Lytle L, et al: Away-from-home family dinner sources and associations with weight status, body composition and related biomarkers of chronic disease among adolescents and their parents, *Journal of the American Dietetic Association* 111(112):1892–1897, 2011.

Green L, Kreuter M: *Health promotion and planning: an educational and environmental approach*, Mountain View, CA, 1991, Mayfield.

Hendrick PA, Ahmed OH, Bankier SS, et al: Acute low back pain information online: an evaluation of quality, content, accuracy and readability of related websites, *Manual Therapy* 17: 318–324, 2012.

Hochbaum G: *Public participation in medical screening programs: a socio-psychological study*, Washington, DC, 1958, U.S. Public Health Service.

The Keystone Center: *The Keystone forum on away-from-home foods: opportunities for preventing weight gain and obesity*, Washington, DC, 2006, Author.

Kupferberg N, Protus B: Accuracy and completeness of drug information in Wikipedia: an assessment, *Journal of the Medical Library Association* 99:310–313, 2011.

Loef M, Walach H: The combined effects of healthy lifestyle behaviors on all cause mortality: a systematic review and meta-analysis, *Preventative Medicine* 55:163–170, 2012.

Marchetta CM, Denny CH, Floyd L, et al: Alcohol use and binge drinking among women of childbearing age —United States, 2006-2010, *Morbidity and Mortality Weekly Report* 61:534–538, 2012.

McCrory MA, Fuss PJ, Hays NP, et al: Overeating in America: association between restaurant food consumption and body fatness in healthy adult men and women, *Obes Res* 92:564–571, 1999.

McEwen M, Pullis B: *Community-based nursing: an introduction*, St. Louis, 2009, Saunders.

McGinnis JM, Foege WH: Actual causes of death in the United States, *JAMA* 270:2207–2212, 1993.

McGinnis JM, Foege WH: The immediate and the important, *JAMA* 291:1263–1264, 2004.

Merriam-Webster Online Dictionary: *Health*, March 2009. Available from <www.merriam-webster.com/dictionary/health>. Accessed March 23, 2009.

Medscape. *Help me make it through the night (shift)*. Available from http://www.medscape.com/viewarticle/757050. Accessed March 2013.

Mokdab AH, Marks JS, Stroup DF, et al: Actual causes of death in the United States 2000, *JAMA* (291):1238–1245, 2004.

Montano D, Kasprzyk D: Theory of reasoned action, theory of planned behavior, and the integrated behavioral model. In Glanz KR, editor: *Health behavior and health education: theory, research, and practice*, ed 4, San Francisco, 2008, Jossey-Bass, pp 67–96.

National Sleep Foundation: *Drowsy driving: facts and stats*, 2013. Available from <http://drowsydriving.org/about/facts-and-stats/>. Accessed March 2013.

National Sleep Foundation: *How much sleep do we really need?* n.d. Available from <http://www.sleepfoundation.org/article/how-sleep-works/how-much-sleep-do-we-really-need>. Accessed January 28, 2010.

National Heart, Lung, and Blood Institute. Portion Distortion. February 2013. Accessed January 2014. http://www.nhlbi.nih.gov/health/public/heart/obesity/wecan/portion/index.htm

Office of Applied Studies: *The NSDUH report: alcohol dependence or abuse and age at first use*, Rockville, MD, Substance Abuse and Mental Health Services Administration, October 2004.

Ogden C, Carroll MD, Flegal KM: *Prevalence of obesity in the United States: 2009-2010*, 2012. NCHS Data Brief #82. Available from <http://www.cdc.gov/obesity/data/adult.html>. Accessed March 2013.

Ogden C, Carroll C, Curtin LR, et al: Prevalence of overweight and obesity in the United States, 1999-2004, *JAMA* 295:1545–1599, 2006.

Ogden C, Carroll M: *Prevalence of obesity among children and adolescents: United States trends 1963-1965 through 2007-2008*, 2010, Centers for Disease Control and Prevention. Available from <http://www.cdc.gov/nchs/data/hestat/obesity_child_07_08/obesity_child_07_08.htm>. Accessed March 2013.

Ogden CL, Lamb MM, Carroll MD, et al: *Obesity and socioeconomic status in adults: United States, 2005-2008*, 2010 NCHS data brief no. 50. Available from <http://www.cdc.gov/nchs/data/databriefs/db50.pdf>. Accessed March 2013.

Oleckno W: *Essential epidemiology*, Prospect Heights, IL, 2002, Waveland Press.

Parse R: Health promotion and prevention: two distinct cosmologies, *Nurs Sci Q*(3)101, 1990.

Pender N: *Health promotion and disease prevention*, ed 3, Stamford, CT, 1996, Appleton & Lange.

Pender N, Murdaugh CL, Parsons MA: *Health promotion in nursing practice*, ed 6, Upper Saddle River, NJ, 2011, Pearson.

Saelens B, Salis JF, Black JB, et al: Neighborhood-based differences in physical activity: an environment scale evaluation, *Research and Practice* (93): 43–54, 2003.

Savitz DR: Methods in chronic epidemiology. In Brownson RC, Remington PL, Davis JR, editors: *Chronic disease epidemiology and control*, Washington, DC, 1998, American Public Health Association, pp 27–54.

Schroder H, Fito M, Cavas M: Association of fast food consumption with energy intake, diet quality, body mass index, and the risk of obesity in a representative Mediterranean population, *Br J Nutr* 98:1274–1280, 2007.

Schwartz J, Byrd-Bredbrenner C: Portion distortion: typical portion sizes selected by young adults, *J Am Diet Assoc* 106:1412–1418, 2006.

Slater DJ, Nicholson L, Chriqui J, et al: Walkable communities and adolescent weight, *American Journal of Preventive Medicine* 44: 164–168, 2013.

U.S. Department of Agriculture and U.S. Department of Health and Human Services. Chapter 3: Foods and food components to reduce. In *Dietary guidelines for Americans, 2010*, ed 7, Washington, DC, 2010, US Government Printing Office, pp 30–32.

U.S. Department of Agriculture, Center for Nutrition Policy and Promotion: *2010 Dietary guidelines for Americans* ed 7, 2010 Author. Available from <http://www.cnpp.usda.gov/dietaryguidelines.htm>. Accessed March 2013.

U.S. Department of Agriculture: *choose my plate.gov*. Available from <http://www.choosemyplate.gov/>. Accessed March, 2013.

U.S. Department of Health and Human Services: *About healthy people*, December 17, 2012. Available from <http://www.healthypeople.gov/2020/about/default.aspx>. Accessed March, 2013.

U.S. Department of Health and Human Services: *Healthy People 2020: topics and objectives*, March 8, 2013. Available from <http://www.healthypeople.gov/2020/topicsobjectives2020/default.aspx>. Accessed March 2013.

U.S. Department of Justice: *Drinking in America: myths, realities and prevention policies*, Available from <http://www.udetc.org/documents/Drinking_in_America.pdf>. Accessed February 28, 2013.

Van der Horst K, Brunner TA, Siegrist M: Fast food and take-away food consumption are associated with different lifestyle characteristics, *Journal of Human Nutrition and Dietetics* 24:596–602, 2011.

Walk Score: *What makes a city walkable? Walkscore: find a walkable place to live*, 2008. Available from <www.walkscore.com/rankings/what-makes-a-city-walkable.shtml>. Accessed January 9, 2014.

Westberg J, Jason H: Fostering healthy behavior: the process. In Woolf SH, Jonas S, Lawrence RS, editors: *Health promotion and disease prevention in clinical practice*, Baltimore, 1996, Williams & Wilkins.

World Health Organization: Health promotion: a discussion document on the concept and principles, *Public Health Rev* 14:245–254, 1986.

World Health Organization: *Mental health*, 2009. Available from <www.who.int/topics/ mental_health/en/>. Accessed March 23, 2009.

Epidemiology

Holly B. Cassells

KEY TERMS

age-adjustment of rates
age-specific rates
analytic epidemiology
attack rates
cause-and-effect relationship
crude rates
descriptive epidemiology
ecosocial epidemiology
epidemiological triangle

epidemiology
incidence rates
morbidity rates
mortality rates
natural history of disease
person-place-time model
prevalence rate
proportionate mortality ratio
rates

risk
risk factors
screening
screening programs
standardization of rates
surveillance
web of causation

OUTLINE

Use of Epidemiology in Disease Control and Prevention
Calculation of Rates
    Morbidity: Incidence and Prevalence Rates
    Other Rates
Concept of Risk
Use of Epidemiology in Disease Prevention
    Primary Prevention
    Secondary and Tertiary Prevention

    Establishing Causality
    Screening
    Surveillance
Use of Epidemiology in Health Services
Epidemiological Methods
    Descriptive Epidemiology
    Analytic Epidemiology

Epidemiology is the study of the distribution and determinants of health and disease in human populations (Harkness, 1995) and is the principal science of public health. It entails a body of knowledge derived from epidemiological research and specialized epidemiological methods and approaches to scientific research. Community health nurses use epidemiological concepts to improve the health of population groups by identifying risk factors and optimal approaches that reduce disease risk and promote health. Epidemiological methods are important for accurate community assessment and diagnosis and in planning and evaluating effective community interventions. This chapter discusses the uses of epidemiology and its specialized methodologies.

USE OF EPIDEMIOLOGY IN DISEASE CONTROL AND PREVENTION

Although epidemiological principles and ideas originated in ancient times, formal epidemiological techniques developed in the nineteenth century. Early applications focused on identifying factors associated with infectious diseases and the spread of disease in the community. Public health practitioners hoped to improve preventive strategies by identifying critical factors in disease development.

Specifically, investigators attempted to identify characteristics of people who had a disease such as cholera or plague and compared them with characteristics of those who remained healthy. These differences might include a broad range of personal factors, such as age, gender, socioeconomic status, and health status. Investigators also questioned whether there were differences in the location or living environment of ill people, in comparison with healthy individuals, and whether these factors influenced disease development. Finally, researchers examined whether common time factors existed (i.e., when people acquired disease). Use of this person-place-time model organized epidemiologists' investigations of the disease pattern in the community (Box 5-1). This study of the amount and distribution of disease constitutes descriptive epidemiology. Identified patterns frequently indicate possible causes of disease that public health professionals can examine with more advanced epidemiological methods.

In addition to investigating the person, place, and time factors related to disease, epidemiologists examine complex relationships among the many determinants of disease. This investigation of the causes of disease, or etiology, is called analytic epidemiology.

Even before the identification of bacterial agents, public health practitioners recognized that single factors were insufficient to cause disease. For example, while exploring the cholera epidemics in London in 1855, Dr. John Snow collected data about social and physical environmental conditions that might favor disease development. He specifically examined the contamination of local water systems. Snow also gathered information about people who became ill—their living patterns, water sources, socioeconomic characteristics, and health status. A comprehensive database helped him develop a theory about the possible cause of the epidemic. Snow suspected that a single biological agent was responsible for the cholera infection, although the organism, *Vibrio cholerae*, had yet to be discovered. He compared the death rates among individuals using one water well with those among people using a different water source. His findings suggested an association between cholera and water quality.

The epidemiologist examines the interrelationships between host and environmental characteristics and uses an organized method of inquiry to derive an explanation of disease. This model of investigation is called the epidemiological triangle because the epidemiologist must analyze the following three elements: agent, host, and environment (Figure 5-1). The development of disease depends on the extent of the host's exposure to an agent, the strength or virulence of the agent, and the host's genetic or immunological susceptibility. Disease also depends on the environmental conditions existing at the time of exposure, which include the biological, social, political, and physical environments (Table 5-1). The model implies that the rate of disease will change when the balance among these three factors is altered. By examining each of the three elements, a community health nurse can methodically assess a health problem, determine protective factors, and evaluate the factors that make the host vulnerable to disease.

Conditions linked to clearly identifiable agents, such as bacteria, chemicals, toxins, and other exposure factors, are readily explained by the epidemiological triangle. However, other models that stress the multiplicity of host and environmental interactions have developed, and understanding of disease has progressed. The "wheel model" is an example of such a model (Figure 5-2). The wheel consists of a hub that represents the host and its human

| BOX 5-1 | **PERSON-PLACE-TIME MODEL** |

Person: "Who" factors, such as demographic characteristics, health, and disease status
Place: "Where" factors, such as geographic location, climate and environmental conditions, and political and social environment
Time: "When" factors, such as time of day, week, or month and secular trends over months and years

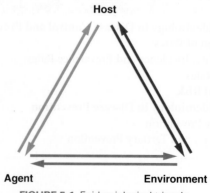

FIGURE 5-1 Epidemiological triangle.

characteristics, such as genetic makeup, personality, and immunity. The surrounding wheel represents the environment and comprises biological, social, and physical dimensions. The relative size of each component in the wheel depends on the health problem. A relatively large genetic core represents health conditions associated with heredity.

Origins of other health conditions may be more dependent on environmental factors (Mausner and Kramer, 1985). This model subscribes to multiple-causation rather than single-causation disease theory; therefore it is more useful for analyzing complex chronic conditions and identifying factors that are amenable to intervention.

EXAMPLE OF THE EPIDEMIOLOGICAL APPROACH

An early example of the epidemiological approach is John Snow's investigation of a cholera epidemic in the 1850s. He analyzed the distribution of person, place, and time factors by comparing the death rates among people living in different geographic sectors of London. His geographic map of cases, shown below, is an early example of the use of geographic information to formulate a hypothesis about the causes of an epidemic. Snow noted that people using a particular water pump had significantly higher mortality rates from cholera than people using other water sources in the city. Although the cholera organism was yet unidentified, the clustering of disease cases around one neighborhood pump suggested new prevention strategies to public health officials (i.e., that cholera might be reduced in a community by controlling contaminated drinking water sources). As an immediate response, in September 1854, Snow persuaded local leaders to remove the handle of the pump, which to this day can be seen on Broadwick Street in London (Snow, 1936).

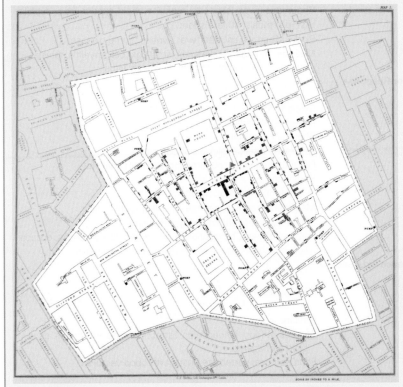

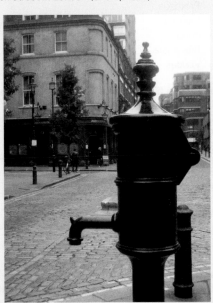

Replica of the famous Broad Street pump. Broadwick Street, London. (Photo courtesy of htt p://commons.wikimedia.org/wiki/File:John_ Snow_memorial_and_pub.jpg, Creative Commons Attribution-Share Alike 2.0 Generic [CC BY-SA 2.0]).

John Snow's map of London neighborhood showing location of cholera case cluster surrounding the Broad Street water pump. (Published by C.F. Cheffins, Lith, Southampton Buildings, London, England, 1854, in Snow J: On the mode of communication of cholera, 2nd ed, London, 1855, John Churchill. Retrieved July 2013 from <htt p://www.ph.ucla.edu/epi/snow/snowmap1_1854_lge.html>.)

Following the discovery of the causative agents of many infectious diseases, public health interventions eventually resulted in a decline in widespread epidemic mortality, particularly in developed countries. The focus of public health then shifted to chronic diseases such as cancer, coronary heart disease, and diabetes during the past few decades. The development of these chronic diseases tends to be associated with multiple interrelated factors rather than single causative agents.

In studying chronic diseases, epidemiologists use methods that are similar to those used in infectious disease investigation, thereby developing theories about chronic disease control. Risk factor identification is of particular importance to chronic disease reduction. **Risk factors** are variables that increase the rate of disease in people who have them (e.g., a genetic predisposition) or in people exposed to them (e.g., an infectious agent or a diet high in saturated fat). Therefore their identification is critical to identifying specific

TABLE 5-1	A CLASSIFICATION OF AGENT, HOST, AND ENVIRONMENTAL FACTORS THAT DETERMINE THE OCCURRENCE OF DISEASES IN HUMAN POPULATIONS
FACTORS	**EXAMPLES**
Agents of Disease—Etiological Factors	
A. Nutritive elements:	
Excesses	Cholesterol
Deficiencies	Vitamins, proteins
B. Chemical agents:	
Poisons	Carbon monoxide, carbon tetrachloride, drugs
Allergens	Ragweed, poison ivy, medications
C. Physical agents:	
Ionizing radiation	Sun exposure, medical imaging
Mechanical	Repetitive motion injury
D. Infectious agents:	
Metazoa	Hookworm, schistosomiasis, onchocerciasis
Protozoa	Amebae, malaria
Bacteria	Rheumatic fever, lobar pneumonia, typhoid, tuberculosis, syphilis
Fungi	Histoplasmosis, athlete's foot
Rickettsia	Rocky Mountain spotted fever, typhus, Lyme disease
Viruses	Measles, mumps, chicken pox, smallpox, poliomyelitis, rabies, yellow fever, human immunodeficiency virus
Host Factors (i.e., intrinsic factors)— Susceptibility or Response Influence Exposure to Agent	
A. Genetic	Cystic fibrosis, Huntington's disease
B. Age	Alzheimer's disease
C. Sex	Rheumatoid arthritis
D. Ethnic group	Tay-Sachs disease, sickle cell disease
E. Physiological state	Fatigue, pregnancy, puberty, stress, nutritional state
F. Prior immunological experience:	Hypersensitivity, protection
Active	Prior infection, immunization
Passive	Maternal antibodies, gamma globulin prophylaxis
G. Intercurrent or preexisting disease	Diabetes, liver dysfunction, hypertension
H. Human behavior	Personal hygiene, food handling, diet, interpersonal contact, occupation, recreation, use of health resources, tobacco use
Environmental Factors (i.e., extrinsic factors)—Influence Existence of the Agent, Exposure, or Susceptibility to Agent	
A. Physical environment	Geology, climate
B. Biological environment	
Human populations	Density
Flora	Sources of food, influence on vertebrates and arthropods, as a source of agents
Fauna	Food sources, vertebrate hosts, arthropod vectors
C. Socioeconomic environment	
Occupation	Exposure to chemical agents
Urbanization and economic development	Urban crowding, tension and pressures, cooperative efforts in health and education
Disruption	Wars, floods

Modified from Lilienfeld DE, Stoley PD: *Foundations of epidemiology*, New York, 1994, Oxford University Press.

prevention and interventionapproaches that effectively and efficiently reduce chronic disease morbidity and mortality. For example, the identification of cardiovascular disease risk factors has suggested a number of lifestyle modifications that could reduce the morbidity risk before disease onset. Primary prevention strategies, such as dietary saturated fat reduction, smoking cessation, and hypertension control, were developed in response to previous epidemiological studies that identified these risk factors (Box 5-2). The web of causation model illustrates the complexity of relationships among causal variables for heart disease (Figure 5-3).

A newer paradigm, ecosocial epidemiology, challenges the more individually focused risk factor approach to understanding disease origins. This ecosocial approach emphasizes the role of evolving macro-level socio-environmental factors, including complex political and economic forces along with microbiological processes, in understanding health and illness (Smith and Lincoln, 2011). Investigating the context of health will

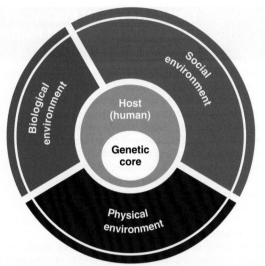

FIGURE 5-2 Wheel model of human-environment interaction. (Redrawn from Mausner JS, Kramer S: *Mausner and Bahn epidemiology: an introductory text*, ed 2, Philadelphia, 1985, Saunders.)

BOX 5-2 CORONARY HEART DISEASE (CHD) RISK FACTORS SUPPORTED BY EPIDEMIOLOGICAL DATA FROM THE FRAMINGHAM STUDY

- Age
- Gender (male)
- Current cigarette smoking
- Hypertension
- High level of low-density lipoprotein (LDL) cholesterol
- Low level of high-density lipoprotein (HDL) cholesterol
- (Diabetes)*
- Family history of premature coronary heart disease[†]

*Diabetes is not included in the Framingham Global Risk Score but is now considered to be a coronary heart disease risk equivalent, meaning that persons with diabetes will be treated as intensively as those with coronary heart disease.

[†]Included in NCEP list of major risk factors but not in the Framingham Global Risk Score.

Data from Executive summary of the third report of the National Cholesterol Education Program (NCEP) expert panel on detection, evaluation, and treatment of high blood cholesterol in adults (adult treatment panel III), *JAMA* 285:2486-2497, 2001. The 2013 recommendations from the American College of Cardiology/American Heart Association indicate the above risk factors predict 10-year cardiovascular disease incidence (rather than CHD as in NCEP ATP III). *Circulation* doi: 10.1161/01.cir.0000437741.48606.98, 2013.

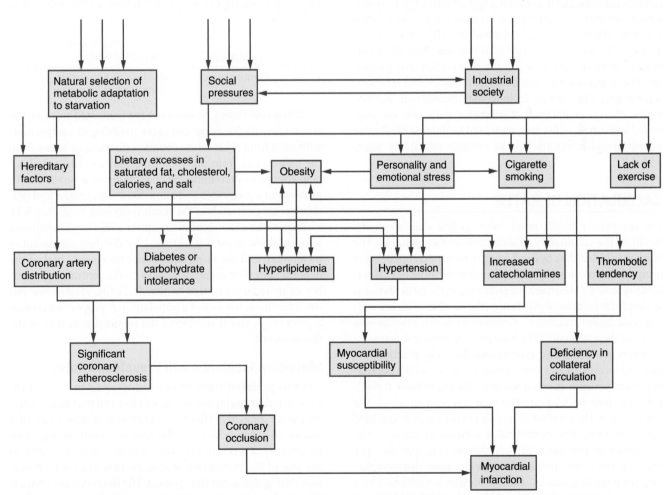

FIGURE 5-3 The web of causation for myocardial infarction: a current view. (From Friedman GD: *Primer of epidemiology*, ed 5, New York, 2004, McGraw-Hill.)

necessitate alternative research approaches, such as qualitative and ecological studies and studies of social institutions and processes. In turn, the examination of social and contextual origins will enlighten the interventions of public health practitioners.

For example, Buffardi, Thomas, Holmes, and colleagues (2008) analyzed the ecosocial and psychosocial correlates of diagnosis of sexually transmitted infections (STIs) among young adults. Specifically, they examined STI diagnosis within "contextual conditions" such as low income, "housing insecurity," childhood physical or sexual abuse, intimate partner abuse, gang participation, personal history of having been arrested, and drug/alcohol use. It was determined that STIs were statistically associated with housing insecurity, exposure to crime, and having been arrested. The researchers concluded that ecosocial or contextual conditions strongly enhance STI risk by increasing sexual risk behaviors and likelihood of exposure to infection.

In another study, Phillips (2011) applied an ecosocial perspective when examining the effects of social/contextual factors on adherence to antiretroviral therapy (ART) among black men who tested positive for human immunodeficiency virus (HIV). He examined both individual factors (e.g., psychological state of mind, psychological distress, illicit drug use) and interpersonal/social contextual factors (e.g., partner status, housing status, patient-provider relationship, social capital [groups/networks]). He concluded that adherence to the medication regimen was strongly associated with homelessness and how well the individual tolerated the ART. Other factors included the individual's state of mind and illicit drug use. Practice implications included the observation that providers should assess social and behavioral factors and intervene accordingly. This would include identification of psychological distress or presence of substance abuse. He also suggested assessment of housing status and facilitation of effective patient-provider relationships to mitigate tolerability issues with ART.

CALCULATION OF RATES

The community health nurse must analyze data about the health of the community to determine disease patterns. The nurse may collect data by conducting surveys or compiling data from existing records (e.g., data from clinic facilities or vital statistics records). Assessment data often are in the form of counts or simple frequencies of events (e.g., the number of people with a specific health condition). Community health practitioners interpret these raw counts by transforming them into rates.

Rates are arithmetic expressions that help practitioners consider a count of an event relative to the size of the population from which it is extracted (e.g., the population at risk). Rates are population proportions or fractions in which the numerator is the number of events occurring in a specified period of time. The denominator consists of those in the population at the specified time period (e.g., per day, per week, or per year), frequently drawing upon demographic data from the U.S. census. This proportion is multiplied by a constant (k) that is a multiple of 10, such as 1000, 10,000, or 100,000. The constant usually converts the resultant number

to a whole number, which is larger and easier to interpret. Thus, a rate can be the number of cases of a disease occurring for every 1000, 10,000, or 100,000 people in the population, as follows:

$$\text{Rate} = \frac{\text{Numerator}}{\text{Denominator}} = \frac{\text{Number of health events in a specified period}}{\text{Population in same area in same specified period}} \times k$$

When raw counts or numbers are converted to rates, the community health nurse can make meaningful comparisons with rates from other cities, counties, districts, or states; from the nation; and from previous time periods. These analyses help the nurse determine the magnitude of a public health problem in a given area and allow more meaningful and reliable tracking of trends in the community over time (Box 5-3).

Sometimes a ratio is used to express a relationship between two variables. A ratio is obtained by dividing one quantity by another, and the numerator is not necessarily part of the denominator. For example, a ratio could contrast the number of male births to that of female births. Proportions can describe characteristics of a population. A proportion is often a percentage, and it represents the numerator as part of the denominator.

Morbidity: Incidence and Prevalence Rates

The two principal types of morbidity rates, or rates of illness, in public health are incidence rates and prevalence rates. Incidence rates describe the occurrence of new cases of a disease (e.g., tuberculosis, influenza) or condition (e.g., teen pregnancy) in a community over a period of time relative to the size of the population at risk for that disease or condition during that same time period. The denominator consists of only those at risk for the disease or condition; therefore, known cases or those not susceptible (e.g., those immunized

TABLE 5-2 EXAMPLES OF RATE CALCULATIONS

MORBIDITY RATES	CRUDE RATES	SPECIFIC RATES
Incidence Rate	**Crude Death Rate**	**Infant Mortality Rate**
$\dfrac{\text{Number of new cases in given time period}}{\text{Population at risk in same time period}} \times 10,000$	$\dfrac{\text{Number of deaths in year}}{\text{Total population size}} \times 100,000$	$\dfrac{\text{Number of infant deaths} < 1 \text{ year of age}}{\text{Number of births in same year}} \times 1000$
$= \dfrac{75}{(4000 - 250 \text{ old cases})} = 0.2$	$\dfrac{1720}{200,000} = .00086$	$\dfrac{300}{45,000} = .00666$
$.02 \times 1000 = 20$ per 1000 per time period	$.0086 \times 100,000 = 860$ per 100,000 per year	$.00666 \times 1000 = 6.66$ per 1000 live births
Prevalence Rate	**Crude Birth Rate**	**Fertility Rate**
$\dfrac{\text{Number of existing cases}}{\text{Total population}} \times 1000 =$	$\dfrac{\text{Number of births in year}}{\text{Total population size}} \times 100,000$	$\dfrac{\text{Number of live births}}{\text{Number of women aged 15–44 years}} \times 1000$
$\dfrac{250}{4000} = .0625$	$\dfrac{2900}{200,000} = .0450$	$\dfrac{35,000}{500,000} = .07$ per women aged 15-44 years
$.0625 \times 1000 = 62.5$ per 1000	$.0145 \times 100,000 = 1450$ per 100,000 per year	$.07 \times 1000 = 70$ per 1000 women aged 15-44 years

against a disease) are subtracted from the total population (Table 5-2):

$$\text{Incidence rate} = \frac{\text{Number of new cases or events occurring in the population in a specified period}}{\text{Population at risk during same specified period}} \times k$$

The incidence rate may be the most sensitive indicator of the changing health of a community, because it captures the fluctuations of disease in a population. Although incidence rates are valuable for monitoring trends in chronic disease, they are particularly useful for detecting short-term changes in acute disease—such as those that occur with influenza or measles—in which the duration of the disease is typically short.

If a population is exposed to an infectious disease at a given time and place, the nurse may calculate the attack rate, a specialized form of the incidence rate. Attack rates document the number of new cases of a disease in those exposed to the disease. A common example of the application of the attack rate is food poisoning; the denominator is the number of people exposed to a suspect food, and the numerator is the number of people who were exposed and became ill. The nurse can calculate and compare the attack rates of illness among those exposed to specific foods to identify the critical food sources or exposure variables.

A prevalence rate is the number of all cases of a specific disease or condition (e.g., deafness) in a population at a given point in time relative to the population at the same point in time:

$$\text{Prevalence rate} = \frac{\text{Number of existing cases in population at a specified point in time}}{\text{Population at same specified point in time}} \times k$$

When prevalence rates describe the number of people with the disease at a specific point in time, they are sometimes called *point prevalences*. For this reason, cross-sectional studies frequently use them. *Period prevalences* represent the number of existing cases during a specified period or interval of time and include old cases and new cases that appear within the same period of time.

Prevalence rates are influenced by: the number of people who experience a particular condition (i.e., incidence) and the duration of the condition. A nurse can derive the prevalence rate *(P)* by multiplying incidence *(I)* by duration *(D)*: (P = I × D). An increase in the incidence rate or the duration of a disease increases the prevalence rate of a disease. With the advent of life-prolonging therapies (e.g., insulin for treatment of type 1 diabetes and antiretroviral drugs for treatment of HIV), the prevalence of a disease may increase without a change in the incidence rate. Those who survive a chronic disease without cure remain in the "prevalence pot" (Figure 5-4). For conditions such as cataracts, surgical removal of the cataracts permits many people to recover and thereby move out of the prevalence pot. Although the incidence has not necessarily changed, the reduced duration of the disease (because of surgery) lowers the prevalence rate of cataracts in the population.

Morbidity rates are not available for many conditions because surveillance of many chronic diseases is not widely conducted. Furthermore, morbidity rates may be subject to underreporting when they are available. Routinely collected birth and death rates, or mortality rates, are more widely available. Table 5-2 provides examples of calculating selected rates.

Other Rates

Numerous other rates are useful in characterizing the health of a population. For example, crude rates summarize the occurrence of births (i.e., crude birth rate), mortality (i.e., crude death rates), or diseases (i.e., crude disease rates) in the general population. The numerator is the number of events, and the denominator is the average population size or the population size at midyear (i.e., usually July 1) multiplied by a constant.

The denominators of crude rates represent the total population and not the population at risk for a given event; therefore, these rates are subject to certain biases in interpretation.

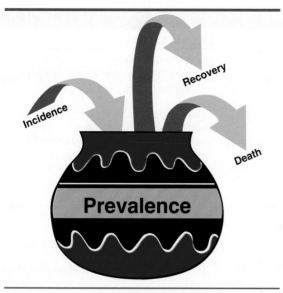

FIGURE 5-4 Prevalence pot: the relationship between incidence and prevalence. (Redrawn from Morton RF, Hebel JR, McCarter RJ: *A study guide to epidemiology and biostatistics,* ed 3, Gaithersburg, MD, 1990, Aspen Publishers.)

TABLE 5-3	COMPARISON OF U.S. MORTALITY RATES—2011 (PRELIMINARY)
DEATH RATE	**RATE PER 100,000**
Crude death rate	806.6
Age-adjusted death rate	740.6
Age-specific death rates (years):	
<1 (infant)	598.3
1-4	26.2
5-14	13.1
15-24	67.6
25-34	104.4
35-44	171.7
45-54	409.2
55-64	848.7
65-74	1845.0
75-84	4750.3
≥85	13,767.3

Modified from National Center for Health Statistics: Deaths: preliminary data for 2011, *Natl Vital Stat Rep* 61(6):1-52, 2012. Available from <http://www.cdc.gov/nchs/data/nvsr/nvsr61/nvsr61_06.pdf>.

Crude death rates are sensitive to the number of people at the highest risk for dying. A relatively older population will probably produce a higher crude death rate than a population with a more evenly distributed age range. Conversely, a young population will have a somewhat lower crude death rate. Similar biases can occur for crude birth rates (e.g., higher birth rates in young populations).

This distortion occurs because the denominator reflects the entire population and not exclusively the population at risk for giving birth. Age is one of the most common confounding factors that can mask the true distribution of variables. However, many variables, such as race and socioeconomic status, can also bias the interpretation of biostatistical data. Therefore, the nurse may use several approaches to remove the confounding effect of these variables on rates.

Age-specific rates characterize a particular age-group in the population and usually consider deaths and births. Determining the rate for specific subgroups of a population and using a denominator that reflects only that subgroup remove age bias:

$$\text{Age specific rate} = \frac{\substack{\text{Number of cases in a specific} \\ \text{age category in population} \\ \text{at a specified time}}}{\substack{\text{Population in the same age} \\ \text{category at the same} \\ \text{specified time}}} \times k$$

To characterize a total population using age-specific rates, one must compute the rate for each category separately. The reason is that a single summary rate, such as a mean, cannot adequately characterize a total population. Specific rates for other variables can be determined in a similar fashion (e.g., race-specific or gender-specific rates) (Table 5-3).

Age-adjustment or **standardization of rates** is another method of reducing bias when there is a difference between the age distributions of two populations. The nurse uses either the direct method or the indirect standardization method. The direct method selects a standard population, which is often the population distribution of the United States. This method essentially converts age-specific rates for age categories of the two populations to those of the standard population, and it calculates a summary age-adjusted rate for each of the two populations of interest. This conversion enables the nurse to compare the two rates as if both had the standard population's age structure (i.e., without the prior problem of age distortion).

The **proportionate mortality ratio** (PMR) method also describes mortality. It represents the percentage of deaths resulting from a specific cause relative to deaths from all causes. It is often helpful in identifying areas in which public health programs might make significant contributions to reducing deaths. In some situations, a high PMR may reflect a low overall mortality or reduced number of deaths resulting from other causes. Therefore the PMR requires consideration in the context of the mortality experience of the population.

$$\text{PMR} = \frac{\substack{\text{Number of deaths resulting from a specific} \\ \text{cause in a specific time period}}}{\substack{\text{Total number of deaths} \\ \text{in same time period}}}$$

Table 5-4 summarizes the advantages and disadvantages of crude, specific, and adjusted rates. Numerous other rates assess particular segments of the population. One that is followed closely by public health professionals is the infant mortality rate, calculated by dividing the number of deaths in infants less than 1 year old by the number of live births for that time period. This rate is considered a particularly sensitive indicator of the health of a community or nation, and reflective of the care provided to women and children. Disparities in infant mortality rates can be seen within subgroups

TABLE 5-4 ADVANTAGES AND DISADVANTAGES OF CRUDE, SPECIFIC, AND ADJUSTED RATES

RATE	ADVANTAGES	DISADVANTAGES
Crude	Actual summary rates Readily calculable for international comparisons (widely used despite limitations)	Populations vary in composition (e.g., age): therefore differences in crude rates are difficult to interpret
Specific	Homogeneous subgroup Detailed rates useful for epidemiological and public health purposes	Cumbersome to compare many subgroups of two or more populations
Adjusted	Summary statements Differences in composition of group "removed," permitting unbiased comparison	Fictional rates Absolute magnitude dependent on chosen standard population Opposing trends in subgroups masked

Modified from Mausner JS, Kramer S: *Mausner and Bahn epidemiology: an introductory text,* ed 2, Philadelphia, 1985, WB Saunders.

of the U.S. population, and the rate has ranked around 35th among developed countries (Organisation for Economic Cooperation and Development [OECD], 2013. Although the U.S. achieved its *Healthy People 2010* goal of 6.91 per 1000, the 2011 rate, 6.05 per 1000, has not significantly declined in the past decade. Black infants experienced an infant mortality rate 2.2 times higher than white infants (11.42 vs. 5.11 per 1000 in 2011) (Centers for Disease Control and Prevention [CDC], 2012). Socioeconomic status and racial disparities, which are frequently associated with inadequate prenatal care, prematurity, adolescent pregnancy, and smoking, are key risk factors. Table 5-5 provides a summary of the major public health rates. A standard epidemiology textbook contains more information.

CONCEPT OF RISK

The concepts of risk and risk factor are familiar to community health nurses whose practices focus on disease prevention. Risk refers to the probability of an adverse event (i.e., the likelihood that healthy people exposed to a specific factor will acquire a specific disease). *Risk factor* refers to the specific exposure factor, such as cigarette smoke, hypertension, high cholesterol, excessive stress, high noise levels, or

TABLE 5-5 MAJOR PUBLIC HEALTH RATES

RATE DENOMINATOR	RATES	USUAL	FACTOR RATE FOR UNITED STATES, 2011
Total population	Crude birth rate = Number of live births during the year/Average (midyear) population	Per 1000 population	14.0
	Crude death rate = Number of deaths during the year/Average (midyear) population	Per 100,000 population	813.0
	Age-specific death rate = Number of deaths among people of a given age group in 1 yr/Average (midyear) population in specified age group	Per 100,000 population	14.1 (5-14 yr) 420.4 (45-54 yr) 1995.6 (65 yr)
	Cause-specific death rate = Number of deaths from a stated cause in 1 yr/Average (midyear) population	Per 100,000 population	186.5 (heart diseases) 175.3 (malignant neoplasms)
Women aged 15-44 yr	Fertility rate = Number of live births during 1 year/Number of women aged 15 to 44 yr in same year	Per 1000 women aged 15-44 yr	68.6
Live births	Infant mortality rate = Number of deaths in 1 yr of children younger than 1 yr/Number of live births in same year	Per 1000 live births	6.6
	Neonatal mortality rate = Number of deaths in 1 yr of children younger than 28 days/Number of live births in same year	Per 1000 live births	4.3
	Maternal mortality rate (puerperal) = Number of deaths from puerperal causes in 1 yr/Number of live births in same year	Per 100,000 live births	12.7[†]
Live births and fetal deaths	Fetal death rate = Number of fetal deaths in 1 yr/Number of live births in same year	Per 1000 live births and fetal deaths	6.1*
	Perinatal mortality rate = Number of fetal deaths (>28 wk plus infant deaths <7 days)/Number of live births and fetal deaths (>28 wk during the same year)	Per 1000 live births and fetal deaths	6.5*

*2006 rate from National Center for Health Statistics: *Health, United States*, 2012. DHHS Publication No: 2012-1232. Available from <http://www.cdc.gov/nchs/data/hus/hus12.pdf>

[†]2007 rate from Centers for Disease Control and Prevention: *Deaths: final data for 2007*. National Vital Statistics Report 58:19. Available from <http://www.cdc.gov/nchs/data/nvsr58/nvsr58_19.pdf>

Modified from Mausner JS, Kramer S: *Mausner and Bahn epidemiology: an introductory text*, ed 2, Philadelphia, 1985, Saunders. Rates from U.S. Department of Health and Human Services/National Center for Health Statistics: *Health, United States, 2011*. DHHS Publication No: 2012-1232. Available from <http://www.cdc.gov/nchs/data/hus/hus11.pdf>.

an environmental chemical. Frequently, the exposure factor is external to the individual. Risk factors may include fixed characteristics of people, such as age, sex, and genetic makeup. Although these intrinsic risk factors are not alterable, certain lifestyle changes may reduce their effect. For example, weight-bearing exercise and taking calcium and hormonal supplements may reduce the risk of osteoporosis for susceptible women.

Epidemiologists describe disease patterns in aggregates and quantify the effects of exposure to particular factors on the disease rates. To identify specific risk factors, epidemiologists compare rates of disease for those exposed with those not exposed. One method for comparing two rates is subtracting the rate of nonexposed individuals from the exposed. This measure of risk is called the *attributable risk*; it is the estimate of the disease burden in a population. For example, if the rate of non–insulin-dependent diabetes were 5000 per 100,000 people in the obese population (i.e., those weighing more than 120% of ideal body weight) and 1000 per 100,000 people in the nonobese population, the attributable risk of non–insulin-dependent diabetes resulting from obesity would be:

$$4000 \text{ per } 100,000 \text{ people } \left(\text{i.e.,} \frac{5000}{100,000} - \frac{1000}{100,000} \right)$$

This means that 4000 cases per 100,000 people may be attributed to obesity. Thus a prevention program designed to reduce obesity could theoretically eliminate 4000 cases per 100,000 people in the population. Attributable risks are particularly important in describing the potential impact of a public health intervention in a community.

A second measure of the excess risk caused by a factor is the *relative risk ratio*. The relative risk is calculated by dividing the incidence rate of disease in the exposed population by the incidence rate of disease in the nonexposed population. In the previous example, a relative risk of 5 was obtained by dividing 5000/100,000 by 1000/100,000. This risk ratio suggests that an obese individual has a fivefold greater risk of diabetes than a nonobese individual. In general, a relative risk of 1 indicates no excessive risk from exposure to a factor; a relative risk of 1.5 indicates a 50% increase in risk; a relative risk of 2 indicates twice the risk; and a relative risk of less than 1 suggests that a factor may have a protective effect associated with a reduced disease rate.

The relative risk ratio forms the statistical basis for the risk factor concept. Relative risks are valuable indicators of the excess risk incurred by exposure to certain factors. They have been used extensively in identifying the major causal factors of many common diseases and they direct public health practitioners' efforts to reduce health risks.

Community health nurses may apply the concept of relative risk to suspected exposure variables to isolate risk factors associated with community health problems. For example, a community health nurse might investigate an outbreak of probable food-borne illness. The nurse may compare the incidence rate among those exposed to potato salad in a school cafeteria with the incidence rate among those not exposed. The relative risk

calculated from the ratio of these two incidence rates indicates the amount of excess risk for disease incurred by eating the potato salad. A community health nurse might also determine the relative risks for other suspected foods and compare them with the relative risk for potato salad. Attack rates are the calculated incidence rates for foods involved in food-borne illnesses. A food with a markedly higher relative risk than other foods might be the causal agent in a food-borne epidemic. The identification of the causal agent, or specific food, is critical to the implementation of an effective prevention program such as teaching proper food-handling techniques.

USE OF EPIDEMIOLOGY IN DISEASE PREVENTION

Primary Prevention

The central goals of epidemiology are describing the disease patterns, identifying the etiological factors in disease development, and taking the most effective preventive measures. These preventive measures are specific to the stage of disease progression or the natural history of disease, from prepathogenesis through resolution of the disease process. When interventions occur before disease development, they are called *primary prevention*. Primary prevention relies on epidemiological information to indicate those behaviors that are protective, or those that will not contribute to an increase in disease, and those that are associated with increased risk.

Two types of activities constitute primary prevention. Those actions that are general in nature and designed to foster healthful lifestyles and a safe environment are called *health promotion*. Actions aimed at reducing the risk of specific diseases are called *specific protection*. Public health practitioners use epidemiological research to understand practices that are likely to reduce or increase disease rates. For example, numerous research studies have confirmed that regular exercise is an important health promotion activity that has positive effects on general physical and mental health. Immunizations exemplify specific protection measures that reduce the incidence of particular diseases.

Secondary and Tertiary Prevention

Secondary prevention occurs after pathogenesis. Those measures designed to detect disease at its earliest stage, namely screening and physical examinations that are aimed at early diagnosis, are *secondary prevention*. Interventions that provide for early treatment and cure of disease are also in this category. Again, epidemiological data and clinical trials determining effective treatments are crucial in disease identification. Mammography, guaiac testing of feces, and the treatment of infections and dental caries are all examples of secondary prevention.

Tertiary prevention focuses on limitation of disability and the rehabilitation of those with irreversible diseases such as diabetes and spinal cord injury. Epidemiological studies examine risk factors affecting function and suggest optimal strategies in the care of patients with chronic advanced disease.

Establishing Causality

As discussed earlier, a principal goal of epidemiology is to identify etiological factors of diseases to encourage the most effective prevention activities and develop treatment modalities. During the last few decades, researchers recognized that many diseases have not one but multiple causes. Epidemiologists who examine disease rates and conduct population-focused research often find multiple factors associated with health problems. For example, cardiovascular disease rates may vary by location, ethnicity, and smoking status. Even infectious diseases often require not only an organism but also certain behaviors or conditions to cause exposure. Determining the extent that these correlates represent associative or causal relationships is important for public health practitioners who seek to prevent, diagnose, and treat disease.

Definitively establishing causality—particularly in chronic disease—is a challenge. The following six criteria establish the existence of a cause-and-effect relationship:

1. **Strength of association:** Rates of morbidity or mortality must be higher in the exposed group than in the nonexposed group. Relative risk ratios, or odds ratios, and correlation coefficients indicate whether the relationship between the exposure variable and the outcome is causal. For example, epidemiological studies demonstrated an higher relative risk for heart disease among smokers than among nonsmokers.
2. **Dose-response relationship:** An increased exposure to the risk factor causes a concomitant increase in disease rate. Indeed, the risk of heart disease mortality is higher for heavy smokers than for light smokers.
3. **Temporally correct relationship:** Exposure to the causal factor must occur before the effect, or disease. For heart disease, smoking history must precede disease development.
4. **Biological plausibility:** The data must make biological sense and represent a coherent explanation for the relationship. Nicotine and other tobacco-derived chemicals are toxic to the vascular endothelium. In addition to raising low-density lipoprotein (LDL) and decreasing high-density lipoprotein (HDL) cholesterol levels, cigarette smoking causes arterial vasoconstriction and platelet reactivity, which contribute to platelet thrombus formation.
5. **Consistency with other studies:** Varying types of studies in other populations must observe similar associations. Numerous studies using different designs have repeatedly supported the relationship between smoking and heart disease.
6. **Specificity:** The exposure variable must be necessary and sufficient to cause disease; there is only one causal factor. Although specificity may be strong causal evidence in the case of infectious disease, this criterion is less important today. Diseases do not have single causes; they have multifactorial origins.

The exposure variable of smoking is one of several risk factors for heart disease. Few factors are linked to a single condition. Furthermore, smoking is not specific to heart disease alone. It is a causal factor for other diseases such as lung and oral cancers. Additionally, smoking is not "necessary and sufficient" to the development of heart disease because there are nonsmokers who also have coronary heart disease. Therefore the causal criterion of specificity more frequently pertains to infectious diseases.

Although these criteria are useful in evaluating epidemiological evidence, it is important to note that causality is largely a matter of judgment. In reality, absolute causality is only rarely established. Rather, epidemiologists more commonly refer to suggested causal and associated factors. The effect of confounding variables makes it difficult to ascertain true relationships between the exposure and outcome variables. Confounding variables are independently related to both the dependent variable and the independent variable. Therefore, confounding variables may mask the true relationship between the dependent and independent variables. For example, Brunner and colleagues (2008) explained the need to control for physical activity when examining the relationship between dietary patterns and coronary heart disease. This is necessary because studies have shown that physical exercise is independently related to both diet (Sanchez et al., 2007) and heart disease (Blair and Morris, 2009) in some populations. The apparent association between fat intake and heart disease may be attributable to the difference in physical activity between those with and without heart disease. Those with heart disease may tend to have a higher fat intake and a lower activity level than those without heart disease. The outcome is not solely attributable to dietary fat.

By measuring the confounding variable, the researcher can statistically account for its effect in the analysis (e.g., by using multiple logistical regression analysis or stratification). A biostatistics text contains a discussion of these methods. Alternatively, matching subjects in treatment and control groups with respect to the confounding variable minimizes the effects of the confounder. Again, standardization for variables such as age is another method for managing spurious associations, which makes true relationships more apparent. An understanding of such relationships facilitates the practitioner's interpretation and application of findings.

Screening

As explained previously, a central aim of epidemiology is to describe the course of disease according to person, place, and time. Observations of the disease process may suggest factors that aggravate or ameliorate its progress. This information also assists in determining effective treatment and rehabilitation options (i.e., secondary or tertiary prevention approaches).

The purpose of screening is to identify risk factors and diseases in their earliest stages. Screening is usually a secondary prevention activity because indications of disease appear *after* a pathological change has occurred. In all forms of secondary and tertiary prevention, the identification of illness prompts the nurse to consider which forms of upstream prevention could have interrupted disease development.

Community health nurses commonly conduct screening programs. Community health nurses may devote a large portion of their work activities to performing physical examinations, promoting client self-examination, or conducting screening programs in schools, clinics, or community settings. Although secondary prevention activities are important and provide vital information on community health status, they focus on detecting existing disease. In contract, primary prevention and anticipatory guidance, which are hallmarks of community health nursing practice, attempt to prevent the development of disease.

There are several guidelines community health nurses should consider for screening programs. First, nurses must plan and execute adequate and appropriate follow-up treatment for patients who test positive for the disease. It is critical that nurses identify how to contact patients with positive findings and where to refer them, and then follow up with patients to determine whether they accessed care. Health fairs have been criticized for the lack of consistent follow-up of screening activities. Second, in the planning phase, the nurse should determine whether early disease diagnosis constitutes a real benefit to clients in terms of improved life expectancy or quality of life. Third, a critical prerequisite to screening is the existence of acceptable and medically sound treatment and follow-up. In the past, public health providers debated the ethical and practical arguments for implementing widespread HIV screening. Concern exists regarding the potential for stigmatic consequences for and discrimination against those who screen positively for a test; therefore, people implementing screening programs should establish procedures for ensuring confidentiality. These procedures, in conjunction with the development of effective antiviral treatments, have encouraged earlier and more widespread identification of HIV-positive individuals.

A screening program's procedures must also be cost-effective and acceptable to clients. Although colonoscopy is a routine and effective screening procedure for colon cancer, it is neither simple nor inexpensive. Although it is recommended periodically for all Americans with no known risk factors beginning at age 50 years, less than 60% of that group have undergone the procedure (CDC, 2012). Frequently, the reason is that the test is relatively expensive and unpleasant. Finally, a nurse should consider whether or not to screen a population on the basis of the significant costs of screening programs and procedures, follow-up for clients who test positive, and subsequent medical care (Box 5-4).

When developing a screening program, the community health nurse also must evaluate issues related to the validity of the screening test. Detecting clients with disease is the purpose of screening, and *sensitivity* is the test's ability to do so correctly. Conversely, *specificity* is the extent to which a test can correctly identify those who do not have disease. To obtain estimates of these two dimensions, the nurse must compare screening results with the best available diagnostic procedure. For a given test, the sensitivity and specificity tend to be inversely related to each other. When a test is highly sensitive, individuals without disease may be incorrectly

---

BOX 5-4   GUIDELINES FOR SCREENING PROGRAMS

- Screen for conditions in which early detection and treatment can improve disease outcome and quality of life.
- Screen populations that have risk factors or are more susceptible to the disease.
- Select a screening method that is simple, safe, inexpensive to administer, and acceptable to clients, and has acceptable sensitivity and specificity.
- Plan for the timely referral and follow-up of clients with positive results.
- Identify referral sources that are appropriate, cost-effective, and convenient for clients.
- Refer to evidenced-based screening recommendations published by the U.S. Preventive Services Taskforce (http://www.uspreventiveservicestaskforce.org/index.html) and other organizations.

---

labeled as testing positive. These false-positive results may cause stress and worry for clients and require further expense in the form of testing to confirm a diagnosis. With a highly sensitive test, specificity may be lower and the test may identify people as having the disease who are in fact disease-free (i.e., more false-positive results). If the sensitivity is low (and the specificity high), more patients who have the disease will have negative test results. These patients will not be diagnosed and thus presumably will receive care later in the disease process.

Optimally, a screening test should be maximally sensitive and specific. To a large extent, this depends on the precision of the test and the stringency of the cutoff point established for determining a positive result. In the past, for example, the tuberculosis skin testing criterion was based exclusively on a skin reaction of 10 mm of induration. As a result, some persons with the disease were missed because their skin reactions were less than 10 mm (false-negative results), and some with 10 mm of reaction were identified as having the disease but further testing showed they did not have it (false-positive results). More recently, risk factors have been considered in addition to induration, creating a more sensitive and specific TB screening algorithm. Currently, high-risk individuals, such as those with HIV disease, are considered to have a positive skin test result with 5 mm of induration, which is more sensitive than the criteria of 15 mm set for those of low risk. Use of the more stringent 5-mm criterion among those with HIV will lead to fewer false-negative results, and use of the 15-mm cut point among low-risk individuals will lead to fewer false-positive results (CDC, 2013). Table 5-6 shows the formula for calculating sensitivity and specificity.

Sensitivity and specificity reflect the *yield* of a screening test, which is the amount of detected disease. One measure of yield is the *positive predictive value* of a test, which is the proportion of true-positive results relative to all positive test results. On the basis of Table 5-6, the formula is $\frac{a}{a+b}$. The positive predictive value depends on the prevalence of undetected disease in a population. Screening for

TABLE 5-6	SENSITIVITY AND SPECIFICITY OF A SCREENING TEST	
SCREENING TEST RESULT	THOSE WITH DISEASE	THOSE WITHOUT DISEASE
Positive	True positives (a)	False positives (b)
Negative	False negatives (c)	True negatives (d)

$$\text{Sensitivity (in percent)} = \frac{\text{True positives}}{\text{All with disease}} = \frac{(a)}{(a+c)} \times 100$$

$$\text{Sensitivity (in percent)} = \frac{\text{True negatives}}{\text{All without disease}} = \frac{(d)}{(b+d)} \times 100$$

a rare disease such as phenylketonuria will yield a lower predictive value and more false-positive results. In phenylketonuria, a low predictive value is acceptable because the false-negative result has very serious consequences. The predictive value is also affected by the nature of the screened population. Screening only the individuals at high risk for a disease will produce a higher predictive value and can be a more efficient way to identify those with health problems. For example, diabetes screening in an American Indian, Mexican-American, or African-American adult population should produce a higher predictive value than screening the general adult population.

Surveillance

In addition to screening, surveillance is a mechanism for the ongoing collection of community health information. Monitoring for changes in disease frequency is essential to effective and responsive public health programs. Identifying trends in disease incidence or identifying risk factor status by location and population subgroup over time allows the community health nurse to evaluate the effectiveness of existing programs and implement interventions targeted to high-risk groups. Again, identifying new cases for calculating incidence rates is particularly useful in evaluating morbidity trends. However, this form of surveillance data is more difficult to collect, and public health practitioners can access the data only for selected diseases. Prevalence rates, mortality data, risk factor data, and hospital and health service data can help indicate a program's successes or deficiencies.

The CDC coordinates a system of data collection among federal, state, and local agencies. These groups compile numerous sets of data and base some of these data sets on the entire population (e.g., vital statistics data) and other collections on subsamples of the population (e.g., the National Health Interview Survey). The completeness of data reporting is variable because not all diseases are reportable. For example, practitioners are required to report only four sexually transmitted infections (i.e., HIV/acquired immunodeficiency syndrome [HIV/AIDS], syphilis, gonorrhea, and chlamydia) to local and state health departments. Furthermore, not all practitioners report cases on a regular basis and not all people with sexually transmitted infections actually seek care. Studies have indicated that practitioners also underreport childhood communicable diseases, such as chickenpox and mumps. The CDC conducts studies that estimate the magnitude of this underreporting problem.

Practitioners have a continuing need for comprehensive and systematically collected surveillance data that describe the health status of national and local subgroups. They use this information to evaluate the impact of programs on specific groups in a community.

HEALTHY PEOPLE 2020

Objectives for Data Collection and Reporting

PHI HP2020–7: Increase the proportion of population-based *Healthy People 2020* objectives for which national data are available for all major population groups.
PHI HP2020–8: Increase the proportion of *Healthy People 2020* objectives that are tracked regularly at the national level.
PHI HP2020–9: Increase the proportion of *Healthy People 2020* objectives for which national data are released within one year of the end of data collection.
PHI HP2020–10: Increase the percentage of vital events (births, deaths, fetal deaths) reported using the latest U.S. standard certificates of birth and death and the report of fetal death.

From U.S. Department of Health and Human Services: *Healthy People 2020: Public health infrastructure*, n.d. Retrieved July 2013 from <http://www.healthypeople.gov/2020/topicsobjectives2020/objectiveslist.aspx?topicId=35>.

For example, the effectiveness of *Healthy People 2020* depends on the availability of reliable baseline and continuing data to characterize health problems and evaluate goal achievement as listed in the *Healthy People 2020* box. *Healthy People 2020* addresses the ongoing need to extend the inclusiveness of such data collection systems (U.S. Department of Health and Human Services [USDHHS], n.d.). For example, simply documenting children's mortality rates resulting from injury is insufficient for the development of specific methods of injury prevention. Data on the number of injured children and the nature of injury (e.g., motor vehicle accidents, drowning, abuse) across the nation would increase the usefulness of surveillance information. The Health Indicators Warehouse compiles indicator data for initiatives like *Healthy People* and the Center for Medicare Services so that health status and service quality can be monitored (National Center for Health Statistics, n.d.).

Nurses need to describe trends in health and illness according to a community's locale, demographics, and risk factor status to intervene effectively on behalf of the people. They must compare the data for their locale with those of a relevant neighboring area (e.g., a census tract, city, county, state, or nation) to gain perspective on the magnitude of a local problem. Ideally, the nurse should have access to surveillance data at several different levels over a period of time. In some instances, community health nurses find it necessary to construct their own surveillance systems that are tailored to specific health conditions or available programs in their community. These smaller data collection systems help nurses evaluate programs when the data are readily accessible and are compatible with data from large city or statewide surveillance systems.

Clinical Example

In 1991, a cluster of neural tube defects (NTDs) occurred in babies born in Brownsville, Texas, within a span of 6 weeks. Further investigation indicated a rate of 27.1 cases per 10,000 live births, in contrast to the U.S. rate of approximately 8 per 10,000. The Brownsville rate was more than three times the national rate and represented an increased risk in Hispanic women. This increased risk was partially attributable to cultural and environmental factors, including lower socioeconomic status and migrant farm work. The investigators implemented a surveillance program which obtained more accurate population-based data. Additionally, the program implemented folic acid supplementation in Texas counties along the Mexican border. NTD rates dropped to 13 per 10,000 following the supplementation effort.

Research suggests that 50% to 70% of NTDs may be preventable with folic acid supplementation. This finding supports the fortification of bread and cereal products; in January 1998, the U.S. Food and Drug Administration mandated the addition of 140 μg of vitamin B per 100 g of most grain products. It is estimated that there has been a 24% reduction in the number of NTDs since grain fortification with folic acid began.

Dietary intake alone may be insufficient; also, the greatest risk to the fetus occurs within the first 3 to 8 weeks of pregnancy, a time when many women do not yet recognize their pregnancies. Therefore, the Centers for Disease Control and Prevention and U.S. Preventive Services Task Force recommend that all women of reproductive age consume 400 μg (0.4 mg) to 800 μg (0.8 mg) daily of synthetic folic acid in addition to dietary sources such as cereal or grain products, leafy green vegetables, and vitamin supplements.

Data from U.S. Preventive Services Task Force Folic Acid for the Prevention of Neural Tube Defects, 2009. Retrieved September 2013 from http://www.uspreventiveservicestaskforce.org/uspstf09/folicacid/folicacidrs.htm.

RESEARCH HIGHLIGHTS

Reducing Infant Mortality Rates Using the Perinatal Periods of Risk Model

The infant mortality rate is an accepted indicator for measuring a nation's health. The rate is representative of the health status and social well-being of any nation. Despite decreases in the past 50 years, infant mortality rates in the United States remain higher than in other industrialized countries. Using overall infant mortality rates to determine the effectiveness of interventions does not help communities focus on particular underlying factors contributing to the rates. Targeting interventions to the factors most responsible for the infant mortality rate should help reduce the rate more rapidly and effectively.

The Perinatal Periods of Risk (PPOR) model was developed to provide direction, focus, and suggestions for effective interventions. The model helps users identify and rank four factors as they contribute to the overall infant mortality rate: (1) mother's health before and between pregnancies, (2) maternal health care systems, (3) neonatal health care systems, and (4) infant health during the first year of life. The PPOR model is based on two major theoretical constructs: age of fetus-infant at death and birth weight. The PPOR model maps each death in a geographic region on the basis of birth weight and age at death, including fetal, neonatal, and postneonatal periods. The lowest birth weight infant deaths are combined into one cell

named the maternal health cell. The three remaining groups are put into cells suggesting the primary preventive focus for that group: maternal health, newborn health, and infant health. Multiple interventions are important in reducing infant mortality, and the PPOR model guides prioritizing interventions based on the cell contributing the most to infant mortality rates (Peck, Sappenfield, and Skala, 2010).

The PPOR model has been used in several programs and research studies to improve mother and infant health. In one intervention study (Chao, et al., 2010) the PPOR model was successfully used to improve birth outcomes in very-high-risk populations in the Antelope Valley area of Los Angeles County. On the basis of assessment findings per PPOR directives, efforts were made to infuse resources into the community and expand case management initiatives for high-risk mothers. Long-term findings indicated that the PPOR model was useful for identifying risk and social factors and that it helped mobilize community partnerships that resulted in widely improved birth outcomes.

Data from Chao SM, Donatoni G, Bemis C, et al: Integrated approaches to improve birth outcomes: perinatal periods of risk, infant mortality review and the Los Angeles mommy and baby project. *Matern Child Health J* 14:827-837, 2010; and Peck MG, Sappenfield WM, Skala J: perinatal periods of risk: a community approach for using data to improve women and infants' health. *Matern Child Health J* 14:864-874, 2010.

As stated, epidemiologists describe the course of disease over time. These secular trends are changes that occur over years or decades, such as the fairly recent, significant decline in lung cancer deaths in men and the gradual increase in lung cancer deaths in women. Frequently, epidemiologists document the associated patterns of treatment and intervention. In many instances, studies conducted by clinical epidemiologists provide this information. Cancer registries are a form of surveillance that document the prevalence and incidence of cancer in a community and document its course, treatment, and associated survival rates. The Surveillance, Epidemiology and End Results (SEER) program of the National Cancer Institute compiles national cancer data from existing cancer registries covering approximately 28% of the U.S. population (National Cancer Institute, 2013).

Public health practitioners need to conduct community surveys of population segments to plan for the segments' health. For example, a survey of the disabled population that assesses prevalence may also evaluate the adequacy of current services and project future needs.

USE OF EPIDEMIOLOGY IN HEALTH SERVICES

Epidemiological approaches, such as the ones presented here, can be used to describe the distribution of disease and its determinants in populations. However, epidemiological principles are also useful in studying population health care delivery and in describing and evaluating the use of community health services. For example, analyzing the ratio of health care providers to population size helps determine the system's ability to provide care. The clients' reasons for seeking care, the clients' payment methods, and the clients' satisfaction with care are also informative. Regardless of whether community health nurses or other health services professionals collect these data, the information is essential for those who strive to improve clients' access to quality health care.

Ultimately, nurses must apply epidemiological findings in practice. It is essential that they incorporate study results into prevention programs for communities and at-risk populations. Furthermore, the philosophy of public health and epidemiology dictates that nurses extend their application into major health policy decisions, because the aim of health policy planning is to achieve positive health goals and outcomes for improved population health.

A goal of policy development is to bring about desirable social changes. Epidemiological factors, history, politics, economics, culture, and technology influence policy development. The complex interaction of these factors may explain the challenges with application of epidemiological knowledge. Lung disease in the United States exemplifies the incomplete progress in implementing effective health policy. In the early 1950s, studies identified and conclusively linked cigarette smoking to lung cancer and heart disease (Doll and Hill, 1952). Beginning in the 1950s, public policies to address this health threat have included cigarette taxes, cigarette package warning labels, smoking restrictions in public areas, the institution of smoke-free workplaces, and restrictions on selling tobacco to minors. Despite the successes of the past 60 years, approximately 20% of Americans continue to smoke with rates particularly high among young adults, suggesting a continued need for focused and effective public health policy. Community health nurses should exercise "social responsibility" in applying epidemiological findings, but doing so will require the active involvement of the consumer. Community health nurses collaborating with community members can combine epidemiological knowledge and aggregate-level strategies to effect change on the broadest scale.

EPIDEMIOLOGICAL METHODS

Two epidemiological methods—descriptive epidemiology and analytic epidemiology—are used by community health nurses. This section describes both and gives examples of how they are used in population health.

Descriptive Epidemiology

Descriptive epidemiology focuses on the amount and distribution of health and health problems within a population.

Its purpose is to describe the characteristics of both people who are protected from disease and those who have a disease. Factors of particular interest are age, sex, ethnicity or race, socioeconomic status, occupation, and family status. Epidemiologists use morbidity and mortality rates to describe the extent of disease and to determine the risk factors that make certain groups prone to acquiring disease.

In addition to "person" characteristics, the place of occurrence describes disease frequency. For example, certain parasitic diseases, such as malaria and schistosomiasis, occur in tropical areas. Other diseases may occur in certain geopolitical entities. For example, gastroenteritis outbreaks often occur in communities with lax water quality standards. Time is the third parameter that helps define disease patterns. Epidemiologists may track incidence rates over a period of days or weeks (e.g., epidemics of infectious disease) or over an extended period of years (e.g., secular trends in the cancer death rate).

These person, place, and time factors can form a framework for disease analysis and may suggest variables associated with high versus low disease rates. Descriptive epidemiology can then generate hypotheses about the cause of disease, and *analytic epidemiology* approaches can test these hypotheses (Box 5-5).

Analytic Epidemiology

Analytic epidemiology investigates the causes of disease by determining why a disease rate is lower in one population group than in another. This method tests hypotheses generated from descriptive data and either accepts or rejects them on the basis of analytic research. The epidemiologist seeks to establish a cause-and-effect relationship between a preexisting condition or event and the disease (see previous section on causality). To determine this relationship, the epidemiologist may undertake two major types of research studies, *observational* and *experimental*.

Observational Studies

Epidemiologists frequently use *observational studies* for descriptive purposes, but they also use them to discover the etiology of disease. The investigator can begin to understand

BOX 5-5 AN EXAMPLE OF DESCRIPTIVE EPIDEMIOLOGY

The **p**erson-**p**lace-**t**ime model is illustrated by two measles outbreaks in Utah:

- *Person:* Initially, an unvaccinated 15-year-old student had contracted measles, likely from a trip to Europe. Subsequently, six more students contracted the illness.
- *Place:* Salt Lake County; three cases were "school transmission" and three cases were "household transmission."
- *Time:* The index case traveled to Europe during March 3-17, 2011. He attended school on March 21 and subsequently became ill. The other cases occurred between April 5 and April 17, 2011.

From Centers for Disease Control and Prevention: Two measles outbreaks after importation— Utah, March-June 2011. *MMWR Morb Mortal Wkly Rep* 62(12):222-225, 2013. Available from <http://www.cdc.gov/mmwr/pdf/wk/mm6212.pdf>.

the factors that contribute to disease by observing disease rates in groups of people differentiated by experience or exposure. For example, differences in disease rates may occur in the obese compared with the nonobese, in smokers compared with nonsmokers, and in those with high stress levels compared with those with low stress levels. These characteristics (i.e., obesity, smoking, and stress) are called *exposure variables*.

Unlike experimental studies, observational studies do not allow the investigator to manipulate the specific exposure or experience or to control or limit the effects of other extraneous factors that may influence disease development. For example, life stress is related to depression. People with low socioeconomic status also have high depression rates. People with low socioeconomic status frequently experience greater life stresses; therefore, the confounding factor of socioeconomic status makes it more difficult to demonstrate the effect of stress on depression. The three major study designs used in observational research are cross-sectional, retrospective, and prospective studies.

Cross-Sectional Studies. Cross-sectional studies, sometimes called prevalence or correlational studies, examine relationships between potential causal factors and disease at a specific time (Figure 5-5). Surveys that simultaneously collect information about risk factors and disease exemplify this design. For example, the National Health and Nutrition Examination Survey (NHANES) has collected cross-sectional data regarding current dietary practices, physical status, and health in adults and children in the United States since the early 1970s (CDC, 2013). Data from the NHANES studies have been analyzed and compared over the years by a number of researchers and have provided important health information.

For example, NHANES studies have tracked contemporary behavior issues such as fast-food consumption in U.S. adults, showing recent declines in the total daily calories consumed from these sources. Although overall fast-food consumption has declined from approximately 13% of daily caloric intake to 11.3% in the period ending 2010, this decline was not shared by all groups with non-Hispanic African Americans consuming more fast food than other groups, as did all persons who were overweight (Fryar & Ervin, 2013). NHANES has conducted interviews and physical examinations on youth, nutrient studies on children, and dietary surveys of older Americans, contributing important data that suggest risk factors that can be examined through more rigorous study designs.

Although a cross-sectional study can identify associations among disease and specific factors, it is impossible to make causal inferences because the study cannot establish the temporal sequence of events (i.e., the cause preceded the effect). For example, the NHANES was unable to determine whether high salt intake precedes hypertension—thus making it a causal factor—or whether they are unrelated. Therefore cross-sectional studies have limitations in discovering etiological factors of disease. These studies can help identify preliminary relationships that other analytic designs may explore further; therefore, they are hypothesis-generating studies.

Retrospective Studies. Retrospective studies compare individuals with a particular condition or disease and those who do not have the disease. These studies determine whether cases, or a diseased group, differ in their exposure to a specific factor or characteristic relative to controls, or a nondiseased group. To make unambiguous comparisons, investigators select the cases according to explicitly defined criteria regarding the type of case and the stage of disease. Investigators also

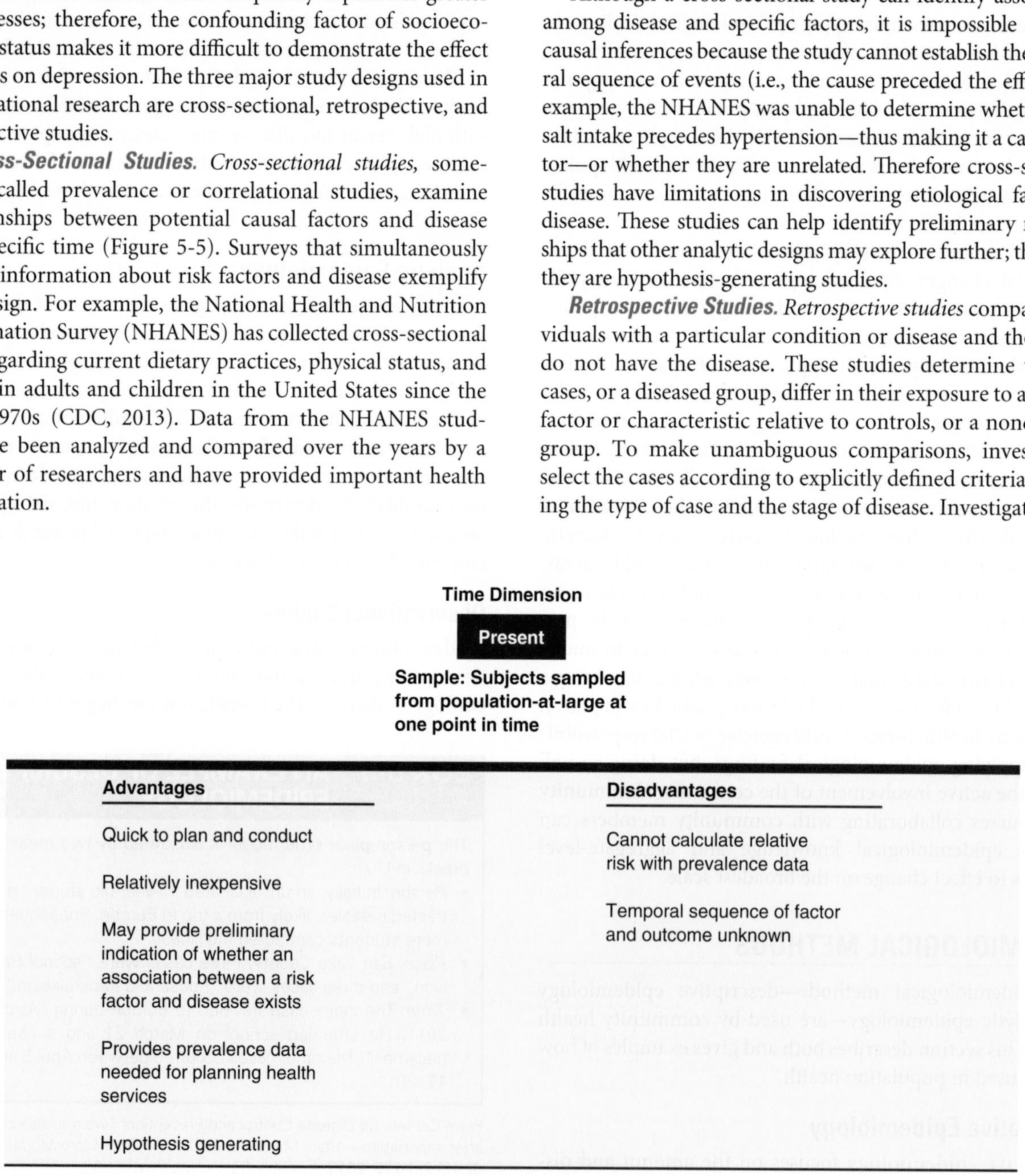

Time Dimension

Present

Sample: Subjects sampled from population-at-large at one point in time

Advantages	Disadvantages
Quick to plan and conduct	Cannot calculate relative risk with prevalence data
Relatively inexpensive	
May provide preliminary indication of whether an association between a risk factor and disease exists	Temporal sequence of factor and outcome unknown
Provides prevalence data needed for planning health services	
Hypothesis generating	

FIGURE 5-5 Cross-sectional, or prevalence, study.

select a control group from the general population that is characteristically similar to the cases (Figure 5-6).

Frequently, people hospitalized for diseases that are not under study become controls if they do not share the exposure or risk factor under study. For example, a researcher may select patients with heart disease to be controls in a study of patients with lung cancer. However, this choice may introduce serious bias because the two groups often share the risk factor of smoking. The methods of data collection must be the same for both groups to prevent further introduction of bias into the study. Therefore it is desirable for interviewers to remain unaware of which subjects are cases and which are controls.

In retrospective studies, data collection extends back in time to determine previous exposure or risk factors. Investigators analyze study data by comparing the proportion of subjects with disease, or cases, who possess the exposure or risk factors with the corresponding proportion in the control group. A greater proportion of exposed cases than of exposed controls suggests a relationship between the disease and the risk factor.

Investigators often use retrospective study designs because these designs address the question of causality better than cross-sectional studies. Retrospective studies also require fewer resources and less data collection time than prospective

studies. Many examples of *retrospective,* or *case-control,* studies exist in the literature. One classic example is Doll and Hill's (1952) investigation of risk factors for lung cancer. They compared exposure rates for cases in which lung cancer was diagnosed with those in the control group, in whom cancer was diagnosed outside the chest and oral cavity. The researchers recorded detailed smoking histories in all subjects. Compared with the controls, a significantly higher proportion of patients with lung cancer smoked. This study yielded the hypothesis that smoking may be etiologically related to lung cancer.

Prospective Studies. *Prospective studies* monitor a group of disease-free individuals to determine whether and when disease occurs (Figure 5-7). These individuals, or the *cohort,* have a common experience within a defined time period. For example, a birth cohort consists of all people born within a given time period. The study assesses the cohort with respect to an exposure factor associated with the disease and thus classifies it at the beginning of the study. The study then monitors the cohort for disease development. The investigator compares the disease rates for those with a known exposure and the disease rates for those who remain unexposed. The study observes subjects prospectively; therefore it summarizes data collected over time by the incidence rates of new

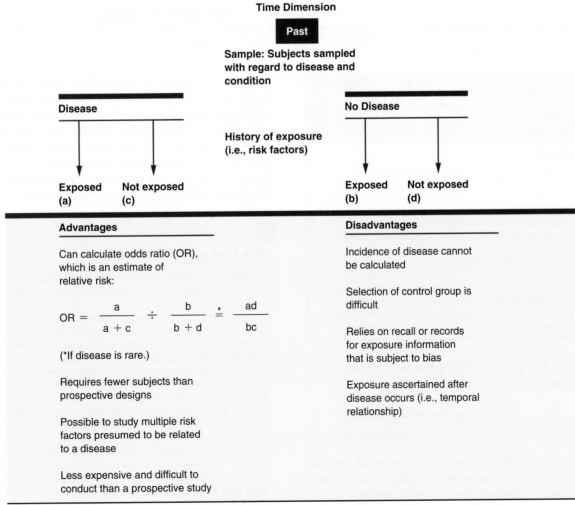

Time Dimension

Past

Sample: Subjects sampled with regard to disease and condition

Disease   No Disease

History of exposure (i.e., risk factors)

Exposed (a)   Not exposed (c)   Exposed (b)   Not exposed (d)

Advantages	Disadvantages
Can calculate odds ratio (OR), which is an estimate of relative risk:	Incidence of disease cannot be calculated
$$OR = \frac{a}{a+c} \div \frac{b}{b+d} \stackrel{*}{=} \frac{ad}{bc}$$	Selection of control group is difficult
(*If disease is rare.)	Relies on recall or records for exposure information that is subject to bias
Requires fewer subjects than prospective designs	Exposure ascertained after disease occurs (i.e., temporal relationship)
Possible to study multiple risk factors presumed to be related to a disease	
Less expensive and difficult to conduct than a prospective study	

FIGURE 5-6 Retrospective, or case-control, study.

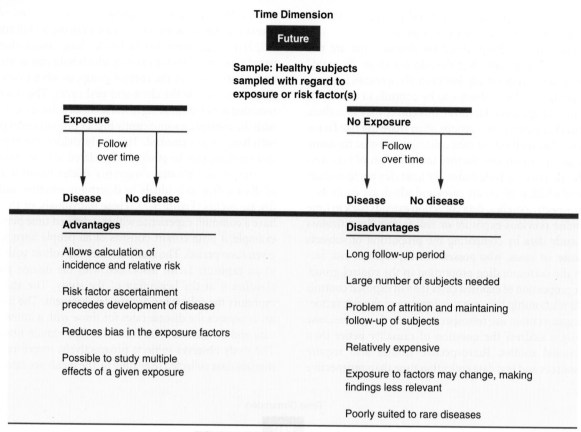

Time Dimension

Future

Sample: Healthy subjects sampled with regard to exposure or risk factor(s)

Exposure	No Exposure
Follow over time	Follow over time
Disease No disease	Disease No disease

Advantages	Disadvantages
Allows calculation of incidence and relative risk	Long follow-up period
Risk factor ascertainment precedes development of disease	Large number of subjects needed
Reduces bias in the exposure factors	Problem of attrition and maintaining follow-up of subjects
Possible to study multiple effects of a given exposure	Relatively expensive
	Exposure to factors may change, making findings less relevant
	Poorly suited to rare diseases

FIGURE 5-7 Prospective, or cohort, study.

BOX 5-6   COMPARISON OF TIME FACTORS IN RETROSPECTIVE AND PROSPECTIVE STUDY DESIGNS

Cohort Study

Girls with bacteriuria → Women with renal disease
Girls with sterile urine → Women without renal disease

Case-Control Study

Girls with bacteriuria ← Women with renal disease
Girls with sterile urine ← Women without renal disease

PAST—————PRESENT (BEGINNING)—————FUTURE

Comparison of time factors in prospective design (i.e., cohort) and retrospective design (i.e., case-control) approaches to studying the possible effect of childhood bacteriuria on renal disease in adult women.

---

cases (Box 5-6). Again, comparing two incidence rates produces a measure of relative risk.

$$\text{Relative risk} = \frac{\text{Incidence rate among exposed}}{\text{Incidence rate among unexposed}}$$

The relative risk indicates the extent of excess risk incurred by exposure relative to nonexposure. A relative risk of 1 suggests no excess risk resulting from exposure, whereas a relative risk of 2 suggests twice the risk of having disease from exposure.

Prospective studies, or *longitudinal, cohort,* or *incidence* studies, are advantageous because they obtain more reliable information about the cause of disease than do other study methodologies. These studies establish a stronger temporal relationship between the presumed causal factors and the effect than do retrospective and cross-sectional studies. Calculations of incidence rates and relative risks provide a valuable indicator of the level of risk that exposure creates.

ETHICAL INSIGHTS

The Tuskegee Syphilis Study

In 1932 the U.S. Public Health Service (PHS) began a longitudinal-experimental study of 600 African-American sharecroppers, 399 of whom had syphilis and 201 who did not. The study was conducted in one of the poorest counties of Alabama, and the subjects were unaware that they had syphilis; they were told they were being treated for "bad blood." Enticed by the promise of free medical care and meals, the subjects joined the study without knowledge of their disease, its treatment, or the study procedures. The experimental group was initially treated with ineffective doses of the treatments of the time, bismuth or mercury, and later with aspirin. Even when penicillin became available in the late 1940s, these subjects were actively denied treatment. For 40 years, these men were followed up by PHS investigators affiliated with the Tuskegee Institute and hospital, who claimed to be observing the differences in the progression of the disease in blacks in comparison with the control group. During the course of the study, many subjects died of syphilis or other causes, numerous wives became infected, and children were born with congenital syphilis.

In 1972, a former venereal disease interviewer, Peter Buxtun, "blew the whistle" on the study, and reports were published in newspapers. Only after the public became outraged about the unethical nature of the study did the Centers for Disease Control and Prevention and the PHS move to end it. In 1973, the National Association for the Advancement of Colored People (NAACP) won a $10 million class action suit on behalf of the subjects. In 1997, President Bill Clinton formally apologized to the few survivors and their families for the harm inflicted on these men and their families in the name of public health research.

The Tuskegee Study raises questions about how a study could proceed without informing and seeking consent of participants, how available treatment could be withheld, and how government researchers could pursue an unethical research plan without periodic review and questioning. Furthermore, the racial and discriminatory issues suggest disturbing questions for researchers and practicing nurses to contemplate, one being that the Tuskegee Study contributes to a legacy of distrust that minorities may harbor toward both the health care delivery system and research programs.

Data from Centers for Disease Control and Prevention: *The Tuskegee timeline,* 2013. Retrieved July 2013 from <http://www.cdc.gov/tuskegee/timeline.htm>; and Infoplease: *The Tuskegee syphilis experiment,* 2005, Pearson Education. Retrieved July 2013 from <www.infoplease.com/ipa/A0762136.html>.

However, certain disadvantages are inherent in the prospective design. It is costly in terms of resources and staff to monitor a cohort over time, and lengthy studies result in subject attrition. Problems arising from the nature of chronic diseases may compound these logistical dilemmas. Frequently, chronic diseases have long latency periods between exposure and symptom manifestation. Furthermore, the onset of chronic conditions may be insidious, making it extremely difficult to document the incidence of disease. In addition, many diseases do not have a unifactorial cause (i.e., single variable) because many interacting factors influence disease. These problems do not negate the benefits of prospectively designed epidemiological studies; rather, they suggest a need to carefully plan and tailor a study specifically to the disease and the study's purpose.

The literature contains numerous prospective studies. In many cases, these studies have been instrumental in substantiating causal links between specific risk factors and disease. A classic example is a Doll and Hill cohort study of subjects who eventually developed lung cancer during the follow-up period (1956). Doll and Hill originally completed questionnaires on a cohort of physicians in Great Britain. Next, they classified the subjects according to several variables, emphasizing the number of cigarettes smoked. In 4½ years, they accessed death certificate data. These data revealed a higher mortality rate resulting from lung cancer and coronary thrombosis among smoking physicians compared with nonsmokers. The death rate for heavy smokers was 166 per 100,000 versus 7 per 100,000 for nonsmokers. Combining these two incidence rates in a measure of excess risk indicated that heavy smokers were 23.7 times more likely to develop lung cancer than nonsmokers:

$$\text{Relative risk} = \frac{166}{100,000} \div \frac{7}{100,000} = 23.7$$

These findings in a prospective study provided strong epidemiological support for smoking as a risk factor for lung cancer.

Another well-known prospective study is the Framingham Heart Study, which has followed an essentially healthy cohort of Framingham, Massachusetts, residents for more than 50 years. Findings from the study suggested that serum cholesterol level and other risk factors are associated with the future development of cardiovascular disease (Kramarow, Lubitz and Francis, 2013). The Framingham Study and subsequent "offspring studies" helped form the basis for later experimental studies aimed at reducing serum cholesterol through diet modification or drug therapy to ultimately lower the incidence rate of coronary heart disease.

The Nurses' Health Study was initiated in 1976 with 122,000 registered nurses, with the intent of examining the long-term consequences of oral contraceptives. The initial cohort still returns questionnaires every 2 years, and data have been collected on diet and nutrition, smoking, hormone use, and menopause as well as various chronic illnesses. In 1989 the Nurses' Health Study II was initiated to study lifestyle issues, contraception, and illness patterns in younger women, and in 2008 a third study was begun looking at similar issues in another cohort.

These studies continue to monitor nurses' changing health status and risk factors and to examine factors associated with the development of numerous health conditions, such as breast cancer and heart disease (Nurses' Health Study, 2013). For example, research using Nurses' Health Study data has determined that regular use of nonsteroidal anti-inflammatory drugs (i.e., acetaminophen) does not reduce the incidence of skin cancer (Jeter et al., 2012) or breast cancer (Eliassen et al., 2009). Similarly, research from the nurses' health studies have shown that although consumption of sugar-sweetened beverages is associated with higher risk of type 2 diabetes, caffeine intake lowers the risk (Bhupatiraju et al., 2013). Last, Arkema and colleagues (2013) used data from the Nurses' Health Study to determine that exposure to ultraviolet-B radiation from the sun is associated with lower risk of rheumatoid arthritis, and a team led by Qi (2012) observed that nurses' body mass index (BMI) values increased proportionally to the number of hours they reported watching television.

Experimental Studies

Another type of analytic study is the experimental design, called the *randomized clinical trial* (Figure 5-8). Epidemiological investigations apply experimental methods to test treatment and prevention strategies. The investigator randomly assigns subjects at risk for a particular disease to an experimental or a control group. The investigator observes both groups for the occurrence of disease over time, but only the experimental group receives intervention, although often the control group receives a placebo. The primary statistical analysis is based on "intention to treat," that is, all subjects remain assigned to the original treatment group, regardless of whether subjects may have decided on their own to discontinue or change their therapy. For example, if a subject in a drug trial who is assigned to the active medication experiences side effects possibly from this medication, and therefore discontinues the medication, this subject still is

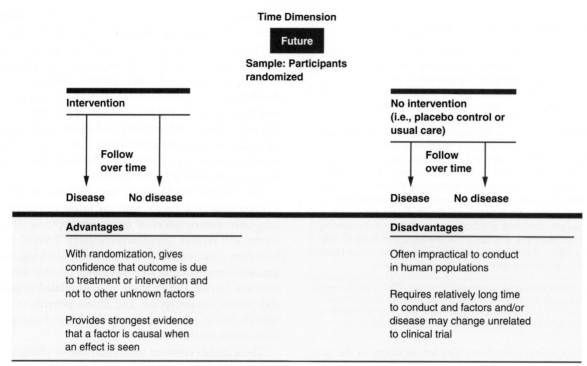

FIGURE 5-8 Experimental study, or clinical trial.

considered within the active drug group for the purpose of statistical testing. The change in category from treatment to no treatment, or vice versa, is called a "crossover" and may decrease the likelihood of finding a significant effect for the active treatment.

Theoretically, it is possible to introduce a harmful exposure or risk factor as the experimental factor; however, ethical considerations usually prohibit the use of human subjects for these purposes. For example, it is unacceptable to require an experimental group to smoke cigarettes in an experiment; therefore the investigator uses case-control or cohort epidemiological designs. This limitation usually restricts experimental epidemiological studies to prophylactic and therapeutic clinical trials. Experimental studies testing vaccines and medications for safety and efficacy are examples.

The experimental design is also useful for investigating chronic disease prevention. Thus experimental studies may help evaluate community health nursing interventions. For example, they may help determine the effectiveness of a sex education program in preventing high rates of teenage pregnancy or the feasibility of an AIDS prevention program among intravenous drug users. Randomized trials were used to evaluate the Nurse-Family Partnership program, which established the long-term positive effects nurse home visits had on high-risk pregnant women and their children in comparison with those who did not receive home visits (Olds et al., 2010).

CASE STUDY

Using an Epidemiological and Public Health Approach to Managing a Food-Borne Outbreak

Nurses working in schools, day-care centers, camps, and other facilities where food is served must be cognizant of safe food-handling principles. Furthermore, they must be aware of the potential for transmitting disease if proper procedures are not followed. Outbreaks of food-borne illness must be assessed and managed, and often it is the community health nurse who initiates and participates in this process. The following is a scenario in which the nurse utilized the nursing process to analyze and intervene in such an epidemic.

Assessment
On Wednesday, October 4, the school nurse at Greenly Elementary School saw 8 students who complained of abdominal cramping, diarrhea, and fever. Parents of the sick students were called, and the students were sent home. On Thursday, the nurse was alerted to a large number of absent students and teachers. Specifically, 62 students and 10 teachers were absent. Most reported diarrhea symptoms. Because the absentee rate of 10% exceeded the average daily rate of 4% for the 620-student school and because the nurse determined that the large number of diarrhea cases suggested an epidemic, the local public health department was notified.

Public health officials arrived at the school and began to assess students still at school and those who were recovering at home. Stool culture specimens were collected and sent to the state laboratory. Results indicated that the organism causing illness was in most cases *Shigella sonnei*, the most commonly found form of the bacteria. Persons with severe symptoms were referred to their physicians for possible antibiotic therapy. Food histories of meals eaten both at school and outside of school were taken.

Friday saw a continuing increase in absenteeism of students and staff reporting gastrointestinal illness. Public health specialists defined the criteria for identifying cases on the basis primarily of positive laboratory results, symptoms of diarrhea or vomiting, fever with nausea or abdominal pain, or all of these. Cafeteria staff were interviewed, and it was determined that one staff member had had diarrhea over the previous weekend but had returned to work on Monday. Public health staff continued to take dietary histories of affected and unaffected persons and constructed rates of illness for all foods served in the cafeteria beginning on Friday of the previous week. These data are displayed in the following table.

Using an Epidemiological and Public Health Approach to Managing a Food-Borne Outbreak—cont'd

From the data, it can be seen that students who ate lunch at school on Tuesday and ate fajitas and salad had higher rates of illness than those who did not. Therefore it was concluded that the outbreak of *Shigella* could be attributed to a food source.

Diagnosis

Determining the likely cause of the outbreak was important in specifying a diagnosis and directing the planning of an intervention. The following diagnosis was formulated:

Increased risk for infectious diarrhea among elementary school children related to inadequate hygiene and food handling practices as evidenced by a 19% increase in reported cases within a 4-day period.

Planning

The school nurse, in conjunction with public health specialists, determined that several groups should be targeted in order to eliminate the further spread of disease. They identified a need to assist families in understanding the nature of the disease, how to care for their children who were ill, and how to prevent the spread at home. Within the school, there was a need to review food-handling practices and the training that cafeteria workers received. Staff, including teachers, also required information about *Shigella* and how it should be prevented in the everyday lives of students. Needs of special ages and developmental levels of children were also important. A formal plan of what needed to be done, by whom, and when was drawn up. Research into the nature and prevention of *Shigella* was gathered from the Centers for Disease Control and Prevention and the local health department, among other sources. Health department staff developed a plan to release information to the public about the prevention of gastrointestinal illnesses, as many of these diseases are easily spread and so many students were already ill.

Long-Term Goal
- An absence of cases of infectious diarrhea

Short-Term Goals
- Treatment and recovery of all identified cases of diarrhea
- Implementation of an effective program of hygienic practices among students and staff
- Implementation of a food-handling program for all cafeteria workers
- Adequate informing of the larger community in order to prevent spread of the epidemic

Intervention

The school nurse took a central leadership role, directing action within the school aimed at staff, students, and student families. Teaching of appropriate hand washing was stressed. Hand-washing facilities were inspected for soap, paper towels, and running water. Food preparation guidelines were reviewed with staff, and policies regarding remaining at home when ill were reiterated. The health department staff provided technical assistance and made recommendations. They informed community physicians about surveillance and reporting requirements and provided information regarding case identification and treatment regimens. Day care centers and preschools were advised to watch for diarrhea outbreaks and to adhere to strict hand-washing and diaper-handling practices, as these facilities tend to be high-risk areas for the transmission of organisms such as *Shigella*. The media were contacted to elicit their help in disseminating correct and useful information to the community.

Evaluation

Immediate evaluation involved monitoring the decline in *Shigella* cases both within the school and in the larger community. The school nurse noted that rates of absenteeism returned to normal on the following Monday. She determined that all classes had received hygiene instruction within the following 2 weeks and that all teachers had received a flyer with specific information about *Shigella*, its care, and its prevention. She observed that bathrooms had filled soap dispensers, that friendly signs reminding students to wash hands were posted near sinks, and that students were given the opportunity to wash hands before lunch and snacks. The public health department, likewise, continued surveillance activities after encouraging physicians to collect and submit stool culture specimens for suspected cases and to report cases to the health department. Rates of diarrhea declined rapidly in the week after the school outbreak. The infection did not spread to other schools or community groups. This outcome can be attributed to successful epidemic management, yet surveillance remains critical if the public's health is to be protected.

Levels of Prevention
Primary
- Teach students and staff about hand washing and hygienic practices.
- Maintain a system that promotes safe food-handling practices.
- Exclude those with symptoms from school or food handling.

Secondary
- Collect stool culture specimens from all symptomatic individuals.
- Treat those with advanced diarrhea symptoms with antibiotics.
- Exclude those with positive culture results from food handling, and those with symptoms from school.
- Advise families and individuals in the care of those with diarrhea.

Tertiary
- Treat and counsel those determined to be carriers of *Shigella*.

Information on *Shigella* infections is available at www.cdc.gov/nczved/dfbmd/disease_listing/shigellosis_gi.html.

NUMBER EXPOSED BY MEAL AND FOOD ITEM (N = 143)

EXPOSURE VARIABLE (FOOD EATEN)	NUMBER WHO ATE		NUMBER WHO DID NOT EAT		
	ILL (A)	NOT ILL (B)	ILL (C)	NOT ILL (D)	ODDS RATIO*
Ate on Monday	47	60	18	18	0.78
Ate on Tuesday:	63	57	3	20	7.37
Fajitas	57	52	8	26	4.56
Salad	44	21	24	54	4.7
Salsa	26	29	40	48	1.07
Tortillas	48	53	16	26	1.47
Beans	29	32	34	48	1.28
Milk	53	56	11	23	1.98
Ate on Wednesday	21	64	43	15	0.11

*Odds ratios were calculated with the formula: ad/bd.

Modified from Texas Department of Health, *Shigella* outbreak in an elementary school, *Dis Prev News* 55(6):1-3, 1995.

VETERANS' HEALTH

An Epidemiological Examination of Suicide Among Veterans

Suicide among our nation's veterans has been recognized as a very serious problem. A 2012 report from the Department of Veterans' Affairs suggested that about 22 veterans die from suicide each day. Among their findings are the following:

- Veterans who die by suicide are much more likely to be male.
- Veterans who take their own lives are generally older than nonveterans who commit suicide (most are older than 50 years).
- The number of suicides has remained fairly stable over the last several years.

The research suggested that the first 4 weeks after the end of service should be a time of intensive monitoring and case management. Among interventions, the researcher encouraged (1) promotion of public education campaigns, (2) evaluation of routine suicide risk assessments, and (3) screening to better identify life stressors and concerns. The goal of screening and public education is to provide assistance earlier, increasing the numbers of veterans who received enhanced follow-up care. This goal is seen as critical to reducing the scope of this tragedy.

Data from Kemp J, Bossarte R: *Suicide data report, 2012*. Department of Veterans Affairs, Suicide Prevention Program, 2012. Available from <http://www.va.gov/opa/docs/Suicide-Data-Report-2012-final.pdf>. Accessed September 2013.

SUMMARY

Epidemiology offers the community health nurse methods to quantify the extent of health problems in the community and provides a body of knowledge about risk factors and their association with disease. At each step of the nursing process, epidemiological applications support the practice of the community health nurse. Compiling descriptive data from surveys or studies contributes to the nurse's understanding of the community's health level. In assessing community problems, epidemiological rates describe the magnitude of disease and provide support for community diagnoses. Epidemiological studies suggest interventions and their potential efficacy, information that is useful in planning prevention and intervention approaches. Evaluation studies using epidemiological methods, either reported in literature or conducted by community health nurses, are essential for providing optimal research-based care.

LEARNING ACTIVITIES

1. Compile a database of relevant demographic and epidemiological data for your community by examining census reports, vital statistics reports, city records, and other sources in libraries and agencies.
2. Using numerators from vital statistics and denominators from census data, compute crude death and birth rates for your community.
3. Compare morbidity and mortality rates for your community with those of the state and the nation. Determine whether your community rates are higher or lower, and hypothesize about reasons for any disparities.
4. Consult *Healthy People 2020* to find the national goals for selected causes of morbidity and mortality. Identify groups at an increased risk for these selected diseases. What are the approaches suggested by these documents for reducing the rates of disease? How can this information be useful in planning for your community?

ⓔ EVOLVE WEBSITE

http://evolve.elsevier.com/Nies

- NCLEX Review Questions
- Case Studies
- Glossary

REFERENCES

Arkema EV, Hart JE, Bertrand KA, et al: Costenbader, KH: Exposure to ultraviolet-B and risk of developing rheumatoid arthritis among women in the Nurse's Health Study, *Ann Rheum Dis* 72:506–511, 2013.

Bhupathiraju SN, Pan A, Malik VS, et al: Caffeinated and caffeine-free beverages and risk of type 2 diabetes, *Am J Clin Nutr* 97:155–166, 2013.

Blair SN, Morris M: Healthy hearts—and the universal benefits of being physically active: physical activity and health, *Ann Epidemiol* 19:253–256, 2009.

Brunner EJ, Mosdol A, Witte DR, et al: Dietary patterns and 15-y risks of major coronary events, diabetes, and mortality, *Am J Clin Nutr* 87(5):1414–1421, 2008.

Buffardi AL, Thomas KK, Holmes KK, et al: Moving upstream: ecosocial and psychosocial correlates of sexually transmitted infections among young adults in the United States, *Am J Public Health* 98(5):1128–1136, 2008.

Centers for Disease Control and Prevention: Prevalence of actions to control high blood pressure—20 states, 2005, *MMWR Morb Mortal Wkly Rep* 56:420–423, 2007.

Centers for Disease Control and Prevention: Cancer screening: United States 2010, *MMWR Morb Mortal Wkly Rep* 60:41–45, 2012. Available from <http://www.cdc.gov/mmwr/preview/mmwrhtmlmm6103a1.htm >.

Centers for Disease Control and Prevention: *About the National Health and Nutrition Examination Survey*, 2013. Available from < www.cdc.gov/nchs/nhanes/about_nhanes.htm>. Accessed March 3, 2013.

Centers for Disease Control and Prevention: *Deaths: preliminary report for 2011*. National Vital Statistics Report. Available from <http://www.cdc.gov/nchs/data/nvsr/nvsr61/nvsr61_06.pdf>.

Centers for Disease Control and Prevention: *Tuberculosis skin testing*, n.d. Available from <http://www.cdc.gov/tb/publications/factsheets/testing/skintesting.htm>. Accessed February 15, 2013.

Centers for Disease Control and Prevention: *The Tuskegee timeline*, 2013. Available from < http://www.cdc.gov/tuskegee/timeline.htm>. Accessed March 3, 2013.

Doll R, Hill AB: Study of the aetiology of carcinoma of the lung, *BMJ* 2:1271–1285, 1952.

Doll R, Hill AB: Lung cancer and other causes of death in relation to smoking, *BMJ* 2:1071–1081, 1956.

Eliassen AH, Chen WY, Spiegelman D, et al: Use of aspirin, other nonsteroidal anti-inflammatory drugs and acetaminophen and risk of breast cancer among premenopausal women in the Nurses' Health Study II, *Arch Intern Med* 169:115–121, 2009.

Friedman GD: *Primer of epidemiology*, ed 4, New York, 1994, McGraw-Hill.

Fryar CD: *Ervin RB: Caloric intake from fast food among adults: United States 2007-2010*. National Center for Health Statistics Data Brief 114, 2013. Available from <http://www.cdc.gov/nchs/data/databriefs/db114.pdf>.

Harkness G: *Epidemiology in nursing practice*, St. Louis, 1995, Mosby.

Jeter JM, Han J, Martinez ME, et al: Non-steroidal anti- inflammatory drugs, acetaminophen and risk of skin cancer in the Nurses' Health Study, *Cancer Causes Control* 223:1451–1461, 2012.

Kramarow E, Lubitz J, Francis R: Trends in the coronary heart disease risk profile of middle-aged adults, *Annals of Epidemiology* 23:31–34, 2013.

Mausner JS, Kramer S: *Mausner and Bahn epidemiology: an introductory text*, ed 2, Philadelphia, 1985, Saunders.

Morton RF, Hebel JR, McCarter RJ: *A study guide to epidemiology and biostatistics*, ed 3, Gaithersburg, MD, 1990, Aspen Publishers.

National Cancer Institute: *Surveillance, epidemiology and end results*, n.d. Available from <http://seer.cancer.gov/>. Accessed March 3, 2013.

National Center for Health Statistics: *Health indicators warehouse*, n.d. Available from <http://www.healthindicators.gov/>. Accessed February 26, 2013.

Nurses' Health Study: *History of the Nurses' Health Study*, 2013. Available from <http://www.channing.harvard.edu/nhs/?page_id=70>.

Olds DL, Kitzman HJ, Cole RE, et al: Enduring effects of prenatal and infancy home visiting by nurses on maternal life course and government spending, *JAMA Pediatrics*164, 419–424, doi:10.1001/archpediatrics.2010.49.

Organisation for Economic Cooperation and Development (OECD): Health: Key tables from OECD, 2013. Available from http://www.oecd-ilibrary.org/social-issues-migration-health/infant-mortality_20758480-table9. Accessed January 5, 2014.

Phillips JC: Antiretroviral therapy adherence: Testing a social context model among black men who use illicit drugs, *J Assoc Nurs AIDS Care* 22:100–127, 2011.

Qi Q, Li Y, Chomistek AK, et al: Television watching, leisure time physical activity and the genetic predisposition in relation to body mass index in women and men, *Circulation* 126:1821–1827, 2012.

Sanchez A, Norman GJ, Sallis JF, et al: Patterns and correlates of multiple risk behaviors in overweight women, *Prev Med* 46:196–202, 2007.

Smith MV, Lincoln AK: Integrating social epidemiology into public health research and practice for maternal depression, *Am Jnl of Public Health* 101:990–994, 2011.

Snow J: *On the mode of communication of cholera*, ed 2, London, 1855, Churchill (Reproduced in Snow on cholera, New York, 1936, Commonwealth Fund).

U.S. Department of Health and Human Services: *Healthy People 2010*, conference ed, Washington, DC, 2000, US Government Printing Office.

U.S. Department of Health and Human Services: *Healthy People 2020*, n.d. Available from <http://www.healthypeople.gov/2020/topicsobjectives2020/default.aspx>. Accessed March 3, 2013.

Xu J, Kochanek K, Murphy S, et al: Deaths: Final data for 2007, *National Vital Statistics Reports* 58(19):1–135, 2010.

Community Assessment

Holly B. Cassells

Upon completion of this chapter, the reader will be able to do the following:

1. Discuss the major dimensions of a community.
2. Identify sources of information about a community's health.
3. Describe the process of conducting a community assessment.
4. Formulate community and aggregate diagnoses.
5. Identify uses for epidemiological data at each step of the nursing process.

aggregate
census tracts
community diagnosis

community of solution
metropolitan statistical areas
needs assessment

social system
vital statistics
windshield survey

The Nature of Community
    Aggregate of People
    Location in Space and Time
    Social System
Healthy Communities

Assessing the Community: Sources of Data
    Census Data
    Vital Statistics
    Other Sources of Health Data
Needs Assessment
Diagnosing Health Problems

The primary concern of community health nurses is to improve the health of the community. To address this concern, community health nurses use all the principles and skills of nursing and public health practice. This process involves using demographic and epidemiological methods to assess the community's health and diagnose its health needs.

Before beginning this process, the community health nurse must define the community. The nurse may wonder how he or she can provide services to such a large and nontraditional "client," but there are smaller and more circumscribed entities that constitute a community than towns and cities. A major aspect of public health practice is the application of approaches and solutions to health problems that ensure that the majority of people receive the maximum benefit. To this end, the nurse works to use time and resources efficiently.

Despite the desire to provide services to each individual in a community, the community health nurse recognizes the impracticality of this task. An alternative approach considers the community itself to be the unit of service and works collaboratively with the community using the steps of the nursing process. Therefore, the community is not only the context or place where community health nursing occurs, it is the focus of community health nursing care. The nurse partners with community members to identify community problems and develop solutions to ultimately improve the community's health.

Another central goal of public health practitioners is primary prevention, which protects the public's health and prevents disease development. Chapter 3 discusses how these "upstream efforts" are intended to reduce the pain, suffering, and huge expenditures that occur when significant segments of the population essentially "fall into the river" and require downstream resources to resolve their health problems. In a society greatly concerned about increasingly high health care costs, the need to prevent health problems becomes dire. In addition to reducing the occurrence of disease in individuals, community health nurses must examine the larger aggregate—its structures, environments, and shared health risks—to develop improved upstream prevention programs.

This chapter addresses the first steps in adopting a community- or population-oriented practice. A community health nurse must define a community and describe its characteristics before applying the nursing process. Then, the nurse can launch the assessment and diagnosis phase of the nursing process at the aggregate level and incorporate epidemiological approaches. Comprehensive assessment data are essential to directing effective primary prevention interventions within a community.

Gathering these data is one of the core public health functions identified in the Institute of Medicine's (2002) report on the future of public health. The community health nurse participates in assessing the community's health and its ability to deal with health needs. With sound data, the nurse makes a valuable contribution to health policy development (Wold et al., 2008).

THE NATURE OF COMMUNITY

Many dimensions describe the nature of community. These include an aggregate of people, a location in space and time, and a social system (Box 6-1).

Aggregate of People

An aggregate is a community composed of people who have common characteristics. For example, members of a community may share residence in the same city, membership in the same religious organization, or similar demographic characteristics such as age and ethnic background. The aggregate of senior citizens, for example, comprises primarily retirees who frequently share ages, economic pressures, life experiences, interests, and concerns. This group lived through the many societal changes of the past 50 years; therefore, they may possess similar perspectives on current issues and trends. Many elderly people share concern for the maintenance of good health, the pursuit of an active lifestyle, and the security of needed services to support a quality life. These shared interests translate into common goals and activities, which also are defining attributes of a common interest community. Communities also may consist of overlapping aggregates, in which case some community members belong to multiple aggregates.

Many human factors help delineate a community. Health-related traits, or *risk factors,* are one aspect of "people factors" to be considered. People who have impaired health or a shared predisposition to disease may join together in a group, or community, to learn from and support each other. Parents of disabled infants, people with acquired immunodeficiency syndrome (AIDS), or those at risk for a second myocardial infarction may consider themselves a community. Even when these individuals are not organized, the nurse may recognize that their unique needs constitute a form of community, or aggregate.

A community of solution may form when a common problem unites individuals. Although people may have little else in common with each other, their desire to redress problems brings them together. Such problems may include a shared hazard from environmental contamination, a shared health problem arising from a soaring rate of teenage suicide, or a shared political concern about an upcoming city council election. The community of solution often disbands after problem resolution, but it may subsequently identify other common issues.

Each of these shared features may exist among people who are geographically dispersed or in close proximity to one another. However, in many situations, proximity facilitates the recognition of commonality and the development of cohesion among members. This active sharing of features fosters a sense of community among individuals.

Location in Space and Time

Regardless of shared features, geographic or physical location may define communities of people. Traditionally, a community is an entity delineated by geopolitical boundaries; this view best exemplifies the dimension of location. These boundaries demarcate the periphery of cities, counties, states, and nations. Voting precincts, school districts, water districts, and fire and police protection precincts set less visible boundary lines.

Census tracts subdivide larger communities. The U.S. Census Bureau uses them for data collection and population assessment. Census tracts facilitate the organization of resident information in specific community geographic locales. In densely populated urban areas, the size of tracts tends to be small; therefore, data for one or more census tracts frequently describe neighborhood residents. Although residents may not be aware of their census tract's boundaries, census tract data help define and describe neighborhood communities.

BOX 6-1   MAJOR FEATURES OF A COMMUNITY

- Aggregate of people
  The "who": personal characteristics and risks
- Location in space and time
  The "where" and "when": physical location frequently delineated by boundaries and influenced by the passage of time
- Social system
  The "why" and "how": interrelationships of aggregates fulfilling community functions

RESEARCH HIGHLIGHTS

Using Community Participatory Research to Assess a Substance Use in a Rural Community

Kulbok and colleagues (2012) employed a Community Participatory Model to guide the assessment of youth substance abuse in a rural Virginia county and the development of a prevention model. They integrated multiple assessment modalities that represent current public health nursing competencies. Specifically, this project engaged local community members and leaders with community health professionals in every step of the project, from planning the assessment to developing and evaluating the intervention. This process allowed public health nurses to integrate their knowledge of the local community with that gained from community partners and to develop a deeper understanding of substance use and its local ecological and cultural context.

Researchers used a geographic information system not only to map the location of youth substance use but also to pinpoint areas where preventive behaviors were more common. These maps helped to specifically target the location for preventive interventions. Perspectives of the youth about key "teen places" were also geographically mapped. The project used the photographic charity Photovoice to capture participants' descriptions of local strengths as well as concerns, and then employed the images to facilitate conversation about the nature of alcohol, tobacco, and substance use in the community. Qualitative data about youth beliefs about substance use were gathered from focus groups. These data were combined with descriptive information about the local population, the community environment, and local social systems and beliefs, to develop a comprehensive picture of the local community. Involvement of a broad range of community members throughout the project planning enabled a more effective, culturally appropriate, and sustainable intervention to be developed for this rural community.

Data from Kulbok PA, Thatcher E, Park E, et al: Evolving public health nursing roles: focus on community participatory health promotion and prevention, *Online J Issues Nurs* 17(2):1, 2012. Available from <http://nursingworld.org/MainMenuCategories/ANAMarketplace/ANAPeriodicals/OJIN/TableofContents/Vol-17-2012/No2-May-2012/Evolving-Public-Health-Nursing-Roles.html>.

A *geographic community* can encompass less formalized areas that lack official geopolitical boundaries. A geographic landmark may define neighborhoods (e.g., the East Lake section of town or the North Shore area). A particular building style or a common development era also may identify community neighborhoods. Similarly, a dormitory, a communal home, or a summer camp may be a community because each facility shares a close geographic proximity. Geographic location, including the urban or rural nature of a community, strongly influences the nature of the health problems a community health nurse might find there. Public health is increasingly recognizing that the interaction of humans with the natural environment and with constructed environments consisting of buildings and spaces, for example, is critical to healthy behavior and quality of life. The spatial location of health problems in a geographic area can be mapped with the use of geographic information system software, assisting the nurse to identify vulnerable populations and public health departments to develop programs specific to geographic communities.

Location and the dimension of time define communities. The community's character and health problems evolve over time. Although some communities are very stable, most tend to change with the members' health status and demographics and the larger community's development or decline. For example, the presence of an emerging young workforce may attract new industry, which can alter a neighborhood's health and environment. A community's history illustrates its ability to change and how well it addresses health problems over time.

Social System

The third major feature of a community is the relationships that community members form with one another. Community members fulfill the essential functions of community by interacting in groups. These functions provide socialization, role fulfillment, goal achievement, and member support. Therefore, a community is a complex social system, and its interacting members constitute various subsystems within the community. These subsystems are interrelated and interdependent (i.e., the subsystems affect one another and affect various internal and external stimuli). These stimuli consist of a broad range of events, values, conditions, and needs.

A health care system is an example of a complex system that consists of smaller, interrelated subsystems. A health care system can also be a subsystem because it interacts with and depends on larger systems such as the city government. Changes in the larger system can cause repercussions in many subsystems. For example, when local economic pressures cause a health department to scale back its operations, many subsystems are affected. The health department may eliminate or cut back programs, limit service to other health care providers, reduce access to groups that normally use the system, and deny needed care to families who constitute subsystems in society. Almost every subsystem in the community must react and readjust to such a financial constraint.

EXAMPLE OF SYSTEMS INTERRELATIONSHIPS

Health problems can have a severe impact on multiple systems. For example, the acquired immunodeficiency syndrome (AIDS) epidemic required significant funds for clients with AIDS and for public education and prevention. It made unrelenting demands on many communities that were already strapped for funds to meet their citizens' basic health needs. In San Francisco, the allocation of funds for AIDS programs initially reduced funding for other programs, such as immunizations, family planning, and well-child care.

HEALTHY COMMUNITIES

Complex community systems receive many varied stimuli. The community's ability to respond effectively to changing dynamics and meet the needs of its members indicates productive functioning. Examining the community's functions and subsystems provides clues to existing and potential health problems. Examples of a community's functions include the provision of accessible and acceptable health services, educational opportunities, and safe, crime-free environments.

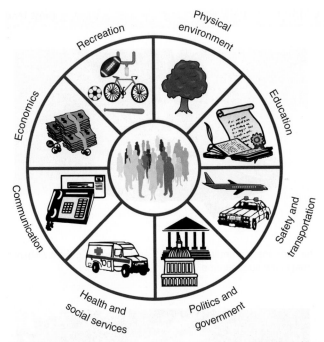

FIGURE 6-1 Diagram of assessment parameters. (Modified from Anderson ET, McFarlane J: *Community as partner: theory and practice in nursing*, ed 6, Philadelphia, 2011, Lippincott Williams & Wilkins.)

The model in Figure 6-1 suggests assessment parameters that can help a nurse develop a more complete list of critical community functions. The community health nurse can then prioritize these functions from a particular community's perspective. For example, a study of Americans' views on health and healthy communities suggested that the public is more concerned with quality-of-life issues than the absence of disease. According to a national study (Healthcare Forum, 1994), the important determinants of a health community include a low crime rate, a good place to bring up children, good schools, a strong family life, good environmental quality, and a healthy economy. These findings are echoed in city-sponsored health surveys across the nation: Ensuring safe and healthy environments that allow for healthy lifestyles, which include activity and nutritious food, is as important to residents as accessing quality health care.

Movements such as *Healthy Cities and Healthy Places* urge community members and leaders to bring about positive health changes in their local environments (World Health Organization, n.d., CDC, 2009). Involving many cities around the nation and world, these models stress the interconnectedness among people and the public and private sectors essential for local communities to address the causes of poor health. In particular, examining the role the "built environment" has on community health (e.g., its physical and environmental design), is an increasing priority (Designing Healthy Communities, 2013). Urban communities are encouraged to consider the health consequences of new policies and programs they introduce by conducting Health Impact Assessments (HIAs) (Pew Charitable Trusts, 2013). These assessments of projects such as the potential impact of zoning decisions, transit systems and sick leave policies serve the important function of bringing a public health perspective to urban and civic initiatives.

Each community and aggregate presumably will have a unique perspective on critical health qualities. Indeed, a community or aggregate may have divergent definitions of health, differing even from that of the community health nurse (Aronson, Norton, and Kegler, 2007). Nevertheless, nurses and health professionals work with communities in developing effective solutions that are acceptable to residents. Building a community's capacity to address future problems is often referred to as developing *community competence*. The nurse assesses the community's commitment to a healthy future, the ability to foster open communication and to elicit broad participation in problem identification and resolution, the active involvement of structures such as a health department that can assist a community with health issues, and the extent to which members have successfully worked together on past problems. This information provides the nurse with an indication of the community's strengths and potential for developing long-term solutions to identified problems.

ASSESSING THE COMMUNITY: SOURCES OF DATA

The community health nurse becomes familiar with the community and begins to understand its nature by traveling through the area. The nurse begins to establish certain hunches or hypotheses about the community's health, strengths, and potential health problems through this down-to-earth approach, called "shoe leather epidemiology." The community health nurse must substantiate these initial assessments and impressions with more concrete or defined data before he or she can formulate a community diagnosis and plan.

Community health nurses often perform a community **windshield survey** by driving or walking through an area and making organized observations. The nurse can gain an understanding of the environmental layout, including geographic features and the location of agencies, services, businesses, and industries, and can locate possible areas of environmental concern through "sight, sense, and sound." The windshield survey offers the nurse an opportunity to observe people and their role in the community. Box 6-2 provides examples of questions to guide a windshield survey assessment. See illustrations depicting an actual "windshield survey" in the photo series in this chapter.

In addition to direct observational methods, certain public health tools become essential to an aggregate-focused nursing practice. The analysis of demographic information and statistical data provides descriptive information about the population. Epidemiology involves the analysis of health data to discover the patterns of health and illness distribution in a population. Epidemiology also involves conducting research to explain the nature of health problems and identify the aggregates at increased risk. The rest of this section provides data sources and describes how the community health nurse can use demographic and epidemiological data to assess the aggregate.

WINDSHIELD SURVEY

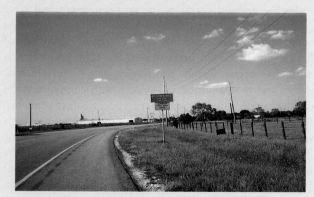

Brookshire is a town of about 3500 in Southeast Texas.

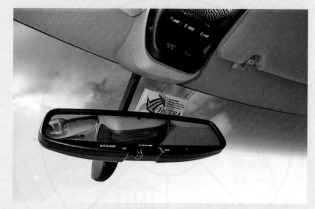

The car's thermometer shows 99°, evidence of a pervasive health threat in the summertime.

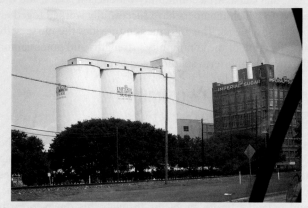

Sugar mills and farms are the source of most jobs.

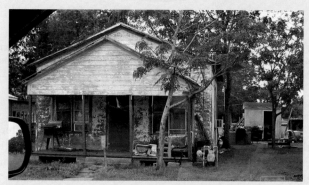

Much of the housing is substandard and suggests low-income families.

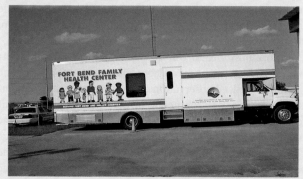

Accessible and affordable health care is a challenge. This van provides services to unskilled workers and area elders.

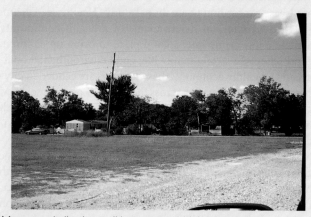

Many people live in small homes on multiple-acre lots.

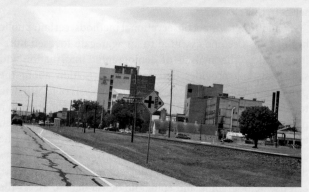

The economy of the town is predominantly agriculture and processing.

Photos courtesy University of Texas Health Science Center at Houston, School of Nursing, Community Health Division.

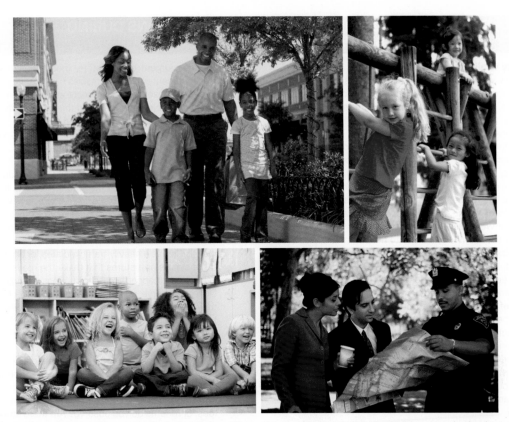

The important determinants of a health community include a low crime rate, a good place to bring up children, good schools, a strong family life, good environmental quality and a healthy economy. (Photos Copyright © 2014 Thinkstock. All rights reserved. Image #76729783, 83273609, 144292431, 178762413.)

Census Data

Every 10 years, the U.S. Census Bureau undertakes a massive survey of all American families. In addition to this decennial census, intermediate surveys collect specific types of information. These collections of statistical data describe the population characteristics of the nation within progressively smaller geopolitical entities (e.g., states, counties, and census tracts). The census also describes large metropolitan areas that extend beyond formal city boundaries, called **metropolitan statistical areas** (MSAs). An MSA consists of a central city with more than 50,000 people and includes the associated suburban or adjacent counties, which yields a total metropolitan area with more than 100,000 people. Adjacent MSAs with their associated cities and counties constitute very large metropolitan regions called combined statistical areas (CSAs). A census tract is one of the smallest reporting units. It usually consists of 3000 to 6000 people who share characteristics such as ethnicity, socioeconomic status, and housing class.

The census is extremely helpful to community health nurses familiarizing themselves with a new community. The census tabulates many demographic variables, including population size, and the distribution of age, sex, race, and ethnicity. The American Community Survey, conducted annually, reports social data such as income, poverty, and occupational factors. Both data sets can be accessed through the use of the Census Bureau's American Factfinder

tools—available at http://factfinder2.census.gov/faces/nav/jsf/pages/index.xhtml—where the nurse can view several variables in combination (e.g., age and ethnicity). One can easily construct a community profile and compare trends with those in other communities. Note that variables that describe the community's health are not part of census data. However, census numbers are frequently used as denominators for morbidity and mortality rates (see the Calculation of Rates section in Chapter 5).

The nurse analyzes and interprets data by comparing current and local census data with previous data and information from various locations, to pinpoint key local differences and changes over time. The nurse can identify the attributes that make each community unique by comparing data for one census unit, such as a census tract or a city, with those of another community or the entire nation. These attributes provide clues to the community's potential vulnerabilities or health risks. For example, a community health nurse may review census reports and discover that a district has many elderly people. This knowledge directs the nurse toward further assessment of the social resources (i.e., housing, transportation, and community centers), health resources (i.e., hospitals, nursing homes, and geriatric clinics), and health problems common to aging people. By identifying the trends in the population over time, the community health nurse can modify public health programs to meet the changing needs of the community.

BOX 6-2 QUESTIONS TO GUIDE COMMUNITY OBSERVATIONS DURING A WINDSHIELD SURVEY

1. **Community vitality:**
   - Are people visible in the community? What are they doing?
   - Who are the people living in the neighborhood? What is their age range? What is the predominant age (e.g., elderly, pre-schoolers, young mothers, or school-aged children)?
   - What ethnicity or race is most common?
   - What is the general appearance of those you observed? Do they appear healthy? Do you notice any people with obvious disabilities, such as those using walkers or wheelchairs, or those with mental or emotional disabilities? Where do they live?
   - Do you notice residents who are well nourished or malnourished, thin or obese, vigorous or frail, unkempt or scantily dressed, or well dressed and clean?
   - Do you notice tourists or visitors to the community?
   - Do you observe any people who appear to be under the influence of drugs or alcohol?
   - Do you see any pregnant women? Do you see women with strollers and young children?

2. **Indicators of social and economic conditions:**
   - What is the general condition of the homes you observe? Are these single-family homes or multifamily structures? Is there any evidence of dilapidated housing or of areas undergoing urban renewal? Is there public housing? What is its condition?
   - What forms of transportation do people seem to be using? Is there public transit? Are there adequate bus stops with benches and shade? Is transportation to health care resources available?
   - Are there any indicators of the kinds of work available to residents? Are there job opportunities nearby, such as factories, small businesses, or military installations? Are there unemployed people visible, such as homeless people?
   - Do you see men congregating in groups on the street? What do they look like, and what are they doing?
   - Is this a rural area? Are there farms or agricultural businesses?
   - Do you note any seasonal workers, such as migrant or day laborers?
   - Do you see any women hanging out along the streets? What are they doing?
   - Do you observe any children or adolescents out of school during the daytime?
   - Do you observe any interest in political campaigns or issues, such as campaign signs?
   - Do you see any evidence of health education on billboards, advertisements, signs, radio stations, or television stations? Do these methods seem appropriate for the people you observed?
   - What kinds of schools and day care centers are available?

3. **Health resources:**
   - Do you notice any hospitals? What kind are they? Where are they located?
   - Are there any clinics? Whom do they serve? Are there any family planning services?
   - Are there doctors' and dentists' offices? Are they specialists or generalists?
   - Do you notice any nursing homes, rehabilitation centers, mental health clinics, alcohol or drug treatment centers, homeless or abused shelters, wellness clinics, health department facilities, urgent care centers, mobile health vehicles, blood donation centers, or pharmacies?
   - Are these resources appropriate and sufficient to address the kinds of problems that exist in this community?

4. **Environmental conditions related to health:**
   - Do you see evidence of anything that might make you suspicious of ground, water, or air pollutants?
   - What is the sanitary condition of the housing? Is housing overcrowded, dirty, or in need of repair? Are windows screened?
   - What is the condition of the roads? Are potholes present? Are drainage systems in place? Are there low water crossings, and do they have warning signals? Are there adequate traffic lights, signs, sidewalks, and curbs? Are railroad crossings fitted with warnings and barriers? Are streets and parking lots well lit? Is this a heavily trafficked area, or are roads rural? Are there curves or features that make the roads hazardous?
   - Is there handicapped access to buildings, sidewalks, and streets?
   - Do you observe recreational facilities and playgrounds? Are they being used? Is there a YMCA/YWCA or community center? Are there any day care facilities or preschools?
   - Are children playing in the streets, alleys, yards, or parks?
   - Do you see any restaurants?
   - Is food sold on the streets? Are people eating in public areas? Are there trash receptacles and places for people to sit? Are public restrooms available?
   - What evidence of any nuisances such as ants, flies, mosquitoes, or rodents do you observe? Are there stray animals wandering in the neighborhood?

5. **Social functioning:**
   - Do you observe any families in the neighborhoods? Can you observe their structure or functioning? Who is caring for the children? What kind of supervision do they have? Is more than one generation present?
   - Are there any identifiable subgroups related to one another either socially or geographically?
   - What evidence of a sense of neighborliness can you observe?
   - What evidence of community cohesiveness can you observe? Are there any group efforts in the neighborhood to improve the living conditions or the neighborhood? Is there a neighborhood watch? Do community groups post signs for neighborhood meetings?
   - How many and what type of churches, synagogues, and other places of worship are there?
   - Can you observe anything that would make you suspicious of social problems, such as gang activity, juvenile delinquency, drug or alcohol abuse, and adolescent pregnancy?

6. **Attitude toward health and health care:**
   - Do you observe any evidence of folk medicine practice, such as a botanical or herbal medicine shop? Are there any alternative medicine practitioners?
   - Do you observe that health resources are well utilized or underutilized?
   - Is there evidence of preventive or wellness care?
   - Do you observe any efforts to improve the neighborhood's health? Planned health fairs? Do you see advertisements for health-related events, clinics, or lectures?

Vital Statistics

The official registration records of births, deaths, marriages, divorces, and adoptions form the basis of data in **vital statistics.** Every year, city, county, and state health departments aggregate and report these events for the preceding year. When compared with those from previous years, vital statistics provide indicators of population growth or reduction. In addition to supplying information about the number of births and deaths, registration certificates record the causes of death, which is useful in determining morbidity and mortality trends. Similarly, birth certificates document birth information (e.g., cesarean delivery, prenatal care, and teen mothers) and the occurrence of any congenital malformations. This information also is important in assessments of the community's health status.

⚖ ETHICAL INSIGHTS

Attending to Nondominant Trends: "Hidden Pockets" of Need

Whereas most public health practitioners are attuned to the leading indicators or dominant trends in data, vital statistics or census data can suggest the existence of small "hidden pockets" of people with special needs. One nurse initially assessed her community as in being an upper-middle-class bracket. She was surprised to find 20 families living below the poverty level and 3 families living without running water. Although these 20 families made up far less than 1% of the community population, they nevertheless necessitated the attention of the community health nurse. Some may view a focus on such a minority segment as insignificant and in conflict with the "Rule of Utility," which posits "the greatest good for the greatest number." However, community health nursing practice combines principles of beneficence and social justice with utilitarianism, and thus, small vulnerable segments of the community are considered legitimate clients of community health nursing. Indeed, social justice not only "gives moral privilege to the needs of the most vulnerable," but also suggests the amelioration of conditions that create social and economic disparities (Boutain, 2012). Furthermore, nurses recognize that this "hidden pocket" is a small piece of the total community and, as such, contributes to its overall health. By attending to these families' health needs, the nurse positively affects the health of the whole.

Other Sources of Health Data

The U.S. Census Bureau conducts numerous surveys on subjects of government interest, such as crime, housing, and labor. Results of these surveys, the census reports, and vital statistics reports are usually available through public libraries and on the Internet. The National Center for Health Statistics (NCHS) compiles annual National Health Interview Survey data, which describe health trends in a national sample. The NCHS publishes reports on the prevalence of disability, illness, and other health-related variables. Specifically, the Behavioral Risk Factor Surveillance System is the world's largest telephone survey of U.S. citizens' health behaviors and risk factors. It tracks trends by nation, state, and year, with the goal of identifying emerging health problems. Data also are used to evaluate achievement of health objectives and develop prevention strategies. The Behavior Risk Factor Surveillance System's website allows one to compile graphs and maps to describe specific risk behaviors by state (http://www.cdc.gov/brfss/).

In addition to these important sources of information, community health nurses can access a broad range of local, regional, and state government reports that contribute to the comprehensive assessment of a population. Local agencies, chambers of commerce, and health and hospital districts collect invaluable information on their community's health. Local health planning agencies also compile and analyze statistical

data during the planning process. The community health nurse can use all of these formal and informal resources in learning about a community or aggregate (Table 6-1). Box 6-3 lists additional information about sources of population health data.

Formal data collection does not exist for all community aspects; therefore many community health nurses must perform additional data collection, compilation, and analysis. For example, school nurses regularly use aggregate data from student records to learn about the demographic composition of their population. They conduct ongoing surveys of classroom attendance and causes of illness, which are essential to an effective school health program. Sometimes the nurse must screen the entire school population to discover the extent of a disease. Thus the school nurse is both a consumer of existent data and a researcher who collects new data for the assessment of the school community.

NEEDS ASSESSMENT

The nurse must understand the community's perspective on health status, the services it uses or requires, and its concerns. Most official data do not capture this type of information. Data collected directly from an aggregate may be more insightful and accurate; therefore community health nurses sometimes conduct community needs assessments. There are several approaches to gathering subjective data; however, a nurse's careful planning of the process will contribute to its reliability and utility regardless of the method. Box 6-4 presents the required steps in conducting a needs assessment.

The strategy chosen for collecting needs assessment data depends on the size and nature of the aggregate, the purpose for collecting information, and the resources available to the nurse. In some cases, the nurse may survey a small sample of clients to measure their satisfaction with a program. In other situations, a large-scale community needs assessment may help the nurse determine gaps in service. Although the process of needs assessment can indicate a program's strengths and weaknesses, it can also raise expectations for new services on the part of community members. Involving community members in the planning of the assessment builds trust and ownership in the process, and subsequently in the improvements that result. With the implementation of the U.S. Patient Protection and Affordable Care Act, nonprofit hospitals must conduct comprehensive community health needs assessments, which create an important opportunity to coordinate with public health agencies to more effectively address local health needs (National Association of County and City Health Officials [NACCHO], 2013).

A first approach to gathering data is to interview *key informants* in the community. These may be knowledgeable residents, elected officials, or health care providers. It is essential that the community health nurse recognize that the views of these people may not reflect the views of all residents. A second approach is to hold a *community forum* to discuss selected questions. It is important for the nurse to carefully plan the meeting in advance to gain the most useful information.

TABLE 6-1 COMMUNITY ASSESSMENT PARAMETERS

PARAMETER	IMPORTANCE TO CHN	SOURCE OF INFORMATION
Geography Topography Climate (e.g., extreme heat or cold)	Influences nature of health problems and access to health care	Almanac Chamber of commerce
Population Size Demographic character (e.g., aged or young) Trends Migration Density	Describes population served; suggests their health risks and needs Suggests growth or decline Increases stress; may increase exposure to communicable disease	Census documents Chamber of commerce
Environment Water (e.g., source, fluoridated) Sewage and waste disposal Air quality (e.g., ozone, pollutants) Food quality and access Housing (e.g., single-family or multifamily dwellings) Animal control (e.g., exposure to rabies and other zoonotic diseases)	Affects quality of life and nature of environmental health problems Reflects community resources Suggests socioeconomic issues	Local and state health departments Newspapers Local environmental action group Census documents
Industry Employment levels Manufacturing White vs. blue collar Income levels	Affects social class, access to health care, and resources Influences nature of health problems	Chamber of commerce Almanac Employment commission Census documents
Education Schools (e.g., physical plant, playground safety) Types of education Literacy rates Special education Health services Sex education School lunch programs (e.g., nutritious diets) After-school programs Day care Access to higher education	Influences socioeconomic status, access to health care, and ability to read and understand health information	Census documents School districts and nurses
Recreation Parks and playgrounds Libraries Public and private recreation Special facilities	Reflects quality of life, resources available to community, and concern for the young and disadvantaged	Parks and recreation departments Newspapers
Religion Churches and synagogues Denominations Community programs Health-related programs and parish health programs Community organizations	Influences values in community by organizing common interests and concerns Reflects involvement of members, community skills, and resources for community needs	Chamber of commerce Newspapers Community center newsletters
Communication Newspapers Neighborhood news Radio and television Telephone Internet Hotlines Medical media Public service announcements	Reflects concerns and needs of the community Contains networks and resources available for health-related use	Local libraries Newspapers Local health department Medical and nursing societies
Transportation Intercity and intracity Handicapped Emergency transport	Affects access to services, food, and other resources Reflects resources available to community	Local bus and train services Local hospital emergency service
Public Services Fire protection Police protection Emergency medical services Rape treatment centers Utilities	Affects community security Reflects available resources	Local police department

TABLE 6-1	COMMUNITY ASSESSMENT PARAMETERS—cont'd	
PARAMETER	**IMPORTANCE TO CHN**	**SOURCE OF INFORMATION**
Political Organization Structure Method for filing positions Responsibilities of positions Sources of revenue Voter registration	Reflects level of citizen activism, involvement, values, and concerns Mechanism for nurse activism and lobbying	Newspapers Local political party organization Local board of elections Local representatives
Community Development or Planning Activities Major issues	Reflects community needs and concerns Affects level of professionals' involvement in issues	Newspapers Local and state planning board Local community organizations
Disaster Programs American Red Cross Disaster plans Potential sources of disaster	Offers a level of preparedness, coordination, and available resources Influences resources and plans	Local American Red Cross office Local emergency coordinating council Local fire department
Health Statistics Mortality Morbidity Leading causes of death Births	Reflects health problems, trends, and state of community health Affects resources needed and CHN services provided	Local and state health department Health facilities and programs National vital statistics reports National Center for Health Statistics reports Morbidity and Mortality Weekly Report
Social Problems Mental health issues Alcoholism and drug abuse Suicide Crime School dropout Unemployment Gangs	Affects health problems and amounts of required services Influences CHN program priorities	Local and state department of social services Local mental health centers Local hotlines Libraries
Health Manpower Number of physicians, dentists, and nurses per population	Influences available health resources and nature of CHN practice	Local and state health planning agencies Health professional organizations Telephone directory Community service director
Health Professional Organizations	Provides support for CHN practice	Public health association
Community Services (e.g., cost and eligibility, accessibility, and acceptability) Institutional care (e.g., hospitals and nursing homes) Mental health care Ambulatory care Preventive health services Nursing services Welfare services	Reflect available resources	Local United Way organization Local voluntary service directory County hospital Local health department Telephone directory

CHN, Community health nursing.

The community health nurse can also mail surveys to community members to elicit information from a more diverse group of people who may be unwilling or unable to attend a community forum. *Focus groups* are a third approach; these can be very effective in gathering community views, particularly for remote and vulnerable segments of a community and for those with underdeveloped opinions (Hildebrandt, 1999). Nurses who conduct focus groups must carefully select participants, formulate questions, and analyze recorded sessions. These sessions can produce greater interaction and expression of ideas than surveys and may provide more insight into an aggregate's opinions. In addition to encouraging community participation in the identification of assets and needs, focus groups may lay the groundwork for community involvement in planning the solutions to identified problems (Clark et al., 2003).

DIAGNOSING HEALTH PROBLEMS

The next step of the nursing process is synthesizing assessment data, in which the nurse examines data and creates a list of all actual and potential problems. Then the nurse develops diagnostic statements about the community's health. These statements, or diagnoses, specify the nature and cause of an actual or potential community health problem and direct the community health nurses' plans to resolve the problem. Muecke (1984) developed a format that assists in writing a

BOX 6-3 RETRIEVAL OF DATA

Current data on U.S. population health are stored in many places. Finding the latest statistics at the local, state, or national level can be a challenging experience for a student, community health nurse, graduate student, or nurse researcher. However, statistics provide a necessary comparison in identifying the health status of an aggregate or population in a community. The following guidelines suggest places to begin a search.

Reference Librarian

The best place to start is in a school or community library or in a large university's health sciences library. Cultivate a relationship with the reference librarian and learn how to access the literature of interest (e.g., government documents) or how to perform computer-guided literature searches.

Government Documents

Local libraries have a listing of government depository libraries, which house government documents for the public. If the government document is not available at a local library, ask the reference librarian to contact a regional or state library for an interlibrary loan. The Library of Congress in Washington, D.C., has a *Directory of U.S. Government Depository Libraries*.

Health, United States, 2012

An annual publication of the National Center for Health Statistics (2012), *Health, United States* reports the latest health statistics for the country. It presents statistics in areas such as maternal-child health indicators (e.g., prenatal care, low birth weight, and infant mortality), life expectancy, mortality, morbidity (e.g., cancer incidence and survival, acquired immunodeficiency syndrome [AIDS], and diabetes),

environmental health indicators (e.g., air pollution and noise exposure), and health system use (e.g., national health expenditures, health insurance coverage, physician contacts, and diagnostic and surgical procedures). Graphs and tables are easy to read and interpret with accompanying texts. Many statistics include a selected number of years to illustrate trends. Some statistics compare themselves with those from other countries and U.S. minority populations. (For more information, visit http://www.cdc.gov/nchs/hus.htm).

Morbidity and Mortality Weekly Report (MMWR)

The Centers for Disease Control and Prevention (CDC) in Atlanta, Georgia, prepares this publication. State health departments compile weekly reports for the publication that outline the numbers of cases of notifiable diseases such as AIDS, gonorrhea, hepatitis, measles (rubeola), pertussis, rubella, syphilis, tuberculosis, and rabies and reports the deaths in 122 U.S. cities by age. It also reports accounts of interesting cases, environmental hazards, disease outbreaks, or other public health problems. Local and state health departments and many local and health sciences libraries house this weekly publication. A subscription is available at http://www.cdc.gov/mmwr/.

Centers for Disease Control and Prevention

The CDC compiles information on a range of topics including health behavior, educational and community-based programs, unintentional injuries, occupational safety and health, environmental health, oral health, diabetes and chronic disabling conditions, communicable disease, immunizations, clinical preventive services, and surveillance and data systems. Data are reported in several publications and on the website: http://www.cdc.gov/.

BOX 6-4 STEPS IN THE NEEDS ASSESSMENT PROCESS

1. Identify aggregate for assessment.
2. Engage community in planning the assessment.
3. Identify required information.
4. Select method of data gathering.
5. Develop questionnaire or interview questions.
6. Develop procedures for data collection.
7. Train data collectors.
8. Arrange for a sample representative of the aggregate.
9. Conduct needs assessment.
10. Tabulate and analyze data.
11. Identify needs suggested by data.
12. Develop an action plan.

Increased risk of _____
(disability, disease, etc.)

among _____ related to
(community or population)

_____ as demonstrated
(etiological statement)

in _____ .
(health indicators)

FIGURE 6-2 Format for community health diagnosis. (Redrawn from Muecke MA: Community health diagnosis in nursing, *Public Health Nurs* 1:23-35, 1984. Used with permission of Blackwell Scientific Publications.)

community diagnosis. The diagnosis consists of four components: the identification of the health problem or risk, the affected aggregate or community, the etiological or causal statement, and the evidence or support for the diagnosis (Figure 6-2). Each of these components has an important role to play in the nursing process. The problem represents a synthesis of all assessment data. The "among" phrase specifies the aggregate that will be the beneficiary of the nurse's action plan and whose health is at risk. The "related to" phrase describes the cause of the health problem and directs the focus of the intervention. All plans and interventions will be aimed at addressing this underlying cause. Last, the health indicators

are the supporting data or evidence, drawn from the completed assessment. These data can suggest the magnitude of the problem and have a bearing on prioritizing diagnoses. Other factors that assist the nurse in ranking the importance of diagnoses include the nature of the diagnosis, its potential impact on a broad range of community residents, and the community's perceptions of the health issue.

With a clear statement of the problem in the form of a diagnosis, the community health nurse is ready to begin the planning phase of the nursing process. Inherent in this phase is a plan for the intervention and its evaluation. Once again, epidemiological data can be useful as a basis for determining success. By comparing baseline data, national and local data, and other relevant indicators, the nurse can construct benchmarks to gauge achievement of program objectives. This step may entail the calculation of incidence rates, if the goal is to reduce the development of disease, or primary prevention. Comparing data with national rates or with prevalence rates found in a local community may be other indicators of success. Reducing the presence of risk factors and documenting patterns of healthy behavior are other objective indices of successful programs.

It is evident that epidemiological data and methods are essential to each phase of the nursing process. The community health nurse compiles a range of assessment data that support the nursing diagnosis. Epidemiological studies support program planning by establishing the effectiveness of certain interventions and their specificity for different aggregates. Finally, epidemiological data are important for the community health nurse's documentation of a program's long-term effectiveness. Box 6-5 provides an evaluation example.

BOX 6-5   EXAMPLE OF OUTCOMES EVALUATION

Example of Community-Based Intervention

Fritz and colleagues (2008) reported on a school-based intervention directed at reducing cigarette smoking among high school–aged adolescents. In this intervention, a team of nurses developed a Computerized Adolescent Smoking Cessation Program (CASCP) consisting of four 30-minute computerized sessions designed to support the student's desire to quit smoking and to decrease the factors that promote continuation of smoking.

In the study, a group of 121 students who were current, self-reported smokers were divided into "experimental" and "control" groups, and the experimental group completed the CASCP program. Evaluation of the data showed that the program was quite effective, in that 23% of the experimental group quit smoking, compared with 5% of the control group. Furthermore, for those in the experimental group who did not quit, nicotine dependence and the number of cigarettes smoked daily decreased. The researchers concluded that the use of a program such as the CASCP can be an effective and inexpensive intervention to help adolescent smokers reduce nicotine dependence and stop smoking.

Data from Fritz DJ, Gore PA, Hardin SB, et al: A computerized smoking cessation intervention for high school smokers, *Pediatr Nurs* 34(1):13-17, 2008.

CASE STUDY

Application of the Nursing Process Assessment and Diagnosis

The following example demonstrates the process of collecting and analyzing data and deriving community diagnoses. It also exemplifies the multiple care levels within which community health nurses function: the individual client, the family, and the aggregate or community levels. In this scenario, the nurse identified an individual client health problem during a home visit, which provided the initial impetus for an aggregate health education program. Data collection expanded from the assessment of the individual to a broad range of literature and data about the nature of the problem in populations. The nurse then formulated a community-level diagnosis to direct the ensuing plan. This was subsequently implemented at the aggregate level and then evaluated.

School nurses frequently address a broad range of student health problems. In the West San Antonio School District, school nurses generally reserve several hours a week for home visits. In a recent case, a teacher expressed concern for a high school junior named "John," whose brother was dying of cancer. In a health class, John shared his personal fears about cancer, which caused his classmates to question their own cancer risks and how they might reduce them.

Assessment

The school nurse visited John's family and learned that the 25-year-old son had testicular cancer. Since his diagnosis 1 year earlier, he had undergone a range of therapies that were palliative but not curative; the cancer was advanced at the time of diagnosis. The nurse spent time with the family discussing care, answering questions, and exploring available support for the entire family.

At a school nurse staff meeting, the nurse inquired about her colleagues' experiences with other young clients with this type of cancer. Only one nurse remembered a young man with testicular cancer. The nurses were not familiar with its prevalence, incidence, risk factors, prevention strategies, or early detection approaches. The nurse recognized the high probability that high school students would have similar questions and could benefit from reliable information.

The school nurse embarked on a community assessment to answer these questions. The nurse first collected information about testicular cancer. Second, the nurse reviewed the nursing and medical literature for key articles discussing client care, diagnosis, and treatment. Epidemiological studies provided additional data regarding testicular cancer's distribution pattern in the population and associated risk factors.

The nurse learned that young men aged 20 to 35 years were at the greatest risk. Other major risk factors were not identified. It was learned that healthy young men do not seek testicular cancer screening and regular health care; they may be apprehensive about conditions affecting sexual function. These factors contribute to delays in detection and treatment. Although only an estimated 7290 new cases of testicular cancer will have been diagnosed in the United States in 2013, it is one of the most common tumors in young men. Furthermore, this cancer is amenable to treatment with early diagnosis (American Cancer Society, n.d.).

On the basis of these facts, the nurse reasoned that a prevention program would benefit high school students. However, to perform a comprehensive assessment, it was important that the nurse clarified what students did know, how comfortable they were in discussing sexual health, and how much the subject interested them. Therefore the nurse approached the junior and senior high school students and administered a questionnaire to elicit this information. The nurse also queried the health teacher about the amount of pertinent cancer and sexual development information the students received in the classroom. The nurse considered the latter an important prerequisite to dealing with the sensitive subject of sexual health. According to the health teacher, the students did receive instruction about physical development and psychosexual issues. Students expressed a strong desire for more classroom instruction on these subjects and more information on cancer prevention. However, they did not have sufficient knowledge of the beneficial health practices related to cancer prevention and early detection.

Key Assessment Data
* Health status of John's brother
* Knowledge, coping, and support resources of family

CASE STUDY—cont'd

Application of the Nursing Process Assessment and Diagnosis

- Testicular cancer, its natural history, treatment and prevention, incidence, prevalence, mortality, and risk factors
- High school students' knowledge about cancer and its prevention
- Students' comfort level discussing sexual health issues

Community Diagnosis

There is an increased risk of undetected testicular cancer among young men related to insufficient knowledge about the disease and the methods for preventing and detecting it at an early stage, as demonstrated by high rates of late initiation of treatment.

Planning

Clarifying the problem and its cause helped the nurse direct the planning phase of the nursing process and determine both long-term and short-term goals.

The long-term goal was:

- Students will identify testicular lesions at an early stage and seek care promptly.

The short-term goals were:

- Students will understand testicular cancer and self-detection techniques.
- Students will exhibit comfort with sexual health issues by asking questions.
- Male students will report regular testicular self-examination.

Planning encompassed several activities, including the discovery of recommended health care practices regarding testicular cancer. The nurse also sought to determine the most effective and appropriate educational approaches for male and female high school students. Identifying helpful community agencies was also an essential part of the process. The local chapter of the American Cancer Society provided valuable information, materials, and consulting services. A nearby nursing school's media center and faculty were also very supportive of the program.

After formalizing her objectives and plan, the nurse presented the project to the high school's teaching coordinator and principal. Their approval was necessary before the nurse could implement the project. After eliciting their enthusiastic support, the nurse proceeded with more detailed plans. She selected and developed classroom instruction methods and activities that would maximize high school students' involvement. The nurse also ordered a film and physical models for demonstrating and practicing testicular self-examination. She prepared group exercises designed to relax students and help them be comfortable with the sensitive subject matter. The nurse scheduled two 40-minute sessions dealing with testicular cancer for the junior-level health class. In a final step of the planning phase, she designed evaluation tools that assessed knowledge levels after each class session and measured the extent to which students integrated these health practices into their lifestyles at the end of their junior and senior years.

The nurse was now ready to proceed with the implementation of a testicular cancer prevention and screening program. She initiated the assessment phase by identifying an individual client and family with a health need, and she extended the assessment to the high school aggregate. Her data collection at the aggregate level, for both the general and local high school populations, assisted in her community diagnosis. The diagnosis directed the development of a community-specific health intervention program and its subsequent implementation and evaluation.

Intervention

The nurse conducted the two sessions in a health education class. At the beginning of the class period, students participated in a group exercise, and the nurse asked them about their knowledge of testicular cancer. The nurse showed a film and led a discussion about cancer screening. In the second session, she demonstrated the self-examination procedure using testicular models and supervised the students while they practiced the procedure on the models. The nurse advised the male students about the frequency of self-examination. With the females, she discussed the need for young men to be aware of their increased risk, drawing a parallel to breast self-examination.

Evaluation

After completing the class sessions, the nurse administered the questionnaires she had developed for evaluation purposes. Analysis of the questionnaires indicated that knowledge levels were very high immediately after the classes. Students were pleased with the frank discussion, the opportunity to ask questions, and the clear responses to a sensitive subject. Teachers also offered positive feedback. Consequently, the nurse became a knowledgeable health resource in the high school.

Intermediate-term evaluation occurred at the end of the students' junior and senior years. The nurse arranged a 15-minute evaluation during other classes, which assessed the integration of positive health practices and testicular self-examinations into the students' lifestyles. At the end of the school year, the prevalence of regular self-assessment was significantly lower than knowledge levels. However, 30% of male students reported regularly practicing self-examinations at the end of 1 year, and 70% reported they had performed self-examination at least once during the past year.

The compilation of incidence data is ideal for long-term evaluation, and it documents the reduction of a community health problem. Testicular cancer is very rare; therefore, incidence data are not reliable and may not be feasible to collect. However, for more prevalent conditions, objective statistics help reveal increases and decreases in disease rates, and these may be related to the strengths and deficiencies of health programs.

Levels of Prevention

The following are examples of the three levels of prevention as applied to this case study.

Primary

- Promotion of healthy lifestyles and attitudes toward sexuality
- Education about sexual health and the care of one's body

Secondary

- Self-examination to detect testicular cancer in its earliest stage
- Referral for medical care as soon as a lump or symptom is discovered
- Medical and surgical care to treat and cure testicular cancer

Tertiary

- Advanced care, including hospice services for those with incurable disease
- Support services and grief counseling to help families cope with loss of a loved one

SUMMARY

Communities form for a variety of reasons and can be homogeneous or heterogeneous in composition. To help them assess the nature of a given community, community health nurses study and interpret data from sources such as local government agencies, census reports, morbidity and mortality reports, and vital statistics. Nurses can gather valuable information about the causes and prevalence of health and disease in a community through epidemiological studies. On the basis of this information, the community health nurse can apply the nursing process, expanding assessment, diagnosis, planning, intervention, and evaluation from the individual client level to a targeted aggregate in the community.

LEARNING ACTIVITIES

1. Walk through a neighborhood, and compile a list of variables that are important to describe with demographic and epidemiological data. Write down hunches or preconceived notions about the nature of the community's population. Compare ideas with the collected statistical data.
2. Walk through a neighborhood, and describe the sensory information (i.e., smells, sounds, and sights). How does each relate to the community's health?
3. Compile a range of relevant demographic and epidemiological data for the community by examining census reports, vital statistics reports, city records, and other library and agency sources.
4. Using the collected data, identify three community health problems, and formulate three community health diagnoses.

ⓔ EVOLVE WEBSITE

http://evolve.elsevier.com/Nies

- NCLEX Review Questions
- Case Studies
- Glossary

REFERENCES

Aronson RE, Norton BL, Kegler MC: "Broad view of health": findings from the California Healthy Cities and Communities Evaluation, *Health Educ Behav* 34(3):441–452, 2007.

Boutain DM: Social justice in nursing: a review of the literature. In de Chesnay M, editor: *Caring for the vulnerable*, Boston, 2012, Jones and Bartlett.

Centers for Disease Control and Prevention: *About Healthy Places*, 2009. Available from <http://www.cdc.gov/healthyplaces/about.htm>. Accessed January 10, 2014.

Clark MJ, Cary S, Diemert G, et al: Involving communities in community assessment, *Public Health Nurs* 20:456–463, 2003.

Designing Healthy Communities: *Response to the built environment*, 2011. Available from <http://designinghealthycommunities.org/built-environment/>. Accessed March 5, 2013.

Healthcare Forum: *What creates health? Individuals and communities respond, a national study conducted by DYG, Inc., for the Healthcare Forum*, San Francisco, 1994, Author.

Hildebrandt E: Focus groups and vulnerable populations: insight into client strengths and needs in complex community health care environments, *Nurs Health Care Perspect* 20(5):256–259, 1999.

Institute of Medicine: *The future of the public's health in the 21st century*, Washington, DC, 2002, National Academies Press.

Muecke MA: Community health diagnosis in nursing, *Public Health Nurs* 1:23–35, 1984.

National Association of County and City Health Officials: *Public Health Infrastructure and Systems*, n.d. Available from <http://www.naccho.org/topics/infrastructure/mapp/chahealthreform.cfm>. Accessed June 9, 2013.

Pew Charitable Trust: *Health impact project: about HIA*, n.d. Available from <http://www.healthimpactproject.org/hia>. Accessed March 5, 2013.

Wold SJ, Brown CM, Chastain CD, et al: Going the extra mile: beyond health teaching to political involvement, *Nurs Forum* 43(4):171–176, 2008.

Community Health Planning, Implementation, and Evaluation

*Diane C. Martins and Patricia M. Burbank**

OBJECTIVES

Upon completion of this chapter, the reader will be able to do the following:

1. Describe the concept "community as client."
2. Apply the nursing process to the larger aggregate within a system's framework.
3. Describe the steps in the Health Planning Model.
4. Identify the appropriate prevention level and system level for nursing interventions in families, groups, aggregates, and communities.
5. Recognize major health planning legislation.
6. Analyze factors that have contributed to the failure of health planning legislation to control health care costs.
7. Describe the community health nurse's role in health planning, implementation, and evaluation.

KEY TERMS

certificate of need
community as client
health planning
Health Planning Model

Hill-Burton Act
key informant
National Health Planning and
    Resources Development Act

Partnership for Health Program
Regional Medical Programs

OUTLINE

Overview of Health Planning
Health Planning Model
    Assessment
    Planning
    Intervention
    Evaluation
Health Planning Projects
    Successful Projects
    Unsuccessful Projects
    Discussion

Health Planning Federal Legislation
    Hill-Burton Act
    Regional Medical Programs
    Comprehensive Health Planning
    Certificate of Need
    National Health Planning and Resources
        Development Act
    Changing Focus of Health Planning
Nursing Implications

Health planning for and with the community is an essential component of community health nursing practice. The term health planning seems simple, but the underlying concept is quite complex. Like many of the other components of community health nursing, health planning tends to vary at the

different aggregate levels. Health planning with an individual or a family may focus on direct care needs or self-care responsibilities. At the group level, the primary goal may be health education, and, at the community level, health planning may involve population disease prevention or environmental hazard control. The following example illustrates the interaction of community health nursing roles with health planning at a variety of aggregate levels.

* The authors would like to acknowledge the contribution of Deborah Godfrey Brown, who co-wrote this chapter for the 4th edition.

Clinical Example

Maria Molina is a registered nurse (RN) in a suburban middle school. During the course of the school year, she noted an increased incidence of sexually transmitted infections (STIs) among the middle school students. After reviewing information in nursing journals, other professional journals, and Internet sources, Maria understood that there was a national increase in sexually transmitted infections among young adolescents. She found that significant numbers of adolescents are initiating sexual activity at age 13 and younger. The school nurse reviewed the Centers of Disease Control and Prevention (CDC, n.d.) site on "Adolescent and School Health—Sexual Risk Behavior." The CDC reported that many young people engage in sexual behaviors that can result in unintended health outcomes. It also reported that among U.S. high school students surveyed in 2011, 47.4% had never had sexual intercourse; 33.7% had had sexual intercourse during the previous 3 months, and, of these latter, 39.8% did not use a condom the last time they had sex; and 15.3% had had sex with four or more people during their lives.

Maria reviewed the reasons for the increased STIs. Her assessment of the problem had several findings. Sexually active teenagers do not use contraception regularly. Also, a variety of sexual misconceptions lead teens to believe they are invulnerable to STIs. Adolescents also find it difficult or embarrassing to obtain contraceptives that protect from not only pregnancy but also STIs. The suburb does not have a local family planning clinic, and area primary care providers are reluctant to counsel teenagers or prescribe contraceptives without parental permission. The nurse also discovered that, several years earlier, a group of parents had stopped an attempt by the local school board to establish sex education in the school system. The parents believed this responsibility belonged in the home.

Maria considered all of these factors in developing her plan of action. She met with teachers, officials, and parents. Teachers and school officials were willing to deal with this sensitive issue if parents could recognize its validity. In meetings, many parents revealed they were uncomfortable discussing sexuality with their adolescent children and welcomed assistance. However, they were concerned that teachers might introduce the mechanics of reproduction without giving proper attention to the moral decisions and obligations involved in relationships. The parents expressed their desire to participate in curriculum planning and to meet with the teachers instead of following a previous plan that required parents to sign a consent form for each student. In support of the parents, Maria asked a nearby urban family planning agency to consider opening a part-time clinic in the suburb.

Implementing such a comprehensive plan is time consuming and requires community involvement and resources. The nurse enlisted the aid of school officials and other community professionals. Time will reveal the plan's long-term effectiveness in reducing teen pregnancy.

This example shows how nurses can and should become involved in health planning. Teen pregnancy is a significant health problem and often results in lower education and lower socioeconomic status, which can lead to further health problems. The nurse's assessment and planned interventions involved individual teenagers, parents and families, the school system, and community resources.

This chapter provides an overview of health planning and evaluation from a nursing perspective. It also describes a model for student involvement in health planning projects and a review of significant health planning legislation.

OVERVIEW OF HEALTH PLANNING

One of the major criticisms of community health nursing practice involves the shift in focus from the community and larger aggregate to family caseload management or agency responsibilities. When focusing on the individual or family, nurses must remember that these clients are members of a larger population group or community and that environmental factors influence them. Nurses can identify these factors and plan health interventions by implementing an assessment of the entire aggregate or community. Figure 7-1 illustrates this process.

The concept of "community as client" is not new. Lillian Wald's work at New York City's Henry Street settlement in the late 1800s exemplifies this concept. At the Henry Street settlement, Miss Wald, Mary Brewster, and other public health nurses worked with extremely poor immigrants.

The increased focus on community-based nursing practice yields a greater emphasis on the aggregate as the client or care unit. However, the community health nurse should not neglect nursing care at the individual and family levels by focusing on health care only at the aggregate level. Rather, the nurse can use this community information to help him or her understand individual and family health problems and improve their health status. Table 7-1 illustrates the differences in community health nursing practice at the individual, family, and community levels. However, before nurses can participate in health care planning, they must be knowledgeable about the process and comfortable with the concept of **community as client** or care focus.

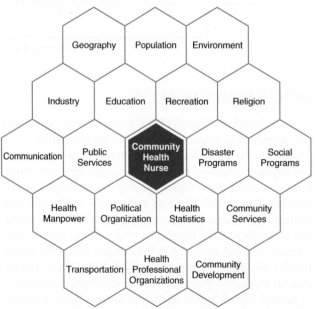

FIGURE 7-1 The community as client. Chapter 6, Table 6-1, provides assessment parameters that help identify the client's assets and needs.

TABLE 7-1		LEVELS OF COMMUNITY HEALTH NURSING PRACTICE		
CLIENT	EXAMPLE	CHARACTERISTICS	HEALTH ASSESSMENT	NURSING INVOLVEMENT
Individual	Lisa McDonald	An individual with various needs	Individual strengths, problems, and needs	Client-nurse interaction
Family	Moniz family	A family system with individual and group needs	Individual and family strengths, problems, and needs	Interactions with individuals and the family group
Group	Boy Scout troop Alzheimer's support group	Common interests, problems, and needs Interdependency	Group dynamics Fulfillment of goals	Group member and leader
Population group	Patients with acquired immunodeficiency syndrome (AIDS) in a given state Pregnant adolescents in a school district	Large, unorganized group with common interests, problems, and needs	Assessment of common problems, needs, and vital statistics	Application of nursing process to identified needs
Organization	A workplace A school	Organized group in a common location with shared governance and goals	Relationship of goals, structure, communication, patterns of organization to its strengths, problems, and needs	Consultant and/or employee application of nursing process to identified needs
Community	Immigrant neighborhood Anytown, USA	An aggregate of people in a common location with organized social systems	Analysis of systems, strengths, characteristics, problems, and needs	Community leader, participant, and health care provider

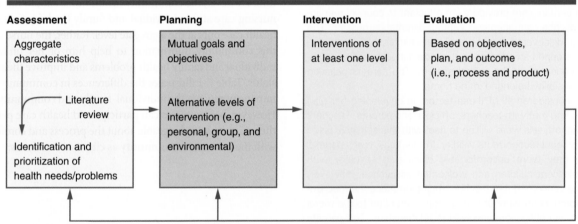

FIGURE 7-2 Health Planning Model.

HEALTH PLANNING MODEL

A model based on Hogue's (1985) group intervention model was developed in response to this need for population focus. The Health Planning Model aims to improve aggregate health and applies the nursing process to the larger aggregate within a systems framework. Figure 7-2 depicts this model. Incorporated into a health planning project, the model can help students view larger client aggregates and gain knowledge and experience in the health planning process. Nurses must carefully consider each step in the process, using this model. Box 7-1 outlines these steps. In addition, Box 7-2 provides the systems framework premises that nurses should incorporate.

Several considerations affect how nurses choose a specific aggregate for study. The community may have extensive or limited opportunities appropriate for nursing involvement.

Additionally, each community offers different possibilities for health intervention. For example, an urban area might have a variety of industrial and business settings that need assistance, whereas a suburban community may offer a choice of family-oriented organizations, such as boys' and girls' "clubs" and parent-teacher associations, that would benefit from intervention.

A nurse should also consider personal interests and strengths in selecting an aggregate for intervention. For example, the nurse should consider whether he or she has an interest in teaching health promotion and preventive health or in planning for organizational change, whether his or her communication skills are better suited to large or small groups, and whether he or she has a preference for working with the elderly or with children. Thoughtful consideration of these and other variables will facilitate assessment and planning.

BOX 7-1   HEALTH PLANNING PROJECT OBJECTIVES

I. Assessment
   A. Specify the aggregate level for study (e.g., group, population group, or organization). Identify and provide a general orientation to the aggregate (e.g., characteristics of the aggregate system, suprasystem, and subsystems). Include the reasons for selecting this aggregate and the method for gaining entry.
   B. Describe specific characteristics of the aggregate.
      1. *Sociodemographic characteristics:* Including age, sex, race or ethnic group, religion, educational background and level, occupation, income, and marital status.
      2. *Health status:* Work or school attendance, disease categories, mortality, health care use, and population growth and population pressure measurements (e.g., rates of birth and death, divorce, unemployment, and drug and alcohol abuse). Select indicators appropriate for the chosen aggregate.
      3. *Suprasystem influences:* Existing health services to improve aggregate health and the existing or potential positive and negative impact of other community-level social system variables on the aggregate. Identify the data collection methods.
   C. Provide relevant information from the literature review, especially in terms of the characteristics, problems, or needs within this type of aggregate. Compare the health status of the aggregate with that of similar aggregates, the community, the state, and the nation.
   D. Identify the specific aggregate's health problems and needs on the basis of comparative data collection analysis

and interpretation and literature review. Include input from clients regarding their need perceptions. Give priorities to health problems and needs, and indicate how to determine these priorities.

II. Planning
   A. Select one health problem or need, and identify the ultimate goal of intervention. Identify specific, measurable objectives as mutually agreed upon by the student and aggregate.
   B. Describe the alternative interventions that are necessary to accomplish the objectives. Consider interventions at each system level where appropriate (e.g., aggregate/target system, suprasystem, and subsystems). Select and validate the intervention(s) with the highest probability of success. Interventions may use existing resources, or they may require the development of new resources.

III. Intervention
   A. Implement at least one level of planned intervention when possible.
   B. If intervention was not implemented, provide reasons.

IV. Evaluation
   A. Evaluate the plan, objectives, and outcomes of the intervention(s). Include the aggregate's evaluation of the project. Evaluation should consider the process, product, appropriateness, and effectiveness.
   B. Make recommendations for further action based on the evaluation, and communicate them to the appropriate individuals or system levels. Discuss implications for community health nursing.

BOX 7-2   SYSTEMS FRAMEWORK PREMISES

I. Each system is a goal-directed collection of interacting or interdependent parts, or subsystems.
II. The whole system is continually interacting with and adapting to the environment, or suprasystem.
III. There is a hierarchical structure (suprasystem, system, subsystems).
IV. Each system is characterized by the following:
   A. *Structure:* Arrangement and organization of parts, or subsystems.
      1. Organization and configuration (e.g., traditional vs. nontraditional; greater variability [no right or wrong and no proper vs. improper form]).
      2. Boundaries (open vs. closed; regulate input and output).
      3. Territory (spatial and behavioral).
      4. Role allocation.
   B. *Functions:* Goals and purpose of system and activities necessary to ensure survival, continuity, and growth of system.

1. General.
   a. *Physical:* Food, clothing, shelter, protection from danger, and provision for health and illness care.
   b. *Affectional:* Meeting the emotional needs of affection and security.
   c. *Social:* Identity, affiliation, socialization, and controls.
2. Specific: Each family, group, or aggregate has its own individual agenda regarding values, aspirations, and cultural obligations.
C. Process and dynamics.
   1. *Adaptation:* Attempt to establish and maintain equilibrium; balance between stability, differentiation, and growth; self-regulation and adaptation (equilibrium and homeostasis).
      a. *Internal:* Families, groups, or aggregates.
      b. *External:* Interaction with suprasystem.
   2. *Integration:* Unity and ability to communicate.
   3. *Decision making:* Power distribution, consensus, accommodation, and authority.

Assessment

As discussed in Chapter 6 on Assessment, it is essential to establish a professional relationship with the selected aggregate, which requires that a community health nurse first gaining entry into the group. Good communication skills are essential to making a positive first impression. The nurse should make an appointment with the group leaders to set up the first meeting.

The nurse must initially clarify his or her position, organizational affiliation, knowledge, and skills. The nurse should also clarify mutual expectations and available times. Once entry into the aggregate is established, the nurse continues negotiation to maintain a mutually beneficial relationship.

Meeting with the aggregate on a regular basis will allow the nurse to make an in-depth assessment. Determining sociodemographic characteristics (e.g., distribution of age, sex, and race) may help the nurse ascertain health needs and develop appropriate intervention methods. For example, adolescents need information regarding nutrition, abuse of drugs and alcohol, and relationships with the opposite sex. They usually do not enjoy lectures in a classroom environment, but the nurse must possess skills to initiate small-group involvement and participation. An adult group's average educational level will affect the group's knowledge base and its comfort with formal versus informal learning settings. The nurse may find it more difficult to coordinate time and energy commitments if an organization is the focus group, because the aggregate members may be more diverse.

The nurse may gather information about sociodemographic characteristics from a variety of sources. These sources include observing the aggregate, consulting with other aggregate workers (e.g., the factory or school nurse, a Head Start teacher, or the resident manager of a high-rise senior-citizen apartment building), reviewing available records or charts, interviewing members of the aggregate (i.e., verbally or via a short questionnaire), and interviewing a key informant. A key informant is a formal or informal leader in the community who provides data that are informed by his or her personal knowledge and experience with the community.

In assessing the aggregate's health status, the nurse must consider both the positive and negative factors. Unemployment or the presence of disease may suggest specific health problems, but low rates of absenteeism at work or school may suggest a need to focus more on preventive interventions. The specific aggregate determines the appropriate health status measures. Immunization levels are an important index for children, but nurses rarely collect this information for adults. However, the nurse should consider the need for influenza and/or pneumonia vaccines with the elderly. Similarly, the nurse would expect a lower incidence of chronic disease among children, whereas the elderly have higher rates of long-term morbidity and mortality.

Public health nursing (PHN) competencies include applying systems theory to PHN practice with communities and populations. This includes integrating systems thinking into public health practice and evaluating new approaches to public health practice that integrate organizational and systems theories (Quad Council of Public Health Nursing Organizations, 2013).

A systems analysis is needed when one is assessing the aggregate. The three levels of the system are the subsystem, the system, and the suprasystem. A community health nurse working with incarcerated women in the prison needs to work at the three levels of the system to assist women planning to reunite with their children at release. The system is the group of women, the subsystem consists of the individual women, and the suprasytem would be the department of corrections and/or the state's department of social services.

The aggregate's suprasystem may facilitate or impede health status. Different organizations and communities provide various resources and services to their members. Some are obviously health related, such as the presence or absence of hospitals, clinics, private practitioners, emergency facilities, health centers, home health agencies, and health departments. Support services and facilities such as group meal sites or Meals on Wheels (MOW) for the elderly and recreational facilities and programs for children, adolescents, and adults are also important. Transportation availability, reimbursement mechanisms or sliding-scale fees, and community-based

volunteer groups may determine the use of services. An assessment of these factors requires researching public records (e.g., town halls, telephone directories, and community services directories) and interviewing health professionals, volunteers, and key informants in the community. The nurse should augment existing resources or create a new service rather than duplicating what is already available to the aggregate.

A literature review is an important means of comparing the aggregate with the norm. For example, children in a Head Start setting, day care center, or elementary school may exhibit a high rate of upper respiratory tract infections during the winter. The nurse should review the pediatric literature and determine the normal incidence for this age range in group environments. Furthermore, the nurse should research potential problems in an especially healthy aggregate (e.g., developmental stresses for adolescents or work or family stresses for adults) or determine whether a factory's experience with work-related injury is within an average range. Comparing the foregoing assessment with research reports, statistics, and health information will help to determine and prioritize the aggregate's health problems and needs.

The last phase of the initial assessment is identifying and prioritizing the specific aggregate's health problems and needs. This phase should relate directly to the assessment and the literature review and should include a comparative analysis of the two. Most important, this step should reflect the aggregate's perceptions of need. Depending on the aggregate, the nurse may consult the aggregate members directly or may interview others who work with the aggregate (e.g., a Head Start teacher). Interventions are seldom successful if the nurse omits or ignores the clients' input.

During the needs assessment, four types of needs should be assessed. The first is the expressed need or the need expressed by the behavior. This is seen as the demand for services and the market behavior of the targeted population. The second need is normative, which is the lack, deficit, or inadequacy as determined by expert health professionals. The third type of need is the perceived need expressed by the audience. Perceived needs include the population's wants and preferences. The final need is the relative need, which is the gap showing health disparities between the advantaged and disadvantaged populations (Issel, 2009).

Finally, the nurse must prioritize the identified problems and needs to create an effective plan. The nurse should consider the following factors when determining priorities:

- The aggregate's preferences
- Number of individuals in the aggregate affected by the health problem
- Severity of the health need or problem
- Availability of potential solutions to the problem
- Practical considerations such as individual skills, time limitations, and available resources

In addition, the nurse may further refine the priorities by applying a framework such as Maslow's (1968) hierarchy of needs (i.e., lower-level needs have priority over higher-level needs) or Leavell and Clark's (1965) levels of prevention (i.e., primary prevention may take priority for children, whereas tertiary prevention may take higher priority for the elderly).

Assessment and data collection are ongoing throughout the nurse's relationship with the aggregate. However, the nurse should proceed to the planning step once the initial assessment is complete. It is particularly important to link the assessment stage with other stages at this point in the process. Planning should stem directly and logically from the assessment, and implementation should be realistic.

An essential component of health planning is to have a strong level of community involvement. The nurse is responsible for advocating for client empowerment throughout the assessment, planning, implementation, and evaluation steps of this process. Community organization reinforces one of the field's underlying premises, as outlined by Nyswander (1956): "Start where the people are." Moreover, Labonte (1994) stated that the community is the engine of health promotion and a vehicle of empowerment. He describes five spheres of an empowerment model that focus on the following levels of social organization: interpersonal (personal empowerment), intragroup (small-group development), intergroup (community collaboration), interorganizational (coalition building), and political action. Paying attention to collective efforts and support of community involvement and empowerment, rather than focusing on individual efforts, will help ensure that the outcomes reflect the needs of the community and truly make a difference in people's lives.

Labonte's (1994) multilevel empowerment model allows us to consider both macro-level and micro-level forces that combine to create both health and disease. Therefore, it seems that both micro and macro viewpoints on health education provide nurses with multiple opportunities for intervention across a broad continuum. In summary, health education activities that have an "upstream" focus examine the underlying causes of health inequalities through multilevel education and research. This allows nurses to be informed by critical perspectives from education, anthropology, and public health (Israel et al., 2005).

Successful health programs rely on empowering citizens to make decisions about individual and community health. Empowering citizens causes power to shift from health providers to community members in addressing health priorities. Collaboration and cooperation among community members, academicians, clinicians, health agencies, and businesses help ensure that scientific advances, community needs, sociopolitical needs, and environmental needs converge in a humanistic manner.

Planning

As already stated, the nurse should determine which problems or needs require intervention in conjunction with the aggregate's perception of its health problems and needs and on the basis of the outcomes of prioritization. Then the nurse must identify the desired outcome or ultimate goal of the intervention. For example, the nurse should determine whether to increase the aggregate's knowledge level and whether an intervention will cause a change in health behavior. It is important to have specific and measurable goals and desired outcomes. Doing so will facilitate planning the nursing interventions and determining the evaluation process.

Planning interventions is a multistep process. First, the nurse must determine the intervention levels (e.g., subsystem, aggregate system, and/or suprasystem). A *system* is a set of interacting and interdependent parts (*subsystems*), organized as a whole with a specific purpose. Just as the human body can be viewed as a set of interacting subsystems (e.g., circulatory, neurological, integumentary), a family, a worksite, or a senior high-rise can also be viewed as a system. Each system then interacts with, and is further influenced by, its physical and social environment, or *suprasystem* (for example, the larger community).

Second, the nurse should plan interventions for each system level, which may center on the primary, secondary, or tertiary levels of prevention. These levels apply to aggregates, communities, and individuals. Primary prevention consists of health promotion and activities that protect the client from illness or dysfunction. Secondary prevention includes early diagnosis and treatment to reduce the duration and severity of disease or dysfunction. Tertiary prevention applies to irreversible disability or damage and aims to rehabilitate and restore an optimal level of functioning. Plans should include goals and activities that reflect the identified problem's prevention level.

Third, the nurse should validate the practicality of the planned interventions according to available personal as well as aggregate and suprasystem resources. Although teaching is often a major component of community health nursing, the nurse should consider other potential forms of intervention (e.g., personal counseling, policy change, or community service development). Input from other disciplines or community agencies may also be helpful. Finally, the nurse should coordinate the planned interventions with the aggregate's input to maximize participation.

Goals and Objectives

Development of goals and objectives is essential. The goal is generally where the nurse wants to be, and the objectives are the steps needed to get there. *Measurable objectives* are the specific measures used to determine whether or not the nurse is successful in achieving the goal. The objectives are instructions about what the nurse wants the population to be able to do. In writing the objectives, the nurse should use verbs and include specific conditions (how well or how many) that describe to what degree the population will be able to demonstrate mastery of the task.

Because the objectives are specific and can be quantified, they may be used to measure outcomes. Objectives may also be referred to as *behavioral objectives* or *outcomes* because they describe observable behavior rather than knowledge. An example of the goals and measurable objectives for a city with a high rate of childhood obesity is shown in Box 7-3.

Intervention

The intervention stage may be the most enjoyable stage for the nurse and the clients. The nurse's careful preliminary assessment and planning should help ensure the aggregate's positive response to the intervention. Although implementation should follow the initial plan, the nurse should prepare for unexpected problems (e.g., bad weather, transportation problems, poor attendance, or competing events). If the nurse is unable to complete the intervention, the reasons for its failure should be analyzed. Interventions should be included from a range of strategies, including mass media (public service announcements, radio, television, billboards), general information dissemination (e.g., pamphlets, DVDs, CDs, posters), electronic information dissemination (e.g., websites, blogs, tweets, video stream), and public forums (e.g., town meetings, focus groups, discussion groups).

Evaluation

Evaluation is an important component for determining the success or failure of a project and understanding the factors that contributed to its success or failure. The evaluation should include the participant's verbal or written feedback and the nurse's detailed analysis. Evaluation includes reflecting on each previous stage to determine the plan's strengths and weaknesses (process evaluation). Process evaluation is also referred to as formative evaluation. It allows one to evaluate both positive and negative aspects of each experience honestly and comprehensively and whether the desired outcomes were achieved (product evaluation). Product evaluation is summative and can consist of end-of-intervention surveys and other tools that measure whether objectives have been met. Summative evaluation is another term for product evaluation and looks at outcomes. Evaluation should include adequacy, efficiency, appropriateness, and cost benefit. During both process and product evaluations, the nurse may ask the following questions:

- Was the assessment adequate?
- Were plans based on an incomplete assessment?
- Did the plan allow adequate client involvement?
- Were the interventions realistic or unrealistic in terms of available resources?
- Did the plan consider all levels of prevention?
- Were the stated goals and objectives accomplished?
- Were the participants satisfied with the interventions?
- Did the plan advance the knowledge levels of the aggregate and the nurse?

The intervention may have limited impact if the nurse fails to communicate follow-up recommendations to the aggregate upon completion of the project. Although follow-up activity is not necessary for all plans, most require additional interventions within the aggregate using community agencies and resources. A comprehensive health planning project involves a close working relationship with the aggregate and careful consideration of each step. Long-term evaluation may need to be done by those professionals working continuously with the aggregate to determine behavior changes and/or changes in health status.

RESEARCH HIGHLIGHTS

What about the Children Playing Sports? Pesticide Use on Athletic Fields

Children come in contact with athletic fields on a daily basis. How these fields are maintained may have an impact on children's potential exposure to pesticides and associated health effects.

This is a cross-sectional, descriptive study that utilized a survey to assess playing field maintenance practices regarding the use of pesticides. Athletic fields (N = 101) in Maryland were stratified by population density and randomly selected.

A survey was administered to field managers (n = 33) to assess maintenance practices, including the use of pesticides. Analysis included descriptive statistics and generalized estimating equations.

Managers of 66 fields (65.3%) reported applying pesticides, mainly herbicides (57.4%). Managers of urban and suburban fields were less likely to apply pesticides than managers of rural fields. Combined cultivation practice was also a significant predictor of increased pesticide use.

The use of pesticides on athletic fields presents many possible health hazards. Results indicate that there is a significant risk of exposure to pesticide for children engaged in sports activities. Given that children are also often concurrently exposed to pesticides as food residues and from home pest management, we need to examine opportunities to reduce their exposures. Both policy and practice questions are raised.

Data from Gilden R, Friedmann E, Sattler B, et al: Potential health effects related to pesticide use on athletic fields, *Public Health Nurs* 29(3):198-207, 2012.

HEALTH PLANNING PROJECTS

Successful Projects

Student projects have used this health planning model with group, organization, population group, and community aggregates. Table 7-2 describes interventions with these aggregates at the subsystem, aggregate system, and suprasystem levels.

BOX 7-3   PROGRAM GOALS AND OBJECTIVES FOR REDUCTION OF CHILDHOOD OBESITY

Goal
Reduce the rate of childhood obesity in the city of New Bedford.

Objectives
1. The percentage of children whose body weight exceeds the 98th percentile for age and height will be reduced to 5%.
2. All the children will be invited to join a 5, 2, 1 program:
   - Five fruits and vegetables per day
   - Two-hour limit on TV, video games, and computer per day
   - One hour of physical activity per day
3. The food pyramid will be taught to all school nurses and health educators by the end of the school year.
4. The food pyramid will be presented and distributed to parents at all the summer health fairs.

TABLE 7-2   INTERVENTIONS BY TYPE OF AGGREGATE AND SYSTEM LEVEL

PROJECT	TYPE OF AGGREGATE	SYSTEM LEVEL FOR INTERVENTION
Rehabilitation group	Group, organization	Subsystem and aggregate system
Textile industry	Population group	Aggregate system and suprasystem
Crime watch	Group, organization, and population group	Aggregate system and suprasystem
Bilingual students (case study)	Community	Aggregate system and suprasystem

Textile Industry

Clinical Example

A nursing student studied a textile plant that had approximately 470 employees but did not have an occupational health nurse. The student nurse collected data and identified three major problems or needs by collaborating with management and union representatives. First, the student nurse observed that the most common, costly, and chronic work-related injury in plant workers was lower back injury. Second, some employees had concerns about possible undetected hypertension. Third, the first-aid facilities were disorganized and without an accurate inventory system. The student nurse planned and implemented interventions for all three areas.

On the suprasystem level, the student nurse formulated plans with the company's physicians and lobbied management to enact an employee training program on proper lifting techniques. The student nurse proposed creating specific and concise job descriptions and requirements to facilitate potential employees' medical assessments. In addition, the student nurse organized and clearly labeled the first-aid supplies and developed an inventory system. On the aggregate system level, the student nurse planned and conducted a hypertension screening program. Approximately 85% of the employees underwent screening, and 10 people had elevated blood pressure readings. These 10 people were referred for follow-up care, and hypertension was subsequently diagnosed in several of them.

In evaluating the project, management representatives recognized that a variety of nursing interventions could improve or maintain workers' health. Consequently, management hired the student nurse upon graduation to be the occupational health nurse.

Crime Watch

Clinical Example

Another nursing student was concerned with the rising incidence of crime in a community and organized a crime watch program. The student nurse met periodically with the police and local residents, or aggregate system. Interventions included posting crime watch signs in the neighborhood and establishing more frequent police patrols at the suprasystem level. Evaluation of the program revealed that the residents had greater awareness of and concern for neighborhood safety.

Rehabilitation Group

Clinical Example

After working at a senior citizens center for a few weeks, a student nurse began a careful assessment of the center's clients. The student nurse interviewed the center's clients and visited its homebound clients served by social workers and the Meals on Wheels (MOW) program. Several of the homebound clients identified a need for socialization and rehabilitation. The center had recently purchased a van equipped to transport handicapped people in wheelchairs, which was a necessary factor in fulfilling this need.

After the student nurse assessed the clients' health and functional status and determined mutual goals, four of these homebound clients expressed a desire to attend a rehabilitation program at the center. The student nurse and the center's management initiated a weekly program based on the clients' needs, which included van transportation, a coffee hour, a noontime meal, an exercise class, and a craft class. Although some members were initially reluctant to participate and one man withdrew from the group, the group ultimately functioned very well. Evaluating this new program showed clearly that the student nurse made progress in meeting the goals of increased socialization and rehabilitation among elders at the center.

Unsuccessful Projects

Project failure is usually caused by problems with one or more steps of the nursing process. Usually the student does not discover problems until the evaluation phase. The following unsuccessful projects illustrate failures at different steps in the nursing process. Table 7-3 summarizes the identified problem areas for these examples.

Group Home for Developmentally Delayed Adults

Clinical Example

A nursing student worked with an aggregate of six women living in a group home for developmentally delayed citizens. The nursing student observed that the clients were all overweight, and she decided to establish a weight reduction program. She proceeded to meet with the women, chart their weight, and discuss their food choices on a weekly basis. After 8 weeks, her evaluation revealed that none of the women had lost weight and a few had actually gained weight. During the assessment phase the student failed to consider the women's perceptions of need. The women did not consider their weight a priority health problem, and their boyfriends provided positive reinforcement regarding their appearance.

Safe Rides Program

Clinical Example

One student nurse assessed a university student community through a questionnaire and identified a drinking and driving problem. Of those she surveyed, 77% admitted to driving under the influence of alcohol, and 16.5% stated they had been involved in an alcohol-related car accident. After identifying the problem and determining student interest, the student nurse worked with the campus alcohol and drug resource center to plan and implement a program called Safe Rides. In this program, student volunteers would work a hotline and dispatch "on-call" drivers to pick up students who were unsafe to drive.

TABLE 7-3	UNSUCCESSFUL PROJECTS
PROJECT	PROBLEMATIC STEP OF NURSING PROCESS
Group home for developmentally delayed	Assessment (i.e., mutual identification of health problems and needs)
Safe Rides program	Planning (i.e., mutual identification of goals and objectives)
Manufacturing plant	Evaluation (i.e., recommendations for follow-up)
	Implementation

The student nurse resolved many potential complications before implementation (e.g., liability coverage for all participating individuals and expense funds for gasoline). The student nurse formulated a 12-hour training program that lasted 3 weeks to prepare student volunteers for the Safe Rides program. By the end of the semester, Safe Rides was ready to begin. However, the student nurse graduated at the semester's end, and her commitment had been the program's prime motivating force. Although others were committed and involved, the student nurse did not arrange for a replacement to coordinate and continue the program upon her departure. The Safe Rides program required ongoing coordination efforts, and no one fully implemented the program in the student nurse's absence.

Manufacturing Plant

Clinical Example

Even careful planning cannot always eliminate potential obstacles. For example, one student nurse chose to work in an occupational setting involving heavy industry. The occupational health nurse and the nurse's personnel supervisor both approved the student nurse's entry into the organization. After reviewing the literature, working with the nurse for several weeks, and assessing the organization and its employees, the student nurse concluded that back injury risk was a primary problem. She planned to reduce the risk factors involved in back injuries by distributing information about proper body mechanics in a teaching session.

The personnel manager resisted this plan. Although he recognized the need for education, he was initially unwilling to allow employees to attend the session on company time. The student nurse and manager reached a compromise by allowing attendance during extended coffee breaks. The personnel manager, however, canceled the program before the student nurse could implement the class; negotiations for a new union contract were forming, and there was high probability of a strike. This situation led management to deny any changes in the usual routine.

The student nurse proceeded appropriately and received clearance from the proper officials, but she could not anticipate or circumvent union problems. The student nurse could only share her information and concern with the nurse and the personnel manager and encourage them to implement her plan when contract negotiations were complete.

Discussion

Each of these projects attempted to address a particular level of prevention. Most of these examples focused on primary prevention and health promotion because they were conducted by students and limited by time available due to the length of the academic semester. Table 7-4 lists these projects and their prevention levels. However, the full-time community health nurse working with an aggregate (e.g., in the occupational health setting) would target interventions for all three levels of prevention at a variety of system levels. It is useful to view nursing interventions with aggregates within a matrix structure to address all intervention opportunities. The matrix in Table 7-5 gives examples of how the occupational health nurse may intervene at all system levels and all prevention levels.

TABLE 7-4	LEVEL OF PREVENTION FOR EACH PROJECT	
PRIMARY PREVENTION	**SECONDARY PREVENTION**	**TERTIARY PREVENTION**
Textile industry	Textile industry	Rehabilitation group
Crime watch	Group home for developmentally delayed	
Manufacturing plant		
Safe Rides program		

In practice, most interventions occur at the individual level and include all prevention levels. Interventions at the aggregate level are usually less common. For many community health nurses, time does not allow intervention at the suprasystem level. However, schools and schoolchildren are integral parts of the community system. Factors that affect the community's health also affect schoolchildren's health. For school nurses in these school districts, interventions at the suprasystem level may become a reality and improve the health of the community and the students. The suprasystem intervention can be used to reduce hunger and food insufficiency for all schoolchildren in a district. A school nurse working with students in the school office may note that the students are presenting with dizziness, headaches, or abdominal pain in the morning and may keep intervention at the individual level by treating the symptoms presented (e.g., with acetaminophen or food). However, the school nurse my investigate why the students are presenting with the symptoms especially on Monday mornings and may realize that lack of food in the homes is an issue. The nurse then would work to develop a breakfast program for the school district. This strategy is a good example of refocusing upstream by addressing the real source of problems.

These projects illustrate the variety of available opportunities for aggregate health planning. In addition, they exemplify the application of the nursing process within various aggregate types, at different systems levels, and at each prevention level. These examples demonstrate the vital importance of each step of the nursing process:

1. Aggregate assessments must be thorough. The textile industry project exemplifies this point. Assessments should elicit answers to key questions about the aggregate's health and demographic profile and should compare this information with information for similar aggregates presented in the literature.
2. The nurse must complete careful planning and set goals that the nurse and the aggregate accept. The rehabilitation group project illustrates the importance of mutual planning.
3. Interventions must include aggregate participation and must meet the mutual goals. The Crime Watch project exemplifies this point.
4. Evaluation must include process and product evaluation and aggregate input.

TABLE 7-5	OCCUPATIONAL HEALTH: LEVELS OF PREVENTION FOR SYSTEM LEVELS		
SYSTEM LEVEL	**PRIMARY PREVENTION**	**SECONDARY PREVENTION**	**TERTIARY PREVENTION**
Subsystem	Yearly physical examination for each employee	Regular blood pressure monitoring and diet counseling for each employee with elevated blood pressure	Referral for job retraining for employee with a back injury
Aggregate and group system	Incentive program to encourage departments to use safety devices	Weight reduction group for overweight employees	Support group for employees who are recovering from problems with alcohol or drug use
Suprasystem	Health fair open to the community and employees	Counseling and referral of community members with elevated blood pressure or cholesterol on the basis of health fair findings	Media advertising to encourage people with substance abuse problems to seek help and use community resources that provide assistance

Health Planning Models in Public Health

According to Issel (2009), many planning programs to address public health problems began as environmental planning of water and sewer systems. Additional population-based planning became necessary with the advent of immunizations. Blum (1974) was the first to suggest how public health planning should be done. Perspectives on health planning range from systematic problem solving and an epidemiological approach to a social awareness approach.

Beginning in the mid-1980s the CDC began to develop and promote systematic methods for health planning in public health. These models were important for a structured approach to public health planning.

The PRECEDE-PROCEED model (Figure 7-3) provides a structure for assessing health and quality-of-life needs. It also assists in designing, implementing, and evaluating health promotion and public health programs to meet those needs. PRECEDE (*Predisposing, Reinforcing, and Enabling Constructs in Educational Diagnosis and Evaluation*) assesses the diagnostic and planning process to assist in the development of focused public health programs. PRO-CEED (*Policy, Regulatory, and Organizational Constructs in Educational and Environmental Development*) guides the implementation and evaluation of the programs (Green & Kreuter, 2005).

The PRECEDE-PROCEED framework is an approach to planning that examines factors contributing to behavior change. They are:

Predisposing factors: The knowledge, attitudes, behavior, beliefs, and values before intervention that affect willingness to change.

Enabling factors: The environment or community of an individual that facilitates or presents obstacles to change.

Reinforcing factors: The positive or negative effects of adopting new behavior (including social support).

These factors require that individuals be considered in the context of their community and social structures, and not in isolation, in the planning of communication or health education strategies (Green and Kreuter, 2005).

PATCH. The Planning Approach to Community Health (PATCH) model was based on Green's PRECEDE (Green et al., 1980; Green and Kreuter, 2005). This model encouraged the idea that health promotion is a process that

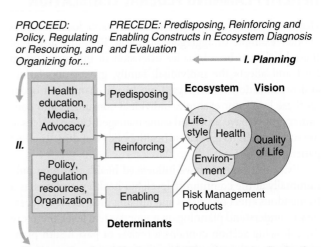

FIGURE 7-3 Green's PRECEDE-PROCEED Model. Green's website provides assistance in guiding use and applications of this model, at http://www.lgreen.net/index.html. (From Green LW, Kreuter MW: *Health program planning: an educational and ecological approach,* ed 4, 2004, McGraw-Hill).

enables the population to have more control of its own health. An essential element of the PATCH model is community participation. Another element is the use of data to develop comprehensive health strategies. The PATCH model achieved this through mobilizing the community, collecting health data, selecting health priorities, developing a comprehensive intervention plan, and evaluating the process (Issel, 2009).

APEX-PH Program. The Assessment Protocol for Excellence in Public Health (APEX-PH) program began in 1987 as a cooperative project of the American Public Health Association (APHA), the Association of Schools of Public Health (ASPH), the Association of State and Territorial Health Officials (ASTHO), the CDC, the National Association of County and City Health Officials (NACCHO), and the United States Conference of Local Health Officers (USCLHO). The APEX-PH is a voluntary process for organizational and community self-assessment, planned improvements, and continuing evaluation and reassessment. It is a true self-assessment and is intended to be more of a public endeavor involving the community as well as the public organizations (CDC, 2009).

MAPP Model. More recently, the CDC and NACCHO have released the MAPP (Mobilizing for Action Through Planning and Partnerships) model. The MAPP model is a health planning model that helps public health leaders facilitate community priorities about health issues and identify sources to address them. The first phase of MAPP is to mobilize the community, the second is to guide the community toward a shared vision for long-range planning, and the third is to conduct four assessments: identifying community strengths, local health system, health status, and forces of change within the population (NACCHO, 2009).

HEALTH PLANNING FEDERAL LEGISLATION

Health planning at the national, state, and local levels is another example of aggregate planning. Planning at any of these levels can be a broader extension of the suprasystem level and affects the individual, family, group, population, and organization levels. Again, upstream change can occur on these levels; for example, individual consumers and consumer groups have protested some managed-care practices at the suprasystem level because health policy can directly affect patient care.

Historically, nurses have influenced health planning only minimally at the community level, but health planning has a tremendous effect on nurses and nursing practice. It is necessary to understand planning on a suprasystem level; therefore the following section contains a review of past health planning efforts with projections for the future.

Hill-Burton Act

In 1946, Congress passed the Hospital Survey and Construction Act (Hill-Burton Act, PL 79-725) to address the need for better hospital access. This act provided federal aid to states for hospital facilities. A state had to submit a plan documenting available resources and need estimates to qualify for hospital construction and modernization funds under the Hill-Burton Act (Sultz and Young, 2006). In addition, each state had to designate a single agency for the development and implementation of the hospital construction plan. The Hill-Burton Act caused the expenditure of vast sums of money and resulted in an increase in the number of beds, especially in general hospitals. Although the act and its amendments focused only on construction, they improved the quality of care in rural areas and introduced systematic statewide planning (Gourevitch, Caronna, and Kalkut, 2005).

Regional Medical Programs

The Hill-Burton Act provided construction-related planning, but it did not address coordination and care delivery directly. In response to recommendations from Dr. Michael DeBakey's national commission, the Heart Disease, Cancer, and Stroke Amendments of 1965 (PL 89-239) were enacted. This legislation was more comprehensive and established regional medical programs.

The Regional Medical Programs (RMPs) intended to make the latest technology for the diagnosis and treatment of heart disease, cancer, stroke, and related diseases available to community health care providers through the establishment of regional cooperative arrangements among medical schools, research institutions, and hospitals. The goals of these cooperative arrangements were to improve the health manpower and facilities available to the communities. The intent was to avoid interfering with methods of financing, hospital administration, patient care, or professional practice.

Although RMPs have been credited with the regionalization of certain services and the introduction of innovative approaches to organization and care delivery, some observers believed the reforms were not comprehensive enough. The RMPs did not partner with the existing federal and state programs; therefore, there were gaps and duplication in service delivery, personnel training, and research (Kovner, 2002).

Comprehensive Health Planning

Congress signed the Comprehensive Health Planning and Public Health Services Amendments of 1966 (PL 89-749) into law to broaden the previous legislation's categorical approach to health planning. Combined with the Partnership for Health Amendments of 1967 (PL 90-174), these amendments created the Partnership for Health Program (PHP). The PHP provided federal grants to states to establish and administer a local agency program to enact local comprehensive health care planning. The PHP's objectives were promoting and ensuring the highest level of health for every person and not interfering with the existing private practice patterns (Shonick, 1995).

To meet these objectives, the PHP formulated a two-level planning system. Under this system, each state had to designate a single health planning agency, or "A" agency. To play a statewide coordinating role, the "A" agency had to partner with an advisory council, which consisted largely of health care consumers. Meanwhile, the local "B" agencies formulated plans to meet designated local community needs, which could be any public or nonprofit private agency or organization. "A" agencies were to encourage the formation of local, comprehensive, health planning "B" agencies, and federal grants were made available for that purpose (Shonick, 1995).

Although the comprehensive health plans were the first of these programs to mandate consumer involvement, they may have failed in their basic intent. The possible failure may have resulted from funding shortage, conflict avoidance in policy formulation and goal establishment, political absence, and provider opposition (e.g., American Medical Association, American Hospital Association, and major medical centers) (Shonick, 1995).

Certificate of Need

In response to increased capital investments and budgetary pressures, state governments developed the idea of obtaining prior governmental approval for certain projects through the use of a certificate of need (CON). New York State passed the first CON law in 1964, which required government approval of hospitals' and nursing homes' major capital investments. Eventually all states supported this CON requirement, and it ultimately became a component of health legislation (PL 93-641). In practice, state CON programs differ in structure and goals. These differences include program focus, decision-making levels, review standard scope, and appeals process exemption (Sultz and Young, 2006).

National Health Planning and Resources Development Act

Given the perceived failure of the comprehensive health planning programs, the federal government focused on a new approach to health planning. The government was greatly concerned with the cost of health care, which escalated dramatically following the end of World War II; the uneven distribution of services; the general lack of knowledge of personal health practices; and the emphasis on more costly modalities of care. The National Health Planning and Resources Development Act of 1974 (PL 93-641) (Endicott, 1975) combined the strengths of the Hill-Burton Act, RMPs, and the comprehensive health planning program to forge a new system of single-state and area-wide health planning agencies (Harlow, 2006).

The goals and purposes of the new law were to increase accessibility to as well as acceptability, continuity, and quality of health services; control over the rising costs of health care services; and prevention of unnecessary duplication of health resources. The new law addressed the needs of the underserved and provided quality health care. The provider and consumer were to be involved in planning and improving health services, and the law placed the system of private practice under scrutiny.

At the center of the program was a network of local health planning agencies, which developed health systems plans for their geographic service areas. The local agencies then submitted these plans to a state health planning and development agency, which integrated the plans into a preliminary state plan. The state agency presented this preliminary plan to a statewide health coordinating council for approval. The law required that the council consist of at least 16 governor-appointed members and that 50% of these members represent health system agencies and 50% represent consumers. One major function of this council was to prepare a state health plan that reflected the goals and purposes of the act. Once the council formulated a tentative plan, they presented it at public hearings throughout the state for discussion and possible revisions (Thorpe, 2002).

Despite careful deliberations by health planners with input from consumers, not all states accepted the health system plan at the grass roots level. A number of problems were encountered, and in time, the legislation failed to effect major change in the health care system. A significant problem was that the legislation had grandfathered the entire health care system (i.e., health care delivery methods did not change). Although legislation mandated consumer involvement in the health system agency, it was often difficult to implement this aspect. Additionally, despite the mandated efforts by CON and required reviews, costs continued to rise, and the health care system remained essentially unchanged (Thorpe, 2002).

Changing Focus of Health Planning

Health planning legislation is heavily influenced by the politics of the administration in power at any given time. The Reagan administration encouraged competition within the health care system. During the 1980s, the administration emphasized cost shifting and cost reduction with greater state power, less centralization of functions, and less national control. This approach represented the government's philosophical shift and combined it with a funding cutback from the Omnibus Budget Reconciliation Act in 1981. The result was a curtailment on federal health planning efforts at that time (Mueller, 1993). The cutbacks caused health system agencies to redefine their roles, and the federal government recommended eliminating these agencies.

A reduction in federal funding and the influence of medical lobbies caused the closure of some health system agencies. Those that remained open experienced a decrease in staff, a resulting drop in overall board functioning, and a reordering of priorities. In an effort to compensate for the decrease in federal funding, some health system agencies sought nonfederal funding or built coalitions to provide the necessary power base for change. Although the administration did not renew federal health planning legislation in the 1980s, it used other regulatory approaches to control costs. These included basing payments to Medicare on diagnosis-related groups (DRGs), and, in the 1990s, the requirement by many individual states that their Medicaid recipients enroll in health maintenance organizations (HMOs).

The Clinton administration's plan for health care reform included mechanisms to revitalize planning at the national level. The failure of Congress to pass the plan in 1994 gave planning efforts back to state and local agencies. As a result, most states have become very involved in various aspects of health planning. Indeed, there is considerable variation as many have statewide health plans, local health plans, and some other type of local health planning (American Health Planning Association [AHPA], 2009).

At the beginning of the twenty-first century, 36 states and the District of Columbia still required CON reviews for selected expenditures that include nursing homes, psychiatric facilities, and expensive equipment (AHPA, 2009). However, within these programs, requirements for approval are more liberal, expedited reviews are conducted, and certain projects are exempted from review, weakening the CON cost-containment mandate. Newer high-technology services (i.e., lithotripsy, gamma knives, and positron emission tomography) still need CON review in most states. Furthermore, it is anticipated that state CON programs will continue to assume a stronger role because states must increasingly monitor and report the quality of, cost of, and access to health care that managed care promised.

Comprehensive Health Reform

The Patient Protection and Affordable Care Act of 2010 has several elements that involve health planning (Kaiser Family Foundation, 2010). Provisions from that act include:

- Creation of task forces on preventive services and community preventive services to develop, update, and disseminate evidence-based recommendations on health care delivery

- Establishment of the National Prevention, Health Promotion, and Public Health Council, an agency that is to be charged with development of a national strategy to improve the nation's health
- Creation of an innovation center within the Centers for Medicare and Medicaid Services
- Development of a national quality improvement strategy that will seek to improve delivery of health care services and population health
- Provision of billions of dollars for funding community health centers, school-based clinics and the National Health Service Corps to improve access to care
- Establishment of an Independent Payment Advisory Board to make proposals to reduce the growth in Medicare spending
- Establishment of a workforce advisory committee to develop a national workforce strategy and to suggest ways to enhance the workforce supply by supporting education of health professionals through scholarships and loans

Many of these provisions will not be implemented for several years, so their impact will not be realized for some time.

Patient Protection and Affordable Care Act (PL 111-148)

On March 23, 2010, President Obama signed comprehensive health reform, the Patient Protection and Affordable Care Act (ACA), into law. On June 28, 2012, the U.S. Supreme Court rendered a final decision to uphold the health care law. This law will require most U.S. citizens and legal residents to have health insurance.

This Act puts individuals, families and small business owners in control of their health care. It reduces premium costs for millions of working families and small businesses by providing hundreds of billions of dollars in tax relief—the largest middle class tax cut for health care in history. It also reduces what families will have to pay for health care by capping out-of-pocket expenses and requiring preventive care to be fully covered without any out-of-pocket expense. For Americans with insurance coverage who like what they have, they can keep it. It keeps insurance companies honest by setting clear rules that rein in the worst insurance industry abuses. And it bans insurance companies from denying insurance coverage because of a person's pre-existing medical conditions while giving consumers new power to appeal insurance company decisions that deny doctor-ordered treatments covered by insurance. (U.S. Department of Health and Human Services, 2013)

The U.S. government provides a website to understand the impact of this legislation for consumers from pregnant women to the elderly, at http://www.hhs.gov/healthcare/rights/index.html, as well as a timeline for the ACA at http://www.hhs.gov/healthcare/facts/timeline/index.html. The Kaiser Family Foundation (2013) offers a video that will be helpful for all patients.

The *Healthy People 2020* objectives support this notion. To help achieve improved health status for all, health planning needs a coordinated approach that combines public and private cooperation with an emphasis on supplies and services. Advances in planning models and the sophistication level of planners will impact future health planning efforts.

GETTING INVOLVED IN HEALTH PLANNING

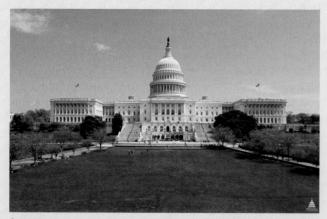

Student nurses can support the health planning process to improve aggregate health care with awareness of, and involvement in, the political process. This involvement can consists of following health care legislation at the state and national levels, being an informed voter, contacting legislators on issues of concern, and participating in special events. (Photo from Architect of the Capital, Retrieved from http://www.aoc.gov/capitol-buildings/about-us-capitol-building.)

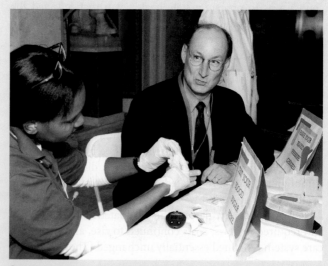

Student nurses also provide blood glucose screenings, with appropriate educational information regarding normal ranges, diet-controlled diabetes, and appropriate referral and treatment when necessary. (Courtesy Michael Salerno.)

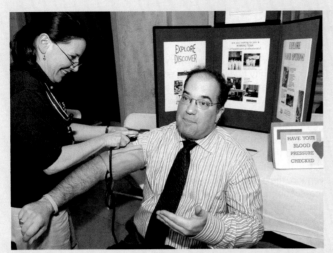

Student nurses attend "Higher Ed Day" at the statehouse to highlight their accomplishments and their participation in the improvement of the health of the state's residents. This student nurse is taking an individual's blood pressure while providing educational information about hypertension identification, referral, and treatment. (Courtesy Michael Salerno.)

Rhode Island Board of Governors
for Higher Education
301 Promenade Street
Providence, Rhode Island 02908–5748

Telephone 401 222-6560
Facsimile 401 222-6111
TDD 401 222-1350

R I B G H E

April 14, 2005

Professor Debby Godfrey Brown
Nursing
University of Rhode Island
White Hall, Room 233
Kingston, RI 02881

Dear Professor Brown:

During the 2004 session of the General Assembly, legislative leaders appropriated $800,000 to increase enrollment in our three nursing programs. This decision proved to be a prudent investment. Your participation in Higher Education Day at the State House received rave reviews. The blood pressure and glucose screenings were services that virtually every legislator and policymaker could identify with. Thank you for your participation and please extend my thanks to the future nurses as well.

Sincerely,

Jack R. Warner

They knew we were here! Positive feedback helps the student nurses recognize the importance of their participation and nursing actions. In addition, their role modeling can have an influence on other legislation, such as funding for their nursing program.

CASE STUDY　APPLICATION OF THE NURSING PROCESS

José Mendez, a bilingual community health nursing student, worked with the school system in a community that had a large Portuguese subsystem. His primary responsibility was for students enrolled in the town's bilingual program. His contacts included the school nurse and the program teachers.

Assessment

José included the specific group of students, the members of the school system's organizational level, and the population group of the town's Portuguese-speaking residents in his assessment of the aggregate's health needs. José identified the subsystem's lack of primary disease prevention, specifically related to hygiene, dental care, nutrition, and lifestyle choices, by observing the children, interviewing teachers and community residents, and reviewing the literature. José's continued assessment and prioritization revealed that the problem was related to a lack of knowledge and not a lack of concern.

Diagnosis
Individual
- Inadequate preparation at home regarding basic hygiene, dental care, nutrition, and healthy lifestyles

Family
- Developing strengths toward self-care regarding basic hygiene, dental care, nutrition, and healthy lifestyles

Community
- Inadequate resources for communicating basics of hygiene, dental care, nutrition, and healthy lifestyles to the Portuguese community

Planning
The teachers and staff of the bilingual program helped contract and set goals, which reinforced the need for mutuality at this step in

the process. A variety of alternative interventions were necessary to accomplish the following goals:

Individual
Long-Term Goal
- Students will regularly practice good hygiene, preventive dental care, good nutrition, exercise, and adequate sleep habits.

Short-Term Goal
- Students will learn the basics of good hygiene, preventive dental care, good nutrition, exercise, and adequate sleep habits.

Family
Long-Term Goal
- Families will regularly practice and teach their children good hygiene, preventive dental care, good nutrition, exercise, and adequate sleep habits.

Short-Term Goal
- Families will learn the basics of good hygiene, preventive dental care, good nutrition, exercise, and adequate sleep habits.

Community
Long-Term Goal
- Systematic programs will provide families and their children with education and information regarding the basics of good hygiene, preventive dental care, good nutrition, exercise, and adequate sleep habits.

Short-Term Goal
- Bilingual personnel will translate information into Portuguese, and program teachers will distribute it to families. This information will cover the basics of good hygiene, preventive dental care, good nutrition, exercise, and adequate sleep habits.

CASE STUDY APPLICATION OF THE NURSING PROCESS—cont'd

Intervention
- Sometimes nursing students' projects are more limited than the planning stage's ideal; in this case, interventions assessed only one grade level.

Individual
- The student nurse taught children many healthy lifestyle basics, including nutrition, hygiene, and dental care. Classes presented information in Portuguese and English.

Family
- All parents received a summary of the class content in both languages and in pictures.

Community
- The local teachers communicated the student nurse's activities to their state-level coordinators, and the coordinators incorporated the student nurse's materials into the bilingual program throughout the state.

Evaluation
Individual, Family, Community
This community health planning project had an impact on the individuals in the specific aggregate and had broader implications for the family systems and the community suprasystem. The outcomes, or product, were hugely successful. Mutually identified goals and objectives influenced the development of the process and incorporated input from a variety of sources. The student nurse believed the resources and support for the bilingual program were adequate. Although the student nurse addressed only primary prevention, the continuing nature of the project will allow the teachers, the school nurse, and the families to assess problems related to the program's content. Future implementation may address secondary and tertiary prevention.

Questions
1. How would you evaluate this project?
2. How would you determine process and product evaluation?
3. What would you do differently?

NURSING IMPLICATIONS

Nurses must work collaboratively with health planners to improve aggregate health. Nurses can influence health planning at the local, state, or community level by fusing current technology with their knowledge of health care needs and skills gained through working with individuals, families, groups, and population groups. This is an example of "upstream interventions." Indeed, nurses may become directly involved in the planning process by participating in CON reviews or gaining membership on health planning councils. Even as students, nurses can begin to participate by engaging in aggregate-level projects, such as those outlined in this chapter, and by tracking health care legislation and contacting their legislators about important issues.

Increased nursing involvement is one method of strengthening local and national health planning. Nurses can use the Health Planning Model presented in this chapter to facilitate a systematic approach to improve aggregate health care. Nurses can assess aggregates from small groups through population groups; identify the group's health needs; and perform planning, intervention, and evaluations by applying this model. The health of individuals, families, and groups would improve if nurses reemphasized the larger aggregate.

SUMMARY

Community health nurses are responsible for incorporating health planning into their practice. Nurses' unique talents and skills, augmented by the comprehensive application of the nursing process, can facilitate population health improvement at various aggregate levels. Health planning policy and process constitute part of the knowledge base of the baccalaureate-prepared nurse. Systems theory provides one framework for nursing process application in the community. Interventions are possible at subsystem, system, and suprasystem levels using all three levels of prevention.

LEARNING ACTIVITIES

1. Review the Affordable Care Act and your state's plans for action.
2. You are working with U.S. Veterans who have served in Iraq/Afghanistan. Refer to the U.S. Department of Veteran's Affairs website (http://www.va.gov/health/) to review some health issues you should consider in your assessment.
3. Select one of the following community diagnoses from your community: Increased rates of violence, asthma, lead poisoning, STIs, pediculosis, infected tattoos/piercings, childhood obesity, hunger and food insufficiency, homelessness. Write a plan on how to address that diagnosis, including goals and objectives. What resources will be needed?
4. Attend a state or local health planning meeting. Observe the number of health care providers and consumers in attendance. Compare the meeting's issues with the goals of improving care quality and reducing health care costs.
5. Review the American Planning Association's Planning and Community Health Research Center Plan. Discuss which plans and policies and plans improve the built environment in your community.

Ⓔ **EVOLVE WEBSITE**

http://evolve.elsevier.com/Nies

- NCLEX Review Questions
- Case Studies
- Glossary

REFERENCES

American Health Planning Association: *National directory of health planning, policy, and regulatory agencies*, ed 20, Falls Church, VA, 2009, AHPA.

American Planning Association: Planning and Community Health Research Center. Available at <http://www.planning.org/nationalcenters/health/>. Accessed April 30, 2013.

Blum HL: *Planning for health*, New York, 1974, Human Sciences Press.

Centers for Disease Control and Prevention: *Adolescent and school health: sexual risk behavior*, n.d. Available from <http://www.cdc.gov/HealthyYouth/sexualbehaviors/>. Accessed March 11, 2013.

U.S. Social Security Administration: Compilation of the Social Security laws: comprehensive health planning and public health services amendments of 1966: *PL 89–749*, 1966. Available from <http://uscode.house.gov/statutes/1966/1966-089-0749.pdf>. Accessed March 15, 2013.

Endicott KL: National Health Planning and Resources Development Act of 1974: PL 93–641, *Public Health Reports* 90(3):i2, 1975. Available from <http://www.ncbi.nlm.nih.gov/pmc/articles/PMC1435675/>. Accessed March 15, 2013.

Gilden R, Friedmann E, Sattler B, et al: Potential health effects related to pesticide use on athletic fields, *Public Health Nursing* 29(3): 198–207, 2012.

Gourevitch MN, Caronna CA, Kalkut G: Acute care. In Kovner AR, Knickman JR, editors: *Jonas and Kovner's health care delivery system in the United States*, ed 8, New York, 2005, Springer.

Green LW, Kreuter MW: *Health promotion planning: an educational and ecological approach*, ed 4, New York, 2005, McGraw-Hill.

Green LW, Kreuter MW, Deeds SG, et al: *Health education planning: a diagnostic approach*, Palo Alto, CA, 1980, Mayfield Publishing.

Harlow JM: Government and other types of oversight. In Garber KM, editor: *The U.S. health care delivery system: fundamental facts, definitions, and statistics*, Chicago, 2006, American Hospital Association.

Heart Disease, Cancer, and Stroke Amendments of 1965: PL 89–239, 1965.

Hogue C: An epidemiologic approach to distributive nursing practice. In Hall JE, Weaver BR, editors: *Distributive nursing practice: a systems approach to community health*, ed 2, Philadelphia, 1985, Lippincott Williams & Wilkins.

Hospital Survey and Construction Act of 1946 (Hill-Burton Act): PL 79–725.

Israel BA, Eng E, Schulz AJ, editors: *Methods in community-based participatory research for health*, San Francisco, 2005, Jossey-Bass.

Issel LM: *Health program planning and evaluation*, ed 2, Sudbury, MA, 2009, Jones and Bartlett.

Kaiser Family Foundation: *Health reform source*, 2010. Available from <http://healthreform.kff.org/the-animation.aspx?source=QL>. Accessed March 11, 2013.

Kovner AR: Hospitals. In Kovner A, Jonas S, editors: *Health care delivery in the United States*, ed 7, New York, 2002, Springer.

Labonte R: Health promotion and empowerment: reflections on professional practice, *Health Educ Q* 21:253–268, 1994.

Leavell HR, Clark EG: *Preventive medicine for the doctor in his community*, New York, 1965, McGraw-Hill.

Maslow AH: *Toward a psychology of being*, New York, 1968, Van Nostrand Reinhold.

Mueller K: *Health care policy in the United States*, Lincoln, NE, 1993, University of Nebraska Press.

National Association of County and City Health Officials (NACCHO): *MAPP*, 2009: Available from <www.naccho.org/topics/infrastructure/MAPP/index.cfm>. Accessed May 31, 2009.

Nyswander DB: Education for health: some principles and their application, *Health Educ Mono* 14:65–70, 1956.

Partnership for Health Amendments of 1967: PL 90–174, 1967.

Quad Council of Public Health Nursing Organizations: American Public Health Association: PHN Section, ACHNE, APHN, ANA: *Quad council PHN competencies*, 2013. Available from <http://quadcouncilphn.org/>. Accessed March 11, 2013.

Shonick W: *Government and health services*, New York, 1995, Oxford University Press.

Silverstein NG: Lillian Wald at Henry Street: 1893–1895, *ANS Adv Nurs Sci* 7:1–12, 1985.

Sultz HA, Young KM: *Health care USA: understanding its organization and delivery*, ed 5, Boston, 2006, Jones and Bartlett.

Thorpe K: Cost containment. In Kovner A, Jonas S, editors: *Health care delivery in the United States*, ed 7, New York, 2002, Springer.

U.S. Department of Health and Human Services: *The health care law and you*, n.d. Available from <http://www.healthcare.gov/law/index.html>. Accessed March 11, 2013.

U. S. Department of Veteran's Affairs, Veteran's Health Administration. Available at <http://www.va.gov/health/default.asp>. Accessed April 30, 2013.

Community Health Education

Cathy D. Meade

OBJECTIVES

Upon completion of this chapter, the reader will be able to do the following:

1. Describe the goals of health education within the community setting.
2. Examine the nurse's role in community education within a sociopolitical and cultural context.
3. Select a learning theory, and describe its application to the individual, family, or aggregate.
4. Examine innovative and effective teaching and learning strategies that exemplify community-centered health education for the individual, family, or aggregate.
5. Compare and contrast Freire's approach to health education with an individualistic health education model.
6. Examine the importance of community engagement for impacting health disparities.
7. Outline a systematic process for developing culturally and literacy relevant health education materials, messages, media, and programs.
8. Relate and apply factors that enhance the suitability of health education materials, messages, media, and programs for an intended audience.
9. Prepare an appropriate and meaningful teaching plan and evaluation criteria for the individual, family, and/or group.

KEY TERMS

cognitive theory
community empowerment
community-based participatory
   methods
culturally effective care
health disparities

health education
health literacy
humanistic theories
learner verification
learning
materials and media

participatory action research (PAR)
Paulo Freire
problem-solving education
social learning theory

OUTLINE

Connecting with Everyday Realities
Health Education in the Community
Learning Theories, Principles, and Health Education Models
   Learning Theories
   Knowles's Assumptions about Adult Learners
   Health Education Models
   Models of Individual Behavior
   Model of Health Education Empowerment
   Community Empowerment
The Nurse's Role in Health Education
Enhancing Communication

Framework for Developing Health Communications
   Stage I: Planning and Strategy Development
   Stage II: Developing and Pretesting Concepts, Messages, and Materials
   Stage III: Implementing the Program
   Stage IV: Assessing Effectiveness and Making Refinements
Health Education Resources
   Literacy and Health
   Assess Materials: Become a Wise Consumer and User
   Assess Relevancy of Health Materials
Social Media

CONNECTING WITH EVERYDAY REALITIES

The nurse may be tempted to ask the following questions:

- Why does she keep smoking? She is pregnant.
- Why doesn't the 63-year-old man get his colonoscopy? His fecal occult blood test (I-FOBT) was abnormal.
- Why doesn't the teen take his diabetic medications (insulin) each day?
- Why are those parents late in immunizing their kids?
- Why don't more women attend the clinic's cervical cancer screenings? They're free!

- Why does the community have such an alarming rate of obesity?

Although these questions show the nurse's desire and good intentions to understand the link between health behavior and health education, they do not yield actionable answers or empower individuals, families, or groups. In fact, such questions do not address critical key root health issues but, rather, create a "blaming the victim" approach as recounted by Israel and colleagues (1994). Instead, the nurse should try to reframe the questions to get at reasons that help explain the behavior and that lend themselves to nursing actions. Consider these questions the nurse might ask instead:

- What life stressors get in the way of the expectant mom's quitting smoking for good? What stage of quitting might she be in? What social support factors could be deployed to help her quit?
- What structural factors might be preventing the man from getting a follow-up test (colonoscopy)? Is transportation a problem? Are the instructions clear? Might he view the colonoscopy procedure as scary? What beliefs might the man have about the tests, for example, "that it has to do with my manhood"? Does he have money for the prep? What can I do to verify that he understands the importance of the test?
- How does the young man with diabetes like to learn? What makes it difficult for him to remember to take his insulin? Are the needles a concern? Does he have worries about how his diabetes might affect his soccer game? What can I do to better connect my instructions to what is important to him in his everyday school and sports activities?
- What types of impediments affect timely immunization of the family's kids? What have they heard about immunizations? Could any religious factors account for their beliefs? Might the family be worried about side effects of the immunizations that they heard about from their relatives? How could I do a better job of explaining the importance of childhood immunizations in light of their concerns?
- What outreach methods might better attract the women to the free cancer screening? Could a promotora help to engage women and help them navigate the process? Are the materials language-specific?
- What social, physical, cultural, language, linguistic, or structural factors should be considered when developing nutrition messages? What role can I play to develop links with schools, grocery stores, churches, and community centers to better reach families with nutritional interventions? How can community capacity be strengthened to advocate for greater access to healthier food in their grocery stores?

HEALTH EDUCATION IN THE COMMUNITY

Historically, teaching has been a significant nursing responsibility since Florence Nightingale's (1859) early work. Gardner (1936) emphasized that health teaching is one of the most fundamental nursing principles and that "a nurse, in even the most obscure position must be a teacher of no mean order." There is much support for the nurse's involvement in health education and health communications, including nurse practice acts, professional statements of the American Nurses Association (2007), the American Hospital Association's Patient Care Partnership (2003), the Joint Commission on Accreditation of Healthcare Organizations (2012), Quad Council of Public Health Nursing Organizations (2011), *Healthy People 2020* objectives (U.S. Department of Health and Human Services [USDHHS], n.d.), and national and enhanced standards on culturally and linguistically appropriate services (CLASs) to advance health equity initiatives (USDHHS, Office of Minority Health [OMH], 2000, 2010).

Health education is an integral part of the nurse's role in the community for promoting health, preventing disease, and maintaining optimal wellness (Box 8-1). Moreover, the community is a vital link for the delivery of effective health care and offers the nurse multiple opportunities to provide appropriate health education within the context of a setting that is familiar to community members (Meade et al., 2009, 2011).

The role of the nurse as health educator is especially important in light of the increasing diversity and demographically changing population in the United States, technological advancements in health care, and the need to reduce the disconnect between scientific discovery and the delivery of interventions in the community (Chu et al., 2008; Freeman, 2004; Kulbock et al., 2012). More than ever before, health education activities and services are taking place outside the walls of hospitals, in such settings as missions, Young Men's/Women's Christian Associations (YMCA/YWCAs), beauty and barber shops, grocery stores, homeless shelters, Veterans of Foreign Wars (VFW) halls, churches, community-based clinics, health maintenance organizations, schools, worksites, shopping malls, senior centers, adult education centers, mobile health units, homes, and libraries. At the core

---

BOX 8-1 HEALTH EDUCATION ROLES AND ACTIVITIES OF THE NURSE IN THE COMMUNITY

- Advocate
- Caregiver
- Case manager
- Collaborator
- Community care agent
- Consultant
- Counselor
- Culture broker
- Educator
- Facilitator of health-promoting behaviors
- Information agent and broker
- Innovator
- Liaison
- Mediator
- Navigator
- Negotiator
- Policy analyst, policy maker, or change agent
- Promoter of collaborative partnerships
- Promoter of self-care and self-efficacy
- "Recognizer" of the dimensions of health choices
- Referral resource
- Researcher
- Sensitizer
- Social activist

Based on data from Clark (2007); Quad Council of Public Health Organizations (2011); Redman (2007); and Stallings, Rankin, and London (2005).

of health education is the development of trusting relationships based on nurturing and healing interactions, the use of community-based participatory methods that highlight community strengths, and the creation of sustainable collaborations and partnerships (Gwede et al., 2010; Leung, Yen, and Minkler, 2004; Luque et al., 2010; Martinez et al., 2008; Meade et al., 2011; Minkler, 2012; Olshansky et al., 2005; Smedley et al., 2003; Wells et al., 2012).

Health education is any combination of learning experiences designed to predispose, enable, and reinforce voluntary behavior conducive to health in individuals, groups, or communities. Its goal is to understand health behavior and to translate knowledge into relevant interventions and strategies for health enhancement, disease prevention, and chronic illness management. Health education aims to enhance wellness and decrease disability; attempts to actualize the health potential of individuals, families, communities, and society; and it includes a broad and varied set of strategies aimed at influencing individuals within their social environment for improved health and well-being (Green and Kreuter, 2004).

Kleinman (1978) described a social and cultural community health care system as one that bridges external factors (e.g., economical, political, and epidemiological) to internal factors (e.g., behavioral and communicative). This view of a sociocultural health care system firmly grounds health education activities within sociopolitical structures, especially within local environmental settings, and views the *community* as client (Coleman et al., 2009; Hunter et al., 2012; Kobetz et al., 2009; Martyn et al., 2009; Meade et al., 2007, 2011; Villarruel et al., 2007). As such, because the community level is often the location of health prevention and health promotion programs, it is a significant and enriching venue for obtaining positive health outcomes. Nurses are uniquely qualified to influence the health and well-being of community members' health behaviors through original and inventive activities that incorporate culturally, linguistically, and educationally relevant health education and messaging. Nurses in population-focused settings can bring together their knowledge, competencies, and skills and take on leadership roles to expertly assess assets and needs, and can put forward solutions to complex, multicausal community concerns (Kulbock et al., 2012; Meade et al., 2007; Watters, 2003).

It is paramount that community nurse educators address the myriad sociopolitical conditions that affect community health by placing value on the contributions of community members' strengths. Sustained cognitive and behavioral changes often rely heavily on engaging learners in becoming partners in their own health behavior and practice. For example, take a look at the community interventions directed toward empowerment and participatory approaches as remarked by the following writers: D'Souza and colleagues (2013), who carried out qualitative work to improve the reproductive health status of married women in mining communities in India; Rutherford (2011), who peeled away the layers of the homeless conditions in Calgary by conducting 7 months of participant observations; Cashman and associates (2008), who illustrated how community members could meaningfully take part in data collection and data analyses; and Bungay and colleagues (2013), who forged a community-academic research partnership that combined health education, medical referrals, sexually transmitted infection (STI) testing using self-swab techniques, and a point-of-care human immunodeficiency virus (HIV) screening test to support the health of commercial sex workers. In short, nurses have significant roles in providing contextually appropriate health education, which involves practical, relevant, and scientifically sound methods that fit the lives and learning needs of an intended population.

LEARNING THEORIES, PRINCIPLES, AND HEALTH EDUCATION MODELS

Learning Theories

Learning theories are helpful in understanding how individuals, families, and groups learn. The field of psychology provides the basis for most of these theories and illustrates how environmental stimuli elicit specific responses. Such theories can aid nurses to recognize the mechanisms that potentially modify knowledge, attitude, and behavior. Bigge and Shermis (2004) assert that learning is an enduring change that involves the modification of insights, behaviors, perceptions, or motivations. Although psychology textbooks describe learning theories in great detail, the following broad categories relate to the nursing application in a community setting: stimulus-response (S-R) conditioning (i.e., behavioristic), cognitive, humanistic, and social learning. ⓔ Resource Tool 8A Learning Theories and Their Relationship to Health Education, on the book's Evolve website at http://evolve.elsevier.com/Nies, outlines these learning theories.

RESEARCH HIGHLIGHTS

Linking Theory to Practice: An Example of a Sexually Transmitted Infection/Human Immunodeficiency Virus Risk Reduction Intervention in a Primary Care Setting

Reducing sexually transmitted infections (STIs)/human immunodeficiency virus (HIV) is a national imperative. Responding to this priority, the "Sister to Sister: Respect Yourself! Protect Yourself! Because You Are Worth It!" program was created. This counseling theory–based intervention consists of a single 20-minute one-on-one nurse-led intervention and addresses three key themes: family/community, caring, and self-worth. The intervention consists of counseling strategies, videos, condom demonstration, and client role-plays to support behavioral change through practice (Jemmott et al., 2008).

As background, this educational, skill-based HIV risk-reduction intervention was previously designed and evaluated through a randomized controlled trial among African-American women (Jemmott, Jemmott, and O'Leary, 2007). Based on the social cognitive theory and theory of planned behavior, the curriculum targets risky sexual behaviors and women's control beliefs about factors that would facilitate and/or hinder their abilities to perform them. The nurses evaluated the effectiveness of four theory-based interventions: skill-building vs. information only, and two methods of intervention delivery (one-on-one vs. group) against a control group among a sample of 564 black women (mean age 27.2 years) seeking outpatient care in a primary care clinic. Primary outcomes were self-reported sexual behaviors, and the secondary outcome was sexually transmitted disease (STD) incidence. Results indicated that the "Sister to Sister" one-on-one brief skill-building and group skill-building interventions were both effective at reducing sexual risk behaviors and STI occurrence, and that these effects lasted at the 12-month follow-up point. Findings showed that the skill-building group intervention did not produce outcomes superior to those of the one-on-one intervention. Even though the group intervention was lengthier and one might posit that greater benefit would be gained from interactions with other group members, the personalized nature of the one-on-one intervention may have been more customized to meet the specific risks of the women. Thus, the researchers concluded that the brief nurse-led one-on-one and group skill-building interventions were effective in reducing STI/HIV sexual risk behaviors and STI incidence. One limitation of the study is that the primary measure was assessed by self-report. Overall, the findings are similar to those of other studies that support the use of cognitive behavioral skill-building interventions for reducing sexual risk behavior among women. Although continued research is necessary to replicate the study with other populations of women in other settings, there is high potential for the application of brief nurse-led theory-based interventions to reduce the spread of sexually transmitted HIV infection.

As a follow-up to this study, Jones and colleagues (2012) report how this evidence-based HIV STD intervention was then prepared for national dissemination using the CDC's Replicating Effective Programs research translation process. Specifically, the research team relied on feedback from their community advisory board and field testing data to convert the protocols into a set of processes and tools for easy adaptation into the clinical setting by health educators, nurses and HIV counselors. This line of research, which has spanned multiple years, demonstrates the importance of involving communities over time in order to sustain the program ideas.

Data from Jemmott JB et al: Sexually transmitted infection/HIV risk reduction interventions in clinical practice settings, *J Obstet Gynecol Neonatal Nurs* 37:137-145, 2008; and Jemmott LS, Jemmott JB, O'Leary A: A randomized controlled trial of brief HIV/STD prevention interventions for African American women in primary care settings: effects on sexual risk behavior and STD rate, *Am J Public Health* 97:1034-1040, 2007; Jones et al: Lessons learned from field-testing a brief behavioral intervention package for African American women at risk for HIV/STDs. *Health Promot Pract* 14:168-173, 2012.

The nurse should remember that theories are not completely right or wrong. Different theories work well in different situations. Knowles (1989) relates that behaviorists program individuals through S-R mechanisms to behave in a certain fashion. **Humanistic theories** help individuals develop their potential in self-directing and holistic manners. Cognitive theorists recognize the brain's ability to think, feel, learn, and solve problems and train the brain to maximize these functions. Although social learning theory is largely a **cognitive theory**, it also includes elements of behaviorism (Bandura, 1977b). **Social learning theory's** premise is based on the idea that behavior explains and enhances learning through the concepts of efficacy, outcome expectation, and incentives.

Clinical Example

Application of Characteristics of Adult Learners to the Development of a Community Support Group

This example illustrates the long-standing value of incorporating theoretical underpinnings in the development of community activities designed to meet specific learning needs. It provides a description of how nurses played an active role in bolstering the community capacity and health of their community. Although this account dates back to the 1980s, it serves as an important reminder of the value of applying learning theories to one's work. It is common for nurses based in the community to be a key educational resource for patients, families, and community members as they cope with health and disease. As discussed later in this chapter, LUNA (Latinas Unidas por un Nuevo Amanecer, Inc., a nonprofit organization), whose mission is to provide support and offer culturally and linguistically relevant education to Hispanic breast cancer survivors and their families, was created more recently and is based on similar tenets.

As background, the author and a colleague began a community education support group for individuals with amyotrophic lateral sclerosis (ALS), more commonly known as Lou Gehrig's disease, on the basis of an identified community need. As background, ALS is an incurable degenerative neuromuscular disease that affects nerve and muscle function and the brain's ability to control muscle movement. (See http://alsawi.org/ for more information about ALS.) The support group was open to family members and friends. At that time, southeast Wisconsin did not have a support group. Community members provided feedback and identified the need for specific education topics and support for people with ALS. This initial dialogue provided the organizing framework for the inception of the first support group, and based on observations and interactions at the monthly meetings, an illustration of Knowles's assumptions follows:

Need to know: At the first support group meetings, the facilitators, both nurses, introduced possible topics by describing the reason for the discussion and the rationale for the selected subjects (e.g., common concerns of patients and family members and informal assessments based on conversations and the literature). To prepare for discussion, group members introduced themselves, and the nurses asked what they hoped to learn from the sessions. In some cases, members were unsure why they might want more information on given topics but indicated that they wanted to listen. Progression of the disease is variable; therefore the need to know was often facilitated by the nurses and other patients who already noted the importance of specific learning tasks (e.g., need for supportive care, assistive walking devices, financial planning, or information on assistive breathing devices).

Self-concept: A comfortable, informal environment allowed patients to express feelings, emotions, and frustrations about the disease. Participants were encouraged to express themselves. Participants cultivated mutual respect and trust for one another as a result of many commonalities. Hugs were common as members began to understand that others had similar situations and concerns. Group members had an opportunity to share and speak about ways that they managed and coped with their disease (e.g., decisions about life support and feeding tubes). Even if their choices were not the same, participants recognized and acknowledged these decisions without imposing their own value judgments. Facilitators and group members soon became equal partners in the learning process. At the core of the meetings was the formation of therapeutic healing and respectful relationships.

Continued

Experiences: Some patients and family members had gone through other difficult life experiences and stressors (e.g., other illnesses or deaths in the family) and helped others cope with the management of ALS. Patients shared their strengths gained from such experiences with other support group members. Additionally, individuals and family members who were going through varying stages of the disease process shared their experiences (e.g., obtaining home care, selecting a computer, and managing swallowing and eating). They shared tips and time-saving strategies with one another and with newly diagnosed families, and learned from those experiences.

Readiness to learn: Family members often take on many roles when someone becomes ill, especially with a chronic illness such as ALS. This redefinition of roles creates new learning opportunities; however, it can hinder learning if it is too overwhelming. For example, the well spouse may assume the roles of caregiver, parent, and financial supporter. It is helpful for nurses to identify resources to help the family cope with new roles (e.g., respite care).

Orientation to learning: Learning a variety of psychomotor skills is necessary to care for the patient with ALS (e.g., suctioning, positioning, using a feeding tube, and toileting). The timeframe for learning such skills varies depending on the course of illness. Presenting information about such skills too early in the course of the disease may cause fear and anxiety. Families may be resistant to learning such tasks until the need is apparent. In some cases, the need may be evident at a crisis point (e.g., a fall, a choking incident, or severe respiratory distress). However, nurse facilitators of support groups can introduce these topics slowly by providing information via educational sessions, newsletter, e-mails, printed brochures, blogs, discussion boards, and one-on-one discussions.

Motivation: Individuals and families often experience a shift in life goals when faced with ALS. Such shifts create new learning opportunities aimed at enhancing quality of life, survivorship, and maintaining self-esteem. For example, a college professor with ALS kept his link to the university. He was highly motivated to continue his research work and supervise his graduate students. To continue his academic work, he learned to manage his breathing by using a ventilator, arranged transportation to the university, obtained nursing care, and created communication methods by using a computer to ensure that his students' work continued.

Today, there are more than seven ALS support/caregiver groups in Wisconsin that grew from just one that was created in response to unmet needs in the community. Also, as a result, the ALS Association (ALSA) Wisconsin Chapter evolved from this local support group and became an official ALSA chapter in 1987. The chapter's mission is to "lead the fight to cure and treat ALS through global, cutting-edge research, and to empower people with Lou Gehrig's disease and their families to live fuller lives by providing them with compassionate care and support."

For more information on services, go to ALS national and state websites.

Knowles's Assumptions about Adult Learners

Knowles (1988, 1989) outlines several assumptions about adult learners. He contends that adults, like children, learn better in a facilitative, nonrestrictive, and nonstructured environment. Nurses who are familiar with these assumptions can develop teaching strategies that motivate and interest individuals, families, and groups and encourage active and full participation in the learning process. Nurses can help create a self-directing, self-empowering learning environment. The following characteristics impact learning: the client's need to know, concept of self, readiness to learn, orientation to learning, experience, and motivation. Table 8-1 expands on these characteristics.

Health Education Models

In addition to learning theories, the application of education theories and principles to situations involving individuals, families, and groups illustrates how ideas fit together, offers explanations for health behaviors or actions, and helps direct community nursing interventions. Such theoretical elements form the basis of understanding health behavior. Theoretical frameworks offer nurses an intervention blueprint that promotes learning and provides them with an organized approach to explaining concept relationships (Padilla and Bulcavage, 1991). Glanz and colleagues (2008) state that theories give educators the power to assess an intervention's strength and impact, and serve to enrich, inform, and complement practice.

What the nurse needs is often not a single theory that would explain all which he or she hears, but rather a framework with meaningful hooks and rubrics on which to hang the new variables and insights offered by different theories. With this customized metatheory or framework, the nurse can triage new ideas into categories that have personal utility in his or her practice and everyday realities. (Green, 1998, p. 2)

Models of Individual Behavior

Two models that explain preventive behavior determinants are the Health Belief Model (HBM), which is presented in Table 8-2 (Becker et al., 1977; Hochbaum, 1958; Kegeles et al., 1965; Rosenstock, 1966), and the Health Promotion Model (HPM) (Pender, Murdaugh, and Parsons, 2010). Both models are multifactorial, are based on value expectancy, and address individual perceptions, modifying factors, and likelihood of action. The HBM is based on social psychology and has undergone much empirical testing to predict compliance on singular preventive measures. The initial purpose of the HBM was to explain why people did not participate in health education programs to prevent or detect disease, in particular, tuberculosis (TB) screening programs (Hochbaum, 1958). Subsequent studies addressed other preventive actions and factors related to adherence to medical regimens (Becker, 1974). Primarily, the HBM is a value expectancy theory that addresses factors that promote health-enhancing behavior. It is disease-specific and focuses on avoidance orientation. The HBM considers perceived susceptibility, perceived severity, perceived benefits, perceived barriers, and other sociopsychological and structural variables. Self-efficacy, defined as the notion that an individual can act successfully on a given behavior to produce the desired outcome (Bandura, 1977a, 1977b), was later added to the HBM (Rosenstock, Strecher, and Becker, 1988; Strecher et al., 1986).

TABLE 8-1   CHARACTERISTICS OF ADULT LEARNERS

CHARACTERISTICS	APPLICATION TO HEALTH EDUCATION
Need to Know Adults must know why they need to learn.	The nurse explores the reasons that individuals, families, and groups want to learn. The nurse helps individuals recognize a need to learn.
Concept of Self Adults have a self-concept that developed from dependence to independence. It moves from others' direction to self-direction. Adults want to be capable of self-direction.	The nurse acknowledges that individuals, families, and groups are able to make choices and decisions. The nurse creates an environment in which patients can express themselves. The nurse recognizes that individuals, families, and groups can learn from their selected actions and can take self-direction and responsibility for such behaviors.
Experience Adults can draw upon many life experiences. Such experiences are enriching and are powerful learning resources.	The nurse assesses individuals, families, and groups for life experiences related to health issues. The nurse helps facilitate connections between previous and present experiences. The nurse allows individuals, families, and groups to share experiences with others in a supportive manner. Experiential methods, problem solving, case methods, and problem-solving discussion can help uncover the learners' experiences. The nurse clarifies previous and present experiences; this is especially helpful with negative and/or positive past experiences.
Readiness to Learn Developmental tasks and social roles affect readiness to learn. The timing of learning experiences with developmental tasks is important.	The nurse assesses and identifies individual, family, and group roles (e.g., caregivers or single parents) and key developmental tasks. The nurse seeks to understand the impact of roles and tasks on learning. The nurse creates role-modeling experiences.
Orientation to Learning Learning is often present-oriented and "now" based. Learning is directed to the immediate need and is problem centered.	The nurse assesses the learning needs of individuals, families, and groups on the basis of their learning priority. The nurse recognizes everyday stresses and hassles and addresses them within the learning context. The nurse provides health information, gives responses to their immediate needs, offers/provides health information, and offers problem-solving skills.
Motivation Internal drivers and factors are powerful motivators (e.g., self-esteem, life goals, quality of life, and responsibility).	The nurse determines individual, family, and group motivators. The nurse assesses for impediments that block motivation (e.g., poor self-esteem or lack of resources) and provides appropriate education, counseling, support, and referrals.

Modified from Knowles MS: *The making of an adult educator: an autobiographical journey,* San Francisco, 1989, Jossey-Bass; and Knowles MS: *The modern practice of adult education: from pedagogy to andragogy,* Chicago, 1988, Cambridge Press.

TABLE 8-2   HEALTH BELIEF MODEL*

COMPONENTS	EXAMPLE AND EXPLANATION
Perceived susceptibility	Belief that disease state is present or likely to occur
Perceived severity	Perception that disease state or condition is harmful and has serious consequences
Perceived benefits	Belief that health action is of value and has efficacy
Perceived barriers	Belief that health action is associated with hindrances (e.g., cost)
Self-efficacy	Belief that actions can be performed to achieve the desired outcome (one's confidence)
Demographics	Age, gender, and race/ethnicity
Cues to action	Influencing factors to get ready for action (e.g., educational materials, text messaging, billboards, newspapers, computer apps, blogs, reminder cues)

*For a more detailed description of the HBM, see Becker (1974).

Champion and Skinner (2008) point out that one of the limitations of the HBM is the variability in measurement of the central HBM constructs, which include the inconsistent measurement of HBM concepts and the failure to establish the validity and reliability of the measures prior to testing. For example, applying similar construct measures across different behaviors, such as barriers for mammography and colonoscopy, may be quite different. The past decades have produced some good examples of HBM scale development (Champion et al., 2008; Joseph et al., 2007; Rawl et al., 2000, 2012), yet caution in the application of the HBM to multicultural settings is merited. It would be important to determine whether the overall assumptions of the HBM—assumptions related to the value of health and illness—are similar to those of the particular racial/ethnic group under study. Although the HBM identifies an array of variables important in explaining individual health, nurses should view these variables within a larger societal perspective. Checking for cultural distinctions is especially critical to the model's usefulness (Janz, Champion, and Strecher, 2002) and is even more important today in light of our demographically changing landscape.

TABLE 8-3	HEALTH PROMOTION MODEL COMPONENTS AND DEFINITIONS*
COMPONENT	**DEFINITION-EXAMPLE**
Individual Characteristics and Experiences	
Prior behaviors	Amount and frequency of same/similar past behaviors
Personal factors (biological, psychological and sociocultural)	Age, gender sex, and race/ethnicity, weight, body fat; Personality, structure; Socioeconomic status
Behavior – Specific Cognitions and Affect	
Activity-related affect	Subjective feeling of emotions prior, during or after health behavior
Interpersonal influences	Interactions with family, peers and nurses: perceptions about the behaviors
Situational factors	Perceptions of compatibility of life context or environmental determinants that make health-promoting options available and engaging
Commitment to plan of action	Intention to carry out a specific health behavior and identification of successful strategies to achieve it
Perceived self-efficacy	Perceived ability to perform the necessary behaviors to achieve an outcome—judgment of personal capability
Immediate competing demands and preferences	Alternative behaviors that get in the way of course of action just before intended occurrence of planned behavior
Perceived benefits of health-promoting behaviors	Perception of positive outcomes that can occur from health-promoting behavior (e.g., feel fit and toned)
Perceived barriers to health-promoting behaviors	Perception of things that obstruct health-promoting behaviors (e.g., money and transportation)
Behavioral Outcome	
Health-promoting behavior	Desired behavioral outcome, such as weight loss, improved decision-making

*For a more comprehensive description and explanation of the HPM, see Pender et al. (2010).

Pender's Health Promotion Model is a competence- or approach-oriented model first appearing in the nursing literature in 1982. The HPM brings together a number of constructs from expectancy-value theory and social cognitive theory within a holistic nursing framework. Unlike the HBM, it does not rely on personal threat as a motivating factor. Rather, it aims to explain why individuals engage in health actions. The central focus of the model is based on eight beliefs that can be assessed by the nurse and that serve as key points for nursing intervention (Pender et al., 2010). It is applicable across the lifespan and has been used to examine the multidimensional nature of persons interacting with their physical and interpersonal environments, in studies that addressed a causal model of commitment to a plan for exercise in a sample of 400 Korean adults (Shin et al., 2005); examined the use of hearing protection devices by 703 construction workers (Ronis, Hong, and Lusk, 2006); explored the factors that enhance health-promoting behaviors of military spouses (Padden et al., 2013); or investigated the efficacy of how a "Girls on the Move" intervention

could improve cardiovascular fitness among urban middle school girls (Robbins et al., 2013). Table 8-3 lists the main components of the HPM and supplies their definitions.

The HBM and HPM can assist community health nurses in examining an individual's health choices and decisions for influencing health-related behaviors. The models offer nurses a cluster of variables that provide interesting insights into explaining health behavior. These variables are helpful cues. The nurse can consider them in planning programs, but should not try to fit an individual into all the categories. Simply put, models are aids that guide nurses in assessing patients and groups for the development, selection, and implementation of relevant educational interventions.

Try applying the model to your own life and health behaviors. Consider the following questions:

- Do you continually strive for improved health?
- Are you or your family susceptible to heart disease or obesity?
- Does a family history of cardiovascular disease motivate you or your family to exercise?
- What are your cholesterol and triglyceride numbers?
- Does looking fit and toned and having energy motivate you to exercise?
- Do work, school, or family responsibilities get in the way of your exercise plans?
- Has a family member, friend, or health provider recently reminded you of the benefits of exercise and encouraged you to start exercising?
- Do you believe you can initiate and incorporate an exercise program into your lifestyle, or do you need external reinforcement and cues?
- Does money, safety, or time pose any impediments to exercise?
- What would make exercise more appealing, such as a "running club"?
- What do you see as the benefits to exercise, for example, looking and feeling better and having more energy?
- In modifying your health behaviors, how important is exercise compared with other behaviors (e.g., getting relief from work and school stresses, cutting down on snacks, spending quality time with your family and friends)?

Think about these questions and consider your answers. Talk about this behavior with your peers and develop an exercise action plan that is personalized to your own priorities, needs, abilities, and interests.

Model of Health Education Empowerment

The HBM and HPM focus on individual strategies for achieving optimal health and well-being. The models are similar in that they are multifactorial, are based on the idea of value expectancy, and address individual perceptions, modifying factors, and likelihood of action. Although such approaches may be quite appropriate in changing individual behaviors, they do not necessarily address the complex relationships among social, structural, and physical factors in the environment, such as lack of social support systems, racism, and inaccessibility of health services (Israel et al., 2005; Minkler and Wallerstein, 2008; Smedley, 2003). Van Wyk (1999) suggests that nurses cannot assign power and control to the individual within the community but, rather, that the "power" must be taken on by the individual and community with the nurse *guiding* this dynamic process. This process includes examination of such factors as education, health literacy, gender, racism, and class and recognition of the structural and foundational changes that are needed to elicit change for socially and politically disenfranchised groups. Thus, knowledge is produced in a social context, and it is inextricably bound to relations of power. Therefore, an appropriate and more relevant health education model may be one that embraces a broader definition of *health* and addresses social, political, and economic aspects of health. Such a theoretical perspective is highly congruent with current community health education practices because it supports learner participation, highlights community engagement, and emphasizes empowerment.

Freire: A Focus on Problem-solving Education

Empowerment and literacy are two concepts that have a common history: The concept of empowerment can be traced back to Paulo Freire, a Brazilian educator in the 1950s who sought to promote literacy among the poorest of the poor, most oppressed members of the population. He based his work on a problem-solving approach to education, which contrasts with what he called the "banking education approach," which often places the learner in a passive role. Problem-solving education allows active participation and ongoing dialogue and encourages learners to be critical of and reflective about health issues. Freire suggested that when individuals assume the role of *objects*, they often become powerless and allow the environment to control them. However, when individuals become *subjects,* they influence environmental factors that affect their lives and community. Thus, community members, or subjects, are the best resources to elicit change (Freire, 2000, 2005).

Freire's methodology, often referred to as *critical consciousness*, involves not only education but also activism on the part of the educator. The basic tenet of Freire's work centers on empowerment, the contextualization of peoples' daily experiences, and collaborative, collegial dialogue in adult education. Freire's work speaks to a variety of action research applications, including those that relate to improving community health of marginalized populations. Freire's approach to health education increases health knowledge through a participatory group process and emphasizes establishing sustainable lateral relationships. This process explores the problem's nature and addresses the problem's deeper issues. The nurse serves as a central resource person and becomes an equal partner with other group members. Listening is a first essential step to understanding the issues. This exchange of ideas and concerns then creates a problem-posing dialogue to identify core problems or generative themes. As this process moves along, the group further delves into the root causes. Finally, the group co-creates relevant action plans that are suitably aligned with their lives (Freire, 2000).

Nurses can use health education as an empowering strategy to help people develop skills in problem solving, critical thinking, networking, negotiating, lobbying, advocacy, policy making, and information seeking to enhance health. Freire's approach may seem similar to health education's emphasis on helping people take responsibility for their health by providing them with information, skills, reinforcement, and support. However, Freire purports that knowledge imparted by the collective group is significantly more powerful than information provided by health educators. This learner-centered approach attempts to uncover the social and political aspects of problems and encourages group members to define and develop action strategies. Hence, there is keen recognition that health and behavior changes are multifaceted and usually do not have immediate solutions; therefore the term problem *posing*, rather than problem *solving*, better describes this empowerment process (Minkler, Wallerstein, and Wilson, 2008). As Steuart and Kark (1962) once stated, "health education must achieve its ends through means that leave inviolate the rights of self-determination of the individuals and their community."

The goal of participatory action research (PAR) is social change. PAR is also quite consistent with the role and responsibilities of nurses who are engaged in community health (Olshansky et al., 2005) and embraces the use of community-based participatory methods. What this means is that participation and action from stakeholders and knowledge about conditions and issues help facilitate strategies reached collectively (e.g., access to care, access to information). As definition, stakeholders are individuals, groups or organizations that have common and direct interests and concern in a topic, situation, or a health outcome. Some examples of the use of PAR include the following projects: English and colleagues (2004) developed the REACH 2010 program to build a public health community capacity program with a tribal community in the Southwest; Edgren and associates (2005) offered suggestions for involving the community in fighting against asthma; and Clements (2012) demonstrated how the use of PAR and photovoice was well suited as a framework within a community psychosocial recovery rehabilitation center in Winnepeg, Canada.

Examples of Empowerment Education and Participatory Methods

1. López and colleagues (2005) relate how photovoice was used as a participatory action research method with African-American breast cancer survivors in rural east North Carolina, referred to as the "inspirational images project." The aim of the study was to use this research method to allow women to convey the social and cultural meaning of silence about breast cancer and to voice their survivorship concerns so that relevant interventions could be developed to meet their needs. The task of the women was to take at least six pictures of people, places, or things that they enjoyed in life; of significant things they encountered as a survivor; and of what they used to cope. Discussion of photographs (e.g., pictures of church) led to discussions including a six-step inductive questioning technique, as suggested by Wallerstein and Bernstein (1988), to help participants frame educational strategies, as follows:

- What do you *SEE* in this photograph?
- What is *HAPPENING* in the photograph?
- How does this relate to *OUR* lives?
- *WHY* do these issues exist?
- How can we become *EMPOWERED* by our new social understanding?
- What can we *DO* to address these issues?

Photovoice offers an important and creative way to facilitate shared knowledge to achieve social change.

2. N. Wilson and colleagues (2008) describe YES! (Youth Empowerment Strategies), an after-school program for underserved elementary and middle school youth. Designed to reduce risky behaviors including drug, alcohol, and tobacco use, YES! combines multiple youth empowerment strategies to bolster youth's capacities and strengths to build problem-solving skills. A number of empowerment education projects, including photovoice and social action projects (e.g., awareness campaigns, projects to improve school spirit), were developed that involved members of the intended audience in the planning and implementation.

3. Luque and associates (2010) report the use of empowering processes based on Freire's popular education principles (Freire, 1968) and social cognitive theory, which focused on the constructs of environment, behavioral capability, observational learning, and self-efficacy (Bandura, 1977a, 1977b) for creating a barbershop training program about prostate cancer. By employing techniques borrowed from empowerment education (Wallerstein and Bernstein, 1988), barbers were engaged in group learning activities and problem-posing exercises designed around preferences and values related to prostate cancer health. Once the training and curriculum were completed among eight barbers, the team worked closely with the barbers to modify and create a supportive workplace environment for new health education tools (easy-to-read posters, brochures, DVD player, prostate cancer display model) to fuel discussions about prostate cancer health and decision making. Once the barbers were trained, structured surveys with barbershop clients (N = 40) were conducted. Results showed a significant increase in participants' self-reported knowledge of prostate cancer and an increased likelihood of discussing prostate cancer with a health care provider ($P < .001$). In conclusion, the barber-administered pilot intervention appeared to be an appropriate and viable communication strategy for promoting prostate knowledge to a priority population in a very convenient and familiar setting.

4. Wells and colleagues (2012) reported on the use of community-based participatory research methods framed within a social construct theoretical framework to develop a low-literacy, navigator-delivered cervical cancer and human papillomavirus (HPV) educational intervention. This program, based on empowerment principles, was designed to reach a rural Hispanic farmworker community in response to three gaps in care identified by a collaborating community clinical partner. The gaps were (1) delays in reporting results of Papanicolaou (Pap) tests to patients; (2) the need for navigated follow-up care for abnormal findings; and (3) the need for enhanced and consistent education about cervical cancer and HPV. The development of the lay navigation program was created on the basis of a long-standing community-academic collaboration between Catholic Mobile Medical Services (CMMS) and the Tampa Bay Community Cancer Network (TBCCN), a community network program funded by the National Cancer Institute. It was informed by formative research conducted with members of the farmworker community. Findings from the pilot are being used to generate knowledge about evidence-based patient navigation programs in community-based settings, develop a set of low-literacy Spanish-language educational teaching cards, and guide the creation of a Spanish-language Virtual Patient Educator (VPE)–"an avatar" to be used with a lay navigator to educate women about cervical cancer and HPV.

Community Empowerment

Community empowerment is a central tenet of community organization, whereby community members take on greater power to create change. It is based on community cultural strengths and assets. An empowerment continuum acknowledges the value and interdependence of individual and political action strategies aimed at the collective while maintaining the community organization as central (Minkler et al., 2008). As such, community organization reinforces one of the field's underlying premises as outlined by Nyswander (1956): "Start where the people are." Meade and Calvo (2001) point out that attention must be given to collective rather than individual efforts to ensure that the outcomes reflect the voices of the community and truly make a difference in people's lives. Furthermore, Labonte (1994) states that the community is an engine of health promotion and a vehicle for empowerment. He describes five spheres of an empowerment model, which focus on the following levels of social organization: interpersonal (personal empowerment), intragroup (small-group development), intergroup (community), interorganizational (coalition building), and political action. A multilevel empowerment model allows us to consider both macro-level and micro-level forces that combine to create both health and disease. Therefore, it seems that both micro and macro viewpoints on health education provide nurses with multiple opportunities for intervention across a broad continuum.

In summary, health education activities that respond to McKinlay's (1979) call to study "upstream," that is, to examine the underlying causes of health inequalities, through multilevel education and research allow nurses to be informed by critical perspectives from education, anthropology, and public health. For more extensive readings on this topic, see *Methods in Community-Based Participatory Research for Health* (Israel et al., 2005), *Community Organizing and Community Building for Health and Welfare* (Minkler M, 2012), or *Community-Based Participatory Health Research: Issues, Methods and Translation to Practices* (Blumenthal et al., 2013).

To effect change at the community level, nurses should become familiar with and knowledgeable about key concepts central to community organization (Table 8-4). This approach is an effective methodological tool that enables nurses to partner with the community, identify common goals, develop strategies, and mobilize resources to increase community empowerment, capacity, and community competence. Key concepts inherent in community health education programming are empowerment, principle of participation, issue selection, principle of relevance, social capital, and creation of critical consciousness (Minkler et al., 2008).

TABLE 8-4	COMMUNITY ORGANIZATION PRACTICE
KEY CONCEPTS	**APPLICATION TO HEALTH EDUCATION (NURSING ACTIONS)**
Empowerment Help individuals, families, and groups gain insight and mastery over life situations through problem solving and dialogue.	The nurse works with community members in identifying and defining issues and creates mechanisms for discussion and problem solving, and identification of other factors that have an impact on everyday lives.
Principle of Relevancy Know what issues are important to community members (these may differ from the issues important to nurses).	The nurse holds "town hall meetings" and community group discussions to allow members to share concerns and important issues. The nurse encourages the community to define issues (*what is important to them*). The nurse facilitates communications with community members to help them make decisions about health programs and messages.
Principle of Participation Learn by doing.	The nurse encourages group support. The nurse recognizes that active rather than passive participation results in greater likelihood of attitude and behavior changes.
Issue Selection Identify community problems that the community believes are specific, meaningful, and attainable.	The nurse uses problem-solving techniques to help group members identify relevant issues (e.g., group process activities, door-to-door surveys, charlas/talking circles).
Creation of Critical Consciousness Encourage relationships of equality and mutual respect among group members and educators to identify root problems and generate appropriate action plans.	The nurse uses problem-posing dialogue (Freire, 2005) to understand root issues and devises creative and innovative methods to transform situations.
Social Capital Foster relationships (networks) between community members (i.e., trust, engagement)	The nurse encourages community members to work together to improve social networks: they work together on a particular health gap in their community through partnership activities.

Modified from Minkler M, Wallerstein N, Wilson N: Improving health through community organization and community building. In Glanz K, Rimer BK, Viswanath K, editors: *Health behavior and health education: theory, research and practice*, ed 4, San Francisco, 2008, Jossey-Bass, pp. 288-312.

The development of LUNA (Latinas Unidas por un Nuevo Amanecer, Inc.) in Tampa, Florida, as described in the following Clinical Example, illustrates how the basic tenets of community need and organization fueled the development of a locally initiated group. LUNA represents a grassroots initiative to meet the needs of Hispanic breast cancer survivors and serves as a model for nurses, researchers, and community advocates working with underserved groups of cancer survivors.

Clinical Example

Example of Community Empowerment-Collaboration-Participation: LUNA

More than a decade ago (2002), a Latina nurse (Melba Martinez, RN, BSN), who had been diagnosed with breast cancer in 1995, started the first grassroots support group for Latinas in West Central Florida. The group began with five members and within the first year had 38 active members who attended monthly meetings. The group was initiated in response to an unmet need in the Tampa Bay area, that is, lack of education services for Latinas who had been diagnosed with breast cancer and who primarily spoke Spanish. Over the years, LUNA has created a network of more than 200 Latina survivors and has grown and become Latinas Unidas por un Nuevo Amanecer, Inc., a nonprofit organization whose mission is to provide support and offer culturally and linguistically relevant education to Hispanic breast cancer survivors and their families, friends, and caregivers. The organization primarily serves underserved, immigrant, low-income Latinas with limited English proficiency, assists with navigating the health care system, and functions as a community resource. LUNA draws on the tenets of community organization and empowerment fueled by problem-posing education. The three components of the LUNA model are (1) education (e.g., classes and presentations, Spanish cancer information, health care navigation, community outreach), (2) support (e.g., peer to peer, home, hospital and phone visits, communications), and (3) social reintegration (e.g., celebration of life events such as birthdays, cancer camps, walks, and other social events), similar to those of the start-up of the ALS support group previously described.

Outcomes of LUNA

1. Campamento Alegria: The first-ever Spanish-language oncology camp for Latina cancer survivors. A biennial program designed to provide Latinas in whom cancer has been diagnosed a positive and unforgettable experience through a variety of activities that help sustain them through their cancer journey (Martinez et al., 2008). Campamento Alegria aims to serve 100 women who would otherwise not have the opportunity to participate in such activities. There are no fees for the patients/survivors for a 3-day/2-night stay at the retreat facility, meals and related activities, orientation, and reunion meeting.

2. Community education and outreach: Attendance at various community events and health fairs to increase breast cancer screening awareness and provide cancer information and resources in Spanish. These events are popular, and attendance increases each year.

3. Ongoing monthly educational support group meetings: Presentations and classes provided by Spanish-speaking health professionals on various survivorship issues and cancer-related topics.

4. Plans to develop a patient navigator program for Latina patients with newly diagnosed cancer.

Continued

The process for creating LUNA began with one nurse who, through dedication and dialogue with others in the same situation, began taking charge of the situation on the basis of input from other community members. From both her nursing and personal experiences she knew how hard it was for Hispanic women in whom cancer was diagnosed to navigate the health care system, how difficult it is to take time for self-care, and how challenging it was for Hispanic women to talk about their fears. She recognized that Latinas with breast cancer should reach out to one another with understanding and compassion in their own language to move toward self-education and self-actualization. Since its inception, LUNA has partnered with various community-based organizations, hospitals, academic centers, churches, and other social support services to create a strong web of support. For example, LUNA has a strong partnership with researchers from the Tampa Bay Community Cancer Network (TBCCN), a community network program funded by the National Cancer Institute's Center to Reduce Cancer Health Disparities, as well as with local hospitals. LUNA also has worked with researchers to transcreate a stress management program for Latinas undergoing chemotherapy, which is now being evaluated in multisite clinical trial. LUNA represents a ground-up effort, which got its start because someone listened to the needs of Hispanic breast cancer survivors. It serves as an excellent model and reminder for nurses, researchers, and community advocates that the best ideas come from the "soul." For more information, view http://www.lunacancersupport.org/index.php/contact-us.

"Never doubt that a small group of thoughtful, committed citizens can change the world. Indeed, it is the only thing that ever has."— Margaret Mead

Acknowledgments: Melba Martinez, RN, BSN, and Dinorah (Dina) Martinez-Tyson, MA, MPH, PhD.

THE NURSE'S ROLE IN HEALTH EDUCATION

Although learning theories and health education models provide a useful framework for planning health interventions, the nurse's ability to facilitate the education process and become a partner with individuals and communities is inherently significant to the method's application. At the core of health education is the therapeutic relationship between the nurse and individuals, families, and the community. Simply put, nurses hold the process together and are catalysts for change in delivering humanistic care. Nurses activate ideas, offer appropriate interventions, identify resources, and facilitate group empowerment. It is beyond the scope of this chapter to describe multiple communication techniques in detail, but the reader is reminded of the value of establishing inclusion and trust before delivering the health education content.

Clinical Example

Mr. Chen is new to the area and starts to visit the local neighborhood senior center weekly to play cards and have lunch with his brothers, who have lived in the area for a number of years. Adjacent to the senior center (men call it "the club") is a nurse-managed clinic, which was started more than 13 years ago by the college of nursing at the local university. The clinic offers education and free or low-cost screenings on a regular basis. Many community members take advantage of this convenient service for their primary care. Mr. Chen has limited resources, so this community resource provides him with valuable access to health care services and information. On his first visit to the clinic, his blood pressure is 174/92 mm Hg. He states that the public hospital that cared for him in another city treated him for high blood pressure for more than 7 years, that doctors prescribed several medications 6 months earlier, and that he received many written materials to read (they were all in English). Although he reads somewhat in English, he tells the nurse that it would have been nice to see materials in his familiar language.

The nurse's assessment reveals that Mr. Chen takes his medication only when he does not "feel so good." He said his doctor advises him to take his medicines regularly, and he states that he takes them faithfully when he does not feel well. He tells the nurse that he remembers getting some educational booklets about his medications and "blood," but he found them too long and tiring to read. The nurse's educational assessment reveals that Mr. Chen has completed 8 years of schooling, does not read much, enjoys television over print, and likes to learn from pictures or from other people in groups. He states that he would really like to get his health information in easy English but would mostly prefer to get some easy materials in Chinese. His reading skills have not been verified by health providers. Yet it seems that he has taken the health instruction literally (e.g., he interprets "take regularly" to mean take consistently when "I don't feel right" vs. take the pills on a regular schedule).

To facilitate learning, the nurse establishes a teaching plan with Mr. Chen's input. This plan involves communicating health instructions in more relevant ways (e.g., using pictures, drawings, mnemonics, videotapes), providing word cards for him in Chinese with the help of the local translation services, and putting him in touch with county financial resources to assist in buying his medicines. The nurse also establishes a follow-up plan with a bilingual nurse to verify Mr. Chen's understanding of how to take his meds by asking him to repeat back in his own words when/how he takes his meds (teach-back methods). She also plans to develop a series of health education group classes for seniors at "the club" about health and wellness, with high blood pressure as one of the topics of discussion.

ENHANCING COMMUNICATION

The critical step of *inclusion* establishes the base for possible health action; it sets the relationship. What this means is that the nurse needs to be especially cognizant of those first introductory oral exchanges and interactions. Inclusion may simply entail greeting individuals, families, and groups in a warm fashion, offering comfort, and attending to their immediate concerns or worries. Education does not begin with the first instructional word. Rather, education begins with establishing an atmosphere conducive to learning, whereby a therapeutic trusting relationship forms the foundation for a healing relationship. If the nurse attends to *inclusion* first, individuals, families, and groups next begin to *trust* the nurse and thereby trust the *content* of the health education message. This trust is evident through active participation in and commitment to the education process.

It is important to note that the ongoing enhancement and refinement of nursing knowledge and skills to provide culturally effective care is critical to community health education. Nurses are fundamental in responding to diverse community members' everyday health concerns with meaningful and understandable information. This involves taking time to get to know individuals, their families, and their experiences.

Meleis (1999) describes culturally competent care as care that exhibits sensitivity to individuals based on their vast experiences and their responses, which are due to their backgrounds, sexual orientation, socioeconomic status, ethnicity, literacy, and cultural background. She depicts several properties that make up the "essence of health nurses" who deliver culturally competent care. First, they possess an explanatory system that values diversity. This is a system that is not drained by the constant attempt to interpret symbols but rather is energized by the variations. Second, they show expert assessment skills to discern different and similar patterns of responses that help in planning appropriate educational interventions. Third, culturally competent nurses are aware of the diversity of communication patterns and how language and communication influence "trust within the relationship." Culturally effective professionals also recognize how marginalization may increase health risks for individuals and that using the expertise of insiders in the culture is a highly valued skill.

For more information on the provision of culturally appropriate health care, consult the OMH's national standards for Culturally and Linguistically Appropriate Services (CLASs) (USDHHS OMH, 2000,) and the updated, enhanced 15 standards (USDHHS OMH, 2010) that represent a comprehensive series of guidelines to advance health equity, improve quality, and help eliminate health disparities. View https://www.thinkculturalhealth.hhs.gov/ to learn more about the enhanced standards. The standards were created in response to growing concerns about health inequities and the need for health care systems to reach increasingly diverse patient populations. The standards reinforce the ability of nurses and organizations to understand and respond well to the cultural and linguistic needs brought by patients and community members to the health care setting. Several standards have particular relevance to community nursing. For example, Standard 1 signifies the importance of providing effective, equitable, understandable, and respectful quality care and services, in light of diverse cultural health beliefs and practices, preferred languages, health literacy, and other communication needs. Standard 13 reinforces the need to partner with the communities to design, implement, and evaluate policies, practices, and services to ensure appropriateness. To learn more about these standards and their application to nurses, visit "Culturally competent nursing care: A cornerstone of caring," at

https://ccnm.thinkculturalhealth.hhs.gov/. And remember: cultural competency is an ongoing journey that requires an openness to acknowledge what one does not know and the willingness to seek better ways to get the job done. It is a process, not simply a program.

⚖ ETHICAL INSIGHTS

Ethical Issues Related to Health Education and Health Literacy

Health literacy—Do community members understand the plethora of printed and electronic health messages communicated to them in terms of language, ease of reading, and linguistics? To address the national problem of health literacy, nurses should assess their roles as educators, information brokers, advocates, facilitators, collaborative problem solvers, and navigators. Nurses should consider the impact that the multitude of demands of the health care system has on client autonomy.

Individual vs. collective/societal rights and responsibility for health—What communication factors should the nurse consider when balancing the health education needs of the individual against those of the collective (e.g., family and community)? What communication gaps can be bridged by the development and implementation of health information that is relevant culturally, linguistically, and in terms of literacy?

Social justice and equity—Do all community members enjoy equity in their access to health education and information? Does health information take into account the diversity of a demographically changing country? What types of materials are available for non–English-speaking clients? What strategies, programs, and interventions can be implemented to reduce the discovery to delivery disconnect? How can nurses reduce the demands of the health care system and implement navigation strategies?

Allocation of resources—In what way do policies promote and/or hinder promotion of health literacy? Do national/local government and corporate/institutional policies impact the availability, accessibility, and equitable distribution of information resources? In what way do current policies reward and support patient education? How can the nurse get involved in shaping and redirecting health policy and moving policy into practice? This includes policies at the institutional, community, local, and national levels.

Cultural effectiveness—What skills, knowledge, and experiences are necessary to the planning of health education within the context of people's history and everyday realities? The nurse should assess his or her abilities to approach health education tasks with confidence, compassion, competence, and cultural humility (Marks, 2009; USDHHS, 2000, 2010).

Consider health literacy as an ethical issue of concern in the community and how it contributes to health equity.

FRAMEWORK FOR DEVELOPING HEALTH COMMUNICATIONS

Within the community, the nurse's intended audience may be an individual, family, group, or many segments of the community. Using a systematic approach to the development, design, and delivery of health education programs provides the nurse with an organized, user-friendly way to deliver health messages. Although nurses may select and use a variety of educational models, theoretical frameworks, and teaching and learning principles, the National Cancer Institute suggests using the "Framework for Developing Health Communications" to create a variety of health education messages and programs (USDHHS, 2008). See ⓔ **Resource Tool 8B**, Framework for Developing Health Communications, on the book's Evolve website at http://evolve.elsevier.com/Nies.

This organizing framework has four stages (simplified from six) and is depicted by a circular loop that offers the opportunity for continuous assessment, feedback, and improvement. The framework has been used widely by the author to develop cancer education materials and media on such topics as smoking, prostate cancer, breast and cervical cancer, stress management, and clinical trials (Brandon et al., 2012; Jacobsen et al., 2002, 2012; Meade, McKinney, and Barnas, 1994; Luque et al., 2010; Quinn et al., 2006; Schapira, Meade, and Nattinger, 1997; Simmons et al., 2011; Wells et al., 2012). This framework can be easily adapted to the design and development of all types of health education topics, such as diabetes, hypertension, HIV, and nutrition.

This framework is based on the principles of social marketing and health education, and on mass communication theories and relies on intended audience assessment to guide the process. It is highly congruent with Freire's model of empowerment education, which encourages ongoing dialogue with potential consumers and users of health education services. Although this model focuses on communication strategies aimed at the programmatic level, the basic elements are applicable to individual, family, and group systems. The nurse should not expect to apply the model in a linear manner but rather to move back and forth between the stages. These stages mirror the nursing process (assessment, planning, implementation, and evaluation) and provide a sequential and organized path for continuous assessment, feedback, and improvement so as to achieve a successful communication program. The ideas contained in this Framework for Developing Health Communications model are a practical schema for planning and implementing health education communications programs (see the box "Launching a Breast Education and Outreach Screening Program"). See Figure 8-1.

Stage I: Planning and Strategy Development

The planning stage provides the foundation for a communication program's planning process and is crucial in setting the stage for creating salient communications. Understanding the intended audience's learning needs and targeting the program or message to the audience are pivotal to activating effective health education. This step reinforces Freire's philosophical tenets of ascertaining the intended audience's needs and creating open dialogue. This stage also reduces expensive alterations once the program is under way.

Questions to Ask

- Who is the intended audience?
- What is known about the audience and from what sources?
- What are the communication and education objectives and goals?
- What evaluation strategies will the nurse use?
- What are the issues of most concern? (Note: these may not necessarily be health issues but may be important ones to link to the health issue when planning, e.g., safety, transportation)
- What is the health issue of interest?

Collaborative Actions to Take

- Review available data from health statistics, census data, local sources, libraries, newspapers, and local or community stakeholders.
- Get community partners involved.
- Obtain new data (e.g., interviews, surveys, and focus groups using problem-posing dialogue format).
- Determine the intended group's needs and perceptions of health problems (i.e., identify audiences).
- Determine the community's assets and strengths:
  - Physical (e.g., gender, age, and health history)
  - Behavioral (e.g., lifestyle characteristics and health-related activities)
  - Demographic (e.g., income, years of schooling, language, and cultural characteristics)
  - Psychographics (e.g., beliefs, values, and attitudes)
- Identify issues behind the issues and identify health knowledge gaps.
- Establish goals and objectives that are specific, attainable, prioritized, and time specific.
- Assess resources (e.g., money, staff, and materials).

LAUNCHING A BREAST EDUCATION AND OUTREACH SCREENING PROGRAM

The H. Lee Moffitt Cancer Center and Research Institute, or Moffitt, formed a partnership with Suncoast Community Health Centers, Inc., or Suncoast, in rural Hillsborough County, Florida. The partnership initially brought breast cancer education and screening services to Hispanic migrant and seasonal farmworkers and low-income rural women via Moffitt's Lifetime Cancer Screening Mobile Unit. Initiated by a cancer center physician who visited Suncoast, a federally funded, community-based center located about 30 miles south of Tampa, he was struck by the center's services and impressed with the clinic's dedication to reaching medically underserved populations. Suncoast consisted of multiple comprehensive federally qualified health care clinics, in Plant City, Ruskin, Brandon, and Dover, Florida, and offered a wide range of primary health care services. yet it did not have mammography facilities. Moffitt was expanding its community outreach initiatives through mobile outreach services. Moffitt was a freestanding, private, nonprofit institution located at the University of South Florida campus in Tampa. A National Cancer Institute–designated comprehensive cancer center in Florida, Moffitt is widely known for state-of-the-art treatment, novel research, and ambulatory services, and advanced screening modalities. After a series of meetings between Suncoast and Moffitt's Lifetime Cancer Screening Center, the groups formed a partnership based on a mutual shared goal—to improve the breast health of high-risk and medically underserved women. Both parties determined that the goal was to develop and offer the community culturally appropriate education, accessible mammography service, and follow-up care.

TABLE 8-5   TEACHING-LEARNING FORMATS

TEACHING FORMAT	APPLICATION TO HEALTH EDUCATION
Brainstorming session	Allows participants the freedom to generate ideas and discuss them in a group setting. Cultivates creativity. Fosters empowerment to allow members to identify the issue and find solutions.
Community-wide programs	Can reach large numbers of community members through a systematic plan. May include individual or group approaches with a defined intended audience.
Demonstration	Effective in learning perceptual motor skills. Aids in visual identification.
Group discussion	Members can learn from each other and receive support. Nurses can personalize teaching content to group needs. Ideal for groups combining patients and families. Nurses, health professionals, or lay members can lead the groups. Facilitator must be comfortable with group method and familiar with group characteristics.
Lecture	Varying group sizes can use formal oral presentations. Group members share expertise and experiences. Presenter must be comfortable and possess speaking ability. Requires organizational skills and ability to highlight key points in interesting and creative ways. A combination of lecture media may enhance learning. Audience participation is linked to the presenter's speaking style and ability. Audience feedback is limited.
Indivdual discussion	Allows individual assessment and identification of cultural barriers, physical impairments, learning needs, literacy, and anxiety. Promotes the tailoring of health education plans. Ideal to capture "teachable moments." Does not allow sharing and support from others. High cost in terms of staff time.
Role playing	Effective in influencing attitudes and opinions. Encourages problem-solving and critical thinking skills. Enhances learner participation. Some members may be hesitant to become involved.
Task force committee/ community organizing meetings	Joins individuals with diverse backgrounds and expertise to achieve a goal. May represent many interests and perspectives.
Talking circles/charlas	May be held in convenient settings such as missions, homes, or service settings: engages people in small group discussions (Strickland, 1999).
Town hall meetings	Can offer shared experience in a familiar setting.

Data from Stallings et al (2005); Redman (2007); and USDHHS (2008).

Stage II: Developing and Pretesting Concepts, Messages, and Materials

The nurse's decisions in stage I can help guide him or her in selecting appropriate communication channels and producing effective and relevant materials. Consider how to reach the intended audience and use interesting and engaging supporting materials and media. *Channel* refers to how the nurse reaches communication sites (i.e., churches, clinics, missions, nurses, or community-based organizations). *Format* refers to how the nurse communicates the health message (e.g., through individual or group discussion) (Table 8-5). Keep in mind that materials and media are the program's tools, not the program itself (Table 8-6). Education is a human activity and should not focus on audiovisuals exclusively. To ensure that messages are relevant and meaningful, the nurse can employ qualitative research methods (pretesting, learner verification) to obtain feedback about the understandability and acceptability of the materials. Learning now what works and does not work saves a lot of time and money later!

Questions to Ask

- What channels are best?
- What formats should be used?
- Are there existing resources?
- How can the nurse present the message?
- How will the intended audience react to the message?
- Will the audience understand, accept, and use the message?
- What changes can improve the message?

DESCRIPTION OF HEALTH ISSUE AND INTENDED AUDIENCE

Despite progress in the fight against cancer, many communities continue to bear a disproportionate share of the cancer burden. Cancer disparities very likely arise from the complex interplay of factors—that is, low socioeconomic status, low levels of education and literacy, social injustice, and poverty—that impede awareness about screening and follow-up care. Together, these factors affect access to care and cancer survival and yield an uneven distribution of cancer morbidity and mortality, which substantially impacts marginalized populations (Albano et al., 2007; American Cancer Society, 2013; Brookfield et al., 2009; Chu et al., 2007). Meade and colleagues (2009) suggest that in the development of cancer outreach and screening programs, it is absolutely critical to layer on additional levels of understanding of and sensitivity to the social, cultural, and political conditions of home countries, language and literacy needs, obstacles to basic health care access, cultural significance of gender and age roles, culturally mediated etiologic perceptions of

Continued

DESCRIPTION OF HEALTH ISSUE AND INTENDED AUDIENCE—cont'd

disease, illness experiences, religiosity, and the sociopolitical nature of immigration situations. Such factors affect the design and meaning of health communication and health education. Our assessment revealed that many women did not appear for breast screenings because of a "fear of cancer" and uncertainty of how to navigate the health care system. Typically, many women did not seek preventive health care; but rather sought care for episodic acute illnesses. The lack of mammography screening and education for rural Hillsborough County's medically underserved women represented a health service gap. In particular, individuals may face a number of potential factors that get in the way to acceptable mammography services. These factors may reflect limited access points to health care, low awareness of the importance of the screening and language, literacy, and linguistic concerns. Educational and communication interventions and tools that address (1) unique value systems, (2) relevant and specific cultural and linguistic factors, and (3) access issues—as well as capitalize on the strengths of the women—were warranted (Meade et al., 2009). Our experiences reminded us that women want and need health information about breast health but that they also experience everyday struggles. As such peer outreach/navigation can help to deconstruct those concerns and better engage community members in their health.

What was required in Hillsborough County was the delivery of a culturally relevant health service in a geographically convenient area. Women aged 40 years and older were eligible for this service. The initial intended audience was primarily Hispanic migrant and seasonal farmworkers but also grew to include women from other diverse ethnic backgrounds (i.e., Haitian, rural white).

Goal: To prevent premature death and disability from breast cancer through early detection, screening, and culturally and linguistically relevant education.

Objectives: To increase education, mammograms, clinical breast examinations, and follow-up programs among medically underserved women in rural Hillsborough County.

TABLE 8-6   MATERIALS AND MEDIA

MEDIA	CONSIDERATIONS IN HEALTH EDUCATION SETTINGS
Audio response system (ARS)	Allows high interactivity and participation among audience. Offers a data collection and assessment tool. Helps to assess immediate understanding (Davis et al., 2012).
Audiotapes	Do not require reading. Portable and small. Individuals can use them at home in a comfortable setting and can replay and use them at their own pace. Economical. Helpful for individuals with visual difficulties or low literacy skills.
Bulletin boards	Inexpensive and easy to develop. Direct attention to a specific message; use few words.
Exhibits and displays	Graphics offer appeal. Placement in high-traffic areas (e.g., waiting rooms and examination rooms) reaches wide audiences.
Flip charts, chalkboards and whiteboards	Excellent format to enlarge teaching concepts or cue reader to salient points; graphics and diagrams may be added. Chalkboards are reusable; flip charts have replacement pads, so inexpensive.
Games and simulations	Involve patients in a fun manner; involve the entire family. Highly effective with children.
Graphics	Can convey important points in salient and visual fashion.
Drawings and visuals	Can aid understanding for low-literacy audiences. Visual messages should be pretested to ensure acceptability and understanding.
Interactive media	A variety of computer programs, talking touch screens, interactive kiosks, computer-assisted instructive media, mobile tablet technology-based, etc. Algorithms and branching decisions aid patients in decision making, problem solving, and fact acquisition (Woolfe et al., 2005; Yost et al., 2009). Interactive patient education is becoming more common via kiosks in waiting rooms. Nurses should assess patients' computer comfort level. Software development may be time intensive and costly.
Models and real objects	Bring the teaching concept to the patient in a familiar way.
Demonstrations	Helpful when conveying psychomotor skills; encourage patient involvement and tactile learning (e.g., penis model for condom placement or breast model to show breast self-examination). No reading needed.
Storytelling/theater	Reading is minimal. Encourages questions and elicits insights (Werle, 2004). Helpful in individual and group instruction. Nurses can incorporate models and real objects into displays or fairs.
Overhead /data projector presentations	Useful in small- and large-group settings. Highlight key points and help patient focus ideas. Use of color and advance organizers, large type, and key points is recommended; avoid busy and cluttered overheads. Can be prepared in advance. Inexpensive.

TABLE 8-6	MATERIALS AND MEDIA—cont'd
MEDIA	**CONSIDERATIONS IN HEALTH EDUCATION SETTINGS**
Photographs, picture books, pictographs, and slide series (i.e., PowerPoint slides); photo-essay and photovoice Prezi presentations	Help promote understanding by showing realistic images and real situations. Help patients make connections to their lives. Photographs may appear alone or in combination with other photographs or slides or may be placed in an album and (Choi, 2011; Houts et al., 2006; Machtinger et al., 2007; Quinn et al., 2008; Roberts et al., 2009) PowerPoint slides are easily updated. Helpful for patients with limited literacy skills; offer visual presentation of concepts. Effective with an individual and with small groups (i.e., self-study or reflection). Easily updated.
Printed materials (brochures, leaflets, or booklets)	Portable, widely available, and economical. Useful in reinforcing health concepts and interactions. Patients can set and adjust the pace and refer back to information later. Can be effective with individuals, families, groups, or community-wide dissemination. Materials written at simple levels can be effective and acceptable for both low-level and high-level readers (Doak et al., 1998; Meade and Byrd, 1989). Tailored materials are a promising strategy for health education (Hawkins et al., 2008). Nurses should assess issues of readability, design, layout, cultural relevance, and appropriateness of content.
Programmed materials, self-help guides, slides, and tape programs	May involve printed materials combined with visuals to allow self-pacing. Helpful for learning facts. Nurse should assess individual or group to determine whether independent learning style is preferred. Storytelling (Larkey et al., 2009).
Teaching cards	Portable, use few words, and offer visual interpretations. Can be easily personalized.
Flash cards	The nurse can create them economically and update them easily. Effective with individual, small-group, or family instruction.
Radio and newspapers	Reach large audiences within the community. Effective in conveying general health information in a user-friendly manner. Nurses can play an active role in disseminating health information.
Television and cable television	Reach large audiences within the community. Can help enhance community members' general health and well-being. Effective in influencing attitudes and behaviors. Offer a familiar medium for viewer to learn about health topics. Nurses can play key roles in reaching the community.
Telephones/ smartphones	Automated phone systems: reminder phone calls (Rubin et al., 2006). Telephone coaching (Sepulveda et al., 2008); telenursing (Jönsson and Willman, 2008)
Videotapes, DVDs/telenovela	Combine audio and visual media to convey realistic images (Meade, 1996). Videotapes/DVDs should incorporate a role modeling concept. Used in stress management materials (Jacobsen et al., 2002); for prostate cancer education (Sheehan, 2009); and for deaf audiences (Pollard et al., 2009). Expensive to produce and update; require access to audiovisual equipment and viewing sites. Videotapes/DVDs may be costly to produce and purchase but with computerized digital editing, are easily updated. Telenovella-storytelling (Cueva et al., 2013)
Online resources (i.e., Internet, simple dial-up services, information, databases, bulletin board chat services, and World Wide Web)	Electronic information sources can link individuals, families, and groups to health. Can reach large audiences rapidly. World Wide Web sites should be evaluated by nurses/providers for accuracy, credibility, and relevancy. New technologies and innovations can help consumers find health information, advice, and support, especially at-risk groups (Vishwanath et al., 2013).
Podcasts	Portable video technology that uses media broadcasts and can be accessed via the Internet and viewed on a personal computer or on a handheld device, such as an iPod or an MP3 player (Abreu et al., 2008).
Social media	Online interactive discussions, blogs, social bookmarking, social news, social networking sites (Vyas et al., 2012; Bender et al., 2012; CDC, 2010; Koskan et al., under review; Vyas et al., 2012 Ramanadhan et al., 2013; Chou et al., 2013).

Data from U.S. Department of Health and Human Services: *Making health communication programs work: A planner's guide, pink book,* Bethesda, MD, 2008, Office of Cancer Communications, National Cancer Institute. Available from <http://www.cancer.gov/cancertopics/cancerlibrary/pinkbook>.

Collaborative Actions to Take

- Identify messages and materials.
- Decide whether to use existing materials or produce new ones.
- Select channels and formats.
- Develop relevant materials with the target audience.
- Pretest the message and materials and obtain audience feedback (e.g., through interviews, questionnaires, focus groups, and readability testing). Pretesting helps ensure comprehension, acceptability, and cultural relevance.

SELECTING CHANNELS AND METHODS

Nurses selected a combination of channels to communicate health information about breast cancer, screenings, and early detection methods (e.g., community-based clinics, missions, social service agencies, health events, and fairs). Nurses conducted individual interactions at the mobile or stationary site at the screening center.

Nurses collected a variety of health materials and media about breast cancer from national, state, and local sources and determined that many of the printed materials were not culturally or educationally suited for the individuals the nurses were serving; for example, the materials were geared toward high reading levels, and few Spanish-language or Haitian Creole materials were available.

DEVELOPING MATERIALS

Grants from Avon, National Alliance of Breast Cancer Organizations (NABCO), Susan G. Komen for the Cure Florida Suncoast Affiliate, and National Cancer Institute supported the development of English, Spanish, and Creole materials to educate women about breast health. Additionally, although translators were sporadically present, it became apparent that bilingual/bicultural staff was necessary. Ongoing dialogue with community members and clinics helped refine the screening process, the education component, and follow-up services to ensure effectiveness, efficiency, appropriateness, and timely follow-up.

Stage III: Implementing the Program

At the third stage, the nurse introduces the health education message and program to the intended audience and reviews and revises necessary components. The nurse also analyzes the program and health message for effectiveness and tracks the mechanisms using process evaluation. This way of organizing the implementation process examines the procedures and tasks involved in the program or message, such as monitoring media, identifying the intended audience's interim reactions, and addressing internal functioning (e.g., work schedules and expenditures).

IMPLEMENTATION

The mass media publicizes the services and disseminates human-interest stories, especially during October—Breast Cancer Awareness Month. The outreach workers posted flyers at a variety of sites (e.g., beauty shops, laundromats, missions, churches, grocery stores, churches, unemployment offices, and community centers). Twice per month, the mobile unit traveled to rural areas. There, staff greeted women and answered questions about the mammography procedure and follow-up.

Questions to Ask

- How should the health education program/message be launched?
- How do we maintain interest and sustainability?
- How can we use process evaluation?
- What are the strengths of the health program?
- How can we keep on track within the timeline and budget?
- How can we find out whether we have reached the intended audience?
- How well did each step work (i.e., process evaluation)?
- Are we maintaining good relationships with our community partners?

Collaborative Actions to Take

- Work with community organizations, adult education centers, businesses, media, and other health agencies to enhance effectiveness.
- Monitor and track progress.
- Establish process evaluation measures (e.g., follow-up with users of the service, number of community members who used the service, and expenditures).

Stage IV: Assessing Effectiveness and Making Refinements

Outcome evaluation examines whether changes in knowledge, attitudes, and behavior did or did not occur as a result of the program. Together with the process evaluation, the data inform how well the program is functioning and direct future modifications. The nurse prepares for a new development cycle using information gained from audience feedback, communication channels, and the program's intended effect. This stage helps to continually refine the health message and respond to the intended audience's needs. New information helps to validate the program's strengths and allows for necessary modifications. Feedback is necessary to continually refine the message and direct new messages.

Questions to Ask

- What was learned?
- How can outcome evaluation be used to assess effectiveness?
- What worked well, and what did not work well?
- Has anything changed within the intended audience?
- How might we refine the methods, channels, or formats?
- Overall, what lessons were learned, and what modifications could strengthen the health education activity?

Collaborative Actions to Take

- Conduct outcome evaluations (e.g., randomized experiment, evaluation studies, definition of data needed for data collection).
- Reassess and revise goals and objectives.
- Modify unsuccessful strategies or activities.
- Generate continual support from businesses, health care agencies, and other community groups for ongoing collaboration and partnerships.

ASSESSING EFFICIENCY

Process Evaluation

A number of newspapers/flyers, television, and radio advertisements publicized the free or low-cost mammography service and highlighted the importance of breast health. Also, several human-interest stories emerged, which communicated the screening services to a wider audience. Since the onset of the program, increases in the number of staff involved in the program, the number of volunteers, and the number of funded projects that support the program enhanced its breadth and depth and sparked the development of new initiatives. Most notably, the Tampa Bay Community Cancer Network (TBCCN), an NCI-funded community network program center, a partnership of 23 community organizationshas increased the number of committed key stakeholders who have identified other areas of community need and outreach such as a need for cervical cancer navigation and increased colorectal cancer screening uptake (Wells et al., 2012b; Gwede et al., 2013). As a result of an additional community partner needs assessment, (Gwede et al., 2010), additional cancer education workshops, health events, and cancer services have been broadened and evaluated.

For example, funding for a Patient Research Navigation Program, further augmented outreach efforts. Designed to eliminate barriers to cancer diagnosis and treatment, this project generated new knowledge for the advancement of an evidence-based, culturally and literacy appropriate lay navigation program for community members who had a breast/colorectal cancer abnormality by evaluating timeliness to resolution of abnormality and enhancing timeliness to diagnosis and delivery of cancer care (Roetzheim et al., 2012; Lee et al., 2013; Wells et al., 2008; Wells et al., 2011.)

Outcome Evaluation

During the mammography screening program's initial years, fewer than 200 women received mammography screening per year. The number of women screened approached more than 1000 per year in subsequent years. Currently, mammography services are provided at stationary screening sites at the cancer center (women use vouchers), and funding opportunities and institutional support sustain the program. The number of community partners has grown considerably, a reflection of enhanced community capacity and awareness. Regular health events are scheduled, continual refinement of screening services and follow-up are ongoing.

FEEDBACK

Reports describing process and outcome evaluation and analysis provide a point of reference for continual improvements. Such reports apply knowledge and outline methods to enhance and improve the service's efficiency and effectiveness.

The mammography program has incorporated a network of outreach and educational components to reach rural migrant and seasonal farmworkers and other low-income women in south and east Hillsborough County. Although the program provided desired links to screening services and has formed successful community partnerships, it is important to develop and refine community empowerment strategies through outreach and education to sustain and widely disseminate the program. Building on this successful model of education and outreach (Meade et al., 2002b; Meade et al., 2009), the administrators of the program applied lessons learned for outreach to other high-risk populations, (e.g., Haitian and African-American men and women) in the development of colorectal cancer screening initiatives (Gwede et al., 2013). A key lesson learned here is that community outreach, based on trust, respect and mutual commitment, can fuel community-identified research priorities and lead to the testing and evaluating of evidence based interventions for community benefit.

Instructions: Think about a target group that you are currently working with and planning to deliver/create a health education program or message. Complete the exercise by asking yourself the following questions:

Questions to Ask

Action Plan

• **What is the overall intended message/goal?** (What are my reasons for planning this message? How do I know that it is needed or wanted by the audience?)

• **Who is the intended audience?** (Write a brief statement describing the characteristics of the group.)

• **What are the benefits of this message to the group?**

• **What channels will I use to deliver the message?** (Provide a rationale.)

• **Will I need to create materials?** (Are there available materials that are appropriate for the group?)

• **How will I know if my message gets across to the audience?** (Did the audience respond? How many people were reached? Who responded?)

• **Was there change?** (What are the reasons the message was or was not effective? What can be modified to strengthen the message?)

FIGURE 8-1 Planning your health education message.

- Provide justification for continuing or ending the program.
- Summarize the health education program or message in an evaluation report.

The reader is encouraged to think about how health education messages or programs can be planned using this model. The exercise in Figure 8-1 can be helpful to organize your ideas.

HEALTH EDUCATION RESOURCES

A variety of health education materials and resources are available from local, state, and national organizations and agencies. Such associations provide helpful information about services, educational materials, and links to support groups or self-help groups. Often, printed and electronic materials are available for free or for a nominal cost. Nurses can help individuals, families, and groups find and access materials, services, or equipment loan programs and can become knowledgeable about community resources. Additionally, identifying gaps in services may help nurses create new materials. Some examples of resources are as follows:

- Local and regional hospitals, clinics, libraries, adult education centers, health education centers, media outlets, and businesses
- Local and state governmental sources (e.g., health departments and social service agencies); check the Internet for listings
- Community-based organizations (i.e., advertised, non-advertised, and those recommended by community leaders and stakeholders, National Association of Community Health Centers, parish nursing associations, faith-based organizations, social service agencies)
- Universities and colleges, community colleges, and academic nursing centers
- Professional organizations (e.g., American Public Health Association, National Association of Hispanic Nurses, National Black Nurses Association, National Student Nurses Association, Society for Behavioral Medicine)
- Commercial organizations (e.g., pharmaceutical companies, medical supply companies, and patient and health education companies); printed and electronic sources are often available
- Federal government sources (e.g., National Institutes of Health [NIH]; National Cancer Institute; National Heart, Lung, and Blood Institute; OMH; CDC; National AIDS Clearinghouse; and Office on Smoking and Health)
- Voluntary agencies and their local affiliates (e.g., American Cancer Society, American Heart Association, Amyotrophic Lateral Sclerosis Association, Susan G. Komen®, Livestrong™ Foundation, American Diabetes Association, American Council for Drug Disorders, American Dairy Council, Alzheimer's Association, and American Lung Association)
- Internet searches
- Medline Plus Health Information (i.e., a service of the National Library of Medicine for patient and consumer information), at medlineplus.gov

Can you think of another organization that you or a family member recently obtained information from relating to a health need? University or college libraries often provide information on beginning and advanced search strategies and are one of the most credible and accessible sources of information. The National Library of Medicine, at www.nlm.nih.gov/hinfo.html, maintains extensive health-related bibliographies and offers links to the databases Medline Plus Health Information (http://www.nlm.nih.gov/medlineplus/), Household Products Database, Office of the Surgeon General, NIH Senior Health, and much more.

The nurse can locate many health resources through a variety of search engines on the Internet. As the World Wide Web continues to evolve as a major source of information exchange, an assessment of the quantity, quality, and broad nature of information must be undertaken. Key to the plethora of resources is gauging the appropriateness of the materials and media in consideration of literacy (see next section).

Literacy and Health

Clinical Example

A 2-year-old is diagnosed with an inner ear infection and is prescribed an antibiotic. Her mother understands that her daughter should take the prescribed medication twice a day. After carefully studying the label on the bottle and deciding that it does not tell how to take the medicine, she fills the teaspoon and pours the antibiotic into her daughter's ear (Parker et al., 2003).

The nurse in a community setting who sees a sick child at the pediatric clinic might ask the following questions:

- Do the parents have an understanding of the names of the medicines for their baby, how they work, and how and when to give them?
- In what manner might teach-back methods (described later in this chapter) help the parents have a good understanding of how to administer the antibiotic?
- Will the parents know what to do if their infant gets a fever?
- Is the information in their preferred language?
- Do the parents know how to read a thermometer? Did I show them? Were they able to "show me back"?
- Does the family know who to call and under what conditions, if their baby's condition worsens? Does the family have an understanding of what constitutes *worsen?* Will the parents know what action to take in case of a very high fever at 1:00 AM? Will they have the critical literacy skills to manage similar situations?

In her 1944 text, *The Public Health Nurse in the Community*, Rue stated that the community's illiteracy level is an important factor in health program planning. This factor remains a significant issue in planning health education programs and materials. Low literacy is a problem of great magnitude in the United States and has serious implications across the continuum of health care. Consider the following clinical example.

As background, the conceptual definitions of health literacy have evolved greatly over time. At one point, "literacy" was operationally defined as the ability to read and write at the fifth-grade level in any language and was measured on a continuum (National Literacy Act, 1991). *Health literacy,* on the other hand, is about empowerment, that is, having access to information, knowledge, and innovations. It is viewed as increasingly important for social, economic, and health development and is a key public health issue in the delivery of effective safe health care (Baur, 2011; Chinn, 2011; Eichler, Wieser, and Brugger, 2009; Kickbush, 2001; Mancuso, 2009; National Adult Literacy Survey, 2009; Nielsen-Bohlman et al., 2004; Nutbeam, 2008; Peerson and Saunders, 2009). For example, health literacy skills entail knowing when and where to go for health screenings, reading labels on prescription bottles, understanding public health messages about text messaging while driving, completing health insurance forms, recognizing how to read food labels, and being aware of the expectations of clinical trials.

Health literacy is a constellation of skills needed to perform basic reading tasks required to function in the health care environment for accessing, understanding, and using information to make health decisions, such as reading a food label. It is further identified that patients with the most health care needs are often the least able to read and understand information so as to function successfully in the health care system (American Medical Association, 1999). The recognition of this topic as a serious health issue subsequently resulted in the naming of specific topics, goal, and objectives in the *Healthy People 2020,* entitled Health Communication and Health Information Technology (IT). The objectives in this topic area describe many ways in which health communication and health IT can have a positive impact on health, health care, and health equity. Examples especially pertinent to health education actions taken by nurses include delivering accurate, accessible, and actionable health information that is targeted or tailored to increasing health literacy skills, providing personalized self-management tools and resources, and following sound principles in the design of programs and interventions that result in healthier behaviors. See http://www.healthypeople.gov/2020/topicsobjectives2020/ for more information.

Nutbeam (2000) proposes three levels for intervention that have individual and population benefits: (1) functional/basic literacy (focus on increasing basic reading/writing skills), (2) communicative/interactive literacy (focus on enhancing abilities to extract information and apply in new settings and with providers), and (3) critical literacy (focus on advancing skills to analyze information critically and use the information to control and manage life situations). Too often, he asserts, the provider's focus is on basic literacy rather than on critical literacy. The latter, he asserts, increases community members' empowerment abilities to successfully manage their everyday situations.

In 2004, the Institute of Medicine (IOM) published a landmark report titled *Health Literacy: A Prescription to End Confusion* that relates that millions of U.S. adults are unable to read and act on the plethora of health instructions and messages (Nielsen-Bohlman et al., 2004). The definition of health literacy adopted by the IOM report is consistent with the *Healthy People 2020* program as follows: "the capacity to obtain, interpret and understand basic health information and services and the competence to use such information and services to enhance health." The IOM report lists a series of recommendations that offer the nurse a blueprint of action. Several recommendations emphasize the need for clear communication, stress the importance of involving consumers in the development of the health communications process, and relate the need to create culturally and linguistically appropriate health information. For more details on the report and other health literacy–related resources, go to the IOM's website, www.iom.edu, and search for the term *health literacy.* Pause for a moment now, and consider the skills needed to read the words on this page, the skills needed to assimilate the information, and the skills needed to ultimately apply the information to your interactions with community members.

Nutbeam (2008), on the other hand, emphasizes that health literacy from public health and health promotion perspectives should be conceptualized as an "asset." In this manner, strategies to promote literacy move beyond mere transmission of content to the promotion of skills that develop confidence in how to act on the information. This viewpoint regards health literacy as a critical component of empowerment by improving people's access to health information and their capacity to use it. Moreover, Peerson and Saunders (2009) hold that implicit in understanding the broad concepts of health literacy is that motivation and behavioral activation must be considered separate entities. Simply put, having knowledge does not necessarily equate to action. Therefore, the quality of provider interactions and a greater awareness of and sensitivity to the possible impact of low literacy on individuals and communities is paramount (Nutbeam, 2008).

Early research shows serious disparities between the reading levels of materials and patients' reading skills (Meade, 1999; Meade and Byrd, 1989; Meade, et al., 1994; Mohrmann et al., 2000). Additionally, materials often fail to incorporate the intended audience's cultural beliefs, values, languages, and attitudes (Doak et al., 1998; Makosky et al., 2009; Meade et al., 2003; Meade et al., 2009; Nielson-Bohlman et al., 2004; Powe et al., 2007). Studies show that low literacy increases the use of health care services and costs (Eichler et al., 2009; Guerra, Krumholz, and Shea, 2005; Howard, Gazmararian, and Parker, 2005), decreases self-esteem and increases shame and stigma (Waite et al., 2008; Wolf et al., 2007), and adversely affects diabetes, medication, blood pressure control, dialysis maintenance, and nicotine dependence (Davis et al., 2006a; Green et al., 2013; Jahan, 2008; Pandit et al., 2009; Schillinger et al., 2009; Stewart et al., 2013); and that women who had abnormal Pap smears and who were perceived by their physician to have low literacy were significantly less likely to present for follow-up (Lindau, Basu, and Leitsch, 2006).

Additional studies reveal that health literacy may impact participation in research and may pose barriers to obtaining informed consent (Donovan-Kicken et al 2012; Kilbridge et al., 2009; Simon et al., 2009), may lead to health care and linguistic isolation that places individuals at risk for the development of health complications (Donelle, Arocha, and Hoffman-Goetz, 2008), and may impede patient-provider communication (Sudore et al., 2009) and impact the number of questions asked at medical visits (Aboumater et al., 2013).

Clearly, the past few decades have seen unprecedented advances in translating research findings into public health practices to reduce health risks, yet such successes have not been realized by all members of society representing various age, race and ethnic, and socioeconomic groups. Community members who are unable to read well enough to cope with the persistent reading demands of an increasingly complicated health care system continue to fall behind more literate groups in adopting and using health education and promotion procedures and interventions (e.g., affordable care act information) (Meade et al., 2007; Murphy-Knoll, 2007; Nutbeam, 2008; Long et al., 2014). Too often, health instructions not read and interventions poorly understood influence self-care abilities and health and wellness. Although the exact relational mechanisms between literacy and health are unclear, it is known that individuals with very low literacy skills are at an increased risk for poor health, which contributes to health disparities. Paasche-Orlow and Wolf (2007) describe a conceptual causal model that aims to explain associations between limited health literacy and health outcomes, and which center on three distinct aspects of care: 1) access and utilization of health care; 2) patient-provider relationships; and 3) self-care.

The authors point out that the relationship of literacy to health outcomes is not necessarily linear—as people exist within a sociocultural network, and suggest that health literacy be viewed as a "risk factor to be managed in clinical care."

A number of systematic reviews of health literacy studies conducted over the past decade show evidence of the high prevalence of limited health literacy, increasingly complex medical systems, and need for high-level navigation skills for self-management of acute and chronic disease and promotion of health (Chinn, 2011; Dewalt et al., 2004; Eichler et al., 2009; Mancuso, 2009; Nielsen-Bohlman et al., 2004; Paasche-Orlow et al., 2005). Furthermore, the World Health Organization (WHO) Commission on Social Determinants (2007) identifies literacy as a key determinant in health inequities. This being the case, nurses are ideally qualified and skilled to promote health in the community and address health literacy through the implementation of multiple techniques, as explained in the upcoming sections.

The Doaks (Leonard and Cecilia), who brought the literacy issue to the forefront in public health, describe the health community as a written culture. Unfortunately, many written instructions are "over the heads" of patients. There is a serious mismatch between the readability levels of health instructions and the reading skills of patients, but nurses can adapt the literacy levels of their instructions and reduce this mismatch. Techniques to reduce this mismatch are cogently outlined in the book *Teaching Patients with Low Literacy Skills* (Doak, Doak, and Root, 1996), which offers practical suggestions for preparing and evaluating materials. This book is not currently in print, but all chapters can be accessed through the Harvard health literacy website, at http://www. hsph.harvard.edu/healthliteracy/resources/teaching-patients-with-low-literacy-skills/; this is a very helpful resource. The author has used the information contained in this book in the development of educational materials, community-based programs, and research interventions.

What steps can nurses employ to address health literacy in the community setting? Within Stage I of the Framework for Developing Health Communications model, the nurse can use assessment skills to determine the reading level of the intended audience. For example, the nurse could employ a number of informal and formal assessment measures to assess an individual's literacy skills. Informal measures include asking a series of simple questions to provide a better indication of his or her reading skills. For example: *Do you enjoy reading? What do you read? How often do you read? Where do you get your health information?* Although years of schooling completed can serve as a gauge of literacy, previous studies suggest that a three- to four-grade–level difference often exists between an individual's literacy level and years of education completed. The nurse could ask patients to read a paragraph from a health document aloud. Skilled readers enjoy reading, are fluent readers, understand content, interpret the meaning of words, and look up unfamiliar words. Limited readers read slowly, miss the intended meaning, take words literally, tire quickly from reading, and skip over uncommon words. Also, the nurse should ask the patients a few questions about the information they read. Readers should be able to answer questions about the material's content. Although these strategies are especially helpful to individuals with low literacy, people at all literacy levels prefer and better understand simply written, concise materials and are more motivated by materials that are relevant to their learning needs (Doak et al., 1998; Doak LG et al., 1996).

There has been ongoing attention to the development of literacy screening questions, but validation studies are needed before they become routine in clinical care (Chin et al, 2011; Mancuso, 2009). Some formal instruments that have been used in health care settings to estimate academic skills include the Wide Range Achievement Test, Level IV (Wilkinson and Robertson, 2006) and the Rapid Estimate of Adult Literacy in Medicine (REALM—assesses ability to read common terms in English and is used as a brief literacy-screening tool; Davis et al., 1993, 2006b). See **Resource Tool 8C**, on the book's Evolve website at http://evolve.elsevier.com/Nies, for the REALM screening instrument.

Also, please note that there is now a short form of the REALM (only seven terms—see http://www.ahrq.gov/professionals/quality-patient-safety/quality-resources/tools/literacy/realm.pdf). Although these instruments take only a few minutes to administer, they are unavailable in Spanish. The Test of Functional Health Literacy in Adults, long and short forms (TOFHLA and S-TOFHLA; Parker et al., 1995) have been used in a variety of health settings with English-speaking/reading subjects (Cordasco et al., 2009; Ginde et al., 2008; Jackson and Eckert, 2008; Paasche-Orlow and Wolf, 2010; Schillinger et al., 2006) and to some degree with Spanish-speaking subjects (Brice et al., 2008). Yet, Robinson and colleagues (2011), who administered the S-TOFHLA to 612 rural older adults with heart failure, found that inaccurate categorization of patients with low or marginal health literacy may occur when the test's time limits (7 minutes) are enforced. These findings reinforce that some health literacy instruments may not be useful with patients who have undetected and/or declining cognitive impairment.

Building on their prior work (Chew et al., 2004; Wallace et al., 2006), Morris and colleagues (2006) developed the Single Item Literacy Screener (SILS): "How often do you need to have someone help when you read instructions, pamphlets, or other written material from your doctor or pharmacy (1 = never; 2 = rarely; 3 = sometimes; 4 = often; 5 = always)?" This particular item was found to be reasonably successful in detecting health literacy (in comparison with the TOFHLA), but only moderately sensitive. Yet, it focuses on only one aspect of health literacy, which is reading materials. In 2006, Lee and associates reported on the Short Assessment of Health Literacy for Spanish-speaking Adults (SAHLSA), a word recognition tool that requires the subject to read out loud from a list of 50 medical terms and associate each term with another word of similar meaning. Another short assessment tool, called the Newest Vital Sign (NVS) was created by Weiss and colleagues (2005). This tool, available in English and Spanish as a six-question assessment tool based on an ice cream nutrition label, is a quick (3- to 5-minute) assessment. Henrich (2012), who used the NVS in a primary care setting among a diverse population, suggests that health literacy be considered the sixth vital sign.

Later efforts have centered on the development of tools that measure print literacy, numeracy and oral literacy, and Internet-seeking abilities (using a total of 10 questions; Bann et al., 2012) or assess general health skills across the dimensions of functional, communicative and critical health, with such questions as "do you need help to fill out official forms?" (using a total of 14 items; Chinn and McCarthy, 2013). Other tools under development are very specific to content and language, such as the Chinese health literacy scale for diabetes (Leung et al., 2012).

As one can see, there are many formal tools to measure reading level or word recognition, which in turn may be helpful to gauge an individual's health literacy. Yet the time needed to administer them in community-based settings greatly limits their use. Most importantly, these collective findings underscore that formal assessments should be secondary to the nurse's informal and ongoing assessments, which allow for verification of understanding about specific health content within a specific health context. Nurses need to be astute in their assessment of people's skills and also to continually monitor the demands of the health care environment and make organizational adjustments as needed. Furthermore, Meade and Calvo (2001) continue to suggest asking patients and community members a series of simple questions on the topic of years of schooling that will help to gauge health literacy, followed by ongoing learner verification and teach-back methods. In this manner, health literacy can be viewed both from both content and context outlooks.

Ongoing research is needed to develop a relevant health literacy index (Kickbush, 2001; Mancuso, 2009; Nielsen-Bohlman et al., 2004). Yet the promising news here is that health literacy can be realized through health education (Nutbeam, 2009). Key to implementing effective health education strategies is recognizing that health literacy needs to be viewed within its context, that is, the physical and social environment of health care settings (Rudd , 2013). As such, nurses play pivotal roles in their community outreach and engagement activities for conveying knowledge, deciphering motivations, adapting health education messages, making information accessible, promoting health decisions, and facilitating empowering processes to increase the useful uptake of information. As Sykes and colleagues (2013) point out, health literacy goes beyond merely the motivation and development of skills within the individual or community, also entailing a number of collaborative efforts at a structural level. It needs to become an organizational value integrated into all aspects of community planning and health operations and to be viewed as a relationship between individuals and environments (Koh et al, 2013; Rudd, 2013).

Helpful Tips for Effective Teaching

- Assess reading skills using informal and formal methods.
- Determine what your patient/community member wants to know.
- Identify motivating factors for learning new information.
- Stick with the essentials. Limit the number of concepts or key points. Focus on important critical and survival skills.
- Set realistic goals and objectives. Take cues from your patients about what they want to learn and how to help them learn.
- Use clear and concise language. Avoid technical terms, if possible. For example, substitute *problem* for *complication*. Use *high blood pressure* instead of *hypertension*, or use *chance* instead of *possibility*. Do not needlessly simplify if the intended meaning is lost. Although the words *insulin* and *infection* are polysyllabic words, people with diabetes are often quite familiar with them (Box 8-2).
- Consider developing a glossary or vocabulary list for common words on the health topic. For example, in teaching a family about dental health, create a list of common words about the topic and words that might substitute well (e.g., flossing, toothbrush, cavity, decay, check-ups, x-rays).
- Space your teaching out over time, if possible. Incorporate health education activities into other activities. For example, ask women about their smoking habits at each prenatal visit. Relate teaching to their everyday concerns. Introduce HPV education into women's and men's health visits.

BOX 8-2 PATIENT COMMUNICATION: PROSTATE CANCER AND TREATMENT OPTIONS

Version A (harder to grasp – passive)
The doctor has recently communicated to the patient that he has localized prostate cancer, commonly labeled stage II. In addition to managing the anxieties associated with a life-threatening illness, patients with this disease must carefully consider the available treatment modalities and account for the potential effect each one may have on quality of life. Patients must seriously evaluate the benefits and adverse side effects of each treatment modality and determine the most efficacious intervention for their lifestyle.

Version B (easier to grasp – active)
You have just been told that you have early stage prostate cancer. Choosing a treatment is hard, but it is important. Besides dealing with fears that often go along with having cancer, get to know about your treatment options:

- Learn about how each treatment and how it may affect your life and your family.
- Get to know the benefits and side effects of each treatment.
- Ask questions. Write them down. Talk it over with your family.
- Choose the best treatment for you.

- Personalize health messages. Use the active voice. For example, instead of saying, "It is important that patients read labels if they want to cut down on fat and sodium intake," say, "Read the labels on foods to know what is in them. This will help you cut down on your fat and salt intake." See ⓔ **Resource Tool 8D**, Patient Communication: Testicular Self-Examination (TSE), on the book's Evolve website at http://evolve.elsevier.com/Nies.
- Incorporate methods of illustration, demonstration, and real-life examples. Connect the health message to everyday events and real-life situations.
- Give and get. Review information often. Ask the patient questions before, during, and after teaching.
- Summarize often. Provide the patient with feedback. Obtain feedback from the patient.
- Be creative. Use your imagination to convey difficult concepts (e.g., use picture cards, drawings, objects, streaming videos, DVDs, audiobooks, podcasts, flip charts, multimedia decision aids, photographs, storytelling).
- Use appropriate resources and materials to enhance teaching and convey ideas (e.g., videotapes, computer-based mobile tablet interactive programs, iPods, and bulletin boards).
- Put patients at ease. Focus on inclusion and trust before delivering content.
- Praise patients, but do not patronize them. Let them know what they are doing right. Focus on their strengths and assets and what they bring to the teaching encounter.
- Be encouraging throughout the educational steps. We all like to be told what we are doing right.
- Allow time for patients and family members to think and ask questions.
- Remember that comprehension and understanding require time and practice. Ongoing feedback helps refocus the teaching encounter and can keep you on track.

TABLE 8-7 COMPONENTS OF LEARNER VERIFICATION (CHECKS THE SUITABILITY OF THE MESSAGE WITH LEARNERS)

COMPONENTS	DESCRIPTION
Attraction	Readers should be attracted to the message. For example, the cover should stimulate interest, and when possible, pictures should foster an identification that "tells me that this is important for my situation." Examples: • Is this material attractive/pleasing to you? • Overall, would you be likely to pick up and read this brochure?
Comprehension	Readers should be able to summarize the main points in their own words, not the vocabulary of the instruction. Examples: • What do you feel is the main point? • Are there any words that are not clear?
Acceptability	Readers need to perceive that the information is culturally acceptable for their lifestyle, situation, and background. Examples: • Is there anything that bothers you about this booklet? • In your opinion, who is this booklet for?
Persuasion	Readers need to feel that the instruction is significant for them. Example: • Do you think that the message in this booklet is important for you?
Self-efficacy	Is the message doable, and does the reader feel confident in carrying it out? Example: • Do you think you could do what is suggested in this booklet (e.g., cut down on cigarettes)?

Modified from Doak CC, Doak LG, Root JH: *Teaching patients with low literacy skills,* ed 2, Philadelphia, 1996, Lippincott Williams & Wilkins. (Chapter 10 on learner verification can now be accessed at the Harvard health literacy website: http://www.hsph.harvard.edu/healthliteracy/resources/teaching-patients-with-low-literacy-skills/).

- Employ "teach-back" methods. This means asking patients to state in their own words (i.e., teach back) key concepts, decisions, or instructions just discussed (Negarandeh et al., 2012; Wilson FL et al., 2008).
- Conduct learner verification (a process that checks suitability of information) to ensure understanding (Table 8-7).
- Evaluate the teaching plan, and keep adding new information to the interaction.

Assess Materials: Become a Wise Consumer and User

Materials are collected, stored, and disseminated within community sites. In many instances, nurses distribute pamphlets, but patients either do not read them or review them only superficially.

People of this country have had so much pamphlet materials passed out to them free that some have lost respect for free literature. Health educators may have contributed to this delinquency by passing out health literature carelessly and indiscriminately. The nurse who expects the pamphlet to take the place of the health teacher is employing weak measures in the health education program. (Rue, 1944, p. 215)

This statement continues to be true today. Moreover, many of today's pamphlets are even more complex and lengthier because of technological advances and health care innovations. Thus, it is important that nurses evaluate health materials, including websites, before they disseminate them to or share them with individuals, families, or the general public. Health materials should strengthen previous teaching and should be used as an adjunct to health instruction.

Assessing the Relevancy of Health Materials

It is critical that nurses find and use materials, documents, and media that are appropriate for the intended target audience in community health education initiatives. Questions that the nurse should ask include the following:

- Do the materials match the intended audience?
- Are the materials appealing and culturally and linguistically relevant?
- Do they convey accurate and up-to-date information?
- Are the messages clear and understandable?
- Do the messages promote self-efficacy and motivation?

🄔 Resource Tool 8C Rapid Estimate of Adult Literacy in Medicine (REALM) screening instrument on the book's Evolve website at http://evolve.elsevier.com/Nies, provides an assessment guide for reviewing health materials that the author has used for gauging the appropriateness of materials. The nurse can use this guide in critiquing printed materials. Similarly, the nurse can make slight modifications in the tool and assess other types of health resources (e.g., videotapes/DVDs, blogs, websites, and multimedia interactive modules). To use the tool, gather a few materials/media that are commonly used in the clinical setting where you are based. In a group or individually, begin to assess each category and critically assess the suitability for your intended audience. The tool allows the nurse to review health materials systematically for appropriateness for the intended target audience. The material assessment should focus on the following criteria: format-layout, type, verbal content, visual content, and aesthetic quality. This activity probably will take 15 minutes. It can also be used as a group activity with patients or community members. The feedback your users offer about the tools may surprise you!

CASE STUDY

Application of the Nursing Process

The following case study and teaching plan provide an example of selected teaching approaches and learning needs for the individual, family, and community.

Emma Jackson, aged 33 years, receives ongoing health care at her neighborhood's community-based clinic, a federally funded community clinic. She visits the nurse practitioner, and the nurse confirms that Mrs. Jackson is 2 months pregnant. She is married and has an 8-year-old son. Emma tells the nurse she smokes and wants to quit but she has been unable to quit since her last pregnancy. She tells the nurse, "I smoke when I get stressed. I have so many things on my mind." Her husband is also a smoker and has tried to quit at times as well. The nurse refers Mrs. Jackson to a community nursing student named Irene Green for counseling, education, and follow-up.

Assessment

Irene recognizes that smoking during pregnancy is detrimental for the unborn infant, unhealthy for Mrs. Jackson, and harmful for the 8-year-old child, who breathes the secondhand smoke (USDHHS, 2004). Irene also knows that smokers often experience stages of readiness in their attempts to quit and that relapse is often part of the process (Prochaska and DiClemente, 1983). She notes that family and community support systems are important.

Irene assesses Mrs. Jackson on an individual level, as follows:
- Smoking history, smoking patterns, and previous attempts to quit
- Support systems (e.g., family, friends, and peers)
- Perceived barriers to quitting
- Perceived benefits to quitting
- Perceived priority in addressing this health issue vs. other everyday stresses
- Perceived effect of smoking behavior on family communication patterns

- Confidence and perceived efficacy in ability to quit
Assessment of other groups includes families, neighborhoods, churches, community organizations, and environmental messages that promote smoking cessation.

Diagnosis
Individual
- Health concerns related to smoking and personal stressors/triggers
- Desire for more information about ways to quit and stay smoke free

Family
- Effect and impact of smoking on family dynamics

Community
- Need for information about community programs and social support resources

Planning
Individual
Long-Term Goal
- Mrs. Jackson will quit smoking.

Short-Term Goals
- Mrs. Jackson will recognize that continued smoking is unhealthy for herself, her unborn infant, her young child, and her family.
- Mrs. Jackson will become aware of ways to enhance her confidence during smoking cessation.
- Mrs. Jackson will identify situations and stressors that influence her smoking patterns.
- Mrs. Jackson will learn two strategies to cope with stressful situations and will apply those strategies.

Continued

CASE STUDY—cont'd

Application of the Nursing Process

Family

Long-Term Goal

- Mr. and Mrs. Jackson will quit smoking and become a smoke-free family.

Short-Term Goals

- Mr. and Mrs. Jackson will acknowledge the benefits of a smoke-free environment.
- Mr. Jackson will recognize the need to quit smoking.
- The couple will recognize the need to support each other in smoking cessation.
- Mr. and Mrs. Jackson will identify and discuss specific supportive actions during the smoking cessation phases. The couple will enlist the support of another person or network.

Community

Long-Term Goals

- The community will support and endorse a smoke-free environment and publicize these efforts through billboards and other media.
- Community agencies and organizations will integrate smoking cessation and relapse programs and messages into their existing health-related activities.
- Cigarette advertising will cease.

Short-Term Goals

- A coalition of community members will develop and implement policies to support smoking cessation and relapse strategies.
- A consortium of health care agencies and community-based organizations will recognize the need to develop partnerships in creating smoking cessation strategies for the community and for high-risk groups.

Intervention

Individual

Planning interventions encourage self-expression, promote the use of adaptive coping mechanisms, offer positive reinforcement, disseminate appropriate smoking cessation strategies, and provide culturally and educationally relevant materials and media. The nurse applies the "five As" approach to smoking cessation counseling (Ask, Advise, Assess, Assist, and Arrange). Irene offers empowerment strategies to help Mrs. Jackson cope with her smoking cessation attempts and identifies daily hassles and stressors. Irene gives personalized smoking cessation messages and culturally and educationally appropriate materials and initiates a follow-up plan that is acceptable and doable on the basis of ongoing assessment and feedback (American College of Obstetrics and Gynecology, 2010; Brandon et al., 2012; Quinn et al., 2006; USDHHS, 2004).

Family

Planning and interventions recognize the need for strong support systems within families. Irene provided education and counseling to promote family self-care and recognized that she must address and incorporate Mr. Jackson's support, or lack thereof, into the care plan. Irene makes links to community resources (e.g., health classes, support groups, and networking with other expectant mothers who have quit or are attempting to quit) to build Mrs. Jackson's support system.

Community

Planning and interventions implemented on an aggregate level identify key community leaders, agencies, legislators, and lay members who are committed to supporting smoking cessation/relapse initiatives at a sociopolitical level (e.g., creating smoking cessation/relapse initiatives at various community channels). Program initiatives assist community members in defining issues and solutions to the effects of smoking on individuals, families, and community groups. Developing coalitions and partnerships among community-based organizations, health care groups, governmental agencies, and intended audience members through dialogue and increased awareness is essential.

Evaluation

Evaluation is systematic and continuous and focuses on the individual, family, and community.

Individual

An evaluation of Mrs. Jackson's smoking habits occurs within the health system and the community (clinics and Women, Infants, and Children [WIC] Service). These groups address both process (decrease in number of cigarettes smoked) and outcome (quit or not quit) end points. Mrs. Jackson experiences an increase in her coping skills and support system, which is evident in her personalized care plan.

- Irene tailors smoking cessation messages to Mrs. Jackson to fit her everyday life.
- Irene provides Mrs. Jackson with follow-up (e.g., telephone, letter, and follow-up visits).

Family

Care plans include supporting pattern development with family or significant other in smoking cessation initiatives.

- Irene assesses family health patterns and screens for other at-risk behaviors.
- Irene identifies and addresses family support and communication patterns in the care plan.

Community

Irene introduces smoking cessation and relapse programs and smoking prevention initiatives to at least two channels of dissemination (e.g., churches, schools, worksites, and community-based clinics).

- Smoking cessation/relapse messages are infused throughout the community by means of radio, television, and billboards.
- Community task forces and coalitions demonstrate a collaborative partnership among lay members, community leaders, organizers, and legislators to address smoking-related health issues.

Format/Layout

- Is the information organized clearly? Does it make sense?
- Do headers or advance organizers cue the reader? Headers help the reader visualize what is next.
- Is there a 50%/50% allocation of white and black space? This proportion gives the reader "breathing space."
- Is the information easy to read and uncluttered?

Type

- Is the type or font a readable size? Consider the age of your intended group and whether visual difficulties are likely.

Verbal Content

- Is the information current, accurate, and relevant to the intended group?

- Is the information culturally acceptable?
- Are difficult terms defined?
- Does the text reflect the racial and ethnic diversity of the intended audience?
- What is the reading level?

Visual Content

- Are the graphics accurate, current, and relevant to the intended group?
- Does cueing help the reader connect the printed words and pictures?
- Will the reader understand the intended meanings of the pictures?
- Is the information culturally acceptable?
- Are the pictures on the cover reflective of the material inside?
- Do the pictures reflect the target audience's racial and ethnic diversity?

Aesthetic Quality and Appeal

- Is the material appealing and engaging?
- Are there helpful special features (e.g., glossary, space for notes, and useful telephone numbers)?

Assessment of Reading Level

Part of the written material's assessment is reading level. Many formulas are available to estimate the printed text's readability and grade level, including the SMOG readability formula.

Readability formulas are objective, quantitative tools that measure sentence and word variables. However, they do not consider factors such as motivation, experience, and need for information (Meade and Smith, 1991). Nor do they determine the effects of visuals or design factors that could influence readability and comprehension of, for instance, cancer education information (Friedman and Hoffman-Goetz, 2006). These formulas do estimate reading ease and provide guidelines for assessing and rewriting health information. Two of the most commonly used formulas are the Flesch-Kincaid and the SMOG formulas (Wang et al., 2012). The Flesch-Kincaid Formula (Flesch, 1948) is a broad estimate of reading and is programmed into most computer software programs' grammar editing tools. To test a document's readability on your computer using the Flesch-Kincaid formula, search the term "readability statistic." You will be directed to a series of file and option tabs to reach grammar and spelling, and then readability statistics. The SMOG formula is shown in Resource 8D and is frequently used to calculate the readability estimate of health materials.

Learner Verification

The best way to identify material suitability is to deliver the materials to the intended audience and obtain feedback about acceptability, understanding, and usefulness. Learner verification engages intended members in dialogue and helps uncover unsuitable aspects of the material

(i.e., content, visuals, or format) (Doak LG et al., 1996). If the nurse discovers a need for new educational materials or media, he or she can incorporate Freirean principles to produce empowering products. The Freire approach supports learner participation in the development process, ensures that the learner is the active subject of the educational experience, and allows learners to define content and outcomes.

The process of learner verification helps identify the likelihood that the message is well suited to the audience. It involves verifying whether certain elements work well together to result in a good match of information for the learner. See Table 8-7 for a description of the specific elements and sample questions associated with each one.

For example, the author and colleagues have used learner verification processes on many occasions, for example, to develop a series of education toolboxes on breast and cervical cancer and prostate cancer for Hispanic migrant and seasonal farmworker and African-American women and men. After holding a series of focus groups with members of the intended audience to elicit themes about health, illness, cancer, and prevention, we conducted learner verification measures. Through systematic questions and interviewing processes, we were able to collect information in the intended audience's own words to help shape and refocus the cancer issues (breast, cervical, and prostate) from their own perspective (African-American men and women and Hispanic men and women farmworkers). Such verifying checks help assess the understanding of words and pictures; the acceptability of music, narrator, and pictures; the efficacy and persuasion of the message; and the overall attractiveness of the tools (e.g., videotape, DVD, website, flip chart, and booklet). For example, we found that the word *prevention* was a term many men found it difficult term to grasp. What we found was that tuning up one's car was a familiar concept that could similarly be used to convey the importance of ongoing check-ups as in maintaining prostate health. Similarly, the author and her colleagues used this approach to adapt smoking-relapse prevention materials for pregnant and postpartum women (Quinn et al., 2006), to develop stress management tools for Latinas undergoing chemotherapy (Meade, 2009), and to create biobanking education materials (Meade et al., 2012).

Another useful example can be seen in the study by Hunter and colleagues (2012), who used learner verification techniques to clarify terminology, translation, preferred content, and illustrations for cervical cancer content for Mexican immigrant women. Their findings challenged the common simplification approaches often linked to teaching learners with low literacy and reinforced the need of learners to know more about their anatomy. Overall, the process of learner verification fits well within the framework of community-based participatory research methods, as outlined earlier in this chapter, and can be a very helpful qualitative tool for the nurse to use in gauging the suitability of his or her health education efforts.

SOCIAL MEDIA

Nurses should consider the role of social media channels in connecting communities with reliable health information. Nurses should also think about how mobile health and e-health technologies might improve health outcomes of communities. *Social media* refers to interactive Internet-based communication channels that allow users to create, share, comment on, and modify online content (Ahlqvist et al. 2010; Fox and Bernhardt, 2010; Ventura et al., 2012). Social media platforms might include blogs, online discussion boards, microblogs such as Twitter, and video-sharing sites such as YouTube, Vimeo, and Flickr. In light of the growing number of community members (both here in the U.S. and globally), who have mobile phones and use social media, such platforms may lend themselves to reaching diverse community constituents with important public health messages (O'Mara, 2012). Social media sites have the potential to facilitate interactive communications, increase the sharing of health information, and personalize and reinforce health messages, all of which in turn can empower community members to make informed health decisions (CDC, 2010). For example, Strasser and colleagues (2012) explored the use of social media (e.g., Facebook) to reduce intimate partner violence among gay men in Atlanta; Vyas and others (2012) found that short message service (SMS[texting]) was a promising tool to reach Latino teens with public health interventions; and Bender and colleagues (2012) related that online support via social media may be a helpful strategy to meet the unmet supportive care needs of testicular cancer survivors, especially young survivors.

The results of a systematic review conducted by Koskan and colleagues (under review), using a series of terms related to cancer and social media, found a lag between social media channel development and the use of these communication channels in cancer care. Results identified the existence of a number of published descriptive studies on the topic of social media and cancer (e.g., type of cancer content posted on sites, user preferences) yet highlighted the lack of published intervention studies. Their findings reinforced that the role of social media in cancer care (and most likely other areas of health) is an exceptionally fertile area for future research and has practice implications. In particular, nurses in community health education settings are well poised to explore the utility of novel digital technology to connect individuals, families, and groups to reliable and credible information, which has meaning for their everyday health concerns and needs.

SUMMARY

Teaching is a significant component of community health nursing, affecting virtually every nursing activity. The goal of health education is to facilitate a process that allows individuals, families, and groups to make well-informed decisions about health practices. An understanding of learning and the theoretical frameworks that explain behaviors and health actions is inherent in community health education. No single theory explains human behavior; the nurse must apply multiple theories and approaches.

Nurses must be knowledgeable about sociopolitical, cultural, environmental, and ecological forces affecting community health to ensure the success of health education strategies. Furthermore, relevant health education (classes, talking circles, support groups, individual/family instruction, health fairs, etc.) is based on the meeting of individual variables and social, structural, political, cultural, and economic factors within the larger community context. To create meaningful education interventions, nurses need to assess their audience(s) and their characteristics thoroughly, and to employ systematic approaches when delivering health messages and programs. Implementing social action strategies, such as advocating health-promoting lifestyles, creating an environment for problem-posing dialogue, and providing links to appropriate health resources, supports the philosophy of critical consciousness. Nurses can facilitate the principle of social justice by mastering health information delivery and committing themselves to creating empowerment strategies that equip individuals, families, and communities with knowledge and navigation skills for healthy lifestyles and environments.

The nurse can use a variety of methods, materials, media, and innovative technologies to support their health education activities, including electronic and digital information. The nurse should review and evaluate these resources for their cultural, linguistic, and literacy suitability. Embracing the notion that health education is an ongoing interactive process influenced by many internal and external factors is strategic to meeting the needs of individuals, families, and communities. The nurse can make important contributions to the prevention of disease and the promotion of personal and community health with knowledge, spirit, and an ongoing community mindset and commitment to empowerment and engagement strategies.

LEARNING ACTIVITIES

1. In groups of three to four students, discuss how theoretical frameworks help explain health behavior. Identify the strengths and limitations of models that focus on individual health determinants versus models that encompass sociopolitical, environmental, and structural factors.

2. Discuss the role of the nurse in health education. Outline specific activities and roles that the nurse can perform with regard to health education issues. Share with one another personal experience(s) relating to cultural effectiveness that might enhance/impede the education role.

3. Identify a specific intended group in the community that you are interested in (e.g., medically underserved, homeless, seniors, pregnant women, new immigrants, deaf children, middle-school children).

   a. Describe the group's characteristics, learning needs, and strengths.

   b. Identify your methods for obtaining this information.

   c. Next, describe the application of Freire's empowerment education model to address health education priorities. How would you engage them in determining learning priorities?

4. Identify an issue of concern among community members (e.g., obesity, access to care). Discuss sociopolitical issues that impact this issue and how it relates to health. Outline specific community-based participatory activities and roles that the community nurse can take on that can address this health issue. Identify at least two ways to promote community engagement on this topic. What educational resources might the nurse use?

5. Select a health education brochure or health website. Apply the assessment criteria presented to assess its appropriateness for an intended audience. Evaluate the relative strengths of the printed material or website and potential areas for improvement using learner verification questions. Describe how you and your group can make it more relevant for your audience. How could you involve your audience in its assessment?

ⓔ EVOLVE WEBSITE

http://evolve.elsevier.com/Nies
- NCLEX Review Questions
- Case Studies
- Glossary
- Resource Tools
  - 8A: Learning Theories and Their Relationship to Health Education
  - 8B: Framework for Developing Health Communications
  - 8C: Rapid Estimate of Adult Literacy in Medicine (REALM) screening instrument
  - 8D: Patient Communication: Testicular Self-Examination (TSE)

REFERENCES

Aboumatar HJ, Carson KA, Beach MC, et al: The impact of health literacy on desire for participation in healthcare, medical visit communication, and patient reported outcomes among patients with hypertension, *J Gen Intern Med* 28:1469–1476, 2013.

Abreu DV, Tamura TK, Sipp JA, et al: Podcasting: contemporary patient education, *Ear Nose Throat J* 87(208):210–211, 2008.

Ahlqvist T, Bäck A, Heinonen S, et al: Road-mapping the societal transformation potential of social media, *Foresight* 12:3–26, 2010.

Albano JD, Ward E, Jemal A, et al: Cancer mortality in the United States by education level and race, *J Natl Cancer Inst* 99:1384–1394, 2007.

American Cancer Society: *Cancer facts and figures 2013*, Atlanta, 2013, Author.

American College of Obstetricians and Gynecologists: *Smoking cessation during pregnancy*. Available from <http://www.acog.org/Resources_And_Publications/Committee_Opinions/Committee_on_Health_Care_for_Underserved_Women/Smoking_Cessation_During_Pregnanc>, 2010.

American Hospital Association: *The patient care partnership*, Chicago, 2003, Author.

American Medical Association: Ad Hoc Committee on Health Literacy for the Council on Scientific Affairs: Health literacy: report of the council on scientific affairs, *JAMA* 281:552–557, 1999.

American Nurses Association (ANA): *Public health nursing: scope and standards of practice*, Washington, DC, 2007, American Nurse Publishing.

Bandura A: Self-efficacy: toward a unifying theory of behavioral change, *Psychol Rev* 84:191–215, 1977a.

Bandura A: *Social learning theory*, Englewood Cliffs, NJ, 1977b, Prentice Hall.

Bann CM, McCormack LA, Berkman ND, et al: The health literacy skills instrument: a 10-item short form, *J Health Commun* 17:191–202, 2012.

Baur C: Calling the nation to act: implementing the national action plan to improve health literacy, *Nurs Outlook* 59:63–69, 2011.

Becker MH, editor: *The health belief model and personal health behavior*, Thorofare, NJ, 1974, Charles B. Slack.

Becker MH, Maiman LA, Kirscht JP, et al: The Health Belief Model and prediction of dietary compliance: a field experiment, *J Health Soc Behav* 18:348–366, 1977.

Bender JL, Wiljer D, To MJ, et al: Testicular cancer survivors' supportive care needs and use of online support: a cross-sectional survey, *Support Care Cancer* 20(11):2737–2746, 2012. Epub 2012 March 3.

Bigge ML, Shermis SS: *Learning theories for teachers*, ed 6, Boston, 2004, Allyn & Bacon Classics.

Blumenthal DS, DiClemente RJ, Braithwaite R, et al: *Community-based participatory health research: issues, methods and translation to practices*, ed 2, Springer, 2013.

Brandon TH, Simmons VN, Meade CD, et al: Self-help booklets for preventing postpartum smoking relapse: a randomized trial, *Am J Public Health* 102:2109–2115, 2012.

Brice JH, Travers D, Cowden CS, et al: Health literacy among Spanish-speaking patients in the emergency department, *J Natl Med Assoc* 100:1326–1332, 2008.

Brookfield KF, Cheung MC, Lucci J, et al: Disparities in survival among women with invasive cervical cancer: a problem of access to care, *Cancer* 115:166–178, 2009.

Bungay V, Kolar K, Thindal S, et al: Community-based HIV and STI prevention in women working in indoor sex markets, *Health Promot Pract* 24:247–255, 2013.

Cashman SB, Adeky S, Allen AJ, et al: The power and the promise: working with communities to analyze data, interpret findings, and get to outcomes, *Am J Public Health* 98:1407–1417, 2008.

Centers for Disease Control and Prevention: *The health communicator's social media toolkit*, Atlanta, 2010, Author.

Champion VL, Monahan PO, Springston JK, et al: Measuring mammography and breast cancer beliefs in African American women, *J Health Psychol* 138:27–37, 2008.

Champion VL, Skinner CS: The health belief model. In Glanz K, Rimer BK, Visnawath K, editors: *Health behavior and education: theory, research, and practice*, ed 4, San Francisco, 2008, Jossey-Bass, pp 45–65.

Chew LD, Bradley KA, Boyko EJ: Brief questions to identify patients with inadequate literacy, *Fam Med* 36:588–594, 2004.

Chin J, Lee EH, Son HJ, et al: The process-knowledge model of health literacy: evidence from a componential analysis of two commonly used measures, *J Health Communication* 16(Suppl 3):222–241, 2011.

Chinn D, McCarthy C: All aspects of health literacy scale (AAHLS): developing a tool to measure functional, communicative and critical health literacy in primary healthcare settings, *Patient Educ Couns* 90:247–253, 2013.

Chinn D: Critical health literacy: a review and critical analyses, *Soc Sci Med* 73:60–67, 2011.

Choi J: Literature review: using pictographs in discharge instructions for older adults with low literacy skills, *J Clin Nurs Nov* 20:2984–2996, 2011 (epub 2011).

Chou WY, Prestin A, Lyons C, et al: Web 2.0 for health promotion: reviewing the current evidence, *Am J Public Health*, 2013. Jan;103(1).

Chu KC, Miller BA, Springfield SA: Measures of racial/ethnic health disparities in cancer mortality rates and the influence of socioeconomic status, *J Natl Med Assoc* 99(1092-1100):1102–1104, 2007.

Chu KC, Chen Jr MS, Dignan MB, et al: Parallels between the development of therapeutic drugs and cancer health disparity programs: implications for disparities reduction, *Cancer* 113:2790–2796, 2008.

Clark MJD: *Community health nursing: advocacy for population health*, ed 5, Englewood Cliffs, NJ, 2007, Prentice Hall.

Clements K: Participatory action research and photovoice in a psychiatric nursing/clubhouse collaboration exploring recovery narrative, *J Psychiatr Ment Health Nurs* 19:785–791, 2012.

Coleman CL, Jemmott L, Jemmott JB, et al: Development of an HIV risk reduction intervention for older seropositive African American men, *AIDS Patient Care STDS* 8:647–655, 2009.

Cordasco KM, Asch SM, Franco I, et al: Health literacy and English language comprehension among elderly inpatients at an urban safety-net hospital, *J Health Hum Serv Adm* 32:30–50, 2009.

Cueva M, Kuhnley R, Slatton J, et al: Telenovela: an innovative colorectal cancer screening health messaging tool, *Int J Circumpolar Health*, 2013. Aug 5;72:21301.

D'Souza MS, Karkada SN, Somayaji G, et al: Women's well-being and reproductive health in Indiana mining community: need for empowerment, *Reprod Health*, 2013. April 19;10:24.

Davis JL, McGinnis KE, Walsh ML, et al: An innovative approach for community engagement: using an audience response system, *J Health Dispar Res Pract*, 2012. 5:pii: 1.

Davis TC, Long SW, Jackson RH, et al: Rapid estimate of adult literacy in medicine: a shortened screening instrument, *Fam Med* 25:56–57, 1993.

Davis TC, Wolf MS, Bass PF, et al: Low literacy impairs comprehension of prescription drug warning labels, *J Gen Intern Med* 21:847–851, 2006a.

Davis TC, Wolf MS, Arnold CL, et al: Development and validation of the Rapid Estimate of Adolescent Literacy in Medicine (REALM-Teen): a tool to screen adolescents for below-grade reading in health care settings, *Pediatrics* 118:1707–1714, 2006b.

Dewalt DA, Berkman ND, Sheridan S, et al: Literacy and health outcomes: a systematic review of the literature, *J Gen Intern Med* 19:1228–1239, 2004.

Doak CC, Doak LG, Root JH: *Teaching patients with low literacy skills*, ed 2, Philadelphia, 1996, Lippincott Williams & Wilkins. Also available from. <http://www.hsph.harvard.edu/healthliteracy/files/2012/09/doakintro.pdf>.

Doak CC, Doak LG, Friedell GH, et al: Improving comprehension for cancer patients with low literacy skills: strategies for clinicians, *CA Cancer J Clin* 48:151–162, 1998a.

Doak LG, Doak CC, Meade CD: Strategies to develop effective cancer education materials, *Oncol Nurs Forum* 23:1305–1312, 1996b.

Donelle L, Arocha JF, Hoffman-Goetz L: Health literacy and numeracy: key factors in cancer risk comprehension, *Chronic Dis Can* 29:1–8, 2008.

Donovan-Kicken E, Mackert M, Guinn TD, et al: Health literacy, self-efficacy, and patients' assessment of medical disclosure and consent documentation, *J Health Commun* 27:581–590, 2012.

Edgren KK, Parker EA, Israel BA, et al: Community involvement in the conduct of a health education and research project: community against asthma, *Health Prom Pract* 6:263–269, 2005.

Eichler K, Wieser S, Brugger U: The costs of limited health literacy: a systematic review, *Int J Public Health* 54:313–324, 2009.

English KC, Wallerstein N, Chino M, et al: Intermediate outcomes of a tribal community public health infrastructure assessment, *Ethn Dis* 14, 2004. S1–61-S1-69.

Flesch RR: A new readability yardstick, *J Appl Psychol* 32:221–223, 1948.

Fox S, Bernhardt JM: Health Communication 2.0: The promise of peer participation. In Rutten LF, Moser RP, Kreps GL, editors: *Building the evidence base in cancer communication*, Cresskill, NJ, 2010, Hampton Press, pp 257–270.

Freeman HP: Poverty, culture, and social injustice: determinants of cancer disparities, *CA Cancer J Clin* 54:72–77, 2004.

Freire P: *Pedagogy of the oppressed*. New York, 1970, Herder and Herder (translated from original 1968 manuscript by Myra Bergman Davis) (Bloomsbury Academic 30th anniversary ed, 2000).

Freire P: *Education for critical consciousness*, New York, 1973, (Continuum reprint, 2005).

Friedman DB, Hoffman-Goetz L: A systematic review of readability and comprehension instruments used for print and web-based cancer information, *Health Educ Behav* 33:352–373, 2006.

Gardner MS: *Public health nursing*, ed 3, New York, 1936, Macmillan (University of Michigan reprint, 2009).

Ginde AA, et al: Multicenter study of limited health literacy in emergency department patients, *Acad Emerg Med* 15:577–580, 2008.

Glanz K, Rimer BK, Viswanath K, editors: *Health behavior and health education: theory, research and practice*, ed 4, San Francisco, 2008, Jossey-Bass.

Green JA, Mor MK, Shields AM, et al: Associations of health literacy with dialysis adherence and health resource utilization in patients receiving maintenance hemodialysis, *Am J Kidney Dis* 62(1):73–80, 2013.

Green L: Introduction to behavior change and maintenance: theory and measurement. In Schumaker S, Schron EB, Ockene JK, editors: *The handbook of health behavior change*, New York, 1998, Springer.

Green LW, Kreuter MW: *Health program planning: an educational and ecological approach*, ed 4, New York, 2004, McGraw-Hill.

Guerra CE, Krumholz MA, Shea JA: Literacy and knowledge, attitudes and behavior about mammography in Latinas, *J Health Care Poor Underserved* 16:152–166, 2005.

Gwede CK, William CM, Thomas KB, et al: Exploring disparities and variability in perceptions and self-reported colorectal cancer among three ethnic subgroups of US Blacks, *Oncol Nurs Forum* 37:581–591, 2010.

Gwede CK, Davis SN, Quinn GP, et al: Meade CD and the Tampa Bay Community Cancer Network (TBCCN) partners. (2013). Making It work: provider perspectives on improving communication strategies for colorectal cancer screening in federally qualified health centers, *J Cancer Educ*, 2013. Dec:28(4):777-83.

Gwede CK, Menard JM, Martinez-Tyson D, et al: Community Cancer Network community partners. Strategies for assessing community challenges and strengths for cancer disparities participatory research and outreach, *Health Promotion Practice*, 2010. Nov;11(6):876-87.

Hawkins RP, Kreuter M, Resnicow K, et al: Understanding tailoring in communicating about health, *Health Educ Res*, 2008. 2008 Jun;23(3):454-66. Epub 2008 March 17.

Heinrich C: Health literacy: the sixth vital sign, *J Am Acad Nurse Pract* 24:218–223, 2012.

Hochbaum GM: *Public participation in medical screening programs: a sociopsychological study*, US Public Health Service Pub No 572, Washington, DC, 1958, US Government Printing Office.

Houts PS, Doak CC, Doak LG, et al: The role of pictures in improving health communication: a review of research on attention, comprehension, recall, and adherence, *Patient Educ Couns* 61:173–190, 2006.

Howard DJ, Gazmararian J, Parker RM: The impact of low health literacy on the medical costs of Medicare managed care enrollees, *Am J Med* 118:371–377, 2005.

Hunter J, Kelly PJ: Imagined anatomy and other lessons from learner verification interviews with Mexican immigrant women, *J Obstet Gynecol Neonatal Nurs* 41:E1–E12, 2012.

Israel BA, Checkoway B, Schulz A, et al: Health education and community empowerment: conceptualizing and measuring perceptions of individual, organization, and community control, *Health Educ Q* 32:149–170, 1994.

Israel BA, Eng E, Schultz AMJ, et al: *Methods in community-based participatory research for health*, San Francisco, 2005, Jossey-Bass.

Jackson RD, Eckert GJ: Health literacy in an adult dental research population: a pilot study, *J Public Health Dent* 68:196–200, 2008.

Jacobsen PB, Meade CD, Stein KD, et al: Efficacy and costs of two forms of stress management training for cancer patients undergoing chemotherapy, *J Clin Oncol* 20:2851–2862, 2002.

Jacobsen PB, Phillips KM, Jim HS, et al: Effects of self-directed stress management training and home-based exercise on quality of life in cancer patients receiving chemotherapy: a randomized controlled trial, *Psycho-Oncology* 22(6):1229–1235, 2012.

Jahan S: Poverty and infant mortality in the Eastern Mediterranean region: a meta-analysis, *J Epidemiol Community Health* 62:745–751, 2008.

Janz NK, Champion VL, Strecher VJ: The health belief model. In Glanz K, Rimer BK, Lewis FM, editors: *Health behavior and education: theory, research and practice*, ed 2, San Francisco, 2002, Jossey-Bass, pp 45–66.

Jemmott LS, Jemmott JB, O'Leary A: A randomized controlled trial of brief HIV/STD prevention interventions for African American women in primary care settings: effects on sexual risk behavior and STD rate, *Am J Public Health* 97:1034–1040, 2007.

Jemmott LS, Jemmott JB, Hutchinson MK, et al: Sexually transmitted infection/HIV risk reduction interventions in clinical practice settings, *J Obstet Gynecol Neonatal Nurs* 37:137–145, 2008.

Joint Commission on Accreditation of Healthcare Organizations: Comprehensive accreditation manual for hospitals (CAMH), *Oak Brook Terrace*, 2012. Joint Commission Resources.

Jones PL, Baker JL, Gelaude D, et al: Lessons learned from field-testing a brief behavioral intervention package for African American women at risk for HIV/STDs, *Health Promot Pract* 14:168–173, 2012.

Jönsson AM, Willman A: Implementation of telenursing within home healthcare, *Telemed J E Health* 14:57–62, 2008.

Joseph CL, Peterson E, Havstad S, et al: A web-based, tailored asthma management program for urban African American high school students, *Am J Respir Crit Care Med* 175:888–895, 2007.

Kegeles SS, Kirscht JP, Haefner DP, et al : Survey of beliefs about cancer detection and Papanicolaou tests, *Public Health Rep* 80:815–823, 1965.

Kickbush IS: Health literacy: addressing the health and education divide, *Health Prom Intern* 16:289–297, 2001.

Kilbridge KL, Fraser G, Krahn M, et al: Lack of comprehension of common prostate cancer terms in an underserved population, *J Clin Oncol* 27:2015–2021, 2009.

Kleinman A: Concepts and a model for the comparison of medical systems as cultural systems, *Soc Sci Med* 12:85–93, 1978.

Knowles MS: *The modern practice of adult education: from pedagogy to andragogy*, rev ed. Chicago, 1988, Cambridge Press.

Knowles MS: *The making of an adult educator: an autobiographical journey*, San Francisco, 1989, Jossey-Bass.

Kobetz E, Menard J, Barton B, et al: Patnè en Aksyon: Addressing cancer disparities in Little Haiti through research and social action, *Am J Public Health* 99:1163–1165, 2009.

Koh HK, Brach C, Harris LM, et al: A proposed 'health literate care model' would constitute a systems approach to improving patients' engagement in care, *Health Aff (Millwood)* 32:357–367, 2013.

Koskan A, Klasko L, Davis S, et al: **Usage and Taxonomy of Social Media in Cancer-Related Research Studies: A Systematic Review (under revision)**

Kulbok PA, Thatcher E, Park E, et al: Evolving public health nursing roles: focus on community participation health promotion and prevention, *Online J of Issues in Nurs* 17:1–14, 2012.

Labonte R: Health promotion and empowerment: reflections on professional practice, *Health Educ Q* 21:253–268, 1994.

Larkey LK, Lopez AM, Minnal A, et al : Storytelling for promoting colorectal cancer screening among underserved Latina women: a randomized pilot study, *Cancer Control* 16:79–87, 2009.

Leung MW, Yen IH, Minkler M: Community-based participatory research: a promising approach for increasing epidemiology's relevance in the 21st century, *Intern J Epidemiol* 33:499–506, 2004.

Leung AY, Lou VW, Cheung MK, et al: Development and validation of Chinese health literacy scale for diabetes, *J Clin Nurs* 22(15-16):2090–2099, 2012.

Lindau ST, Basu A, Leitsch SA: Health literacy as a predictor of follow-up after an abnormal Pap smear: a prospective study, *J Gen Intern Med* 21:829–834, 2006.

Long SK, Kenney GM, Zuckerman S, et al: The health reform monitoring survey: addressing data gaps to provide timely insights into the affordable care act, *Health Aff (Millwood)*, 2014. Jan;33(1):161-7. Epub 2013 Dec 18.

Lopéz EDS, Eng E, Robinson N, et al: Photovoice as a community-based participatory action method. In Israel BA, Eng E, Schulz AJ, Parker EA, editors: *Methods in community-based participatory research for health*, San Francisco, CA, 2005, Jossey-Bass, pp 326–358.

Luque JS, Rivers B, Kambon M, et al: Barbers against prostate cancer: a feasibility study for training barbers to deliver prostate cancer education in an urban African American community, *J Cancer Educ*, 2010. Feb 10. [Epub ahead of print].

Machtinger EL, Wang F, Chen LL, et al: A visual medication schedule to improve anticoagulation control: a randomized, controlled trial, *Comm J Qual Patient Saf* 33:625–635, 2007.

Makosky Daley C, Cowan P, Nollen NL, et al: Assessing the scientific accuracy, readability, and cultural appropriateness of a culturally targeted smoking cessation program for American Indians, *Health Promot Pract* 10:386–393, 2009.

Mancuso JM: Assessment and measurement of health literacy: an integrative review of the literature, *Nurs Health Sci* 11:77–89, 2009.

Marks R: Ethics and patient education: health literacy and cultural dilemmas, *Health Promot Pract* 10:328–332, 2009.

Martinez D, Aguado Loi CX, et al: Development of a cancer camp for adult Spanish-speaking survivors: lessons learned from Camp Alegria, *J Cancer Educ* 23(1):4–9, 2008.

Martyn KK, Loveland-Cherry CJ, Villarruel AM, et al: Mexican adolescents' alcohol use, family intimacy, and parent-adolescent communication, *J Fam Nurs* 15:152–170, 2009.

McKinlay JB: Epidemiological and political determinants of social policies regarding the public health, *Soc Sci Med* 13A:541–558, 1979.

Meade CD: Producing videotapes for cancer education: methods and examples, *Oncol Nurs Forum* 23:837–846, 1996.

Meade CD: Improving understanding of the informed consent process and document, *Semin Oncol Nurs* 15:124–137, 1999.

Meade CD: *Creating educational tools: from concept to product*, Montreal, Canada, 2009, Society for Behavioral Medicine (abstract).

Meade CD, Byrd JC: Patient literacy and the readability of smoking education literature, *Am J Public Health* 79:204–206, 1989.

Meade CD, Smith CF: Readability formulas: cautions and criteria, *Patient Educ Couns* 17:153–158, 1991.

Meade CD, Menard J, Luque J, et al: Creating community-academic partnerships for cancer disparities research and health promotion, *Health Promotion Practice* 12:456–462, 2011.

Meade CD, Calvo A: Developing community-academic partnerships to enhance breast health among rural and Hispanic migrant and seasonal farmworkers, *Oncol Nurs Forum* 28:1577–1584, 2001.

Meade CD, Calvo A, Rivera M: Screening and community outreach programs for priority populations: considerations for oncology managers, *J Oncol Manag* 11(5):14–22, 2002b.

Meade CD, Calvo A, Rivera M: Focus groups in the design of prostate cancer screening information for Hispanic farmworkers and African American men, *Oncol Nursing Forum* 30:967–975, 2003.

Meade CD: Menard J, Martinez D, et al: Impacting health disparities through community outreach: utilizing the CLEAN look (culture, literacy, education, assessment, networking), *Cancer Control* 14:70–77, 2007.

Meade CD, Menard J, Thervil C, et al: Addressing cancer disparities through community engagement: improving breast health among Haitian women, *Oncol Nurs Forum* 36:716–722, 2009.

Meade CD, McKinney WP, Barnas G: Educating patients with limited literacy skills: the effectiveness of printed and videotaped materials about colon cancer, *Am J Public Health* 84:119–121, 1994.

Meade CD, Arevalo M, Quinn GP, et al: Community Cancer Network partners, Enhancing awareness about biobanks: processes for developing multi-lingual educational aids about biospecimen donation. Poster presentation at the European Association of Communication in Healthcare. Scotland, UK, 2012, St. Andrews University.

Meleis AI: Culturally competent care, *J Transcult Nurs* 10:12, 1999.

Minkler M, editor: *Community organizing and community building for health and welfare*, ed 3, New Brunswick, NJ, 2012, Rutgers University Press.

Minkler M, Wallerstein N, editors: *Community-based participatory research for health: from process to outcomes*, ed 2, San Francisco, 2008, Jossey-Bass.

Minkler M, Wallerstein N, Wilson N: Improving health through community organization and community building. In Glanz K, Rimer BK, Visnawath K, editors: *Health behavior and education: theory, research, and practice*, ed 4, San Francisco, 2008, Jossey-Bass, pp 288–312.

Mohrmann CC, Coleman EA, Coon SK, et al: An analysis of printed breast cancer information for African American women, *J Cancer Educ* 15:23–27, 2000.

Morris NS, MacLean CD, Chew LD, et al: Single item literacy screener: evaluation of a brief instrument to identify limited reading ability, *BMC Fam Pract* 21, 2006.

Murphy-Knoll L: Low health literacy puts patients at risk: the Joint Commission proposes solutions to National Problem, *J Nurs Care Qual* 22:205–209, 2007.

The National Literacy Act of 1991: *PL 102–173* [Go to http://eric.ed.gov/?id=ED341851, 1991. to download full-text document (28 pages)].

National Center for Education Statistics: *Technical report and data file user's manual for 2003 National Assessment of Adult Literacy*, NCES 2009476, August 11. Available from http://nces.ed.gov/pubsearch/pubsinfo.asp?pubid=2009476, 2009.

Negarandeh R, Mahmoodi H, Noktehdan H, et al: Teach back and pictorial image educational strategies on knowledge about diabetes and medication/dietary adherence among low health literate patients with type 2 diabetes, *Prim Care Diabetes Nov 26*, 2012. [Epub ahead of print].

Nielson-Bohlman L, Panzer A, Kindig D, editors: *Health literacy: a prescription to end confusion*, Washington, DC, 2004, National Academies Press.

Nightingale F: *Notes on nursing*, New York, 1859, Appleton-Century-Crofts.

Nutbeam D: The evolving concept of health literacy, *Soc Sci Med* 67:2072–2078, 2008.

Nutbeam D: Defining and measuring health literacy: what can we learn from literacy studies? *Int J Public Health* 54(5):303–305, 2009.

Nyswander DB: Education for health: some principles and their application, *Health Educ Mono* 14:65–70, 1956.

Olshansky E, Sacco D, Braxter B, et al: Participatory action research to understand and reduce health disparities, *Nurs Outlook* 53:121–126, 2005.

O'Mara B: Social media, digital video and health promotion in a culturally and linguistically diverse Australia, *Health Promot Int* 28(3):466–476, 2012.

Paasche-Orlow MK, Wolf MS: The causal pathways linking health literacy to health outcomes, *Am J Health Behav* 31(Suppl):S19–S26, 2007.

Paasche-Orlow MK, Parker RM, Gazmararian JA, et al: The prevalence of limited literacy, *J Gen Intern Med* 20:175–184, 2005.

Paasche-Orlow MK, Wolf MS: Promoting health literacy research to reduce health disparities, *J Health Communication* 15(S2):34–41, 2010.

Padden DL, Connors RA, Posey SM, et al: Factors influencing a health promoting lifestyle in spouses of active duty military, *Health Care Women Int* 34(8):674–693, 2013.

Padilla GV, Bulcavage LM: Theories used in patient/health education, *Semin Oncol Nurs* 7:87–96, 1991.

Pandit AU, Tang JW, Bailey SC, et al: Education, literacy, and health: mediating effects on hypertension knowledge and control, *Patient Educ Couns* 75:381–385, 2009.

Parker EA, Israel BA, Williams M, et al: Community action against asthma: examining the partnership process of a community-based participatory research project, *J Gen Intern Med* 18:558–567, 2003.

Parker RM, Baker DW, Williams MV, Nurss JR: The test of functional health literacy in adults: a new instrument for measuring patients' literacy skills, *J Gen Intern Med* 10:537–541, 1995.

Peerson A, Saunders M: Health literacy revisited: what do we mean and why does it matter? *Health Promot Int* 24:285–296, 2009.

Pender NJ, Murdaugh CL, Parsons MA: *Health promotion in nursing practice*, ed 6, Englewood Cliffs, NJ, 2010, Prentice Hall.

Pollard RQ, Dean RK, O'Hearn A, et al: Adapting health education material for deaf audiences, *Rehabil Psychol* 54:232–238, 2009.

Powe BD, Ross L, Wilkerson D, et al: Testicular cancer among African American college men: knowledge, perceived risk, and perceptions of cancer fatalism, *Am J Mens Health* 1:73–80, 2007.

Prochaska JO, DiClemente CC: Stages and processes of self-change of smoking: toward an integrative model of change, *J Consult Clin Psychol* 51(3):390–395, 1983.

Quad Council of Public Health Organizations: *Core competencies for public health nurses*, Washington DC, 2011, Author.

Quinn G, Ellison BB, Meade C, et al: Adapting smoking relapse-prevention materials for pregnant and postpartum women: formative research, *Matern Child Health J* 10:235–245, 2006.

Quinn GP, Thomas KB, Hauser K, et al: Evaluation of educational materials from a social marketing campaign to promote folic acid use among Hispanic women: insight from Cuban and Puerto Rican ethnic subgroups, *J Immigr Minor Health* 11(5):406–414, 2009.

Ramanadhan S, Mendex SR, Rao M, et al: Social medial use by community-based organizations conducting health promotion: a content analysis, *BMC Public health*, 2013. Dec 5 13(1): 1129 (Epub ahead of print).

Rawl SM, Champion VL, Menon U, et al: The impact of age and race on mammography practices, *Health Care Women Int* 21:583–597, 2000.

Rawl SM, Skinner CS, Perkins SM, et al: Computer-delivered tailored intervention improves colon cancer screening knowledge and health beliefs of African Americans, *Health Educ Res* 5:868–885, 2012.

Redman BK: *The practice of patient education: a case study approach*, ed 10, St. Louis, 2007, 2007 Elsevier.

Roberts NJ, Mohamed Z, Wong PS, et al: The development and comprehensibility of a pictorial asthma action plan, *Patient Educ Couns* 74:12–18, 2009.

Robbins LB, Pfeiffer KA, Vermeesch A, et al: "Girls on the move" intervention protocol for increasing physical activity among low-active underserved urban girls: a group randomized trial, *BMC Public Health* 13, 2013.

Robinson S, Moser D, Pelter MM, et al: Assessing health literacy in heart failure patients, *J Card Fail* 17(11):887–892, 2011.

Roetzheim RG, Lee JH, Ferrante JM, et al: Diagnostic resolution of cancer screening abnormalities at community health centers, *J Health Care Poor Underserved* 23:1280–1293, 2012. 2013.

Ronis DL, Hong O, Lusk SL: Comparison of the original and revised structures of the Health Promotion Model in predicting construction workers' use of hearing protection, *Res Nurs Health* 29:3–17, 2006.

Rosenstock I: Why people use health services, *Milbank Mem Fund Q* 44:94–127, 1966.

Rosenstock IM, Strecher VJ, Becker MH: Social learning theory and the health belief model, *Health Educ Q* 15(2):175–183, 1988.

Rubin A, Migneault JP, Marks L, et al: Automated telephone screening for problem drinking, *J Stud Alcohol* 67:454–457, 2006.

Rudd RE: Needed action in health literacy, *J Health Psychol*, 2013. Aug;18(8):1004–10. Epub 2013 Jan 24.

Rue CB: *The public health nurse in the community*, Philadelphia, 1944, Saunders.

Rutherford GE: Peeling the layers: a grounded theory of professional co-learning with residents of a homeless shelter, *J Interprof Care* 25:352–358, 2011.

Schapira MM, Meade C, Nattinger AB: Enhanced decision-making: the use of a videotape decision-aid for patients with prostate cancer, *Patient Educ Couns* 30:119–127, 1997.

Schillinger D, Barton LR, Karter AJ, et al: Does literacy mediate the relationship between education and health outcomes? A study of a low-income population with diabetes, *Public Health Rep* 121:245–254, 2006.

Schillinger D, Handley M, Wang F, et al: Effects of self-management support on structure, process, and outcomes among vulnerable patients with diabetes: a three-arm practical clinical trial, *Diabetes Care* 32:559–566, 2009.

Sepulveda AR, Lopez C, Macdonald P, et al: Feasibility and acceptability of DVD and telephone coaching-based skills training for carers of people with an eating disorder, *Int J Eat Disord* 41:318–325, 2008.

Sheehan CA: A brief educational video about prostate cancer screening: a community intervention, *Urol Nurs* 29:103–111, 2009.

Shin Y, Yun S, Pender NJ, Jang H, et al: Test of the health promotion model as a causal model of commitment to a plan for exercise among Korean adults with chronic disease, *Res Nurs Health* 28:117–125, 2005.

Simmons VN, Quinn G, Litvin EB, et al: Transcreation of validated smoking relapse-prevention booklets for use with Hispanic populations, *J Health Care Poor Underserved* 22:886–893, 2011.

Simon MA, Dong X, Nonzee N, Bennett CL: Heeding our words: complexities of research among low-literacy populations, *J Clin Oncol* 27:1938–1940, 2009.

Smedley BD, editor: *Unequal treatment: confronting racial and ethnic disparities in health care*, Washington, DC, 2003, National Academies Press.

Stallings KD, Rankin SH, London F: *Patient education in health and illness*, ed 5, Lippincott, 2005, Williams & Wilkins.

Steuart GW, Kark SO: *A practice of social medicine: a South African team's experiences in different African communities*, Edinburgh, 1962, Livingstone.

Stewart DW, Adams CE, Cano MA, et al: Associations between health literacy and established predictors of smoking cessation, *Am J Public Health*, 2013. May 16. [Epub ahead of print].

Strasser SM, Smith M, Pendrick-Denney D, et al: Feasibility study of social media to reduce intimate partner violence among gay men in metro Atlanta, *Georgia. West J Emerg Med* 13(3):298–304, 2012.

Strecher VJ, DeVellis BM, Becker MH, et al: The role of self-efficacy in achieving health behavior change, *Health Educ Q* 13:73–92, 1986.

Strickland CJ, Squeoch MD, Chrisman NJ, et al: Health promotion in cervical cancer prevention among the Yakama Indian women of the Wa'Shat Longhouse, *J Transcult Nurs* 10:190–196, 1999.

Sudore RL, Landefeld CS, Pérez-Stable EJ, et al: Unraveling the relationship between literacy, language proficiency, and patient-physician communication, *Patient Educ Couns* 75:398–402, 2009.

Sykes S, Wills J, Rowlands G, et al: Understanding critical health literacy: a concept analysis, *BMC Public Health* 13:150, 2013.

U.S. Department of Health and Human Services: *Making health communication programs work: a planner's guide, pink book*, Bethesda, MD, 2008, Office of Cancer Communications, National Cancer Institute. Available from <http://www.cancer.gov/cancertopics/cancerlibrary/pinkbook>.

U.S. Department of Health and Human Services: *National action plan to improve health literacy*. Available from <http://www.health.gov/communication/hlactionplan/>, 2010b.

U.S. Department of Health and Human Services, Centers for Disease Control and Prevention, National Center for Chronic Disease Prevention and Health Promotion: *The health consequences of smoking: a report of the Surgeon General*, Atlanta, 2004, Office on Smoking and Health.

U.S. Department of Health and Human Services, Public Health Services: *Healthy People 2020*, n.d. Available from https://www.healthypeople.gov/2020/default.aspx.

U.S. Department of Health and Human Services, Public Health Services, Office of Minority Health (OMH): *The national culturally and linguistically appropriate services (CLAS) standards*. Available from <http://minorityhealth.hhs.gov/templates/browse.aspx?lvl=2&lvlid=15>, 2000.

U.S. Department of Health and Human Services, Public Health Services, Office of Minority Health (OMH): *Enhanced national culturally and linguistically appropriate services (CLAS) standards*. Available from https://www.thinkculturalhealth.hhs.gov/content/clas.asp view *The Blueprint* and *National CLAS Standards* https://www.thinkculturalhealth.hhs.gov/pdfs/EnhancedCLASStandardsBlueprint.pdf.

Van Wyk NC: Health education as education of the oppressed, *Curationis* 22:29–34, 1999.

Ventura F, Ohlén J, Koinberg I: An integrative review of supportive e-health programs in cancer care, *Eur J Oncol Nurs* 12, 2012. Nov 14 [Epub ahead of print].

Villarruel AM, Jemmott JB, Jemmott LS, Ronis DL, et al: Predicting condom use among sexually experienced Latino adolescents, *West J Nurs Res* 29:724–738, 2007.

Viswanath K, McCloud R, Minsky S, et al: Internet use, browsing, and the urban poor: implications for cancer control, *J Natl Cancer Inst Monogr* 47:199–205, 2013.

Vyas AN, Landry M, Rojas AM, et al: Public health interventions: reaching Latino adolescents via short message service and social media, *J Med Intern Res* 14:e99, 2012.

Waite KR, Paasche-Orlow M, Rintamaki LS, et al: Literacy, social stigma, and HIV medication adherence, *J Gen Intern Med* 23:1367–1372, 2008. 9: 503–516, 2013.

Wallace LS, Rogers ES, Roskos SE, et al: Brief report: screening items to identify patients with limited health literacy skills, *J Gen Intern Med* 21:874–877, 2006.

Wallerstein N, Bernstein E: Empowerment education: Freire's ideas adapted to health education, *Health Educ Q* 15:379–394, 1988.

Weiss BD, Mays MZ, Martz W, et al: Quick assessment of literacy in primary care: the newest vital sign, *Ann Fam Med* 3:514–522, 2005.

Wells KJ, Battaglia TA, Dudley DJ, et al: Patient navigation: state of the art or is it science? *Cancer* 113:1999–2010, 2008.

Wells KJ, Meade CD, Calcano E, et al: Innovative approaches to reducing cancer health disparities: The Moffitt Cancer Center patient Navigator research program, *Journal of Cancer Education*, 2011. Dec;26(4):649–57.

Wells KJ, Rivera MI, Proctor SS, et al: Creating a patient navigation model to address cervical cancer disparities in a rural Hispanic farmworker community, *J Health Care Poor Underserved* 23:1712–1718, 2012a.

Wells KJ, Quinn GP, Meade CD, et al: Development of a cancer clinical trials multi-media intervention: clinical trials: are they right for you? *Patient Education and Counseling* 88(2):232–240, 2012b.

Werle GD: The lived experience of violence: using storytelling as a teaching tool with middle school students, *J Sch Nurs* 20(2):81–87, 2004.

Wilkinson GS, Robertson GJ: *Wide Range Achievement Test 4 professional manual*, Lutz, FL, 2006, Psychological Assessment Resources.

Wilson FL, Baker LM, Nordstrom CK, et al: Using the teach-back and Orem's self-care deficit nursing theory to increase childhood immunization communication among low-income mothers, *Issues Compr Pediatr Nurs* 31:7–22, 2008.

Wilson N, Minkler M, Dasho S, et al: Getting to social action: the Youth Empowerment Strategies (YES!) project, *Health Promot Pract* 9:395–403, 2008.

Wolf MS, Williams MV, Parker RM, et al: Patients' shame and attitudes toward discussing the results of literacy screening, *J Health Commun* 12:721–732, 2007.

Woolf SH, Chan EC, Harris R, et al: Promoting informed decision choice: transforming health care to dispense knowledge for decision making, *Ann Intern Med* 143:293–300, 2005.

World Health Organization Commission on the Social Determinants of Health: *Achieving health equity: from root causes to fair outcomes*, Geneva, 2007, World Health Organization. Available from <http://whqlibdoc.who.int/publications/2007/interim_statement_eng.pdf>.

Yost KJ, Webster K, Baker DW, et al: Bilingual health literacy assessment using The Talking Touchscreen/Lapantalla Parlanchina: development and pilot testing, *Patient Educ Couns* 75:295–301, 2009.

9

Case Management

Karyn Leavitt Grow and Jean Cozad Lyon

OBJECTIVES

Upon completion of this chapter, the reader will be able to do the following:

1. Define case management and care management, and compare the differences.
2. Discuss the philosophy and guiding principles of case management.
3. Identify the origin and purpose of case management.
4. Identify the case management process.
5. Discuss the roles and characteristics of case management in a reformed health care environment.
6. Incorporate case management concepts into clinical practice settings.
7. Identify educational preparation and skills recommended for case managers.

KEY TERMS

care management
case management
client-centered case management

continuum of care
patient-centered medical home

system-centered case management
utilization review

OUTLINE

Overview of Case Management
  Care Management
  Care Coordination
Origins of Case Management
  Public Health
  Case Management in Mental Health
  Case Management and the Elderly
  Disease-Specific Case Management
  Patient-Centered Medical Home
Purpose of Case Management
Utilization Review and Managed Care
Trends that Influence Case Management
  Changes in Health Care Reimbursement
  Access to Health Care for More Americans

Education and Preparation for Case Managers
  Nurse Case Managers
Case Manager Services
Case Manager Roles and Characteristics
  Case Identification
  The Referral Process
Application of Case Management in Community Health
  Community Case Management Models
  Public Health Clinic Settings
  Occupational Health Settings
  High-Risk Clinic Settings
Research in Case Management
International Case Management

OVERVIEW OF CASE MANAGEMENT

Case management is a term that describes a wide variety of patient care coordination programs in acute hospital and community settings. The term *case management* applies to community health settings that include patient-centered medical homes (PCMHs), occupational health, geriatric services, ambulatory care clinics, mental health settings, and outpatient primary care settings. Patient populations of all ages receive case management services.

Since the late 1980s and the 1990s, a variety of case management programs have emerged (Huber, 2002). From 1990 to 2005, case management evolved rapidly in response to changes in the health care environment and an increase in the number of managed care programs. Client service use reflects a greater emphasis on health care costs. Third-party payers evaluate the appropriate use of health care resources such as diagnostic tests, laboratory tests, length of hospital visits, and duration of home health care services. Managed care organizations (MCOs) may deny reimbursement to health care providers that exceed the expected costs. Health care providers, interested in close monitoring of resources, introduced various forms of case management programs.

More recently, health care evolved from a quantity-driven delivery system to a quality-driven system. In 2001, the Institute of Medicine (IOM) published a report, *Crossing the Quality Chasm.* It recommended a redesign of the health care system to provide care that is safe, efficient, effective, timely, equitable, and patient centered. The report names care coordination as an essential function to reach these goals and improve health care quality (IOM, 2001). The Institute for Healthcare Improvement's (IHI) Triple Aim Initiative is a framework of goals to optimize health system performance. The framework includes improving the patient experience, improving the health of populations, and reducing the per capita cost of health care. Additionally, the Centers for Medicare and Medicaid (CMS) have initiated reimbursement initiatives to providers to improve the quality of health care. The functions and principles of case management are in accord with these quality health care doctrines.

Case management has emerged as an intervention strategy for quality improvement initiatives. A single definition of case management does not exist. The Case Management Society of America (CMSA) (2010) offers the following definition of case management:

> *Case management is a collaborative process of assessment, planning, facilitation, care coordination, evaluation, and advocacy for options and services to meet an individual's and family's comprehensive health needs through communication and available resources to promote quality cost-effective outcomes. (p. 8)*

The philosophy statement published by CMSA (2010) reads as follows:

> *The underlying premise of case management is based in the fact that, when an individual reaches the optimum level of wellness and functional capability, everyone benefits: the individuals being served, their support systems, the health care delivery systems, and the various reimbursement sources. Case management serves as a means for achieving client wellness and autonomy through advocacy, communication, education, and identification of service facilitation. (p. 10)*

CMSA has now published the *Case Management Adherence Guide* (Rogers et al., 2012). The purpose of this guide is to provide a resource for every case manager in engaging patients in active participation in:

- Patient knowledge
- Patient involvement in care
- Patient empowerment
- Improved adherence
- Improved coordination of care (CMAG, 2012, p. 1)

According to the American Nurses Credentialing Center (ANCC, 2009), a subsidiary of the American Nurses Association (ANA), *nursing case management* is "a dynamic and systematic collaborative approach to provide and coordinate health care services to a defined population. The framework includes five components: assessment, planning,

---

BOX 9-1   POSSIBLE CASE MANAGEMENT FUNCTIONS

- Identifying the target population
- Determining screening and eligibility
- Arranging services
- Monitoring and follow-up
- Assessing
- Planning care
- Reassessing
- Assisting clients through a complex, fragmented health care system
- Care coordination and continuity

---

implementation, evaluation and interaction." Many labels describe case management within a profession. Terms used in addition to case management include care coordination, care management, geriatric care management (GCM), and integrated care management. Multiple case management labels cause further confusion among health care professionals and health care consumers. Case management takes on many forms, depending on the level, discipline, organization, situation, and basic client care needs being addressed (White and Hall, 2006).

Some hospitals, health maintenance organizations (HMOs), and other insurance companies inaccurately use the term *case management* to describe "utilization management," "managed care," or the method of monitoring and controlling service use within a system or care episode to control cost. Case management programs, however, aim to provide a service delivery approach to ensure the following: cost-effective care, alternatives to institutionalization, access to care, coordinated services, and patient's improved functional capacity (Lyon, 1993) (Box 9-1). These goals apply to community health and acute care settings. A subset of case management is care management.

Care Management

Care management consists of programs that apply systems, science, incentives, and information to improve medical practice and to allow clients and their support systems to participate in a collaborative process with a goal of improving medical, social, and mental health conditions more effectively. Care management is an emerging concept that is evidence-based, patient centered, and clinical care focused.

The overall goal of care management is to improve the coordination of services provided to clients who are enrolled in a care management program. Examples of groups of people who may be served by care management services are the elderly, children from low-income families who receive Medicaid services, and groups of people with chronic illnesses.

Patient-centered medical homes are another example of care management. The American Academy of Family Physicians (AAFP) defines the patient-centered medical home as follows:

> *Transition away from a model of symptom and illness based episodic care to a system of comprehensive coordinated primary care for children, youth and adults. Patient centeredness refers to an ongoing, active partnership with a personal primary care*

physician who leads a team of professionals dedicated to providing proactive, preventive and chronic care management through all stages of life. These personal physicians are responsible for the patient's coordination of care across all health care systems facilitated by registries, information technology, health information exchanges, and other means to ensure patients receive care when and where they need it. With a commitment to continuous quality improvement, care teams utilize evidence-based medicine and clinical decision support tools that guide decision making as well as ensure that patients and their families have the education and support to actively participate in their own care. Payment appropriately recognizes and incorporates the value of the care teams, non-direct patient care, and quality improvement provided in a patient-centered medical home. (AAFP, 2008)

Care Coordination

Care coordination was identified in the Institute of Medicine (IOM) report *Crossing the Quality Chasm* as an essential function in improving health quality (IOM, 2001). It has also been recognized as an approach to integrate fragmented health care, improve the transitions of care between providers, and decrease the unnecessary utilization of resources and costs. Care coordination programs are those

that target chronically ill persons at risk for adverse outcomes and expensive care and that meet their needs by filling the gaps in health care. They (1) identify the full range of medical, functional, social, and emotional problems that increase patients' risk of adverse health events; (2) address those needs through education in self-care, optimization of medical treatment, and integration of care fragmented by setting or provider; and (3) monitor patients for progress and early signs of problems. Such programs hold the promise of raising the quality of health care, improving health outcomes, and reducing the need for costly hospitalizations and medical care. (Chen, 2000)

There are many definitions of care coordination. In its 2005 report *Closing the Quality Gap: A Critical Analysis of Quality Improvement Strategies, Volume 7: Care Coordination,* the Agency for Health Care Research and Quality (AHRQ) defines *care coordination* as:

The deliberate organization of patient care activities between two or more participants (including the patient) involved in a patient's care to facilitate the appropriate delivery of health care services. Organizing care involves the marshaling of personnel and other resources needed to carry out all required patient care activities, and is often managed by the exchange of information among participants responsible for different aspects of care. Care coordination is a process component and function of case management. (McDonald et al., 2005)

ORIGINS OF CASE MANAGEMENT

Case management has a long history with the mentally ill, elderly patients, and the community setting (Steinberg and Carter, 1983). Public health, mental health, and long-term care settings have implemented and studied case management services and have reported them in their literature for many years (Mahn and Spross, 1996; Weil and Karls, 1985).

Public Health

Community service coordination, which was a forerunner of case management, appeared in public health programs in the early 1900s. During this time, health care providers reported these community service and case management programs in the nursing literature. Programs focused on community education in sanitation, nutrition, and disease prevention became prevalent. Lillian Wald and Mary Brewster conducted many of these programs at the Henry Street Settlement House in New York City. The Metropolitan Life Insurance Company later expanded nursing services for individuals, families, and the community to include disease prevention and health promotion (Conger, 1999).

The concept of continuum of care originated after World War II to describe the long-term services required for discharged psychiatric patients (Grau, 1984). Service coordination evolved into case management, a term that first appeared in social welfare literature during the early 1970s.

Case Management in Mental Health

During the late 1960s and early 1970s, mental health care emphasized moving patients from mental health institutions back into the community (Crosby, 1987; Pittman, 1989). The Community Mental Health Center Act of 1963 placed federal approbation on deinstitutionalization, which emphasized the importance of community mental health services. Mental health providers began to move patients from large state institutions to the community.

Several problems resulted from the deinstitutionalization of mentally ill patients. In 1977, Congress acknowledged that many disabled people had been deinstitutionalized without basic needs, proper follow-up, or health care monitoring. Congress further recognized that a systematic approach to service delivery could have prevented many state hospital readmissions. Case management in community mental health helped avoid client service fragmentation (Pittman, 1989).

Case Management and the Elderly

Specific elderly services recognized that age-generic programs do not adequately assist older people. Many older people have special, population-specific health care needs. Thus, case management services frequently target the elderly population, specifically homebound individuals or those with complex problems. However, not all older people who subscribe to multiple services require a case manager. Older adults may not need a case manager if they possess adequate functional status and can coordinate and access services for themselves, if they have family support, or if they have formal or informal caregivers who provide these functions for them. The elderly who have support require information about options, available services, and follow-up assistance (Lyon et al., 1995).

The Hartford Institute for Geriatric Nursing

The Hartford Institute for Geriatric Nursing (HIGN) was started in 1996 with the mission of shaping the quality of health care of older adults through the development of nursing excellence. The HIGN is the geriatric section of New York

> ## BOX 9-2   PRINCIPLES OF A PATIENT-CENTERED MEDICAL HOME
>
> The patient-centered medical home has the following seven characteristics:
> - The patient's relationship with the primary care physician
> - The physician-led, team-based care
> - The patient as a "whole person" who requires comprehensive care at various stages of life
> - Integration and coordination of care
> - Quality and safety
> - Improved access to care
> - A payment system that accurately reflects the efforts and care provided by the team

University (NYU) College of Nursing. To achieve the objective of shaping the care provided to the geriatric population, HIGN has developed ConsultGeriRN, an application available on the Apple iPad that is designed to help health care professionals with decision making in providing the best quality care for older adults (HIGN, n.d.).

Disease-Specific Case Management

Case management services are often provided for individuals who are identified as having medical conditions that are high-cost or high-volume acute and chronic illnesses. Examples are chronic obstructive pulmonary disease and chronic cardiac conditions such as congestive heart failure. The goal of disease-specific case management is to keep the individuals as healthy as possible and stable in their home environments. One particular goal is to decrease the frequency and length of hospital stays and consequently reduce health care costs.

Patient-Centered Medical Home

As previously mentioned, the patient-centered medical home is a recent model of care developed to provide collaborative, quality-driven, safe primary care. The PCMH utilizes care coordination and case management processes to provide comprehensive, patient-centered, cost-effective, quality care (Henderson, Princell, and Martin, 2012). In 2007, the report *Joint Principles of the Patient-Centered Medical Home,* sponsored by four medical professional organizations, described the seven principles or characteristics of the PCMH, which are listed in Box 9-2 (Patient-Centered Primary Care Collaborative, 2007).

PURPOSE OF CASE MANAGEMENT

Case management is client centered and system centered. Client-centered case management helps the client or patient proceed through a complex, fragmented, and often confusing health care delivery system and achieves specific client-centered goals. System-centered case management recognizes that health care resources are finite. The upward spiral in health care costs leads third-party payers such as Medicare, managed care organizations, and insurance companies to demand cost-effective health care. Hospitals are reimbursed for care provided on the basis of value-based purchasing. Client consumers insist on cost-effective, quality care. This demand forces health care providers to reevaluate the way they administer care, to emphasize quality improvement, and to focus on decreasing cost. Health care resources then become allocated to those populations with the greatest needs.

Case management is used to promote and integrate the coordination of clinical services, linking patients to community services and agencies. Case managers monitor resources used by clients, support collaborative practice and continuity of care, and enhance patient satisfaction (Yamamoto and Lucey, 2005).

For the hospitalized patient, health care service coordination begins either upon hospital admission or shortly thereafter and continues after the patient's discharge for an unspecified time. The patient's physical and psychosocial status and the plan's success will determine the length of the case manager's evaluation and intervention (Lyon, 1993; Lyon et al., 1995)

⚖ ETHICAL INSIGHTS
Ethical Issues in Case Management

> There are several ethical issues that a case manager should take into consideration when working with populations. Examples are as follows:
> 1. Right to privacy. Confidentiality of clients served must be maintained. Communicating patient information to others who are involved with the client's care must be done only with the client's knowledge and permission.
> 2. Health care resources are expensive and limited. The case manager must use appropriate, reliable, and accessible resources for individual clients or groups of clients with the same identified needs.
> 3. Respect for the client's rights to be informed about his or her care and services and to choose to receive services or not.
> 4. Clients have the right to know what resources are available to them and have the right to select providers of the resources.

UTILIZATION REVIEW AND MANAGED CARE

Equity and cost-effectiveness require management and allocation of available resources in a hospital, community, city, state, or particular health care client population. Utilization review (UR), as defined by CMSA, consists of the evaluation of medical appropriateness or medical necessity of care. This review ensures that patients receive the "right care at the right time" to improve clinical outcomes and lower costs (Stricker, n.d.).

System-centered case management rations and sets priorities for those in a larger group or population who could benefit from specific services.

Case management programs are often motivated by the need to evaluate, use, and allocate health care resources. Many case management programs evolved from utilization review departments. These departments showed that monitoring service use alone is insufficient for managing patient populations with diverse resource needs. Over time, the utilization review nurses assumed the additional case manager responsibilities.

TRENDS THAT INFLUENCE CASE MANAGEMENT

Numerous trends have influenced case management programs. During the 1970s, hospitals billed Medicare, Medicaid, and other third-party payers for client services and received reimbursement. Health care costs skyrocketed and rapidly became the basis for discussion and concern throughout the health care industry and the country. In 1983, PL 98-21 of the Social Security Amendments introduced the prospective payment system (PPS) in the acute care setting. Under the PPS, health care providers receive a fixed amount of money based on the relative cost of resources they use to treat Medicare patients within each diagnosis-related group. Other third-party payers followed this example and negotiated reimbursement schedules through preferred provider programs or managed care contracts (U.S. Department of Commerce, 1990).

Health care costs continue to escalate, the population is aging, and the elderly population is growing. Many elderly suffer from chronic illness and require health care resources.

Changes in Health Care Reimbursement

Title III of the Patient Protection and Affordable Care Act (Public Law 111-148), passed by Congress in March 2010, includes provisions requiring improvement in the quality and efficiency of health care. The Centers for Medicare and Medicaid (CMS), has established a value-based purchasing program for hospitals, launched in the fall of 2013. The program links Medicare payments to quality performance on common, high-cost conditions such as cardiac care, surgical care, and pneumonia care. The Physician Quality Reporting Initiative (PQRI), which has been extended through 2014, has incentives for physicians to report Medicare quality data. Physicians began to receive feedback reports from the initiative in 2012. Long-term care hospitals, inpatient rehabilitation facilities, and hospice providers will participate in value-based purchasing, and quality measure reporting starts in 2014, with financial penalties for nonparticipating providers (Public Law 111-148, 2010).

Access to Health Care for More Americans

The Patient Protection and Affordable Care Act removes many barriers to health care for Americans. With insurance coverage available to people through employers or purchased through health care access networks, more Americans will be insured and will have access to health care. The anticipated increase in the number of people seeking access to health care is expected to provide more challenges to health care providers. These changes open up opportunities for nurses working in case manager or care coordination roles to identify issues and further develop and expand their roles in working with diverse patient populations. These issues have influenced, and continue to influence, the introduction of case management services to control costs and distribute health care resources in a variety of settings.

EDUCATION AND PREPARATION FOR CASE MANAGERS

It is essential to determine what classification of health care provider is best qualified to provide case management services. Traditionally, case managers were social workers (SWs) who assumed the role of discharge planner. Client health care needs have become more complex, the need for ongoing patient assessment has emerged, and available resources have become more numerous and diverse; therefore nurses have become case managers. Several health care organizations exclusively employ SWs in case manager roles, others exclusively employ nurses in case management, and others use a combination of SWs and nurses, depending on the client population's needs. Combining the strength and knowledge of the nurse's clinical background with the SW's community service background can efficiently move a client through the complex health care system (Lyon et al., 1995).

Nurse Case Managers

Although both nurses and SWs have proved themselves to be excellent case managers, this chapter focuses on the nurse case manager in discussing educational requirements. A nurse case manager's optimum education level is debatable. The basic nursing education for case managers required by employers can vary. Some require a baccalaureate degree, and others do not. In some settings, a master's degree is required. Some programs are more interested in prior experience, continuing education, and case management certification than in the entry-level nursing degree. Education and experience requirements may vary, depending on the program's geographic location, specific client needs, and available staff.

Nurses with master's degrees and a focus in case management are readily available in urban settings. This gives facilities the opportunity to hire case managers who are academically prepared in theory and clinical experience. Rural areas that do not have master's-level academic programs are at a great disadvantage in recruiting and hiring qualified nurses. To fill the case manager role, rural facilities promote nurses to case management positions, provide them with continuing education programs, and offer them necessary job-related experience. Although this is not the ideal solution, it is often the only option for smaller facilities that are smaller or in more remote parts of the United States.

Regardless of the educational requirements in the individual case management program, case managers need a minimum skill level to ensure success in the role. These skills include sound knowledge of reimbursement structures; knowledge of available resources within the institution, organization, or community; working knowledge of the identification and evaluation of quality outcomes; the ability to perform cost-benefit ratios; and an understanding of financial strategies. In addition to the required knowledge, the nurse case manager needs flexibility, creativity, excellent communication skills, and the ability to work autonomously.

Case Manager Certification Options

There are two options for case managers to become certified. The certifications are offered by the CMSA and by the ANCC.

Case Management Society of America. The CMSA offers Certified Case Manager Certification (CCMC). The certification granted is the Certified Case Manager (CCM) credential. Following are the requirements for applicants (Commission for Case Manager Certification, 2009):

- Possess a good moral character
- Meet acceptable standards of practice
- Provide a job description for each case management position held
- Meet the continuum of care requirement
- Hold an acceptable license or certification based on a postsecondary degree program in a field that promotes the psychosocial or vocational well-being of the persons being served
- Ensure that the license or certification grants the ability to practice without the supervision of another licensed professional
- Perform the following essential activities of case management:
  1. Assessment
  2. Coordination
  3. Planning
  4. Monitoring
  5. Implementation
  6. Evaluation
  7. Outcomes
  8. General

American Nurses Credentialing Center. The ANCC offers certification in nursing case management. To be eligible to take the certification examination, applicants must:

- Hold a current, active registered nurse (RN) license within a state or territory of the United States or the professional, legally recognized equivalent in another country
- Have practiced the equivalent of 2 years full time as an RN
- Have a minimum of 2000 hours of clinical practice in case management nursing within the last 3 years
- Have completed 30 hours of continuing education in case management nursing within the last 3 years

Other Certifications. Several other certifications in specialty case management are available: disability management, health care quality, utilization management, managed care, and case management administrator certification. Case management professionals who are interested in obtaining certification should carefully research the options available for certification and should select the credentialing program that fits their work performed, education, and future career goals (CMSA, 2005).

CASE MANAGER SERVICES

Although case management programs differ in structure and design, case managers provide some services regardless of the program's location. There appears to be a consensus in the literature that four core functions or activities delineate case management—assessment, planning, facilitation, and advocacy—which are achieved through collaboration with the client and other health professionals (CMSA, 2010). The focus of each of these functions varies depending on the case management model.

Examples of care coordination include assisting the client or family member with medical appointments, equipment acquisition, home meal delivery, home follow-up services (e.g., home health or public health nursing), appointment transportation, and medical insurance or Medicare form completion. The types of services differ depending on the location of the case management program, the population of clients, and the scope of case management services. Some case managers in managed care environments monitor whether the patient keeps medical appointments and follows the prescribed course of treatment.

The coordination of health care services for hospitalized patients begins at admission or shortly thereafter and continues after discharge for an unspecified time (Ethridge and Lamb, 1989; Lyon, 1991). Depending on the setting, community case management services continue for varying lengths of time. Some programs continue service coordination indefinitely for populations such as the high-risk elderly and the chronically ill. Other programs move clients' case management status from active to inactive when patients no longer require services. However, the status becomes active again if their conditions change. Case management services continue in the home health care setting until the client is discharged from the program. Care coordination in the primary health care delivery setting is increasingly being provided in the patient-centered medical home. It is widely recognized that early intervention on the part of a case manager and appropriate referrals prevent costly complications and can result in better health outcomes (Thurkettle and Noji, 2003).

CASE MANAGER ROLES AND CHARACTERISTICS

The individual case manager's role will vary depending on the specific program's services. The role functions of case managers are defined by the CMSA as including assessment, planning, facilitation, and advocacy, achieved through collaboration with the client and others involved in the client's care (CMSA, 2010).

The ANCC describes the practice of a nurse case manager as follows:

Nurse case managers actively participate with their clients to identify and facilitate options and services, providing and coordinating comprehensive care to meet patient/client health needs, with the goal of decreasing fragmentation and duplication of care, and enhancing quality, cost-effective clinical outcomes. Nursing case management is a dynamic and systematic collaborative approach to provide and coordinate health care services to a defined population. Nurse case managers continually evaluate each individual's health plan and specific challenges and then seek to overcome obstacles that affect outcomes. A nurse case manager uses a framework that includes interaction, assessment, planning, implementation, and evaluation. Outcomes are evaluated to determine if additional actions such as reassessment or revision to a plan of care are required to meet clients' health needs. To facilitate patient outcomes, the nurse case manager may fulfill the roles of advocate, collaborator, facilitator, risk manager, educator, mentor, liaison, negotiator, consultant, coordinator, evaluator, and/or researcher. (ANCC, 2009)

Nurse case managers must be flexible. The health care environment experiences rapid change, and new regulations and reimbursement schedules frequently emerge. The health care provider must respond to these changes rapidly to remain competitive. It is an ideal job for the self-directed nurse who enjoys being involved in a larger health care team within the organization and in the larger community. CMSA (2010) defines the Standards of Case Management Practice (Box 9-3).

CASE IDENTIFICATION

Identification of case management clients occurs in many ways, and each program should determine the criteria for eligibility for case management services. These criteria depend on the services provided, the service's location, the population served, and whether the service is in an acute care or community setting. Some programs are diagnosis based and use many community health care resources; for example, clients with chronic obstructive pulmonary disease often require numerous hospitalizations. Programs may focus on a particular population (e.g., the elderly) and establish criteria to identify which clients to target for services (e.g., the high-risk elderly who are chronically ill or frail and would benefit from case management services).

All clients referred for case management must undergo screening to determine their appropriateness for inclusion in the program. Not all referred clients need the services of a nurse case manager. Often, a nurse can arrange community services or instruct the client and family in the most appropriate follow-up based on client need and program design. The screening instrument must be comprehensive enough to determine which clients meet the program's criteria and user friendly enough to allow the screener to evaluate the clients rapidly to determine their appropriateness for the program. The screener should refer clients to more suitable services within the community if they are not appropriate candidates for a particular case management program. For example, a nurse may refer a client who has tested positive for human immunodeficiency virus (HIV) to a case management program for high-risk clients in the community, but the program may not accept clients with HIV and acquired immunodeficiency syndrome (AIDS) because the community already has a program for HIV-positive clients. Instead, the nurse should refer the client to a case management program that focuses exclusively on comprehensive service coordination for clients with HIV and AIDS.

THE REFERRAL PROCESS

The nurse may perform program referrals in a variety of ways. In the acute care hospital setting, referrals are usually based on patient diagnosis or other criteria that trigger a nurse case manager referral (e.g., patient rehospitalization). Internal mechanisms alert the case manager of the patient's admission (e.g., a computerized list).

A variety of tools are used to identify people who would benefit from case management services. They include health-risk screening tools, evidence-based criteria, risk stratification through data management, and referrals from hospitals, health care providers, and families. Information is collected by the case manager and analyzed to determine whether the individual being referred is a candidate for case management services (CMSA, 2005; Rogers et al., 2012).

In community settings, referrals originate from a variety of sources, such as a client's family, a primary care provider, and a hospital case manager. These referrals may be written or verbal. Staff in community agencies can also make service referrals; for example, the American Heart Association or American Cancer Society may receive calls from clients and families requesting information and assistance.

APPLICATION OF CASE MANAGEMENT IN COMMUNITY HEALTH

Case management can be used in all community health settings, with interventions at the primary, secondary, and tertiary levels of prevention, according to the community program and population served. Nurses working as case managers in the community setting have diverse roles and responsibilities.

Community Case Management Models

Some case managers provide services exclusively in the community setting after discharge. Proponents argue that discharge planning and case management should be two separate and distinct functions with separate staff, procedures, and accountability. Supporters of this model believe case management's purpose is much broader than discharge planning and includes planning alternative to institutionalization, which ensures cost-effective care, access to comprehensive care, coordinating services, and improved client functional capacity (Simmons and White, 1988).

Public Health Clinic Settings

Depending on the services provided in the public health setting, the nurse has an opportunity to provide education, screening, and referrals as needed to the clients served. Examples of primary prevention include an antepartum clinic, where the nurse interacts with women and can teach about pregnancy, diet, and exercise during pregnancy.

Working with parents in pediatric settings, the nurse case manager can teach nutrition, growth, and development and provide anticipatory guidance (primary level of prevention). The nurse can also screen children for growth and development and make referrals as needed to the Women, Infants, and Children (WIC) program, and other specialty programs available in the area for the clients' needs (secondary prevention).

Nurses can also serve as case managers working with elderly clients, providing nutrition education (primary prevention), screening for hypertension (secondary prevention), and even assisting with medication management and care of chronic diseases (tertiary prevention). The opportunities for community health nurses to provide case management services are vast, depending upon the location, the populations served, and the resources available in the community.

Occupational Health Settings

More employers are providing health screening and education to their employees to keep their work forces healthy. Community health nurses who work in occupational health settings are in a position to provide primary prevention in health education classes designed to meet the needs of the employees. These classes can be designed on the basis of the health status of workers and to prevent the types of injuries to which they are prone. The nurse in this setting can also provide primary prevention by offering influenza vaccines and other immunizations to keep the employees healthy.

Secondary prevention can be provided to employees through screening clinics for hypertension and other potential chronic illnesses or health problems to which the employees may be more susceptible because of the nature of work performed. Referrals can be made as needed for follow-up with these employees. The occupational health nurse would continue to follow these employees and case-manage any health issues that could affect the employees' ability to perform the duties of their jobs.

Case management for tertiary prevention can include keeping in touch with injured employees and monitoring their recovery, therapy, or other services that are provided to the employees in the process of returning to health and their jobs. The occupational health nurse who provides case management services to these employees offers them education, referrals as needed, and assistance in their recovery process.

High-Risk Clinic Settings

There are many examples of health care settings that provide services to high-risk clients in which the nurse serves as case manager. A few examples are HIV clinics, settings that provide health care services to high-risk perinatal clients, clients who have received transplants, dialysis settings, oncology clinics, and infusion centers. The case management services offered by the nurse are determined by the specific needs of the clients seen in these settings. The models of case management are also developed for the needs of the clients.

Clients with Chronic Diseases

The community health nurse who interacts with clients with chronic diseases can be instrumental in monitoring the client in the community, monitoring medication management, assessing clients to identify problems early, and intervening with physicians to modify therapy. With patients who have chronic obstructive pulmonary disease, hypertension, or congestive heart failure, early intervention on the part of the nurse can decrease the need for hospitalization and, if the patient is hospitalized, ensure early hospitalization with a shorter stay.

Home Health and Hospice Settings

The community health nurse working in home health or hospice services is often assigned a case load of clients for whom he or she provides case management services. In both of these settings, the nurse case manager provides primary, secondary, and tertiary prevention to clients. These services are designed on the basis of the individual needs of clients and their families. Coordination of care, referrals, assessment, medication management, patient and family education, and the development of plans of care are just a few of the nursing functions that are provided through a case management model.

RESEARCH IN CASE MANAGEMENT

Case management research is increasing in the last decade, much of as a result of the quality reforms in health care and the role of case management in these reforms. A literature search in *PubMed* and the *Cumulative Index to Nursing and Allied Health* (CINAHL) found many categories of case management research. These include disease management; evidence-based practice; roles and functions; models; transitions of care; and roles in quality improvement initiatives. Specific research evaluating case management and quality improvement examined the roles of case management in transitions of care and readmissions, core measures, hospital-acquired conditions, and patient satisfaction. Other research evaluated the effect of case management on geriatric populations, disabled populations, and end-of-life situations. The documented studies describe the implemented programs and evaluate the program outcomes. An example is given in the Research Highlights box.

RESEARCH HIGHLIGHTS

Geriatric Care Management for Low-Income Seniors: A Randomized Controlled Trial

Counsell et al. (2007) conducted a randomized clinical control study of 951 adults 65 years or older with annual incomes less than 200% of the federal poverty level whose primary care physicians were randomly assigned to the intervention group (474 patients) or usual care (477 patients) in community-based health centers. The intervention consisted of 2 years of home-based care management by a nurse practitioner and social worker, who collaborated with the primary care physician and a geriatrics interdisciplinary team and were guided by 12 care protocols for common geriatric conditions. Results of the study showed that integrated and home-based geriatric care management resulted in improved quality of care and reduced acute care utilization among a high-risk group, in comparison with community-based care. Improvements in health-related quality of life issues were mixed, and physical function outcomes did not differ between the groups.

Case management programs in all settings require further study. Terms used in case management programs should be defined for comparison in various clinical sites. Programs with similar organizational structures and services can then be compared among settings. Critical to the success of case management programs are the inclusion of costs and cost savings and the evaluation of quality outcomes. The researcher or case manager must report the program's description as well as the case manager's role and professional background. Well-defined patient and program outcomes are essential to the evaluation of case management programs. With the implementation of well-designed research with measurable outcomes, management in health care settings across the continuum of care can identify the most cost-effective programs for specific populations served.

INTERNATIONAL CASE MANAGEMENT

As more Americans are traveling outside of the United States in search of affordable health care, a new need for case management has emerged. There is a now a need for international case management with great potential and new opportunities. New challenges are emerging in the need for ongoing consumer-relevant quality in the international case management arena (The PCM Editorial Review Board, 2008).

CASE STUDY   APPLICATION OF THE NURSING PROCESS

The following case study is an example of a comprehensive case management program. Case management programs and the served populations are diverse; this is only one example of case management implementation.

Judy, the case manager at an HIV early intervention program in Reno, Nevada, received a call from Don, a white man aged 29 years. Don had just moved from a neighboring state, where he recently discovered he was HIV positive. A clinic administered his HIV test, and he did not receive any health services. He found the HIV clinic's phone number in the phone book and did not have a local health care provider. He was a construction worker before he moved, but the company laid him off. He moved to Reno to find work because new building and growth abounded in the area. He moved into a local motel and paid rent for the following 2 weeks. He did not have health insurance, but he was eligible for continued health insurance coverage through the Consolidated Omnibus Budget Reconciliation Act (COBRA). Unfortunately, he could not afford to pay the COBRA premium because he was unemployed. He felt desperate, alone, isolated, and depressed, and he needed help.

Judy performed an intake screening and assisted Don in receiving needed services. She scheduled appointments with the clinic's health care providers and met with him to identify the services he needed. Judy completed her assessment after Don attended the clinical appointment and met with her for case management.

Assessment

Don was HIV positive, but he did not have any symptoms of AIDS. He took medication, ate well, maintained good physical condition and dentition, and owned a car. Although he had limited finances,

he had paid his rent for 2 weeks. He did not have health insurance and could not afford medications or laboratory tests. Judy developed the following plan:

Individual

Judy used Ryan White grant funds to finance Don's services through the clinic. She applied for housing assistance and scheduled an appointment with the clinic's social worker to discuss his financial situation and job prospects. The pharmacist provided his medications, which were funded by the clinic; explained the drugs in detail; and offered to answer questions.

Family

Don was estranged from his family. His mother, who lived 2000 miles away, was aged 65 years, widowed, and retired. Don had not visited his two siblings in 10 years and chose not to have family contact. Although Don had friends at his last job, he had not made friends in Reno. Before moving, he was in a relationship with a woman for 2 years. After the relationship ended, he did not know where she lived.

Community

Judy knew Don could access a solid network of community services. Don was new in the community, and he did not have social support; therefore Judy identified that he needed to contact job placement services and to attend an HIV support group.

Diagnosis

Judy worked with Don and discussed his disease process and provided him with information about HIV; together they developed a plan on how to proceed in obtaining services in the community.

CASE STUDY APPLICATION OF THE NURSING PROCESS—Cont'd

Individual

- Insufficient knowledge related to HIV, including knowledge of the disease, medications, and available resources
- Inadequate income from unemployment

Family

- Lack of family and social support
- Poor family communication patterns

Community

- Adequate services through the HIV clinic
- Coordination of services through case management from Judy and care management from the HIV clinic

Planning

Judy and Don made the following plan, which is open for modification, based on the established goals that she and Don identified.

Individual

Short-Term Goals

- Don will find employment within 2 months. If his employer does not provide health care benefits, the clinic program will continue to provide them.
- If Don does not find work and cannot pay rent, local HIV funding will be used to provide housing assistance.

Long-Term Goal

- The clinic will provide health care services, medications, laboratory tests, and other outpatient services.

Family

Short-Term Goal

- Don was not interested in communicating with his family. Judy respected his wishes and did not pursue the issue in the short term.

Long-Term Goal

- Judy will ask Don again whether he is interested in having contact with his family. Judy will offer Don the opportunity of family counseling to explore his feelings about his family and allow Don to determine whether he wants to communicate with any of his family members.

Community

Short-Term Goal

- Judy will collect information on available community resources to share with Don.

Long-Term Goal

- Judy will evaluate Don's involvement in using community resources. As needed, Judy will offer Don more options in terms of resources that are available and appropriate.

Intervention

Individual

Acting as his case manager, Judy connected Don with job opportunities, housing, and community support groups. Judy explained the available programs and allowed Don to choose his services.

Don had to attend his scheduled clinic appointments, take his medication, and contact his case manager regularly.

Family

Judy knows that Don is estranged from his family. As appropriate, Judy will continue to approach Don about exploring his feelings about his family with a professional counselor. If Don is interested in making contact with any of his family members, Judy will assist in the coordination of this process.

Community

The plan supplemented the services that Don could not afford. The plan focused on Don's individual needs for health care, employment, housing, and support groups. Judy will provide Don with available services in the community. As new programs become available, Judy will contact Don to explain the services and make referrals to services that both she and Don believe are appropriate.

Evaluation

Individual

Judy evaluated the results of Don's comprehensive case management plan on a continuing basis. If Don obtained employment in construction, he could support himself adequately and would require financial assistance primarily with his medications. If he did not find a job, or if his health status changed and he was unable to work in construction, then Judy would need to modify the plan.

Family

Judy evaluated Don's interest in getting in touch with his family. She will assist him in getting referred for family therapy. When and if Don wishes to contact any of his family, Judy will assist him in making arrangements.

Community

Judy will need to connect Don with community support groups to establish friendships and gain social support.

SUMMARY

Case management programs will continue to emerge in all health care settings. These programs will change as health care reform measures are initiated and the needs of the population change. A common need among all programs is to collect data on the efficacy of programs, measuring client and program outcomes to ensure that the services that are offered are meeting targeted goals.

Staff who work as case managers should consider obtaining certification to develop common knowledge and skills among case management providers and better validate the services provided.

LEARNING ACTIVITIES

1. Contact case management programs in the community and acute care setting.
2. Interview case management program directors. Ask them about their program's structure and process, the program's acceptance criteria, and their referral sources.

3. Ask the directors what data they collect on their clients and what is reported to their administration.
4. Ask the directors about their program's required education and experience levels for case managers.
5. Spend a day with a case manager, and ask about his or her various roles and services.
6. Participate in a client/family interview.

ⓔ **EVOLVE WEBSITE**

http://evolve.elsevier.com/Nies

- NCLEX Review Questions
- Case Studies
- Glossary

REFERENCES

American Academy of Family Physicians (AAFP): 2008. Available from < http://www.aafp.org/about/policies/all/pcmh.html >.

American Nurses Credentialing Center: *Case management nursing*, 2009. Available from <www.nursingworld.org>.

Case Management Society of America: Philosophy of case management, 2005. Available from <www.cmsa.org/ABOUTUS/DefinitionofCaseManagement/tabid/104/Default.aspx>.

Case Management Society of America: *Standards of practice for case management*, Little Rock, AR, 2010, Author.

Center for Health Care Strategies, Inc.: *Fact Sheet: Care management definition and framework*, Hamilton, NJ, 2007, Author.

Chen A, Brown R, Archibald N, et al: *Best practices in coordinated care*, March 2000. Available from <http://www.cms.hhs.gov/DemoProjectsEvalRpts/downloads/CC_Full_Report.pdf>.

Commission for Case Manager Certification: *Certified Case Manager (CCM) certification requirement*, 2009. Available from <www.ccmcertification.org>. Accessed March 1, 2013.

Conger MM: Nursing case management: a managed care organizational strategy. In Conger MM, editor: *Managed care: practice strategies for nursing*, Thousand Oaks, CA, 1999, Sage Publications.

Counsell SR, Callahan CM, Clark DO, et al: Geriatric care management for low-income seniors, *JAMA* 298:2623–2633, 2007.

Crosby RL: Community care of the chronically mentally ill, *Journal of Psychosocial Nursing* 25(1):33–37, 1987.

Ethridge PA: Nursing HMO: Carondelet St. Mary's experience, *Nurs Manage* 22(7):22–27, 1991.

Ethridge PA, Johnson S: The influence of reimbursement on nurse case management practice: Carondelet's experience. In Cohen EL, editor: *Nurse case management in the 21st century*, St. Louis, 1996, Mosby.

Ethridge PA, Lamb GS: Professional nursing case management improves quality, access, and costs, *Nurs Manage* 20(3):30–35, 1989.

Grau L: Case management and the nurse, *Geriatr Nurs* 5(8):372–375, 1984.

Greenberg E: State of the science paper #3: care coordination, *Case Management Society of America*, 2006.

Hartford Institute for Geriatric Nursing (HIGN): *Hartford Institute history*, n.d. Available from <www.hartfordign.org/About/History>. Accessed April 14, 2013.

Henderson S, Princell C, Martin CO: The patient centered medical home: this primary care model offers RNs new practice—and reimbursement—opportunities, *American Journal of Nursing* 112(12):54–59, 2012.

Huber DL: The diversity of case management models,, *Lippincott's Case Manag* 7(6):212–220, 2002.

Institute for Healthcare Improvement: *IHI triple aim initiative*, 2013. Available from http://www.ihi.org/offerings/Initiatives/TripleAim/Pages/default.aspx.

Institute of Medicine: *Crossing the quality chasm*, 2001. Available from <http://www.iom.edu/Reports/2001/Crossing-the-Quality-Chasm-A-New-Health-System-for-the-21st-Century.aspx>.

Lyon JC: *Descriptive study of models of discharge planning and case management in California (doctoral dissertation)*, San Francisco, 1991, University of California.

Lyon JC: Models of nursing care delivery and case management: clarification of terms, *Nurs Econ* 11(3):163–169, 1993.

Lyon JC, et al: *Case management for high risk elderly*. Paper presented at the 123rd annual meeting of the American Public Health Association, San Diego, 1995.

Mahn VA, Spross JA: Nursing case management as an advanced practice role. In Hamric AB, Spross JA, Hanson CM, editors: *Advanced nursing practice: an integrative approach*, Philadelphia, 1996, Saunders.

McDonald K, Sundaram V, Bravata D, et al.: *Closing the quality gap: a critical analysis of quality improvement strategies, Vol. 7: Care coordination* AHRQ Technical Reviews No. 9.7, Rockville, MD, 2005, Agency for Healthcare Research and Quality.

Patient-Centered Primary Care Collaborative: *Joint principles of the patient-centered medical home*, 2007. Available from <http://www.aafp.org/dam/AAFP/documents/practice_management/pcmh/initiatives/PCMHJoint.pdf>.

Patient Protection and Affordable Care Act, Title III: Improving the quality and efficiency of healthcare. Public Law 111–148, 2010. Available from <www.gpo.gov>.

PCM Editorial Review Board: The PCM journal "think tank" on case management predictions for 2009, *Prof Case Manag* 13:299–301, 2008.

Pittman DC: Nursing case management: holistic care for the deinstitutionalized mentally ill, *J Psychosoc Nurs* 27(11):23–27, 1989.

Public Law 111-148, 2010. Available from <http://www.gpo.gov/fdsys/pkg/PLAW-111publ148/pdf/PLAW-111publ148.pdf>.

Rogers S, Aliotta S, Commander C: *Case management adherence guide*, Little Rock, AR, 2012, Case Management Society of America.

Shea SC: *Improving medication adherence: how to talk with patients about their medications*, Philadelphia, 2006, Lippincott Williams & Wilkins.

Shea SC: The "Medication Interest Model": an integrative clinical interviewing approach for improving medication adherence—part I: clinical applications, *Prof Case Manag* 6(13):305–315, 2008.

Simmons WJ, White M: Case management and discharge planning: two different worlds. In Volland P, editor: *Discharge planning: an interdisciplinary approach to continuity of care*, Owings Mills, MD, 1988, National Health Publication.

Steinberg RM, Carter GW: *Case management and the elderly* Lexington, MA, 1983, Lexington Books DC Health.

Stricker P: *The role of utilization management in case management*. n.d. Available from <http://cmsa.org/individual/newsevents/healthtechnologyarticles/tabid/649/default.aspx>.

Thurkettle MA, Noji A: Shifting the healthcare paradigm: the case manager's opportunity and responsibility, *Lippincott's Case Manag* 8(4):160–165, 2003.

U.S. Department of Commerce/International Trade Administration: *Health and medical services: US industrial outlook*, Washington, DC, 1990, Author.

Weil M, Karls J: *Case management in human service practice*, San Francisco, 1985, Jossey-Bass.

White P, Hall ME: Mapping the literature of case management nursing, *J Med Libr Assoc* 94 (2 Suppl), 2006 E99E106.

Yamamoto L, Lucey C: Case management "within the walls": a glimpse into the future, *Crit Care Nurs Q* 28(2):162–178, 2005.

Policy, Politics, Legislation, and Community Health Nursing

*Anita W. Finkelman**

OBJECTIVES

Upon completion of this chapter, the reader will be able to do the following:

1. Discuss how the structure of government impacts the policy development process.
2. Describe the legislative, judicial, and administrative (executive) processes involved in establishing federal, state, or local health policy.
3. Examine the power of nursing to influence and change health policy.
4. Discuss current health policy issues.
5. Identify the social and political processes that influence health policy development.
6. Discuss the nurse's role in political activities.
7. Discuss nursing's involvement in private health policy.

KEY TERMS

administrative agencies
Clara Barton
coalition
Florence Nightingale
government
health policy
institutional policies
Lavinia Dock
laws

Lillian Wald
lobby
lobbyist
Mary Wakefield
nursing policy
organizational policies
organizations
policy
policy analysis

political action committees
politics
public health law
public policy
Ruth Watson Lubic
social policy
Sojourner Truth
statutes

OUTLINE

Overview: Nurses' Historical and Current Activity in Health Policy
Definitions
A Major Paradigm Shift
Structure of the Government of the United States
Overview of Health Policy
    Public Health Policy
    Health Policy and the Private Sector
    The Legislative Process: How a Bill Becomes a Law
Major Legislative Actions and the Health Care System
    Federal Legislation
    Role of State Legislatures
Public Policy: Blueprint for Governance
    Policy Formulation: The Ideal

    Policy Formulation: The Reality
    Steps in Policy Formulation and Analysis
The Effective Use of Nurses: A Policy Issue
Nurses' Roles in Political Activities
The Power of One and Many
    Nurses as Change Agents
    Nurses and Coalitions
    Nurses as Lobbyists
    Nurses and Political Action Committees
    Nurses and Campaigning
    Nurses and Voting Strength
    Nurses in Public Office
Health Care Reform and Restructuring of the Health Care Industry
Nurses and Leadership in Health Policy Development

---

*The author would like to acknowledge the contributions of Linda Thompson Adams and Deborah M. Tierney, who wrote this chapter for the previous edition.

This chapter addresses the interrelationships of the processes through which health policies are determined and instituted. Politics and legislation are the routes through which public health policies are established. Policy, politics, and legislation are the forces that determine the direction of health programs at every level of government, as well as the private sector. These programs are crucial to the health and well-being of the nation, the state, the community, and the individual. Nurses influence the maintenance and improvement of the health of individuals, groups, and communities by contributing to policy and legislative advancement.

The health care delivery system, including nursing practice and research, is profoundly influenced by policies set by both government and private entities. Nurses who understand the system of health policy development and implementation can effectively interpret and influence policies that affect nursing practice, the health of individuals, families, groups, communities, and populations, and, when required, offer an international health perspective.

OVERVIEW: NURSES' HISTORICAL AND CURRENT ACTIVITY IN HEALTH CARE POLICY

The more a nurse knows about the political process, the more he or she tends to become involved. Individual nurses may become politically active on a local, state, or national level. Nurses may work collectively within a group such as the National Student Nurses Association, the American Nurses Association (ANA), and state boards of nursing to lobby for health causes. There are about 3 million employed registered nurses (Kaiser Foundation, 2011). Together nurses can be patient advocates, change agents, and policy makers. Lawmakers respect nurses and thus are usually effective as consultants in both the legislative and executive branches at state and federal levels. It is the hallmark of the U.S. system of government that citizens have the right to have an influential voice in the governance of the community. Nurses are able to communicate concerns about conditions and issues in health care, the health care needs of individuals and communities, as well as the profession of nursing. United, nurses can influence political leaders to make changes to the health care system that are beneficial to all. Nurses experienced in the political arena can mentor novices to it.

Many individual nurses in the past and present have been instrumental in working with legislation and politics. A few exemplary nurses who had an impact on public health are:

Florence Nightingale was the first nurse to exert political pressure on a government (Hall-Long, 1995). She transformed military health and knew the value of data in influencing policy. She was a leader who knew how to use the support of followers, colleagues, and policy makers. As discussed in Chapter 2, Nightingale collected and analyzed data about health services and outcomes, an activity that now is a critical element of public health.

Sojourner Truth became an ardent and eloquent advocate for abolishing slavery and supporting women's rights. Her work helped transform the racist and sexist policies that limited the health and well-being of African Americans and women. She fought for human rights and lobbied for federal funds to train nurses and physicians (Mason, Leavitt, and Chaffee, 2007).

Clara Barton was responsible for organizing relief efforts during the U.S. Civil War. In 1882, she successfully persuaded Congress to ratify the Treaty of Geneva, which allowed the Red Cross to perform humanitarian efforts in times of peace. This organization has had a lasting influence on national and international policies (Hall-Long, 1995; Kalisch and Kalisch, 2004).

Lavinia Dock was a prolific writer and political activist. She waged a campaign for legislation to allow nurses to control the nursing profession instead of physicians. In 1893, with the assistance of Isabel Hampton Robb and Mary Adelaide Nutting, she founded the politically active American Society of Superintendents of Training Schools for Nurses, which later became the National League for Nursing (Kalisch and Kalisch, 2004). She was also active in the suffrage movement, advocating that nurses support the woman's right to vote (Lewinson, 2007).

Lillian Wald's political activism and vision were shaped by feminist values. Working in the early 1900s, she recognized the connections between health and social conditions. She was a driving force behind the federal government's development of the Children's Bureau in 1912. Wald appeared frequently at the White House to participate in the development of national and international policy (Mason et al., 2007).

Mary Breckenridge worked to develop nursing in rural Kentucky in the 1920s, establishing the Frontier Nursing Service.

Susie Walking Bear Yellowtail (1930-1960) was a Native American nurse who walked from reservation to reservation, working to improve health services for this population. She also established the Native American Nurses Association.

Florence Wald was a nursing leader in establishing hospice care in the United States—modeled after similar services offered in the United Kingdom—in the 1970s.

Dr. Ruth Watson Lubic is a nurse-midwife who crusaded for freestanding birth centers in this country. After developing the birth center model through the Maternity Center Association in New York City, Dr. Lubic expanded the model to Washington, DC, where the infant mortality rate was twice the national average. In 1993, Lubic was awarded the MacArthur Fellowship Grant and, in 2001, the Institute of Medicine's Lienhard Award (Institute of Medicine, 2001; Lyttle, 2000).

DEFINITIONS

Policy denotes a course of action to be followed by a government, business, or institution to obtain a desired effect. *Merriam-Webster's Dictionary* defines policy as "a definite course or method of action selected from among alternatives and in light of given conditions to guide and determine present and future decisions" (Merriam-Webster, 2014). Policy encompasses the choices that a society, segment of society, or organization makes regarding its goals and priorities and the ways it allocates its resources to attain those goals. Policy choices reflect the values, beliefs, and attitudes of those designing the policy (Mason et al., 2007).

Public policy denotes precepts and standards formed by governmental bodies that are of fundamental concern to the state and the whole of the general public. The field of public policy involves the study of specific policy problems and governmental responses to them. Political scientists involved in the study of public policy attempt to devise solutions for problems of public concern. They study issues such as health care, pollution, and the economy. Public policy overlaps comparative politics in the study of comparative public policy with international relations in the study of foreign policy and national security policy, and with political theory in considering ethics in policy making. See the examples in Table 10-1.

Health policy is a statement of a decision regarding a goal in health care and a plan for achieving that goal. For example, to prevent an epidemic, a program for inoculating a population is developed and implemented, and priorities and values underlying health resource allocation are determined.

Nursing policy specifies nursing leadership that influences and shapes health policy and nursing practice. Nursing, and therefore nursing leadership, is shaped dramatically by the impact of politics and policy. Effective nursing leadership is a vehicle through which both nursing practice and health policy can be influenced and shaped.

Institutional policies are rules that govern worksites and identify the institution's goals, operation, and treatment of employees.

Organizational policies are rules that govern organizations and their positions on issues with which the organization is concerned (Mason et al., 2007).

Social policy is policy associated with individuals and communities. In very general terms, social policy can be defined as the branch of public policy that advances social welfare and enhances participation in society. Social safety nets, however, often contribute to social exclusion, especially in urban settings, instead of being universally accessible. In most Western societies, social protection usually depends on contributory social insurance schemes to which only regular job holders have access (either in their own right or as dependents). In the United States, this is particularly evident with respect to the way the health care system and Social Security retirement benefits work. Social justice argues that all individuals and groups receive fair treatment in society as well as impartially share in the benefits of that society (Almgren, 2007).

Administrative agencies are departments of the executive branch with the authority to implement or administer particular legislation.

Laws are rules of conduct or procedure; they result from a *combination* of legislation, judicial decisions, constitutional decisions, and administrative actions.

Public health law focuses on legal issues in public health practice and on the public health effects of legal practice. Public health law typically has three major areas of practice: police power, disease and injury prevention, and the law of populations. Statute, ordinance, or code prescribes sanitary standards and regulation for the purpose of promoting and preserving the community's health. Public health law consists of legislation, regulations, and court decisions enacted by government at the federal, state, and local levels to protect the public's health. This includes case law and treaties.

Statutes are any laws passed by a legislative body at the federal, state, or local level.

Organizations are associations that set and enforce standards in a particular area; a group of individuals who voluntarily enter into an agreement to accomplish a purpose.

A *professional association* (also called a professional body, professional organization, or professional society) is a nonprofit organization seeking to further a particular profession, the interests of individuals engaged in that profession, and the public interest. It is a volunteer group that seeks to join large numbers of individuals who have a significant wealth of knowledge and experience in a particular field. There are also pooled funds for lobbying purposes (Thomas, 1997). The roles of these professional organizations are viewed as maintaining the control and oversight of the professional occupation as well as safeguarding the public trust. There is an element of protecting the interests of the professional practitioners, as in a cartel or labor union. Inherent in these organizations is the promotion of general standards for the performance of its members and the expectation of continued professional development.

Many professional bodies are involved in the development and monitoring of professional educational programs and the updating of skills, and thus they perform professional certification to indicate that a person possesses qualifications in the subject area. Sometimes membership in a professional body is synonymous with certification,

TABLE 10-1	**TERMINOLOGY EXAMPLE**
TOPIC	**EXAMPLE**
Public policy	A local or regional effort to prevent the sale of tobacco or alcohol to minors. Public policy directs that the right to health of the majority must be preserved over individual freedoms and corporate interests.
Public health law	New York State Public Health Law §2164: "Every person in parental (statute) relation to a child in this state shall have administered to such child an adequate dose of an immunizing agent against poliomyelitis, mumps, measles, diphtheria, rubella, varicella, *Haemophilus influenza* type B, and hepatitis B..."
Common law	The Supreme Court decision in *Roe v Wade*, making first-trimester abortion legal, is an example of how common law becomes enforceable.
Regulation	Reporting of communicable diseases to state and local health departments, which then report them to the Centers for Disease Control and Prevention.
Treaty	Multilateral treaty: Treaty to eliminate all forms of discrimination against women.

though not always. Membership in a professional body, as a legal requirement, can in some professions form the primary formal basis for gaining entry to and setting up practice within the profession. Professional bodies also act as learned societies for the academic disciplines underlying their professions.

A MAJOR PARADIGM SHIFT

Policy is based on values, and the first step in forming policy is identification of the issue. Therefore, it would seem rational to define "health" as the starting point for any policy annexed to health care issues. Historically, health was defined in the context of infectious diseases. Current definitions encompass prevention and management of chronic conditions. The World Health Organization (WHO) considers health to be the state of complete physical, mental, and social well-being and not merely the absence of disease or infirmity. Despite this broad definition, it is only in the most recent decades that the WHO is refocusing on its initial definition as it attempts to deal with environmental issues such as nuclear contamination and industrial toxins in industrialized nations and the exploration of carcinogenic commercial products such as tobacco products. On a global level, the WHO is working to eliminate antibiotic-resistant bacteria and find a way to solve the human immunodeficiency virus (HIV) pandemic. The emergence of HIV has changed the global health paradigm from the traditional notions of containment and treatment to a more comprehensive approach of social intervention. Thus there is a realization that health is a basic human right and that health problems are linked to government actions, and, hence affect human rights.

Human rights violations occur when governments fail to provide their people with the infrastructure, services, and information necessary to promote health, reduce risk, and control disease. For example, for every year of education women have, their infant mortality is decreased by 10%; yet education of women is not a global reality.

On a national level, an example of changing emphasis is the Centers for Disease Control and Prevention (CDC). It is committed to achieving true improvements in people's lives by accelerating health impact and reducing health disparities. Box 10-1 describes this shift. All people, and especially those at greater risk of health disparities, will achieve their optimal lifespan with the best possible quality of health in every stage of life. However, a shift in the paradigm of health concepts would necessitate a substantial reallocation of resources because the vast majority of health spending is directed at medical care and biomedical research and, as such, reflects a viewpoint of health care as a commodity. If one considers that in 2011 47.9 million people in the United States younger than 65 years had no health insurance and 11.7% of children are uninsured, it becomes clear that the health and human rights relationship is not yet reflected in our health policies (Kaiser Family Foundation, 2012). In addition, many people are underinsured. Their insurance coverage is not at the level it should be to cover full services

BOX 10-1	SHIFTS IN PHILOSOPHY AT THE CENTERS FOR DISEASE CONTROL AND PREVENTION
FROM	**TO**
Disease orientation	Health protection focus
Designing and implementing sponsored programs	Informing and guiding health system actors
Allocating agency resources	Leveraging resources to steer larger health system
Emphasis on clinical prevention	Focus on prevention and health protection
Transaction-based relationships	Partnerships and strategic alliances
Program requirements	Incentives for participation/ cooperation
Collecting and analyzing health data	Creating integrated health information systems
Issuing advisories and guidelines	Building decision-support system

From Centers for Disease Control and Prevention: *State of the CDC: fiscal year 2008*. Available from <www.cdc.gov/about/stateofcdc/FY08/cd/SOCDC/SOCDC2008.pdf>.

or longer-term needs. The economics of health care are discussed further in Chapter 12.

The publication of *Healthy People 2000* by U.S. Surgeon General C. Everett Koop in 1990 led to a resurgence of interest by the federal government in the health and welfare of Americans. However, fiscal resources for public health interventions declined, and only marginal progress was made in meeting the goals. In early 2000, *Healthy People 2010* marked the beginning of the new millennium and an enhanced focus on population-based health promotion strategies (U.S. Department of Health and Human Services [USDHHS], 2000). Many *Healthy People 2010* objectives directly or indirectly involve health policy. The most recent update, *Healthy People 2020* enhances the focus on the social determinants of health and adds even greater emphasis on health policy (USDHHS, 2013) (see the *Healthy People 2020* box).

Virtually all of the areas of *Healthy People 2020* have multiple policy-related objectives, and the *Healthy People* box lists only a few of them. Building on previous iterations, the updated 2020 version has four "over-arching goals" for 2020: attain high-quality, longer lives free of preventable disease, disability, injury, and premature death; achieve health equity, eliminate disparities, and improve the health of all age groups; create social and physical environments that promote good health for all; and promote quality of life, health development, and health behaviors across all life stages. The *Healthy People 2020* box describes *Healthy People* content related to public health infrastructure. Another forward-looking recommendation is making *Healthy People 2020* into a Web-accessible database that is searchable and interactive and allows users to tailor the document to the public's needs. The intent is that enhanced focus on social determinants represents a "deliberate shift away from the perception that access to health care services will ever solve all of our health care problems" (USDHHS, 2013).

HEALTHY PEOPLE 2020

Content Related to Public Health Infrastructure

Goal

To ensure that Federal, State, Tribal, and local health agencies have the necessary infrastructure to effectively provide essential public health services.

Overview

Public health infrastructure is fundamental to the provision and execution of public health services at all levels. A strong infrastructure provides the capacity to prepare for and respond to both acute (emergency) and chronic (ongoing) threats to the nation's health. Infrastructure is the foundation for planning, delivering, and evaluating public health.

Why Is Public Health Infrastructure Important?

Public health infrastructure includes 3 key components that enable a public health organization at the Federal, Tribal, State, or local level to deliver public health services. These components are:

- A capable and qualified workforce
- Up-to-date data and information systems
- Public health agencies capable of assessing and responding to public health needs

These components are necessary to fulfill the following 10 Essential Public Health Services:

1. Monitor health status to identify and solve community health problems.
2. Diagnose and investigate health problems and health hazards in the community.
3. Inform, educate, and empower people about health issues.
4. Mobilize community partnerships and action to identify and solve health problems.
5. Develop policies and plans that support individual and community health efforts.
6. Enforce laws and regulations that protect health and ensure safety.
7. Link people to needed personal health services and assure the provision of health care when otherwise unavailable.
8. Ensure competent public and personal health care workforces.
9. Evaluate effectiveness, accessibility, and quality of personal and population-based health services.
10. Research for new insights and innovative solutions to health problems.

Understanding Public Health Infrastructure

Public health infrastructure is key to all other topic areas in *Healthy People 2020*. It allows for and supports key goals of *Healthy People,* including the:

- Improvement of health

- Creation of environments that promote good health
- Promotion of healthy development and behaviors

Public health infrastructure, along with the 10 essential functions of public health, influences—and is influenced by—a number of factors, including the social and political environment. As such, public health infrastructure provides a useful framework for addressing the social determinants of health.

Emerging Issues in Public Health Infrastructure

Increasing attention to public health infrastructure has led to the identification of a number of emerging issues.

Tribal Public Health Infrastructure

Each Tribe is an independent government that must adopt local strategies to meet its public health challenges; interventions must be tailored to the cultural beliefs and practices of each Tribe. There are many ways Tribal entities are served through the Indian Health Service, Tribal Epidemiology Centers, and national organizations; however, challenges remain.

Disparities in the Public Health Workforce

As minority populations in the United States increase, the country will need a more diverse public health workforce. Hispanics, American Indians and Alaska Natives, and African Americans are underrepresented in the public health workforce.

Accreditation of Public Health Agencies

In an effort to standardize services and improve performance, public health agencies are moving toward a voluntary national accreditation program. This program will highlight agencies' commitment to service and quality and provide a standard toward which all public health agencies can work.

Public Health Systems Research

Expanding the evidence base for community interventions and for the effective organization, administration, and financing of public health services is critical to the future development of public health infrastructure. The emerging field of public health systems and services research is playing an important role in the development of this evidence base; its role should be supported and expanded over the decade, with a strong focus on translating research into practice.

Public Health Law

Novel policies are being developed to address legal and political challenges resulting from new and re-emerging infectious diseases and increasing levels of chronic disease. New centers devoted to the study of public health law are adding to the body of knowledge in this critical area.

From U.S. Department of Health and Human Services: *Healthy People 2020*, April 10, 2013 Public Health Infrastructure, retrieved from <http://www.healthypeople.gov/2020/topicsobjectives2020/overview.aspx?topicid=35>.

STRUCTURE OF THE GOVERNMENT OF THE UNITED STATES

Government is the structure of principles and rules determining how a state, country, or organization is regulated. Among its purposes are regulation of conditions beyond individual control and provision of individual protection through a population-wide focus. These tasks are accomplished through passage and enforcement of laws. Requirements of childhood immunizations for school attendance, disease vector control, and sewage treatment are examples of regulations to protect the health of the population.

Government can also be viewed as the sovereign power vested in a nation or state. *Sovereign power* is the independent and supreme authority of the nation or state. Historical documents describe the government's responsibility for health in the United States and the subsequent authority to enact laws (including health laws). These documents reflect the values of

TABLE 10-2	GOVERNMENT BRANCHES
BRANCH OF GOVERNMENT	**INCLUDES**
Executive branch	The president, the vice president, and the administrative agencies
Legislative branch	The Senate and the House of Representatives (Congress)
Judicial branch	At the federal level: district courts, circuit courts, and the Supreme Court
	At the state level: state and county courts

BOX 10-2 AN EXAMPLE OF THE PRESIDENT'S RESPONSE TO A HOUSE BILL (A PRESIDENT MAY OR MAY NOT RESPOND TO A BILL)

State Children's Health Insurance Program (SCHIP)

H.R. 2 (and related bills H.R. 57, H.R. 72, and S. 275) became Public Law 111-3, The Children's Health Insurance Reauthorization Act of 2009. This was signed into law by President Barack Obama on February 4, 2009. It went into effect on April 1, 2009. This bill:

- Allows certain state plans under Titles XIX (Medicaid) or Title XXI (State Children's Health Insurance Program, referred to in this Act as CHIP) of the Social Security Act (SSA) that require state legislation to meet additional requirements imposed by this Act additional time to make required plan changes.
- Provides for coordination of CHIP funding for the 2009 fiscal year.
- Amends SSA Title XXI to reauthorize the CHIP program through FY2013 at increased levels.

See http://thomas.loc.gov/home/thomas.php for more information.

BOX 10-3 ADMINISTRATIVE AGENCIES

One of the most dramatic changes in American government since the ratification of the Constitution is the growth of administrative agencies. Federal administrative agencies have broad power. They exercise all of the powers of government: executive, legislative, and judicial.

The U.S. Food and Drug Administration (FDA) is one such administrative agency. Its power is in regulating the pharmaceutical industry as well as the food industry.

---

the country's founders. They give the government the authority to enact laws, but they also limit that power. The earliest of these statements was the Mayflower Compact, through which the Pilgrims committed themselves to making "just and equal laws" for the general good. The Declaration of Independence later established the doctrine of inalienable rights, life, liberty, and the pursuit of happiness. However, it was not until the representatives of the individual states signed the Constitution of the United States that the federal government realized its sovereign power. At the same time that its power was realized, a limit to that power was placed on the federal government. The drafters of the Constitution sought to balance the need to empower the new federal government to "establish Justice, insure domestic Tranquility, provide for the common defense, promote the general Welfare, and secure the Blessings of Liberty" for its people but with limits on that power. That balance is achieved in several important ways.

The federal government is a government of limited powers, which means that for a federal action to be legitimate, it must be authorized. Only those actions that are within the scope of the Constitution, the supreme law of the land, are authorized. The Constitution separates governmental powers among the branches of government (Table 10-2).

Some examples of the separation of powers doctrine that are written into the U.S. Constitution are as follows:

- The legislature is prohibited from interfering with the courts' final judgments.
- The Supreme Court cannot decide a "political question"; the issue must be an actual case or controversy.
- Congress must present a bill to the President before it can become law (Box 10-2).
- The President needs consent of the Senate to appoint Supreme Court Justices or to make treaties.
- The President and members of Congress are elected; the Judiciary is appointed.

The Constitution not only set forth the responsibilities of the federal government, but it also provided for the individual citizen's rights and freedoms. These are contained in the first ten Amendments, which were added after the original Articles of the Constitution were ratified in 1787. These ten amendments, added in 1791, are known as the Bill of Rights. The rights guaranteed in the Bill of Rights, such as those of free speech and freedom of religion, applied only to the laws and actions of the *federal* government. It would take another 72 years for these rights to be guaranteed within the states.

"Liberty interests" and "privacy rights" have been found to exist by Supreme Court determinations and have become guiding principles in setting policy and enacting legislation. Note that these rights are applicable only to state or federal government's interaction with people. Violations of restrictions on rights such as free speech do not apply to nongovernmental entities, unless a specific law states otherwise.

The balance of powers is an important concept in the U.S. government. *Federalism* is the relationship and distribution of power between the national and the state governments. This balance flows directly from the text of the Constitution: "The powers not delegated to the United States by the Constitution, nor prohibited by it to the States, are reserved to the States respectively, or to the *people*." Box 10-3 highlights one of the changes in the federal government since the Constitution, the development of administrative agencies. This development has had a major impact on government functioning.

States retain powers not delegated to the federal government; therefore much of public health law is under state jurisdiction and, as a result, varies considerably from state to state. These powers to enact laws for the public welfare are referred to as the states' "police powers." Additionally, states may delegate these powers to local governments. In the United States, legislative activities of the three levels of government (federal, state, and local) may vary greatly in their expectations, actions, and results. The state legislatures, for the most part, are directly involved in health care, yet the federal government influences health policy, directly and indirectly, through the financing of health care for many groups (e.g., Medicare, Medicaid), regulation activities (e.g., approval of drugs), and setting of standards (e.g., air quality).

Decisions affecting the public's health are made not only at every level of government but also in each branch of government. The separation and balance of powers, referred to as *checks and balances*, is as important to health as it is to the economic or military status of the country.

The legislative branch (i.e., Congress at the federal level; legislature, general assembly, or general court at the state level) enacts the statutory laws that are the basis for governance. The executive branch administers and enforces the laws, which are broad in scope, through regulatory agencies. These agencies, in turn, define more specific implementation of the statutes through rules and regulations (i.e., regulatory or administrative law). The judiciary body provides protection against oppressive governance and against professional malpractice, fraud, and abuse. Its function through the courts, both state and federal, is to determine the constitutionality of laws, interpret them, and decide on their legitimacy when they are challenged. Decisions of the U.S. Supreme Court are binding law for the nation. Decisions of an individual state's highest court are binding law within that state alone. The courts also have jurisdiction over specific infractions of laws and regulations.

OVERVIEW OF HEALTH POLICY

Public Health Policy

To review, *public policy* refers to decisions made by legislative, executive, or judicial branches of one of the three levels of government (local, state, or federal). These decisions are intended to direct or influence actions, behaviors, or decisions of others. Public health policies influence health care through the monitoring, production, provision, and financing of health care services. Everyone, from health care providers to consumers, is affected by health policies. Likewise, health policy influences corporations, employers, insurers, colleges of nursing, hospitals, clinics, producers and retailers of medical technology and equipment, as well as senior care facilities.

The authority for the protection of the public's health is largely vested with the states, and most state constitutions specifically delineate their responsibility. Municipal subdivisions of states, such as counties, cities, and towns, generally have the power of local control of the services, conferred by the state legislature. The responsibilities of local, state, and federal governments for health services may differ under varying circumstances, sometimes complicating attempts to determine the locus of political decision making. The supremacy of the state prevails in most instances; therefore, the state is a critical arena for political action. An example is the state's authority to license health professionals and health care institutions.

Each state establishes policies or standards for goods or services that affect the health of its citizens. However, if the federal government or the local government imposes a higher standard than the state requires, the lower standard is negated by the higher standard. An example would be standardization of pasteurized milk. A state may hold to one standard, whereas interstate commerce, which is under federal jurisdiction, may dictate a higher standard that must be met by that state.

The federal government has a strong influence on the health services available in each state. Constitutionally, this authority is derived from the federal role in interstate commerce and through broad interpretation of the "general welfare" clause (e.g., Medicare and Medicaid). States vary considerably in resources allocated to provide health programs; therefore, significant de facto authority derives from the promise of revenues or threats to remove funding (e.g., funds for interstate highway repair are often tied to air quality requirements). Federal funds typically fund most health care programs fully or partially.

Compliance by states with federal program standards is voluntary, but the advantage of the revenue, which is withheld from the states that fail to comply, is seldom ignored. Programs such as a statistical reporting system of sexually transmitted infections and control are standardized across the country in response to the indirect but marked effect of federal funding.

Health Policy and the Private Sector

In addition to the public policy-making sector, health policies can also be made through the private sector. For example, an insurance company or an employer will determine what illnesses and preventive care is covered by the insurance program, what drugs are included in the formulary, and how much to charge for an insurance policy. The private sector includes employers, professional organizations (e.g., American Hospital Association), nonprofit health care organizations (e.g., American Heart Association), and for-profit corporations that deliver, insure, or fund health care services outside government control. In particular, health insurance companies and managed care organizations (MCOs) are increasingly setting policies that impact a large number of individuals.

In the private sector, health policy evolves differently from in the public sector. One difference is that private health policy is largely influenced by theories of economics and business management, as compared with the social and political theories that predominate in the public sector. In the private sector economics is central, whereas in the public sector economics is but one of many factors. In the private sector decisions can be swift and are often proactive, whereas in the public sector decisions are slow, deliberate, and more reactive. Private sector needs are determined by consumerism, market trends, and economics. Public sector needs are determined by voting shifts, electoral realignment, and term limits (Pulcini et al., 2000). Box 10-4 provides the history of several critical examples of government-funded health care legislation.

The Legislative Process: How a Bill Becomes a Law

As stated in the previous section, there is a balance of powers within the government at both state and federal levels. The three branches of government, executive, judicial, and legislative, form a three-legged stool that is in equilibrium. Along with a separation of powers of the three branches of government, there is an additional mechanism that balances the power of the Congress: bicameralism (consisting of two houses). Bicameralism ensures that the power to enact laws is shared between the House of Representatives and the Senate. The procedure through which legislation must pass to eventually become law is similar for all legislative bodies in the country. Once a

concept has been drafted into legislative language, it becomes a bill, is given a number, and moves through a series of steps. The bill's passage is sometimes smooth, but, more often than not, the bill is extensively altered through amendments or even "killed" (dropped from or stopped in the process).

In Congress and in the 49 states that have bicameral legislatures, a bill must succeed through the two legislative bodies, that is, the House of Representatives and the Senate (Figure 10-1). Nebraska, which has a single-house legislature, is the exception. A bill that has moved successfully through the legislative process has one final hurdle, which is the chief executive's approval. The approval may be a clear endorsement, in which case the governor or president signs it. If the executive neither signs nor vetoes it, the bill may become law by default. An explicit veto conclusively kills the bill, which then can be revived only by a substantial vote of the legislature to override the veto. This is another example of the checks and balances of the government process.

Issues that find their way into the legislative arena are commonly controversial, and proponents and opponents quickly align themselves. Defeating a bill is much easier than getting one passed; therefore, the opposition always has the advantage.

Health legislation, which usually requires preventive action (e.g., toxic waste management) or creates a new service (e.g., nursing center organizations for Medicare recipients), is

---

BOX 10-4 HISTORY OF SEVERAL EXAMPLES OF GOVERNMENT-FUNDED HEALTH CARE LEGISLATION

- **1965:** The Social Security Act established both Medicare and Medicaid. Medicare was a responsibility of the Social Security Administration (SSA), whereas federal assistance to the state Medicaid programs was administered by the Social and Rehabilitation Service (SRS). SSA and SRS were agencies in the Department of Health, Education, and Welfare (HEW).
- **1977:** The Health Care Financing Administration (HCFA) was created under HEW to effectively coordinate Medicare and Medicaid.
- **1980:** HEW was divided into the Department of Education and the Department of Health and Human Services (HHS).
- **2001:** HCFA was renamed the Centers for Medicare and Medicaid Services (CMS). CMS is the federal agency that administers the Medicare and Medicaid programs.
- **2010:** Patient Protection and Affordable Care Act was a very comprehensive attempt to improve access to care by providing health insurance to most of the nation's uninsured.

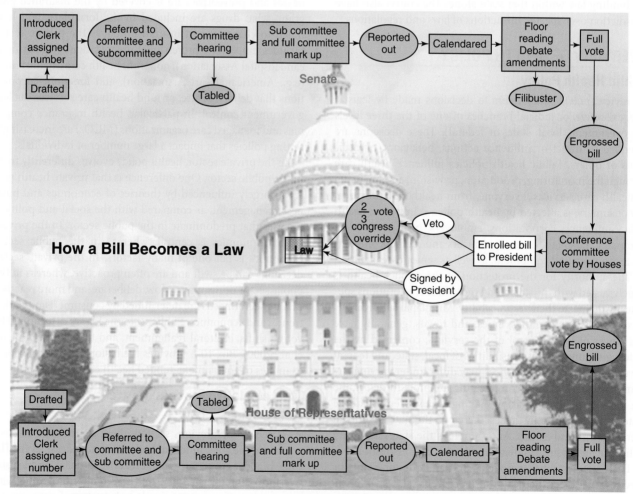

FIGURE 10-1 How a bill becomes a law at the federal level. (Retrieved October 19, 2009, from public-domainclip-art.blogspot.com/2007_09_01_archive.html.)

at a disadvantage from several standpoints. Few elected officials are knowledgeable about the health care field. Typically, they have staff who have more expertise in this area, and it is the staff who write legislation. Although health is readily recognized as a national resource, it is not easily quantified into the economic terms that make the issue easy to grasp. Other disadvantages are the backgrounds, biases, and ambitions of each legislator. Despite these obstacles, good health laws can be passed when concerned nurses and other health care workers understand the legislative process and use it effectively. Nurses should educate their elected officials and function as expert tutors for them. In addition, this is yet another mode of intervention that nurses may perform on behalf of clients.

MAJOR LEGISLATIVE ACTIONS AND THE HEALTH CARE SYSTEM

An examination of the major legislative actions that federal and state governments have taken and recognition of their influence on health and health care delivery are critical to understanding the evolution of the health care system in the United States. Throughout the twentieth century, the U.S. Congress enacted bills that had a major influence on the private and public health care subsystems. Legislation pertaining to health increased in scope in each decade of the twentieth century, with the goal of improving the health of populations and coping with changing health care needs. During the last two decades, concerns about an increase in health care costs and the growth of managed care stimulated even more legislation. Indeed, health care reform/health insurance reform was a major issue during the 2008 and 2012 presidential elections. Furthermore, Congress continues to debate numerous bills and amendments proposed to help reduce costs, increase access, and improve quality. The Supreme Court also reviewed a major case related to the health care reform legislation, tying all levels of government to this landmark legislation—administrative, legislative, and judicial. The Court decision did not lead to major changes in the health care reform law; however, other legal cases related to health care reform may be initiated.

Federal Legislation

This section describes some of the landmark federal laws that have influenced health services and health care professionals. They are listed in Table 10-3.

Pure Food and Drugs Act of 1906: This act established a program to supervise and control the manufacture, labeling, and sale of food. Subsequent legislation included meat and dairy products, pharmaceuticals, cosmetics, toys, and household products. Since 1927, the U.S. Food and Drug Administration (FDA) has administered elements of this act.

Children's Bureau Act of 1912: The Children's Bureau was founded to protect children from the unhealthy child labor practices of the time and to enact programs that had a positive effect on children's health. In 1921, the Sheppard-Towner Act extended children's health care programs by providing funds for the health and welfare of infants.

Social Security Act of 1935 and its amendments (1965, 1972): The Social Security Act and its subsequent amendments have had a far-reaching effect on health care for many groups. The Social Security Administration (SSA) provides welfare for high-risk mothers and children. Benefits were later expanded to include health care provisions for older adults and the handicapped. This major governmental action was the enactment of legislation for Medicare and Medicaid.

Medicare, Title XVIII Social Security Amendment (1965): This federal program, administered by the Centers for Medicare and Medicaid Services (CMS; formerly Health Care Financing Administration [HCFA]), pays specified health care services for all people 65 years of age and older who are eligible to receive Social Security benefits. People with permanent disabilities and those with end-stage renal disease are also covered. The objective of Medicare is to protect older adults and the disabled against large medical outlays. The program is funded through a payroll tax

TABLE 10-3	CRITICAL FEDERAL LEGISLATION RELATED TO HEALTH CARE
YEAR(S)	**LEGISLATION OR OTHER GOVERNMENT ACTION**
1906	Pure Food and Drugs Act
1912	Children's Bureau Act
1921	Sheppard-Towner Act
1935	Social Security Act
1944	Public Health Act
1945	McCarren-Ferguson Act
1946	Hill-Burton Act
1953	Establishment of the Department of Health, Education and Welfare as a cabinet-status agency; in 1980 establishment of U.S. Department of Education as separate from Department of Health and Human Services
1956	Health Amendments Act
1964	Nurse Training Act
1965	Social Security Act amendments: Title XVIII Medicare; Title XIX Medicaid
1970	Occupational Safety and Health Act
1972	Social Security Act amendments: Professional Standards Review Organization; further benefits under Medicare and Medicaid, including dialysis
1973	Health Maintenance Act
1974	National Health Planning Resources Act
1981, 1987, 1989, 1990	Omnibus Budget Reconciliation Acts
1982	Tax Equity and Fiscal Responsibility Act
1985	Consolidated Omnibus Budget Reconciliation Act
1988	Family Support Act
1990	Health Objectives Planning Act
1996	Health Insurance Portability and Accountability Act
1996	Welfare Act
2003	Nurse Reinvestment Act
2004	Medicare Reinvestment Act
2008	Mental Health Parity and Addictions Equity
2010	Patient Protection and Affordable Care Act

of most working citizens. Individuals or providers may submit payment requests for health care services and are paid according to Medicare regulations. See Chapter 12 for more information on Medicare.

Medicaid, Title XIX Social Security Amendment (1965): This combined federal and state program provides access to care for the poor and medically needy of all ages. Each state is allocated federal dollars on a matching basis (i.e., 50% of costs are paid with federal dollars). Each state has the responsibility and right to determine the services to be provided and the dollar amount allocated to the program. Basic services (e.g., ambulatory and inpatient hospital care, physical therapy, laboratory, radiography, skilled nursing, and home health care) are required to be eligible for matching federal dollars. States may choose from a wide range of optional services, including drugs, eyeglasses, intermediate care, inpatient psychiatric care, and dental care. Limits are placed on the amount and duration of service. Unlike Medicare, Medicaid provides long-term care services (e.g., nursing home and home health) and personal care services (e.g., chores and homemaking). In addition, Medicaid has eligibility criteria based on level of income. Table 10-4 provides the U.S. Department of Health and Human Services (HHS) poverty guidelines for 2013. The Medicaid population has complex needs, and managed care organizations may not always be able to provide optimum services to these beneficiaries. See Chapter 12 for more information on Medicaid.

Public Health Act of 1944: The Public Health Act consolidated all existing public health legislation into one law. Since then, many new pieces of legislation have become amendments. Some of its provisions, either in the original law or in amendments, provided for or established the following:

- Health services for migratory workers
- Family planning services
- Health research facilities
- National Institutes of Health (NIH)
- Nurse training acts
- Traineeships for graduate students in public health
- Home health services for people with Alzheimer's disease
- Prevention and primary care services
- Rural health clinics
- Communicable disease control

McCarren-Ferguson Act of 1945: The McCarren-Ferguson Act has had a major influence on the insurance industry through giving states the exclusive right to regulate health insurance plans (Knight, 1998). No federal government agency is solely responsible for monitoring insurance, as this supervision is in the hands of state governments. Some federal agencies are involved in insurance reimbursement; however, the structure of the benefit program for federal employees and military personnel, Medicare, and Medicaid allows Congress to pass laws that can override state health insurance laws if the laws do not meet certain criteria.

Hill-Burton Act of 1946: The Hill-Burton Act authorized federal assistance in the construction of hospitals and health centers with stipulations about services for the uninsured. As a result, hospitals with obligations to care for the uninsured were built in towns and cities across the United States. Through these measures, hospital care became more accessible, but by the late 1990s, the high cost of health care, combined with decreasing lengths of stay and increasing use of primary care, forced the closure of many of the hospitals built with Hill-Burton funds.

Health Amendments Act of 1956: The Health Amendments Act, Title II, authorizes funds to aid registered nurses (RNs) in full-time study of administration, supervision, or teaching. In 1963, the Surgeon General's Consultant Group on Nursing noted that there were still too few nursing schools, nursing personnel were not put to good use, and there was limited nursing research. As a result, in 1964, the Nurse Training Act provided funds for loans and scholarships for full-time study for nurses and funds for construction of nursing schools. Since this time, additional legislation has funded nursing education; even the Patient Protection and Affordable Care Act of 2010 provides some funding opportunities.

Occupational Safety and Health Act of 1970: The Occupational Safety and Health Act focuses on the health needs and risks in the workplace and environment. It continues to provide critical programs important to the workplace and the community. See Chapter 30 for more information on both the Occupational Safety and Health Act and the Occupational Safety and Health Administration.

Health Maintenance Organization (HMO) Act of 1973: The HMO Act provided grants for HMO development. The act required that employers offer federally qualified HMOs as a health care coverage option to employees and established that states were responsible for the oversight of HMOs. Although initially it was not successful in stimulating

TABLE 10-4	2013 FEDERAL POVERTY GUIDELINES* FOR THE 48 CONTIGUOUS STATES AND THE DISTRICT OF COLUMBIA		
FAMILY SIZE	GROSS YEARLY INCOME ($)	GROSS MONTHLY INCOME ($)	APPROXIMATE HOURLY INCOME ($)
1	11,490	958	5.52
2	15,510	1,293	7.46
3	19,530	1,628	9.39
4	23,550	1,963	11.32
5	27,570	2,298	13.25
6	31,590	2,633	15.19
7	35,610	2,968	17.12
8	39,630	3,303	19.05
Over 8 add per child	+4,020	+$335	+$1.93

Federal Poverty Guidelines: Typically, in January or February of each year the federal government releases an official income level for poverty called the Federal Poverty Income Guidelines, often informally referred to as the "federal poverty level." The benefit levels of many low-income assistance programs are based on these poverty guidelines.

From *Fed Regist* 78(16):5182-5183, 2013.

HMO growth, this legislation has had a long-term effect on the growth of managed care.

National Health Planning and Resources Act of 1974: The National Health Planning and Resources Act assigned the responsibility for health planning to the states and local health systems agencies. In addition, it required health care facilities to obtain prior approval from the state for expansion in the form of a certificate of need (CON).

Omnibus Budget Reconciliation Acts (1981, 1987, 1989, and 1990): The Omnibus Budget Reconciliation Acts were each enacted in response to the huge federal deficit. They have influenced funding for nursing homes, home health agencies, and hospitals and have set up guidelines and regulations about several issues, including a move from process to outcome evaluation, use of restraints, and prescription drugs for Medicaid recipients.

Tax Equity and Fiscal Responsibility Act of 1982: The Tax Equity and Fiscal Responsibility Act was a major amendment to the Social Security Act of 1935, establishing the prospective payment system (PPS) for Medicare, the diagnosis-related group (DRG) system. This law changed health care radically by introducing a new reimbursement method. See Chapter 12 for more information on DRGs.

Consolidated Omnibus Budget Reconciliation Act of 1985: COBRA is a federal law that affects health care delivery and reimbursement. It requires all hospitals with emergency services that participate in Medicare to treat any client in their emergency services, whether or not that client is covered by Medicare or has the ability to pay. This legislation includes requirements for Medicaid services for prenatal and postnatal care to low-income women in two-parent families in which the primary spouse is unemployed. Another important requirement of COBRA focuses on the problem of the loss of health insurance when a person loses his or her job. With the growing number of unemployed, COBRA is even more important. Employers who terminate an employee must continue benefits for the employee and dependents for a specified period if the employee had health benefits before the termination. COBRA is an example of how a federal law can affect state health care practices. The federal government must determine who receives federal Medicare funds; therefore COBRA provides the opportunity for the federal government to legislate health care delivery at the state level.

Family Support Act of 1988: The Family Support Act expanded coverage for poor women and children and required states to extend Medicaid coverage for 12 months to families who have increased earnings but are no longer receiving cash assistance. This act also required states to expand Aid to Families with Dependent Children (AFDC) coverage to two-parent families in which the principal wage earner is unemployed.

Health Objectives Planning Act of 1990: The Health Objectives Planning Act was initiated in response to the 1979 report *Healthy People: The Surgeon General's Report on Health Promotion and Disease Prevention.* After that report, the federal government began to take a directive approach in identifying and monitoring national health care goals.

Healthy People 2000, Healthy People 2010, and *Healthy People 2020* are also results of this Act.

Health Insurance Portability and Accountability Act of 1996: The Health Insurance Portability and Accountability Act (HIPAA) addressed several issues. The law offered protections for patient privacy and confidentiality. Critical insurance issues were the portability of coverage and limits on the restrictions health plans place on coverage for preexisting conditions. This law established that insurers cannot set limits on coverage of longer than 12 months. This is a complex law, but it has been important for consumers with preexisting conditions. It should be noted that 2010 health care reform legislation has eliminated HIPAA applicability to preexisting conditions, and this change goes into effect in 2014.

Welfare Reform Act of 1996: The Welfare Reform Act placed restrictions on eligibility for AFDC Medicaid, and other federally funded welfare programs. The Welfare Reform law decreased the number of people on welfare and forced many individuals to take low-paying jobs, many of which do not offer health insurance. Between 1994 and March 1999, welfare rolls dropped 47% (DeParle, 1999). Many individuals, particularly underserved women and children, subsequently lost Medicaid coverage. In 2012 this became the Temporary Assistance for Needy Families (TANF).

The State Child Health Improvement Act (SCHIP) of 1997: This has been a critical law, providing insurance for children and families who cannot afford health insurance. This law has been very important to children's health. The law was extended several times and then it was not renewed by the Bush administration. The program was renewed by the Obama administration in the Children's Health Insurance Reauthorization Act of 2009. See Box 10-2 (referred to as CHIP or SCHIP if "state" is included).

Medicare Modernization Act of 2003: The Medicare Modernization Act was the most significant law in 40 years for senior health care. After being implemented in January 2006, the law provided seniors and people living with disabilities with some prescription drug benefit coverage, more choices, and better benefits.

Nurse Reinvestment Act of 2003: The Nurse Reinvestment Act is significant because it is a response to the critical nursing shortage that has been present across the country. Funding is provided to increase enrollments and the number of practicing nurses.

Mental Health Parity and Addictions Equity Act of 2008: A similar act was passed in the 1990s, but it was not an effective law. Improving over the earlier law, this act mandates that if a group health plan includes medical/surgical benefits and mental health benefits and/or substance use disorder benefits, the financial requirements (e.g., deductibles and copayments) and treatment limitations (e.g., number of visits or days of coverage) that apply to mental health benefits must be no more restrictive than the predominant financial requirements or treatment limitations that apply to substantially all medical/surgical benefits.

Patient Protection and Affordable Care Act of 2010: The Patient Protection and Affordable Care Act of 2010, also called the Health Care Reform Act, is an extremely complex and comprehensive piece of legislation. One of the primary intents of the act is to reduce the number of uninsured Americans, and a number of provisions directly address this intent. For example, it requires all U.S. citizens and legal residents to have qualifying health coverage, either provided through employers, individually purchased, or provided by federal plans (i.e., Medicare, Medicaid, CHIP). It also dramatically changes eligibility requirements for Medicaid, allowing coverage of childless adults with incomes up to 133% of the federal poverty line, and expands CHIP. Furthermore, it subsidizes premiums for lower- and middle-income families and requires coverage of dependent adult children up to age 26 for those with group policies (Kaiser Family Foundation, 2010).

The Health Care Reform Act includes significant insurance changes. For example, it (1) establishes high-risk pools to provide health coverage to individuals with preexisting conditions; (2) prohibits insurers from placing lifetime limits on the dollar value of coverage; (3) prohibits insurers from disallowing coverage for some individuals because of preexisting health conditions and dropping policyholders when they get sick; and (4) requires health plans to provide some types of preventive care and screenings without consumer cost-sharing (i.e., copayments or coinsurance). The legislation creates programs to foster nonprofit, member-run health insurance companies that can offer health insurance, to establish state-based health insurance exchanges through which individuals and small businesses can buy coverage, and to permit states to form compacts that will allow insurers to sell policies in any participating state.

There has been considerable confusion and debate on how the act will be implemented and funded. This is an ongoing process because its implementation will not be full for several years. Indeed, most of the provisions were not implemented until 2014, and some will not be implemented for several years beyond that. Funds for government-financed elements (i.e., Medicare, Medicaid, CHIP) will be provided through a combination of new fees and taxes and a variety of cost-saving measures. For example, there will be taxes on indoor tanning and new Medicare taxes for people in high-income brackets. The Act requires fees for pharmaceutical companies and medical devices as well as penalties for individuals who do not obtain health insurance. To cut costs, there will be significant cuts to the Medicare Advantage program and modifications and reductions in Medicare spending. It also enhances efforts to reduce administrative costs, streamline care, and reduce fraud and abuse.

Until passage of the Patient Protection and Affordable Care Act of 2010, the focus of federal legislation has been on either prevention of illness through influencing the environment, such as the Occupational Safety and Health Act of 1970, or provision of funding to support programs that influence health care, as demonstrated in the Social Security Act of 1935. Beginning with the Sheppard-Towner Act of 1921 and continuing to the present, federal grants have increased the involvement of state and local governments in health care. The involvement of the federal government through fiscal allocations to state and local governments provided money for programs not previously available

to states and local areas. Similar services became available in all states. Funds supporting these services were accompanied by regulations that applied to all recipients. Many state and local government programs were developed on the basis of availability of federal funds. The involvement of the federal government through funding has served to standardize public health policy in the United States (Pickett and Hanlon, 1990).

The health reform legislation of 2010 was strongly influenced by the rising numbers of uninsured and underinsured U.S. citizens. Although it is anticipated that about 32 million additional citizens will have insurance, these changes do not mean that the country now has universal health care coverage. The United States continues to be the only major developed country to not have universal health care coverage. As mentioned, it will take a number of years to fully implement the act, and the long-term effects will not be known for at least a decade. Further legal and legislative challenges to some provisions are anticipated.

Role of State Legislatures

State governments are also directly involved in health care policy, legislation, and regulation. State governments focus particularly on financing and delivery of services and oversight of insurance. The latter has become important as managed care has grown. The Institute of Medicine (IOM) (1988) report *Future of Public Health* noted that it is the state's responsibility to see that functions and services necessary to address the mission of public health are in place throughout the state. The IOM framed the public health enterprise in terms of three functions: assessment, policy development, and assurance. The Association of State and Territorial Health Officials (ASTHO) (2009) described the public health services of states and expanded on the three core functions of public health as the basis. The state health care basic public health services should include: (ASTHO, 2009, p. 11):

- Running statewide prevention programs (e.g., tobacco use, newborn screening)
- Budgeting and tracking a basic level of public health services across the state
- Providing specialized professional series (e.g., disease outbreak specialists)
- Analyzing statewide data to target public health threats and diseases
- Investigating outbreaks, environmental hazards and other threats across the state
- Verifying that resources are used effectively and equitably throughout the state
- Licensing and regulating health care, food service and other facilities
- Laboratory services for infectious disease and biological and chemical agents

PUBLIC POLICY: BLUEPRINT FOR GOVERNANCE

Policy is directed by values. It articulates the guiding principles of collective endeavors, establishes direction, and sets goals. It influences and, in turn, is influenced by politics.

Policy directives may become realized or obstructed at any stage in the political process.

Policy Formulation: The Ideal

In ideal circumstances, authorized authoritative bodies (e.g., state health departments, USDHHS, the Centers for Medicare and Medicaid Services [CMS]) rationally determine actions to create, amend, implement, or rescind health care policy. These groups decide what is right, or best, and then develop the political strategies to effect the desired outcomes. Whether a particular policy is advocated or adopted depends on the degree that a group or society as a whole may benefit without harm or detriment to subgroups. Of all the seemingly endless limitless factors that may influence policy formation, group need and group demand should be the strongest determinants. The premises supporting the goals of health policy should be equitable distribution of services and the guarantee that the appropriate care is given to the right people, at the right time, and at a reasonable cost.

Policy Formulation: The Reality

In the real world, policy for health care exemplifies both conflict and social change theories. Health policy is the product of continuous interactive processes in which interested professionals, citizens, institutions, industries, and other interested groups compete with one another for health care dollars and policy initiatives. They also compete with one another for the attention of various branches of government. The most obvious and prominent among these is the legislative branch, although policy is also made through regulatory mechanisms and court decisions. Health policy may also be derived from the recommendations of fact-finding commissions established by the legislative or executive branch or nongovernmental organizations such as the IOM and may also be influenced by judicial decisions.

Health policy is rarely created through discrete, momentous determinations in relation to single problems or issues. It often evolves slowly because changes in the social beliefs and values that underlie established policy develop within the context of actual service delivery. Once a direct health care service is offered, especially an official tax-funded service, discontinuing is often difficult. Existing programs create tradition by establishing vested interest and a sense of entitlement on the part of the public. An example is the annual updating of the childhood and adolescent vaccination schedule recommended by the Centers for Disease Control and Prevention (CDC). This is also an example of cooperation between professional organizations and government agencies to promote the well-being of individuals and communities (Box 10-5).

Steps in Policy Formulation and Analysis

The tangible formulation of public policy begins with the most critical step, which is defining the issue or describing the problem and placing it on the legislative agenda. This process includes cost-benefit analysis. Health policy analysis

BOX 10-5 RECOMMENDED CHILDHOOD AND ADOLESCENT IMMUNIZATION SCHEDULE: UNITED STATES

The Advisory Committee on Immunization Practices (ACIP) annually reviews the recommended childhood and adolescent immunization schedule to ensure that the schedule is current with changes in vaccine formulations and reflects revised recommendations for the use of licensed vaccines, including those newly licensed. It is the only federal government body that provides written recommendations for the routine administration of vaccines for children and adults in the civilian population. Recommendations and format of the childhood and adolescent immunization schedule for January 2009 were approved by ACIP, the American Academy of Family Physicians, and the American

From Centers for Disease Control and Prevention: Recommended immunization schedules for persons 0–18 years—United States, 2009, *MMWR Morb Mortal Wkly Rep* 57(51, 52):Q1-Q3, 2009. Available from <http://www.cdc.gov/vaccines/schedules/hcp/index.html>.

determines those who benefit and those who experience a loss as the result of a policy. These considerations are critical in order to develop health policies that are as fair as possible to all who are affected. Then legislation is finalized, typically developed by legislative staff. The bill then winds its way through the bill process in the legislative body at either the state or federal level. If the bill is passed and is signed by either a governor or the president, it becomes law. The next step is the commitment of resources, most often through the passage of legislation, and the development of regulations, which is done by a governmental agency assigned to ensure implementation of a bill that becomes law. A regulatory schedule for the implementation of the law is formulated. Then, an evaluation process is designed that satisfies regulatory and legislative remedies should they be needed. Analysis of health policy is an objective process that identifies the sources and consequences of policy decisions in the context of the factors that influence them.

A 30-day window of opportunity is typical for public input into the development of regulations. Written comments about a political issue are made part of the public record. To facilitate correspondence, websites have been set up to promote contacting agencies, governmental organizations, and political figures. Nurses need to be aware of some of the important websites. Furthermore, many legislators may have their own web pages so that the nurse can easily access their offices.

The Internet can provide almost unlimited access to information. However, access to information does not ensure its quality or credibility. The user is responsible for evaluation of the information and separation of quality information from misinformation. Nurses need to be information and communication technology literate. *Technology literacy* is the ability of an individual, working independently and with others, to responsibly, appropriately, and effectively use technology tools to access, manage, integrate, evaluate, create, and communicate information. Technology fluency builds upon technology literacy and is demonstrated when nurses apply technology to real-world experiences, adapt to changing technologies, modify current as well as create new technologies, and personalize technology to meet personal needs, interests, and learning style.

THE EFFECTIVE USE OF NURSES: A POLICY ISSUE

The Health Resources and Services Administration (HRSA) provides general resources and information to the public and for use in the development of policy by the government. The nursing workforce development programs administered by the HRSA through Public Health Service Act Title VIII funding provide federal support for nurse workforce development. Title VIII provides the largest source of federal funding for nursing education at the undergraduate and graduate levels and favors institutions that educate nurses for practice in rural and medically underserved communities. These programs provide loans, scholarships, traineeships, and programmatic support for nursing students and also for nurses who are continuing their education in graduate programs.

An issue that is vital to effective health care delivery relates to nurse staffing. The current nursing shortage has been a topic of concern of nurses for many years and is now a health care crisis. This crisis has taken a strange course as a result of the economic crisis in the United States. Many nurses who were due to retire did not; some nurses who were working part-time returned to full-time work; and some nurses who had not been nursing returned to the field. These changes reduced the shortage and have also had a negative impact on new graduates obtaining positions. In addition, in some areas of the country, hospital administrators decided that as there are more new graduates, they could focus on hiring graduates with bachelor's degrees instead of associate degree graduates—who have therefore had more difficulty obtaining jobs. Compounding the problem is the fact that nursing colleges and universities across the nation are struggling to expand enrollment to meet the rising demand for nursing care. A shortage of nursing faculty and changing demographics contribute to the concern that all 50 states will experience a shortage of nurses in the next few years. The Nurse Education, Expansion, and Development Act of 2009 was introduced to amend Title VIII funding to authorize capitation grants for nursing schools to increase the number of faculty and students. The health care reform legislation of 2010 also includes some assistance for nursing education.

NURSES' ROLES IN POLITICAL ACTIVITIES

The Power of One and Many

Registered nurses are the largest health care professional group. One in 44 women voters is a registered nurse. Why are nurses not more politically active? In 1997, Winter and Lockhart found that there are many factors contributing to

---

BOX 10-6   RESPONSES TO POLICY ACTIVISM SURVEY

Positive Influences and the Importance of Mentorship

"I became involved in politics through a relationship with a professor who felt strongly about an issue."

"I have found communication among peers to be informative and often inspiring. That has motivated my involvement in health care issues."

"I became aware of the potential role nurses could play related to policy as an undergrad. I had a few dynamic professors who were very inspiring by their involvement and passion related to various issues. At that point I didn't consider myself as someone to get involved but I think it ignited a spark for 'someday'...."

"My exposure to professors who were actually involved in different 'causes' and not just teaching the course made a huge difference in my perspective on getting involved. The continual role model/mentor is also a huge inspiration."

"...nurses who take an interest in current events and enjoy discussing their opinions regarding public policies."

"I think if you don't get exposed to that 'spark' throughout your career, it goes out. An inspiring speaker at a professional meeting will get me every time!"

"I was inspired by my professor who was past president for New York State Nurses Association."

"It would be great if one of the clinical nurse specialists at my hospital were to ask some nurses in a unit what they thought about something and how we could try to change or fix it. We just need that little nudge and some guidance to kindle that passion."

Negative Experiences Influencing Awareness

"I became more aware of the policies from my institution, from preceptors, and when I had a problem. I was more aware as a novice because I was scared to do something that was going to get me into trouble."

"I became more involved at the institutional level after being 'wronged' by administration in regard to a policy, procedure, or benefit."

"I was usually unaware of a policy until it affected me directly; therefore the need to know became paramount."

---

the political activism of nurses. Factors identified that facilitate political involvement include being raised in a family that was politically active and having positive role models who exemplified the importance of involvement in health policy, social issues, etc. Hindrances to political action included lack of resources, the slow nature of the political process, time constraints, perceived lack of support from peers and society, gender issues, administrative structure, negative experiences, frustration, burnout, and apathy. More effort needs to be given to educate nurses about the importance of being informed on health policy issues and to encourage them to be politically active. Exposure to positive role models is particularly important. Nurses must obtain the tools to overcome factors that impede involvement. Nurses most often identify positive role models as the major influence that assisted them to become politically active in the profession. Therefore, mentorship at the student level up to expert level is important. Box 10-6 describes responses to a survey used by Winter and Lockhart (1997) about what methods were useful in developing awareness in the profession, policy, and politics.

TABLE 10-5	SOURCES FOR LEGISLATIVE INFORMATION	
GOVERNMENT LEVEL	INFORMATION AVAILABLE	LOCATION
Federal	Background of members of Congress	Congressional Directory
	Congressional committee assignments	Government documents section of selected public or
	Congressional terms of service	university libraries
	Congressional news	*Congressional Quarterly Weekly Report*
	House/Senate vote tabulations	U.S representative or senator (may have local office)
	Bills in process or legislated (bill number needed)	
	Health and nursing issues in Congress	*The American Nurse*
		ANA
		600 Maryland Ave SW
		Suite 100
		Washington, DC 20024
		(202) 554-4444
	American Nurses Association Political Action	*The American Nurse*
	Committee (ANA-PAC)	ANA (see above)
	Public health issues in U.S. Congress	*The Nation's Health*
		American Public Health Association (APHA)
		1015 15th St NW
		Washington, DC 20005
		(202) 789-5600
State	Bills in process or legislated (bill number needed)	State representative or senator (may have local office)
	Health and nursing issues in state legislature	State nurses association (SNA) (for location, see April
	State political action committees for nursing	directory issue of the *American Journal of Nursing*)
		National League for Nursing

Nurses as Change Agents

The public, as well as the government, recognizes the nursing profession as indispensable, necessary, and a valuable national resource. In their advocacy role, nurses are seen as professionals whose knowledge, skills, and caring concern are used to promote both the individual's and the community's well-being. Nurses have a unique status in caring for patients; they are interpreters of the health care system to the public, and government-funded programs influence their professional activities. The private business sector is also involved. Therefore, public health nurses must know how to participate in the political process. To do this effectively, they need a sound knowledge of the community, state, and national government organization and function and a clear understanding of how these bodies collectively interact to influence policy. Nurses must know how to influence the creation of health care legislation and how to contribute to the election and appointment of key officials.

Although there are more nurses than physicians, hospital administrators, insurance administrators, or other health care professionals, nursing traditionally has not been seen as a having major political influence because of a lack of public policy consensus within the nursing community. Unity within professional organizations, coalitions, and lobbying efforts is changing this perception. Policy is fundamental to governance; therefore nurses need to know about the formation of public policy and the acts of government and its agencies. Tables 10-5 and 10-6 give sources of information on these issues.

Nurses and Coalitions

When two or more groups join to maximize resources, increasing their influence and improving their chances of success in achieving a common goal, they have formed a coalition.

TABLE 10-6	SOURCES FOR ELECTORAL INFORMATION	
GOVERNMENT LEVEL	INFORMATION AVAILABLE	LOCATION
State	State government operations	Secretary of State (state capitol)
	Political subdivisions	Office of Lieutenant
	Legislative information telephone number	Governor (state capitol)
	State election laws and procedures	
	Campaign finance reports	
County or municipal	Similar to state as appropriate to local government	County clerk (county courthouse)
	Political jurisdictions for each household address	City clerk (city hall)
General	Government information	County clerk (county court-house)
	Political jurisdictions for each household address	City clerk (city hall)
	Names of current office holders in local jurisdictions	

Coalitions of health care providers often work on issues such as family violence and fluoridation of water supplies. An outstanding example of such cooperative action is the establishment of rehabilitation programs for health professionals whose practice has been impaired by substance abuse or mental health problems.

Nursing and consumer groups often form coalitions to advance their shared interests in health promotion. The

ANA joined 16 other organizations (e.g., American College of Nurse Practitioners, American Red Cross, Department of Veterans Affairs, and Sigma Theta Tau) in the 1990s to form a coalition called Nurses for a Healthier Tomorrow. This organization has grown to a membership of 43 organizations. Responding to concerns about a potentially dangerous shortage of nurses, this coalition hopes to raise funds for a national advertising campaign designed to recruit new nurses and encourage existing ones to remain in the profession. The campaign focuses on the message that nurses are essential to the health care team and that they save health care dollars. The campaign shows that an increased demand exists for nurses, both in specialty areas and outside the hospital (NHT, 2013).

Nurses as Lobbyists

A lobbyist is a person who, voluntarily or for a fee, represents himself or herself, another individual, an organization, or an entity before the legislature. A lobbyist typically represents special interest groups. The term derives from the fact that lobbyists usually stay in the areas (lobbies) next to the Senate and House chambers, seeking to speak with legislators and their aides as they walk to and from the chambers, or as lobbyists await legislative action that might affect their interests.

To lobby is to try to influence legislators; it is an art of persuasion. Influencing lawmakers to pass effective health legislation requires the participation of individual nurses and nursing organizations. There are currently more than 100 national nursing organizations. Many also have state chapters. Professional organizations make advocacy easier for members through the use of the Internet. Policy action centers are now part of many organizations' websites. E-mail alerts can be sent instantly to members residing in targeted districts to contact their legislators on a particular bill or issue. By entering one's postal zip code and pushing a button, one can sign a template letter and send it to one's legislator.

The goal of the first contact with an official is to establish that the nurse is a concerned constituent as well as a credible source of information on health issues. The image of nurses caring for people is a definite advantage at this point. Nurses are considered the most ethical of all health care providers and are considered to be trustworthy (Robert Wood Johnson Foundation, 2012). In communities in which nurses have already established strong political credentials, their colleagues will be more readily accepted. An individual who establishes a reputation as a reliable and accurate resource as a lobbyist has substantial influence.

Legislators rely heavily on lobbyists to educate them on issues, and they usually want to hear from all sides before taking a position on an issue. The official must trust the lobbyists to give accurate, though predictably biased information. Information needs to be timely and up-to-date.

Each official represents a constituency with varied needs and interests, and each vote must be weighted within this context. The positions taken by legislators will not always be to an individual or organization's liking. Evaluation of their performance should be based on their overall voting pattern, not just on individual votes. Many organizations

regularly tally and publish the records of each federal legislator on all issues related to nursing and health. This information can be helpful in evaluating elected officials. Collective action by nursing and health care organizations is critical to meeting their goals. Professional associations monitor legislative activity related to relevant health issues and link the process to their membership. This continual surveillance of the legislative environment is critical because even seemingly minor amendments can have profound effects on health issues. Thorough legislative surveillance requires the participation of people who are knowledgeable about nursing, health care, and the political intricacies of the legislative process. Some of the nursing organizations that have fulltime lobbyists who work in Congress are the ANA, the American Academy of Nursing (AAN), and the National League for Nursing. State associations also work with state legislators. State legislative contacts become the eyes, ears, and voices of their professional organizations. These associations can then provide testimony and comment on relevant state and federal issues. However, regardless of the effectiveness of association lobbyists in promoting the interests of nurses and society, they always need grassroots cooperation to truly influence decisions. In the final analysis, a sufficiently high number of communications from individual constituents, via e-mail messages, telephone calls, and letters, has the greatest influence. Lobbying is an ongoing activity for health policy issues influencing nursing and health care delivery. Lobby basics (Box 10-7) provide an overview of the lobbying process.

Nurses and Political Action Committees

Political action committees (PACs) have been important sources of collective political influence since the 1970s. These nonpartisan entities promote the election of candidates believed to be sympathetic to their interests. PACs are established by professional associations, businesses, and labor organizations and are highly regulated by federal and state laws that stipulate how they may contribute financially to campaigns. The advantage of a PAC is that small donations from many members add up to a significant donation to a campaign fund in the name of the organization. This gains the attention of the candidate and earns good will for the group.

Valid concern exists about the correlation of major PAC contributions and legislators' votes on special interest legislation. However, as long as PACs are a reality of political life, nurses need to recognize their power and support those that are committed to electing candidates sympathetic to health care issues. Most national associations of health care providers, including nursing organizations, have PACs. Among the more powerful are those representing hospitals, nursing homes, health insurers, home health agencies, and pharmaceutical companies. A PAC that makes major political contributions is the American Medical Political Action Committee, sponsored by the American Medical Association. State medical associations also have strong PACs. This means that organized medicine has a powerful influence on national and state elections and on health care legislation at both levels.

BOX 10-7   ABCs OF LOBBYING ON A STATE LEVEL

Before the Meeting

- Appointments will have been made with your legislator(s) for the Lobby Day. Tell the staff that you are a constituent and what issue(s) you would like to discuss with your representative. If your legislator is unavailable, you may have a scheduled appointment with a member of the legislative staff.
- If possible, put together a delegation of nurses to attend the meeting. A number of individuals from the legislator's district who are concerned about the same issue will make a big impression. Take along students from their districts, because legislators are impressed with their participation.

Preparing for the Meeting

- Establish your agenda and goals. For example, focus on educating the legislators on the profession of nurse midwifery, the legislation that this group would like them to sponsor, the concerns about the malpractice insurance crisis, and the benefit to women's and children's health. Nurse practitioners would focus on the cost-benefit of NPs as primary care providers in all settings, including health care homes.
- Research your legislator's stance prior to the meeting. It is important that you know your official's position so that you can present your stance more effectively and can have an intelligent discussion.
- Meet with the delegation (e.g. midwives, NPs) that will participate in the lobbying. It is important that you review what each person will say during the meeting. Select someone as the group leader, and make a list of points to be made and questions to be asked by each person.

- Prepare materials. Review the packet of information you will leave with your legislator. It is important to include your name and phone number in the packet so that your legislator will have a contact person for more information. Leaving a business card would be appropriate.

During the Meeting

- Be on time for your meeting.
- Be concise and diplomatic. Keep your presentation short and to the point.
- Be a good listener. Look for indications of your legislator's views, and watch for opportunities to provide useful information in order to strengthen or counter particular views.
- Stress why the issues concern you and others in your district.
- Don't be intimidated. Your legislator is in office to serve you. It is important to have a general knowledge of the issues, but you don't have to know every little detail. If he/she asks a question that you do not know the answer to, simply say that you do not know but are willing to find out. Find out the best way to get the information to him/her (fax, e-mail, or a follow-up phone call).

After the Meeting

- Write a follow-up letter. After your visit, write a letter thanking your legislator for his/her time.
- Stay in contact with your legislator. Remember: your goal is to strengthen Advance Practice Nurse relationships with your legislators.

Modified from New York State Association of Licensed Midwives (NYSALM): *The Voice of Midwives* letter.

Nurses and Campaigning

Helping someone win an election is a sure way of gaining influence. All candidates are grateful for campaign assistance and usually remember to thank those who have helped. Although campaign contributions are commonly thought of as financial, they can also take the form of participation in campaign activities. Nurses are frequently unable to contribute much money, but they can provide these invaluable services. For the novice, veteran campaigners are eager to help develop the necessary skills. Initially, a volunteer can address or stuff envelopes for mailings. The volunteer can also invite friends and neighbors for a social gathering to meet the candidate, thereby providing an opportunity to discuss issues of concern with constituents. Telephone banks help a candidate identify supporters, opponents, and the critical undecided voters. This last group can make a difference on election day and is courted by all candidates. The telephone interviews are highly structured and easily handled by inexperienced campaign workers. Direct contact with potential voters may occur later in the form of house-to-house block walks or poll work on election day. The confidence that this process requires comes with experience and a strong commitment to the candidate and the cause. Hosting a social function to allow nurse colleagues to meet the candidate is a welcome contribution to the campaign. Nurses are substantial in number, and their voting record is humanistic; therefore, they are valued as a political force. Government employees may be

restricted by policies that limit or disallow political activism. Nurses employed at any level of government should be aware of such prohibitions.

Nurses and Voting Strength

With around 3 million members, nurses make up the largest profession in health care (ANA, 2009; HRSA, 2010). Therefore, if every registered nurse voted, the influence of registered nurses on health policy would be tremendous. If the nursing profession is to meet the challenges of the twenty-first century and work as a profession to positively influence the health of populations, political action is necessary, and an understanding of the factors that motivate or impede political action is needed (Winter and Lockhart, 1997).

Nurses in Public Office

President Barack Obama named Mary Wakefield, PhD, RN, administrator of the HRSA on February 20, 2009. HRSA is an agency of the USDHHS. HRSA works to fill in the health care gaps for people who live outside the economic and medical mainstream. The agency uses its $7 billion annual budget (fiscal year [FY] 2008) to expand access to quality health care in partnership with health care providers and health professions training programs. Dr. Wakefield has served on the Medicare Payment Advisory Commission, as chair of the National Advisory Council for the Agency for Healthcare Research and Quality, as a member of President Clinton's Advisory Commission on Consumer Protection and Quality in the Health Care Industry, and as a member of the National Advisory Committee to HRSA's Office of Rural Health Policy (HRSA, 2010). Obama's announcement included the following comments about Mary Wakefield: "As a nurse, a PhD, and a leading rural health care advocate, Mary Wakefield brings expertise that will be instrumental in expanding and improving services for those who are currently uninsured or underserved. Under her leadership, we will be able to expand and improve the care provided at the community health centers, which serve millions of uninsured Americans and address severe provider shortages across the country" (HRSA, 2010).

Other women who have been active in the federal government are Carolyn Davis, who in 2001 served as the administrator of the Health Care Financing Administration (renamed the Centers for Medicare and Medicaid Services); Shirley Chater, Commissioner of the Social Service Administration; and Patricia Montoya, Commissioner for Children, Youth, and Families. Virginia Trotter Betts, who served as the President of the ANA, was also the Senior Advisor on Nursing and Policy to the Secretary of HHS in Washington, DC.

Likewise, Dr. Beverly Malone resigned as President of the ANA in 1999 to assume the position of Deputy Assistant Secretary of the HHS. In this capacity, she advised the Assistant Secretary for the HHS, Dr. David Satcher, in program and political matters, policy and program development, and setting of legislative priorities. Lastly, Janet Heinrich is Associate Administrator of the HRSA's Bureau of Health Professionals, and Michele Richardson is the senior advisor for national workforce diversity in the Bureau of Health Professions (NLN, 2010).

In the 112th Congress, the number of nurses increased by four, reaching a total of seven. This is a major achievement for nursing. It provides direct voice for nursing concerns and also nursing expertise related health care in general. The Congressional Nursing Caucus provides a nonpartisan forum for the discussion of issues that impact the nursing profession. It also allows members of Congress, nurses and non-nurse members, who care about these issues to come together to address them.

In the future, more nurses need to run for public office at all three levels of government. Whether serving as political appointees or career bureaucrats, nurses have much to offer. New nurses should accept the challenge of helping advance the nursing practice and the nation's health.

HEALTH CARE REFORM AND RESTRUCTURING OF THE HEALTH CARE INDUSTRY

Health care reform was a major topic of discussion during the 2008 presidential election. With the election of President Obama and significant Democratic majorities in both the Senate and the House, it appeared that health care reform would pass easily. After the failed attempt at comprehensive reform during the early years of the Clinton presidency, politicians recognized some of the major concerns and issues and addressed them proactively. For example, strong opposition from many health care provider groups (e.g., physicians) and the health care industry groups (e.g., insurers, pharmaceutical

companies, hospitals) led to failure of the Clinton plan. In 2009, Congressional leaders early on sought ways to attract leaders of these groups and persuade them to support reform measures, although passage of health care reform was not easy and there continues to be variable support for the initiatives in the legislation.

A great deal of debate on what should be included in reform was evident throughout 2009. Major items of contention included whether to require all Americans to purchase coverage (i.e., a health insurance mandate), whether there would be a "government option" whereby people could elect to be covered by an extension of Medicare (or another, similar program sponsored and funded by the government), whether government funds would pay for abortions, and how all of the changes and mandates would eventually be financed. After much public and private debate, in March 2010, the House of Representatives rather reluctantly passed the bill that the Senate had approved in late 2009, and President Obama signed it into law on March 23, 2010.

Although the 2010 Patient Protection and Affordable Care Act is extremely controversial, and the long-term effects of its implementation are unclear, health care reform is a nursing issue, and few nurses will argue with the statement that reform is needed in the health system in the United States. In virtually every practice arena, nurses see the inequalities and inadequacies that diminish the nation's level of wellness. Recognition of these problems is important to discussions of reform, and changing policies and targeting popular beliefs that create barriers to reform are essential in correcting the inequalities and inadequacies.

These are some of the areas targeted by the Health Care Reform Act. For example, insurers will no longer be able to drop coverage for those who are seriously ill because the act prohibits health insurance plans for placing lifetime limits on coverage and prohibits insurers from rescinding coverage for those who are diagnosed with chronic or life-threatening conditions. Additionally, mechanisms to reduce administrative costs are encouraged (Kaiser Family Foundation, 2010).

Popular sentiments about governmental control over health care have mirrored attitudes concerning the government's role in general; this was very evident during the debates over reform. The politically viable range of cost-control measures available to public programs has been limited to cutbacks in payments to providers rather than limits on the demand for clinical services or limits on individual choice.

In addition to overall health care reform, one of the issues that is vital to effective health care delivery relates to nurse staffing. Staffing has been a topic of concern of nurses for many years because inadequate and inappropriate staffing can threaten patients' safety as well as the nurses' health and commitment to the profession. Inappropriate staffing also contributes to pressure experienced by nurses because of increasing patient care intensity, growing complexity of care, and fatigue. The Registered Nurse Safe Staffing Act of 2013 (H.R. 1821) was introduced in Congress to address these concerns, and this is not the first time legislation related to staffing has been introduced. According to the Congress-monitoring website GovTrack (n.d.), the chance that the bill will pass both the

THE REGISTERED NURSE SAFE STAFFING ACT OF 2013 (H.R. 1821)

The American Nurses Association (ANA) applauds the introduction of federal legislation that empowers registered nurses (RNs) to drive staffing decisions in hospitals and, consequently, protect patients and improve the quality of care.

The Registered Nurse Safe Staffing Act of 2013 (H.R. 1821), crafted with input from ANA, has sponsors from both political parties who co-chair the House Nursing Caucus, namely Rep. David Joyce (R-OH) and Rep. Lois Capps (D-CA), who is a nurse.

If passed, the legislation would require hospitals to establish committees that would create unit-by-unit nurse staffing plans based on multiple factors, such as the number of patients on the unit, severity of the patients' conditions, experience and skill level of the RNs, availability of support staff, and technological resources.

The safe staffing bill also would require hospitals that participate in Medicare to publicly report nurse staffing plans for each unit. It would place limits on the practice of "floating" nurses by ensuring that RNs are not forced to work on units if they lack the education and experience in that specialty.

Additionally, it would hold hospitals accountable for safe nurse staffing by requiring the development of procedures for receiving and investigating complaints; allowing imposition of civil monetary penalties for knowing violations; and providing whistle-blower protections for those who file a complaint about staffing.

From Advance Healthcare Network for Nurses: *ANA lauds introduction of Registered Nurse Safe Staffing Act in Congress,* May 9, 2013. Available from <http://nursing.advanceweb.com/News/National-News/ANA-Lauds-Introduction-of-Registered-Nurse-Safe-Staffing-Act-in-Congress.aspx>.

RESEARCH HIGHLIGHTS

National Sample of Registered Nurses

The Division of Nursing, a component of the Health Resources and Services Administration (HRSA), helps direct policy through the National Sample Survey of Registered Nurses. Conducted nine times since 1977, this survey was done most recently in March 2008, and preliminary findings were released in 2010. The national survey looks at trends in demographics, employment, education, and compensation among registered nurses (RNs). Here are some of the findings:
- Number of licensed RNs in the United States grew by almost 5.3% between 2004 and 2008, to a new high of slightly more than 3 million.
- Average age of RNs climbed to 47.0 years, the highest average age since the first comparable report was published in 1980.
- Average annual earning for RNs was $66,973.
- Real earnings (comparable dollars over time) have grown almost 16% since 2004.
- The share of RNs whose initial nursing education was a bachelor's degree in nursing rose from 31% to 33.7% between 2004 and 2008.
- Employment in nursing rose to almost 85% of RNs with active licenses, the highest since 1980.
- The number of RNs with master's or doctorate degrees rose to more than 400,000, an increase of 32% from 2000.

Data from Health Resources and Services Administration: *The registered nurse population: initial findings from the 2008 national sample survey of registered nurses,* Washington, DC, 2010, Author.

House of Representatives and the Senate is zero. However, the fact that nursing keeps trying to get national legislation on this critical topic is very important. See Box 10-8 for highlights of the Bill.

At the same time the United States is implementing health care reform, the country is also coping with the health problems of today's military veterans. When these soldiers are discharged, they continue to require care, often for complex physical and mental issues. According to the Kaiser Family Foundation (2012):

> Given the growing need for providing health care and related benefits to the nation's service members, policymakers will continue to focus on strengthening both the Department of Defense [DoD] Military Health System and the Department of Veterans Affairs (VA) health care system, which operate in parallel and in conjunction with each other. There is also greater emphasis in policy circles on ensuring a "seamless transition" process for service members moving from active duty into the VA health care system. Areas of focused attention include coordination between health and other benefits offered by the DoD and the VA, improving care for injured service members, and easing the transition from combat service to other military or civilian life.

Nurses encounter veterans in all types of community and public health settings. Knowledge about these problems and health policies changes is important to providing effective care in the community.

NURSES AND LEADERSHIP IN HEALTH POLICY DEVELOPMENT

As the role of nurses in changing health care policy increases in importance, more nurses are needed who are equipped for this challenge. A strong cadre of nursing leaders who have the vision for change is essential to promoting nursing's policy agenda. National fellowships and internships are available for nurses who are interested in taking leadership roles (Sharp, 1999).

The Robert Wood Johnson Health Policy Fellowship is a 1-year career development program for midcareer health professionals. The goal of this program is to help its fellows gain an understanding of the health policy process and contribute to the formulation of new policies and programs. Robert Wood Johnson Health Policy fellows are selected from academic faculties from diverse disciplines, including medicine, dentistry, nursing, public health, health services administration, economics, and social services. After an extensive orientation on the legislative and executive branches of government, the fellows work with a member of Congress or on a congressional health committee (Sharp, 1999).

The President's Commission on White House Fellowships offers 20 fellowships each year to professionals including nurses early in their careers; the average age is 33 years. The White House fellows participate in an education program that involves working with government officials, scholars, journalists, and private-sector leaders to explore U.S. policy in action. Nurses who have been White House fellows may work at the Centers for Medicare and Medicaid Services and the Office of Science and Technology Policy, among others (Sharp, 1999). These fellowship programs are competitive, but strong leaders are desperately needed.

Nursing should also incorporate private health policy into its policy agenda. Nurses can influence private health care organizations from internal and external positions. From an internal perspective, nurses hold important management positions in health care organizations. This placement allows them to have direct involvement in policy setting. Nurses also support and use nursing research that demonstrates positive clinical and economic outcomes. All of these activities serve to validate the importance of nursing within the health system (Pulcini et al., 2000).

External strategies that nurses can use to influence private health policy include participation in discussions regarding quality care and cost of care (Pulcini et al., 2000). Nurses should monitor the quality ratings of health care organizations and suggest changes that would improve care. Nurses also are developing entrepreneurial practices to provide lower-cost services for underserved groups. Nurses need to do more to request that nursing services be reimbursable under all types of health care coverage plans and programs. Interprofessional care is a key topic today, and nurses need to work with other health care providers to build teams that can influence private policy.

SUMMARY

Historically, nurses have been able to make significant differences in the quality of life experienced by the members of the communities in which they serve. By understanding how government works, how bills become laws, and how legislators make decisions, nurses can influence policy decisions through individual efforts such as electronic letter writing, social networking, participation in political campaigns, and selection of candidates who support policies conducive to improving the health and welfare of all citizens. When organized in lobbying groups, coalitions, and PACs, or when holding office, nurses can be a powerful force that brings about change in the delivery and quality of the health care of aggregates.

LEARNING ACTIVITIES

1. Look at a current public health issue that affects your community, including an understanding of the causes, effect on the public, and possible solutions. Influence its resolution through any of the following activities:
   a. Write a succinct letter to the editor of a local newspaper.
   b. Write a position paper and submit it to the "opinion page" of a local newspaper.
   c. Write to elected or appointed officials whose jurisdiction may be influential on the issue.
   d. Meet with an elected or appointed official to discuss the issue in groups of two or three. Write a one-page summary of your "talking points" to leave with the official.
   e. Call in to a radio talk show about the issue.
   f. Volunteer to speak on the issue to appropriate consumer or professional groups.
2. With a group of two or three, meet with an elected official for a 15-minute appointment to ask about the official's concerns and priorities. Remember to refer to the "ABCs of Lobbying" prior to meeting with the official.
3. Invite an elected official who is sympathetic to nurses to speak to the local chapter of the National Student Nurses Association to discuss the political process and health policy.
4. Invite an elected official to spend a day engaging in appropriate activities with a public health nurse or nursing student. Take black-and-white photos for press use.
5. Participate in a group organized around a public health issue (e.g., disposable diapers, toxic waste, or fluoride).
6. Serve as a volunteer in a campaign for a candidate who is supportive or potentially supportive of public health or nursing issues, or volunteer for a political party.
7. Review your state's legislative agenda. Identify bills that relate to health care, and from those bills, identify any bills that might affect community or public health. Discuss the bills in small groups—their impact in general and how nursing might be involved.
8. Visit the American Nurses Association website and explore its political action section, at http://nursingworld.org/Main MenuCategories/Policy-Advocacy. What type of information is available?
9. Visit the American Public Health Association website for information about policy outcome evaluation, at http://www.apha.org/programs/cba/CBA/resources/Policy+Evaluation.htm. Review the various evaluation programs to gain an understanding of policy outcome evaluation.

ⓔ EVOLVE WEBSITE

http://evolve.elsevier.com/Nies

- NCLEX Review Questions
- Case Studies
- Glossary

REFERENCES

Almgren G: *Health care, politics, policy and services*, New York, 2007, Springer.

American Nurses Association: ANA advises on health care reform, *Capital Update* 11(8):1, 1993.

American Nurses Association (ANA): . Accessed March 1, 2010 www.nursingworld.org/Function/ menucategory/aboutANA.aspx, 2009.

Association of State and Territorial Health Officials: *Public health: an essential component of health reform*, 2009. http://www.astho.org/Programs/Health-Reform/State-Public-Health-and-Health-Reform-Packet/.

Centers for Disease Control and Prevention: *State of the CDC: fiscal year*, 2008. Available from <www.cdc.gov/about/stateofcdc/FY08/cd/SOCDC/SOCDC2008.pdf>.

DeParle J: States struggle to use windfall born of shifts in welfare law, *New York Times*, August 29, 1999.

de Vries C, Vanderbilt M: Nurses gain ground during reform debate, *Am Nurse* 26(10):2–3, 1994.

GovTrack: H.R. 1821: Registered Nurse Safe Staffing Act of 2013, n.d. Available from <http://www.govtrack.us/congress/bills/113/hr1821>. Accessed August 30, 2013.

Hadley EH: Nursing in the political and economic marketplace: challenges for the 21st century, *Nurs Outlook* 44(1):6–10, 1996.

Hall-Long BA: Nursing's past, present, and future political experiences, *Nurs Health Care Perspect* 16(1):24–28, 1995.

Health Resources and Services Administration: *The registered nurse population: initial findings from the national 2008 sample survey of registered nurses*, Washington, DC, 2010, Author.

Henry J, Kaiser Family Foundation: *Military and veterans' health care*, 2012. http://www.kaiseredu.org/Issue-Modules/Military-and-Veterans-Health-Care/Background-Brief.aspx.

Institute of Medicine: *Biographical information: 2001 Lienhard Award Recipient Ruth Watson Lubic*, 2001. Available from <www.iom.edu/subpage.asp?id=5046>.

Institute of Medicine: *Future of public health*, Washington, D.C, 1998, The National Academies Press.

Kaiser Family Foundation: *Focus on health reform*, 2010. Available from <www.kff.org/healthreform /upload /8061.pdf 2010b>.

Kaiser Family Foundation: *The uninsured: a primer*, 2012. Available from <http://www.kff.org/uninsured/7451.cfm>.

Kaiser Family Foundation: *Total employed nurses in 2011*, 2011. Available from <http://statehealthfacts.org/comparemaptable.jsp?ind=438&cat=8>.

Kalisch PA, Kalisch BJ: *American nursing: a history*, ed 4, Philadelphia, 2004, Lippincott Williams & Wilkins.

Knight W: *Managed care: what it is and how it works*, Gaithersburg, MD, 1998, Aspen Publishers, Inc.

Lewinson SB: A historical perspective on policy, politics and nursing. In Mason DJ, Leavitt JK, Chaffee MW, editors: *Policy and politics in nursing and health care*, ed 5, Philadelphia, 2007, Saunders.

Litman T: *Health, politics and policy*, ed 3, Albany, NY, 1997, Delmar.

Lyttle B: Humanizing childbirth, *Am J Nurs* 100(10):52–53, 2000.

Mason DJ, Leavitt JK, Chaffee MW: *Policy and politics: a framework for action. Policy and politics in nursing and health care*, ed 5, St. Louis, 2007, Saunders.

Merriam-Webster: *Merriam-Webster Dictionary*, 2014. Retrieved from http://www.merriam-webster.com/dictionary/policy.

National League for Nursing http://www.nln.org/newsletter/aug092010.htm

Nurses for a Healthier Tomorrow: Mission/purpose, 2013. http://www.nursesource.org/mission.html.

Pickett G, Hanlon JJ: *Public health administration and practice*, ed 9, St. Louis, 1990, Mosby.

Pulcini J, Mason DJ, Cohen SS, et al: Health policy and the private sector: new vistas for nursing, *Nurs Health Care Perspect* 21(1):22–28, 2000.

Robert Wood Johnson: *Enduring trust: nurses again top Gallup's poll on honesty and ethics*, 2012. Retrieved from http://www.rwjf.org/en/blogs/human-capital-blog/2012/12/enduring_trust_nurs.html.

Sharp N: Wanted: nurse leaders to craft health policy, *Nurse Pract* 24(10):85–86, 1999.

Thomas J: Introduction, *Library Trends* 46(2), 1997.

U.S. Department of Health and Human Services: *Healthy People 2010*, Conference ed. Washington, DC, 2000, Author.

U.S. Department of Health and Human Services: *Centers for Medicare and Medicaid Services: FY 2005 budget in brief*, 2004. Available from <www.dhhs.gov/budget/05budget/centersformed.html#med>.

U.S. Department of Health and Human Services: Office of Disease Prevention and Health Promotion, *Healthy People 2020*, 2013. Accessed January 22, 2014 at http://www.healthypeople.gov/2020/about/history.aspx.

U.S. Department of Health and Human Services, Health Resources and Services Administration: Accessed March 1, 2010.

U.S. Department of Health and Human Services: *Secretary's Advisory Committee on National Health Promotion and Disease Prevention for 2020: Healthy People 2020, phase I report*, 2009. Available from <www. healthypeople.gov/HP2020/advisory/PhaseI/PhaseI.pdf>.

Winter MK, Lockhart JS: From motivation to action: understanding nurses' political involvement, *Nurs Health Care Perspect* 18(5):244–250, 1997.

Upon completion of this chapter, the reader will be able to do the following:

1. Describe the organization of the public health care subsystem at the federal, state, and local levels.
2. Compare and contrast the scopes of the private health care subsystem and the public health care subsystem.
3. Describe the roles of the members of the interprofessional health care team.
4. Examine the impact of the Institute of Medicine reports on quality care in the health care delivery system.
5. Discuss the relationship of critical health care issues to the health care organization and health care providers.
6. Discuss future concerns for the health care delivery system.

accreditation
alternative therapies
client rights
community health center
health care reform

managed care
managed care organizations
Medicaid
Medicare
outcomes measures

public health
quality care
telehealth

Overview: The Health Care System
Components of the Health Care System
    Private Health Care Subsystem
    Public Health Subsystem
    Health Care Providers
Quality Care
    The Institute of Medicine Reports Examine Quality
    Accreditation
    Current Status of Health Care Quality

Critical Issues in Health Care Delivery
    Managed Care
    Information Technology
    Consumerism, Advocacy, and Client Rights
    Coordination and Access to Health Care
    Disparity in Health Care Delivery
    Globalization and International Health
    Health Care Reform: Impact on the Health Care System
Future of Public Health and the Health Care System

OVERVIEW: THE HEALTH CARE SYSTEM

The health care system of the United States is dynamic, multifaceted, and not comparable with any other health care system in the world. It is regularly praised for its technological breakthroughs, frequently criticized for its high costs, continues to experience major problems with its quality, and often is difficult for those most in need to access. This chapter describes landmark health care legislation, the components of the health care system, critical health care organization (HCO) and provider issues, and the role of government in public health and health care reform, and presents a futuristic perspective.

COMPONENTS OF THE HEALTH CARE SYSTEM

The current health care system consists of private and public health care subsystems (Figure 11-1). The private health care subsystem includes personal care services from various sources, both nonprofit and profit, and numerous voluntary agencies. The major focus of the public health subsystem is prevention of disease and illness. These subsystems are not always mutually exclusive, and their functions sometimes overlap.

With the rapid growth of technology and increased demands on the private and public health care subsystems, health care costs have become prohibitive. Cost-effectiveness and cost containment have become critical driving forces as health care delivery system changes are made; however, cost-effectiveness often conflicts with the provision of quality care. The Institute of Medicine (IOM) report *Best Care at Lower Costs: The Path to Continuously Learning Health Care in America* "presents a vision of what is possible if the nation applies the resources and tools at hand by marshaling science, information technology, incentives, and care culture to transform the effectiveness and efficiency of care—to produce high-quality health care that continuously learns to be better" (IOM, 2012a, p. ix). Since 1999, the IOM has completed many extensive reports examining the status of health care in the United States. Some improvement has been seen in the delivery system, but much more needs to be done. This report addresses these critical concerns again.

Community health nursing requires an understanding of the mission, organization, and role of the private and the public health care subsystems and the contexts within which they function to effectively collaborate with health care organizations to reach community health goals. An organizational framework in which private and voluntary organizations and the government work collaboratively to prevent disease and promote health is essential. Public health and community health nurses are in a unique position to provide leadership and facilitate change in the health care system.

Private Health Care Subsystem

Most personal health care services are provided in the private sector. Services in the private subsystem include health promotion, prevention and early detection of disease, diagnosis and treatment of disease with a focus on cure, rehabilitative-restorative care, and custodial care. These services are provided in clinics, physicians' offices, hospitals, hospital ambulatory centers, skilled care facilities, and homes. Increasingly, these private sector services are available through managed care organizations (MCOs).

Private health care services in the United States began with a simple model. Physicians provided care in their offices and made home visits. Patients were admitted to hospitals for general care if they experienced serious complications during the course of their illness. Currently, a variety of highly skilled health care professionals provide comprehensive, preventive, restorative, rehabilitative, and palliative care. Interprofessional teams have become more important. A broad array of services is available, ranging from general to highly specialized with multiple delivery configurations.

Personal care provided by physicians is delivered under the following five basic models:

1. The solo practice of a physician in an office continues to be present in some communities.
2. The single specialty group model consists of physicians in the same specialty, who pool expenses, income, and offices.
3. Multispecialty group practice provides for interaction among specialty areas.
4. The integrated health maintenance model has prepaid multispecialty physicians.
5. The community health center, developed through federal funds in the 1960s, addresses broader inputs into health such as education and housing.

Managed care has become the dominant paradigm in health care, affecting many aspects of health care delivery. Managed care involves capitated payments for care rather than fee-for-service. Health care providers, including physicians, hospitals, community clinics, and home care providers, are integrated in a system such as a health maintenance organization (HMO). See Chapter 12 for a more detailed discussion of managed care and reimbursement.

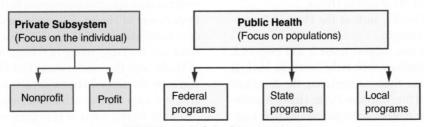

FIGURE 11-1 U.S. health care system.

Though change in the configuration of the health care system is common, some of the newer changes relate more to the community than in the past. For example, more physician practices are joining together to form multispecialty groups, and hospitals are buying practices to expand their market into the community. The solo practice is fading. In addition, there are more advanced nurse practitioners (ANPs) who are assuming primary practice roles in a variety of settings, including community clinics, retail health clinics, and home health, and some who are opening their own practices. Patient-centered medical homes are practices that offer a team approach to care to assist in coordination of care for positive outcomes, providing comprehensive primary care. This model, which is connected to health care reform, is new, and thus its success is unknown. As health care reform legislation is implemented, additional changes will occur.

Voluntary Agencies

Voluntary or nonofficial agencies are a part of the private health care system of the United States and developed at the same time that the government was assuming responsibility for public health. In the United States during the 1700s and early 1800s, voluntary efforts to improve health were virtually nonexistent because early settlers from Western Europe were not accustomed to participating in organized charity. Immigration expanded to include slaves from Africa and people from Eastern Europe, and their well-being received little attention.

Toward the end of the nineteenth century, new immigrants brought a heritage of social protest and reform. Wealthy businesspeople, such as the Rockefellers, Carnegies, and Mellons, responded to the needs and set up foundations that provided health and welfare money for charitable endeavors. District nurses, such as Lillian Wald, established nursing practices in the large cities for the poor and destitute. Services focused not just on illness but also on work conditions, health, communicable diseases, living conditions, and language skills. Even today we see initiatives from philanthropic organizations such as the Gates Foundation, which is very active in health care concerns, particularly from a global perspective.

Voluntary agencies can be classified into those dealing with the following categories of health (Hanlon and Pickett, 1990):

- Specific diseases, such as the American Diabetes Association, American Cancer Society, and National Multiple Sclerosis Society
- Organ or body structures, such as the National Kidney Foundation and the American Heart Association
- Health and welfare of special groups, such as the National Council on Aging and the March of Dimes
- Particular phases of health, such as the Planned Parenthood Federation of America

Philanthropic groups also support research and programs. Many professional organizations, such as the American Medical Association, the American Nurses Association, the American Hospital Association, and the American Public Health Association, as well as many other professional organizations, have a significant role in advocacy and in providing professional expertise.

Voluntary organizations are major sources of help in prevention of disease, promotion of health, treatment of illness, advocacy, consumer education, and research. For example, private and voluntary organizations currently support clients with acquired immunodeficiency syndrome (AIDS). In many cities, the Chicken Soup Brigade provides meals for clients with AIDS who are unable to cook for themselves, and AIDS support groups exist in most larger communities. Services for the homeless such as meals, temporary housing and housing during the winter, medical care, and job support are common in most large cities. Overlap of services often occurs among the numerous private, voluntary, and public agencies. The private and public agencies provide a wide array of services, but sometimes duplication causes them not to be cost-effective. Without voluntary and official agencies, the array of services would be less than what is currently available.

The future is somewhat uncertain for voluntary agencies because major changes are occurring in health care. In the mid-1990s, the Pew Health Professions Commission projected that the emerging health care system would be an amalgam of different public and private forces that would work together to provide integrated, resource-conscious, population-based services (O'Neil and Pew Health Professions Commission, 1998). It was projected that the system would also be more innovative and diverse in how it responded to health needs and more concerned with disease prevention and promotion of health. The Pew Health Professions Commission's projection has not yet been fully realized. As noted by the Agency for Healthcare Research and Quality, the annual National Healthcare Disparities Report, the country continues to have very significant disparities in health care (AHRQ, 2013).

Public Health Subsystem

The U.S. Constitution mandates that the federal government "promote the general welfare of its citizens." The public health subsystem is required by law to address the health of populations. Legal provisions at the local, state, and federal levels of government direct the establishment, implementation, and evaluation of these activities. At the federal level, Congress enacts laws and writes rules and regulations. The various departments of the executive branch implement and administer them. Interpretations of, and amendments to, the Constitution and Supreme Court decisions over time have changed and enlarged the role of the federal government in health activities.

Federal policies and practices have had an increasing influence on local and state governments in meeting health and social problems, and many laws have been enacted to respond to changing health needs. Coordination of federal services under several agencies culminated in the establishment of the Department of Health, Education, and Welfare under President Eisenhower in 1953. In 1979, this department was separated into the Department of Education and the Department of Health and Human Services (USDHHS). The USDHHS is currently the second largest department of the federal government; only the Department of Defense is larger

Public health refers to the efforts organized by society to protect, promote, and restore the people's health. Public health

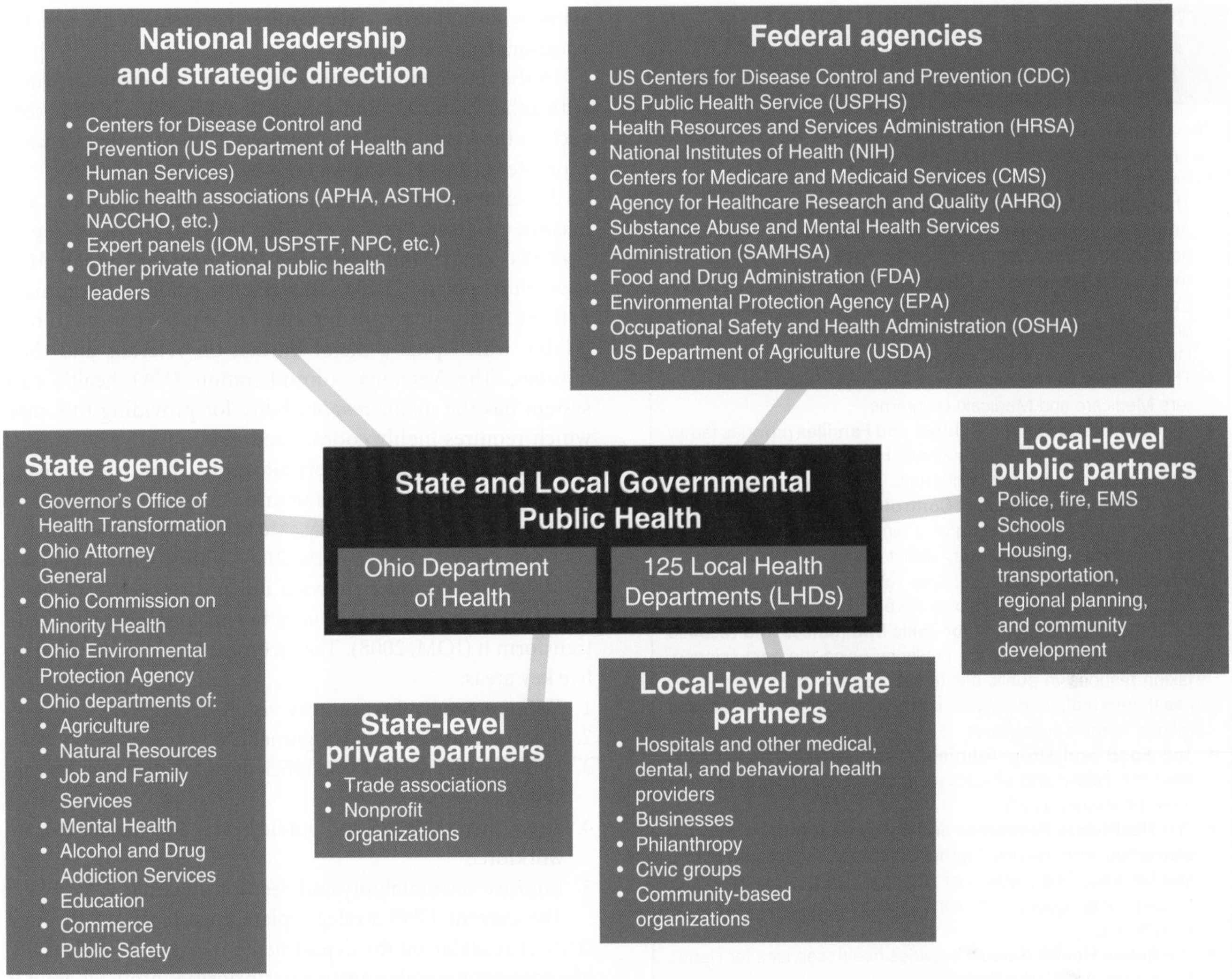

National leadership and strategic direction

- Centers for Disease Control and Prevention (US Department of Health and Human Services)
- Public health associations (APHA, ASTHO, NACCHO, etc.)
- Expert panels (IOM, USPSTF, NPC, etc.)
- Other private national public health leaders

Federal agencies

- US Centers for Disease Control and Prevention (CDC)
- US Public Health Service (USPHS)
- Health Resources and Services Administration (HRSA)
- National Institutes of Health (NIH)
- Centers for Medicare and Medicaid Services (CMS)
- Agency for Healthcare Research and Quality (AHRQ)
- Substance Abuse and Mental Health Services Administration (SAMHSA)
- Food and Drug Administration (FDA)
- Environmental Protection Agency (EPA)
- Occupational Safety and Health Administration (OSHA)
- US Department of Agriculture (USDA)

State agencies

- Governor's Office of Health Transformation
- Ohio Attorney General
- Ohio Commission on Minority Health
- Ohio Environmental Protection Agency
- Ohio departments of:
  - Agriculture
  - Natural Resources
  - Job and Family Services
  - Mental Health
  - Alcohol and Drug Addiction Services
  - Education
  - Commerce
  - Public Safety

State and Local Governmental Public Health

| Ohio Department of Health | 125 Local Health Departments (LHDs) |

Local-level public partners

- Police, fire, EMS
- Schools
- Housing, transportation, regional planning, and community development

State-level private partners

- Trade associations
- Nonprofit organizations

Local-level private partners

- Hospitals and other medical, dental, and behavioral health providers
- Businesses
- Philanthropy
- Civic groups
- Community-based organizations

FIGURE 11-2 The public health system in Ohio. (From Health Policy Institute of Ohio: *Ohio public health basics*, 2012, p. 4. Retrieved from <http://www.hpio.net>.)

programs, services, and institutions emphasize the prevention of disease and address the health needs of the population as a whole. Public health activities typically respond to changing technology and social values, but the goals remain the same (i.e., to reduce the amount of disease, premature death, and disease-produced discomfort and disability).

The public health subsystem is concerned with the health of the population and a healthy environment. The scope of public health is broad and encompasses activities that promote good health. The public health subsystem is organized into multiple levels (i.e., federal, state, and local) to more effectively provide services to those who are unable to obtain health care without assistance and to establish laws, rules, and regulations to protect the public. Figure 11-2 provides an overview of this system, specifically for the state of Ohio.

Federal-Level Subsystem

Most health-related activities at the federal level are implemented and administered by the HHS. This department is directed by the Secretary of Health and Human Services, numerous undersecretaries, and assistant secretaries, and

it is divided into 10 regions as identified on the map on the department's website, at http://www.hhs.gov/about/#.UgE5lt LkuSo. The Surgeon General is the principal deputy to the assistant secretary of HHS. The HHS consists of 11 major agencies (Box 11-1).

In addition to HHS, many federal agencies perform activities related to health. For example, the Department of Education is involved with health education and school health. The Department of Agriculture administers the inspection of meat and milk and provides funds for the Women, Infants, and Children (WIC) program (supplemental nutrition), the food stamp program, and the school-based nutrition program. Other examples of federal agencies of interest to community health are the U.S. Environmental Protection Agency (EPA), the Occupational Safety and Health Administration (OSHA), and the National Institute of Occupational Health and Safety (NIOSH), and the Centers for Disease Control and Prevention (CDC).

Scope of health services of the federal-level subsystem targets the following major health areas: the general population, special populations, and international health. For the general population, federal activities include protection

BOX 11-1 **STRUCTURE OF THE U.S. DEPARTMENT OF HEALTH AND HUMAN SERVICES**

The USDHHS is composed of many agencies that provide different services related to U.S. health care. Among them are the following:

- The **Administration for Community Living** combines the Administration on Aging—agency responsible for coordinating home- and community-based services for older persons and their caregivers—and the Office on Disability and the Administration on Developmental Disabilities in a single agency, with enhanced policy and program support for both cross-cutting initiatives to serve these populations.
- The **Centers for Medicare and Medicaid Services** administers Medicare and Medicaid programs.
- The **Administration for Children and Families** provides family assistance (welfare), child support, Head Start, and other programs to strengthen the family unit.
- The **Centers for Disease Control and Prevention (CDC)** conducts and supports programs directed to prevent and control infectious diseases; they assist states during epidemics. In addition, they provide services related to health promotion and education and professional development and training. The CDC includes the **Agency for Toxic Substances and Disease Registry**, which serves the public by using the best science, taking responsive public health actions, and providing trusted health information to prevent harmful exposures and diseases related to toxic substances.
- The **Food and Drug Administration** provides surveillance over the safety and efficacy of foods, pharmaceuticals, and other consumer goods.
- The **Healthcare Resources and Services Administration** is concerned with the development of health services programs and facilities. The Division of Nursing is in this unit. A major focus of this agency is funding grants for nursing education and training.
- The **Indian Health Service** provides health services for Native Americans and Alaska Natives.
- The **National Institutes of Health (NIH)** perform and support research programs. The focus of their efforts is to develop and extend the scientific knowledge base related to their respective areas. The National Institute for Nursing Research, which is part of NIH, focuses on nursing research.
- The **Substance Abuse and Mental Health Services Administration** awards grants and funds research related to problems with substance abuse and mental health.
- The **Agency for Healthcare Quality and Research** works to improve quality, safety, efficiency, and effectiveness of health care services for all Americans.

against hazards, maintenance of vital and health statistics, advancement of scientific knowledge through research, and provision of disaster relief. In recent years, public health efforts have been directed toward changing behaviors by fostering healthy eating habits, encouraging exercise, and preventing or reducing tobacco, drug, and alcohol use. Other programs have provided nutritional food and food stamps to individuals and families to ensure adequate food intake.

Services for special populations include protection of workers against hazardous occupations and work conditions and health care for military veterans, Native Americans, Alaska natives, federal prisoners, and members of the armed services. In addition, the federal government provides special services for children, older adults, the mentally ill, and the vocationally handicapped.

In the international arena, the federal government works with other countries and international health organizations such as the World Health Organization and the Red Cross to promote various health programs throughout the world.

An example of how services for special populations can become of greater concern is described in the IOM report *Gulf War and Health: Volume 9: Treatment for Chronic Multisymptom Illness* (2013). This report includes recommendations to provide care for chronic multisymptom illness (CMI), which puts a major burden on veterans and their families. The Veterans Administration (VA) health care system has the major responsibility for providing this care, which requires highly coordinated care, effective sharing of information among an interprofessional health care team, and engagement of the veteran and family. Most of this care is provided on an ambulatory care basis in the community.

The IOM report *HHS in the 21st Century: Charting a New Course for a Healthier America* did not recommend major reorganization of the HHS but rather an approach that would transform it (IOM, 2008). The recommendations centered on five key areas:

1. Define a twenty-first century vision.
2. Foster adaptability and alignment.
3. Increase effectiveness and efficiency of the U.S. health care system.
4. Strengthen the HHS and public health and the health care workforce.
5. Improve accountability and decision-making.

The current HHS strategic plan, covering 2010 through 2015, is available on the department's website, at http://www.hhs.gov/secretary/about/priorities/priorities.html, where it is updated periodically. The goals are to:

- Transform health care
- Advance scientific knowledge and innovation
- Advance health, safety, and well-being of the American people
- Increase the efficiency, transparency, and accountability of HHS
- Strengthen the nation's health and human services infrastructure and work force

The HHS is the federal agency that is implementing health care reform. Implementation includes making the rules for implementation of the law, awarding funding to meet the law's requirements, measuring program performance to ensure program integrity, and informing the public of results. This complex legislation requires intricate implementation planning and evaluation, and it will be implemented over several years.

State-Level Subsystem

States are responsible for the health of their citizens and are the central authorities in the public health care system. The organization and activities of public health services vary widely among the states. A health commissioner or secretary of health who is typically appointed by the governor directs most state health agencies. The health officer is usually a physician with a degree and experience in public health. In some states, the health officer directs the health department. Many states have boards of health, which determine policies and priorities for allocation of funds. Staffing of the state agency varies among states; however, in comparison with other state programs, state health programs usually have a large staff.

The state health department, however, does not stand alone. It is highly dependent on the federal level for resources and guidance. For example, funds contributed by the federal government to Medicaid, which is jointly funded by the federal government and states, have been changed over time, increasing and decreasing beneficiaries and services per state. This has had a major impact on services that states can provide to their most vulnerable citizens. Cooperation between the state and federal levels of the health care system has also been brought to the forefront with efforts to plan for bioterrorism, an event that would necessitate cooperation, sharing, and disaster planning. The United States requires an integrated system so that both federal and state levels work to the benefit of all citizens.

According to the scope of health services of the state level subsystem is responsible for its own public health laws; therefore, state policy is widely varied. Factors that affect the level of state services include state-legislated or mandated services, political factors related to division of power between state and local health departments (LHDs), and competition among officials, providers, and the business community.

As discussed in previous chapters, the three core functions of public health are assessment, policy development, and assurance (IOM, 1988). Assessment activities include the collection of data pertaining to vital statistics, health facilities, and human resources; epidemiological activities, such as communicable disease control, health screening, and laboratory analyses; and participation in research projects. In the area of policy development, states formulate goals, develop health plans, and set standards for local health agencies. Assurance activities involve inspection in a variety of areas, licensing, health education, environmental safety, personal health services, and resource development.

Local Health Department Subsystems

LHDs are generally responsible for the direct delivery of public health services and protection of the health of citizens, although not all communities/counties have LHDs. State and local (i.e., city and county) governments delegate the authority to conduct these activities. The organization of LHDs varies widely depending on community size, economics, partnerships with the private health care system, health care facilities, business support, health care needs, transportation, and the number of citizens requiring public health care. Some LHDs function as district offices of the state health department; others are responsible to local government and the state; and still others are autonomous, particularly those in large cities. An LHD may be a separate agency or a division within an agency, such as the HHS.

A health officer or administrator appointed by local government directs the LHD. At least half of the states require that the health officer of an LHD have a medical degree. An interdisciplinary team carries out the activities of the department. Public health nurses and health inspectors represent the two largest groups of professional staff members. Other professional staff members include dentists, social workers, epidemiologists, nutritionists, and health educators.

According to the scope of services of the LHD subsystem is responsible for determining the health status and needs of their constituents. This involves identifying unmet needs and taking actions to meet these needs. Most services to groups and individuals are provided at the local level. These services fall into the following four major categories:

Community health services include control of communicable disease such as surveillance and immunizations, maternal-child health programs, nutrition services, and education. Health promotion education is directed toward changing behavior; individuals are encouraged to eat healthy foods, exercise more, and decrease their use of tobacco, drugs, and alcohol. Other programs provide nutritious food and food stamps to individuals and families. A major activity of LHDs perform preventive screening for potential problems throughout the lifespan of their community members.

Environmental health services include food hygiene such as inspection of food-producing and food-processing plants and restaurants; protection from hazardous substances; control of waste, air, noise, and water pollution; and occupational health. The objective of these activities is to provide a safe environment.

Personal health services provide care to individuals and families in clinics, schools, and prisons. In many areas, home health care services are provided through the LHD.

Mental health services are provided through LHDs in many communities. These services are supported by funds offered by local and regional mental health and mental retardation facilities and programs. See Chapter 24 for more information on community-based mental health care.

LHDs establish local health codes, fund public hospitals such as city and/or county hospitals, and provide services to populations and individuals at risk who often lack health insurance. Programs and services for state health departments and LHDs vary among jurisdictions. The services provided reflect the values of the residents and officials, available resources, and perceived needs of their respective populations within their state and local area. Although the goals of the public health subsystem do not change, the programs and services change to meet the changing needs of the public.

Several provisions of the 2010 health care reform legislation address improvement of quality and access to care. For example, the law promotes establishment of local consortiums of health care providers to coordinate health care services for low-income uninsured and underinsured populations. It also substantially increases funds for community health centers and finances newly developed school-based health centers and nurse-managed health clinics.

Summary of Public Health's Three Levels

In the preceding description of the three government levels that provide public health services (i.e., local, state, and federal), distinctive and overlapping roles have been discussed. The federal government has been assuming a larger role in the protection of the population through regulation and funding. It finances specific programs such as Medicare and categorical programs for mothers and infants and provides direct care to special populations, for example, military veterans. States establish health codes, regulate the insurance industry, and license health care facilities and personnel. States also provide funds for services offered through Medicaid. Direct care activities funded by state health departments may include care in mental hospitals, state medical schools, and associated hospitals. LHDs are the primary agencies that provide direct services to communities, families, and individuals.

Health Care Providers

Providers of health care are individuals, groups, and organizations that deliver or support health care services. This section describes the different types of health care providers, including provider organizations, health care professionals, and nontraditional providers.

Provider Organizations

The following are examples of health care provider organizations:

- Hospital
- Clinic
- Physician practice
- Ambulatory care center
- Home health agency
- Long-term care facility
- Skilled nursing facility
- Rehabilitation center
- Hospice service
- Public health department
- School health clinic
- Birthing center
- Ambulatory surgical center
- Occupational health clinic
- Crisis clinic
- Community health center
- Retail health clinics located in retail stores, supermarkets, pharmacies
- Any other type of organization that provides health care to the community

Health care provider organizations are undergoing tremendous changes. This is particularly true of hospitals, which are merging, consolidating, and closing. These changes have an impact on the entire community health system. With the increasing shift to ambulatory and primary care, hospital stays have shortened, and the patients who are admitted to the hospital are more acutely ill and require more intensive care. Primary care is described in Box 11-2. Consequently, reduced hospital stays result in more home care admissions or more discharges to long-term care facilities for short-term recovery and rehabilitation. This has all had an effect on the need for services in the community.

BOX 11-2 PRIMARY CARE AND PRIMARY PREVENTION

"Primary health care is essential health care based on practical, scientifically sound, and socially acceptable methods and technology made universally accessible to individuals and families in the community through their full participation and at a cost that the community and country can afford to maintain at every stage of their development in the spirit of self-reliance and self-determination.... It is the first level of contact of individuals, the family, and the community with the national health system bringing health care as close as possible to where people live and work." (World Health Organization, 1978)

A physician, nurse practitioner, or physician's assistant may provide primary health care. Generally, the primary care provider's practice is in family medicine, internal medicine, or pediatrics. The primary care provider is responsible for health maintenance and for treatment of common illnesses and may refer clients to specialists as needed.

Primary prevention is a type of intervention that promotes health and prevents disease. Primary prevention includes immunizations and contraception as well as promotion of good nutrition, exercise, and healthy lifestyle choices (e.g., avoidance of tobacco, limitation of alcohol).

How do these definitions compare? The WHO definition and the definition of primary care that is usually used in the United States are similar. Primary prevention is an intervention that is used in primary care services.

⚖ **ETHICAL INSIGHTS**

Universal Health Care

Universal health care has been a topic of interest in the United States for some time. The United States is the only developed country that does not have some form of universal health care. Although the health care reform legislation of 2010 should significantly reduce the number of uninsured individuals, it is estimated that after full implementation in 2017, there will still be about 13 million people without any health care coverage and many with inadequate coverage. Thus, universal health coverage remains an important question. Clients without health coverage have a direct impact on communities, and we should consider the following questions: How do we deal with this question? What additional reforms will be necessary to resolve this question? Is health care a right of all citizens? These are difficult questions particularly in light of the growing problem of health care disparities in the United States.

Health Care Professionals

The interprofessional health care team has been growing and changing over the last few years, with new types of health care professionals added and other members of the team taking on new responsibilities. There is greater emphasis today in all types of health care settings on using interprofessional teams to better coordinate care and ensure effective outcomes. The community particularly needs an interprofessional approach, because clients often have complex needs. This approach was recommended by the IOM in its 2003 report *Health Professions Education*, which identified working on interprofessional teams as a critical health care professions core competency (IOM, 2003d). Even in health care education there is a push to move to more interprofessional education (Interprofessional Professional Education Collaborative [IPEC], 2011; World Health Organization [WHO], 2010). The following is a brief review of the major types of professional and nonprofessional members of the health care team:

Registered Nurse (RN): This appears to be a simple designation that should be familiar to the reader. However, different educational routes exist to obtain a license to practice nursing: diploma, associate degree, and baccalaureate degree. In addition, many nurses now obtain master's degrees and doctorates. These advanced degrees provide them with the opportunity to do more independent practice, teach, and conduct research. RNs practice in all types of health settings. Nurses represent the largest group of professionals providing health services. State legislatures determine licensure requirements and enact nurse practice acts. State boards of nursing are the administrative arm for implementation of these laws and regulations. RNs are the lead professional in home health agencies and provide many services in clinics. They are active in all types of community settings.

Advanced Nurse Practitioner (ANP): This is a nurse who has obtained education beyond a baccalaureate degree and has studied content related to primary care. ANPs specialize in such areas as adult health, pediatrics, neonatology, gerontology, and psychiatric nursing. An ANP may work in a clinic, the community, a private practice, the home, the hospital, or a long-term care facility (i.e., any setting in which health care is provided). With health care reform raising the demand for primary care, it is expected that ANPs will provide more and more primary care, although clearly, clients will need to have choice as to the type of providers they see.

Clinical Nurse Leader (CNL): Clinical Nurse Leader is a new position that requires a master's degree. The CNL is a provider and manager of care at the point of care for individuals and cohorts and does not have a clinical specialty in the master's program. The types of positions that CNLs are taking are variable, though many are in acute care settings.

Clinical Nurse Specialist (CNS): The Clinical Nurse Specialist, who has a master's degree in a specialty area, provides acute care and guides other nursing staff in providing care.

Nurse-Midwife (NM): A Nurse-Midwife is a nurse who has completed an additional educational program focused on midwifery. NMs work in all types of settings in which women's health and obstetrical services are provided, and they may be very active in community health services.

Licensed Practical Nurse (LPN) or Licensed Vocational Nurse (LVN): LPNs and LVNs perform some specific nursing functions and play a critical role in providing direct client care. They have high school degrees and additional training (usually 1 year) and work in all types of settings, typically under the direct supervision of an RN or a physician. They may work in hospitals, long-term care facilities, clinics, and homes.

Physician (MD or DO): A physician has a medical degree; most physicians specialize in a specific area of practice (e.g., internal medicine, surgery, pediatrics, gynecology).

Physician Assistant (PA): The PA is a "physician extender" who provides medical services under the supervision of a licensed physician. The role was developed in the 1960s in response to a shortage of primary care physicians in certain areas. PAs generally work in primary care.

Registered Dietitian (RD): This health care professional assesses the client's nutritional status and needs. RDs work in hospitals, long-term care facilities, clinics, community health, and homes.

Social Worker (SW): SWs assist clients and their families with problems related to reimbursement, access to care, housing, care in the home, transportation, and social problems. They are discharge planners, particularly in acute care facilities or hospitals, often as case managers; however, they work in all types of settings. SWs may also have additional education to specialize in counseling. Social workers work in many community agencies to help clients with a variety of needs, such as housing, ensuring that food is accessible, transportation, vocational assistance, medical equipment, and counseling.

Occupational Therapist (OT): OTs assist clients with impaired functions or disabilities to reach the clients' maximum level of physical and psychosocial independence. They work in all types of settings, including with clients in their homes through home health agencies.

Speech-Language Pathologist: Speech-language pathologists assist clients who need rehabilitative services related to speech and hearing. They work in all types of settings, including with clients in their homes through home health agencies.

Physical Therapist (PT): PTs help clients who are experiencing musculoskeletal problems. These providers focus on maximizing physical functioning and work in all types of settings (e.g., hospitals, long-term care/rehabilitation, home health).

Pharmacist: Pharmacists prepare and dispense medications. Pharmacists have become much more involved in educating clients about medications and in monitoring and evaluating the effects of medications. They work in all types of settings, including the local drug store, where they play a critical role in ensuring safe prescriptions and providing consumer education, and this function has a direct impact on community health. Pharmacists are also collaborating with ANPs in retail located in pharmacies, groceries, and so on.

Respiratory Therapist (RT): RTs provide care to clients with respiratory illnesses. They use oxygen therapy, intermittent positive-pressure respirators, artificial mechanical ventilators, and inhalation therapy. Most RTs work in hospitals and long-term care, but they are becoming more common in home health care.

Chiropractor: Chiropractors are concerned with improving the function of the clients' nervous system by means of various treatment modalities (e.g., spinal manipulation, diet, exercise, and massage). Visits to chiropractors have increased as consumers have become more interested in nontraditional medical interventions. Chiropractors are mostly community based.

Paramedical Technologists: Paramedical technologists work in various medical technology areas (e.g., radiology, nuclear medicine, and other laboratories).

Unlicensed Assistive Personnel (UAP): Members of the health care team know as unlicensed assistive personnel have caused some controversy in last few years; however, the UAP is a critical member of the team. UAPs provide more direct client care, supervised by RNs. The amount of education and training of UAPs is highly variable. UAPs work not only in acute care and long-term care but also for home health agencies under the supervision of RNs.

Nontraditional Health Care Providers

Nontraditional health care providers deliver alternative or complementary therapies. During the last two decades, consumers have become more interested in this type of care and have demanded that it be available.

Although many large medical centers are now developing programs and centers that offer complementary therapies, reimbursement for these services is lagging. The National Institutes of Health (NIH) agreed to conduct research focused on a wide array of alternative therapies and their effects on health and disease. As a result, in 1998, the NIH established the National Center for Complementary and Alternative Medicine (NCCAM) to meet the need. This represents a major change in the scientific and medical communities. Alternative therapies, provided by a variety of health care providers, include massage therapy, herbal therapy, healing touch, energetic healing, acupuncture, and acupressure. Ethnic healers, such as *curanderos,* and folk healers are also found in some communities. Training and licensure requirements vary but will probably become more standard as their care becomes more accepted in established medical practice. Many nurses have incorporated alternative therapies into their practices and are seeking continuing education on this topic.

QUALITY CARE

Quality care has been a concern of consumers and providers for many years, and continues to be the most important concern. Quality care is a difficult concept to define and more difficult to measure. In 1996, President Clinton established the Advisory Commission on Consumer Protection and Quality in the Health Care Industry, and its final report was published in 1999 (President's Advisory Commission on Consumer Protection and Quality in the Health Care Industry, 1999). As identified in this report, "the purpose of the health care system must be to continuously reduce the impact and burden of illness, injury, and disability and to improve the health and functioning of the people of the United States" (para 6). The report strongly supported public-private partnerships, strong leadership with clearly defined goals for improvement, an increase in consumer power and rights, a focus on vulnerable populations, promotion of accountability, reduction in errors and an increase

in health care safety, fostering of evidence-based practice, adaptation of organizations for change, an increase in health care workforce involvement, and investment in information systems.

This report had a major impact, in that it stimulated a series of more in-depth explorations of the health care delivery system, including the IOM's "quality chasm" series. The IOM defines *quality* as "the degree to which health services for individuals and populations increase the likelihood of desired health outcomes and are consistent with current professional knowledge" (IOM, 2001, p. 232; Lohr, 1990, p. 20). This series of reports have had a major impact on the U.S. health care delivery system.

The Institute of Medicine Reports Examine Health Care Quality

To Err Is Human: Building a Safer Health System

The first report, *To Err Is Human: Building a Safer Health System* (IOM, 1999), focused on safety within the health care delivery system. Data indicated that there have been, and continue to be, serious safety problems. Examples include the following (IOM, 1999):

- When data from one study were extrapolated, the findings indicated that at least 44,000 Americans die each year as a result of a medication error, and another study indicated the number could be as high as 98,000.
- In a given year, more people die as a result of medical errors than because of motor vehicle accidents (43,664), breast cancer (41,491), or AIDS (12,113) (CDC, 1999). There are clear problems, and, to date, the focus has been only on hospital errors. This fact, however, does not negate the presence of medical errors in the community's health system, such as home care, long-term care, ambulatory care, primary care and other health care settings, which require further exploration.

To Err Is Human clearly states that there is no one answer to solving this problem. The report defines *safety* as "freedom from accidental injury" and defines *error* as "the failure of a planned action to be completed as intended or the use of a wrong plan to achieve an aim" (IOM, 1999, p. 3). Errors are directly related to outcomes, which is a significant concern in quality improvement efforts. Patient safety is a critical component of quality.

This initiative represents a collaborative effort from a health care professional organization, an accrediting organization, and consumers. Getting the patient involved is a very important strategy; however, the critical next step is listening to the patient. The four key messages from this report are as follows: (1) the magnitude of harm that results from medical errors is great; (2) errors result largely from systems' failures, not individual failures; (3) voluntary and mandatory reporting programs are needed now to improve patient safety; and (4) the IOM committee and others call on health care systems to focus on error reduction as an important part of their operations and to embrace organizational change needed to reorient error-ridden systems and process (Maddox, Wakefield, and Bull, 2001).

Crossing the Quality Chasm

The second major report, *Crossing the Quality Chasm* (IOM, 2001a), focused on the development of a new health care system for the twenty-first century, one that improves care. The first conclusion from the report is that the system is in need of fundamental improvement. The report emphasizes the impact of the rapid change in the health care system: new medical science, new technology, rapid availability of information, and so on. Health care providers cannot keep up, and "performance of the health care system varies considerably" (IOM, 2001a, p. 3). As was noted in *To Err Is Human*, the system is fragmented, is poorly organized, and does not make the best use of its resources.

Another conclusion from the report is the impact that the rise in numbers of chronic conditions has had on the system. With people living longer, mostly because of the advances in medical science and technology, more are living with chronic conditions. Many of these patients also have comorbid conditions—complicated problems that require collaborative treatment efforts. The health care system is ineffective in dealing with these problems. To address these multiple concerns, the report supports changes that were identified by Wagner, Austin, and Von Korff (1996):

1. Need for evidence-based, planned care
2. Reorganization of practices to meet the needs of patients who require more time, a broad array of resources, and closer follow-up
3. Systematic attention to patients' need for information and behavioral change
4. Ready access to necessary clinical expertise
5. Supportive information systems

Most people with chronic illnesses receive the majority of their care in their communities and not in acute care settings. In addition, community health providers must consider programs to prevent many of the chronic illnesses for vulnerable populations. Nurses assume major roles in providing care to these populations—direct care, development of effective health programs, health education, preventive strategies, and evaluation of outcomes in the community.

For an agenda for *Crossing the Quality Chasm*, the report makes the following recommendations directly related to nursing (IOM, 2001, p. 5):

- All health care constituents, including policy makers, purchasers, regulators, health professionals, health care trustees and management, and consumers, commit to a national statement of purpose for the health care systems as a whole and to a shared agenda.
- Clinicians and patients and the health care organizations that support care delivery adopt a new set of principles to guide the redesign of care processes.
- Health care organizations design and implement more effective organizational support processes to make change in the delivery of care possible.
- Purchasers, regulators, health professions, educational institutions, and the HHS create an environment that fosters and rewards improvement by (1) creating an infrastructure to support evidence-based practice, (2) facilitating the use of information technology, (3) aligning payment incentives, and (4) preparing the workforce to better serve patients in a world of expanding knowledge and rapid change.

Leadership by Example

Leadership by Example was an IOM report requested by Congress that examined the federal government's quality enhancement processes (IOM, 2003b). It focused on six government programs: Medicare, Medicaid, the State Children's Health Insurance Program, the Department of Defense's TRICARE and TRICARE for Life programs, the Veterans Administration program, and the Indian Health Services program. These programs cover approximately 100 million people. The report concluded that improvement was needed in several areas. Among the findings:

1. There is a lack of consistent performance measurement across and within programs.
2. The usefulness of quality information has been questioned.
3. There is a lack of a conceptual framework to guide the evaluation.
4. There is a lack of computerized clinical data.
5. There is a lack of commitment to guide decisions.
6. There is a lack of a systematic approach for assessing the quality enhancement activities.

The report noted that federal leadership is needed because the federal government is in a unique position to assume a lead role in developing a national health care quality improvement initiative. The federal government is the largest purchaser of care and has a major impact on many people. It provides direct care to many: military personnel and their families, Native Americans, and veterans. Through these programs, the federal government can establish models to improve care. Furthermore, because the federal government is also a regulator, federal leadership can affect many health care providers who are not in the federal system; for example, health care organizations that accept Medicare or Medicaid funds must comply with federal regulations (IOM, 2001b). Sponsorship of research, education, and training are other areas in which the federal government has a major impact. The report's conclusions recommend that the federal government lead by example and coordinate government roles in improving health care quality.

Who Will Keep the Public Healthy?

The report entitled *Who Will Keep the Public Healthy?* brought public health to the forefront by focusing on issues such as globalization, rapid travel, scientific and technological advances, and demographic changes. It provided an in-depth exploration of the educational needs for improved public health. The report pointed out that to address current and future public health problems, there is a great need for appropriately prepared public health professionals. Eight content areas were identified in this report aimed at public health professionals: informatics, genomics, communication, cultural competence, community-based participatory research, global health, policy and law, and public health ethics. These areas are additions to the long-held core components of public health: epidemiology, biostatistics, environmental health, health services administration, and social and behavioral science (IOM, 2003c).

Health Professions Education

In the report *Health Professions Education*, the education of all health professionals is viewed as a bridge to quality care. This discussion included the need to have qualified, competent staff in order to improve health care. The report indicated that health professions education must change to meet the growing demands of the health care system today. It identified five core competencies that apply to all health care professions: (1) provide patient-centered care, (2) work in interdisciplinary/interprofessional teams, (3) employ evidence-based practice, (4) apply quality improvement, and (5) utilize informatics. The writers of the report noted that all health professionals "should be educated to deliver patient-centered care as members of an interdisciplinary team, emphasizing evidence-based practice, quality improvement approaches, and informatics" (IOM 2003d, p. 3).

Priority Areas for National Action

In *Priority Areas for National Action: Transforming Health Care Quality* the IOM identified 19 priority areas that should be addressed to improve quality. In the first list of priority areas obesity was listed as an "emerging area," but currently it is an active problem requiring multiple interventions directed at prevention when possible. These priority areas were identified to promote care coordination and self-management/health literacy and to enhance the continuum of care across the lifespan. The original 19 areas were changed on the basis of results of the annual quality report.

The Agency for Healthcare Research and Quality (AHRQ) publishes two reports annually, the *National Healthcare Quality Report* and the *National Healthcare Disparities Report*. In 2010, the AHRQ asked the IOM to review versions of these two reports and identify how they could be improved. The IOM had originally developed the framework for the two reports and the list of priority areas to monitor. The IOM noted that reports such as these will not alone improve the quality of health care. They provide direction and description of gaps in care between performance and standards. The IOM (2010d, p. xi) made the following recommendations to the AHRQ:

- Align the content of the reports with nationally recognized priority areas for quality improvement to help drive national action.
- Select measures that reflect health care attributes or processes that are deemed to have the greatest impact on population health.
- Affirm through the contents of the reports that achieving equity is an essential part of quality improvement.
- Increase the reach and usefulness of AHRQ's family of report-related products.
- Revamp the presentation of the reports to tell a more complete quality improvement story.

- Analyze and present data in ways that inform policy and promote best-in-class achievement for all actors.
- Identify measure and data needs to set a research and data collection agenda.

The IOM recommended that the priority areas be changed as follows, although many of the areas in the list are similar to priority areas previously identified (2010, p. 3):

Patient and family engagement: Engage patients and their families in managing their health and making decisions about their care.

Population health: Improve the health of the population.

Safety: Improve the safety and reliability of the U.S. health care system.

Care coordination: Ensure that patients receive well-coordinated care within and across all health care organizations, settings, and levels of care.

Palliative care: Guarantee appropriate and compassionate care for patients with life-limiting illnesses.

Overuse: Eliminate overuse while ensuring the delivery of appropriate care.

Access: Ensure that care is accessible and affordable for all segments of the U.S. population.

Health systems infrastructure capabilities: Improve the foundation of health care systems (including infrastructure for data and quality improvement; communication across settings for coordination of care; and workforce capacity and distribution among other elements) to support high-quality care.

These priority areas include priorities identified by the National Priorities Partnership. This partnership of 52 major national organizations works together for better health and safe, equitable, and value-driven health care system (National Quality Forum, 2013).

The areas identified in the current annual quality report and also in the annual disparities report should be used as a guide by health care providers. A community can use this list to develop its community health focus and thus improve the quality of life and care of its populations.

Keeping Patients Safe: Transforming the Work Environment of Nurses

The IOM report *Keeping Patients Safe: Transforming the Work Environment* is an important report for nurses in all types of settings (IOM, 2004). This critical report addressed critical quality and safety issues with a particular focus on nursing care and nurses and examined these issues from the perspective of the work environment. The report focused on nurses in acute care. It presented methods for designing the work environment so that nurses may provide safer patient care and described concerns related to the nursing shortage, health care errors, patient safety risk factors, the central role of the nurse in patient quality improvement, and work environment threats to patient safety. This report laid the groundwork for other comments and reports from the IOM about nursing, such as *The Future of Nursing: Leading Change, Advancing Health* (2011). The 2004 report emphasizes the major role nurses assume in health care and notes that nurses need to be more effective leaders in quality improvement, but are not prepared to do so. Many of the themes found in the IOM 2011 *Future of Nursing* report originated in the 2004 IOM report. The 2004 report was hardly noticed by nursing, and as a consequence, opportunity to take advantage of this highly supportive report was missed.

Accreditation

Accreditation is one means to assess the quality of services and care of the organization. Specific minimum standards must be met by an organization to obtain accreditation. Many groups provide accreditation for health care providers and health care organizations. The Joint Commission accredits hospitals, home care agencies, long-term care facilities, and ambulatory care centers. The National Committee for Quality Assurance (NCQA) accredits managed care organizations (MCOs) and insurers and uses the Health Plan Effectiveness Data and Information Set (HEDIS) to collect data about more than 90% of health care plans to measure performance and consumer satisfaction. Medicare also uses HEDIS. The American Healthcare Commission also accredits MCOs (NCQA, 2009).

Purchasers of care who are insurers and MCOs are also concerned about the accreditation status of health care organizations when they negotiate reimbursement contracts. Insurers and MCOs are concerned about the accreditation status of health care provider organizations, as are nursing schools that use clinical sites for educational purposes. Health care providers should also be concerned about the accreditation status of their employers. The Consumer Assessment of Healthcare Providers and Systems (CAHPS) is a survey and reporting tool administered by the AHRQ. CAHPS collects data and reports on consumer experience with specific aspects of their health plans. This type of survey provides data that help purchasers of plans compare and contrast plans (AHRQ, 2009).

Current Status of Health Care Quality

Currently, quality care monitoring focuses on improvement. With the improvement approach, outcomes measures have moved to the forefront. Accrediting organizations require outcomes data, which they use to assess overall performance. Practitioners use outcomes to identify the treatment goals with the client. "Report cards" are used to compare and contrast health care organizations and health care plans. These report cards are available to the consumer, providers, and insurers. Quality data are no longer hidden and will continue to be available when new methods are developed to assess improvement on the basis of outcomes (Beyers, 2003; McCarthy, 2002). Medicare has been increasing the number of its quality initiatives. Some of these initiatives, which are described on http://www.cms.gov, are:

- Physician Quality Reporting System
- Quality Improvement Organizations (QIO)
- Development of Quality Measures
- Post Acute Care Reform Plan
- Development of Quality Indicators for Inpatient Rehabilitation Facilities (IRFs)

The IOM developed frameworks to monitor health care quality and health care disparities. As previously discussed, AHRQ collects data about the status of national health care quality using the framework and publishes the report annually on the Internet (access the report at www.ahrq.gov). Despite all these efforts to use evaluation and accreditation to ensure quality care, the United States has not really been all that successful. There is still discussion about what constitutes quality care and how to best assess quality. The number of errors continues to be high, and clients continue to be dissatisfied. Dr. Harvey Fineberg, president of the IOM, commented on the health system:

> *America's health system is neither as successful as it should be nor as sustainable as it must be. The Patient Protection and Affordable Care Act of 2010 (ACA) introduces the prospects for major reforms in payment for and organization of care, in prevention and population health, and in approaches to continuous improvement. Yet it remains under legal assault and a cloud of controversy. Even if it is fully implemented, the ACA will not represent a complete solution to the core dilemma of affordability and performance. The country's political appetite for further reform may be sated, but unless we attend to the major sources of waste and impediments to performance, the United States will remain vulnerable to an excessively costly health system that delivers incommensurate health benefit. (Fineberg, 2012, p. 1020)*

He also noted that the United States has a lower life expectancy than other similar countries, and in comparison with Australia, Canada, Germany, the Netherlands, New Zealand, and Britain, the United States was last in relation to health care quality, access, efficiency, and equity in 2010 (Davis, Schoen, and Stremikis, 2010; Fineberg, 2012).

CRITICAL ISSUES IN HEALTH CARE DELIVERY

Managed Care

Managed care refers to any method of health care delivery designed to reduce unnecessary use of services, improve cost containment or cost-effectiveness, and ensure high-quality care. Managed care is currently the predominant force in health care delivery. It affects health care organizations, health care providers, and reimbursement and has a direct influence on what care is provided and by whom, where, when, and whether it is to be provided. Chapter 12 provides additional information on managed care and reimbursement.

Information Technology

The development of information technology (IT) over the last decade has been phenomenal. Clinical staff members use computers in all health care settings. For example, telehealth is growing, which means that clients can receive care via technology, such as computer, video, or interactive television. The IOM, examining the use of telehealth and its potential impact on health care delivery, noted that "telehealth is a key component in ensuring access to health care services in isolated geographic areas across the United States. More effective deployment of telehealth technologies will enhance our ability to better meet the health care needs of those in rural and frontier parts of the country. However, telehealth is important not just for rural communities, but for any underserved community" (IOM, p. 4, 2012).

The Internet has opened doors for consumers and providers, and health information access has expanded rapidly. Although information availability to millions of people has been enhanced, resulting in an explosion of knowledge regarding health and health issues, the quality of this information is sometimes questionable. Providers must address the source and content of Internet information. There is a drive now to move the health care system to electronic medical records (EMRs), though it will take funding and effort to make this a reality throughout the health care delivery system. Social media has become a more common source of information and could be used to share information about community health, including health promotion and prevention. Individuals share a great variety of information now through social media, and this venue could be used in more organized efforts to get information out to the public. Smartphones are another resource for engaging the community—for example, with applications (apps) that track weight, exercise, and other health issues.

Fineberg (2012, p. 1025) identified potential uses of health information, and a number of them on this list relate directly to community health:

- Personal health, diet, and activity monitoring and motivation
- Real-time clinical decision support
- Remote professional consultation and care
- Monitoring and advising of patients with chronic disease
- Quality assurance
- Performance assessment of providers and institutions
- Comparative outcomes research
- Comparative health assessments across populations, communities, cities, and states
- Public health surveillance for disease outbreaks, environmental risks, and potential bioterrorism

Consumerism, Advocacy, and Client Rights

The growth of managed care increased the strength of consumerism. Over the past decade, the baby boomer generation has been subsidizing the health care system and paying more in premiums than it has taken out in claims. However, growing concern exists that, as this generation ages, it will demand more care than previous generations. Consumers are now critical of the health care system and demand changes as they encounter problems. Health care organizations, individual providers, and insurers, including MCOs, recognize the importance of the consumer voice and the need for explanations. *Client-* or *customer-centered health care* is a term that has become commonly used in health care, and more effort has been made to provide the consumer with information.

Client rights are now an important health care issue that individual states and the federal government have been addressing through legislation. In 1999, the U.S. House and Senate passed bills that focused on client rights in the managed care environment, but more needs to be done to improve client rights. Client rights issues that are vitally important are information disclosure, physician and provider choice, direct access to specialists, reimbursement for emergency care, and reimbursement denial.

Coordination and Access to Health Care

The social justice foundation of public health is yet to be realized because many inequalities in access to health care still exist. "Nearly 48 million nonelderly Americans were uninsured in 2011, a decline of 1.3 million since 2010. Decreasing the number of uninsured is a key goal of the 2010 Patient Protection and Affordable Care Act (ACA), which will provide Medicaid or subsidized coverage to qualifying individuals with incomes up to 400% of poverty beginning in 2014. Characteristics of uninsured people reflect a wide range of incomes, races, and occupations, although children, minorities, the poor, and those with less education are overrepresented" (Kaiser Family Foundation, 2012).

Health care providers often function in isolation from one another and provide fragmented services. Although multiple services are available for the wellness–serious illness continuum, coordination is lacking. Services range from office-clinic, home care, adult day care, acute care institutions, and specialized institutions to skilled nursing facilities. The services provided by one agency or one provider do not help the individual transit, or move, across boundaries and receive services offered by others. "Handoffs," when patients are transferred from one provider (e.g., individual provider, unit, agency) to another, are a time of increased risk for errors, reducing the quality of care. In addition, the services tend to be geographically separated, and each agency has different criteria for access. The focus of services has not kept pace with the changing needs of individuals and populations. Millions of Americans lack access to health care services, and inadequate financial resources are a deterrent to available health services. Interprofessional teams can address many of these concerns and improve care in the community.

The current health care system continues to be pluralistic and competitive, and it provides fragmented and uncoordinated care. Private care agencies and institutions are in competition with one another for clients, health professionals, and resources. Even with recent reforms, two hospitals in the same geographic area may be competing for the same clients while other communities may not have a hospital at all, may have only minimal services, or may lack essential services, such as obstetrics. Hospital home care programs are in direct competition with private or public home care agencies. Hospitals diversify services to become economically viable; therefore, they compete with ambulatory care providers for the ambulatory market. Public health services can be viewed as indirectly competing for resources. This fragmentation and duplication must be overcome to provide coordinated, collaborative, and accessible service to all citizens.

Disparity in Health Care Delivery

Disparity in health care delivery is certainly related to the number of uninsured and underinsured, but it is also more than this. The IOM (2002) report *Unequal Treatment: Confronting Racial and Ethnic Disparities in Health Care* addressed potential causes of disparities in health care. The report observed that bias and stereotyping on the part of health care providers might contribute to differences in care. Disparities in care were particularly found in cancer, cardiovascular disease, human immunodeficiency virus (HIV)/AIDS, diabetes, and mental illness. To address this problem, more cross-cultural education for health care professionals, including nurses, is needed to improve awareness of cultural and social factors and their impact on health care. The annual AHRQ disparities report provides critical information on the status of health care disparities. Additional information on this critical problem is found in Chapter 10.

Globalization and International Health

The world today had no real boundaries. The Internet, along with the ease of travel has made this absence of boundaries a reality. With increasing travel there is also greater ease to sharing of illnesses. Also, given the political status of many areas of the world, there are increased risks for types of terrorism, such as bioterrorism. Preparing for these possibilities requires plans and steps that focus on these problems. The federal government and also states have plans to respond to events that may affect the health of populations. The Centers for Disease Control and Prevention has been very active in responding to the need for preparedness. Immunizations are also a population-focused intervention to respond to risk of infectious diseases that are now easy to share worldwide. The Internet and growing collaborative global initiatives provide the United States and other countries opportunities to share information and development for improvement. The World Health Organization is one organization that focuses on these concerns, and the International Council of Nurses (ICN) offers a global nursing perspective. Some schools of nursing are providing international experiences for students to broaden global knowledge.

Health Care Reform: Impact on the Health Care System

The United States appeared to be ready for health care reform when the Clinton administration took office (Skocpol, 1994). By 1990, support for reform had reached a 40-year high in the polls, and the election of Bill Clinton in 1992 brought the health care debate onto the national agenda. Believing reform of the health care system to be part of his election mandate, the new president assembled an ambitious plan to produce legislation for national reform of the health care system. The process was initially supported by diverse sectors of the system, but some participants began to distance themselves and ultimately opposed reform. This was true in the case of many major power constituents (i.e., businesses, physicians, and insurance companies). Ultimately, the bills failed.

With the Obama administration, a great deal of effort has been made at the federal level to achieve major health care reform. As discussed, when fully implemented, the Patient Protection and Affordable Care Act of 2010 will dramatically influence virtually all components of the country's health care system. Significant reforms will be seen in private health insurance in addition to changes in Medicare and Medicaid. Additionally, it is anticipated that about 75% of uninsured citizens will obtain health coverage. How exactly these changes will influence health, health care economics, and health care delivery, however, remains to be seen. Additional content on health care reform can be found in Chapters 10 and 12.

⚖ ETHICAL INSIGHTS

Limited Health Care for Some

The health care system in the United States is complex, with social policies that favor pluralism, free choice, and free enterprise. The private sector personal care subsystem provides the majority of care to individuals. The private sector includes nonprofit agencies, for-profit agencies, and voluntary organizations. The public health subsystem provides limited personal care services for socially marginalized populations but, for the most part, subsidizes the private sector through Medicare and Medicaid reimbursement to provide these services.

FUTURE OF PUBLIC HEALTH AND THE HEALTH CARE SYSTEM

Many changes are occurring in the health care system. With the implementation of the health care reform legislation, the health care system is required to set limits on the care provided; identify criteria for the use of technology; and determine which conditions will be treated, which interventions are effective, and who should receive the care. The health care reform debate is not over, because now we have to respond to implementation issues and then evaluate outcomes long term. Questions that continue to be important are:

- What health care services should be provided?
- Who should have access to health care services?
- Who should pay for health care services?
- How should health care be delivered?
- What is the role of the government?

The importance of health promotion, disease prevention, and a population-based approach to health care is becoming increasingly recognized. The IOM reports indicate a need for improvement in all sectors of the health care delivery system. There is recognition of the need for an electronic medical record, which, to be effective, would have to incorporate care provided in the community. The growing concern over bioterrorism and roles of health care organizations, practitioners, and the government must address the community health components of the system. There is also the problem of changing climate, which can lead to major community health and safety concerns in relation to weather disasters. Local, state, and national political leaders must begin to grapple with the health of the population and the need to reduce the levels of health care expenditures in a voluntary environment.

Futurists rarely identify the public health subsystem as a component of the health care system, but this situation is changing. Indeed, the history of the public health subsystem's involvement with the poor and disenfranchised is a major influence on inattention to their problems. Furthermore, focus on environmental influences, such as air quality, on the population is critical for the future health of any nation.

Nursing has also been involved in change. The IOM report *The Future of Nursing* (2011) also focuses on the nursing profession and how it might fit into the change process. The key messages in this report are (IOM, 2011, p. 4):

1. Nurses should practice to the full extent of their education and training.
2. Nurses should achieve higher levels of education and training through an improved education system that promotes seamless academic progression.
3. Nurses should be full partners, with physicians and other health professionals, in redesigning health care in the United States.
4. Effective workforce planning and policy making require better data collection and an improved information infrastructure.

This report offers eight recommendations. Many of the report's recommendations are having a major impact on nursing, such as the drive to increase the number of nurses with bachelor's of science nursing degrees by developing more RN-BSN opportunities. Community health has been one area of health care that often has required a BSN for its entry positions, though with the nursing shortage this situation has been moderated some. Increasing the number of nurses with BSN degrees would help fill empty positions in community health that require a BSN degree. The role of the ANP, as commented on earlier, is also expanding. The IOM report discusses change, emphasizing the following principles of change, which focus on quality, access, and cost or value:

- The need for patient-centered care
- The need for stronger primary care services
- The need to deliver more care in the community
- The need for seamless, coordinated care
- The need for reconceptualized roles for health professionals
- The need for interprofessional collaboration

All of these principles apply to community health nursing.

Predicting future trends in human values is more difficult than predicting scientific discoveries or the patterns of disease. However, Koop (1989) stated that the ultimate test of the public health subsystem is whether it effectively serves the people by their measurements, not those of the public health profession. The past two decades have brought a significant shift in thinking about the future of the health care system.

Consumer rights and further efforts to control or limit health care costs while improving access will be critical issues to be resolved in the future. How these decisions, and implementation of health care reform law, will affect public health is unclear.

SUMMARY

The health care system is complex and changes quickly. Federal, state, and local legislation and policies affect the system, and understanding the legislation and its effect on the health care delivery system is critical for any nurse. In addition, the development of managed care demonstrated how important it is for health care providers to understand the reimbursement system and to learn how to advocate for their clients.

The many different types of health care organizations and health care providers also affect the health care system. Interprofessional care will be necessary for providers to achieve success in the system and to ensure that the client receives cost-effective, quality care. There are many concerns about health care, including cost, access, the number of uninsured, quality, and health care fraud and abuse. Resolving these problems will not be an easy task, but it must be done. Understanding the system helps as health care providers learn to function in the rapidly changing system.

LEARNING ACTIVITIES

1. Describe the organization of the state and local health departments.
2. Visit the local health department, and learn what services are provided. How do these services relate to *Healthy People 2020* objectives?
3. Identify regional and state health services.
4. Visit a voluntary agency. Determine the services it offers and how the agency collaborates with the local public health agency. Does the agency have a website? If so, visit it and find out what information is available to consumers and professionals.
5. Review the current national health care quality report and the national disparities report on the Internet. They can be accessed at http://www.ahrq.gov/research/findings/nhqrdr/index.html. What frameworks or matrices are used to structure the report? What is the status of health care quality and disparities? What can you learn that would impact planning for health care services in a community? Also review the associated *National Healthcare Disparities Report*.
6. Discuss how critical health care issues (e.g., managed care, quality care, fraud and abuse, diversity, and disparity) affect health care organizations in the community.
7. Cite examples of health care consumerism in the local community. What are their histories?
8. Give a personal reaction to health care fraud and abuse. How should the principles found in the Code for Nurses apply in practice?

9. Visit the following site on health care reform: http://www.hhs.gov/healthcare/rights/index.html. Review the elements of the law and current status. Discuss implications for nursing in the community. Also review http://www.helpingyoucare.com/21950/hhs-provides-tool-to-find-out-how-the-presidents-health-care-law-benefits-you-your-state. HHS provides this site for comparisons.

ⓔ **EVOLVE WEBSITE**

http://evolve.elsevier.com/Nies

- NCLEX Review Questions
- Case Studies
- Glossary

REFERENCES

Agency for Healthcare Research and Quality: 2012 National Healthcare Disparities Report, 2013. Available from http://www.ahrq.gov/research/findings/nhqrdr/nhdr12/index.html.

Agency for Healthcare Research and Quality: *Consumer assessment of health plans*, 2009. Available from <www.ahrq.gov>. Accessed January 10, 2009.

American Hospital Association: *Hospital statistics*, Chicago, 1999, Author.

Beyers M: Viewpoint: report cards are here to stay, *Patient Care Manag* 19(1):10–11, 2003.

Centers for Disease Control and Prevention, National Center for Health Statistics: Births and Deaths: Preliminary Data for 1998, *National Vital Statistics Reports* 47(25):6, 1999.

Centers for Disease Control and Prevention: National Center for Health Statistics: Deaths: final data for 2006, *Natl Vital Stat Rep* 57(14), 2009. Available from <www.cdc.gov/nchs/data/nvsr/nvsr57/ nvsr57_14.pdf>.

Davis K, Schoen C, Stremikis K: *Mirror, mirror on the wall: how the performance of the U.S. health care system compares internationally, 2010 update*, New York, 2010, Commonwealth Fund.

Fineberg H: A successful and sustainable health system—how to get there from here, *New England Journal of Medicine* 366(11):1020–1027, 2012.

Hanlon G, Pickett J: *Public health administration and practice*, ed 9, St. Louis, 1990, Mosby.

Institute of Medicine: *The future of public health*, Washington, DC, 1988, National Academies Press.

Institute of Medicine: *To err is human: building a safer health system*, Washington, DC, 1999, National Academies Press.

Institute of Medicine: *Crossing the quality chasm*, Washington, DC, 2001a, National Academies Press.

Institute of Medicine: *Envisioning the national health care quality report*, Washington, DC, 2001b, National Academies Press.

Institute of Medicine: *Unequal treatment: confronting racial and ethnic disparities in health*, Washington, DC, 2002, National Academies Press.

Institute of Medicine: *Health professions education: a bridge to quality*, Washington, DC, 2003a, National Academies Press.

Institute of Medicine: *Leadership by example*, Washington, DC, 2003b, National Academies Press.

Institute of Medicine: *Who will keep the public healthy?* Washington, DC, 2003c, National Academies Press.

Institute of Medicine: *Health professions education*, Washington, DC, 2003d, National Academies Press.

Institute of Medicine: *Priority areas for national action: transforming health care quality*, Washington, DC, 2003e, National Academies Press.

Institute of Medicine: *Keeping patients safe: transforming the work environment of nurses*, Washington, DC, 2004, National Academies Press.

Institute of Medicine: *HHS in the 21st century: charting a new course for a healthier America*, Washington, DC, 2008, National Academies Press.

Institute of Medicine: *Future directions for the national healthcare quality and disparities reports*, Washington, DC, 2010, The National Academies Press.

Institute of Medicine: *The future of nursing: leading change, advancing health*, Washington, DC, 2011, The National Academies Press.

Institute of Medicine: *Best care at lower costs: the path to continuously learning health care in America*, 2012a, National Academies Press.

Institute of Medicine: *The role of telehealth in an evolving health care environment: workshop summary*, Washington, DC, 2012b, The National Academies Press.

Institute of Medicine: *Gulf War and health: volume 9: treatment for chronic multisymptom illness*, Washington, DC, 2013, The National Academies Press.

Interprofessional Professional Education Collaborative (IPEC): *Core competencies for interprofessional collaborative practice: report of an expert panel*, 2011. Available from <www.aacn.nche.edu/education-resources/IPECReport.pdf>.

Kaiser Family Foundation: *Focus on health reform* 2010. Available from <www.kff.org/healthreform/upload/ 8061.pdf 2010b>.

Kaiser Family Foundation: *Five facts about the uninsured population*, 2012. Available from <from http://www.kff.org/uninsured/upload/7806-05.pdf>.

Knight W: *Managed care: what it is and how it works*, Gaithersburg, MD, 1998, Aspen.

Koop CE: An agenda for public health, *J Public Health Policy* 10:7, 1989.

Lohr K, editor: *Medicare: a strategy for quality assurance*, Washington, DC, 1990, The National Academy Press.

Maddox P, Wakefield M, Bull J: Patient safety and the need for professional and educational change, *Nurs Outlook* 49(1):8–13, 2001.

McCarthy M: U.S. government releases nursing home report cards, *Lancet* 360:1670, 2002.

National Committee for Quality Assurance: *National Committee for Quality Assurance: Accreditation*, 2009. Available from <www.ncqa.org/tabid/66/Default.aspx>.

National Quality Forum: *National Priorities Partnership*, 2013. Available from http://www.qualityforum.org/Setting_Priorities/NPP/National_Priorities_Partnership.aspx.

O'Neil EH and the Pew Health Professions Commission: *Recreating health professional practice for a new century*, San Francisco, 1998, The Commission.

President's Advisory Commission on Consumer Protection and Quality in the Health Care Industry: *Quality first: better health care for all Americans*, Washington, DC, 1999, U.S. Government Printing Office.

Skocpol T: From social security to health security? *J Health Polit Policy Law* 19:239, 1994.

Stanton TH: Fraud and abuse enforcement in Medicare: finding middle ground, *Health Aff* 20(4):28–38, 2001.

U.S. Department of Health and Human Services: *Healthy People 2010*, Washington, DC, 2000, US Government Printing Office.

U.S. Department of Health and Human Services: *Computations for the 2009 annual update of the HHS Poverty Guidelines for the 48 contiguous states and the District of Columbia*, 2009. Available from <aspe.hhs.gov/poverty/09poverty.shtml>.

Wagner E, Austin B, Von Korff M: Organizing care for patients with chronic illness, *Milbank Q* 74(4):511–542, 1996.

World Health Organization: *Framework for action on interprofessional education and collaborative practice*, 2010. Available from <http://www.who.int/hrh/resources/framework_action/en/index.html>.

World Health Organization: *Declaration of Alma Ata*, 1978. Available from http://www.who.int/publications/almaata_declaration_en.pdf.

Economics of Health Care

*Anita W. Finkelman**

OBJECTIVES

Upon completion of this chapter, the reader will be able to do the following:

1. Discuss factors that influence the cost of health care.
2. Identify terms used in the financing of health care.
3. Discuss public financing of health care.
4. Discuss private financing of health care.
5. Discuss health insurance plans.
6. Describe trends in health care financing.
7. Describe the effects of economics on health care access.
8. Identify the future of health care economics.

KEY TERMS

access
actuarial classifications
adverse selection
ambulatory care
capitated reimbursement
carrier
carve-out service
coinsurance
co-payment
cost containment
cost shifting
current procedural terminology codes

deductible
diagnosis-related group
effectiveness
flexible spending account
gatekeepers
health care providers
health insurance plans
health maintenance organization
  (HMO)
indemnity plan
managed care groups
managed care plans

mandates
Medicaid
Medicare
Medigap insurance
outcomes
out-of-pocket expenses
preferred provider organization (PPO)
premiums
primary care provider
prospective payment system

OUTLINE

Factors Influencing Health Care Costs
  Historical Perspective
  Use of Health Care
  Lack of Preventive Care
  Lifestyle and Health Behaviors
  Societal Beliefs
  Technological Advances
  Aging of Society
  Pharmaceuticals
  Shift to For-Profit Health Care
Health Care Fraud and Abuse
Public Financing of Health Care
  Medicare
  Medicaid
  Governmental Grants

Philanthropic Financing of Health Care
Health Care Insurance Plans
  Historical Perspective
  Types of Health Care Plans
  Reimbursement Mechanisms of Insurance Plans
  Prospective Reimbursement
  Covered Services
Cost Containment
  Historical Perspective of Cost Containment
  Current Trends in Cost Containment
Trends in Health Financing
  Cost Sharing
  Health Care Alliances
  Self-Insurance
  Flexible Spending Accounts

*The author would like to acknowledge the contributions of Carrie Morgan and Melanie McEwen, who wrote this chapter for the previous edition.

OUTLINE — cont'd

Health Promotion and Disease Prevention: Impact on
    Health Care Costs
Health Care Financing Reform
    Access to Health Care
    Historical Perspectives
    Societal Perceptions
    Health Care Reform—2010

**Roles of the Community Health Nurse in the Economics
    of Health Care**
    Researcher
    Educator
    Provider of Care
    Advocate
Best Care at Lower Cost

Economics represents the science of allocation of resources. Resources are commonly known as goods or services, for example, health care services. Economics affects all aspects of health care. Nurses have traditionally avoided the arena of health care economics, preferring to focus on the actual, direct care of the client. So strong is the feeling of social justice that some nurses express a reluctance to be informed of the individual client's health care financing source for fear that this knowledge will influence their care. Community health nurses who deal with the medically underserved have had more experience in this area. However, even these nurses may have only rudimentary knowledge.

Health care costs continue to rise and consume a greater percentage of our nation's resources. Nursing can no longer ignore the intricacies of health care financing. The health of individuals, families, and aggregates is influenced by economics. Economically disadvantaged individuals who have difficulty obtaining the basics, such as food and shelter, are less likely to have access to health care. The 2010 passage of the Patient Protection and Affordable Care Act (PL 111-148), however, should dramatically influence health care access. Indeed, when health care reform is fully implemented, almost all citizens will have health insurance, provided by their employers, through private purchase, or, for those from low income groups, through state and federal government sources (e.g., Medicare, Medicaid, Children's Health Insurance Plan [CHIP]). This change, however, is not to universal health care coverage.

This chapter focuses on the economics of health care. It specifically discusses factors that influence health care costs, terminology of health care financing, and trends in health care economics and their impact on community health. This chapter also addresses the future of health care financing. Box 12-1 presents terms and definitions that are important to the discussion of these topics.

FACTORS INFLUENCING HEALTH CARE COSTS

Historical Perspective

Until the 1930s, the predominant method of individual health care financing in the United States was self-payment. Health care providers charged a fee for the services they rendered, and the patient paid these out-of-pocket expenses. The price of the service was under the control of the provider and generally represented the cost of providing that service. A certain amount of "charity" services was expected. The assumption was that those who could pay would pay and those who could not pay should receive care and pay what they could. The concept of public financing of health care for a specific aggregate was restricted and varied from geographic area to area until the term *public health* came into common use.

The following types of hospitals existed:

1. Public hospitals, which received public funds and served the health care needs of the entire population regardless of ability to pay
2. Private hospitals, which cared mainly for those whose ability to pay was greater than that of the general population
3. For-profit hospitals, which were limited in number, received funds from investors, and cared for those who could definitely pay

Over time there has been growth in private and for-profit hospitals, resulting in large national hospital corporations that then expanded into offering more nonacute services.

This system worked well as long as those who could pay outnumbered those who could not. During the Great Depression, with more than 25% of the population out of work, the number of those capable of paying for health care was greatly reduced. Because public financing of health care was limited, hospitals, physicians, and other providers of health care went bankrupt.

In 1929, schoolteachers in Dallas, Texas, negotiated a prepaid health provision contract with Baylor Hospital. The teachers paid a sum of money each month, which guaranteed them access to health care through the hospital. The concept of insurance for health care proved extremely successful for Baylor Hospital. By 1939, this insurance plan had grown to include other groups and hospitals and became Blue Cross-Blue Shield (Momanyi, 2014).

Health insurance, or the idea of paying a small fee for guaranteed health care, appealed to the public. Societal concerns were mainly focused on sick care and acquisitions of curative therapies whenever needed. A public view that health insurance would provide freedom from fear that illness would impoverish them developed and prevails today. Health care providers envisioned guaranteed payment for their services (Higgins, 1997). During World War II, faced with a limited workforce and governmental restrictions on wages, employers began to see health insurance as a means of supplying workers' benefits without granting a wage increase.

BOX 12-1 TERMINOLOGY USED IN HEALTH CARE FINANCING

The financing of health care has given rise to new terminology. Nurses, as providers of care and consumers of services, need to be knowledgeable about these terms to improve their understanding of health care financing.

Terms Pertaining to Consumers

Access—Ability to obtain health care services in a timely manner, at a reasonable cost, by a qualified practitioner, and at an accessible location.

Carve-out service—A service (e.g., mental health care) provided within a standard benefit package, but delivered exclusively by a designated provider or group.

Charges—The posted prices of provider services.

Coinsurance—Cost sharing required by a health plan whereby the individual is responsible for a set percentage of the charge for each service.

Co-payment—Cost sharing required by the health plan whereby the individual must pay a fixed dollar amount for each service.

Deductible—Cost sharing whereby the individual pays a specified amount before the health plan pays for covered services.

Fee schedule—List of predetermined payment rates for medical services.

Flexible spending account (FSA)—A mechanism by which an employee may pay for uncovered health care expenses through payroll deductions.

Gatekeeper—Person in a managed care organization who decides whether a patient will be referred for specialty care. Doctors, nurses, nurse practitioners, and physician assistants function as gatekeepers.

Health care provider—An individual or institution that provides medical services (e.g., physicians, hospitals, or laboratories).

Health maintenance organization (HMO)—A managed care plan that acts as an insurer and sometimes a provider for a fixed prepaid premium. HMOs usually employ physicians.

Health plan—An insurance plan that pays a predetermined amount for covered health services.

Indemnity plan—A health plan that pays covered services on a fee-for-service basis.

Managed care plan—A health plan that uses financial incentives to encourage enrollees to use selected providers who have contracted with the plan.

Medicaid—Joint federal- and state-funded programs that provide health care services for low-income people.

Medicare—A health insurance program for people who are older than 65 years of age, are disabled, or have end-stage renal disease.

Medicare Advantage—Part of Medicare by which recipients may choose to enroll in a coordinated care plan, private fee-for-service, or medical savings account plan created by the Balanced Budget Act of 1997.

Medigap insurance—Privately purchased individual or group health insurance plan designed to supplement Medicare coverage.

Out-of-pocket expenses—Payment made by the individual for medical services.

Point-of-service (POS) plan—A managed care plan that combines prepaid and fee-for-service plans. Enrollees may choose to use the services of an uncontracted provider by paying an increased co-payment.

Portability—The guarantee that an individual changing jobs continues to receive health care coverage with the new employer without a waiting period or having to meet additional deductible requirements.

Preferred provider organization (PPO)—A health plan that contracts with providers to furnish services to the enrollees of the plan. Usually no insurance copayment is required.

Premium—Amount paid periodically to purchase health insurance benefits.

Primary care provider—A generalist physician, typically a family physician, internist, gynecologist, or pediatrician, who provides comprehensive medical services.

Terms Pertaining to Providers

Ambulatory care—Medical services provided on an outpatient basis in a hospital or clinic setting.

Capitation—Payment mechanism that pays health care providers a fixed amount per enrollee to cover a defined set of services over a specified period regardless of actual services provided.

Care management—Process used to improve quality of care by analyzing variations in and outcomes for current practice in the care of specific health conditions.

Cost containment—Reduction of inefficiencies in the consumption, allocation, or production of health care services.

Customary charge—Physician payment based on a median charge for a given service within a 12-month period.

Diagnosis-related group (DRG)—A system of payment classification for inpatient hospital services based on the principal diagnosis, procedure, age and gender of the patient, and complications.

Effectiveness—Net health benefit provided by a medical service or technology for a typical patient in community practice.

Full capitation—A stipulated dollar amount established to cover the cost of all health care services delivered for a person.

Maximum allowable costs—Specified cost level established by the health plan.

Outcome—The consequences of a medical intervention in a patient.

Physician's current procedural terminology (CPT) codes—A list of codes for medical services and procedures performed by physicians and other health care providers that has become the health care industry's standard for reporting physician procedures and services.

Practice guidelines—An explicit statement of what is known and believed about the benefits, risks, and costs of particular courses of medical action intended to assist decisions made by practitioners, patients, and others about appropriate health care for specific and clinical conditions.

Utilization review—A formal prospective, concurrent, or retrospective assessment of the medical necessity, efficiency, and appropriateness of health care services.

Terms Pertaining to Third-Party Payers

Actuarial classification—Classification of enrollees that is determined by use of the mathematics of insurance, including probabilities, to ensure adequacy of the premium to provide future payment.

Administrative costs—Costs that the insurer incurs for utilization review, marketing, medical underwriting, agents' commissions, premium collection, claims processing, insurer profit, quality assurance activities, medical libraries, and risk management.

Adverse selection—Procedure in which a larger proportion of people with poorer health status enroll in specific plans or options. Plans that enroll a subpopulation with lower-than-average costs are favorably selected.

Capital cost—Depreciation, interest, leases and rentals, taxes, and insurance on tangible assets.

Carrier—An organization that contracts with the CMS to administer claims processing and make Medicare payments to health care providers.

Cost contract—Arrangement between a managed health care plan and the CMS for reimbursement of the costs of services provided.

Cost shifting—The cost of uncompensated care is passed on to the insured, resulting in higher costs for those with insurance coverage.

Mandate—A state or federal statute or regulation that requires coverage for certain health services.

Risk assessment—Statistical method used to estimate claims costs of enrollees.

To extend this same "insurance" to the general population, the Social Security Act of 1935 was amended in 1965 to create Medicare and Medicaid. Medicare provided indemnity insurance to those over the age of 65 years, and Medicaid, a state-administered health plan, provided a source for financing health care for some of the poor and the disabled.

As a result of these health care resources, the majority of the population was protected by indemnity health care insurance from various sources. The indemnity plans lacked an incentive for limitation of use and had few or no provisions for health promotion. The emphasis was placed on illness care, providers received a fee only when a service was rendered, and all costs of services were reimbursed. Insulated from rising health care costs, health care consumers demanded complex and technologically advanced services whenever illness struck. These demands for costly services represented the major driving force in rising health care costs.

By the 1980s, the first efforts to curtail health care costs were made by the federal government. With institution of the prospective payment system (PPS), hospital reimbursement for Medicare patients was based on a classification system that identified costs according to diagnosis and client characteristics. The PPS prompted an evolution toward managed care, dramatically altering health care financing through the end of the twentieth century and into the first decade of the twenty-first century. Despite containment efforts, however, costs of health care have continued to rise.

The spiraling health care costs, starting from the mid-1960s and persisting into the twenty-first century, were fueled by the presence of technological advances, society's sense of entitlement to these therapies, a guaranteed payer, and the prevailing medical orientation toward curative measures. Prior to implementation of Medicare and Medicaid, national health expenditures represented less than 5% of the gross domestic product (GDP). Forty years later, however, costs have risen exponentially.

Use of Health Care

According to economic principles, the existence of a desirable product, the demand for the product, and the availability of financial funding influence the use of the product. Health care is the product, and the demand for this product increases when funding is available. In an attempt to reduce unnecessary utilization, insurance plans began to limit coverage for certain services and people; thus the move toward "managed care." Restrictions on use of health care, such as the establishment of a "gatekeeper," limited patient provider choice, requirement of preauthorization for some services, limited coverage for preexisting illnesses, and exclusion of those participants whose use was deemed exorbitant, have been instituted. These restrictions have had only limited success in curbing health care costs. Consumers were activated by these changes made by managed care, protesting them, and in many instances alterations were made. In 2010, spending for health care in the United States was more than double that of other developed countries (i.e., those in the Organization for Economic Cooperation and Development [OCED]). Indeed,

average per capita spending in that year was $3625 (9.5% of GDP) for OCED countries, compared with $8233 (17.6% of GDP) in the U.S. (OCED, 2012). Because the approach in the U.S. health care system is reimbursement with multiple insurers, both private and public, expenses for health care vary according to types of care and sources of funding.

Lack of Preventive Care

Until recently, little to no incentive has existed to prevent illness or promote health. Curative measures have traditionally been the focus of health care. Soaring health care costs and an improved knowledge of health have heightened the public's awareness of their obligation to assume responsibility for their health by amending many unhealthy behaviors. As a result, more people are demanding preventive health care from the provider and their health care contractors. Public financing of health care has increased funding for such preventive care as screening tests, periodic examinations, and immunizations. Use of these preventive health services has increased, but disparities persist in relation to ethnic background and economic status (National Center for Health Statistics [NCHS], 2009). There continues to be a gap between the amount of funding available for preventive treatment modalities and funding for curative treatments.

Lifestyle and Health Behaviors

A healthy lifestyle does not ensure good health but has been shown to contribute to longevity and productivity (Harvard Medical School, 2009). The five leading causes of death and illness can be positively affected by changes in lifestyle. Studies have now found that a low-fat diet, exercise, maintaining of an optimal body weight, smoking cessation, and stress reduction can modify or even prevent most chronic illnesses. Smoking cessation reduces the incidence of lung cancer. Seat belt use decreases the severity of injuries incurred during moving vehicle accidents. Effective treatment of illness must be coupled with a change in lifestyle. In the near future, access to expensive and unique medical treatment will probably be influenced less by the patient's ability to pay and more by the person's commitment to compulsory lifestyle changes. For example, legislation has levied "sin taxes" on products whose use has been associated with chronic illnesses. The Commonwealth of Kentucky has the highest rate of adult smoking in the country. To offset the cost of Medicaid care, the legislature levied a $0.30 per package cigarette tax. This income is utilized to fund care for, prevention of, and research on chronic illness (Commonwealth of Kentucky Department of Revenue, 2005).

Old movies dramatize the change in lifestyle that has taken place in the past 30 years. The current "smoke-free" environment appears shocking when contrasted to the nonchalant attitude toward smoking that was pervasive in the 1940s and '50s. The advent of the Health Belief Model and Pender's Health Prevention Model has given rise to numerous studies into methods of achieving lifestyle changes. The total effects of these changes are just now being seen. Meanwhile, the health care system must continue to contend with the results of years of unhealthy lifestyles.

Health care funding is changing to provide more funding for preventive services. Some insurance plans provide monetary incentives, such as reduction in insurance premiums, for those who participate in behavioral changes toward a healthier lifestyle. Medicare will pay for many screening procedures performed for specific persons at specified times (Centers for Medicare and Medicaid Services [CMS], 2010b). Funding for behavioral changes, however, is often limited, inadequate, or unavailable. Weight loss programs, support groups for smoking cessation, and participation in relaxation programs are not usually considered reimbursable treatment regimens, but more expensive pharmaceutical interventions are reimbursable.

Societal Beliefs

With the advent of such wonders as penicillin, society began to believe that the eradication of disease was just a few years away. More and more resources were dedicated to this elusive search. Armed with the belief that disease would soon be eliminated, society had limited interest in preventive care. The general belief was that making more money available for health care would lead to better health care and the greater likelihood that illness would be cured. Society has viewed insurance as an economic shield protecting against all disease and illness. The belief in cure rather than prevention, combined with this financial safety net, encouraged society to become a passive participant in health care. The feeling "I don't have to worry, I have insurance" became the pervasive societal thought (Sloan, 2004).

Health care professionals also were slow to embrace preventive care. Most efforts were directed toward curing illness. With what seemed to be an unending source of financing for curative care, illness prevention seemed counterproductive.

As health care costs accelerated at an alarming rate and technological advances did not keep up with the increase in illnesses, the health of society had to become a collaborative effort between society itself and the health care industry. Although the United States spends more money on health care than any other industrialized country, it ranks significantly behind many other countries in health status indicators (NCHS, 2009; OECD, 2012). People still expect the health care industry to cure them when they are ill, but there is now an increase in preventive care interest, including interest in health education, health promotion, and behavioral changes. Research into barriers and facilitators to lifestyle changes has increased, but it is not funded at the same level as curative measures (OECD, 2008; 2012). As discussed in Chapter 11, the United States continues to spend more money on health care and yet to have lower quality health care, than many other countries (Fineberg, 2012).

Technological Advances

Modern society has come to expect miraculous technological advances. In response to this expectation, and supplied with funding from various sources, technological advances have become too numerous to mention. The United States leads the world in laboratory and clinical research. People come from all over the world for education and to train in leading American centers for excellence (Weintraub and Shine, 2004). The United States exceeds other industrialized countries in the availability and use of these technological advances. Such advances can save the lives of people who would otherwise die.

These advances, although remarkable, are expensive, with the result that 20% of the population consumes 80% of the health care resources. As the health care dollar shrinks, these advances raise ethical questions involving health care access and rationing. Restriction on technology can significantly reduce the cost of health care, but the delays, inconvenience, and limitations to care with rationing would be strongly resisted by most Americans. An example of a growing technology area is telehealth:

> Telehealth has already started to play an even more important role, especially as we move away from the traditional fee for service system and toward new models of care, including accountable care organizations (ACOs), patient-centered medical homes (PCMHs), and other strategies that focus on outcomes. At the same time, the costs of telehealth technologies are dropping and [they are] becoming even easier to use. These technologies are becoming more widely prevalent in the marketplace, more accessible, and consequently, can be adopted more easily than perhaps 5 or 10 years ago. The pace of technological innovation is accelerating, but the cost of innovation is falling. (Institute of Medicine [IOM], 2012a, p. 7)

Telehealth has implications for community health as it expands care and access to specialists into the community. A key to success will be the cost factor.

Aging of Society

Health care expenditures rise with age, dramatically so at older ages. According to the latest population projections, individuals older than 65 years constituted about 12.8% of the total population in 2011; this proportion is expected to almost double by the year 2050 (U.S. Census Bureau, 2012). As people live longer the percentage of those older than 85 years is also increasing. Therefore, the number of those consuming the greatest amount of health care resources will rise more rapidly than the number of those who provide the monetary support for these resources. For example, the cost of care for Alzheimer's disease and related dementias is considerable, and the rate of such dementias is expected to rise as baby boomers age, with the expectation that cost for this care—which in 2010 was between $159 and $215 billion, depending on what factors were included—is expected to double by 2040 if no effective treatment or cure is found for the diseases (NIH-supported study, 2013).

Pharmaceuticals

A relatively new phenomenon that has influenced health care economics is the utilization of drugs, both over-the-counter and prescription drugs. New drugs are improving health outcomes and quality of life. These new drugs and new uses for older drugs are curing some illnesses, preventing or delaying other chronic diseases, and hastening recovery from yet other illnesses. As a result, during the last several decades, costs of prescription drugs have risen dramatically and have become a significant part of health expenditures. Seniors in particular are affected, because many have chronic illnesses that require daily medications.

In 2003, to help alleviate the costs of prescriptions for seniors, Medicare added a pharmaceutical benefit for enrollees. With implementation of the Medicare Prescription Drug and Modernization Act, all Medicare recipients are eligible to purchase insurance coverage to offset the costs of prescription drugs. As with other health care services, once a funding source has been established, utilization and costs increase. For 2006, the U.S. expenditure for pharmaceuticals was 1.5 times that of other industrialized countries, and these expenditures continue to rise (OCD, 2008).

Shift to For-Profit Health Care

The final contributor to the increase in health care costs is a national shift from nonprofit health care to for-profit health care. This has given rise to the term "health care industry." More and more large, for-profit organizations are taking over smaller community organizations. As the emphasis is on profit, mechanisms of achieving higher reimbursement have been developed, which have had an effect on health care costs.

Health Care Fraud and Abuse

Health care fraud has been an ongoing problem. The billions of dollars spent on health care and the struggles for control between providers, consumers, and health care organizations have increased the risk of fraud and abuse. The Federal Bureau of Investigation (FBI) estimates that health care fraud costs the U.S. $80 billion annually (FBI, 2012). The FBI is the primary agency that handles this fraud. Though all areas of health care and all payers experience fraud, Medicare and Medicaid have the highest levels (National Health Care Anti-Fraud Association [NHCAA], 2007). A number of actions have been taken to address this problem. Among them are the False Claims Act Amendments (1986), which allow private citizens to collect a percentage of recovered funds if they report fraudulent Medicare claims and monies are recovered as a result (Stanton, 2001). The Health Insurance Portability and Accountability Act (HIPAA) contains a set of provisions that address fraud, including a Fraud and Abuse Control Program, the Medicare Integrity Program, and the Health Care Fraud and Abuse Data Collection Program. Each of these programs is designed to address concerns over health care fraud. In addition, HIPAA legislation dramatically raised funding for fraud enforcement activities (Michael, 2003).

Major health care fraud and abuse incidents have influenced the most vulnerable of the population (i.e., the mentally ill and older adults). In recent years, overbilling and unnecessary visits in home health care were reported across the United States, resulting in widespread reforms to Medicare reimbursement for home health services (Infante and McAnaney, 2004).

BOX 12-2   MEDICARE FRAUD

What is fraud?
- Billing Medicare for services not received
- Billing Medicare for services other than those received
- Use of another's Medicare card to obtain services
  Be suspicious if providers tell you:
- Medicare wants you to have this service.
- They know how to get Medicare to pay for service.
- The more services provided, the cheaper they are.
  Be suspicious if providers:
- Change co-payment of Medicare-approved services.
- Advertise "free" consultations to those with Medicare.
- Claim they represent Medicare.
- Use pressure to persuade you of the need for high-priced services.
- Use telemarketing as a marketing tool.
  Whenever you receive a Medicare payment notice, review it for errors. Make sure Medicare was not billed for services not received.

Modified from Centers for Medicare and Medicaid Services: *Medicare fraud: detection and prevention tips*, n.d. Available from <www.medicare.gov/Fraud Abuse/Tips.asp>.

President Obama's health care reform legislation includes provisions to reduce fraud and abuse in public programs. It encourages screening of providers and enhanced oversight for initial claims for durable medical equipment suppliers. The law requires Medicare and Medicaid program providers and suppliers to establish compliance programs and develops a database to share fraud and abuse information among federal and state programs. Finally, it increases penalties for submitting false claims and increases funding for antifraud activities (Kaiser Family Foundation, 2010). Box 12-2 describes consumer tips related to health care fraud and abuse.

PUBLIC FINANCING OF HEALTH CARE

As the popularity and benefits of employer-provided insurance plans were recognized, it became evident that the health care of some segments of society was being neglected. The 1960s, with a pervasive thrust for social justice in the public and political arenas, presented the ideal opportunity for governmental participation in health care financing. In 1965, the federal government enacted the first movement toward universal health care coverage. Titles XVIII and XIX of the Social Security Act created Medicare and Medicaid, respectively.

Medicare

Medicare is a federal entitlement program that is totally funded by the federal government (Figure 12-1). This program is intended to help cover the costs of health care for people 65 years of age and older and people who are disabled or have end-stage renal disease. Medicare is divided into four parts. Medicare Part A is basically hospital insurance. Services covered by Medicare Part A include inpatient care in hospitals and skilled nursing facilities (not unskilled or long-term care). It also covers hospice care and some home health care. Most U.S. residents are eligible for premium-free Medicare Part A benefits when they reach age 65, on the basis of their own or their

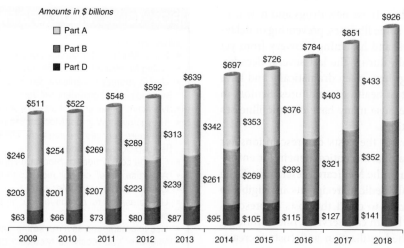

FIGURE 12-1 Overall Medicare spending, 2009-2018. (Adapted from Kaiser Family Foundation: *Update on Medicare spending and financing and highlights from the 2009 Medicare trustees' report*. Avenue from http://kff.org/health-reform/report/update-on-medicare-spending-and-financing data from Board of Trustees of the Federal Hospital Insurance and Federal Supplementary Medical Insurance Trust Funds: *2009 annual report*, Washington, DC, 2009, Author.)

spouse's employment. Although Medicare Part A is an entitlement program, the enrollee must pay a deductible for health services. The Part A deductible is the beneficiary's only cost for up to 60 days of Medicare-covered inpatient hospital care in a benefit period. Beneficiaries have to pay an additional co-payment per day for days 61 through 90, and this co-payment increases per day for hospital stays beyond the ninetieth day in a benefit period. The CMS website provides current information on costs for beneficiaries.

Those individuals who are eligible for Medicare Part A may purchase Medicare Part B for a monthly fee. Medicare Part B is medical insurance that helps pay for out-of-pocket costs related to physician services, hospital outpatient care, durable medical equipment, and other services, including some home health care. The monthly premium paid by beneficiaries enrolled in Medicare Part B has changed over time. In addition to the monthly premium, Part B requires subscribers to pay deductibles and coinsurance (CMS, 2010b). The CMS website provides current information on these costs.

Medicare Part C, also known as the Medicare Advantage Plans, is optional "gap" coverage provided by private insurance companies that are approved by, and under contract with, Medicare, and may include health maintenance organizations (HMOs) and preferred provider organizations (PPOs). Covered services vary by plan and may include vision, hearing, and dental care as well as other services and supplies not covered by Medicare Parts A, B, and D. Costs vary by plan, and to be eligible, the individual must have Medicare Parts A and B and must live in the service area of the plan (CMS, 2010b).

Medicare Part D was initiated in 2006 to help defray the costs of prescription drugs. Like Parts B and C, Medicare Part D is optional, and if eligible Medicare recipients choose this option they must enroll in an approved prescription drug plan. Most participants in Medicare Part D pay a monthly premium, a yearly deductible, and co-payments, with out-of-pocket costs based on the plan selected and drugs used. In addition to these costs, the enrollee is responsible for cost

that can vary of prescription drug costs once the total costs reach a certain amount in a year. This is termed the "coverage gap" or "donut hole." When the enrollee's out-of-pocket total for drugs reaches a particular level, Medicare will pay 95% of the costs of any further prescription drugs. The CMS website provides current information on the amounts to be paid.

Medicaid

Title XIX of the Social Security Act established the Medicaid Program. Medicaid is a public welfare assistance program that finances health care coverage for the indigent and children. Eligibility for this program, a joint venture with state and federal funding, depends on the size and income of the family, and priority participation is given to children, pregnant women, and the disabled.

The federal government sets baseline eligibility requirements for Medicaid. State governments that wish to provide care to more citizens through this program can lower the eligibility requirements. For example, the federal government may set 100% of poverty as an eligibility requirement, but an individual state may set the requirement as 110% of poverty. This means that a family living in that state can have an income slightly above the federal standard and still qualify for Medicaid.

The federal government mandates covered services, but state governments may provide more services. Mandated services covered by Medicaid for eligible recipients include inpatient and outpatient hospital care, pregnancy-related care, vaccines for children, family planning services, rural health clinic services, home health care, laboratory and radiography services, and Early and Periodic Screening, Diagnosis, and Treatment (EPSDT) services for children younger than 21 years. Care provided by pediatric and family nurse practitioners is covered. Optional services that states may elect to provide include optometrist services and glasses, intermediate care facilities for the mentally disabled, rehabilitation, physical therapy, and hospice (Kaiser Family Foundation, 2009a).

Medicaid and CHIP currently (2011) provide coverage to some, but not all, low-income individuals and people with disabilities. Medicaid and CHIP cover 17.6% of the nonelderly population by primarily covering four main categories of low-income individuals: children, their parents, pregnant women, and individuals with disabilities. Individuals who do not fall into one of these groups—most notably adults without dependent children—are now generally ineligible for public coverage regardless of their income. Adults without dependent children comprise the majority of the uninsured population largely because they are the least likely to qualify for Medicaid. (Kaiser Family Foundation, 2012, p. 3)

Aside from Medicaid, many children younger than 18 years are eligible for the CHIP. Established in 1997 and reauthorized in 2009, CHIP is a program that provides insurance for children of low socioeconomic families who do not qualify for Medicaid. Like Medicaid, the program is administered by the states, which share the cost with the national government. President Obama's health care reform plan requires expansion of Medicaid and CHIP to cover many of those who were previously uninsured. The final decision as to whether Medicaid will be expanded in a state will be made by the state. The law provides federal payment of services for newly eligible Medicaid beneficiaries from 2014 to 2016, after which the federal government will pay 90% of the cost for several more years. Given that Medicaid is currently jointly funded by states and the federal government, this is a change, but it would affect only newly enrolled beneficiaries during this period. The requirement for states to decide whether they will participate has caused some states to consider not participating. This situation is due to politics. If states opt out of participating, there are implications for how the law is implemented in those states to provide insurance options because the law requires health care insurance coverage. The final outcome is not yet known.

Governmental Grants

Unlike individual health care services, governmental grants are directed toward funding large populations and different aggregates. Historically, the bulk of health promotion and disease preventive measures have been limited to this arena of public health care. All three levels of government provide the major contribution of funding for these programs. On the national level the U.S. Department of Health and Human Services (USDHHS, also called HHS) administers this funding.

A variety of funding grants are available through the HHS (USDHHS, 2007). These health grants are administered through the public health department at each governmental level or community. A large part of the federal government funding provided to the states through "block grants." These are "blocks" of funds provided to the states to impact the health of the public as a whole. There are specific restrictions on how these monies can be spent, including limitations on the population that receives the services and what types of programs are to be funded. The states use these monies to provide for the care of the public within these restrictions. Depending on the health needs of the state, these monies may be spent to provide direct aggregate care, but most often they are used for health promotion activities that are directed at

a larger percentage of the population. Each level of government may make funds available for a specific health need of the members of the community.

To ensure that the needs of the community are being addressed, health care providers and programs may be required to compete for these funds. Proposals, grant applications, or requests must be submitted, reviewed, and prioritized. Funds are allocated on the basis of need and program merit. This type of funding is directed toward the population in general and not to specific individuals. When the funding is no longer provided, the programs cease, leading to lack of continuity of care. Currently, the funding priorities are closely related to the achievement of the *Healthy People 2020* objectives. Limitations on the amounts provided are related to available governmental resources.

PHILANTHROPIC FINANCING OF HEALTH CARE

A limited amount of the nation's health care bill is paid by philanthropic sources whose priorities are usually capricious and oriented toward research or disease. Eligibility for services through these associations is generally limited to the specific disease or population of interest, as with the American Heart Association. Few direct services are rendered, and these services are approved on individual case considerations. Ancillary health care needs such as transportation, parental housing, or wigs may be addressed. Informational and research activities constitute the majority of services provided by these types of organizations. The organizations fund many educational programs that increase awareness of specific diseases, screening procedures, and preventive measures.

An example of philanthopic national organizations is the Shriners-operated health care institutions designed to provide specialty care for a specific population group. These services and all costs related to this care, including transportation, are often provided to the eligible person free of charge. The only requirement for this care is sponsorship by a member of the supporting organization.

HEALTH CARE INSURANCE PLANS

Historical Perspective

During the 1930s, in an effort to provide care and avoid bankruptcy, health care providers began to establish health insurance plans. One of the most recognizable of these plans is Blue Cross and Blue Shield. Those enrolled in the plan, called *enrollees,* paid a monthly fee for a guarantee of health care. Providers delivered services to the enrollees and collected payment from the health insurance plan. The insurance plan paid fees plus its administrative costs from money collected from the enrollees.

During World War II, when prices and wages were frozen, industries began to offer health care insurance as a fringe benefit to employees. In 1953, as a further employer incentive to offer health care coverage to employees, money spent on health insurance was declared tax-exempt. Over the years, workers' union groups began to negotiate for these benefits. With more available financial resources, the health care expenditures increased. Reimbursement based on operational costs represented a strong incentive for health care expansion (Higgins, 1997). Reasons for lack of health care insurance were costs, change in employment, change in marital status, and death of spouse or parent (NCHS, 2008). Even though the United States has an employer-based insurance system, only 61% of businesses provided health insurance coverage for employees in 2012 (Kaiser Family Foundation, 2012). Smaller businesses typically find it more costly to provide coverage, and some businesses do not provide coverage for part-time employees. This situation will change with health care reform because more employers will be required to provide coverage options.

Types of Health Care Plans

The early Blue Cross and Blue Shield was an example of an indemnity plan. This plan paid all of the costs of covered services provided to the enrollee. The enrollee enjoyed free choice of provider and services. Indemnity plans preserve the enrollee's right of choice and allow the person to manage his or her own health care. These plans lack incentives for cost containment. Although indemnity plans are still available, the monthly cost of enrollment has increased to exorbitant amounts, making the plans cost prohibitive. In an effort to support these plans these incentives while preserving freedom of choice, mechanisms of cost sharing were introduced. These cost-sharing methods include co-payment, deductible amounts, and coinsurance. All of these methods represented efforts to have the enrollee share in the cost of medical care.

As health care costs escalated, variations in health care insurance plans were developed. Industries, the major providers of insurance coverage, began to look for a more economical means of providing health care to their employees. Kaiser Permanente decided to assemble their own health care programs. They built hospitals, hired physicians, and provided health care services to their employees. In an effort to market this concept, Dr. Paul Elwood coined the phrase health maintenance organization (HMO) (Higgins, 1997). HMOs were designed to provide more comprehensive care, but this type of program lacks enrollee freedom of choice. Preventive care is covered and encouraged, but care is somewhat restricted, and HMOs are encouraged to reduce costs by providing only the most necessary services. This loss of choice led to a decrease in popularity of HMOs. In the United States, the number of HMO plans peaked in the mid-1990s, when about 31% of the population was enrolled in them, and they continue to represent a small portion of the plans.

In an effort to compete with the HMO, physicians and hospitals organized the independent practice model (IPM). The IPM was a separate entity that provided services to enrollees of one insurance company. This model evolved into the preferred provider organization (PPO). These types of insurance plans negotiated with health care providers for services at a reduced rate in exchange for a guaranteed increase in consumers. A negotiated reimbursement rate allows the cost of the plan to be somewhat controlled. Plan enrollees are offered cost incentives for choosing health care from within the plan's network of health care providers. Because they receive a specific amount of reimbursement, regardless of the rendered services, providers have an incentive to be cost-conscious of the services provided (Ginsburg, 2004). PPOs are more flexible than HMOs, but to receive full benefits, the covered individual must use network providers. PPOs are the most common type of insurance plan in the United States.

Point-of-service (POS) plans combine elements of the HMO and the PPO. In POS plans, the covered individual designates an in-network physician as the primary health care provider (PCP). If the individual goes outside the network for care, he or she will be responsible for most of the costs unless referred by the PCP. POS plans were common during the early years of the twenty-first century, but interest dropped off over time.

Private Insurance

Costs of private health insurance are staggering, often prohibitively high, so it is not a popular choice. However, individuals who are not employed but still working, such as consultants and other freelance workers, may be forced to pay private health insurance fees in order to get insurance coverage. They represent a small segment of the population.

Health Insurance–Purchasing Cooperatives

Multistate networks or alliances are health insurance–purchasing cooperatives that establish purchasing pools responsible for negotiating health insurance arrangements for employers, employees, and state Medicaid recipients. These alliances use the volume of health consumers that they represent as leverage to negotiate contracts for health care coverage. Provider membership in the alliance is voluntary but exclusive. If the provider is located in an area in which the alliance is the predominant insurance plan, the provider is financially forced to join and to accept the negotiated reimbursement.

Cafeteria Plans

Another means of providing the enrollee with choice, but at the same time allowing the plan to control prices, is a "cafeteria plan." Insurance providers may offer the enrollee or consumer a wide variety of choices. Employers may specify the amount of money that will be contributed toward health care. The consumers may then customize their health care coverage according to their needs and willingness to pay. By choosing the types of services they want covered and the provider of these services, consumers have some control over their own health care costs. Consumers assume financial responsibility for any costs that exceed the employer's contributing amount (Clark, 2003).

Reimbursement Mechanisms of Insurance Plans
Retrospective Reimbursement

When insurance plans were initially offered, the customary method of reimbursement was a fee for the service rendered, or retrospective reimbursement. Calculation of the fee was based on the cost of providing the service. Included in this "umbrella" of costs were such things as salaries, supplies, equipment, building depreciation, utilities, and taxes. Cost-based reimbursement encouraged inflated prices and fraud.

Physicians were encouraged to overtreat patients, and participants were encouraged to overuse the health care system.

Prospective Reimbursement

Prospective reimbursement (i.e., the PPS), a concept derived from the HMO method of payment, seemed to be an effective financial alternative to cost-based reimbursement. Prospective reimbursement meant that care, no matter what the provider's cost, would be reimbursed according to a predetermined amount. The government introduced this method of reimbursement for Medicare in 1983, and an immediate savings was noted. The prospective reimbursement rates are based on diagnoses and patient characteristics. These factors are represented by codes, following the *International Classification of Diseases, Tenth Edition,* or ICD-10 (Centers for Disease Control and Prevention [CDC], 2010). Physician services are given current procedural terminology (CPT) codes. Coding of the patient's illness can result in an increase in reimbursement. Specialists in coding, as well as computer programs, are employed by both third-party payers and service providers. Third-party payers' code specialists scrutinize the claims for the appropriate data to support the code. Service provider code specialists are paid to ensure that the code is as accurate as possible to obtain the higher reimbursement. The appropriateness of services is based on the diagnosis code. For example, spirometry is appropriate (reimbursable) when the patient's diagnosis code indicates a variety of pulmonary and nonpulmonary conditions. Specialists in coding can quickly identify these codes, thus increasing payment for services. Physician visits, or CPT codes, are reimbursed on the basis of the documentation of the degree of "medical decision making" and time spent with the patient. Computerized medical record programs increase the ability to ensure that the visit can be reimbursed at the highest rate possible. This development has changed health care practices to the utilization of services that are low in costs and higher in reimbursement. High-cost services are limited or are not offered.

Figure 12-2 illustrates how the nation's health care dollar was spent in 2011. For determination of the prospective amount, Medicare depended on the diagnosis-related group (DRG) to calculate the reimbursement. The amount to be paid to the provider was determined according to the client's primary and secondary diagnoses, age, gender, and complications. This amount was deemed sufficient cost for health care ascertained to be adequate for treatment. If the provider, at first limited to hospitals but later other type of providers, could provide the treatment for less than this amount, a profit was made. If the required services cost more than this amount, then the provider took a loss (Rozzini, Sabatini, and Trabucchi, 2005).

Implementation of the PPS led to a reduction in Medicare costs but did not result in overall health care cost savings as intended. Hospitals developed cost shifting as a means of supplementing the loss of Medicare funding. Private insurance's reimbursement continued to be cost based. Therefore, hospitals could include the loss from caring for Medicare patients in their cost. Private insurance companies were paying for the cost of providing care to their enrollees and to Medicare patients.

Only a few years after implementation of the PPS by Medicare, private health care plans followed the government's lead. In an effort to ensure appropriate reimbursement, more

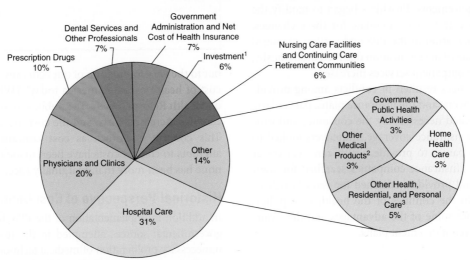

The Nation's Health Dollar ($2.7 Trillion), Calendar Year 2011: Where It Went

[1] Includes Research (2%) and Structures and Equipment (4%).
[2] Includes Durable (1%) and Non-durable (2%) goods.
[3] Includes expenditures for residential care facilities, ambulance providers, medical care delivered in non-traditional settings (such as community centers, senior citizens centers, schools, and military field stations), and expenditures for Home and Community Waiver programs under Medicaid.
Note: Sum of pieces may not equal 100% due to rounding.
SOURCE: Centers for Medicare & Medicaid Services, Office of the Actuary, National Health Statistics Group.

FIGURE 12-2 The Nation's Health dollar, Calendar Year 2011: Where It Went. (From Department of Health and Human Services, Centers for Medicare and Medicaid Services, Office of Actuary, National Health Statistics Group. Available from <https://www.cms.gov/Research-Statistics-Data-and-Systems/Statistics-Trends-and-Reports/NationalHealthExpendData/downloads/PieChartSourcesExpenditures2011.pdf>.)

sophisticated methods of calculating the relative cost of health care were developed. Actuarial classifications ensured that adequate premiums were charged for the projected health care needs of those enrolled, and other means of cost control began to emerge. Managed care groups negotiated with health care providers to render care for a specified amount of reimbursement based on community ratings modified by group-specific demographics (Turner, 1999). Prospective reimbursement created incentives to control costs but also led to instances of undertreatment and underuse of the system.

Covered Services

Insurance plans have always designated the types of services for which a plan would be financially responsible. When first developed, health insurance was meant to be a means of protecting an individual or family from economic catastrophe should a serious illness occur. Once an employee's fringe benefits included health insurance coverage, expanded benefit packages were developed. The scope of covered services began to widen to include such things as physician's office visits, medication, and dental costs. Unions began to negotiate for such expansion of covered medical services in lieu of additional wages.

When health care costs increased, so did the price of enrollment into the insurance plans. Industries began to refuse to pay these higher premium rates. Workers became disgruntled when their employers passed the cost of increased rates to them. To curtail the escalating premium price, insurance companies began to limit the covered services and dictate the conditions under which these services would be covered. Sites of care delivery changed. More treatments were required to be delivered outside the hospital, or in ambulatory care centers. The patient was held financially responsible for "uncovered" services. Providers were pressured to comply with these requirements. Providers began to modify the delivery of health care to accommodate for these changes. Following implementation of the PPS and various managed care options, the rate of hospitalization declined dramatically, and the number of outpatient services increased.

All of these changes resulted in conflicts among providers, patients, employers, and the insurance plans, particularly when services deemed necessary by the consumer and provider were denied insurance coverage. Employers looked to the insurance companies to provide health care services at a reasonable price. Insurance companies searched for ways to control costs, and providers searched for ways to deliver needed care within the confines of the health care policy. Table 12-1 describes some of the advantages and disadvantages of insurance reimbursement plans.

COST CONTAINMENT

Limiting health care costs is an imperative. All recent presidents, including Clinton, Bush, and Obama, have recognized that spiraling health care costs have eroded an already suffering economy. Early in his presidency, President Obama stated that "one of the greatest threats not just to the well-being of our families and the prosperity of our businesses,

TABLE 12-1	CONSUMER ADVANTAGES AND DISADVANTAGES OF INSURANCE REIMBURSEMENT PLANS	
TYPE	**ADVANTAGES**	**DISADVANTAGES**
Indemnity Fee for service	No gatekeeper	High premiums
	Unlimited choice of providers	Potential for overuse
	Full access to all services	No incentive for cost containment
Managed care	"Credentialed" providers promote quality assurance	
Health maintenance organization (HMO)	Comprehensive care	Restricted to plan provider
	Lower premium	Potential for lower quality care to maximize costs
	No deductibles or co-payment	
Preferred provider organization (PPO)	Greater selection of providers than with HMO	Gatekeeper
	Expedited provider reimbursement	Additional cost for out-of-plan provider
	Lower premiums	Potential for lower quality care to maximized costs
Point of service (POS)	More flexibility	Deductible
	Comprehensive services with plan	20%-50% co-payment for out-of-plan services
		Primary care provider referral needed for specialized care

but to the very foundation of our economy ... is the exploding cost of health care in America today" (White House Forum on Health Reform, 2009). The public's increasing demand for care has increased costs, and the costs need to be controlled. This concept is known as cost containment. Numerous attempts to control costs have been made over the years, but none has been more than marginally successful.

Historical Perspective of Cost Containment

In addition to implementation of the PPS, health insurers and governmental sources attempted in the mid-1980s to curtail unnecessary proliferation of medical technology by requiring a certificate of need (CON) for additions to current health care buildings or services. To further reduce use, hospital records were reviewed for the appropriateness of care provided. Admission and treatment of hospitalized patients were reviewed by peer standard review organizations (PSROs). Physicians and other medical personnel reviewed the hospital records and counseled the attending physician about unnecessary or excessively lengthy stays in the hospital as well as unwarranted services.

⚖ ETHICAL INSIGHTS

Cost Containment: How Will You Make Decisions?

You are the gatekeeper, meeting with others in your community health organization to determine what services to provide to clients. You have $400,000 to divide among the needs. Who of the following clients will receive the required treatment? Who will not?

1. A child with broken leg needs physical therapy (estimated cost: $10,000).
2. A 55-year-old man requires knee replacement surgery and physical therapy (estimated cost: $40,000).
3. A 76-year-old woman requires hip replacement (estimated cost: $40,000).
4. A 32-year-old woman with leukemia requires a bone marrow transplant (estimated cost: $350,000).
5. The community clinic needs new equipment for laboratory tests (estimated cost: $60,000).
6. There is need for a new nurse who can act as a case manager for patients with complex diseases (estimated cost: $75,000 per year).

Questions to Consider

1. How does the American Nurses Association *Code of Ethics* apply to this case?
2. What factors should be considered in the decision?
3. How much does the cost of treatment affect the decision?
4. How much does the age of the patient affect the decision?
5. Is social justice a factor in the decision?

The cost reduction, as a result of prospective payment and other efforts, gave rise to the managed care revolution. Unable to shift costs to other entities, and with a predetermined reimbursement rate, providers searched for the most cost-effective mechanism of care provision. Greater ability to predict the cost of care enabled health care plans to negotiate the best value for their premiums.

Current Trends in Cost Containment

The managed care form of health care financing changed economic incentives and forced health care providers to rethink health management decisions. Treatment recommendations may be tied more to "Can you afford this?" rather than "This is best for you." Costs of the service rendered, rather than enhancement of revenue through service provision, must be considered. These economic or cost-containment incentives can be divided into the following broad categories: capitated reimbursement, access limitation, and rationing.

Capitated Reimbursement

The growing visibility of managed care models and their associated success in cost containment through the use of prospective reimbursement to influence provider practice gave rise to various arrangements that link health care financing to service delivery such as managed care. Managed care organizations create partnerships with health care providers

RESEARCH HIGHLIGHTS

Hospital Readmissions from Home Health Care Before and After Change to Prospective Payment System

In an effort to control the Medicare home health expenditure, home health reimbursement was changed from a fee-for-service system to a prospective payment system (PPS). This changed the reimbursement from a per-visit fee to episodes of care. Each episode of care begins on the first billable day and proceeds for a period of 60 days. Reimbursement is based on the diagnosis and type and level of care predicted to be required.

Through the use of a comprehensive evaluative tool, the Outcome and Assessment Information Set (OASIS), a client is placed in a home health resource group (HHRG). Payment for services is based on the HHRG. Another important factor is that payment is received in two parts: 60% at the start of care and 40% after the episode of care is completed. Adjustments in final payment are made according to changes in the client's condition and may result in more or less than anticipated.

Anderson and colleagues (2005) chose to study unplanned hospital readmissions, which are an aspect of adverse change in patient condition or outcome. This study was designed to compare characteristics of clients rehospitalized during home health care before and after the institution of PPS.

The sample size of 76 clients was chosen from a Midwestern U.S., not-for-profit, Medicare-certified, hospital-affiliated home health care agency. This agency served approximately 280 to 300 clients daily. Characteristics of the clients at time of rehospitalization were determined by means of a Hospital Readmission Inventory. This instrument has an interrater reliability of 96%. Closed-case medical records were reviewed.

The sample was matched for characteristics such as age, sex, marital status, referral sources, and length of stay in home health care. For all pre-PPS clients in the sample, the primary diagnosis at hospital discharge and readmission was chronic obstructive pulmonary disease and congestive heart failure. For post-PPS clients, the primary diagnosis at hospital discharge and readmission was circulatory associated. Pre-PPS clients' length of stay was 13 days, compared with 9.01 days for post-PPS clients.

From this study it is difficult to conclude whether PPS has any negative effect on home health care patient outcomes. The data set does confirm that during the first 2 weeks after discharge, there was an increase in the number of different nurses caring for the client, in comparison with the care provided by the same nurse to the home health client. Post-PPS clients were judged to be sicker at the time of rehospitalization and were almost twice as likely to be readmitted for another diagnosis. The investigators concluded that, since the institution of PPS in 2000, the hospital length of stay has decreased, with the result that clients are sicker at time of discharge.

The study shows that the first 2 weeks following hospital discharge are the most critical. Payments for home health services are suspended at the time of readmission, pending a client's return to home health care after rehospitalization. If the client does not return to home health care and the agency has completed five visits, 60% of the payment will awarded. If the agency has not completed the five visits, only 11% of the amount will be awarded. This arrangement might serve as an incentive for agencies to increase the number of visits after the initial hospital discharge but not after the second discharge.

Data from Anderson MA, Clarke MM, Helms LB, et al: Hospital readmission from home health care before and after prospective payment, *J Nurs Scholarsh* 37(1):73-79, 2005.

using financial incentives to prevent overuse. Statistical norms, practice parameters, and population data determine the capitated, or maximum, payment for services. This is the maximum reimbursement amount that the health care provider will receive for the provision of care. The actual cost of provision of care does not affect the reimbursement. Health care providers must provide appropriate medical care while being cognizant of health care costs. As a reward for conservative practices, health care providers may receive a specified amount of money or a percentage of the agreed reimbursement if services are delivered below the limit set by the third-party payer. Providers whose services are inadequate or exceed this limit may be excluded from the network.

Cost Containment Through Access Limitation

All third-party payers, or insurance plans, control access to health care through designation of covered services. Managed care organizations designate the type of covered services and specify the conditions under which the service is covered. Some services may only be accessed upon approval or referral from physicians who are used as gatekeepers. The enrollee must choose a primary care provider and consult this provider for a referral before seeking specialty services. Without this referral, the enrollee is financially responsible for the service. Even with the referral, choices may be limited to the providers who have contracted with the managed care plan.

Managed care plans may require that less costly health care modalities or medications be used. Exceptions to these modalities require justification. More technologically advanced and expensive treatments may be accessed under the most stringent conditions. Preauthorization requirements determine the medical necessity of the service. The process is so complex that the client may not be aware that the service is not covered until the reimbursement for the service is denied.

Cost Containment Through Rationing

Rationing is best described as determining the most appropriate use of health care or directing the health care where it can do the most good. The following clinical example dramatizes the problem.

Clinical Example

A middle-aged woman was diagnosed with ovarian cancer. She was covered by Medicaid, lived alone in subsidized housing, and had a distant relative in another state. Following surgery some years ago, she used home health services through the city home health agency. After conventional and high-dose chemotherapy failed, her physician recommended autologous bone marrow transplantation, which was considered experimental at the time. The procedure was approved and performed. Medical costs exceeded $200,000, but the patient died 2 months later.

Was this a wise use of medical resources? Health care is not an exact science; too many variables exist. What appears to be the best course of action for one is not the best course of action for another. Making accurate treatment decisions is

difficult, and the ramifications of a mistake are great. Complex socioeconomic factors also must be considered. Health care providers and third-party payers, including the federal government, are currently investigating the outcomes of health care practices to determine what methods, if any, can be instituted to improve the accuracy of these choices. Research into the area of treatment outcomes has led to major changes in treatments, many of which are very costly. This situation presents a dilemma when decisions must be made as to their use.

TRENDS IN HEALTH FINANCING

The public's demand for affordable health care has created a new environment for health care financing. Competition among health care providers and third-party payers has led to new and innovative health care. Outpatient services, patient education packages, electronic health records, and telehealth are just a few of these innovations. Increased competition has required insurance plans to be sensitive to the needs of the employee organizations and their enrollees. Individualized plans of covered services can be created. Enrollees can choose the plan that provides them with the services they desire at a selected cost. Health care providers advertise to ensure that the consumer selects an insurance plan that includes their services. Some providers, such as hospitals, campaign for inclusion in a plan.

There is no doubt that health care costs will continue to increase.

In 2014, national health spending is projected to rise to 7.4 percent, or 2.1 percentage-points faster than in the absence of reform, as the major coverage expansions from the Affordable Care Act (ACA) are expected to result in 22 million fewer uninsured people (compared to estimates that exclude the law's impacts). Increases in Medicaid spending growth of 18.0 percent and private health insurance growth of 7.9 percent both contribute to this overall acceleration in national health spending in 2014. Conversely, out-of-pocket spending is projected to decline 1.5 percent as third-party coverage will cover expenses previously paid by consumers out of pocket. Because the newly insured populations are anticipated to be relatively younger and healthier than currently insured individuals they are expected to devote a greater proportion of their spending to prescription drugs and physician and clinical services, and a smaller proportion of their spending to more acute care, such as hospital care. Consequently, prescription drug spending growth is projected to reach 8.8 percent in 2014 (4.7 percentage-points faster than in the absence of reform) and spending on physician and clinical services is projected to grow at 8.5 percent (3.2 percentage-points faster than in the absence of reform). On the other hand, hospital spending growth is projected to reach 6.7 percent, just 1 percentage-point faster than in the absence of reform. (CMS, 2012)

Cost Sharing

Aware of the amount that the employer is willing to contribute for basic coverage, a third-party payer or insurance plan may propose several options, giving the employee freedom to choose services desired. Employees willing to pay may be able to increase the covered services not provided by the basic plan. This arrangement is known as *cost sharing*. Cost sharing may also require the consumer to pay a greater portion of the bill for covered services in return for lower premiums. Enrollees may opt to pay a higher premium for the freedom to choose providers, or elimination of the gatekeeper. This can result in increased consumer control of health care.

Health Care Alliances

The creation of powerful regional or statewide insurance purchasing pools, or health alliances, is seen as one of the means of reform for the health care industry. The alliance would define basic benefits that all insurers would have to offer to everyone at the same price regardless of health status. These alliances would not regulate insurance prices. Health alliances would collect premiums and help consumers choose among competing insurers and plans. The consumer's choice would be based on published, simple, standard information about benefits and outcomes of the different available plans. Plans would have to compete by offering better outcomes or lower cost. Insurers would have to contract with providers who find ways of delivering cost-efficient care. Medicare is currently participating in health care alliances. Enrollees are given a choice between traditional Medicare, Parts A and B, and Medicare Advantage.

Self-Insurance

Some organizations have used health care information collected by insurance plans to self-insure their employees. This development has enabled industries and other types of organizations to reduce the administrative cost of insurance. Unlike the large industrial HMOs, self-insured status organizations administer their own health care plan and purchase health care services from an established insurance plan. In these cases the organizations or businesses are relying on a healthy employee population that will require less health care. The organization or business that uses self-insurance takes a risk and needs to ensure that it can cover any major costs. Health care reform will require that there be sufficient funds to cover these costs.

Flexible Spending Accounts

Another source of funding for uncovered services is the flexible spending account (FSA). The employee determines how much he or she will have to spend for uncovered services and arranges to have this amount deducted from his or her paycheck. When these services are incurred, the employee pays for them with this account. The employee continues to pay into the account until the estimated amount is reached. If the employee overestimates the cost, the remaining amount is forfeited. If the cost of the services exceeds the estimate, only the amount estimated will be paid. Health care reform legislation limits the amount of money that can be put into FSAs.

Health Promotion and Disease Prevention: Impact on Health Care Costs

"We can agree that if we want to bring down skyrocketing costs, we'll need to modernize our system and invest in prevention," stated President Obama (White House Forum on Health Reform, 2009). Unfortunately, reimbursement for health promotion and disease prevention continues to be limited. Most health insurance plans, both private and public, pay for screening procedures. However, funding or reimbursement for treatment modalities such as support groups for smoking cessation, home safety evaluation, and relaxation techniques is not common. Obesity is one of this nation's most common health problems, yet the costs of weight loss programs are not reimbursed.

Research into barriers and facilitators to changes in lifestyle continues to be funded well below curative treatment research. Lifestyle change interventions are slow to be developed and even more difficult to implement and evaluate (Reid et al., 2009). For example, research into weight loss strategies found that documenting all food intake was effective in initial and sustained weight loss (Hollis et al., 2008). Until these types of interventions are directly financed, they most likely will not become widely implemented. With rise in obesity there have been state proposals, and some have been initiated, to incentivize healthy eating habits, such as taxing the sale of sodas and putting calorie counts on restaurant menus. This type of approach relies heavily on policy and subsequent legislation, and causes some people to protest because they consider it invasion of their personal decisions. Some businesses have taken these steps themselves, such as restaurants that have added calorie and nutritional information to their menus.

HEALTH CARE FINANCING REFORM

It has been estimated that in 2011, more than 48 million nonelderly Americans were uninsured (Kaiser Family Foundation, 2012). Certain racial/ethnic groups have higher rates of underinsurance. The ranking of such groups from highest to lowest rate of non-insurance is: Hispanic, American Indian, Black/non-Hispanic, Asian, multiracial, White/non-Hispanic (Kaiser Family Foundation, 2012). Underinsurance is also a problem, as the underinsured cannot fully cover their health needs.

Lack of insurance is the major factor associated with lack of access to medical care. Uninsured adults are more than three times as likely as insured adults to go without needed medical care (NCHS, 2010). In order to appreciate the potential impact of health care reform, one can look at the issue of lack of insurance among young adults. "The uninsured rate among young adults, ages 19 to 25, has improved slightly in the last year. The share of young adults that were uninsured decreased from 30.0% in 2010 to 27.9% in 2011, due in part to the ACA provision allowing them to remain on a parent's private health plan until age 26. The change in coverage for this age group accounted for about 40% of the overall decline in the number of uninsured. However, young adults continue to have a high uninsured rate" (Kaiser Family Foundation, 2012, p. 9).

The Affordable Care Act (ACA) calls for each state to set up an "exchange," or marketplace, where small businesses (those with 100 or fewer employees) and people not covered through their employers could shop for health insurance at competitive rates. Some of those insured through the exchanges would pay for the insurance coverage themselves, while others with relatively low incomes would receive subsidies to help defray the cost of the premiums. As envisioned, the exchanges, which are to be operational by 2014, will offer four levels of plans—platinum, gold, silver, and bronze— that would vary in price. States have flexibility in how the insurance exchanges would operate, and in fact, states can opt out of setting up an exchange. A federally operated exchange would operate in those states that do not set up one themselves. (IOM, 2012b)

The IOM notes that health literacy and communication will be key factors in success as consumers try to figure out the new legislation and use the exchanges to obtain insurance if their employers are not providing this information directly. The success of this process will impact access to health care.

Access to Health Care

Access to health care is a complex situation that is defined by the circumstances of the individual. The primary concern is inadequate access to health care, which leads to unnecessary illness. Most Americans want to believe that the best possible health care will be available for them and their family members at any time regardless of their age, sex, race, or ability to pay. Anything that obstructs this pursuit can be considered a barrier to health care.

Financial support for health care, through either private insurance coverage or participation in government programs, is the mechanism that is largely responsible for access. Lack of a source for health care financing due to lack of insurance coverage, preexisting conditions, unapproved care, and physicians who do not participate in the health plan available to the patient, represent the most common factors attributed to difficulty in obtaining care. Other impediments to health care access are physical barriers, including structural inaccessibility, lack of appropriate equipment, hours of operation, convenient transportation, inadequate services when needed, and inability to communicate.

Inequality in the distribution of health care services represents another type of physical barrier. Even those with insurance coverage may be unable to locate participating health care providers. Opportunities to seek health care, especially preventive health care, during work hours is often discouraged by employers, although this situation is gradually changing as some employers recognize that preventive care can reduce overall costs. Rural areas and inner cities have been recognized as medically underserved for many years. Government incentives for increasing available medical services in these areas have not solved the problem.

Sociological barriers to health care access exist among poor and ethnic Americans. Poor outpatient diagnosis and treatment, increased use of emergency departments for primary care, and reluctance to hospitalize are possible explanations. Language and fear of reprisals have become important sociological barriers. Many of the poor and uninsured are illegal aliens, and seeking medical attention, even during illnesses, may have severe repercussions. Disparities are discussed later in the text.

Historical Perspective

National health insurance is not a new concept. European countries began a social model of health insurance in the early 1900s. In 1916, President Theodore Roosevelt advocated enactment of a form of national medical coverage. President Franklin Roosevelt wanted national health insurance to be part of the Social Security Act of 1935, but that provision did not pass (Higgins, 1997). During the administration of President Lyndon Johnson, however, a modified form of national health insurance, Medicare and Medicaid, was instituted.

Before the 1930s, most Americans were uninsured. Most health care providers considered it their duty to donate time and services to charity. Hospitals and clinics maintained charity wards. Society believed that those who could, and those who could not, should help themselves. The enactment of governmental entitlement programs, coupled with the availability of health care insurance as a benefit of one's occupation, helped change this belief. Quickly, the pervasive societal view was that those who could not help themselves should get government assistance or go to work (Higgins, 1997).

As discussed earlier in the 1960s Medicare and Medicaid brought about national health insurance coverage for older adults, the disabled, and those, especially children, living below the poverty level. Expansion of Medicaid with CHIP in the 1990s expanded care coverage for children of the "working poor," or those whose employers did not provide insurance.

During the 1992 presidential campaign, Bill Clinton promised to reform America's health care system, ensure universal coverage, and reduce medical care costs without damaging the economy. At that time, it was thought that basic health care coverage for all individuals could be achieved over several years. After a year of debate and numerous proposals, the Clinton plan eventually failed to reach a consensus because of widespread opposition from various health care provider groups and organizations as well as lack of support of the public.

Societal Perceptions

Social justice, in the form of equal health care for all, is a concept that most Americans support. Most people state that health care should be one of those necessities available to all without consideration of what it costs; however, when discussion turns to actually do this, many people get concerned about the implications. Efforts to provide universal coverage through increased governmental involvement in health care have failed because of a number of factors, including rejection of much higher taxes, objection to paying for care for noncitizens, concerns over access and availability, and fears of rationing.

The current dilemma is how to provide health care to all Americans in a way that is acceptable and affordable. Other countries provide their citizens with universal health care, but there are aspects of this care that are unpopular with U.S. society. The most concerning or pressing problem relates to funding sources, because significant tax increases would be necessary to provide coverage for all. Waiting several months for nonemergency treatment, lack of choice of treatment, and inaccessibility or unavailability of diagnostic and treatment modalities are not acceptable to most Americans. Indeed, most Americans want assurance that all of the health care services that they and their families need, now and in the future, will be available no matter what the condition, age of the patient, job status, or ability to pay.

Health Care Reform—2010

During the 2008 presidential campaign, health care reform was a key issue. The election of President Obama and Democratic Party majorities in both houses of Congress helped pave the way for significant changes in health care financing. After hundreds of deliberations that were often contentious, and after more than a year of debate, Congress passed the Patient Protection and Affordable Care Act (PL111-148), also known as the Health Care Reform Act, which was signed into law March 23, 2010. Although the Act does not ensure "universal coverage" per se, the Congressional Budget Office (CBO) estimated that when fully implemented, it will ensure that an additional 32 million people will have access to health insurance coverage (Kaiser Family Foundation, 2010).

The Health Care Reform Act is an extremely complex piece of legislation, and the final version of the bill exceeded 2000 pages. There are many health-related provisions of the law. Examples of these provisions are: mandating that all citizens obtain health insurance; expanding Medicaid eligibility; subsidizing insurance premiums for low-income purchasers; prohibiting denial of coverage for preexisting conditions; and establishing health insurance exchanges. Costs for expansion of coverage and subsidies will be offset by a combination of taxes and fees, reduction in payments for Medicare and Medicaid services and prescription drugs, and enhanced efforts to reduce Medicare fraud and abuse. Box 12-3 outlines some of the major provisions covered in the health care reform legislation.

A few of the provisions of the Health Care Reform Act were implemented in 2010, but most do not take effect until 2014. The law will not be fully implemented until 2018. Furthermore, the law remains very controversial, and legislative and legal challenges are anticipated. All health care providers and consumers should remain alert to both short- and long-term changes in health care financing and health care delivery that will result. Additional information about this law can be found in Chapter 10.

ROLES OF THE COMMUNITY HEALTH NURSE IN THE ECONOMICS OF HEALTH CARE

Researcher

Nurses need to be engaged in research about the provision of efficient, cost-effective health care. Nurses are in a pivotal role to investigate culturally sensitive treatment modalities, health education, disease prevention, and factors to change behaviors. Health promotion and disease prevention are more cost-effective than curative treatment modalities. Community health nurse researchers need to investigate, develop, and evaluate the effectiveness of health promotion and disease prevention. Research on health promotion intervention outcomes, program cost/benefit analysis, and health informatics are just a few of these areas.

Educator

Health education is the foundation of community health nursing practice. Community health nurses agree that knowledge empowers clients to actively participate in their health care.

BOX 12-3   HIGHLIGHTS OF THE PATIENT PROTECTION AND AFFORDABLE CARE ACT (P.L. 111-148)

Individual Mandate—Requires U.S. citizens and legal residents to have qualifying health coverage.

Employer Requirements—Requires employers with more than 50 employees to offer coverage or vouchers for full-time employees; requires employers with more than 200 employees to enroll employees into health insurance plans offered by the employer.

Expansion of Medicaid—Expands Medicaid to all individuals under age 65 with incomes up to 133% of the federal poverty line.

Expansion of CHIP—Requires states to maintain current income eligibility levels for children enrolled in the Children's Health Insurance Plan (CHIP) until 2019.

Premium and Cost-Sharing Subsidies to Individuals—Creates insurance exchanges to provide premium credits and subsidies to individuals and families with incomes between 133% and 400% of the federal poverty level.

Changes to Private Insurance—Establishes a temporary national high-risk pool to provide health coverage to individuals with preexisting medical conditions; establishes a process for reviewing increases in health plan premiums and requires justification of increases; provides dependent coverage for children up to age 26 years for all individual and group policies; prohibits health plans from placing lifetime limits on the dollar amount of coverage and from rescinding coverage; establishes a website to help residents identify health coverage options; permits states to form health care choice compacts and allow insurers to sell policies in any state participating in the compacts.

Cost Containment Provisions—Requires rules to simplify health insurance administration by adopting a single set of rules for payment, verification, and claims status; restructures payments to Medicare Advantage plans; reduces waste, fraud, and abuse in public programs by allowing providers to have screening-enhanced oversight periods for new providers and suppliers; increases penalties for submitting false claims.

Prevention and Wellness—Improves prevention by covering preventive services and eliminating cost sharing for preventive services in Medicare and Medicaid; requires qualified health plans to provide preventive services, recommended immunizations, preventive care for infants, children, and adolescents, and additional preventive care and screening for women; provides grants for small employers who establish wellness programs; requires chain restaurants and foods sold from vending machines to disclose the nutritional content of each item.

Modified from The Henry J. Kaiser Family Foundation: *Summary of new health reform law (#8061)*, April 2010. This information was reprinted with permission from the Henry J. Kaiser Family Foundation. The Kaiser Family Foundation is a non-profit private operating foundation, based in Menlo Park, California, dedicated to producing and communicating the best possible analysis and information on health issues.

Funding for this education is provided primarily through public governmental plans. Educational plans for individuals are almost nonexistent. In the area of health care economics, the nurse needs to demonstrate the value of this education. Outcome measures for health education need to be established.

Provider of Care

Any service delivered by the nurse needs to be appropriate, necessary, and cost-effective. Nurses in all areas of practice need to be cost-conscious. Judicious application of the nursing process is imperative. An accurate assessment is the foundation for an appropriate nursing diagnosis. Goals for care, jointly established between members of the community and the community health nurse, will guide the choice of interventions. Evaluation, using previously developed outcome measures, will lead to appropriate modifications of the plan.

Nurses can serve as program service providers, health education providers, and health program participants. Nurses need to participate in the grant proposal process, design, and evaluation for these programs. They need to be familiar with and participate in the statistical information gathering process that serves as the basis for determining community health need.

Advocate

Nurses must become more involved in the economics of health care. Too often, nurses are cognizant of the effects of changes in health care economics but feel powerless to act. Increasing knowledge of health care funding and policy making will empower nurses to advocate for the type of funding that provides appropriate care to obtain the greatest good. The large number of nurses gives our occupation potential political clout. Nurses need to utilize this political power to influence health care funding. Nurses need to advocate for increase in health promotion/disease prevention funding from both public and private sectors. Nurses need to plan programs, seek funding, and evaluate program effectiveness through outcome measures. Nurses need to constantly seek sources of funding for health programs through any available sources.

BEST CARE AT LOWER COST

In 2012, the IOM published a report entitled *Best Care at Lower Cost: The Path to Continuously Learning Health Care in America*. Building on its earlier work in relation to quality care (discussed in Chapter 11), the IOM was asked to examine a critical concern. "Health care in America presents a fundamental paradox. The past 50 years have seen an explosion in biomedical knowledge, dramatic innovation in therapies and surgical procedures, and management of conditions that previously were fatal, with ever more exciting clinical capabilities on the horizon. Yet, American health care is falling short on basic dimensions of quality, outcomes, costs, and equity" (IOM, 2013, Ab-1). Among the factors that are pushing this examination is the fact that there is an estimated $750 billion waste of resources in the health care system, meaning that the United States loses this amount of money that could be spent on improved health care outcomes. We need best care at lower cost, not higher cost. Compared with other countries, the United States is paying more for less—poorer outcomes. The system has to manage the complexity that continues to grow and at the same time slow down ever-escalating costs. Citizens want quality care that is evidence-based, but the system is not managing this well.

SUMMARY

Health care economics is influencing health care practice at all levels. Nurses in community health must become aware of the economics of health care to practice in this new era. Patient outcomes are quickly being seen as a measurement for health care financing. As the health care system evolves toward health promotion and disease prevention, nursing will play a pivotal role. Community health nurses, whose domain of practice has encompassed these areas, will be in the forefront of this change. This chapter has presented the basics of health care economics and its importance in providing effective, quality care in all settings, including the community. An understanding of these elements is essential to the practice of nursing. This is an ever-changing field with innovations and changes coming every day. To be effective, the nurse must be attentive to these developments.

LEARNING ACTIVITIES

1. Learn more about changes in health care reimbursement due to health care reform by visiting http://www.cms.gov/cciio/index.html. http://cciio.cms.gov/resources/factsheets/ehb-2-20-2013.html This CMS website is the Center for Consumer Information and Insurance Oversight. What type of information is provided? What is the value of this information to consumers?

2. Evaluate a family's health care coverage. Investigate the type of coverage and the ability of this coverage type to meet the needs of the family. Is there another type of insurance coverage that would meet more of the family's needs? What prohibits their ability to obtain this coverage?

3. Investigate the Health Care Reform Act from the points of view of the consumer, health care provider, and third-party payer and community health. How will it affect the concerns of each of these constituents?

4. Examine the status of health care reform implementation in your state. How has the community been informed about changes? Has this been effective? How is it impacting community health in your state?

5. Interview public health nurses employed in a public health department about their perception of funding for health promotion/disease prevention.

6. Interview an official from your LHD about finances. Identify strengths and weaknesses. Consider solutions for one of the weaknesses.

7. In small groups review the Institute of Medicine report *U.S. Health in International Perspective: Shorter Lives, Poorer Health* (2013). Divide up the content. Discuss this report from perspectives of the health care delivery system, quality care, diversity, and cost of care. The report is fully accessible and can be downloaded from http://www.iom.edu/Reports/2013/US-Health-in-International-Perspective-Shorter-Lives-Poorer-Health.aspx.

ⓔ EVOLVE WEBSITE

http://evolve.elsevier.com/Nies

- NCLEX Review Questions
- Case Studies
- Glossary

REFERENCES

Centers for Disease Control and Prevention (CDC): *International classification of diseases, tenth revision, clinical modification (ICD-10-CM)*, 2010. Available from <http://www.cdc.gov/nchs/icd/icd10cm.htm#10update>.

Centers for Medicare and Medicaid Services (CMS): *National health expenditure projections, 2010–2021*, 2010a. Available from <https://www.cms.gov/Research-Statistics-Data-and-Systems/Statistics-Trends-and-Reports/NationalHealthExpendData/index.html>.

Centers for Medicare and Medicaid Services (CMS): *Medicare and you, 2010*, 2010b. Available from <http://www.medicare.gov/Publications/Pubs/pdf/10050.pdf>.

Centers for Medicare and Medicaid Services: *Medicare fraud: detection and prevention tips*, n.d. Available from <www.medicare.gov/Fraud Abuse/Tips.asp.>.

Centers for Medicare and Medicaid Services (CMS): *National health expenditures projections: 2011-2021*, 2012. Available from <https://www.cms.gov/Research-Statistics-Data-and-Systems/Statistics-Trends-and-Reports/NationalHealthExpendData/NationalHealthAccountsProjected.html>.

Clark K: Cost cure-all? Or unhealthy shift? Employers seek to pass on the workers more of the burden of soaring medical costs, *US News World Rep* 135(21):38–39, 2003.

Commonwealth of Kentucky Department of Revenue: *Tobacco taxes*, 2005. Available from <revenue.ky.gov/business/tobaccotax.htm>.

Congressional Research Service: *U.S. Health Care Spending—comparison with other OCED countries*, 2007. Available from <http://digitalcommons.ilr.cornell.edu/cgi/viewcontent.cgi?article=1316&context=key_workplace>.

Federal Bureau of Investigation: *Health care fraud*, 2012. Available from <http://www.fbi.gov/about-us/investigate/white_collar/health-care-fraud>.

Fineberg H: A successful and sustainable health care system—how to get there from here, *New England Journal of Medicine* 366:1020–1027, 2012.

Ginsburg P: Controlling health care costs, *N Engl J Med* 351:1591–1593, 2004.

Harvard Medical School: *Harvard's Men's Health Watch*. The numbers game: Risk factors, lifestyle and longevity 13:2009 8.

Higgins W: How did we get this way? *Health Care Econ* 11:35, 1997.

Hollis J, Gullion C, Stevens V, et al: Weight loss during the intensive intervention phase of weight loss maintenance trial, *J Prevent Med* 35(2):118–126, 2008.

Infante M, McAnaney K: Home health agencies can avoid fraud charges with compliance plans, *Hosp Home Health* 21(5):49–51, 2004.

Institute of Medicine: *The role of telehealth in an evolving health care environment: a workshop summary*, Washington, DC, 2012a, National Academies Press.

Institute of Medicine: *Facilitating state health exchange communication through the use of health literate practices: workshop summary*, Washington, DC, 2012b, National Academies Press.

Institute of Medicine: *Best care at lower cost: the path to continuously learning health care in America*, Washington, DC, 2013, National Academies Press.

Kaiser Family Foundation: *Medicaid: a primer*, 2009a. Available from <http://www.kff.org/medicaid/upload/ 7334–03.pdf>.

Kaiser Family Foundation: *Employer medical benefits, 2009: annual survey*, 2009b. Available from <http://ehbs. kff.org/pdf/2009/7936.pdf>.

Kaiser Family Foundation: *Focus on health reform*, 2010. Available from <http://www.kff.org/healthreform/upload/8061.pdf 2010b>.

Kaiser Family Foundation: *The uninsured: a primer*, 2012. Available from <http://kff.org/uninsured/report/the-uninsured-a-primer-key-facts-about-health-insurance-on-the-eve-of-coverage-expansions/>.

Michael JE: What home healthcare nurses should know about fraud and abuse, *Home Healthcare Nurse* 21(8):523–530, 2003.

Momanyi B: Blue cross and blue shield of texas handbook of texas online. http://www.tshaonline.org/handbook/online/articles/djbcz, accessed January 11, 2014. Published by the Texas State Historical Association.

National Health Care Anti-Fraud Association: *Health care fraud: a serious and costly reality for all Americans*, 2007. Available from <http://www.nhcaa.org/eweb/docs/nhcaa/PDFs/about nhcaafinal.pdf>.

National Center for Health Statistics: Health: *United States, 2009*, 2010. Available from <http://www.cdc.gov/nchs/data/hus/hus09.pdf#126>.

NIH-supported study finds U.S. dementia care costs as high as $215 billion in 2010. *NIH News*, April 3, 2013. Available from <http://www.nih.gov/news/health/apr2013/nia-03.htm>.

Organization for Economic Co-operation and Development: *Health data 2010*, 2012. Available from <http://www.oecd.org/els/healthpoliciesanddata/oecdhealthdata2012-frequentlyrequesteddata.htm>.

Reid G, van Teijlingen E, Douglas F, et al: The reality of partnership working when undertaking an evaluation of a national well men's service, *J Mens Health* 6(1):36–49, 2009.

Rozzini R, Sabatini T, Trabucchi M: Diagnosis related groups and hospital costs in elderly dependent patients, *J Am Geriatr Soc* 53:174–175, 2005.

Sloan T: Consumer-driven to nowhere: study throws cold water on recent efforts to beat health care cost inflation, *Mod Healthcare* 34(49):21, 2004.

Stanton T: Fraud-and-abuse enforcement in Medicare: finding middle ground, *Health Affairs* 20(4):28–42, 2001.

Turner SO: *The nurse's guide to managed care*, Gaithersburg, MD, 1999, Aspen.

U.S. Census Bureau: *U.S. population projections: 2000-2050*, 2012. Available from <www.census.gov/.../projections/files/analytical-document09.pdf>.

U.S. Census Bureau: *Current population survey, 2011*, 2012. Available from <http://www.census.gov/population/age/data/2011.html>.

U.S. Department of Health and Human Services: *Grants and funding*, 2007. Available from <www.hhs.gov/grants/index.shtml>.

Weintraub W, Shine K: Is a paradigm shift in US healthcare reimbursement inevitable? *Circulation* 109:1448–1455, 2004.

White House Forum on Health Reform: *Report*, March 5, 2009. Available from <www.whitehouse.gov/assets/documents /White_House_Forum_on_Health_Reform_Report.pdf>.

Cultural Diversity and Community Health Nursing

Carrie L. Buch*

OBJECTIVES

Upon completion of this chapter, the reader will be able to do the following:

1. Critically analyze racial and cultural diversity in the United States.
2. Analyze the influence of sociocultural, political, economic, ethical, and religious factors that influence the health of culturally diverse individuals, groups, and communities.
3. Identify the cultural aspects of nursing care for culturally diverse individuals, groups, and communities.
4. Apply the principles of transcultural nursing to community health nursing practice.

KEY TERMS

biomedical
cultural competence
cultural imposition
cultural negotiation
cultural stereotyping
culture
culture-bound syndrome
culture shock
culture specific

culture universal
culturological assessment
dominant value orientation
ethnocentrism
Leininger's theory of culture care diversity and universality
magicoreligious
naturalistic
norms

poverty
religion
socioeconomic status
spirituality
subculture
transcultural nursing
value
yin-yang theory

OUTLINE

Cultural Diversity
Transcultural Perspectives on Community Health Nursing
Population Trends
Cultural Perspectives and *Healthy People 2020*
    Addressing Racial and Ethnic Disparities in Health Care
Transcultural Nursing
Overview of Culture
    Culture and the Formation of Values
    Culture and the Family

Culture and Socioeconomic Factors
    Distribution of Resources
    Education
Culture and Nutrition
    Nutrition Assessment of Culturally Diverse Groups
    Dietary Practices of Selected Cultural Groups
    Religion and Diet
Culture and Religion
    Religion and Spirituality
    Childhood and Spirituality

* The author would like to acknowledge the contribution of Margaret M. Andrews, who wrote this chapter for the fourth edition.

OUTLINE—con'd

Culture and Aging
Cross-Cultural Communication
  Nurse-Client Relationship
  Space, Distance, and Intimacy
  Overcoming Communication Barriers
  Nonverbal Communication
  Language
  Touch
  Gender
Health-Related Beliefs and Practices
  Health and Culture
  Cross-Cultural Perspectives on Causes of Illness
  Biomedical Perspective
  Folk Healers
  Cultural Expressions of Illness
  Cultural Expression of Pain
  Culture-Bound Syndromes
Management of Health Problems: A Cultural Perspective
  Cultural Negotiation

Management of Health Problems in Culturally Diverse Populations
  Providing Health Information and Education
  Delivering and Financing Health Services
  Developing Health Professionals from Minority Groups
  Enhancing Cooperative Efforts with the Nonfederal Sector
  Promoting a Research Agenda on Minority Health Issues
Role of the Community Health Nurse in Improving Health for Culturally Diverse People
  Culturological Assessment
  Cultural Self-Assessment
  Knowledge about Local Cultures
  Recognition of Political Issues of Culturally Diverse Groups
  Providing Culturally Competent Care
  Recognition of Culturally Based Health Practices
Resources for Minority Health
  Office of Minority Health
  Indian Health Service

CULTURAL DIVERSITY

Cultural diversity is a multifaceted and complex concept that refers to the differences among people, especially those related to values, attitudes, beliefs, norms, behaviors, customs, and ways of living. It is essential that all nurses understand how cultural groups view life processes, how cultural groups define health and illness, how healers cure and care for members of their respective cultural groups, and how the cultural background of the nurse influences the way in which care is delivered. Nurses in community health settings also need to understand the diversity or differences that occur in families, groups, neighborhoods, communities, and public and community health care organizations.

TRANSCULTURAL PERSPECTIVES ON COMMUNITY HEALTH NURSING

Nurses' knowledge of culture and cultural concepts improves the health of the community by enhancing their ability to provide culturally competent care. Cultural competence is respecting and understanding the values and beliefs of a certain cultural group so that one can function effectively in caring for members of that cultural group. Culturally competent community health nursing requires that nurses understand the lifestyle, value system, and health and illness behaviors of diverse individuals, families, groups, and communities. Nurses should also understand the culture of institutions that influence the health and well-being of communities. Nurses who have knowledge of, and an ability to work with, diverse cultures are able to devise effective interventions to reduce risks in a manner that is culturally congruent with community, group, and individual values.

The "Standards of Practice for Culturally Competent Nursing Care" established by the Expert Panel on Global Nursing and Health (2010) provide important guidelines to help nurses provide culturally competent care. The 12 standards are:

1. Social Justice
2. Critical Reflection
3. Knowledge of Cultures
4. Culturally Competent Practice
5. Cultural Competence in Health Care Systems and Organizations
6. Patient Advocacy and Empowerment
7. Multicultural Workforce
8. Education and Training in Culturally Competent Care
9. Cross-Cultural Communication
10. Cross-Cultural Leadership
11. Policy Development
12. Evidence-Based Practice and Research

In the United States, metaphors such as *melting pot* describe the cultural diversity that characterizes the population. Although there is a tendency to identify the federally defined racial and ethnic minority groups when referring to the cultural aspects of community health nursing, all individuals, families, groups, communities, and institutions, including nurses and the nursing profession, have cultural characteristics that influence community health. When planning and implementing health care, community health nurses need to balance cultural diversity with the universal human experience and common needs of all people.

POPULATION TRENDS

The population of the United States is becoming increasingly diverse. In recent years, the populations within the federally defined minority groups have grown faster than the population as a whole. In 1970, minority groups accounted for 16% of the population. By 2010, this share had increased to 36% (U.S. Census Bureau, 2011). Assuming that current trends continue, the U.S. Census Bureau (2012) projects that, by 2025, more than half of all children will be minorities and that, by 2050, minorities will account for 54% of the total population. For the first time in U.S. history, minorities will make up a majority of the total population.

Furthermore, the numbers of certain minority groups, such as Hispanics, are growing considerably faster than those of whites and other groups. If current demographic trends continue, the United States will have the following population composition by the year 2060: white, 44%; Hispanic, 30%; African American, 15%; Asian, 9%; and American Indians and Alaska Natives, 2% (U.S. Census Bureau, 2012).

Although the nursing profession has representatives from diverse groups, minorities are generally underrepresented. Currently about 82.2% of registered nurses (RNs) in the United States are white/non-Hispanic. Estimates for each minority group are as follows: African American, 5.6%; Hispanic, 3.9%; Asian and Pacific Islander, 5.8%; and Native American and Alaska Native, 0.6% (Health Resources and Services Administration [HRSA], 2010). Additionally, each minority group is distributed differently around the country. African American nurses are more likely to be found in the South, Hispanics in the West or South (i.e., especially states bordering Mexico), and Asian and Pacific Islanders in the West or Northeast. Native American and Alaska Native nurses are predominantly in states with Native American reservations.

The United States has grown and achieved its success largely through immigration. Since 1991, more than 13 million legal immigrants have come to United States (U.S. Department of Homeland Security, 2006). In 2010, the U.S. population included almost 40 million foreign-born individuals, or 12.9% of the total population. Among those foreign born, 53.1% were born in Latin America, 28.2% in Asia, 12.1% in Europe, and the remaining 9% in other regions of the world (U.S. Census Bureau, 2012). The number of immigrants and refugees in the United States is projected to continue to increase.

In addition, people from other countries continue to seek treatment in U.S. hospitals, particularly for cardiovascular, neurological, and cancer care. Furthermore, U.S. nurses have the opportunity to travel abroad to work in a variety of health care settings in the international marketplace. In the course of a nursing career, it is possible to encounter foreign visitors, international university faculty members, international high school and university students, family members of foreign diplomats, immigrants, and refugees. Moreover, members of some cultural groups desire culturally relevant health care that incorporates their specific beliefs and practices. A growing expectation exists among members of certain cultural groups that health care providers will respect their "cultural health rights." However, this expectation frequently conflicts with the unicultural, Western biomedical worldview taught in most U.S. educational programs. Therefore, a serious conceptual problem exists within nursing, in that nurses are expected to know, understand, and meet the health needs of these culturally diverse individuals, groups, and communities without adequate preparation.

♥ HEALTHY PEOPLE 2020

Selected Objectives Related to Cultural Health

- Increase the proportion of all degrees awarded to members of underrepresented racial and ethnic groups among the health professions, allied and associated health profession fields, the nursing field, and the public health field
- Reduce the proportion of adults who are obese
- Reduce the overall cancer death rate
- Reduce the rate of new cases of end-stage renal disease (ESRD)
- Reduce the rate of lower extremity amputations in persons with diabetes
- Reduce coronary heart disease and stroke deaths
- Reduce pregnancy rates among adolescent females
- Reduce low birth weight (LBW) and very low birth weight (VLBW)
- Reduce human immunodeficiency virus incidence among adults and adolescents
- Reduce hospitalizations for sickle cell disease among children age 9 years and under
- Achieve and maintain effective vaccination coverage levels for universally recommended vaccines among young children
- Reduce past-month use of illicit substances
- Reduce firearm-related deaths
- Improve health, fitness, and quality of life through daily physical activity

From U.S. Department of Health and Human Services: *Healthy People 2020*: *topics and objectives,* Available from http://www.healthypeople.gov/2020/topicsobjectives2020/default.aspx.

CULTURAL PERSPECTIVES AND HEALTHY PEOPLE 2020

Healthy People 2020, identifies priority areas and objectives. By developing a set of national health targets, which includes eliminating racial and ethnic disparities in health U.S. health officials, together with state and local officials and members of the private sector, set goals to improve the quality and increase the years of healthy life for all Americans (U.S. Department of Health and Human Services [USDHHS], 2013).

The *Healthy People 2020* objectives embrace and focus on ways to close the gaps in health outcomes. Particularly targeted are racial and ethnic disparities in areas such as diabetes, acquired immunodeficiency syndrome (AIDS), heart disease, infant mortality rates, cancer screening and management, and immunizations. The objectives bring focus on disparities among racial and ethnic minorities, women, youth, older adults, people of low income and education, and people with disabilities (USDHHS, 2013). The *Healthy People 2020* box lists selected objectives from *Healthy People 2020* specific to cultural health issues.

The aims of *Healthy People 2020* are the promotion of healthy behaviors, promotion of healthy and safe communities, improvement of systems for personal and public health, and prevention and reduction of diseases and disorders. The initiative is a tool for monitoring and tracking health status, health risks, and use of health services.

Addressing Racial and Ethnic Disparities in Health Care

As in many nations, people in the United States who come from various racial, ethnic, cultural, and socioeconomic backgrounds often experience marked disparities in health care. The occurrence of many diseases, injuries, and other public health problems is disproportionately higher in some groups; access to health care may be more restricted, and the overall quality of health care is deemed inferior, for people from certain racial, ethnic, and cultural populations. Although the overall health of the U.S. population has improved during the past several decades, research reveals that all people have not shared equally in those improvements. For example, 17% of Hispanic adults and 16% of African American adults report that they are in fair or poor health, compared with 10% of non-Hispanic whites (Agency for Healthcare Research and Quality, 2013).

Primary care provides the foundation for the health care system, and research indicates that having a usual source of care increases the chance that people will receive adequate preventive care and other important health services. Data from the Agency for Healthcare Research and Quality (2013) reveal the following facts:

- Cancer mortality rates are 35% higher in African Americans than in whites.
- African Americans are 13% less likely to undergo coronary angioplasty and one-third less likely to undergo bypass surgery than are whites.
- Thirty percent of Hispanics and 20% of African Americans lack a usual source of health care (compared with fewer than 16% of whites).
- Hispanic children are nearly three times as likely as non-Hispanic white children to have no usual source of health care.
- African Americans (16%) and Hispanic Americans (13%) are more likely to rely on hospitals or clinics for health care than are whites (8%).

During the past two decades, health disparities have become the focus of numerous federal, state, and local government studies, and one of the major goals of *Healthy People 2020* is to achieve health equity, eliminate disparities, and improve the health of all groups (USDHHS, 2013). Therefore, it is essential to look at how to overcome these and other identified factors that contribute to poorer health among members of some minority groups. A survey by the Commonwealth Fund (2007) found that disparities in health care can be reduced or even eliminated when adults have health care insurance and a *medical home,* which is defined as "a health care setting that provides patients with timely, well-organized care and enhanced access to providers." According to the survey, when adults have insurance and a medical home, "their access to needed care, receipt of routine preventive screenings, and management of chronic conditions improve substantially."

TRANSCULTURAL NURSING

In 1959, Madeleine Leininger, a nurse-anthropologist, used the term transcultural nursing to define the philosophical and theoretical similarities between nursing and anthropology. In 1968, Leininger proposed her theory-generated model, and, in 1970, she wrote the first book on transcultural nursing, *Nursing and Anthropology: Two Worlds to Blend* (Leininger, 1970). According to Leininger (1978), transcultural nursing is "a formal area of study and practice focused on a comparative analysis of different cultures and subcultures in the world with respect to cultural care, health and illness beliefs, values, and practices with the goal of using this knowledge to provide culture-specific and culture-universal nursing care to people" (p. 493). Culture specific refers to the "particularistic values, beliefs, and patterning of behavior that tend to be special, 'local,' or unique to a designated culture and which do not tend to be shared with members of other cultures" (Leininger, 1991, p. 491), whereas culture universal refers to the commonalities of values, norms of behavior, and life patterns that are similarly held among cultures about human behavior and lifestyles and form the bases for formulating theories for developing cross-cultural laws of human behavior" (Leininger, 1991, p. 491).

Although many nurse-scholars have developed theories of nursing, Leininger's theory of culture care diversity and universality is the only one that gives precedence to understanding the cultural dimensions of human care and caring. Leininger's theory is concerned with describing, explaining, and projecting nursing similarities and differences focused primarily on human care and caring in human cultures. Leininger used worldview, social structure, language, ethnohistory, environmental context, and the generic or folk and professional systems to provide a comprehensive and holistic view of influences in cultural care and well-being. The following three models of nursing decisions and actions may be useful in providing culturally congruent and competent care (Andrews and Boyle, 2008; Leininger, 1978, 1991, 1995; Leininger and McFarland, 2002):

1. Culture care preservation and maintenance
2. Culture care accommodation and negotiation
3. Culture care repatterning and restructuring

Among the strengths of Leininger's theory is its flexibility for use with individuals, families, groups, communities, and institutions in diverse health systems. Leininger's Sunrise Model depicts the theory of cultural care diversity and universality and provides a visual representation of the key components of the theory and the interrelationships among its components (Figure 13-1).

The term *cross-cultural nursing* is sometimes used synonymously with *transcultural nursing*. The terms *intercultural nursing* and *multicultural nursing* and the phrase "ethnic people of color" are also used. Since Leininger's early work, many nurses have contributed significantly to the advancement of nursing care of culturally diverse clients, groups, and communities, and some of their contributions are mentioned in this chapter.

One of the major challenges that community health nurses face in working with clients from culturally diverse

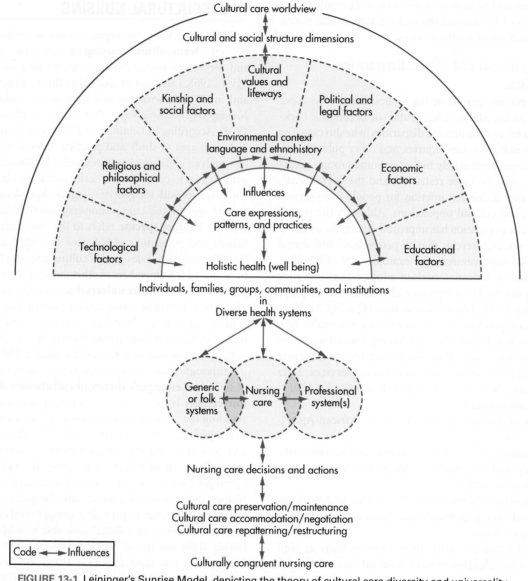

FIGURE 13-1 Leininger's Sunrise Model, depicting the theory of cultural care diversity and universality. (From Leininger MM: *Culture, care, diversity, and universality: a theory of nursing,* New York, 1991, National League for Nursing Press.)

backgrounds is overcoming individual ethnocentrism, which is a person's tendencies to view his or her own way of life as the most desirable, acceptable, or best and to act in a superior manner toward individuals from another culture. Nurses also must beware of cultural imposition, which is a person's tendency to impose his or her own beliefs, values, and patterns of behavior on individuals from another culture. When clients' cultural values and expressions of care differ from those of the nurse, the nurse must exercise caution to ensure that mutual goals have been established.

OVERVIEW OF CULTURE

In 1871, the English anthropologist Sir Edward Tylor was the first to define the term *culture.* According to Tylor (1871), culture is the complex whole, including knowledge, beliefs, art, morals, law, customs, and any other capabilities and habits

acquired by virtue of the fact that one is a member of a particular society. Culture represents a person's way of perceiving, evaluating, and behaving within his or her world, and it provides the blueprint for determining his or her values, beliefs, and practices. Culture has four basic characteristics:

1. It is learned from birth through the processes of language acquisition and socialization.
2. It is shared by members of the same cultural group.
3. It is adapted to specific conditions related to environmental and technical factors and to the availability of natural resources.
4. It is dynamic.

Culture is an all-pervasive and universal phenomenon. However, the culture that develops in any given society is always specific and distinctive, encompassing the knowledge, beliefs, customs, and skills acquired by members of that society. Within cultures, groups of individuals share beliefs, values, and attitudes that are different from those of other groups within the same culture. Ethnicity, religion, education, occupation, age, sex, and individual preferences and variations bring differences. When such groups function within a large culture, they are termed *subcultural groups*.

The term subculture is used for fairly large aggregates of people who share characteristics that are not common to all members of the culture and that enable them to be a distinguishable subgroup. Ethnicity, religion, occupation, health-related characteristics, age, sex, and geographic location are frequently used to identify subcultural groups. Examples of U.S. subcultures based on ethnicity (e.g., subcultures with common traits such as physical characteristics, language, or ancestry) include African Americans, Hispanics, Native Americans, and Chinese Americans. Subcultures based on religion include members of the more than 1200 recognized religions, such as Catholics, Jews, Mormons, Muslims, and Buddhists. Those based on occupation include health care professionals (e.g., nurses and physicians), career military personnel, and farmers. Those based on health-related characteristics include the blind, hearing impaired, and mentally challenged. Subcultures based on age include adolescents and older adults, and those based on sex or sexual preference include women, men, lesbians, and gay men. Those based on geographic location include Appalachians, Southerners, and New Yorkers. Lastly, military veterans are another, very common subculture that shares distinct needs and values (see the Veterans' Health box).

Culture and the Formation of Values

According to Leininger (1995), value refers to a desirable or undesirable state of affairs. Values are a universal feature of all cultures, although the types and expressions of values differ widely. Norms are the rules by which human behavior is governed and result from the cultural values held by the group. All societies have rules or norms that specify appropriate and inappropriate behavior. Individuals are rewarded or punished as they conform to, or deviate from, the established norms.

VETERANS' HEALTH

Culture and Veterans

The military is a unique culture influenced by factors such as training, the command hierarchy, and deployment to theaters of war. Veterans are impacted greatly by the war in which they served and the public's response to that war. The cohort of veterans who served in WWII is different from those who served in Afghanistan, with each group having their own combat experiences. The following list presents generational differences from a military perspective, using war theater, age, and cultural demographics to describe the groups of veterans.

World War II (born between 1901 and 1924)
- Known as the GI Generation or The Greatest Generation
- Were enthusiastically supported by Americans
- Had a very unified mission

Korean War (born between 1925 and 1942)
- Known as the Silent Generation
- Received no welcome from a war-weary public, and the war was quickly forgotten
- Have a lot in common with the GI Generation:
  - Raised in traditional homes during the Great Depression
  - May resist efforts to downsize because they view "decluttering" as wasteful
  - Learned to follow orders and rarely questioned authority
  - Accept that life is sometimes not fair
  - Are quiet about emotions and feelings and may be resistant to therapy for mental health issues
  - May have experienced exposure to extreme cold, suffering frostbite that still affects their health and function

Vietnam War (born between 1943 and 1960)
- Known as the baby boomers
- Are a very diverse and large group
- Dealt with crowds and competition at every phase of life owing to the great number of people in this generation—the largest group of veterans

- Fought a shadowy guerilla army, with no clarity as to who was friend or foe
- Returned to an often hostile public and peers
- Experienced recreational use of drugs and the sexual revolution, and were the first generation influenced by TV
- Have been active in the women's and gay rights movements
- Expect to be actively involved in their health care
- Value individuality, autonomy
- Distrust authority
- As the first "me" generation, may experience feelings of regret or guilt over lost relationships
- May have been exposed to Agent Orange, a defoliant that causes neurodegenerative effects and cancer
- Have high rates of hepatitis C

Gulf War/Operation Enduring Freedom (OEF)/Operation Iraqi Freedom (OIF) (born between 1964 and 1980)
- Known as Generation X or the Millennials (two different groups)
- Have the highest education levels of any veterans age group
- Work to live rather than live to work
- Came of age in times of great economic uncertainty
- Are technologically savvy
- Feel more entitled to success
- Are diverse
- Are open-minded
- Were welcomed home as heroes
- Were exposed to toxic agents, resulting in "Gulf War sickness"—fibromyalgia, depression, cognitive difficulties
- May have respiratory illnesses from exposure to oilfield fires and smoke
- Gulf war veterans are more than twice as likely as other veterans to experience amyotrophic lateral sclerosis (ALS)
- Veterans of OEF/OIF endured multiple and long deployments, resulting in significant increases in rates of posttraumatic stress disorder (PTSD) and suicide

Modified from a chart created by Bridgette Crotwell Pullis, PhD, RN, CHPN; data from Doka K: Generational cohorts: a military perspective. In Doka KJ, Tucci AS, editors: *Improving care for veterans facing illness and death*, Washington, DC, 2013, Hospice Foundation of America, pp. 47-53.

Values and norms, along with the acceptable and unacceptable behaviors associated with them, are learned in childhood.

Every society has a dominant value orientation, a basic value orientation that is shared by the majority of its members as a result of early common experiences. In the United States, the dominant value orientation is reflected in the dominant cultural group, which is made up of white, middle-class Protestants, typically those who came to the United States at least two generations ago from northern Europe. Members of the dominant cultural group are sometimes referred to as white Anglo-Saxon Protestants (WASPs), a term that reflects their ancestry and religious beliefs. In the United States, the dominant cultural group places emphasis on educational achievement, science, technology, individual expression, democracy, experimentation, and informality.

Although an assumption is sometimes made that the term *white* refers to a homogeneous group of Americans, a rich diversity of ethnic variation exists among the many groups that constitute the dominant majority. Countries of origin include those of eastern and western Europe (e.g., Ireland, Poland, Italy, France, Sweden, and Russia). The origins of people in Canada, Australia, New Zealand, and South Africa can ultimately be traced to western Europe. Appalachians, Amish, Cajuns, and other subgroups are also examples of whites who have cultural roots that are recognizably different from those of the dominant cultural group.

Values and norms vary, sometimes significantly, among various cultural groups. According to Kluckhohn and Strodtbeck (1961), several basic human problems exist for which all people must find a solution. They identified the following five questions related to values and norms:

1. What is the character of innate human nature (human nature orientation)?
2. What is the relationship of the human to nature (person-nature orientation)?
3. What is the temporal focus (i.e., time sense) of human life (time orientation)?
4. What is the mode of human activity (activity orientation)?
5. What is the mode of human relationships (social orientation)?

Human Nature Orientation

Innate human nature may be good, evil, or a combination of good and evil. Some believe that life is a struggle to overcome a basically evil nature; they consider human nature to be unalterable or able to be perfected only through great discipline and effort. For others, human nature is perceived as fundamentally good, unalterable, and difficult or impossible to corrupt.

According to Kohls (1984), the dominant U.S. cultural group chooses to believe the best about a person until that person proves otherwise. Concern in the United States for prison reform, social rehabilitation, and the plight of less fortunate people around the world is a reflective perception of the belief in the fundamental goodness of human nature. Recent scientific advances, such as the advent of stem cell research and genome studies, have necessitated consideration

of ethical quandaries regarding human nature. Questions emerge as to whether science can or should pursue activities that could alter the basic human orientation.

Person-Nature Orientation

The following three perspectives examine the ways in which the person-nature relationship is perceived:
- Destiny, in which people are subjugated to nature in a fatalistic, inevitable manner
- Harmony, in which people and nature exist together as a single entity
- Mastery, in which people are intended to overcome natural forces and to put them to use for the benefit of humankind

Most Americans consider humans and nature clearly separated; this is an incomprehensible perspective for many individuals of Asian heritage. The idea that a person can control his or her own destiny is alien to many individuals of culturally diverse backgrounds. Many cultures believe that people are driven and controlled by fate and can do very little, if anything, to influence it. Americans, by contrast, have an insatiable drive to subdue, dominate, and control their natural environment.

For example, the reader should consider three individuals in whom hypertension has been diagnosed, each of whom embraces one of the values orientations described. The person whose values orientation is destiny may say, "Why should I bother watching my diet, taking medication, and getting regular blood pressure checks? High blood pressure is part of my genetic destiny and there is nothing I can do to change the outcome. There is no need to waste money on prescription drugs and health checkups." The person whose values orientation embraces harmony may say, "If I follow the diet described and use medication to lower my blood pressure, I can restore the balance and harmony that were upset by this illness. The emotional stress I've been feeling indicates an inner lack of harmony that needs to be balanced." The person whose values orientation leads to belief in active mastery may say, "I will overcome this hypertension no matter what. By eating the right foods, working toward stress reduction, and conquering the disease with medication, I will take charge of the situation and influence the course of my disease."

Time Orientation

People can perceive time in the following three ways:

The focus may be on the past, with traditions and ancestors playing an important role in the client's life. For example, many Asians, Native Americans, East Indians, and Africans hold particular beliefs about ancestors and tend to value long-standing traditions. In times of crisis, such as illness, individuals with a values orientation emphasizing the past may consult with ancestors or ask for their guidance or protection during the illness.

The focus may be on the present, with little attention paid to the past or the future. Individuals with this focus are concerned with the current situation, and they perceive the future as vague or unpredictable. Nurses may have difficulty encouraging such individuals to prepare for the future (e.g., to participate in primary prevention measures).

The focus may be on the future, with progress and change highly valued. Individuals with a future focus may express discontent with the past and present. In terms of health care, they may inquire about the "latest treatment" and the most advanced equipment available for a particular problem.

The dominant U.S. cultural group is characterized by a belief in progress and a future orientation. This combination implies a strong task or goal focus. The group has an optimistic faith in what the future will bring. Change is often equated with improvement, and a rapid rate of change is usually normal.

Activity Orientation

There are different values orientations concerning activity. Philosophers have suggested the following three perspectives:

Being, in which a spontaneous expression of impulses and desires is largely nondevelopmental in nature

Growing, in which the person is self-contained and has inner control, including the ability to self-actualize

Doing, in which the person actively strives to achieve and accomplish something that is regarded highly

The person with a doing orientation often directs the doing toward achievement of an externally applied standard, such as a code of behavior from a religious or ethical perspective. The Ten Commandments, Pillars of Islam, Hippocratic oath, and Nightingale pledge are examples of externally applied standards.

The dominant cultural value is action oriented, with an emphasis on productivity and being busy. As a result of this action orientation, Americans have become proficient at problem solving and decision making. Even during leisure time and vacations, many Americans value activity.

Social Orientation

Variations in cultural values orientation are also related to the relationships that exist with others. Relationships may be categorized in the following three ways:

Lineal relationships: These exist by virtue of heredity and kinship ties. These relationships follow an ordered succession and have continuity through time.

Collateral relationships: The focus is primarily on group goals, and family orientation is important. For example, many Asian clients describe family honor and the importance of working together toward an achievement of the group versus a personal goal.

Individual relationships: These refer to personal autonomy and independence. Individual goals dominate, and group goals become secondary.

The social orientation among the dominant U.S. cultural group is toward the importance of the individual and the equality of all people. Friendly, informal, outgoing, and extroverted members of the dominant cultural group tend to scorn rank and authority. For example, nursing students may call faculty members by their first names, clients may call nurses by their first names, and employees may fraternize with their employers.

When making health-related decisions, clients from culturally diverse backgrounds rely on relationships with others in various ways. If the cultural values orientation is lineal, the client may seek assistance from other members of the family and allow a relative (e.g., parent, grandparent, or elder brother) to make decisions about important health-related matters. If collateral relationships are valued, decisions about the client may be interrelated with the influence of illness on the entire family or group. For example, among the Amish, the entire community is affected by the illness of a member because the community pays for health care from a common fund. Members join together to meet the needs of the client and family for the duration of the illness, and the roles of many in the community are likely to be affected by the illness of a single member.

In another example, there are approximately 11.5 million undocumented residents living in the United States as of January 2011 (Hoefer, Rytina, and Baker, 2012). These individuals often create their own social groups in which they seek to protect themselves from being discovered by immigration authorities. These groups fear that attempting to access the health care system may lead to deportation, and they often have "underground" or private access to home remedies and pharmaceuticals for their health care. As a result, they often enter the formal health care system via emergency departments when their health status has declined considerably.

A values orientation that emphasizes the individual is predominant among the dominant cultural majority in the United States. Decision making about health and illness is often an individual matter, with the client being responsible, although members of the nuclear family may participate to varying degrees.

Culture and the Family

The family remains the basic social unit in the United States. Although various ways exist to categorize families, the following are commonly recognized types of constellations in which people live together in society:

- Nuclear (i.e., husband, wife, and child or children)
- Nuclear dyad (i.e., husband and wife alone, either childless or with no children living at home)
- Single parent (i.e., either mother or father and at least one child)
- Blended (i.e., husband, wife, and children from previous relationships)
- Extended (i.e., nuclear plus other blood relatives)
- Communal (i.e., group of men and women with or without children)
- Cohabitation (i.e., unmarried man and woman sharing a household with or without children)
- Gay (i.e., same-gender couples with or without children)

In addition to structural differences in families cross-culturally, accompanying functional diversity may exist. For example, among extended families, kin residence sharing has long been recognized as a viable alternative to managing scarce resources, meeting child care needs, and caring for a handicapped or older family member.

The family constellations associated with teen parenting are unique and provide a special socialization context for infants. For example, Hispanic teen mothers receive more child care help from grandmothers and peers than do white teen mothers. Among African Americans and Puerto Ricans, the presence of the maternal grandmother ameliorates the negative consequences of adolescent childbirth on the infant. In addition, grandmothers are more responsive and less punitive in their interactions with the infant than their daughters (Andrews and Boyle, 2008). Three-generational households can have an influence on the infant's development: by influencing the mother's knowledge about development and providing other more responsive social interactions with the infant.

Families from diverse backgrounds are often characterized as being more conservative in terms of sex roles and parenting values and practices than white families. For example, traditional Japanese-American and Mexican-American families are family centered, enforce strict gender and age roles, and emphasize children's compliance with authority figures. Children of culturally diverse backgrounds are involved in family interactions that differ from those of children from the dominant U.S. cultural group. The values of children of immigrants typically evolve, depending on how far removed they are from the country of origin. These children may detach from their cultural traditions, becoming more individually focused or autonomous—often to the dismay of the elders in the family. Often the language of the ancestors is forgotten or, in certain subcultures, forbidden to be spoken, so that the children may assimilate to the dominant culture.

Relationships that may seem apparent sometimes warrant further exploration by nurses interacting with clients from culturally diverse backgrounds. For example, the dominant cultural group defines siblings as two people with the same mother, the same father, the same mother and father, or the same adoptive parents. In some Asian cultures, a sibling relationship is defined as involving infants who are breastfed by the same woman. In other cultures, certain kinship patterns, such as maternal first cousins, are sibling relationships. In some African cultures, anyone from the same village or town may be called "brother" or "sister."

When providing care for infants and children, the nurse must identify the primary provider of care because this individual may or may not be the biological parent. For example, among some Hispanic groups, female members of the nuclear or extended family (e.g., sisters or aunts) are sometimes the primary providers of care. In some African American families, the grandmother may be the decision maker and primary caregiver of the children.

CULTURE AND SOCIOECONOMIC FACTORS

No single indicator can adequately capture all facets of economic status for entire populations, but measures such as median or average annual income, employment rate, poverty rate, and net worth are most often used. The economic status of most individuals, especially children, is better reflected by the pooled resources of family or household members than by their individual earnings or incomes. Socioeconomic status (SES) is a composite of the economic status of a family or unrelated individuals based on income, wealth, occupation, educational attainment, and power. It is a means of measuring inequalities based on economic differences and the manner in which families live as a result of their economic well-being. Most families with racially or ethnically diverse backgrounds have a lower SES than the population at large, with a few exceptions (e.g., Cuban Americans and subgroups of Asian Americans).

Poverty is another factor that dramatically influences health and well-being. National poverty data are calculated through the use of the official U.S. Census Bureau definition of poverty, which has remained standard since its initial introduction in the mid-1960s. Under this definition, poverty is determined by comparing pretax cash income with the poverty threshold, which adjusts for family size and composition. Table 13-1 provides an overview of the poverty thresholds according to size of family and number of related children

TABLE 13-1	POVERTY THRESHOLDS ($) FOR 2012 BY SIZE OF FAMILY AND NUMBER OF RELATED CHILDREN UNDER 18 YEARS								
	RELATED CHILDREN UNDER 18 YEARS								
SIZE OF FAMILY UNIT	**NONE**	**ONE**	**TWO**	**THREE**	**FOUR**	**FIVE**	**SIX**	**SEVEN**	**EIGHT OR MORE**
One person under 65 years	11,945								
One person 65 years and over	11,011								
Two people: Householder under 65 years	15,374	15,825							
Two people: Householder 65 years and over	13,878	15,765							
Three people	17,959	18,480	18,498						
Four people	23,681	24,069	23,283	23,364					
Five people	28,558	28,974	28,087	27,400	26,981				
Six people	32,847	32,978	32,298	31,647	30,678	30,104			
Seven people	37,795	38,031	37,217	36,651	35,594	34,362	33,009		
Eight people	42,271	42,644	41,876	41,204	40,249	39,038	37,777	37,457	
Nine people or more	50,849	51,095	50,416	49,845	48,908	47,620	46,454	46,165	44,387

Note: The poverty thresholds are updated each year with the use of the change in the average annual Consumer Price Index for All Urban Consumers (CPI-U).

From U.S. Census Bureau: *Poverty thresholds by size of family and number of children, 2012.* Available from https://www.census.gov/hhes/www/poverty/data/threshld/index.html.

under age 18 years residing in the home. The poverty guidelines are issued each year by the USDHHS. The guidelines are a simplification of the poverty threshold for administrative purposes, such as determining financial eligibility for federal programs (e.g., Head Start, National School Lunch, Medicaid, Aid to Families with Dependent Children) (U.S. Census Bureau, 2012).

According to the U.S. Census Bureau (2012), the poverty rate in 2011 was 15%. The distribution of the poor varies considerably on the basis of certain factors such as age, race or ethnicity, and marital status. For example, 27.6% of the African American population, 12.3% of the Asian population, and 25.3% of the Hispanic population live in poverty. In addition, children under 6 years of age are particularly vulnerable to poverty, with 24.5% of all U.S. children in this age-group being poor.

Distribution of Resources

Status, power, and wealth in the United States are not distributed equally throughout society. Rather, a small percentage of the population enjoys most of the nation's resources, primarily through ownership of multibillion-dollar corporations, large pieces of real estate in prime locations, and similar assets. The U.S. population has traditionally been divided into the following three social classes: upper, middle, and lower. SES may be calculated by considering a variety of factors, but it is customarily determined by examining factors such as total family income, occupation, and educational level.

A disproportionate number of individuals from the racially and ethnically diverse subgroups are members of the lower socioeconomic class, whereas a larger percentage of members of the dominant cultural group belong to the upper and middle socioeconomic classes. The United States has socioeconomic stratification; therefore, the idealization of America as the land of opportunity often applies more to members of the upper and middle classes than to those of the lower class. The outcome of social stratification is social inequality. For example, school systems, grocery stores, and recreational facilities vary significantly between the inner city, which has a high percentage of minority residents, and the suburbs, where the residents are overwhelmingly WASP.

For many years, health care settings have been the subject of study and concern regarding distribution of resources, with members of racial and ethnic minority groups compellingly pointing out the inequalities. Because financing of health care in the United States largely relies on a combination of federally funded insurance (i.e., Medicare) and employer-provided health insurance, those from the highest SES groups and elders tend to receive the best health care. In contrast, those from low SES groups (i.e., those without health insurance or with Medicaid) tend to receive less health care. Thus, in the United States, SES largely determines access to health care as well as the quality of care received.

Education

One of the components considered in determining SES is educational level. Educational attainment is perhaps the single most important factor. In recent years, there has been an improvement in the level of education among those who have historically been less educated (e.g., elders, women, minorities). For example, women now have a higher rate of high school completion than men. Also, dropout rates for both African Americans and Hispanics are steadily declining (National Center for Educational Statistics, 2012).

CULTURE AND NUTRITION

Long after assimilation into U.S. culture has occurred, many members of various ethnic groups continue to follow culturally based dietary practices and eat ethnic foods. Often, neighborhood food markets and ethnic restaurants are established soon after the arrival of a new group of immigrants to the United States. The ethnic restaurant is commonly a place for members of cultural group to meet and mingle, and customers from the dominant cultural group may be of secondary interest. Food is an integral part of cultural identity that extends beyond dietary preferences.

Nutrition Assessment of Culturally Diverse Groups

Factors that must be considered in a nutrition assessment include the cultural definition of food, frequency and number of meals eaten away from home, form and content of ceremonial meals, amount and types of food eaten, and regularity of food consumption. Twenty-four-hour dietary recalls or 3-day food records traditionally used for assessment may be inadequate when dealing with clients from culturally diverse backgrounds. Standard dietary handbooks may fail to provide culture-specific diet information because nutritional content and exchange tables are usually based on Western diets. Another source of error may originate from the cultural patterns of eating. For example, among low-income urban African American families, elaborate weekend meals are frequent, whereas weekday dietary patterns are markedly more moderate.

Although community health nurses may assume that *food* is a culture-universal term, they may need to clarify its meaning with the client. For example, certain Latin American groups do not consider greens, an important source of vitamins, to be food and fail to list intake of these vegetables on daily records. Among Vietnamese refugees, dietary intake of calcium may appear inadequate because low consumption rates of dairy products are common among members of this group. However, they commonly consume pork bones and shells, providing adequate quantities of calcium to meet daily requirements.

Food is only one part of eating. In some cultures, social contacts during meals are restricted to members of the immediate or extended family. For example, in some Middle Eastern cultures, men and women eat meals separately, or women are permitted to eat with their husbands but not with other males. Among some Hispanic groups, the male breadwinner is served first, then the women and children eat. Etiquette during meals, use of hands, type of eating utensils (e.g., chopsticks or special flatware), and protocols governing the order in which food is consumed during a meal all vary cross-culturally.

Dietary Practices of Selected Cultural Groups

Cultural stereotyping is the tendency to view individuals of common cultural backgrounds similarly and according to a preconceived notion of how they behave. However, not all Chinese like rice, not all Italians like spaghetti, and not all Mexicans like tortillas. Nevertheless, aggregate dietary preferences among people from certain cultural groups can be described (e.g., characteristic ethnic dishes and methods of food preparation, including use of cooking oils); the reader is referred to nutrition texts on the topic for detailed information about culture-specific diets and the nutritional value of ethnic foods.

Religion and Diet

Cultural food preferences are often interrelated with religious dietary beliefs and practices. As indicated in Table 13-2, many religions have proscriptive dietary practices, and some use food as symbols in celebrations and rituals. Knowing the client's religious practice as it relates to food makes it possible to suggest improvements or modifications that will not conflict with religious dietary laws.

Fasting and other religious observations may limit a person's food or liquid intake during specified times. For example, many Catholics fast or abstain from meat on Ash Wednesday and each Friday of Lent, Muslims refrain from eating during the daytime hours for the month of Ramadan but are permitted to eat after sunset, and Mormons refrain from ingesting all solid foods and liquids on the first Sunday of each month.

CULTURE AND RELIGION

According to the *Yearbook of American and Canadian Churches*, more than 226 million people in North America are affiliated with organized religion (National Council of Churches, 2005). A 2013 Gallup Poll found that 90% of Americans report that they believe in God (Gallup, 2013). Furthermore, about 66% note that they are members of a church, synagogue, or mosque. The largest religious groups are Protestant, 41%; Catholic, 24%; Jewish, 2%; Mormon, 2%; and other, 12%. The largest specific Protestant denominations are, in order, Baptist (other than Southern Baptist), Methodist, Southern Baptist, Lutheran, and Presbyterian.

Although the nurse cannot be an expert on each of the estimated 1200 religions practiced in the United States, knowledge of health-related beliefs and practices and general information about religious observances are important in providing culturally competent nursing care. For example, when planning home visits or scheduling clinic visits for members of a specific religious group, the nurse should consult the group's religious calendar and work around designated holy days. The nurse should also know the customary days of religious worship observed by members of the religion. Most Protestants worship on Sundays, whereas Muslims' holy day of worship

TABLE 13-2	DIETARY PRACTICES OF SELECTED RELIGIOUS GROUPS
RELIGION	**DIETARY PRACTICE**
Hinduism	All meats are prohibited.
Islam	Pork and intoxicating beverages are prohibited.
Judaism	Pork, predatory fowl, shellfish, other water creatures (fish with scales are permissible), and blood by ingestion (e.g., blood sausage and raw meat) are prohibited. Blood by transfusion is acceptable. Foods should be kosher (meaning "properly preserved"). All animals must be ritually slaughtered by a shochet (i.e., quickly with the least pain possible) to be kosher. Mixing dairy and meat dishes at the same meal is prohibited.
Mormonism (Church of Jesus Christ of Latter-day Saints)	Alcohol, tobacco, and beverages containing caffeine (e.g., coffee, tea, colas, and select carbonated soft drinks) are prohibited.
Seventh-Day Adventism	Pork, certain seafood (including shellfish), and fermented beverages are prohibited. A vegetarian diet is encouraged.

extends from sunset on Thursday to sunset on Friday, and Jews and Seventh-Day Adventists' holy day extends from sunset on Friday to sunset on Saturday. Roman Catholics may worship in the late afternoon or evening of Saturday or all day Sunday. Some religions may meet more than once weekly.

As an integral component of the individual's culture, religious beliefs may influence the client's explanation of the cause of illness, perception of its severity, and choice of healer. In times of crisis, such as serious illness and impending death, religion may be a source of consolation for the client and family and may influence the course of action believed to be appropriate.

Religion and Spirituality

Religious concerns evolve from, and respond to, the mysteries of life and death, good and evil, and pain and suffering. Nurses frequently encounter clients who find themselves searching for a spiritual meaning to help explain illness or disability. Some nurses find spiritual assessment difficult because the topic is abstract and personal, whereas others feel comfortable discussing spiritual matters. Comfort with personal spiritual beliefs is the foundation for effective assessment of spiritual needs in clients.

Although religions offer various interpretations of many of life's mysteries, most people seek a personal understanding and interpretation at some time in their lives. Ultimately, this personal search becomes a pursuit to discover a supreme being (e.g., Allah, God, Yahweh, or Jehovah) or some unifying truth that will render meaning, purpose, and integrity to existence.

An important distinction must be made between religion and spirituality. Religion refers to an organized system of beliefs concerning the cause, nature, and purpose of the universe, especially belief in or the worship of a god or gods. As already stated, more than 1200 religions are practiced in the United States. Spirituality, in contrast, is born out of the individual's unique life experience and personal effort to find purpose and meaning in life. Box 13-1 provides suggested guidelines for assessing the spiritual needs of culturally diverse clients.

SHARED BELIEFS AMONG VARIOUS RELIGIONS: THE "GOLDEN RULE"

Buddhism: "Hurt not others in ways that you yourself would find hurtful." (Udana-varga 5:18)

Christianity: "Whatsoever you would that men should do to you, do you even so to them." (Matthew 7:12)

Confucianism: "Do not do to others what you do not want them to do to you." (Analects 15:23)

Hinduism: "One should not behave towards others in a way which is disagreeable to oneself." (Mahabharata 5:1517; Mencius Vii.A.4)

Islam: "Not one of you is a believer until he loves for his brother what he loves for himself." (Number 13 of Al-Nawawi's Forty Hadiths)

Judaism: "Thou shalt love thy neighbor as thyself." (Leviticus 19:18)

Taoism: "Regard your neighbor's gain as your own gain and your neighbor's loss as your own loss." (T'ai Shang Kan Ying P'ien)

Religion may influence decisions regarding prolongation of life, euthanasia, autopsy, donation of a body for research, disposal of a body and body parts including fetus, and type of burial. The nurse should use discretion in asking clients and their families about these issues and gather data only when the clinical situation necessitates that the information be obtained. The nurse should encourage clients and families to discuss these issues with their religious representative when necessary. Before dealing with potentially sensitive issues, the nurse should establish rapport with the client and family by gaining their trust and confidence in less sensitive areas.

Childhood and Spirituality

Serious illness during childhood is especially difficult. Children have spiritual needs that vary according to the child's developmental level and the religious climate that exists in the family. Parental perceptions about the illness of their child may be partially influenced by religious beliefs. For example, some parents may believe that a transgression against a religious law is responsible for a congenital anomaly in their offspring. Other parents may delay seeking medical care because they believe that prayer should be tried first. Certain types of treatment (e.g., administration of blood or medications containing caffeine or other prohibited substances and selected procedures) may be perceived as cultural taboos, which are to be avoided by children and adults.

CULTURE AND AGING

Values held by the dominant U.S. culture, such as emphasis on independence, self-reliance, and productivity, influence aging members of society. Americans define people 65 years and older as "old" and limit their work. In some other cultures, people are first recognized as being unable to work and then identified as being old. In some cultures the wisdom, not the productivity, of the older adult is valued; the diminution of one's activity level and the reduction of physical stamina associated with growing old are accepted more readily without loss of status among culture members. Retirement is also culturally defined, with some older adults working as long as physical health continues and others continuing to be active but assuming less physically demanding jobs.

The main task of older adults in the dominant culture is to achieve a sense of integrity in accepting responsibility for their own lives and having a sense of accomplishment. Individuals who achieve integrity consider aging a positive experience, make adjustments in their personal space and social relationships, maintain a sense of usefulness, and begin closure and life review. Not all cultures value accepting responsibility for an individual's own life. For example, among Hispanics, Asians, Arabs, and other groups, older adults are often cared for by family members who welcome them into their homes when they are no longer able to live alone. The concept of placing an older family member in an institutional setting to be cared for by strangers is perceived as an uncaring, impersonal, and culturally unacceptable practice by many cultural groups.

Older adults may develop their own means of coping with illness through self-care, assistance from family members, and social group support systems. Some cultures have developed attitudes and specific behaviors for older adults that include humanistic care and identification of family members as care providers. Older adults may have special family responsibilities (e.g., the older Amish adults provide hospitality to visitors, and older Filipino adults spend considerable time teaching the youth skills learned during a lifetime of experience).

Older adult immigrants who have made major lifestyle adjustments in the move from their homeland to the United States or from a rural to an urban area, or vice versa, may need information about health care alternatives, preventive programs, health care benefits, and screening programs for which they are eligible. These individuals may also be in various stages of culture shock, the state of disorientation or inability to respond to the behavior of a different cultural group because it holds sudden strangeness, unfamiliarity, and incompatibility for the newcomer's perceptions and expectations (Leininger and McFarland, 2002).

Several examples of how being an elderly immigrant influences health can be found in the nursing literature. Wilmoth and Chen (2003) studied living arrangements and symptoms of depression among middle-aged and older immigrants and concluded that immigrants had significantly more depressive symptoms than nonimmigrants. Furthermore, immigrants who lived alone or with family had more depressive symptoms than those who lived with a spouse.

CROSS-CULTURAL COMMUNICATION

Verbal communication and nonverbal communication are important in community health nursing and are influenced by the cultural background of the nurse and client. *Cross-cultural, or intercultural, communication* refers to the communication process between a nurse and a client with different cultural backgrounds as each attempts to understand the other's point of view from a cultural perspective.

Nurse-Client Relationship

From the introduction of the nurse to the client through termination of the relationship, communication is a continuous process for the community health nurse. First impressions are important in all human relationships; therefore cross-cultural considerations concerning introductions warrant a few brief remarks. To ensure a mutually respectful relationship, the nurse should introduce himself or herself and indicate how the client should refer to the nurse (i.e., by first name, last name, or title). Having done so, the nurse should ask the client to do the same. This enables the nurse to address the client in a manner that is culturally appropriate, thereby avoiding potential embarrassment. For example, some Asian and European cultures write the last name first; confusion can be avoided in an area of sensitivity (i.e., the client's name).

TABLE 13-3	**FUNCTIONAL USE OF SPACE**
ZONE	**REMARKS**
Intimate zone (0 to 1.5 feet)	Visual distortion occurs. Best for assessing breath and other body odors.
Personal distance (1.5 to 4 feet)	Perceived as an extension of the self, similar to a "bubble." Voice is moderate. Body odors are inapparent. Visual distortion does not occur. Much of the physical assessment will occur at this distance.
Social distance (4 to 12 feet)	Used for impersonal business transactions. Perceptual information is much less detailed. Much of the interview will occur at this distance.
Public distance (>12 feet)	Interaction with others is impersonal. Speaker's voice must be projected. Subtle facial expressions are imperceptible.

Data from Hall E: Proxemics: the study of man's spatial relations. In Galdston I, editor: *Man's image in medicine and anthropology,* New York, 1963, International Universities Press.

Space, Distance, and Intimacy

Sense of spatial distance is significant because culturally appropriate distance zones vary widely. For example, the nurse may back away from clients of Hispanic, East Indian, or Middle Eastern origin who invade personal space with regularity in an attempt to bring the nurse closer into the space that is comfortable to them. Although the nurse is uncomfortable with clients' close physical proximity, clients are perplexed by the nurse's distancing behaviors and may perceive the community health nurse as aloof and unfriendly. Table 13-3 summarizes the four distance zones identified for the functional use of space that are embraced by the dominant cultural group in the United States, including most nurses.

Overcoming Communication Barriers

Nurses tend to have stereotypical expectations of the client's behavior. In general, nurses expect behavior to consist of undemanding compliance, an attitude of respect for the health care provider, and cooperation with requested behavior throughout the examination. Although clients may ask a few questions for clarification, slight deference to recognized authority figures (e.g., health care providers) is expected. However, individuals from culturally diverse backgrounds may have significantly different perceptions about the appropriate role of the individual and family when seeking health care. If nurses find themselves becoming annoyed that a client is asking too many questions, assuming a defensive posture, or otherwise feeling uncomfortable, they may pause for a moment to examine the source of the conflict from a cross-cultural perspective.

During illness, culturally acceptable "sick-role" behavior may range from aggressive, demanding behavior to silent passivity (Cockerham, 2009). Complaining, demanding behavior during illness is often rewarded with attention among

Jewish and Italian-American clients, whereas Asian and Native American clients are likely to be quiet and compliant during illness. Furthermore, during an interview, Asian clients may provide the nurse with the answers they think the nurse wants to hear, behavior that is consistent within their cultural value for harmonious relationships with others. The nurse should attempt to phrase questions or statements in a neutral manner that avoids foreshadowing an expected response. Appalachian clients may reject a community health nurse whom they perceive as prying or nosy because a cultural ethic of neutrality mandates that people mind their own business and avoid assertive or argumentative behavior.

Nonverbal Communication

Unless the nurse makes an effort to understand the client's nonverbal behavior, he or she may overlook important information such as that conveyed by facial expressions, silence, eye contact, touch, and other body language. Communication patterns vary widely cross-culturally, even for seemingly "innocent" behaviors such as smiling and shaking hands. For example, among many Hispanic clients, smiling and shaking hands are considered an integral part of sincere interaction and essential to establishing trust, whereas a Russian client may perceive the same behavior from the nurse as insolent and frivolous.

Gender issues also become significant. For example, among some groups of Middle Eastern origin, men and women do not shake hands or touch each other in any manner outside the marital relationship. However, if the nurse and client are both female, a handshake is usually acceptable.

Wide cultural variation exists in the interpretation of silence. Some individuals find silence extremely uncomfortable and make every effort to fill conversational lags with words. In contrast, Native Americans consider silence essential to understanding and respecting the other person. A pause after a question signifies that what the speaker has asked is important enough to be given thoughtful consideration. In traditional Chinese and Japanese cultures, silence may mean that the speaker wishes the listener to consider the content of what has been said before continuing. The English and Arabs may use silence out of respect for another person's privacy, whereas the French, Spanish, and Russians may interpret it as a sign of agreement. Asian cultures often use silence to demonstrate respect for elders.

Eye contact is among the most culturally variable nonverbal behaviors. Although most nurses have been taught to maintain eye contact while talking with clients, individuals from culturally diverse backgrounds may misconstrue this behavior. Asian, Native American, Indochinese, Arab, and Appalachian clients may consider direct eye contact impolite or aggressive, and they may avert their own eyes during the conversation. Native American clients often stare at the floor when the nurse is talking. This culturally appropriate behavior indicates that the listener is paying close attention to the speaker.

In some cultures, including Arab, Hispanic, and some African American groups, modesty for women is interrelated with eye contact. For a Muslim woman, modesty is achieved in part by avoiding eye contact with men, except for her husband, and keeping the eyes downcast when encountering members of the opposite sex in public situations. In many cultures, the only women who smile and establish eye contact with men in public are prostitutes. Hasidic Jewish men also have culturally based norms concerning eye contact with women. Such a man may avoid direct eye contact and turn his head in the opposite direction when walking past or speaking to a woman. The preceding examples are intended to be illustrative and are not exhaustive; nor do they represent values, actions, and beliefs of all members of the cultural groups described.

Language

To assess non–English-speaking clients, the nurse may need the help of an interpreter. Interviewing a non–English-speaking person requires a bilingual interpreter for full communication. Even the person from another culture or country who has a basic command of English may need an interpreter when faced with the anxiety-provoking situation of becoming ill, encountering a strange symptom, or discussing sensitive topics such as birth control, gynecological concerns, and urological problems. The nurse may be tempted to ask a relative or friend of another client to interpret because this person is readily available and is anxious to help. However, doing so is disadvantageous because it violates confidentiality for the client, who may not want personal information shared with another. Furthermore, the friend or relative, although fluent in ordinary language, is likely to be unfamiliar with medical terminology, clinical procedures, and medical ethics.

Whenever possible, the nurse should use a bilingual team member or trained medical interpreter. This person knows interpreting techniques, has a health care background, and understands clients' rights. The trained interpreter is also knowledgeable about cultural beliefs and health practices, can help bridge the cultural gap, and can provide advice concerning the cultural appropriateness of recommendations.

Although the nurse is in charge of the client-nurse interaction, the interpreter is an important member of the health care team. Whenever feasible, the nurse should ask the interpreter to meet the client before the visit to establish rapport and learn about the client's age, occupation, educational level, and attitude toward health care. This knowledge enables the interpreter to communicate on the client's level.

The nurse should allow more time for visits with culturally diverse clients who require an interpreter. With the third person repeating everything, it can take considerably longer than interviewing English-speaking clients. The nurse will need to focus on the major points and prioritize data.

Line-by-line and summarization are interpretation styles. Translation line-by-line ensures accuracy, but it takes more time. The nurse and client should speak only a sentence or two and then allow the interpreter time to interpret. The nurse should use simple language, not medical jargon that the interpreter must simplify before translating. Summary translation is faster and useful for teaching relatively simple health techniques with which the interpreter is already familiar. The nurse should be alert for nonverbal cues as the client talks because they can give valuable data. A good interpreter will also note nonverbal messages and communicate those to the community health nurse. Box 13-2 summarizes suggestions for the selection and use of an interpreter.

Although use of an interpreter is ideal, the nurse may find himself or herself in a situation with a non–English-speaking client in which no interpreter is available. Box 13-3 provides some suggestions for overcoming language barriers when an interpreter is not available.

BOX 13-2 OVERCOMING LANGUAGE BARRIERS: USE OF AN INTERPRETER

- Before locating an interpreter, the nurse should know what language the client speaks at home because it may be different from the language spoken publicly (e.g., French is sometimes spoken by aristocratic or well-educated people from certain Asian or Middle Eastern cultures).
- The nurse should avoid interpreters from a rival tribe, state, region, or nation (e.g., a Palestinian who knows Hebrew may not be the best interpreter for a Jewish client).
- The nurse should be aware of the gender difference between the interpreter and client to avoid violation of cultural mores related to modesty.
- The nurse should be aware of the age difference between the interpreter and client.
- The nurse should be aware of socioeconomic differences between the interpreter and client.
- The nurse should ask the interpreter to translate as closely to verbatim as possible.
- An interpreter who is not a relative may seek compensation for services rendered.

Touch

Touching the client is a necessary component of a comprehensive assessment. Although benefits exist in establishing rapport with clients through touch, including the promotion of healing through therapeutic touch, physical contact with clients conveys various meanings cross-culturally. In many cultures (e.g., Arab and Hispanic), male health care providers may be prohibited from touching or examining all or certain parts of the female body. During pregnancy, the client may prefer female health care providers and may refuse to be examined by a man. The nurse should be aware that the client's significant other also might exert pressure on health care providers by enforcing these culturally meaningful norms in the health care setting.

Touching children may also have variable meanings cross-culturally. For example, Hispanic clients may believe in *mal ojo* (evil eye), in which an individual becomes ill as a result of excessive admiration by another. Many Asians believe that personal strength resides in the head and consider touching the head disrespectful. The nurse should approach palpation of the fontanelle of an infant of Southeast Asian descent with sensitivity. The nurse may need to rely on alternative sources of information (e.g., assessing for clinical manifestations of increased intracranial pressure or signs of premature fontanelle closure). Although it is the least desirable option, the nurse may need to omit this part of the assessment.

Gender

Violating norms related to appropriate male-female relationships among various cultures may jeopardize the therapeutic nurse-client relationship. Among Arab Americans, a man

---

BOX 13-3 OVERCOMING LANGUAGE BARRIERS WHEN AN INTERPRETER IS NOT AVAILABLE

- The nurse should be polite and formal.
- The nurse should greet the client using his or her last or complete name. The nurse should gesture to himself or herself and say his or her name. The nurse should offer a handshake or nod and smile.
- The nurse should proceed in an unhurried manner. The nurse should pay attention to efforts by the client or family to communicate.
- The nurse should speak in a low, moderate voice. The nurse should remember that he or she may have a tendency to raise the volume and pitch of his or her voice when the listener appears not to understand, and the listener may perceive that the nurse is shouting or angry.
- The nurse should use words that he or she may know in the client's language. Doing so indicates that the nurse is aware of and respects the client's culture.
- The nurse should use simple words, such as "pain" instead of "discomfort." The nurse should avoid medical jargon, idioms, and slang. He or she should avoid using contractions such as "don't," "can't," and "won't." The nurse should use nouns repeatedly instead of pronouns. For example, the nurse should say, "Do you take medicine?" instead of "You have been taking your medicine, haven't you?"

- The nurse should pantomime words and simple actions while verbalizing them.
- The nurse should give instructions in the proper sequence. For example, he or she should say, "First, wash the bottle. Second, rinse the bottle," instead of "Before you rinse the bottle, sterilize it."
- The nurse should discuss one topic at a time. He or she should avoid use of conjunctions. For example, the nurse should ask, "Are you cold [while pantomiming]?" and then "Are you in pain?" instead of, "Are you cold and in pain?"
- The nurse should determine whether the client understands by having the client repeat instructions, demonstrate the procedure, or act out the meaning.
- The nurse should write out several short sentences in English and determine the client's ability to read them.
- The nurse should try a third language. Many Indo-Chinese people speak French. Europeans often know three or four languages. The nurse should try Latin words or phrases.
- The nurse should ask who among the client's family and friends could serve as an interpreter.
- The nurse should obtain phrase books from a library or bookstore, make or purchase flash cards, contact hospitals for a list of interpreters, and use both formal and informal networking to locate suitable interpreters.

is never alone with a woman, except his wife, and is usually accompanied by one or more other men when interacting with women. This behavior is culturally significant, and failure to adhere to the cultural code (i.e., set of rules or norms of behavior used by a cultural group to guide their behavior and interpret situations) is viewed as a serious transgression, often one in which the lone male will be accused of sexual impropriety. The best way to ensure that cultural variables have been considered is to ask the client about culturally relevant aspects of male-female relationships, preferably at the beginning of the interaction before an opportunity arises to violate culturally based practices.

HEALTH-RELATED BELIEFS AND PRACTICES

One of the major aspects of a comprehensive cultural assessment concerns the collection of data related to culturally based beliefs and practices about health and illness. Before determining whether cultural practices are helpful, harmful, or neutral, the nurse must first understand the logic of the belief system underlying the practice and then be sure to grasp fully the nature and meaning of the practice from the client's cultural perspective.

Health and Culture

The first step in understanding the health care needs of clients is to understand personal culturally based values, beliefs, attitudes, and practices. Sometimes this step requires considerable introspection and may necessitate that the nurse confront his or her own biases, preconceptions, and prejudices about specific racial, ethnic, religious, sexual, or socioeconomic groups. The next step is to identify the meaning of health to the client, remembering that concepts are derived, in part, from the way in which members of their cultural group define health.

Considerable research has been conducted on the various definitions of health that may be held by various groups. For example, Jamaicans define health as having a good appetite, feeling strong and energetic, performing activities of daily living without difficulty, and being sexually active and fertile. For traditional Italian women, health means the ability to interact socially and perform routine tasks such as cooking, cleaning, and caring for oneself and others. On the other hand, some individuals of Hispanic origin believe that coughing, sweating, and diarrhea are a normal part of living rather than symptoms of ill health, because the frequency of these problems in the clients' country of origin is high. Individuals may define themselves or others in their group as healthy even though the nurse identifies symptoms of disease.

Cross-Cultural Perspectives on Causes of Illness

For clients, symptom labeling and diagnosis depend on the extent of the difference between the individual's behaviors and those the group defines as normal. Other issues that the nurse should consider include the client's beliefs about the causation of illness, level of stigma attached to a particular set of symptoms, prevalence of the disease, and meaning of the illness to the individual and family.

Throughout history, humankind has attempted to understand the cause of illness and disease. Theories of causation have been formulated on the basis of religious beliefs, social circumstances, philosophical perspectives, and level of knowledge. Disease causation may be viewed from the following three major perspectives: biomedical (i.e., sometimes used synonymously with the term *scientific*), naturalistic (i.e., sometimes used synonymously with the term *holistic*), and magicoreligious.

Biomedical Perspective

The biomedical (i.e., scientific) theory of illness causation is based on the following beliefs:

1. All events in life have a cause and effect.
2. The human body functions more or less mechanically (i.e., the functioning of the human body is analogous to the functioning of an automobile).
3. All life can be reduced or divided into smaller parts (e.g., the human person can be reduced into body, mind, and spirit).
4. All of reality can be observed and measured (e.g., with intelligence tests and psychometric measures of behavior).

Among the biomedical explanations for disease is the germ theory, which posits that microscopic organisms such as bacteria and viruses are responsible for many specific disease conditions. Most educational programs for nurses and other health care providers embrace biomedical, or scientific, theories that explain the causes of physical and psychological illnesses.

Naturalistic Perspective

Another way in which clients may explain the cause of illness is from the naturalistic (i.e., holistic) perspective. This viewpoint is found most frequently among Native Americans, Asians, and others who believe that human life is only one aspect of nature and a part of the general order of the cosmos. Individuals from these groups believe that the forces of nature must be kept in natural balance or harmony to maintain health and well-being. A combination of worldviews is possible, and many clients are likely to offer more than one explanation for the cause of their illness. As a profession, nursing largely embraces the biomedical-scientific worldview, but some aspects of holism have begun to gain popularity. These include a wide variety of techniques for management of chronic pain (e.g., hypnosis, therapeutic touch, and biofeedback). Many nurses hold a belief in spiritual power and readily credit supernatural forces with various unexplained phenomena related to clients' health and illness states.

Numerous Asians subscribe to the yin-yang theory, in which health is believed to exist when all aspects of the person are in perfect balance. Rooted in the ancient Chinese philosophy of Tao, the yin-yang theory states that all organisms and objects in the universe consist of yin or yang energy forces. The origin of the energy forces is within the autonomic nervous system, where balance between the opposing forces is maintained during health. Yin energy represents the female and negative forces (e.g., emptiness, darkness, and cold), whereas yang forces are male and positive, emitting fullness, light, and warmth. Foods are classified as hot and cold in this theory and are transformed into yin and yang energy when metabolized by the body. Yin foods are cold, and yang foods are hot. Cold foods are eaten when one has a hot illness, and hot foods are eaten when one has a cold illness. The yin-yang theory is the basis for Eastern or Chinese medicine.

The naturalistic perspective posits that the laws of nature create imbalance, chaos, and disease. Individuals embracing the naturalistic view use metaphors such as the healing power of nature, and they may call the earth "Mother." For example, from the perspective of the Chinese, illness is seen not as an intruding agent but rather as a part of life's rhythmic course and an outward sign of the disharmony that exists within.

Many Hispanic, Arab, African American, and Asian groups embrace a hot-cold theory of health and illness, an explanatory model with its origin in the ancient Greek humoral theory. Blood, phlegm, black bile, and yellow bile, the four humors of the body, regulate basic bodily functions and are described in terms of temperature, dryness, and moisture. The treatment of disease consists of adding or subtracting cold, heat, dryness, or wetness to restore the balance of the humors.

Beverages, foods, herbs, medicines, and diseases are classified as hot or cold according to their perceived effects on the body, not on their physical characteristics. Illnesses believed to be caused by cold entering the body include earache, chest cramps, paralysis, gastrointestinal discomfort, rheumatism, and tuberculosis. Illnesses believed to be caused by overheating include abscessed teeth, sore throats, rashes, and kidney disorders.

According to the hot-cold theory, the individual as a whole, rather than a specific ailment, is significant. Those who embrace the hot-cold theory maintain that health consists of a positive state of total well-being, including physical, psychological, spiritual, and social aspects of the person. Paradoxically, the language used to describe this artificial dissection of the body into parts is a reflection of the biomedical-scientific perspective, not a naturalistic or holistic one.

Magicoreligious Perspective

Another way in which people explain the causation of illness is from a magicoreligious perspective. The basic premise of this explanatory model is that the world is seen as an arena in which supernatural forces dominate. The fate of the world and those in it depends on the action of supernatural forces for good or evil. Examples of magical causes of illness include the belief in voodoo or witchcraft among some African Americans and others from circum-Caribbean countries. Faith healing is based on religious beliefs and is most prevalent among selected Christian religions, including Christian Scientists. Various healing rituals may be found in many religions—Roman Catholicism, Mormonism (i.e., Church of Jesus Christ of Latter-day Saints), and others (Andrews, 2008).

Folk Healers

All cultures have their own recognized symptoms of ill health, acceptable sick-role behavior, and treatments. In addition to seeking help from the nurse as a biomedical-scientific health care provider, clients from many groups may seek help from folk or religious healers.

Numerous types of folk healers exist, each with a unique scope of practice. Hispanic clients may turn to a *curandero* (male folk healer) or *curandera* (female folk healer), spiritualist, *yerbo* (herbalist), or *sabador* (healer who manipulates muscles and bones). In many instances, people from diverse cultures combine folk healing and biomedicine. Among the main reasons for seeking care from folk healers is the perception that biomedical practitioners (e.g., physicians and nurses) fail to provide holistic care and use medicines that are not natural.

Some African American clients may mention having received assistance from a *hougan* (voodoo priest or priestess), spiritualist, or "old lady" (an older woman who has successfully raised a family and specializes in child care and folk remedies). Likewise, Native American clients may seek assistance from a shaman or a medicine man or woman. Clients of Asian descent may mention that they have visited herbalists, acupuncturists, or bone setters.

Each culture has its own healers, most of whom speak the native tongue of the client, make house calls, and cost significantly less than healers practicing in the biomedical-scientific health care system. In addition to folk healers, many cultures rely on lay midwives (e.g., *parteras* for Hispanic women) or other health care providers to meet the needs of pregnant women.

In some religions, spiritual healers may be found among the ranks of the ordained or official religious hierarchy ranks and are called priest, bishop, elder, deacon, rabbi, brother, or sister. Other religions have a separate category of healer (e.g., Christian Science "nurses" [not licensed by states] or practitioners) (Andrews, 2008).

A comprehensive discussion of the variety of healing beliefs and practices used by the numerous cultural groups is beyond the scope of this chapter. However, the nurse should be aware of alternative practices and folk healers that are used by the groups for which they care. The nurse should also be aware that most indigenous healing practices are innocuous, regardless of whether they are effective.

Cultural Expressions of Illness

A wide cultural variation exists in the manner in which certain symptoms and disease conditions are perceived, diagnosed, labeled, and treated. The disease that is grounds for social ostracism in one culture may be reason for increased status in another. For example, epilepsy is contagious and untreatable among Ugandans, a cause for family shame among Greeks, a reflection of a physical imbalance among Mexican Americans, and a sign of having gained favor by enduring a trial by God among the Hutterites.

Bodily symptoms are also perceived and reported in a variety of ways. For example, individuals of Mediterranean descent tend to report common physical symptoms more often than people of northern European or Asian heritage. The Chinese do not have a translation for the English word *sadness,* yet all people experience the feeling of sadness at some time in their lives. To express emotion, Chinese clients sometimes somaticize their symptoms. For example, a client may complain of cardiac symptoms because the center of emotion in the Chinese culture is the heart. If the client has experienced a loss through death or divorce and is grieving, he or she may describe the loss in terms of a pain in the heart. Although some biomedical-scientific clinicians may refer to this pain as a psychosomatic illness, others will recognize it as a culturally acceptable somatic expression of emotional disharmony.

Cultural Expression of Pain

Pain, an extensively studied symptom, is used here to illustrate the manner in which symptom expression may reflect the client's cultural background. Pain is a universally recognized phenomenon and an important aspect of assessment for clients of various ages. It is also a private, subjective experience that is greatly influenced by cultural heritage. Expectations, manifestations, and pain management are all embedded in a cultural context. The definition of pain, like that of health or illness, is culturally determined.

The term *pain* is derived from the Greek word for penalty, a fact that helps explain the long association between pain and punishment in Judeo-Christian thought. The meaning of painful stimuli for individuals, the way people define their situation, and the influence of personal experience combine to determine the experience of pain.

Much cross-cultural research has been conducted on pain (Ludwig-Beymer, 2008; Zborowski, 1969). Pain has been found to be a highly personal experience that depends on cultural learning, the meaning of the situation, and other factors unique to the individual. Health care professionals have identified silent suffering as the most valued response to pain. The majority of nurses have been socialized to believe that, in virtually any situation, self-control is better than open displays of strong feelings.

Studies of nurses' attitudes toward pain reveal that the ethnic background of clients is relevant to the nurses' assessment of physical and psychological pain. Nurses view Jewish and Spanish clients as experiencing suffering the most and Anglo-Saxon Germanic clients as experiencing suffering the least. In addition, nurses who infer relatively greater client pain tended to report their own experiences as more painful. In general, nurses with an eastern or southern European or African background tend to infer greater suffering than do nurses of northern European background. Years of experience, current position, and area of clinical practice are unrelated to inferences of suffering (Ludwig-Beymer, 2008).

In addition to expecting variations in pain perception and tolerance, a nurse should expect variations in the expression of pain. Individuals turn to their social environments for validation and comparison. A first important comparison group is the family, which transmits cultural norms to its children.

Culture-Bound Syndromes

Clients may have a condition that is culturally defined, known as a culture-bound syndrome. Some of these conditions have no equal from a biomedical or scientific perspective, but others, such as anorexia nervosa and bulimia, are examples of health problems found primarily among members of the dominant U.S. cultural group. Table 13-4 presents selected examples from among more than 150 culture-bound syndromes that have been documented by medical anthropologists.

TABLE 13-4	SELECTED CULTURE-BOUND SYNDROMES	
GROUP	**DISORDER(S)**	**REMARKS**
Whites	Anorexia nervosa	Excessive preoccupation with thinness, self-imposed starvation
	Bulimia	Gross overeating, then vomiting or fasting
African Americans	Blackout	Collapse, dizziness, or inability to move
	Low blood	Not enough blood or weakness of the blood that is often treated with diet
	High blood	Blood that is too rich in certain components from ingesting too much red meat or rich foods
	Thin blood	In women, children, and the elderly; renders the individual more susceptible to illness in general
	Diseases of hex, witchcraft, or conjuring	Sense of being doomed by a spell, part of voodoo beliefs
Chinese or Southeast Asians	Koro	Intense anxiety that the penis is retracting into the body
Greeks	Hysteria	Bizarre complaints and behavior because the uterus leaves the pelvis and goes to another part of the body
Hispanics	Empacho	Food forms into a ball and clings to the stomach or intestines, causing pain and cramping
	Fatigue	Asthma-like symptoms
	Mal ojo (evil eye)	Fitful sleep, crying, and diarrhea in children caused by a stranger's attention; sudden onset
	Pasmo	Paralysis-like symptoms of face or limbs; prevented or relieved by massage
	Susto	Anxiety, trembling, and phobias from sudden fright
Native Americans	Ghost	Terror, hallucinations, and sense of danger
Japanese	Wagamama	Apathetic childish behavior with emotional outbursts

MANAGEMENT OF HEALTH PROBLEMS: A CULTURAL PERSPECTIVE

After a symptom is identified, the first effort at treatment is often self-care. In the United States, an estimated 70% to 90% of all illness episodes are treated first, or exclusively, through self-care, often with significant success. The availability of over-the-counter medications, a relatively high literacy level, and influence of the mass media in communicating health-related information to the general population have contributed to the high percentage of self-treatment. Home treatments are attractive because of their accessibility in comparison with the inconvenience associated with traveling to a physician, nurse practitioner, and pharmacist, particularly for clients from rural or sparsely populated areas. Furthermore, home treatment may mobilize the client's social support network and provide the sick individual with a caring environment in which to convalesce.

However, the nurse should be aware that not all home remedies are inexpensive. For example, urban African American populations in the Southeast sometimes use medicinal potions that cost much more than an equivalent treatment with a biomedical intervention.

Various nontraditional interventions are gaining the recognition of health care professionals in the biomedical-scientific health care system. Acupuncture, acupressure, therapeutic touch, massage, biofeedback, relaxation techniques, meditation, hypnosis, distraction, imagery, and herbal remedies are interventions that clients may use alone or in combination with other treatments.

Cultural Negotiation

Cultural negotiation refers to the process in which messages, instructions, and belief systems are manipulated, linked, or processed between the professional and lay models of health problems and preferred treatment. In each act, the nurse gives attention to eliciting the client's views regarding a health-related experience (e.g., pregnancy, complications of pregnancy, or illness of an infant).

Katon and Kleinman (1981) describe negotiation as a bilateral arrangement in which two principal parties attempt to work out a solution. The goal of negotiation is to reduce conflict in a way that promotes cooperation. Cultural negotiation is used when conceptual differences exist between the client and the nurse, a situation that may occur for one or more of the following reasons:

- The nurse and client may be using the same words but applying different meanings to them.
- The nurse and client may apply the same term to the same phenomenon but have different notions of its causation.
- The nurse and client may have different memories or emotions associated with the term and its use.

In cultural negotiation, the nurse provides scientific information while acknowledging that the client may hold different views. If the client's perspective indicates that behaviors would be helpful, positive, adaptive, or neutral in effect, the nurse should include them in the plan of care. However, if the client's perspective would result in behaviors that may be harmful, negative, or nonadaptive, the nurse should attempt to shift the client's perspective to that of the practitioner (Spector, 2008).

Pregnancy and childbirth are social, cultural, and physiological experiences; therefore, an approach to culturally sensitive nursing care of childbearing women and their families must focus on the interaction between cultural meaning and biological functions. Childbirth is a time of transition and social celebration that is of central importance in any society; it signals realignment of existing cultural roles and responsibilities, psychological and biological states, and social relationships. Child rearing is also a period during which culturally bound values, attitudes, beliefs, and practices permeate virtually all aspects of life for the parents and child (Andrews and Boyle, 2008). Careful assessment and attention to culturally based practices are particularly important during these occasions.

Clinical Example

Bobby Jackson, 24, ducked in to the Pontiac Health Department to get out of the January wind and settled in to one of the hard plastic chairs in the waiting room for a nap. Because everyone is required to leave the overnight shelter by 7 AM each morning, he has a long 14 hours to fill until the shelter opens for the night. Since his discharge from the army, Bobby hasn't been able to find work, other than odd jobs shoveling walkways for strangers or washing windshields for stopped cars. Typically he spends any money he makes on a bottle, or a fix—anything to calm his nerves and stop the flashbacks.

Amy Butler, RN, has worked at the Health Department for six months. She has noticed the young African American man asleep in the waiting room several times recently, and she knows that the army boots and flak jacket he usually wears are not warm enough for the Michigan winters. Today, she observed him twitching and trembling while he slept. Although a colleague suggested, "Ignore him, he's just a street person," Amy approached him after he awoke to offer the services of the Health Department.

When asked by Amy, Bobby explained that he had served in Operation Iraqi Freedom. Although Bobby was very polite, like many combat veterans, he seemed reluctant to seek assistance. As with every vet she cares for, Amy looked him in the eye and thanked him for his service. Then, she reminded him that he is entitled to health care and other benefits through the Veterans Administration (VA). She also gave him contact information for the VA clinic a few miles away, the local Veterans Center, so he can connect with other vets, and a flyer from the Michigan Veterans Trust Fund, which provides for temporary basic living needs of veterans. Then she pointed out the Alano club across the street, where recovering alcoholics would be available to help Bobby with his substance abuse problem. Finally, she made an appointment for Bobby to be evaluated by the Health Department's Nurse Practitioner for possible elevated blood pressure and frostbite.

Before he left, Bobby promised to follow up with the VA and report back to the Health Department within one week.

Created by Kathleen Walsh Spencer, DNP, MA, ACNS-BC.

MANAGEMENT OF HEALTH PROBLEMS IN CULTURALLY DIVERSE POPULATIONS

The factors responsible for the health disparity between minority and white populations are complex and defy simplistic solutions. Health status is influenced by the interaction of physiological, cultural, psychological, and societal factors that are poorly understood for the general population and even less so for minorities. Despite the shared characteristic of economic disadvantage among minorities, common approaches for improving health are not recommended because of the variations in cultural beliefs and practices that exist among the different minority populations. Rather, solving problems among minorities necessitates activities, programs, and data collection that are tailored to meet the unique health care needs of many different subgroups. Solutions to health care problems among culturally diverse populations include the following recommendations that are the cornerstone of public health nursing (Keller, Strohschein, and Schaffer, 2011):

- Focus on the health of entire populations
- Reflect community priorities and needs
- Establish caring relationships with the communities, families, and individuals that make up the population
- Remain grounded in social justice having compassion and respect for the worth of all people especially the vulnerable
- Provide care for the whole person: mental, physical, emotional, social, spiritual and environmental aspects
- Promote health through strategies based on epidemiological evidence (evidence-based practice)
- Collaborate with community resources to reach health care goals

Providing Health Information and Education

Minority populations need more information about their health risks and treatment options. This is demonstrated by the following facts (American Cancer Society, 2012; USDHHS, 2006):

- African Americans have the highest mortality rate and shortest survival rate for many cancers.
- African Americans receive less information about cancer and heart disease than nonminority groups.
- African Americans tend to underestimate the prevalence of cancer, give less credence to the warning signs, obtain fewer screening tests, and receive a diagnosis at later stages of cancer than whites.
- Many professionals and laypeople, both minority and white, do not know that heart disease is as common in African American men as in white men and that African American women die of coronary heart disease at a higher rate than white women.
- Mexican Americans have a higher incidence of overweight and obesity than non-Hispanic whites.

Programs to increase public awareness about health problems have been well received in several areas. For example, the Healthy Mothers, Healthy Babies Coalition, which provides an education program in both English and Spanish, has contributed to greater awareness of measures to improve the health status of mothers and infants. In addition, increased knowledge among African Americans of hypertension as a serious health problem is one of the accomplishments of the National High Blood Pressure Education program. The success of these efforts indicates that carefully planned programs have a beneficial effect, but efforts must continue and must expand to reach even more of the target population and focus on additional health problems.

Planning Health Information Campaigns

Sensitivity to cultural factors is often lacking in the health care of minorities. Key concepts for the nurse to consider in designing a health information campaign include meeting the language and cultural needs of each identified minority group, using minority-specific community resources to tailor educational approaches, and developing materials and methods of presentation that are commensurate with the educational level of the target population. Furthermore, the powerful influences of cultural factors over a lifetime in shaping people's attitudes, values, beliefs, and practices concerning health require health information programs to be sustained over a long period. The following are examples of ways in which the nurse can interweave these concepts into health promotion efforts:

- The nurse should involve local community leaders who are members of the targeted cultural group to promote acceptance and reinforcement of the central themes of health promotion messages.
- Health messages are more readily accepted if they do not conflict with existing cultural beliefs and practices. Where appropriate, messages should acknowledge existing cultural beliefs.
- The nurse should involve families, churches, employers, and community organizations as a support system to facilitate and sustain behavioral change to a more healthful lifestyle. For example, although hypertension control in African Americans depends on appropriate treatment (e.g., medication), blood pressure can be improved and maintained by family and community support of activities such as proper diet and exercise.
- Language barriers, cultural differences, and lack of adequate information on access to care complicate prenatal care for Hispanic and Asian women who have recently arrived in the United States. Through the use of lay volunteers to organize community support networks, programs have been developed to disseminate culturally appropriate health information.

Health Education

Although printed materials and other audiovisual aids contribute to the educational process, client education is inherently interpersonal. The success of educational efforts is often determined by the credibility of the source and is highly dependent on the skill and sensitivity of the nurse in communicating information in a culturally appropriate manner. Education programs are particularly critical and necessary for several health problems with the greatest influence on minority health, such as hypertension, obesity, and diabetes. For example, if patients with diabetes could improve their self-management skills through education, a significant number of complications (e.g., ketoacidosis, blindness, and amputations) could be avoided, saving human misery and health care dollars.

Delivering and Financing Health Services

Innovative models for delivering and financing health services for minority populations are needed. According to community health experts, models should increase flexibility of health care delivery, facilitate minorities' access to services, and improve efficiency of service and payment systems. One of the most commonly used indicators of the adequacy of health services for a population is the distribution of health care providers; however, this is an inadequate measurement. The following observations exemplify the problems associated with health services for minorities:

- The disparities in death rates between minorities and whites remain despite overall increases in health care access and use.
- Language problems hinder refugees and immigrants when they seek health care.
- African Americans with cancer postpone seeking diagnosis of their symptoms longer than whites and delay initiation of treatment once diagnosed (American Cancer Society, 2012).
- The infant mortality rate among African American women is more than twice as high as the infant mortality rate among white women (USDHHS, 2006).

Models of Health Promotion

In most health models, SES is assumed to affect health status through environmental or behavioral factors. These models posit that poor families may not have the economic, social, or community resources needed to remain in good health. For example, poverty is thought to affect children's well-being by affecting health and nutrition, the home environment, caregiver interactions with children, caregiver mental health, and neighborhood conditions. The deficits associated with poverty may lead to an inadequate diet, which results in poor growth and delayed development. Likewise, poor housing raises the risk for exposure to many illnesses and infections; overcrowding results in increased risk for infectious diseases such as tuberculosis, meningitis, influenza, and related conditions; and community violence threatens the safety and well-being of children. The combined effect of these stressors is thought to provide the foundation for a cycle of hopelessness and depression among family members, who in turn may engage in risky health behaviors (e.g., smoking, substance abuse, and poor dietary habits resulting in obesity and high cholesterol levels) and unfavorable family interactions.

Although many Latino children live in poverty, they enjoy relatively good health in comparison with children in other low socioeconomic groups. This finding has been called an epidemiological paradox. The assumption is that if the family promotes beneficial health behaviors among its members, these behaviors will become integrated into the culture. Healthy lifestyle behaviors become an integral component of the family identity, traditions, and history.

Continuity of Care

Continuity of care is associated with improved health outcomes and is presumably greater when a client is able to establish an ongoing relationship with a care provider. Many of the leading causes of death among minorities (e.g., cancer, cardiovascular disease, and diabetes) are chronic rather than acute problems; therefore they require extended treatment regimens. Consider the following:

- Refugees are eligible for special refugee medical assistance during their first 18 months in the United States. However, after this period, refugees who cannot afford private health insurance and are ineligible for Medicaid or state medical assistance may become medically indigent.
- Many Native Americans and Alaska Natives live in areas where the availability of health care providers is half the national average.

Health Care Financing Problems

As mentioned previously, problems associated with financing health care tend to be more common in minority groups than in the dominant cultural group. Consider the following (National Center for Health Statistics, 2008):

- Economic inequalities cause members of minority groups to rely disproportionately on Medicaid for their health care needs.
- Older minority people are less likely than whites to supplement Medicare with additional private insurance.
- Proportionately, three times as many Native Americans, African Americans, Hispanics, and certain Asian and Pacific Islander groups as whites live in poverty.
- In 2008, 30.4% of Hispanics lacked insurance coverage, compared with 17% of African Americans and 9.9% of whites.

To better manage health problems and reduce the disparity in health indicators, these issues of financing must be addressed. Failure to address them will result not only in continued inequity in access to services but also in continued poor health among minority groups.

Developing Health Professionals from Minority Groups

The need to increase the number of health professionals from minority groups has been recognized for decades. With few exceptions, minorities are underrepresented as students and practitioners of the health professions. Although the number of minority nursing students has been steadily increasing, there still are proportionately more white nursing students.

Differences in the availability of health personnel resources in minority communities are apparent, regardless of the minority group being considered. Communities located in urban-metropolitan areas have significantly more professional resources. Among the factors that contribute to the imbalances in minority representation in health professions are the size of a minority population, number of cultural subgroups, and demographic features. Efforts to encourage more students from minority groups are ongoing, and government and private foundations offer grants, scholarships, and low-cost loans to recruit and retain students from underserved minority groups in nursing and other health care professions. Minority and nonminority health professional organizations, academic institutions, state governments, health departments, and other organizations from the public and private sectors should work together to develop strategies to improve the availability and accessibility of health care professionals to minority communities (Sullivan Commission, 2004).

Enhancing Cooperative Efforts with the Nonfederal Sector

Activities to improve minority health should involve participation of organizations at all levels (i.e., community, municipal, state, and national). Community involvement in developing health promotion activities can contribute to their success by providing credibility and visibility to the activities and facilitating their acceptance. Changes in health behavior frequently depend on personal initiative and are most likely to be triggered by efforts from locally based sources.

However, not all minority communities have the ability to identify their own health problems and initiate activities to address them. Support from the state and federal governments and private sector assistance are needed to assist with identifying and solving health-related problems afflicting the minority community. Assistance may be provided to minority communities in the following ways:

1. The use of technical assistance to identify high-risk groups
2. Assistance with planning, implementing, and evaluating programs to address identified needs
3. Specialized community services (e.g., federally funded projects for infants and frail older adults)
4. Programs supported by businesses and industries (e.g., health promotion programs organized by unions)

The private sector can also serve as an effective channel for programs targeted to minority health projects. National organizations concerned with minorities, such as the National Urban League and the National Alliance for Hispanic Health, include health-related issues in their national agendas and are actively seeking effective ways to improve the health of minorities. Organizations such as these have a powerful potential for effecting change among their constituencies because they have strong community-level, grass-roots support.

Promoting a Research Agenda on Minority Health Issues

The National Center on Minority Health and Health Disparities (NCMHD) (http://ncmhd.nih.gov/) was developed in 2000 to assist in the investigation of factors affecting minority health. Its mission is to promote minority health and to ultimately eliminate health disparities. The NCMHD conducts and supports research that examines risk factor prevalence and treatment services. It also reviews health education

interventions, preventive services interventions, and sociocultural factors that influence health and outcomes of care.

For further information on current research related to culture and community health nursing, the reader should search library databases for reports of completed studies. Electronic bulletin boards also may be valuable when one is searching for research in progress and for communicating with researchers studying a particular phenomenon of interest. An example of recent nursing research related to culturally competent care is described in the Research Highlights box.

RESEARCH HIGHLIGHTS

Nutritional Patterns of Recent Immigrants

Edmonds (2005) examined the nutritional patterns of 23 women who had recently immigrated from Honduras to assist in understanding health-related nutritional issues in this Hispanic subgroup. She determined that the Honduran women had made both positive and negative changes in their diets since coming to the United States. Rice, beans, natural fruit juices, tortillas, bananas, beef, and eggs were reported as the typical foods eaten every day in Honduras. Positive changes in diets included eating a greater variety of fruits and vegetables, cooking with less grease, baking more frequently than frying, and using vegetable oil rather than lard. The women also ate more meat and dairy products. Negative changes noted were more skipped meals and eating foods high in fat and calories (e.g., fast foods). Research suggests that classes be taught in Women, Infants, and Children (WIC) programs and other venues that would support the Hondurans' traditional diet and focus on how to eat nutritionally in fast-food restaurants, eat a balanced diet, plan meals and cook ahead, and read food labels.

Data from Edmonds VM: The nutritional patterns of recently immigrated Honduran women, *J Transcult Nurs* 16(3):226-235, 2005.

ROLE OF THE COMMUNITY HEALTH NURSE IN IMPROVING HEALTH FOR CULTURALLY DIVERSE PEOPLE

This chapter provides data detailing the health care problems of culturally diverse individuals, families, groups, and communities. Given the complexity of the problems and the wide variation in incidence and distribution of these problems within specific subgroups, no simple method exists for providing culturally sensitive community health nursing care to all clients. However, the following strategies may assist the community health nurse when working with culturally diverse clients:

- Conduct a "culturological" assessment.
- Conduct a cultural self-assessment.
- Seek knowledge about local cultures.
- Recognize the political issues of culturally diverse groups.
- Provide culturally competent care.
- Recognize culturally based health problems.

Culturological Assessment

All nursing care is based on a systematic, comprehensive assessment of the client; therefore the community health nurse must gather cultural data on clients from racially and ethnically diverse backgrounds. A culturological assessment refers to a systematic appraisal or examination of individuals, groups, and communities regarding their cultural beliefs, values, and practices to determine explicit nursing needs and intervention practices within the cultural context of the people being evaluated (Leininger, 1995). The term culturological is a descriptive reference to cultural phenomena in their broadest sense.

Culturological assessments are as vital as physical and psychological assessments. Culturological assessments tend to be broad and comprehensive because they deal with cultural values, belief systems, and ways of living now and in the recent past. In conducting a culturological assessment, the community health nurse should be involved in determining and appraising the traits, characteristics, or smallest units of cultural behavior as a guide to nursing care. The following sections summarize major data categories pertaining to the culture of clients and offer suggested questions that the nurse may ask to elicit needed information.

Brief History of Ethnic and Racial Origins of the Cultural Group with Which the Client Identifies

- With what ethnic group or groups does the client report affiliation (e.g., Hispanic, Polish, Navajo, or a combination)? To what degree does the client identify with the cultural group (e.g., "we" concept of solidarity or a fringe member)?
- Where has the client lived (i.e., country and city) and when (i.e., during what years)? If the client has recently relocated to the United States, knowledge of prevalent diseases in the country of origin may be helpful.

Values Orientation

- What are the client's attitudes, values, and beliefs about birth, death, health, illness, and health care providers?
- Does culture influence the manner in which the client relates to body image change resulting from illness or surgery (e.g., importance of appearance, beauty, strength, and roles in cultural group)?
- How does the client view work, leisure, and education?
- How does the client perceive change?
- How does the client value privacy, courtesy, touch, and relationships with individuals of different ages, of different social class, or caste, and of the opposite sex?
- How does the client relate to people in a different cultural group (e.g., withdrawal, verbal or nonverbal expression, or negative or positive attitude)?

Cultural Sanctions and Restrictions

- How does the client's cultural group regard expression of emotion and feelings, spirituality, and religious beliefs? How are dying, death, and grieving expressed in a culturally appropriate manner?
- How is modesty expressed by men and women in the client's cultural group? Does the client's cultural group have culturally defined expectations about male-female relationships, including the nurse-client relationship?

- Does the client have restrictions related to sexuality, exposure of body parts, or certain types of surgery (e.g., amputation, vasectomy, or hysterectomy)?
- Does the client have restrictions against discussion of dead relatives or fears related to the unknown?

Communication

- What language does the client speak at home? What other language does the client speak or read? In what language would the client prefer to communicate with you?
- What is the written and spoken English fluency level of the client? Remember that the stress of illness may cause clients to use a more familiar language and temporarily forget some English.
- Does the client need an interpreter? If so, make sure to use an interpreter who is fluent in medical language and is not a relative or friend of the client.
- What are the rules (i.e., linguistics) and modes (i.e., style) of communication?
- Is it necessary to vary the technique of communication during the interview and examination to accommodate the client's cultural background (e.g., tempo of conversation, eye contact, sensitivity to topical taboos, norms of confidentiality, and style of explanation)?
- How does the client's nonverbal communication compare with that of individuals from other cultural backgrounds? How does it affect the client's relationship with the nurse and with other members of the health care team?
- How does the client feel about health care providers who are not of the same cultural background (e.g., African American, middle-class nurse, or Hispanic of a different social class)? Does the client prefer to receive care from a nurse of the same cultural background, sex, or age?

⚖ ETHICAL INSIGHTS

Disclosure Of HIV/AIDS Status

Ortiz (2005) examined the experiences of 19 Latinas who disclosed they were living with human immunodeficiency virus (HIV)/acquired immunodeficiency syndrome (AIDS). She described how the women decided to disclose their HIV status to partners, family members, friends, and employers. Four categories emerged: timing of the disclosure, the need to disclose, controlling disclosure, and supportive disclosing. These factors were influenced by the Latinas' relationship with others, the perceived risks to the women and others, the need to disclose, the wish to give support to themselves or others, and the desire to control who should know and when. Ortiz concluded that nurses should be knowledgeable of the realities of Latinas' lives and to be able to incorporate that knowledge into comprehensive care plans that will help them maximize the utilization of appropriate resources.

Data from Ortiz CE: Disclosing concerns of Latinas living with HIV/AIDS, *J Transcult Nurs* 16(3):210-217, 2005.

Health-Related Beliefs and Practices

- To what cause(s) does the client attribute illness and disease (e.g., divine wrath, imbalance in hot-cold or yin-yang, punishment for moral transgressions, hex, or soul loss)?

- What does the client believe promotes health (e.g., eating certain foods, wearing amulets to bring good luck, exercise, prayer, ancestors, saints, or intermediate deities)?
- What is the client's religious affiliation (e.g., Judaism, Islam, Pentecostalism, West African voodooism, Seventh-Day Adventism, Catholicism, or Mormonism)?
- Does the client rely on cultural healers (e.g., curandero, shaman, spiritualist, priest, minister, or monk)? Who determines when the client is sick and when the client is healthy? Who determines the type of healer and treatment that should be sought?
- In what types of cultural healing practices does the client engage (e.g., herbal remedies, potions, massage, wearing talismans or charms to discourage evil spirits, healing rituals, incantations, or prayers)?
- How does the client perceive biomedical-scientific health care providers? How do the client and family perceive nurses? What are the expectations of nurses and nursing care?
- What constitutes appropriate "sick-role" behavior? Who determines what symptoms constitute disease and illness? Who decides when the client is no longer sick? Who cares for the client at home?
- How does the client's cultural group view mental disorders? Do they show differences in acceptable behaviors for physical versus psychological illnesses?

Nutrition

- What nutritional factors are influenced by the client's cultural background?
- What meanings does the client attach to food and eating? With whom does the client usually eat? What types of foods does the client usually eat? What does the client define as food? What does the client believe defines a "healthy" versus an "unhealthy" diet?
- How does the client prepare foods at home (e.g., type of food preparation; cooking oils used; length of time foods, especially vegetables, are cooked; amount and type of seasoning added to various foods during preparation)?
- Do religious beliefs and practices influence the client's diet (e.g., amount, type, preparation, or delineation of acceptable food combinations, such as kosher diets)? Does the client abstain from certain foods at regular intervals, on specific dates determined by the religious calendar, or at other times?
- If the client's religion mandates or encourages fasting, what does the term *fast* mean to the client (e.g., refraining from certain types or quantities of foods, eating only during certain times of the day)? For what period of time is the client expected to fast? Does the religion allow exemption from fasting during illness, and, if so, is the client believed to have an exemption?

Socioeconomic Considerations

- Who constitutes the client's social network (i.e., family, peers, and healers)? How do they influence the client's health or illness status?
- How do members of the client's social support network define *caring* (e.g., being continuously present, doing things for the client, or looking after the client's family)? What are the roles of various family members during health and illness?
- How does the client's family participate in the client's nursing care (e.g., bathing, feeding, touching, and being present)?
- Does the cultural family structure influence the client's response to health or illness (e.g., beliefs, strengths, weaknesses, and social class)? Does a key family member have a role that is significant in health-related decisions (e.g., grandmother in many African American families or eldest adult son in Asian families)?
- Who is the principal wage earner in the client's family? What is the total annual income? This is a potentially sensitive question that should be asked only if necessary. Does the family have more than one wage earner? Does the family have other sources of financial support (e.g., extended family or investments)?
- What influence does economic status have on lifestyle, place of residence, living conditions, ability to obtain health care, and discharge planning?

Organizations Providing Cultural Support

- What influence do ethnic and cultural organizations have on the client's receiving health care (e.g., National Association for the Advancement of Colored People, African American Political Caucus, churches, schools, Urban League, and community-based health care programs and clinics)?

Educational Background

- What is the highest educational level the client has obtained? Does the client's educational background affect the client's knowledge level concerning the health care delivery system, how to obtain the care needed, teaching and learning skills, and written material that is distributed in the health care setting (e.g., insurance forms, educational literature, information about diagnostic procedures and laboratory tests, and admissions forms)?
- Can the client read and write English, or does he or she prefer another language? If English is the client's second language, are materials available in the client's primary language?
- What learning style is most comfortable or familiar? Does the client prefer to learn through written materials, oral explanation, or demonstration?

Religious Affiliation

- How does the client's religious affiliation influence health and illness (e.g., death, chronic illness, body image alteration, and cause and effect of illness)?
- What is the role of the client's religious beliefs and practices during health and illness?
- What is the role of significant religious representatives during health and illness? Does the client have recognized religious healers (e.g., Islamic imams, Christian Scientist practitioners or nurses, Catholic priests, Mormon elders, and Buddhist monks)?

Cultural Aspects of Disease Incidence

- Does the client have specific genetic or acquired conditions that are more prevalent in a specific cultural group (e.g., hypertension, sickle cell anemia, Tay-Sachs disease, or lactose intolerance)?
- Are any socioenvironmental diseases more prevalent among the client's specific cultural group (e.g., lead poisoning, alcoholism, acquired immunodeficiency syndrome [AIDS], drug abuse, or ear infections)?
- Do diseases exist against which the client has an increased resistance (e.g., skin cancer in a darkly pigmented individual)?

Biocultural Variations

- Does the client have distinctive physical features that are characteristic of a particular racial group (e.g., skin color or hair texture)? Does the client have variations in anatomy that are characteristic of a particular racial or ethnic group (e.g., body structure, height, weight, facial shape and structure [nose, eye shape, and facial contour], or upper and lower extremity shape)?
- How do anatomical and racial variations affect the assessment?

Developmental Considerations

- Does the client have distinct growth and development characteristics that vary with his or her cultural background (e.g., bone density, psychomotor patterns of development, or fat folds)?
- What factors are significant in assessing children from the newborn period through adolescence (e.g., expected growth on standard grid, culturally acceptable age for toilet training, introduction of various types of foods, sex differences, discipline, and socialization to adult roles)?
- What is the cultural perception of aging (e.g., is youthfulness or the wisdom of old age more highly valued)?
- How are older people handled culturally (e.g., cared for in the home of adult children or placed in institutions for care)? What are culturally acceptable roles for older adults?
- Does the older adult expect family members to provide care, including nurturance and other humanistic aspects of care?
- Is the older adult isolated from culturally relevant supportive people or enmeshed in a caring network of relatives and friends?
- Has a culturally appropriate network replaced family members in performing some caring functions for older adults?

Cultural Self-Assessment

Community health nurses can engage in a cultural self-assessment. Through identification of health-related attitudes, values, beliefs, and practices that are part of the personal cultural meaning brought to the nurse-client interaction, the nurse can better understand the cultural aspects of health care from the perspective of the client, family, group, or community. Everyone has ethnocentric tendencies that must be brought to a level of conscious awareness so that efforts can be made to temper ethnocentrism and view reality from the perspective of the client.

Knowledge about Local Cultures

Community health nurses can learn about the cultural diversity characteristics of the subgroup or subgroups that are most prevalent within their communities. The nurse cannot know about all health-related beliefs and practices of the diverse groups served, but he or she can study select ones. The nurse can accomplish this cultural study through a review of nursing, anthropology, sociology, and related literature on culturally diverse groups; in-service programs held at community health agencies, educational institutions in the community, or organizations serving minority groups; enrollment in courses on transcultural or cross-cultural nursing and medical anthropology; and interviews with key members of the subgroups of interest, such as clergy members, nurses, and physicians, to obtain information about the influence of culture on health-related beliefs and practices.

Recognition of Political Issues of Culturally Diverse Groups

Awareness of the political aspects of health care for culturally diverse groups and communities can help community health nurses influence legislation and funding priorities aimed at improving health care for specific populations. Recognized for their leadership role in community health matters involving culturally diverse groups, community health nurses may be invited by political leaders to participate in political decision making that affects the health of a targeted subgroup. Community health nurses should also be active politically, both individually and collectively, to influence legislation affecting culturally diverse individuals, groups, and communities, and they should offer to serve on key community committees, boards, and advisory councils that impact the health of culturally diverse groups.

Providing Culturally Competent Care

When caring for individuals and families from culturally diverse backgrounds, the community health nurse can assess, diagnose, implement, and evaluate nursing care in a manner that is culturally congruent, competent, relevant, and appropriate. To provide this culturally appropriate nursing care, the nurse must create a relationship of mutual respect by becoming aware of the cultural similarities and differences between herself or himself and the client. A guideline for gathering cultural data has been presented, and the nurse may use this guideline or a similar one to identify significant areas in which the nurse and client differ. Knowledge about biocultural variations in health and illness is particularly important when the nurse is conducting cultural assessments.

Recognition of Culturally Based Health Practices

As discussed previously, the community health nurse should attempt to understand the nature and meaning of culturally based health practices of clients, groups, and communities. Once the practices are understood, the nurse can make a determination regarding their appropriateness in a particular context. Generally, the nurse should decide whether a cultural practice is useful, neutral, or harmful to the client, group, or community. The nurse should encourage or "tolerate" helpful and neutral practices, whereas he or she should discourage harmful practices.

However, the classification of some cultural healing practices is not so easily determined. For example, many Southeast

Asians practice coining, which is the rubbing of a coin over body surfaces to expel "bad winds" that are believed to cause illness. Community health nurses are faced with an ethical dilemma when coining is practiced on young children, because it leaves abrasions on the skin and may be viewed by some as child abuse. This practice is not useful, so the nurse must make the decision whether it is neutral or harmful. An argument for the practice's being neutral is that abrasions usually heal quickly, so no harm is done to the child as a result. Further-more, the practice is meaningful to parents who have much confidence in the healing powers associated with coining.

The argument can also be made that the practice is harm-ful. The red marks and skin abrasions caused by the coining place the child at increased risk for skin infection. Given that the child may require antibiotics or other medication for a respiratory disorder, encouragement of coining as the only treatment may prevent the child from receiving needed medi-cal intervention and may delay medical treatment. As a solu-tion, the community health nurse may suggest that parents combine traditional treatment with Western biomedicine (i.e., they can use coining in conjunction with a biomedical intervention). Therefore the healing will occur in a manner that has involved the use of both folk and professional health care systems.

RESOURCES FOR MINORITY HEALTH

Community health nurses will find federal resources for improv-ing the health care of the federally defined minority populations through the USDHHS. Within the USDHHS, the Office of Minority Health (OMH) and the Indian Health Service (IHS) divisions are concerned with health promotion, disease preven-tion, service delivery, and research for minority groups.

Office of Minority Health

The OMH coordinates federal efforts to improve the health status of racial and ethnic minority populations (i.e., African Americans, Hispanics, Native Americans and Alaska Natives, and Asians and Pacific Islanders). Directed by the deputy assistant secretary for minority health, the OMH was estab-lished by the Disadvantaged Minority Health Improvement Act of 1990 (PL 101-527), which was signed by President George H. W. Bush on November 6, 1990. Under the direc-tives of the act, the OMH is charged with duties to:

- Establish short- and long-range goals and objectives relat-ing to disease prevention, health promotion, service deliv-ery, and research on the health of minority people.
- Promote increased participation of disadvantaged people, including minorities, in health service and health promo-tion programs.
- Create a national minority health resource center.
- Support research, demonstrations, and evaluations of new and innovative models that increase understanding of disease risk factors and support better information dis-semination, education, prevention, and service delivery to minority communities.
- Promote minority health–related activities in the corpo-rate and voluntary sectors.

- Develop minority-focused health information and health promotion materials and teaching programs.
- Assist providers of primary care and preventive services in obtaining assistance of bilingual health professionals when appropriate.

As the focal point for minority health efforts, the OMH plays a key role in major initiatives launched by the secretary of the USDHHS. Table 13-5 lists some of these initiatives.

Indian Health Service

The IHS is responsible for providing federal health services to Native Americans and Alaska Natives. Federal Indian health services are based on a special government-to-government relationship and laws that Congress has passed pursuant to its authority to regulate commerce with the Indian Nations as specified in the Constitution and other documents.

TABLE 13-5	FEDERALLY SPONSORED INITIATIVES TO IMPROVE THE HEALTH OF MINORITY GROUPS
INITIATIVE	**DESCRIPTION**
Health Resources and Services Administration Health Disparity Collaboratives (HDC)	HDC is a broad, multiyear plan to improve the health status of underserved populations. It seeks to ensure that clients receive evidence-based care, and it encourages clients to be active participants in their own care.
Racial and Ethnic Approach-es to Community Health (REACH 2010)	This program was launched in 1999 to eliminate health disparities in six priority areas: cardiovascular diseases, immunizations, breast and cervical cancer screening and management, diabetes, hu-man immunodeficiency virus /acquired immunodeficiency syndrome (AIDS), and infant mortality. REACH 2010 supports community coalitions in designing, implementing, and evaluating community-driven strategies to eliminate health disparities.
National Breast and Cervical Cancer Early Detection Program (NBCCEDP)	NBCCEDP provides breast and cervical cancer screening, diagnosis, and treatment to low-income, medically under-served, and uninsured women (emphasizing recruitment of minority women).
Ryan White Comprehensive AIDS Resources Emergency (CARE) Act B	Ryan White CARE Act provides services to persons living with HIV disease, primarily racial and ethnic minorities.
National Center on Minority Health and Health Disparities (NCMHD)	NCMHD leads, coordinates, supports, and assesses the National Institutes of Health's research efforts to reduce and ultimately eliminate health disparities.

The primary responsibility of the IHS is to elevate the health status of Native Americans and Alaska Natives to the highest level possible. The mission is to ensure quality, availability, and accessibility of a comprehensive, high-quality health care delivery system, providing maximum involvement of Native Americans and Alaska Natives in defining their health needs, setting health priorities for their local areas, and managing and controlling their health programs.

The IHS also acts as the principal federal health advocate for Native Americans by ensuring that they have knowledge of, and access to, all federal, state, and local health programs to which they are entitled as American citizens. The IHS carried out its responsibilities through development and operation of a health services delivery system designed to provide a broad-spectrum program of preventive, curative, rehabilitative, and environmental services. This system integrates health services delivered directly through IHS facilities and staff with those purchased by IHS through contractual arrangements. Tribes are also actively involved in program implementation.

The 1975 Indian Self-Determination Act (PL 93-638), as amended, builds on IHS policy by giving tribes the option of staffing and managing IHS programs in their communities and provides funding for improvement of tribal capability to contract under the act. The 1976 Indian Health Care Improvement Act (PL 94-437), as amended, was intended to elevate the health care status of Native Americans and Alaska Natives to a level equal to that of the general population through a program of authorized, higher-resource levels in the IHS budget. Appropriated resources were used to expand health services, build and renovate medical facilities, and step up the construction of safe drinking water and sanitary disposal facilities. It also established programs designed to increase the number of Native American health professionals for Native American needs and to improve health care access for Native Americans living in urban areas.

The operation of the IHS health care delivery system is managed through local administrative units called service units. A service unit is the basic health organization for a geographic area served by the IHS program, just as a county or city health department is the basic health organization in a state health department. These are defined areas usually centered on a single federal reservation in the continental United States or a population concentration in Alaska. The IHS serves approximately 50% of the total Native American and Alaska Native population in the United States, primarily those residing on reservations.

CASE STUDY   APPLICATION OF THE NURSING PROCESS

Community health nurse Maria Gonzales visited the home of 5-year-old Nguyen Van Nghi, who was discharged from the hospital on the previous day. The pediatrician had diagnosed pneumonia and "suspected failure to thrive" in the child because the child's growth fell below the third percentile on a standard growth chart for height and weight, and he performed poorly on a screening test used to identify developmental delays for a 5-year-old child.

Residing in the home were the child's parents, four siblings, grandmother, aunt, uncle, and three cousins. Although the child's father and uncle spoke some English, other members of the household communicated in a language unfamiliar to Maria, which "sounded like Chinese." When Maria approached the child, he did not look at her or speak to her, even when she called him Nguyen (pronounced "we'en").

Assessment

In a brief survey of the Nguyens' home, Maria noted that the home and furnishings were modest but very clean. The pantry held a considerable amount of food, including rice and dried noodles. The small refrigerator smelled of fish and contained some vegetables that Maria did not recognize. She did not see any green vegetables, milk, or other dairy products.

During her initial assessment of Nghi, Maria observed multiple tender, ecchymotic areas with petechiae between the ribs on the front and back of the body, resembling strap marks. Suspecting child abuse, Maria told the family that she would return later in the day with an interpreter. She located an interpreter who spoke Mandarin Chinese and briefed him about her concerns with child abuse. When Maria and the interpreter returned to the client's home, she instructed the interpreter to ask the parents for an explanation of the bruises. The interpreter told Maria that the family was Vietnamese and could not understand his Chinese dialect. Both the interpreter and the child's father knew a little French and awkwardly managed to communicate.

The interpreter advised the nurse that, in the Vietnamese culture, the person's family name is given first, followed by the middle name and then the first name. Only a few different family names exist among the Vietnamese; therefore it is common practice to call people by their given first name. At this point, Maria also learned that the child was actually 4 years old, because the Vietnamese consider a newborn to be 1 year old at birth.

The interpreter explained that a Vietnamese healer performed *cao gio,* or coining, to exude the "bad wind" from Nghi. *Cao gio* is performed by applying a special menthol oil to the painful or symptomatic part of the body and then rubbing a coin over the area with firm, downward strokes. When Nghi's condition seemed to worsen after his hospital discharge, his grandmother persuaded his parents that Western biomedicine had failed and that their son required the stronger power of folk healing.

Diagnosis

- Maria must set priorities and focus on selected cultural data categories because they seem most relevant for the Nguyen family at present.

Individual

- High risk for Nghi's pneumonia to worsen
- Potential for child abuse/neglect
- Possible physical and/or developmental delay (low weight/height for age)

Family

- Increased risk for poor health outcomes related to distrust of Western health care practices
- Increased risk for nutritional deficits

Community

- Potential for poor health of area Vietnamese immigrants related to limited knowledge of good nutritional practices and general health promotion

Planning
Individual

Short-Term Goals

- Nghi's pneumonia will resolve.
- Nghi will show no more evidence of the practice of "coining."

CASE STUDY   APPLICATION OF THE NURSING PROCESS—cont'd

Long-Term Goal
- Nghi's height and weight will increase proportionally to at least the 50th percentile for age.

Family

Short-Term Goals
- Family members will cease the practice of "coining."
- Caregivers will recognize the importance of completing the antibiotic therapy as prescribed.

Long-Term Goal
- A family nutritional assessment will be completed, and adjustments will be made to their diet to provide needed nutrients.

Community

Long-Term Goal
- Leaders of the area's Vietnamese community will work with area health care providers to promote good nutritional practices.

Intervention
Individual

Through the interpreter, Maria was able to communicate with the Nguyen family that it was vital for Nghi to take all of the prescribed antibiotics. She also attempted to convey the potentially harmful effect of the practice of coining and suggested that that procedure be stopped. She set a follow-up appointment for the following day.

Family

Maria was able to bring a Vietnamese interpreter for the follow-up appointment. So, in addition to reiteration of the importance of taking the medications, she was able to teach about basic nutritional principles and perform additional nutritional assessments. Although Nghi was not as small as initially thought, he was still below the 50th percentile for his age. Maria gave nutritional pamphlets written in Vietnamese to the parents and provided them with information on where to find low-cost foods in the neighborhood.

Community

Working with the health department's social worker and the Vietnamese interpreter, Maria visited several area markets to gather information on diet and nutritional practices of Vietnamese immigrants. They decided that they would seek a small grant to develop more teaching materials on nutrition for this population.

Evaluation
Individual

By the third follow-up visit, Maria determined that, although Nghi still had a residual cough, his chest was clearing. In addition, there was no evidence of coining. Furthermore, Maria was shown that the family's refrigerator now contained whole milk and some leafy green vegetables. It was decided that she would return in 6 weeks for a follow-up visit to weigh and measure Nghi.

Family

The presence of the interpreter who spoke Vietnamese and who was familiar with the culture was vital. And, by the third visit, most of the family members appeared to be at ease with Maria. Mrs. Nguyen asked a number of questions about nutrition and other health issues and requested that Maria monitor the heights and weights of the other children.

Community

The health department's social worker was able to identify a small grant to develop and purchase teaching materials for the Vietnamese population. The nurse and social worker applied for the funds and are eagerly waiting to hear the outcome.

Levels of Prevention
The following are examples of three levels of prevention as applied to the case study.

Primary Prevention
- Nutritional education for the Nguyen family
- Health education targeted at developing comfort with the U.S. health care system and Western medicine
- Education related to potentially harmful practices (e.g., coining)

Secondary Prevention
Monitoring the height and weight of Nghi and his siblings

Tertiary Prevention
Evaluation of resolution of pneumonia

SUMMARY

To provide community health nursing for individuals, groups, and communities representing the hundreds of different cultures and subcultures found in the United States, the nurse should include cultural considerations in nursing care. Guidelines for gathering data from clients of culturally diverse backgrounds have been suggested in this chapter and are interwoven throughout the text. Knowledge about culture-specific and culture-universal nursing care is foundational and is an integral component of community health nursing.

LEARNING ACTIVITIES

1. Examine the vital statistics of a community, and compare differences in morbidity and mortality rates for whites and racial and ethnic subgroups. What data are available according to racial and ethnic heritage? What data are missing?

2. Visit an inner-city grocery store and compare its quality, prices, customer services, and variety of products with those of a suburban grocery store.

3. Select a client from a racially or ethnically diverse background, and conduct a cultural assessment.

4. Interview someone from a racial or ethnic background different from your own to determine beliefs about illness causation, use of the lay and professional health care delivery systems, and culturally based treatments.

5. Dine at an ethnic restaurant. While dining, notice the type of cultural heritage in restaurant decor and information about the culture available from the menu, placemats, or elsewhere in the restaurant. Ask the owner or manager about the history of the restaurant.

6. Attend religious services at a church, temple, synagogue, or place of worship for a religion unfamiliar to you.

7. Interview an official representative (e.g., priest, elder, monk, or bishop) of a religion unfamiliar to you. Ask

about health-related beliefs and practices, healing rituals, support network for the sick, and dietary practices.

8. Watch prime-time television and note the racial and ethnic diversity that is present during the commercials. During the program, note the roles played by racially and ethnically diverse characters. Are they heroes or heroines or the "bad guys"? What are their occupations, SES, religions, and lifestyles?

9. Skim a popular magazine for references to racially and ethnically diverse subgroups. What is being written? Is the nature of the article favorable or unfavorable?

ⓔ EVOLVE WEBSITE

http://evolve.elsevier.com/Nies

- NCLEX Review Questions
- Case Studies
- Glossary

REFERENCES

Agency for Healthcare Research and Quality: *Addressing racial and ethnic disparities in health care: fact sheet*, AHRQ 00–P041 Rockville, MD, 2013, Author. http://www.ahrq.gov/research/findings/factsheets/minority/disparit/index.html.

American Cancer Society: *Cancer facts & figures for African Americans: 2011-2012*, 2012. Available from <http://www.cancer.org/research/cancerfactsfigures/cancerfactsfiguresforafricanamericans/cancer-facts-figures-af-am-2011-2012>.

Andrews MM: Religion, culture and nursing. In Andrews MM, Boyle JS, editors: *Transcultural concepts in nursing care*, ed 5, Philadelphia, 2008, Lippincott Williams & Wilkins.

Andrews MM, Boyle JS, editors: *Transcultural concepts in nursing care*, ed 5, Philadelphia, 2008, Lippincott Williams & Wilkins.

Cockerham WC: *Medical sociology*, ed 11, Upper Saddle River, NJ, 2009, Prentice Hall.

The Commonwealth Fund: *Closing the divide: how medical homes promote equity in health care: results from the Commonwealth Fund 2006 healthcare quality survey*, 2007. Available from <www.commonwealthfund.org/Content/Publications/Fund-Reports/2007/Jun/Closing-the-Divide-How-Medical-Homes-Promote-Equity-in-Health-Care-Results-From-The-Commonwealth-F.aspx>.

Edmonds VM: The nutritional patterns of recently immigrated Honduran women, *J Transcult Nurs* 16(3):226–235, 2005.

Expert Panel on Global Nursing & Health: *Standards of practice for culturally competent nursing care*, 2010. Available from <http://www.tcns.org/files/Standards_of_Practice_for_Culturally_Compt_Nsg_Care-Revised_.pdf>.

Gallup Poll: *Religion*, 2013. Available from <www.gallup.com/poll/1690/Religion.aspx>.

Health Resources and Services Administration: *The registered nurse population: findings from the 2008 national sample survey of registered nurses*, 2010. Available from <http://bhpr.hrsa.gov/healthworkforce/rnsurveys/rnsurveyfinal.pdf>.

Hoefer M, Rytina N, Baker B: *Estimates of the unauthorized immigrant population residing in the United States, January 2011*, 2012. Available from <http://www.dhs.gov/xlibrary/assets/statistics/publications/ois_ill_pe_2011.pdf>.

Katon W, Kleinman A: Doctor-patient negotiation and other social science strategies in patient care. In Eisenberg L, Kleinman A, editors: *The relevance of social science for medicine*, Boston, 1981, D. Reidel.

Keller L, Strohschein S, Schaffer M: Cornerstones of public health nursing, *Public Health Nursing* 28(3):249–260, 2011.

Kluckhohn F, Strodtbeck F: *Variations in value orientations*, Evanston, IL, 1961, Row, Peterson.

Kohls LR: *Survival kit for overseas living*, Yarmouth, ME, 1984, Intercultural Press.

Leininger MM: *Nursing and anthropology: two worlds to blend*, New York, 1970, Wiley.

Leininger MM: *Transcultural nursing: concepts, theories, and practice*, New York, 1978, Wiley.

Leininger MM: *Culture, care, diversity, and universality: a theory of nursing*, New York, 1991, National League for Nursing Press.

Leininger MM: *Transcultural nursing: concepts, theories, research and practice*, ed 2, New York, 1995, McGraw-Hill.

Leininger MM, McFarland MR: *Transcultural nursing: concepts, theories, research and practice*, ed 3, New York, 2002, McGraw-Hill.

Ludwig-Beymer PA: Transcultural aspects of pain. In Andrews M, Boyle JS, editors: *Transcultural concepts in nursing care*, ed 5, Philadelphia, 2008, Lippincott Williams & Wilkins.

National Center for Educational Statistics: *Fast facts: status dropout rate*, 2012. Available from <nces.ed.gov/fastfacts/display.asp?id=16>.

National Center for Health Statistics: *People without health insurance coverage by race and ethnicity*, 2008. Available from <www.cdc.gov/Features/dsHealthInsurance/>.

National Council of Churches: *Yearbook of American and Canadian churches*, New York, 2005, Office of Minority Health.

Ortiz CE: Disclosing concerns of Latinas living with HIV/AIDS, *J Transcult Nurs* 16(3):210–217, 2005.

Spector R: *Cultural diversity in health and illness*, ed 7, Upper Saddle River, NJ, 2008, Prentice Hall.

Sullivan Commission: *Missing persons: minorities in the health professions: report of the Sullivan Commission on diversity in the healthcare workforce*, 2004. Available from <http://www.aacn.nche.edu/media-relations/SullivanReport.pdf>.

Tylor EB: *Primitive culture*, London, 1871, Murray.

U.S. Census Bureau: *Foreign-born populations in the United States, 2010*, 2012. Available from <http://www.census.gov/prod/2012pubs/acs-19.pdf>.

U.S. Census Bureau: *Income, poverty, and health insurance coverage in the United States, 2011*, 2012. Available from <http://www.census.gov/hhes/www/poverty/data/incpovhlth/2011/table3.pdf>.

U.S. Census Bureau: *Overview of race and Hispanic origin: 2010*, 2011. http://www.census.gov/prod/cen2010/briefs/c2010br-02.pdf.

U.S. Census Bureau: *U.S. Census Bureau projections show a slower growing, older, more diverse nation a half century from now*, Press release, December 12 2012. Available from <http://www.census-.gov/newsroom/releases/archives/population/cb12-243.html>.

U.S. Department of Health and Human Services: *Fact sheet*: Protecting the health of minority communities, 2006. Available from <http://www.hhs.gov/news/factsheet/minorityhealth.html>.

U.S. Department of Health and Human Services: *Healthy People 2020: topics and objectives*, 2013. Available from <http://www.healthypeople.gov/2020/topicsobjectives2020/default.aspx>.

U.S. Department of Homeland Security: *Yearbook of immigration statistics, 2004*, Washington DC, 2006, US Department of Homeland Security, Office of Immigration Statistics.

Wilmoth JM, Chen PC: Immigrant status, living arrangements, and depressive symptoms among middle-aged and older adults, *J Gerontol B Psychol Sci Soc Sci* 58B(5):S305–S313, 2003.

Zborowski M: *People in pain*, San Francisco, 1969, Jossey-Bass.

Environmental Health

Diane Santa Maria*

OBJECTIVES

Upon completion of this chapter, the reader will be able to do the following:

1. Describe areas of environmental health, environmental health problems, and related human health risks.
2. Apply the basic concepts of critical theory to environmental health nursing problems.
3. Describe the importance of air, water, and food quality as a determinant of health.
4. Identify social, cultural, economic, and political factors that contribute to pollution and impact environmental problems.
5. Develop an understanding of the risk assessment and risk management role of nurses.
6. Explain laws and regulations relevant to environmental health and how government agencies use them to address environmental issues.

KEY TERMS

Air Quality Index
biosolids
built environment
climate change
critical theory
environmental health
environmental justice

food desert
food safety
global warming
Healthy Home
outdoor air quality
participatory action research
population

sick building syndrome
social capital
waste management
water quality
work-related exposures

OUTLINE

A Critical Theory Approach to Environmental Health
Areas of Environmental Health
    The Built Environment
    Work-Related Exposures
Outdoor Air Quality
Healthy Homes
    Water Quality
    Food Safety
    Waste Management
Effects of Environmental Hazards

Efforts to Control Environmental Health Problems
Emerging Issues in Environment Health
    Nursing Actions
Approaching Environmental Health at the Population Level
Critical Environmental Health Nursing Practice
    Taking a Stand: Advocating for Change
    Asking Critical Questions
    Facilitating Community Involvement
    Forming Coalitions
    Using Collective Strategies

* The author would like to acknowledge the contribution of Bridgette Crotwell Pullis, who wrote this chapter for the previous edition.

The World Health Organization (WHO) (2013) defines environmental health as "all the physical, chemical, and biological factors external to a person and all the related factors impacting behaviors. It encompasses the assessment and control of those environmental factors that can potentially affect health. It is targeted towards preventing disease and creating health-supportive environments." Figure 14-1, from the U.S. Department of Health and Human Services *Healthy People 2020* program, demonstrates these factors.

Environmental health experts believe that the purpose of environmental health is to assure the conditions of human health and provide healthy environments for people to live, work, and play. This can be accomplished through *risk assessment*, prevention, and intervention.

Efforts are made to reduce and eliminate contaminant and contagion threats to human health from air, water, food, and the built environment (Lindland and Kendall-Taylor, 2011). Maintaining a healthy environment is vitally important to promoting the health of populations—particular groups or types of people. A healthy environment improves quality of life and increases years of healthy living. Accumulated evidence shows that the environmental changes of the past few decades have profoundly influenced the status of public health. Globally, environmental factors contribute to nearly 25% of all deaths and increase disease burden (WHO, 2006). The safety, beauty, and life-sustaining capacity of the physical environment are unquestionably of global consequence. Since the beginning of the twenty-first century, it has become apparent that the world must address urgent environmental

difficulties, including extinction of some species, diminishing rain forests, proliferation of toxic waste dumps, progressive destruction of the ozone layer, shortage of landfill sites, consequences of climate change, threats of terrorism, development of deadly chemical and ballistic weapons, adulteration of food by pesticides and herbicides, oceanic contamination through toxic dumping and petroleum spills, overcrowding of urban areas, and traffic congestion.

This chapter uses critical theory to explore the health of communities in relation to the environment. Critical theory is particularly useful in examining environmental health, because it offers a framework for discussion and a basis for describing community health nursing practice (Martins and Burbank, 2011; Stevens and Hall, 1992). Applying critical theory is a way of thinking upstream (see Chapter 3). Critical theory is an approach that raises questions about oppressive situations, involves community members in the definition and solution of problems, and facilitates interventions that reduce health-damaging effects of environments. By applying the nursing process in a critical fashion, nurses can be dynamically involved in the design of interventions that alter the precursors of poor health.

Recognition of the gravity and pervasiveness of environmental hazards can be overwhelming. Looking beyond the individual to recognize the environmental determinants of health can be complicated and alarming. Intervening to improve the quality of air, water, housing, food, and waste disposal and reducing the risks of harmful exposures to environmental toxins require individual, social, economic, and political changes. Nurses are powerful change agents who use their assessment, management, and communication skills to promote environmental health locally and nationally. Nurses are becoming increasingly active in efforts to address environmental health issues and to increase awareness of the effects of the environment on well-being.

A CRITICAL THEORY APPROACH TO ENVIRONMENTAL HEALTH

Critical theory suggests that nurses must be aware of environmental threats or factors that might detrimentally affect the safety and well-being of particular populations or deprive them of access to resources necessary in the pursuit of health. This awareness may include recognizing, supporting, and maintaining positive environmental influences. For instance, a nurse must consider the effects of having access to a safe place to walk on one's ability to maintain healthy levels of physical activity. A 2011 study found that access to recreation facilities is an important correlate of physical activity (Troped et al., 2011). Nurses can help individuals adopt health behaviors by considering not only individual-level issues but those issues in the environment that facilitate or create barriers to healthy living.

Nurses need to ask critical questions about their clients' environments to help discern the contributions of specific hazards to their health. Occupational exposure to environmental hazardous can cause harm to workers as well as their

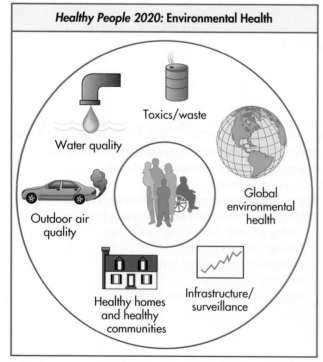

FIGURE 14-1 *Healthy People 2020:* elements of environmental health. (From U.S. Department of Health and Human Services: *Healthy People 2010*, ed 2, Washington, DC, 2000, U.S. Government Printing Office.)

families. For example, farm workers and pesticide applicators who accumulate agricultural chemicals on their skin and clothing take these substances home with them, increasing their children's exposure to toxicants (Thompson et al., 2008). Nurses must provide answers to farm workers who ask questions such as "What do I do if I'm exposed to a pesticide? How long should I wait until after a pesticide application to go back into the field? How do I find out how toxic a certain pesticide is? Where can I get information on a specific pesticide?" Nurses can take an environmental health history. An environmental health history can benefit the client in the following ways:

- Increase awareness of environmental health concerns
- Improve timelines and accuracy of diagnosis
- Prevent disease and aggravation of conditions
- Identify potential environmental hazards

Environmental health histories should be obtained for both adults and children, although the relationship between the environment and children's health is frequently overlooked. Figure 14-2 demonstrates common assessment items of an environmental history. When looking at the community from a critical perspective, nurses have the opportunity to promote population health. In identifying environmental sources of health problems, nurses

must be involved with the affected communities. Rather than impose their views of the problem, nurses should share their ideas and dialogue with community members. For example, nurses should listen to what the community believes is problematic, help raise consciousness about environmental dangers, and help bring about change. If nurses become involved in conducting community assessments and analyses, they can learn how the community members perceive themselves, their health, and their environmental influences.

From a critical standpoint, helping communities become more aware of the environmental effects on health and helping them make needed changes in their environment are legitimate nursing actions. Collective actions have been instrumental in accomplishing positive environmental changes since the 1980s. Some of the mechanisms have included strategic organization, litigation, public hearing testimony, letter-writing campaigns, legislative lobbying, mass demonstrations, and fund-raising. Fund-raising for environmental causes such as the 2012 storms that devastated the Northeast United States and the 2010 earthquake in Haiti facilitated rapid availability of resources, minimized loss of life, and helped restore basic necessities such as clean water and shelter. Public response to "acute" environmental disasters needs to be extended to an

---

1. Do you live next to or near an industrial plant, commercial business, dump site, or nonresidential property?

2. Have you been exposed to hazardous materials at work now or in the past?

3. Which of the following do you have in your home?

    __ air conditioner   __ air purifier   __ central heating (__ gas __ oil)

    __ gas stove   __ fireplace   __ wood stove

    __ humidifier

4. Have you recently acquired new furniture or carpet, refinished furniture, or remodeled your home?

5. Have you weatherized your home recently?

6. Are pesticides or herbicides (bug or weed killers; flea and tick sprays; collars, powders, shampoos) used in your home, garden, or on your pets?

7. Do you (or any household member) have a hobby or craft?

8. Have you ever changed your residence because of a health problem?

9. Does your drinking water come from a private well?

10. Approximately what year was your home built?

11. Has your routine changed recently?

12. Does anyone in your household smoke?

13. Has your home been tested for radon?

FIGURE 14-2 Environmental history assessment.

ongoing, consistent pressure to ensure day-to-day environmental integrity; hence, "chronic" environmental problems need to be addressed more effectively.

A critical perspective can help nurses plan and implement population-level interventions by emphasizing collective strategies for change. Acting collectively can empower nurses to impact environmental health. Assessing environmental health problems, planning and implementing interventions, and evaluating the effectiveness of community-based actions need to be based on a wide lens. Community health nurses should be familiar with physical surroundings and their mutual interaction with cultural realities, social relations, economic circumstances, and political conditions of communities, applying a critical perspective to community health.

AREAS OF ENVIRONMENTAL HEALTH

Environmental health hazards are ubiquitous in communities across the United States and place people at risk for disease or injury. This chapter divides the vast field of environmental health into the following subcategories: the built environment, work-related exposures, outdoor air quality, healthy homes, water quality, food safety, and waste management (Table 14-1). A brief discussion introduces nurses to these seven areas of environmental health, describes how they affect health, and demonstrates basic strategies nurses can use to address them. Table 14-2 provides examples of health problems within each area of environmental health.

It should be noted that a critical perspective does not separate the idea of a safe social environment from a safe physical environment. For example, interpersonal violence is a significant and growing risk, with consequences ranging from bodily injury to psychiatric aftereffects that may last for decades in some individuals. Intergenerational patterns of abuse, hate crimes toward marginalized groups, sexual predators, and hazards of combat might be considered from an environmental health perspective. Issues of violence are discussed in more depth in Chapter 27.

Finally, we must be prepared for the public health effects of terrorism. Terrorism is a word that evokes many images and a range of reactions from rage to grief and loss. Acts of terrorism have drawn the public and political focus to establishing environmental security. Bioterrorism and homeland security are new areas where nurses will have an impact. A critical perspective is needed now more than ever, because security issues are linked

TABLE 14-1	AREAS OF ENVIRONMENTAL HEALTH
AREA	**DEFINITION**
Built environment	Buildings, spaces, and products that are created or modified by people, including homes, schools, workplaces, parks/recreation areas, greenways, business areas, and transportation systems.
Work-related exposure	Occupational exposure to environmental hazards that can cause illness or injury.
Outdoor air quality	The protectiveness of the atmospheric layers, the risks of severe weather, and the purity of the air for breathing purposes.
Healthy home	The availability, safety, structural strength, cleanliness, and location of shelter, including public facilities and family dwellings. This includes indoor air quality.
Water quality	The availability of and accessibility to a clean water supply, the mineral content levels, pollution by toxic chemicals, and the presence of pathogenic microorganisms.
Food safety	The availability, relative costs, variety, safety, and health of animal and plant food sources.
Waste management	The management of waste materials resulting from industrial and municipal processes, human consumption, and efforts to minimize waste production.

TABLE 14-2	EXAMPLES OF ENVIRONMENTAL HEALTH PROBLEMS
AREA	**PROBLEMS**
Built environment	Drunk driving
	Secondhand smoke
	Noise exposure
	Urban crowding
	Technological hazards
Work-related exposure	Asbestos exposure
	Agricultural accidents
	Excessive exposure to x-rays
Outdoor air quality	Gaseous pollutants
	Greenhouse effect
	Destruction of the ozone layer
	Aerial spraying of herbicides and pesticides
	Acid rain
	Nuclear facility emissions
Healthy home	Homelessness
	Rodent and insect infestation
	Presence of lead-based paint
	Sick building syndrome
	Unsafe neighborhoods
	Radon gas seepage in homes and schools
Water quality	Contamination of drinking supply by human waste
	Oil spills in the world's waterways
	Pesticide or herbicide infiltration of groundwater
	Aquifer contamination by industrial pollutants
	Heavy metal poisoning of fish
Food safety	Malnutrition
	Bacterial food poisoning
	Food adulteration
	Disruption of food chains by ecosystem destruction
	Carcinogenic chemical food additives
Waste management	Use of nonbiodegradable plastics
	Poorly designed solid-waste dumps
	Inadequate sewage systems
	Transport and storage of hazardous waste
	Illegal industrial dumping
	Radioactive hazardous wastes

to religious imperatives, moral stances, values, profit motives, health care systems and information, and cultural differences. These issues are also clearly within the scope of community health nursing and are discussed in more detail in Chapter 28.

The Built Environment

The built environment consists of the connections among people, communities, and their surrounding environments that affect health behaviors and habits, interpersonal relationships, cultural values, and customs. There is growing evidence that the built environment directly and indirectly affects health outcomes and disease rates (Figure 14-3). One review of the literature found that neighborhoods that are more walkable are associated with increased physical activity, increased social capital, lower overweight, lower reports of depression, and less reported alcohol abuse (Renalds, Smith, and Hale, 2009). Social capital refers to networks and the associated norms and expected collective benefits derived from cooperation between individuals and groups. Structural characteristics of the built environment, such as street condition, neighborhood deterioration, and the proportion of parks and playgrounds, affect levels of physical activity and obesity (Schulz, et al., 2013). Simply put, having a safe, intact place to walk encourages exercise.

Many people live within areas that require almost daily contact with potential health risks and threats. These include intoxicated or impaired drivers, secondhand smoke, urban crowding, noise exposure, unabated traffic, and the stress of increased mechanization. The type of area one lives in can greatly affect one's health. For example, a research study found that adolescents living in rural working class or mixed-race urban neighborhoods were more likely to be overweight than peers in newer suburbs regardless of their socio-economic status, age, or race/ethnicity (Nelson et al., 2006). Access to equipment and facilities, neighborhood pattern (e.g. rural, exurban, suburban), walkability, and urban sprawl are also associated with obesity outcomes in adolescents (Dunton et al., 2009; Ding, et al., 2011).

Urban sprawl has been defined as the conversion of land to nonagricultural or nonnatural uses at a faster rate than the population growth (Environmental Protection Agency [EPA], 2002). The sprawling development often occurs more rapidly than the expansion of the infrastructure (e.g., schools, sewer systems, water lines) needed for support. Typically, the desire to own one's vehicle, coupled with inadequate public mass transportation systems, contributes to a greater dependence on the automobile. This results in high volumes of traffic and a constant need to build more highways and resources. Consequences of sprawl include air and water pollution, floods, infrastructure expenses, and a decrease in natural areas and forests (EPA, 2002).

One unfortunately common problem associated with living patterns relates to residing near hazardous facilities (e.g., waste incinerators, sewage treatment plants, landfills, refineries, and some correctional facilities). Molitor and colleagues (2011) found that higher levels of pollutants are generally associated with higher poverty. Discriminatory land use ensures that many impoverished and marginalized groups, especially minorities, live in close proximity to industrial contamination (Collins, 2011; Nweke, 2011). People who live near such environmental hazards are in danger of becoming victims of illness and injury related to violence, poisonings and exposures, fires, and malignant and nonmalignant diseases.

Many communities lack sufficient resources to respond when urban development and technological advances jeopardize the health and well-being of families in affected areas. The environmental movement of the 1960s and 1970s succeeded in building political power capable of passing monumental environmental reforms; however, charges that poor and minority communities are dumping grounds for environmental hazards have been substantiated by governmental agencies (EPA, 2004, 2013c).

Difficulties in alerting state and federal officials about environmental health dangers as well as in obtaining compensation for environmental toxin–causing disease and death often result in resident revictimization. Tightly knit social

Other Determinants of Health
(e.g., Genetics, the Social Environment, and the Health Care System)

The Built Environment (Underlying Context)	**Mediating Factors** (Exposure Media)	**Downstream Pathways** (Human Response)	**Health status** (Outcome Indicators)
- Land use patterns - Transportation networks - Infrastructure systems - Public facilities - Buildings	- Environmental toxins - Local climate - Noise level - Crime level - Disasters & accidents - Access to services	- Behavioral; e.g., physical activity, diet behavior, smoking, drinking, drug-taking. - Psychological; e.g., satisfaction, depression/distress, social cohesion. - Physiological; e.g., infection, immune system activation, hormonal response.	- Individual-level; e.g., BMI, perceived health status, well-being. - Population-level; e.g., cause-specific mortality rates, morbidity rates.

FIGURE 14-3 A conceptual model of how the built environment impacts health. (Developed by Fan Y, Song Y: Is sprawl associated with a widening urban–suburban mortality gap? *J Urban Health* 86[5]:708-728, 2009; adapted from a conceptual model Klitzman S, Matte TD, Kass DE: The urban physical environment and its effects on health. In: Freudenberg N, Galea S, Vlahov D, editors: *Cities and the health of the public.* Nashville, TN, 2006, Vanderbilt University Press, p. 364.)

BOX 14-1	LANDMARK FEDERAL ENVIRONMENTAL LEGISLATION

YEAR	LEGISLATION
1970	Clean Air Act
	Poison Prevention Packaging Act
	National Environmental Policy Act
1971	Lead-Based Paint Poisoning Prevention Act
1972	Federal Water Pollution Control Act Amendments
	Noise Control Act
	Clean Water Act
1973	Endangered Species Act
1974	Safe Drinking Water Act
1975	Hazardous Materials Transportation Act
1976	Resource Conservation and Recovery Act
	Toxic Substances Control Act
	Surface Mining Control and Reclamation Act
1980	Low Level Radiation Waste Policy Act
	Comprehensive Environmental Response, Compensation, and Liability Act (i.e., Superfund)
1990	Oil Pollution Act
	Clean Air Act
2003	Healthy Forests Restoration Act
2016	Fuel Economy Standards raised (original legislation: 1975)

structures and a lack of low-cost housing may hinder the mobility of residents and perpetuate the exposure to health hazards. Residents may be unwilling to disrupt family ties and cultural roots to start over elsewhere, or they may be unable to afford a move. These residents may live with uncertainty and conflict. Long-term, community-wide effects of division, animosity, distrust, cynicism, and despair can abound in these situations, negatively affecting social capital.

In the 1990s, the central issues of equity and justice emerged in environmental health policy. In 1994, President Clinton signed Executive Order 12898, which required all federal agencies to develop comprehensive strategies for achieving environmental justice. This directive has served to increase public participation and access to information as well as provision of education about multiple risks and cumulative exposures (EPA, 2005, 2013c) (Box 14-1). Much remains to be done, however, to attain environmental justice in the United States. Nurses are part of the interdisciplinary team made up of urban planners, public health practitioners, and policy makers needed to understand and address issues of the built environment that are critical to establishing health equity.

Clinical Example

In an urban city in the south, the health department is becomingly increasingly concerned about the overweight and obesity rates of young school-age children. At health fairs held around the city, nurses are seeing more children with acanthosis nigricans, elevated blood pressure, high body mass index (BMI), and hypercholesterolemia. Though the public health nurse diligently counsels patients on the benefits of exercise, his patients do not increase their physical activity. When the nurse drives around the neighborhood where many of his patients reside, he realizes there are no recreational parks nearby, the sidewalks are in disrepair, the smokestacks cloud the air, and there appears to be gang-related activity. The nurse considers the impact of the built environment on the ability of his patients to be physically active. In partnership with the school board and neighborhood watch group, the nurse and community members successfully petition for a park to be built within walking distance of the school. Additionally, the partnership is able to establish a "walking school bus," a program where students walk in a group to or from school, as a way for children to increase their physical activity.

Work-Related Exposures

Work-related exposures can happen as a result of poor working conditions and can lead to potential injury or illness. Environmental health problems posed by work-related exposures include such issues as occupational toxic poisoning, machine-operation hazards (e.g., falls, crushing injuries, burns), electrical hazards, repetitive motion injuries, carcinogenic particulate inhalation (e.g., of asbestos, coal dust), and heavy metal poisoning (Centers for Disease Control and Prevention [CDC], 2013; Krieger et al., 2008). Prevention of work-related health problems requires integrated action to improve job safety and the working environment. Occupational and environmental health nurses often collaborate on initiatives to reduce and eliminate work-related exposures, illnesses, and injuries. Nurses can be sure that workers are aware of and know where to access the Safety Data Sheets relevant to their workplace. The U.S. Department of Labor's Occupational Safety and Health Administration (OSHA) (2013) requires chemical manufacturers, distributors, and importers to provide safety data sheets that communicate the hazards of chemical products.

According to the Bureau of Labor Statistics (2012), nearly 3 million nonfatal workplace injuries and illnesses were reported by private industry employers in 2011. This number is down from 2007, when there were 4,002,700 recorded cases of nonfatal illnesses and injuries in the United States (Bureau of Labor Statistics, 2008). The EPA estimates that 10,000 to 20,000 physician-diagnosed pesticide poisonings occur each year among the approximately 2 million U.S. agricultural workers (EPA, 2013). In one year (2010), 476 farm workers died from work-related injuries with tractor overturns being the leading cause of death (CDC, 2013).

These statistics do not reflect unreported health problems. For example, a clerical worker leaves the office every day with back strain and a headache because of ventilation problems in the building. After 5 years on a repetitive hand-movement job task, an employee is diagnosed with carpal tunnel syndrome. An operating room nurse has a miscarriage and recalls that many of her coworkers have also been unable to carry their babies to term. A dry cleaner often leaves work feeling light-headed and dizzy from inhaling solvents at the shop, and one day she has a car accident on her way home. Collective problems related to

EXAMPLES OF ENVIRONMENTAL HEALTH ISSUES AFFECTING COMMUNITIES

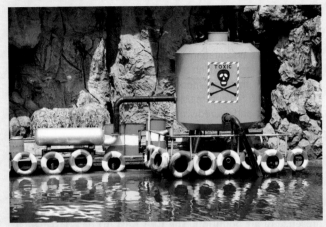

Water pollution from local industry. (Copyright © 2013 Thinkstock. All rights reserved. Image #155251207.)

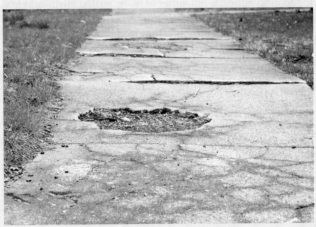

Sidewalks in disrepair. (Copyright © 2013 Thinkstock. All rights reserved. Image #136736843.)

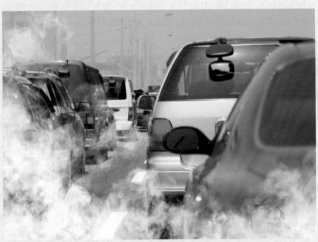

Motor vehicle emissions (primary mobile source of air pollutants). (Copyright © 2013 Thinkstock. All rights reserved. Image #106594948.)

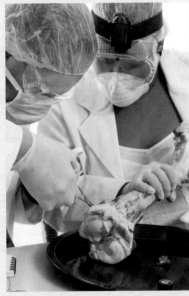

Food safety meat inspection. (Copyright © 2013 Thinkstock. All rights reserved. Image #92400710.)

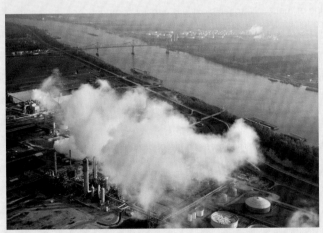

Air pollution from local industry. (Copyright © 2013 Thinkstock. All rights reserved. Image #86504451.)

employment or occupation are often perceived as individualized injuries, and no one "connects the dots." Research is ongoing to determine the outcomes of work-related environmental exposures. For example, the GuLF STUDY (Gulf Long Term Follow-Up Study) is a health study, sponsored by the National Institute of Health (NIH), for individuals who helped with oil spill clean-up after the 2010 Deepwater Horizon disaster in the Gulf of Mexico (NIH, 2014).

Clinical Example

Sanitation workers in an urban area experienced a rising incidence of puncture injuries while transporting hazardous wastes from the public medical center; these puncture injuries caused several cases of hepatitis. When the story became public, members of the city health commission contacted community health nurses and instructed them to politically support the interests of the city and the medical center "at all costs." Subsequently, the sanitation workers' union contacted the community health nursing office and requested information about procedures for safely packaging medical wastes. They also requested that a nurse speak to their membership about immediate measures for preventing further injuries on the job.

The nurses met to resolve the conflict. Most agreed that the sanitation workers had pressing needs for education and support. Despite the city's demand for loyalty, they decided to "choose sides" with the workers and respond to their requests. They collectively drafted a letter to the city health commission and arranged a meeting with the commissioners to discuss their plan to assist the sanitation workers. The health commission held a press conference, which depicted the nurses' actions as mediational efforts that benefited the union and the city. Eventually, the nurses and the commission developed a new medical waste disposal plan, and injured workers received reasonable compensation through an out-of-court settlement.

Outdoor Air Quality

Outdoor air quality refers to the purity of the air and the presence of air pollution. The EPA (2012b) has classified six common air pollutants (Table 14-3). WHO estimates that air pollution is the thirteenth leading cause of mortality worldwide, contributing to approximately 800,000 premature deaths annually. Particulate matter (PM), one common

TABLE 14-3 MAJOR AIR POLLUTANTS

POLLUTANT	SOURCES	EFFECTS
Ozone: A colorless gas that is the major constituent of smog at the earth's surface	Ozone is formed in the lower atmosphere as the result of chemical reactions among oxygen, volatile organic compounds, and nitrogen oxides in the presence of sunlight, particularly during hot weather. Sources of this harmful pollutant include vehicles, factories, landfills, lawn equipment, farm equipment, and industrial solvents.	Ozone can irritate the respiratory tract, impair lung function, and cause throat irritation, chest pain, cough, and susceptibility to lung infection. Individuals with asthma and other existing respiratory conditions are particularly vulnerable. Ozone can also reduce agricultural yields and injure forests and other vegetation.
Carbon monoxide: A colorless and odorless gas that is emitted in the exhaust of motor vehicles and other kinds of engines during combustion of fossil fuels	Carbon monoxide is emitted from the engines of cars, buses, trucks, and other small engines and from some industrial processes. High concentrations can be found in confined spaces (e.g., parking garages, poorly ventilated tunnels, or along roadsides during periods of heavy traffic).	Carbon monoxide reduces the ability of the blood to deliver oxygen to vital tissues, affecting primarily the cardiovascular and nervous systems. Lower concentrations have been shown to adversely affect individuals with heart disease and to affect exercise performance. Higher concentrations can cause symptoms such as dizziness, headaches, and fatigue.
Nitrogen oxides: A light brown gas at lower concentrations; in higher concentrations, a significant component of brown urban haze	Nitrogen dioxide forms from the burning of fuels in utilities, industrial boilers, and the engines of cars and trucks.	Nitrogen dioxide is a major component of smog and acid rain. When concentrations are high, it can increase respiratory illnesses (e.g., chest colds and coughing) in children. For asthmatic people, it may exacerbate breathing difficulty.
Sulfur dioxide: A colorless gas, odorless at low concentrations but pungent at very high concentrations	Sulfur dioxide is emitted from industrial, institutional, utility, and apartment-house furnaces and boilers as well as petroleum refineries, smelters, paper mills, and chemical plants.	Sulfur dioxide is one of the major components of smog. At high concentrations, it can harm humans; asthmatic people are particularly vulnerable. It can also harm vegetation and metals and acidify lakes and streams.
Particulate matter: Droplets from smoke, dust, ash, and condensing vapors that can be suspended in the air for long periods	Particulates are emitted from industrial processes, vehicles, wood smoke, dust from paved and unpaved roads, construction, and agriculture.	Particulates can affect breathing and elicit respiratory symptoms, causing increased respiratory disease and lung damage. Children, elders, and people with heart or lung disease are especially at risk. They can also damage paint, soil, and clothing and reduce visibility.
Lead: A metal found in nature as well as a by-product of industry; can contaminate substances (e.g., soil, dust) that can be directly inhaled	Metals processing is the major source of lead emissions into the air today. Lead is generally found near lead smelters, waste incinerators, utilities, and lead-acid battery manufacturers.	Lead can adversely affect mental development and performance, kidney function, and blood chemistry. Young children are particularly at risk to its effects.

From Environmental Protection Agency: *What are the six common air pollutants?* Retrieved April 20, 2012, from <http://www.epa.gov/airquality/urbanair/>.

pollutant, causes worsening respiratory symptoms, more frequent asthma-related medication use, decreased lung function, recurrent health care utilization, and increased mortality (Anderson, Thurndiyil, and Stolbach, 2012).

Air pollution originates from industry (dry cleaning, factories, oil refineries, coal-burning power plants), modes of transportation (cars, buses, trucks, and planes), and naturally occurring events (volcanic eruptions and windstorms). Tornadoes, electrical storms, smog, gaseous pollutants (e.g., carbon monoxide), excessive hydrocarbon levels, aerial herbicide spraying, and acid rain all contribute to air pollution. Under provisions of the Clean Air Act, the EPA sets the national ambient air quality standards for pollutants considered harmful to humans or the environment.

Ozone is the most common pollutant in the United States and is the primary component of smog. Ozone is formed when nitrogen oxides (created by the burning of fossil fuels in power plants, automobiles, and factories) react with oxygen and sunlight (EPA, 2013f). Ozone, along with other hazardous atmospheric pollutants, causes and/or contributes to asthma, allergic reactions, bronchitis, lung cancer, chronic respiratory disease, and death and harms animal and plant species (Ciencewicki, Trivedi, and Kleeberger, 2008; Sheffield et al., 2011). Furthermore, sulfur dioxide, a by-product of burning coal and other fossil fuels, contributes to acid rain, which affects terrestrial ecosystems by increasing soil acidity, reducing nutrient availability, mobilizing toxic metals, leaching soil chemicals, and altering species composition (EPA, 2012c).Two significant issues related to outdoor air quality are of global concern. First, the amount of protection in the atmospheric layers is diminishing (EPA, 2013e). Chemicals such as chlorofluorocarbons, halons, and carbon tetrachloride, which have been in widespread use for refrigeration, air conditioning, and aerosol propellants, remain in the atmosphere. These molecules cause depletion of the atmosphere's protective ozone layer. The resulting "holes" in the ozone layer allow excess ultraviolet radiation to penetrate, which has harmful effects on many organisms. Long-term problems include increases in rates of skin cancer and cataracts, suppression of immune response, and environmental damage.

Second, there is a disruption in the key processes that break down atmospheric carbon dioxide. The ongoing deforestation of the earth's surface, especially the diminishing of tropical rain forests, not only releases the carbon stored in the biomass but also eliminates sources of photosynthesis (i.e., the process by which plants absorb carbon and release oxygen). The loss of carbon dioxide–consuming resources increases carbon dioxide and traps part of the heat reemitted by the earth. As a result, the earth's surface temperature is rising (i.e., the "greenhouse effect"), with potentially catastrophic ecological consequences. Scientists predict that within a few decades, significant regional climate changes will have occurred, causing sea levels to rise and, in turn, leading to serious coastal wetland loss.

In 1968, the National Air Pollution Control Administration developed the **air quality index** (AQI) to increase public awareness of air pollution (Figure 14-4). The AQI is a number used by government agencies to communicate current and

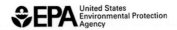

Air Quality Guide for Particle Pollution		
Good	0-50	None
Moderate	51-100	Unusually sensitive people should consider reducing prolonged or heavy exertion
Unhealthy for Sensitive Groups	101-150	People with heart or lung disease, older adults, and children should reduce prolonged or heavy exertion.
Unhealthy	151 to 200	People with heart or lung disease, older adults, and children should avoid prolonged or heavy exertion. Everyone else should reduce prolonged or heavy exertion.
Very Unhealthy Alert	201 to 300	People with heart or lung disease, older adults, and children should avoid all physical activity outdoors. Everyone else should avoid prolonged or heavy exertion.

FIGURE 14-4 Environmental Protection Agency air quality index. (From *Air now: local air conditions and forecasts*, n.d. Retrieved March 1, 2013, from <www.airnow.gov>.)

forecasted air pollution conditions to the public. As the AQI rises, a larger percentage of the population, particularly vulnerable populations, may experience adverse health effects. The AQI fluctuates on the basis of the dilution of air pollutants. Air stagnation can lead to high concentrations of pollutants and haze. Although most air contaminants do not have an associated AQI, many countries monitor ground-level ozone, particulates, sulfur dioxide, carbon monoxide, and nitrogen dioxide to calculate the air quality index (EPA, 2013g). Nurses need to be aware of the AQI and the corresponding recommendations for the public to limit exposure to outdoor air during peak times of high AQI. Additionally, nurses must consider the AQI when making recommendations for physical activity, particularly for asthmatic patients. One study suggests that population-level health benefits from increased physical activity in high-walkability neighborhoods may be offset by the adverse effects of exposure to air pollution (Hankey, Marshall, and Brauer, 2012).

Clinical Example

During a recent summer, a sudden increase occurred in the number of clinic visits from residents of a particular urban neighborhood. The patients were elderly men and women who felt ill after going for a walk and asthmatic children with worsening respiratory symptoms. A nurse at the federally qualified health clinic in the neighborhood suspected that air pollution might be contributing to the increase in health concerns.

The nurse went online to the site www.airnow.gov and searched for the Air Quality Index for the region. She discovered that the region was experiencing a very unhealthy level of outdoor air pollution. She immediately alerted the health care staff that people with heart or lung disease, older adults, and children should avoid all physical activity outdoors and that everyone should avoid prolonged or heavy exertion outdoors. The nurse contacted the local summer camps and nursing homes in the area to alert them of the recommendation. The clinic quickly decided to move their regularly scheduled outdoor picnic to an indoor venue. One week later, the nurse noticed a drop in the number of patients complaining of respiratory distress.

Healthy Homes

A healthy Home refers to the availability, safety, structural strength, cleanliness, location, and indoor air quality of shelter. According to the EPA (2012e), many of the health concerns related to indoor living are a result of exposure to radon, carbon monoxide, molds and dust, secondhand smoke, cooking vapors, lead paint, and rodents. The CDC and Surgeon General have developed a Healthy Home checklist that nurses can use with patients to guide a thorough assessment and develop a care plan to help patients improve the quality of their homes and their indoor air quality (CDC, 2011) (See Ⓔ Resource Tools 14A and 14B, on the book's Evolve website at http://evolve.elsevier.com/Nies, for a Healthy Home Checklist and a Picture of Healthy Home).

Radon causes an estimated 21,000 lung cancer deaths in the United States every year. It is the second leading cause of lung cancer, after active smoking, and the leading cause among nonsmokers (EPA, 2013f). Nine federal agencies are currently working on an initiative to reduce radon exposures and illnesses (EPA, 2013d). Carbon monoxide (CO) is an odorless, colorless toxic gas. It can cause mild flu-like effects such as headaches, dizziness, disorientation, nausea, and fatigue at lower levels of exposure and death at higher levels (EPA, 2012d). Molds, dust, and secondhand smoke exposure can often exacerbate asthma symptoms.

Other health problems related to housing include fire hazards; lack of accommodations for people with disabilities; illnesses caused by overcrowding; psychological effects of architectural design (e.g., low-cost, high-rise housing projects); injuries sustained from collapsed building structures; and exposure deaths from inadequate indoor heating or cooling. Poor housing conditions can contribute to the spread of infectious disease (EPA, 2012e) as well as cardiovascular and respiratory disorders, cancers, allergies, and mental illnesses (Barton et al., 2007; Rauh, Landrigan, and Claudio, 2008). The term sick building syndrome describes a phenomenon in which public structures and homes cause occupants to experience a variety of symptoms, such as headache, fatigue, and exacerbation of allergies. It typically results from poor ventilation and building operations, hazardous building materials, furniture and carpeting substances, and cleaning agents (EPA, 1991). Additionally, volatile organic compounds (VOCs) have been found in soil and soil vapor as a result of industrial spills that contaminate indoor air. One such spill in Endicott, New York, has been linked to congenital cardiac defects, low birth weight, and fetal growth restriction (Farand, Lewis-Michl, and Gomex, 2012).

Other problems may arise related to building structures, composition, and settings. For example, commercial buildings with offices near underground parking garages may cause workers to have carbon monoxide intoxication. Formaldehyde, asbestos, and volatile organic compounds—which are common components of thermal insulation, cement, flooring, furnishings, and household consumer products—have carcinogenic properties. Additionally, "toxic mold" arising from chronically damp wood and improperly sealed areas in homes and offices has been recognized as contributing to respiratory irritation, allergies, and infections in susceptible individuals (EPA, 2012e).

Clinical Example

In a large, northeastern U.S. city, an economic recession led to large company layoffs, leaving many unemployed or underemployed. Because of the loss of income, many families faced tough decisions during the upcoming winter months. Temperatures often went below zero, requiring constant heating. Unfortunately, many people did not have the money to continue to pay their heating bill, fix leaky windows and doors, or buy warm clothes. Some families began to use space heaters and burned scraps of wood that were discarded. Often, this wood came from old abandoned buildings and homes. Other families took to sleeping in their cars.

Soon, hospitals began to see an uptick in patients presenting with respiratory illnesses, carbon monoxide exposure, and burns. The community health nurses in the area met with struggling families to assess their needs and determine a plan to meet their immediate needs. The nurses met with local politicians and church groups to find ways to supply healthy wood for heating, help financially with home utility bills, provide warm clothes for families, and find shelters for homeless families. Within a few months, the local hospitals began to see a decline in home-related injuries and illnesses.

Water Quality

Water quality refers to the water supply's availability, volume, mineral content levels, toxic chemical pollution, and pathogenic microorganism levels. Water quality consists of the balance between water contaminants and the existing capabilities to purify water for human use and plant and wildlife sustenance. Water quality problems include experiencing droughts, dousing reservoirs with chemicals to reduce algae, contaminating aquifers with pesticides and fertilizers, leaching lead from water pipes, and oil spilling from transport tankers or leaking offshore wells. Other sources of water pollution are microbial contamination from poorly managed or maintained septic or sewage systems and animal feedlot wastes (EPA, 2013b). Water pollution can be from point sources (a well-defined source, e.g., factory wastewater discharge) or nonpoint sources (urban runoff, domestic lawn care, and air-to-water transfer).

Advances in water treatment technologies in industrialized countries have controlled many water-related diseases, such as cholera, typhoid, dysentery, and hepatitis A. Nevertheless, disease outbreaks resulting from contamination by untreated groundwater and inadequate chlorination are increasing in both urban and rural areas. In addition, more than 45 million Americans (15%) obtain their drinking water from private water supplies (e.g., wells) that have no treatment or monitoring guidelines (CDC, 2011). Other potential water contaminants include accelerated soil erosion caused by construction, agriculture, and deforestation, which can contribute to high sediment levels in drinking water supplies.

Heavy metal and toxic chemical pollution may also occur during the water treatment process or in the drinking water distribution system. The EPA monitors drinking water for more than 80 organic and inorganic pollutants that have potential health effects in humans, including those who are most vulnerable, such as children and people with weakened immune systems (EPA, 1991). Pesticides, herbicides, and carcinogenic industrial waste infiltrate an increasing amount of groundwater, the underground source of half the U.S. population's drinking water (U.S. Geological Survey, 2005). Additionally, commonly used medications and personal care products that contain endocrine disruptors have been found in water supplies (Wu et al., 2012). This development is particularly tragic because groundwater is uniquely susceptible to long-term contamination. Unlike river or lake water, once groundwater becomes contaminated, it is impossible to cleanse.

Clinical Example

In a Midwestern farm community, there is growing concern about seepage of agricultural pesticides and herbicides into groundwater. Families obtain water from private wells rather than a central municipal source. The families had heard about potential long-term carcinogenic effects of the chemicals, such as pesticides and herbicides, commonly used on the farms in the community. Although family farmers decreased their use of these chemicals, the large-scale agribusiness companies continued to use large amounts of these chemicals.

A community health nurse from the county health department lobbied local officials to begin a comprehensive program to monitor groundwater pollutants and enforce standards for herbicide and pesticide use. However, the powerful agribusiness companies pressured these officials to stand back. Together, some county farmers and nurses organized grassroots information and support groups for the rural families. The families and nurses, in coalition with environmental activist groups in the state, established several projects. These projects included collecting and testing samples from each family well, forming a local organization called "Water Watch" to coordinate actions and communications, and implementing a research project with a local university to track water contamination and health problems of local residents. The organization also disseminated an emergency plan to families whose wells were found to have toxic levels of pesticides, herbicides, or other pollutants.

Food Safety

Food safety refers to availability, accessibility, and relative cost of healthy food free of contamination by harmful herbicides, pesticides, and bacteria. Food safety concerns include malnutrition, bacterial food poisoning, carcinogenic chemical additives (e.g., nitrites, dyes, and cyclamate), improper or fraudulent meat inspection or food labeling, microbial epidemics among livestock (e.g., Escherichia coli), food products from diseased animal sources, and disruption of vital natural food chains by ecosystem destruction. Increased mobility and globalized trade also contribute to global contamination of the food supply. Finally, there are significant disparities in access to healthy and fresh food supplies, with poor minority families being more likely to live in a food desert—a

neighborhood with little to no access to healthy foods (Institute of Medicine [IOM], 2009).

Annually, about 48 million Americans contract gastrointestinal illnesses, resulting in 128,000 hospitalizations and 3000 deaths (U.S. Food and Drug Administration [USFDA], 2011). Potential microbial contaminants of foods include bacteria (e.g., *Shigella salmonella, E. coli, Campylobacter*), parasites (e.g., *Balantidium coli, Cryptosporidium parvum, Entamoeba histolytica*), and viruses (e.g., calicivirus, rotavirus, hepatitis A virus, enterovirus) (FoodSafety.gov, 2009). The federal government utilizes meat inspectors to prevent misbranded meat and meat products from being sold as food and ensure that meat animals are slaughtered and meat products processed under sanitary and humane conditions. The United States currently depends on the Foodborne Diseases Active Surveillance Network (FoodNet) of CDC's Emerging Infections Program to collect data on diseases caused by enteric pathogens transmitted through food (CDC, 2010). Public health nurses play a key role in foodborne illness investigations. See ⓔ **Resource Tool 14C** for Steps in a Foodborne Outbreak Investigation.

Food can also be contaminated by agrichemicals, such as pesticides and fertilizers; materials from mechanical handling devices; detergents; and organic packaging materials. Toxic chemicals from farming and ranching may be introduced into the food chain, increasing risk of reproductive and mutagenic effects in humans (Driehuis et al., 2008; Knobeloch et al., 2009). For instance, farmers spray dioxin-containing weed killers on rangeland. Beef cattle graze on the land, herbicide accumulates in their fatty tissue, and the contaminated meat is sold in markets. The complexity of transfer of these contaminants makes for difficulty in establishing causality and tracing accountability for these health risks.

Unsuitable handling, storage, processing, and transport techniques can damage food and make it unsuitable for consumption. Nurses can council patients on the proper handling of food (Figure 14-5). Furthermore, additives are often used to improve food properties. For example, vitamins and minerals are used to enhance nutritional content; salt, sugars, and monosodium glutamate are used to improve flavor; dyes are used to enhance color; leavening agents, gums, or thickening agents are used to improve consistency; and various preservatives are used to increase shelf life. Many of these additives are not nutritious, and some may be harmful. Additionally, residues from the overuse of antibiotics in

CLEAN SEPARATE COOK CHILL

FIGURE 14-5 Steps to food safety. (From FoodSafety.gov: *Keep food safe,* n.d.. Retrieved March 1, 2013, from <http://www.foodsafety.gov/keep/basics/index.html>.)

animal husbandry remain in meat and milk products, causing consumers to develop resistance, thus rendering these antibiotics ineffective in treating human infections (Hurd and Malladi, 2008).

Another potential threat related to food quality involves "genetically modified" (GM) or genetically engineered foods. GM foods, which have been in existence since the early 1970s, are created by a process in which scientists splice plant or animal genes with particular traits into the DNA of other organisms. This technology has contributed to crops and livestock that grow faster, more resistant to disease and insects, and produce higher yields and greater nutritive value. Often GM crops require less water and fertilizer. There is concern that genetic alteration of food is growing despite the fact that the long-term health effects of eating GM food are unknown. Some believe that allergies and other immunity problems may proliferate because unique antigens are present on GM proteins, and GM foods have unpredictable metabolic processes in animals, humans, and plants (Whitney et al., 2004). Although the U.S. Department of Agriculture and the U.S. Food and Drug Administration set policy for foods produced from new plant varieties and breeding, a number of groups and organizations have called for greater public awareness of the potential risks of genetically engineered foods and are working to require more stringent testing of them. The American Nurses Association was among several professional groups that developed principles of a healthy and sustainable food system (Box 14-2) (American Planning Association, 2010).

Clinical Example

A southwestern U.S. town with a population of 10,000 has three elementary schools. School nurses at all three schools had an influx of children into their offices one afternoon with complaints of gastrointestinal symptoms. After verifying that this was happening at all three schools, the nurses called the county health department to report possible food-borne illness outbreak. The county health nurse came out to the schools that afternoon to investigate the food-borne outbreak. She interviewed the school nurses, the affected and unaffected students, and the cafeteria staff.

After having all students in the school fill out a form describing what they had eaten for lunch, the county nurse was able to determine that the chicken salad was the likely source of contamination. The nurses sent the chicken salad as well as samples of all the ingredients in the salad for laboratory testing. Within 2 days, the nurse received confirmation that the chicken salad had been the source of the illness, related to the use of contaminated celery. The nurse then alerted federal officials. A warning was issued on www.foodsafety.gov to alert officials across the nation. Food inspectors were sent to the factory that prepared and sold the celery. The source of contamination was isolated to three of the five machines used to slice the prepackaged celery. The factory was temporarily shut down for thorough disinfection. The school and county nurses worked together to assess the outbreak, alert the appropriate officials, and stop the outbreak from spreading. They undoubtedly saved thousands from illness and possibly death.

BOX 14-2 HEALTHY AND SUSTAINABLE FOOD SYSTEMS

Health-Promoting
- Supports the physical and mental health of all farmers, workers, and eaters
- Accounts for the public health impacts throughout the entire life-cycle of how food is produced, processed, packaged, labeled, distributed, marketed, consumed, and disposed

Sustainable
- Conserves, protects, and regenerates natural resources, landscapes, and biodiversity
- Meets our current food and nutrition needs without compromising the ability of the system to meet the needs of future generations

Resilient
- Thrives in the face of challenges, such as unpredictable climate, increased pest resistance, and declining, increasingly expensive water and energy supplies

Diverse in
- Size and scale—includes a variable range of food production, transformation, distribution, marketing, consumption, and disposal practices, occurring at different scales, from local and regional to national and global
- Geography—considers geographic differences in natural resources, climate, customs, and heritage

- Culture—appreciates and supports a diversity of cultures, sociodemographics, and lifestyles
- Choice—provides a variety of health-promoting food choices for all

Fair
- Supports fair and just communities and conditions for all farmers, workers, and eaters
- Provides equitable physical access to affordable food that is health-promoting and culturally appropriate

Economically Balanced
- Provides economic opportunities that are balanced across geographic regions of the country and at different scales of activity, from local to global, for a diverse range of food system stakeholders
- Affords farmers and workers in all sectors of the system a living wage

Transparent
- Provides opportunities for farmers, workers and eaters to gain the knowledge necessary to understand how food is produced, transformed, distributed, marketed, consumed and disposed
- Empowers farmers, workers, and eaters to actively participate in decision making in all sectors of the system

Waste Management

Waste management entails the handling of waste materials resulting from industry, municipal processes, and human consumption as well as efforts to minimize waste production. Environmental health problems related to waste management include nonbiodegradable plastics, inefficient recycling programs, unlicensed waste dumps, inadequate sewage systems for growing populations, unsafe dumping of industrial toxins, exportation of radioactive medical wastes, illicit dumping, and nonenforcement of environmental regulations.

American consumers' increasing trash production and the improper treatment, storage, transport, and disposal of waste are a significant concern. Routinely, commercial and institutional wastes are dumped with household waste in the same municipal incinerator, landfill, or sewer system. These commercial enterprises are generally exempt from the strict waste regulation applied to industry, although they often generate the same hazardous materials. Small businesses such as dry cleaners, photography laboratories, pesticide formulators, construction sites, and car repair shops discard a variety of substances that can cause serious public health problems.

Traditionally, U.S. economic development has produced optimal wealth with the assumption that the environmental health consequences would be minor. This notion of sustainable development has proved inadequate, and cumulative hazardous episodes necessitate tough pollution control technologies. The sustainability paradigm has led to a shift from disposing to recycling of biosolids. Biosolids refers to sewage sludge that has been treated for pathogens to meet the regulatory requirements for land application. This has been a cost-effective practice, but more research needs to be conducted on human health risks of biosolid distribution in the ecosystem.

A number of potential health problems are associated with waste management. For example, solid waste landfills accumulate methane gas, a by-product of decomposing organic wastes. Without proper venting, this volatile gas can move through soil and cause fires and explosions in nearby areas. Waste incineration causes particulate air pollution and is ineffective in the combustion of many materials. Improper design, operation, or location of waste site causes hazardous substances to spread through air, soil, and water to poison humans, animals, and plant life. Alarmingly, only a small percentage of hazardous waste actually reaches the designated waste sites; much is disposed of in open pits and in bodies of water, with dangerously uncertain long-term effects. New methods are being developed to estimate long-term rates of leaching of materials in various types of waste sites, based on probability principles (Sanchez and Kosson, 2005).

In 1980, Congress passed the Environmental Response Compensation and Liability Act, which established a revolving fund called the Superfund to clean up several hundred of the worst abandoned chemical waste disposal sites. One of the most notorious sites is the Love Canal in Niagara Falls, New York. For 40 years before the 1960s, more than 80 different types of chemicals, including benzene, dioxin, trichloroethylene, toluene, and chloroform, were dumped in an abandoned canal. Afterward, the covered area became the site for a school and several hundred homes. In the winters of 1976 and 1977, heavy snowfall and rain caused toxic wastes to reach the surface. Subsequently, the inhabitants experienced elevated miscarriage rates, blood and liver abnormalities, birth defects, and chromosome damage.

Clinical Example

In a city on the Mississippi River, an outbreak of shigellosis was traced to a group of high school students who had been swimming in a particular area of the river. The local meatpacking plant was releasing waste material, including human and animal feces, directly into the river. After intervening to contain the *Shigella* outbreak, the local community health nurses began to assess the situation. Their research indicated that the meatpacking facility had been in violation of waste control laws for some time. City officials imposed fines, which the company paid, but the dumping continued. A sign at the riverside prohibited swimming. Frustrated by their attempts to negotiate with the city and the plant, the nurses wrote a letter to the state capital newspaper, which had a large state readership. In the letter, they voiced concern about the community's health and the river's ecological integrity. The paper published their commentary, prompting responses from two local environmental groups, several activist groups, and a national organization concerned with clean water. These groups provided legal support and brought a collective suit against the meatpacking company. Subsequently, the company improved its waste treatment process to avoid legal ramifications.

EFFECTS OF ENVIRONMENTAL HAZARDS

Environmental hazards are ubiquitous, and their effects on the public's health are complex and generally interconnected. Nurses must understand the multiple and complex sequences leading to health concerns (Fig. 14-6). For example, nuclear power plant emissions may contaminate water and air supplies, affecting water quality, atmospheric quality, and radiation risk. Overcrowded housing may exacerbate problems in managing human waste, which may taint foodstuffs and contribute to the spread of communicable disease. Climate change continues to impact humans, the food chain, vegetation, and wildlife.

Effects of environmental hazards may be general or specific. For example, the ramifications of high unemployment, drought, and extensive smog cover affect the public generally.

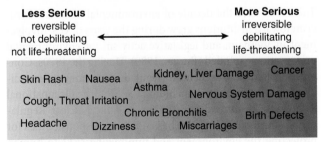

Which Risks are of Greatest Concern?

Less Serious	More Serious
reversible	irreversible
not debilitating	debilitating
not life-threatening	life-threatening

Skin Rash   Nausea   Kidney, Liver Damage   Cancer
Asthma
Cough, Throat Irritation   Nervous System Damage
Chronic Bronchitis   Birth Defects
Headache   Dizziness   Miscarriages

FIGURE 14-6 Degrees of health effects from environmental exposures. (From Environmental Protection Agency: *Air pollution and health risk.* Retrieved March 27, 2013, from <http://www.epa.gov/ttnatw01/3_90_022.html>.)

Other environmental health concerns, such as the housing needs of elderly people who use walkers or canes, the occupational risks of electrical line repair workers, and the mentally incapacitating effects of elevated blood lead values in children, affect the public more specifically.

Environmental health effects can be immediate, long-term, or intergenerational. Burns, gunshot wounds, hurricane damage, and outbreaks of gastrointestinal distress among cafeteria customers are examples of immediate effects from health-damaging environments. Examples of long-term health effects include gradual occupational hearing loss, "black lung" in coal miners, and increased rates of thyroid cancer among young victims of the Chernobyl nuclear reactor accident (Ron, 2007). Intergenerational effects will likely occur with climate change by affecting women of childbearing age.

Certain environmental exposures have been found to have a direct relationship with the development of some cancers, chronic diseases, and other health-related problems (Boyd and Genuis, 2008). Furthermore, oppressive environments may affect health directly. In one case, an American company dumped dangerous waste material in Mexico rather than pay for proper disposal (Schrieberg, 1991). Poor children who lived nearby and scavenged for food in the dump picked up and played with the shiny, brightly colored radioactive medical waste. The severe burns they suffered and the wine-colored spots on their skin were direct effects of the illegally dumped toxic waste.

Effects of environmental risks may also be indirect, such as in the case of global warming (Akhtar et al., 2009; Pan and Kao, 2009). Global warming is the gradual increase in the average temperature of Earth's near-surface air and oceans since the mid-twentieth century and its projected continuation (Easterling, 2011). Rising global temperatures may enhance the quantity and distribution of parasites, insects, and other disease vectors, potentially increasing the prevalence of a variety of infectious diseases (See ⓔ **Resource Tool 14D**). For example, global warming contributed to the entry and propagation of the West Nile virus in the United States (Epstein, 2001). Higher air and water temperatures facilitate the spread of vector-borne diseases transmitted by mosquitoes (e.g., West Nile virus). As a result, 2012 saw more cases of West Nile virus infection (5387) than any year since 2003, with a higher proportion of deaths (243) (CDC, 2012).

EFFORTS TO CONTROL ENVIRONMENTAL HEALTH PROBLEMS

The 1970s were the decade of environmental concern. Cynicism toward institutions grew during the years of U.S. involvement in Vietnam, and legislative activism for environmental preservation exploded (Burger, 1989). During the 1970s, Congress created new agencies to regulate environmental conditions on a national level, including the EPA, the Occupational Safety and Health Administration, and the Nuclear Regulatory Commission. The EPA has enormous responsibilities for protecting the environment and minimizing risks to human health. Among its roles are health surveillance and monitoring; setting standards for air and water quality; evaluating environmental risks; acquiring information; screening new

chemicals; performing basic research and training; and establishing, evaluating, and enforcing regulatory efforts.

The legislative activism of the 1970s was aimed toward a comprehensive national environmental policy. For example, stricter automobile fuel and emissions standards created improvements in air quality, which caused lead levels in urban air to decrease dramatically over the next decade. The momentum to control environmental pollution in the United States slowed in the 1980s and 1990s, with several policy reversals and the defunding of regulatory mechanisms. In recent years, administrative and legislative activity related to the environment have focused on such issues as climate change, oil spills, hazardous waste, and toxic exposures.

Frequently, laws and regulatory structures are weak or nonexistent with regard to environmental health problems. For example, federal mandates for recycling do not exist, although local communities have made great strides in this area. Comprehensive groundwater legislation, similar to adopted measures to preserve marine and surface waters, also does not exist. Additionally, the EPA tends to set priorities for the reduction of environmental problems but does not allocate the resources necessary to accomplish these goals.

RESEARCH HIGHLIGHTS

I PREPARE: Development and Clinical Utility of an Environmental Exposure History Mnemonic

The I PREPARE environmental exposure history mnemonic is a quick reference tool created by Paranzino and colleagues (2005) for primary care providers. A total of 159 health care providers, both students and professionals, were asked to evaluate a prototype of the mnemonic, to suggest new health history questions, and to propose the deletion of less relevant questions. The prototype was formatted as a pocket guide. The goal of this evaluation was to create a practical and clinically relevant mnemonic, rather than to obtain quantitative estimates of its validity. This mnemonic is meant to serve as a mental cue to facilitate the collection and documentation of health information in a systematic manner:

I—Investigate Potential Exposures
P—Present Work
R—Residence
E—Environmental Concerns
P—Past Work
A—Activities
R—Referrals and Resources
E—Educate

Questions to ask are presented for each letter in the mnemonic, except for Referrals and Resources, which provides sources of additional information. A checklist of strategies to prevent or minimize exposures can be used by the health care provider to help clients identify potential exposures. The sequence of I PREPARE makes intuitive sense by cueing the provider to ask specific questions and then provide educational materials to the client. The final version was reprinted on heavy laminated material. The I PREPARE mnemonic increases the repertoire of tools clinicians have available to elicit an appropriate health history. The national improvements in the quality of environmental exposure history are predicated, in part, on the creation of simple and convenient tools for use in clinical practice.

Data from Paranzino GK, Butterfield P, Nastoff T, Ranger C: I PREPARE: Development and clinical utility of an environmental exposure history mnemonic, *AAOHN J* 53(1):37-42, 2005.

Most of the U.S. environmental health efforts have aimed for short-term results rather than anticipating future issues and problems. A crucial need exists in the development of human resources in the area of environmental health. Nurses in all areas of practice should be aware of the implications of the environment for their clients and their health. It is for this reason that nurses need to take and record an environmental health history for every client.

EMERGING ISSUES IN ENVIRONMENT HEALTH

Within the past decade, we are beginning to recognize that our environmental public health infrastructure is quite weak and that the United States is susceptible to many of the same problems that burden the rest of the world. For example, the illegal use of pesticides, medical waste incineration, and the increased incidence of asthma related to air pollution are just a few of the challenges facing the United States today. The manufacturing of methamphetamine in home-based and mobile laboratories continues to rise, and the "cooking process" emits dangerous levels of toxic chemicals into the air. Similarly, the abandoned labs also pose a threat (Grant, Bell, Stewart, 2010). Finally, natural disasters and climate change affects the entire world.

Natural disasters can disrupt and oftentimes overwhelm private and public health systems. Natural disasters, such as the tsunami that struck the coast of Indonesia in December 2004, Hurricane Katrina in August 2005, the devastating earthquakes in the Sichuan Province of China in 2008 and in Haiti in 2010, and superstorm Sandy in 2012 require mobilization of disaster relief units that offer substantial assistance and expertise. Natural disasters such as hurricanes, tornados, and earthquakes frequently receive notable publicity, but other, more insidious disasters, such as droughts, floods, heat waves, and extreme cold, also pose major public health concerns. All of the aforementioned threats can cause significant mortality and morbidity and, therefore, have the potential to burden the health care delivery system.

Global warming is part of a larger issue called climate change that poses significant health hazards. Climate change is the change in weather over a certain period. Weather patterns are greatly affected by atmospheric and oceanic temperature rises. Climate change projections suggest that heat waves and hot weather are likely to increase in frequency, with the overall temperature distribution shifting away from extreme cold (O'Neill and Ebi, 2009). Climate change can have severe adverse health effects, such as health-related illness and death; increases in air pollution; water-, food-, vector-, and rodent-borne diseases; malnutrition; contaminated water supply; and injuries and deaths related to extreme weather and storm surges (Balbus, 2011; Sheffield et al., 2011). There are regional differences in the effects of climate change, although vulnerable populations will be affected the most (See ⓔ **Resource Tool 14E**). For instance, climate change will raise the risks of infant and maternal mortality, birth complications, and poorer reproductive health, especially in developing countries (Rylander, Odland, and Sandanger, 2013).

BOX 14-3 NONGOVERNMENTAL ENVIRONMENTAL ORGANIZATIONS

- Alliance of Nurses for Healthy Environments (http://envirn.org/)
- American Farmland Trust (http://www.farmland.org/)
- Citizens for a Better Environment (http://www.cbezambia.org/)
- Clean Water Action (http://www.cleanwateraction.org/)
- Green America (http://www.greenamerica.org/)
- Environmental Defense Fund (http://www.edf.org/)
- Environmental Working Group (http://www.ewg.org/)
- Greenpeace (http://www.greenpeace.org/usa/en/)
- International Rivers Network (http://www.internationalrivers.org/)
- National Audubon Society (http://www.audubon.org/)
- National Environmental Law Center (http://www.nelconline.org/)
- National Geographic Society (http://www.nationalgeographic.com/about/)
- Natural Resources Defense Council (http://www.nrdc.org/)
- National Wildlife Federation (http://www.nwf.org/)
- Ocean Alliance (http://www.oceanalliance.org/)
- Pesticide Action Network (http://www.panna.org/)
- Rainforest Action Network (http://ran.org/)
- Sierra Club (http://www.sierraclub.org/)
- The Nature Conservancy (http://www.nature.org/)
- Trust for Public Land (http://www.tpl.org/)
- Wilderness Society (http://wilderness.org/)
- World Wildlife Fund (http://worldwildlife.org/)

For further information, see the report by the Institute of Medicine Committee on Enhancing Environmental Health Content in Nursing Practice: *Nursing, health, and the environment*, Washington, DC, 1995, National Academies Press.

Nursing Actions

Nurses must work with the public to promote more stringent and actively enforced environmental legislation and regulations. In the twenty-first century, actions must include not only national but also worldwide environmental policies. Ozone depletion, climate change, fossil fuel burning, marine dumping, abandonment of active land mines in war-torn areas, and destruction of tropical rain forests are among the key global environmental health concerns.

Environmental concerns for clean air, clean water, and freedom from noxious chemicals must become nursing concerns. Community health nurses can be catalysts to neighborhood efforts to produce safe living environments. Community health nursing must expand its theory and practice to incorporate the fact that individual and community health ultimately depends on global environmental integrity. Many organizations work to preserve and protect the environment and could benefit from the active involvement and support of nurses. Box 14-3 lists some of these organizations. Nursing must include an environmental perspective by committing to environmental health promotion initiatives that promote social justice and environmental responsibility.

APPROACHING ENVIRONMENTAL HEALTH AT THE POPULATION LEVEL

In the United States, personal independence and individual responsibility for success and failure are valued. These values can lead nurses to overlook environmental hazards and instead blame individual clients for their health problems. Placing responsibility for the cause and cure of health problems exclusively on the individual reinforces the belief that all individuals are free to exert meaningful control over the quality and length of their lives. Such a perspective absolves society, government, industry, and business from accountability.

Research suggests that changing individual behaviors does not lead to significant reductions in overall morbidity and mortality in the absence of basic social, economic, and political changes (Bhatia and Wernham, 2008). Emphasizing only interventions that address deleterious personal habits through exercise programs, weight-loss regimens, smoking-cessation classes, and stress-reduction tactics fails to take into account the broader environmental origins of disease, injury, and ecological degradation. An attempt to approach health at the aggregate level is the *Healthy People 2020* initiative (USDHHS, 2013). The *Healthy People* box lists selected environmental health objectives of the *Healthy People 2020* initiative.

Interventions designed for individuals must consider the environmental determinants of behavior and health

♥ **HEALTHY PEOPLE 2020**

Selected Objectives for Environmental Health

EH–2: Increase use of alternative modes of transportation for work

EH–3: Reduce air toxic emissions to decrease the risk of adverse health effects caused by mobile, area and major sources of airborne toxins

EH–4: Increase the proportion of persons served by community water systems who receive a supply that meets the regulations of the Safe Drinking Water Act

EH–5: Reduce waterborne disease outbreaks arising from water intended for drinking among persons served by community water systems

EH–8.1: Eliminate elevated blood lead levels in children

EH–12: Increase recycling of municipal solid waste

EH–14: Increase the proportion of persons living in homes at risk that have an operating radon mitigation system

From U.S. Department of Health and Human Services: *Healthy People 2020,* http://www.healthypeople.gov/2020/topicsobjectives2020/objectiveslist.aspx?topicId=12

⚖ ETHICAL INSIGHTS

Protecting Vulnerable Aggregates

Community health nurses have a mandate to assist vulnerable aggregates who have fewer options in protecting themselves from pollution, inadequate housing, toxic poisoning, unsafe products, and other hazards. Non–English-speaking individuals, children, very low-income women and families, undocumented manual laborers, and people from racial and ethnic minorities are just some of the groups in the United States who hold minimal influence with industry, government, business, and other large institutions for environmental changes and compensations for harm from environmental hazards.

outcomes (Bartholomew et al., 2011). Community health nurses who base their practices on theory and evidence are better prepared to respond to collective challenges. These nurses can facilitate community participation in identifying and solving environmental health problems and bringing about changes that improve environments and eliminate hazards.

CRITICAL ENVIRONMENTAL HEALTH NURSING PRACTICE

The National Center for Environmental Health, the CDC, and the American Public Health Association have established three core competencies for environmental health professionals: assessment, management, and communication (Box 14-4). Several clinical examples throughout the chapter illustrate how nurses can focus their efforts by organizing groups of people, taking a stand, and acting as advocates for change. The nurses ask critical questions, stay engaged with the communities they serve, form coalitions, and use various collective strategies. The American Nurses Association highlights 10 critical environmental health principles. In the interest of educating future practitioners about the critical practice of environmental community health nursing, the following sections discuss each of these interventions.

Taking a Stand: Advocating for Change

Nurses must make individual and collective decisions about which interests they want to serve with their specialized knowledge and skills. Nurse may choose to work with vulnerable people or those disproportionally experiencing the consequences of environmental hazards. Vulnerable groups are exposed to more health-damaging effects than less vulnerable groups (Chakraborty and Zandbergen, 2007; EPA, 2013c). Nurses can work toward health equity through the decisions they make, the positions they accept, and the interventions they undertake. Environmental problems are clearly intertwined with social, political, and economic policies, resource barriers, and the interests of those in positions of control. Nurses need to connect the immediate and long-term health problems experienced by particular communities to this larger sphere of influence.

Asking Critical Questions

Community health nurses must also consider the relationships between non-health policies and health policies. They should ask how policies concerning ecological preservation, energy, housing, immigration, civil rights, crime, nutrition, minimum wage, occupational safety, and defense might affect the health and well-being of people. Addressing critical questions such as who has access to resources in this country and whose interests are served in the existing system provides a way to include social, political, and economic factors in environmental nursing assessments. Box 14-5 provides a sample set of questions that are useful in this endeavor. Nurses can ask these critical questions when approaching environmental health problems.

BOX 14-4   CORE ENVIRONMENTAL HEALTH COMPETENCIES

Assessment

Research: The capacity to identify and compile relevant information to solve a problem, and the knowledge of where to go to obtain the relevant information

Data analysis and interpretation: The capacity to analyze data, recognize meaningful test results, interpret findings, and present the results in a meaningful way to different types of audiences

Evaluation: The capacity to evaluate the effectiveness or performance of procedures, interventions, and programs

Management

Problem solving: The capacity to understand and solve problems.

Economic and political issues: The capacity to understand and appropriately utilize information concerning the economic and political implications of decisions.

Organizational knowledge and behavior: The capacity to function effectively within the culture of the organization and to be an effective team player.

Managing work: The capacity to plan, implement, and maintain fiscally responsible programs/projects using appropriate skills, and prioritize projects across the employee's entire workload.

Computer/information technology (IT): The capacity to utilize information technology as needed to produce work products.

Reporting, documentation, and record-keeping: The capacity to produce reports that document actions, keep records, and inform appropriate parties.

Partnering: The capacity to form partnerships and alliances with other individuals and organizations in order to enhance performance on the job.

Communication

Education: The capacity to use the environmental health practitioner's front-line role to effectively educate the public on environmental health issues.

Communication: The capacity to effectively communicate risk and exchange information with colleagues, other practitioners, clients, policy-makers, interest groups, media, and the public through public speaking, print and electronic media, and interpersonal relations.

Conflict resolution: The capacity to facilitate the resolution of conflicts within the agency, in the community, and with regulated parties.

Marketing environmental/public health as a service: The ability to articulate basic concepts of environmental health and public health and convey an understanding of their value and importance to clients and the public.

Data from American Public Health Association: *Environmental Health Competency Project: draft recommendations for non-technical competencies at the local level,* 2013. Retrieved from <http://www.apha.org/programs/standards/healthcompproject/corenontechnicalcompetencies.htm>.

BOX 14-5   CRITICAL QUESTIONS ABOUT ENVIRONMENTAL HEALTH PROBLEMS

- What is the problem?
- Who is defining the problem?
- In what terms is the problem described?
- How are others in the situation viewing the problem?
- What is the history of the problem?
- How did things get the way they are?
- What other situations does this problem directly affect?
- Who does the problem affect?
- Whose health is damaged because things are this way?
- Who benefits from the way things are?
- Whose interests do current solutions serve?
- What are the economic inequities in the situation?
- Who has political power in the situation?
- Who knows about the problem?
- Who needs to know more about the problem?
- How effective are current programs, strategies, and policies?
- What are the barriers to solving the problem?
- What strategies may alleviate the problem?
- How successful have these strategies been?
- What existing groups might deal with this problem?
- What resources are needed to solve the problem?
- How accessible are the resources?
- How can nurses evaluate potential solutions?

be prepared to take leadership positions and join in mutual exchanges with community members that consider each person's experience. The nurse's role changes from presenting solutions and directing lifestyle changes to providing support, information, and expertise to assist in meeting the group goals. Using critical questions, community health nurses can help community members look beyond immediate environmental problems and explore social, cultural, economic, and political circumstances that contribute to them. Nurses can share their knowledge about the scientific basis for health problems, their insights about the historical origins of particular environmental hazards, their technical skills, and their expertise in communicating and organizing. By addressing people's everyday concerns and targeting the problems they identify, nurses situate their efforts in community struggles.

Forming Coalitions

Another very important nursing task that arises from approaching environmental health from a critical perspective involves forming coalitions to produce social change. By initiating dialogue and building a strong base of collective support, nurses join with communities to eliminate hazards and improve public health. Nurses can approach existing community organizations, churches, and family and friendship networks to help mobilize aggregate members who have not previously socialized or acted together. Nurses can then discuss environmental concerns, assess needs, plan actions, secure appropriate resources, and advocate for legislative changes.

Nurses can be instrumental in these efforts by helping community groups make connections with larger, more powerful organizations. Nurses can organize forums whereby community groups meet with scientific experts who can help them

Facilitating Community Involvement

Approaching community health from a critical perspective requires working to improve health conditions and creating the context in which people can identify health-damaging problems in their environments. One important nursing goal is to help people learn from their own experiences and analyze the world with an intention to change it. It is essential that the affected people participate in the process of identifying and working to solve environmental problems. To foster community-based, active participation, nurses must

Asthma is a significant public health problem that disproportionately affects preschool-age, low-income children. Indeed, children from low-income families have significantly higher asthma prevalence rates, hospitalization rates, and emergency department visits than children from middle-income and wealthier families. This problem is even more pronounced among children in urban areas.

A team of public health nurses led by Garwick (2010) used participatory action research (PAR) techniques in working with teachers in an urban Head Start program with multiple sites to address asthma management among the children at their sites. In this project, teachers and managers from 16 Head Start centers were identified to participate in three focus groups. During the focus groups, participants identified asthma management issues and challenges, including: undiagnosed and unreported asthma, coordination of asthma care with parents, medication administration issues, and variability among asthma action plans. As a result of the PAR, a standardized, comprehensive Head Start asthma action plan was developed that outlined strategies the teachers could use to better manage the problem of asthma among the children.

Data from Garwick AW, Seppelt A, Riesgraf M: Addressing asthma management challenges in a multisite, urban Head Start Program, *Public Health Nurs* 27(4):329-336, 2010.

gather evidence about health threats, with business managers whose actions impinge on the economic life of the community, with industry leaders whose companies create ecological hazards, and with legislators who can bring community concerns to lawmaking bodies. Using available institutional resources, skills, and knowledge, nurses can also explore what is happening elsewhere. Making connections with groups in other locales who are struggling for similar environmental changes can enhance collective strength and solidarity. Press releases, media events, interviews, television spots, speeches, newsletters, and leaflets are important means of calling attention to a situation and raising awareness among communities.

Using Collective Strategies

Nurses can use a variety of strategies to intervene at the population level and facilitate improvement in a community's health. Nurses can organize people to change health-damaging environments through combinations of strategies including building coalitions, providing educational forums, facilitating a community needs assessment, disseminating research, and lobbying for legislative changes.

One collective strategy that is an effective population-level community health nursing intervention is participatory action research (Box 14-6). This form of research calls for nurses, community members, and other resource people to work together in identifying health problems, designing the studies, collecting and analyzing the data, disseminating the results, and posing solutions to the problems (Garwick, Seppelt and Riesgraf, 2010; Li et al., 2011). In participatory action research applied to environmental health, community health nurses and community members would gather information on suspected environmental hazards, determine their effects on health, and devise a plan of action to mitigate the threat.

Although nurses have not traditionally used all of these collective strategies to intervene in community health matters, environmental hazards are multiplying geometrically, pushing nurses to expand their skills repertoire. Pioneers such as Hollie Shaner, RN, have embraced that concept and are blazing the path to environmental awareness (Sattler, 2003). In the 1990s, Shaner frequently left her home, where she avidly separated and recycled, to work at a Vermont hospital, where none of the waste was recycled. Shaner was not comfortable throwing everything into a "red bag" and decided that there must be a way to change the environmental unfriendliness of her place of employment. She began voluntarily recycling the hospitals' cardboard and then began to recycle the newspapers, glass, and plastics. In addition, she received a grant from the state of Vermont to maximize her efforts in medical waste reduction. The efforts and savings did not go unnoticed by the hospital, as Shaner received a new job title of clinical waste reduction coordinator, and saved the hospital $175,000 per year.

Shaner also wrote a book for the American Hospital Association on medical waste management. She quickly realized the negative impact the health care industry was having on the environmental health of the communities served. Mercury was being released into the streams from medical waste, and dioxins were being released into the air from medical waste incineration. From this realization, in 1996, Shaner and a small group of other health professionals launched a campaign to lead the health care industry toward environmental stewardship. This campaign, supported by the American Nurses Association, was named Health Care Without Harm. "The goal of the campaign was to reduce the environmental health risks that were being created by the health care industry" (Sattler, 2003, p. 8). The campaign still exists and is building momentum; today there are 433 participating organizations in 52 different countries (Health Care Without Harm, 2013).

CASE STUDY APPLICATION OF THE NURSING PROCESS

In July 2001, the *Metro Pulse* newspaper reported an extensive air pollution problem in the city of Knoxville, Tennessee (Tarr, 2001). The American Lung Association had recently named Knoxville as the ninth most polluted city in the country on the basis of the ozone contamination in the air. The following case study expands on some of the reported facts of the situation to construct hypothetical nursing interventions.

Knoxville's community health nurses and the public health department were aware of increasing rates of asthma in particular

neighborhoods. In the wake of alarming newspaper and research articles about the dangerous incidence of air pollution and related asthma, the nurses decided to make the health issues a priority. The community health nurses and several nursing students assigned to their department researched the topics and uncovered the following information.

Asthma has long been recognized as a condition in which an acute respiratory response may follow inhalation of a material to which a person is sensitized. Scientists now know that air pollution can lead

CASE STUDY   APPLICATION OF THE NURSING PROCESS—cont'd

to nonspecific generalized inflammation. One study found strong evidence that ozone can *cause,* as well as exacerbate, asthma (Sheffield, et.al, 2011). The study found that days with worse AQI values resulted in significantly higher school absences due to respiratory illness, and asthma was more likely to develop in children living in high-ozone communities who actively participated in several outdoor sports than in children in communities not participating in sports.

Indeed, the nation's leading group of pediatricians, the American Academy of Pediatrics (AAP) revised its policy statement on outdoor air pollution and the health hazards to children (Schwartz, 2004). The AAP's Committee on Environmental Health strengthened its warning about the dangers that air pollution poses to children because of the recent studies correlating air pollution with asthma and negative lung growth and function. Estimates are that more than 25 million Americans have asthma (Asthma and Allergy Foundation, 2013).

An economically depressed neighborhood in Knoxville, hypothetically called Trent Park, is situated near numerous railways, freeways, and industrial yards. High numbers of African American, Latino, and Southeast Asian residents live in the older homes that line the streets of Trent Park. Isolated by language and economic circumstances, many Trent Park residents do not know they are exposed to these environmental health hazards.

Assessment

Elena Garcia, an 8-year-old girl who lives in Trent Park, presented to the pediatric primary clinic at the health department at 8 AM in November. Elena had been diagnosed with asthma 2 months ago and was now in mild respiratory distress. Elena explained to the nurse that she had gone trick-or-treating the night before in her neighborhood. It had turned cold that weekend, and she had also played outside in her neighborhood with friends the day before. In addition, the child's mother explained that Elena had recently had a respiratory virus. The nurse realized that Elena and her mother both mentioned several factors, such as her playing outside on a cold afternoon/evening in a polluted neighborhood and a respiratory virus, that could have exacerbated her asthma.

At the clinic visit, the nurse assessed the following:
- Elena's heart rate and cardiovascular status
- Elena's pattern of breathing, which includes rate, rhythm, and effort
- Elena's asthma medication history
- Evidence of diaphoresis, papillary dilation, and fear, which are all features of the adrenergic response to hypoxia
- Elena's global central nervous system function, such as alertness, cooperation, and motor activity
- Elena's environmental health assessment

Diagnosis
Individual
- Ineffective respirations related to environmental exposure to air pollution
- Insufficient knowledge related to precipitating factors that can cause/worsen an asthma attack
- Stress related to ongoing fear of daughter's illness

Family
- Risk for family crisis related to instability caused by the illness
- Insufficient knowledge related to factors that can cause/worsen an asthma attack

Community
- Risk for increased incidence of asthma due to air pollution
- Inadequate programs for asthma screening

Planning

A plan of care was developed at the individual, family, and community levels. Mutual goal setting and contracting are essential if the outcome is to be optimal.

Individual
Long-Term Goals
- Client will modify outdoor time daily according to the Air Quality Index
- Client will reduce exposure to allergy triggers
- Client will avoid secondhand tobacco smoke
- Client will keep pets out of the bedroom
- Client will experience successful maintenance of asthma

Short-Term Goals
- Client will report reduced outdoor time on days with poor AQI values
- Client will keep an asthma diary and identify which allergy triggers are problematic
- Client will remain free of acute asthma attacks

Family
Long-Term Goals
- Family will follow the city's daily AQI
- Family will encourage child to stay indoors on days with high pollution levels
- Family will remove as many allergy triggers from home as possible
- Family will enforce the pets-out-of-the-bedroom policy
- Family will cope effectively with daughter's asthma

Short-Term Goals
- Family will provide encouragement for client to keep an asthma diary

Community
Long-Term Goals
- Citizens will be involved in decision-making process about proposed activities that could pose an environmental hazard
- Citizens will encourage utility companies, government, and industries to reduce air pollution
- Citizens will be encouraged to use mass transit and carpools to reduce vehicle emissions

Short-Term Goals
- Citizens will be alerted about the air pollution problem in the area
- Citizens will be educated about the AQI and its implications for outdoor activity

Intervention
Individual
- Identify Trent Park children with asthma and plan follow-up home visits to provide education on basic pathophysiology, symptoms of distress, and environmental controls needed for successful asthma management
- Add environmental health assessments to child health assessment protocol
- Coordinate with school nurses to ensure they incorporate similar changes into their health assessment protocols
- Prepare and distribute an educational pamphlet with members of Trent Park that details Trent Park residents' air pollution and asthma risks

Continued

CASE STUDY   APPLICATION OF THE NURSING PROCESS—cont'd

- Prepare translations of the pamphlet in languages and reading levels appropriate for Trent Park residents, and mail it to individual households.

Family

- Facilitate the formation of a support group for families with children who have asthma

Community

- Initiate an asthma awareness program for Trent Park community members.
- Coordinate with school nurses to implement an asthma awareness program in Trent Park schools.
- Develop an asthma action team consisting of Trent Park community members.
- Participate in the action team's development of an intervention to reduce asthma-related illness in Trent Park.
- Encourage nursing students and community health nursing faculty from the local university and college programs to participate.
- Lobby state legislatures, municipal officials, local medical associations, local hospitals, and city clinics regarding the project.
- Form broader coalitions with Knoxville churches, local nurses association, several preschool and day care centers, and the Knoxville School Board to design a comprehensive, nonduplicative, cost-effective asthma screening program.
- Train action team members on how to conduct Healthy Home assessments.
- Contact state environmental groups for advice on local efforts, and join in their fight for stricter regulation of air pollutants and toxic wastes.
- Contact local media (e.g., television, radio, and newspaper) about running a series of stories about Knoxville air pollutants and related asthma risks; supply information and contacts for interviews and photographs.

Evaluation

Individual

- Evaluate the child and mother's understanding of asthma treatments at follow-up home visits.
- Facilitate the evaluation of ongoing interventions.
- Track the number of asthma screening tests that Trent Park children receive and their rates of asthma to determine the effectiveness of their efforts in these areas.
- Keep close contact with the school nurses, and organize an after-school educational and screening program at schools that are understaffed.
- Ask school nurses to report on the educational sessions' success.

Family

- Document participation levels at educational programs and family training sessions.
- Document ongoing participation in referrals and support groups.

Community

The action team was able to get funding to provide Healthy Home assessments and asthma screening to at-risk youth in Trent Park.

Levels of Prevention

Primary Prevention

Educating the community regarding air pollution and its relationship to asthma

Secondary Prevention

Screening at-risk populations for asthma

Tertiary Prevention

Follow-up treatment for people with asthma and reduction of air pollutants in the community environment

SUMMARY

This chapter provided a glimpse into the complex world of environmental health from a critical community health nursing perspective. The case study and clinical examples illustrate that nurses must evaluate the broader picture in assessing the environmental health status of communities and the vulnerable aggregates within them. In preventing, minimizing, and resolving environmental health problems, nurses must recognize patterns, detect subtle changes, identify underlying issues, and work collaboratively with a variety of individuals and groups. In the past, environmental threats to health were usually suspected only when other possible causes of illness were ruled out. Nurses can expect this pattern to change dramatically in the twenty-first century as environmental health moves increasingly to the forefront of the public health agenda.

LEARNING ACTIVITIES

1. Identify a health-related problem associated with some aspect of the environment. It may be a problem in a nearby community, a problem publicized in the media, or a difficulty experienced by a family. Examine the problem using the sample series of critical questions listed in Box 14-5. Without sharing the results, present the problem to the group and ask them to discuss it by responding to the same questions. Were there differences or similarities in the initial results and the group's answers? On what points did everyone agree? Why? What questions caused the most disagreement? Why? Now repeat the entire activity by involving people other than nursing students in the group discussion. How did this discussion compare with the previous discussion and responses?

2. Attend meetings that hold environmental hazard discussions. If meetings or public forums are not available in the vicinity, write for information about the state's actions to fight environmental hazards. The reference librarians at colleges or public libraries can suggest ways of contacting sources and will supply addresses. Organizations that are likely to sponsor forums and provide information include those listed in Box 14-3, the Environmental Protection Agency, the National Institute for Occupational Safety and Health, state and municipal agencies for environmental protection and occupational health, environmental caucuses of political parties, the American Public Health Association, the local public health department, farmers' organizations, and labor unions.

3. This chapter described how to use participatory research as an intervention in dealing with ecological hazards. In a group, brainstorm about possibilities for participatory action research projects in the area. Try to identify examples from a variety of environmental health areas. Be creative in planning. How might a nurse mobilize community support and participation in the research? What groups would be approachable? What critical questions might facilitate dialogue about the problem? What kinds of data could be collected, and how could they be used? How could research results be publicized? What ramifications could the completed study have for community members, other communities in the state, and community health nurses in other locales?

4. Nurses may have to supplement their knowledge of collective strategies by reading books about political action and by learning from community members who are experienced in political organizing. Visit a college or public library to investigate books and journal articles outside the nursing literature. Compile a list of references related to one of these political strategies (e.g., grassroots organizing, legislative lobbying, community education, policy analysis, use of the media, coalition building, citizen surveys, public protest, letter-writing campaigns, or consciousness-raising groups). Exchange reference lists with peers to benefit from their efforts. Then choose one or two books of interest and read them.

ⓔ EVOLVE WEBSITE

http://evolve.elsevier.com/Nies
- NCLEX Review Questions
- Case Studies
- Glossary
- Resource Tool 14A: A Healthy Home Checklist
- Resource Tool 14B: Picture of Healthy Home
- Resource Tool 14C: Steps in a Foodborne Outbreak Investigation
- Resource Tool 14D: Potential Health Effects of Climate Change
- Resource Tool 14E: Regional Differences Due to Climate Change

---

REFERENCES

Akhtar AZ, Greger M, Ferdowsian H, et al: Health professionals' roles in animal agriculture, climate change, and human health, *Am J Prev Med* 36(2):182–187, 2009.

American Planning Association: *Principles of a healthy sustainable food system*, 2010. Available from <http://www.planning.org/nationalcenters/health/foodprinciples.htm>.

Anderson JO, Thundiyil JG, Stolbach A: Clearing the air: a review of the effects of particulate matter air pollution on human health, *J Med Toxicol* 8(2):166–175, 2012.

Asthma and Allergy Foundation: *Asthma facts and figures*, 2013. Available from <http://aafa.org/display.cfm?id=8&sub=42>.

Balbus JM: Health implications. In *Climate change: mastering the public health role, a practical guidebook*, Washington, DC, 2011, American Public Health Association, pp 15–30.

Bartholomew LK, Parcel GS, Kok G, et al: *Planning health promotion programs: an intervention mapping approach*, Hoboken, NJ, 2011, Jossey-Bass/Wiley.

Barton A, Basham M, Foy C, et al: The Watcombe housing study: the short term effect of improving housing conditions on the health of residents, *J Epidemiol Community Health* 61:771–777, 2007.

Bhatia R, Wernham A: Integrating human health into environmental impact assessment: an unrealized opportunity for environmental health and justice, *Environ Health Perspect* 116(8):991–1000, 2008.

Boyd DR, Genuis SJ: The environmental burden of disease in Canada: respiratory disease, cardiovascular disease, cancer and congenital affliction, *Environ Res* 106(2):240–249, 2008.

Bureau of Labor Statistics: *Current injury, illness, and fatality data*, 2008. Available from <http://data.bls.gov/search/query/results?cx=01373803619591937764 4%3A6ih0hfrgl50&q=2008+in url%3Abls.gov%2Fiif>.

Bureau of Labor Statistics: *Workplace injuries and illnesses—2011*, 2012. Available from <http://www.bls.gov/news.release/archives/osh_10252012.pdf>.

Burger EJ: Human health: a surrogate for the environment: the evolution of environmental legislation and regulation during the 1970s, *Regul Toxicol Pharmacol* 9:196–206, 1989.

Centers for Disease Control and Prevention: Novel influenza A (H1N1) virus infection—Mexico, March-May 2009, *MMWR Morb Mortal Wkly Rep* 58(21):585–589, 2009.

Centers for Disease Control and Prevention: Preliminary FoodNet data on the incident of infection with pathogens transmitted commonly through food: 10 sites—United States, 2009, *MMWR Surveill Summ* 59(14):418–422, 2010.

Centers for Disease Control and Prevention: *Drinking water*, 2011. Available from <http://www.cdc.gov/healthywater/drinking/private/wells/>.

Centers for Disease Control and Prevention: *Healthy homes*, 2011. Available from <http://www.cdc.gov/healthyhomes>.

Centers for Disease Control and Prevention: *West Nile Virus*, 2013. Available from <http://www.cdc.gov/ncidod/dvbid/westnile/index.htm>.

Centers for Disease Control and Prevention: *Workplace safety and health topics: agricultural safety*, 2013. Available from <http://www.cdc.gov/niosh/topics/aginjury/>.

Chakraborty C, Zandbergen PA: Children at risk: racial/ethnic disparities in potential exposure to air pollution at school and home, *J Epidemiol Community Health* 61:1074–1079, 2007.

Ciencewicki J, Trivedi S, Kleeberger SJ: Oxidants and the pathogenesis of lung disease, *J Allergy and Clin Immunol* 3(122):456–468, 2008.

Collins MB: Risk-based targeting: Identifying disproportionalities in the sources and effects of industrial pollution, *Am J Public Health* 101(S1):S231–S237, 2011.

Ding D, Sallis JF, Kerr J, et al: Neighborhood environment and physical activity among youth: A review, *Amer J Prev Med* 41(4):442–455, 2011.

Driehuis F, Spanjer MC, Scholten JM, et al: Occurrence of mycotoxins in feedstuffs of dairy cows and estimation of total dietary intakes, *J Dairy Sci* 91(11):4261–4271, 2008.

Dunton GF, Kaplan J, Wolch J, et al: Physical environmental correlate of childhood obesity: a systematic review, *Obesity Rev* 10:393–402, 2009.

Environmental Protection Agency: *Indoors air facts No. 4 (revised): sick building syndrome*, 1991. Available from <http://www.epa.gov/iaq/pdfs/sick_building_factsheet.pdf>.

Environmental Protection Agency: *Urban sprawl modeling, air quality monitoring and risk communication: The Northeast Ohio Project*, EPA/625/R-02/016, Washington, DC, 2002, Author.

Environmental Protection Agency: *Ensuring risk reduction in communities with multiple stressors: environmental justice and cumulative risks/impacts*, Washington, DC, 2004, Author.

Environmental Protection Agency: *Highlighting success: the region 9 environmental justice small grant program, fiscal years 1994–99*, EPA 909-R99–002, Washington, DC, 2005, Author.

Environmental Protection Agency: *Air quality index (AQI): a guide to air quality and your health*, 2013g. Available from <http://www.airnow.gov/index.cfm?action=aqibasics.aqi>.

Environmental Protection Agency: *Food safety*, 2012a. Available from <http://www2.epa.gov/safepestcontrol>.

Environmental Protection Agency: *Public water systems: laboratories and monitoring*, 2012b. Available from <http://water.epa.gov/infrastructure/drinkingwater/pws/labmon.cfm>.

Environmental Protection Agency: *The effects of acid rain*, 2012c. Available from <http://www.epa.gov/acidrain/effects/>.

Environmental Protection Agency: *What are the six common air pollutants?* 2012d. Available from <http://www.epa.gov/airquality/urbanair/>.

Environmental Protection Agency: *You're your house and healthy home*, 2012e. Available from <http://yosemite.epa.gov/ochp/ochpweb.nsf/content/Healthy_Homes_Action_Card_English.htm/$File/Healthy_Homes_Action_Card_English.pdf>.

Environmental Protection Agency: *An introduction to indoor air quality*, 2013a. Available from <http://www.epa.gov/iaq/co.html>.

Environmental Protection Agency: *Drinking water contaminants*, 2013b. Available from <http://water.epa.gov/drink/contaminants/>.

Environmental Protection Agency: *Environmental justice*, 2013c. Available from <http://www.epa.gov/environmentaljustice/>.

Environmental Protection Agency: *Federal radon action plan: celebrating success, looking to the future*, 2013d. Available from <http://www.epa.gov/radon/pdfs/FRAP_2013Accomplishments.pdf>.

Environmental Protection Agency: *Ozone layer protection*, 2013e. Available from http://www.epa.gov/ozone/strathome.html.

Environmental Protection Agency: *Radon: health risks*, 2013f. Available from <http://www.epa.gov/radon/healthrisks.html>.

Epstein PR: West Nile virus and the climate, *J Urban Health* 78:367–371, 2001.

Easterling D: Basic Climate change science. In *Climate change: mastering the public health role, a practical guidebook*, Washington, DC, 2011, American Public Health Association, pp 7–14.

Fan Y, Song Y: Is sprawl associated with a widening urban–suburban mortality gap? *Journal of Urban Health* 86(5):708–728, 2009.

Farand SP, Lewis-Michl EL, Gomex MI: Adverse birth outcomes and maternal exposure to trichloroethylene and tetrachloroethylene through soil vapor intrusion in New York State, *Environ Health Persp* 120(4), 2012.

Food Safety.gov: *Causes of food poisoning*, 2013. Available from <http://www.foodsafety.gov/poisoning/causes/index.html>.

Garwick AW, Seppelt A, Riesgraf M: Addressing asthma management challenges in multisite, urban Head Start Program, *Public Health Nursing* 27(4):329–336, 2010.

Grant P, Bell K, Stewart D, et al: Evidence of methamphetamine exposure in children removed from clandestine methamphetamine laboratories, *Pedi emerg care* 26(1):10–14, 2010.

Hankey S, Marshall JD, Brauer M: Health impacts of the built environment: within-urban variability in physical inactivity, air pollution, and ischemic heart disease mortality, *Environ health persp* 120(2):247, 2012.

Health Care Without Harm: *About us*, 2013. Available from <http://noharm.org/us_canada/about/>.

Hurd HS, Malladi S: A stochastic assessment of the public health risks of the use of macrolide antibiotics in food animals, *Risk Anal* 28(3):695–710, 2008.

Institute of Medicine: *Committee on Enhancing Environmental Health Content in Nursing Practice: nursing, health, and the environment*, Washington, DC, 1995, National Academies Press.

Institute of Medicine: *The public health effects of food deserts: workshop summary*, 2009. Available from <http://www.iom.edu/Reports/2009/FoodDeserts.aspx>.

Klitzman S, Matte TD, Kass DE: The urban physical environment and its effects on health. In Freudenberg Nicholas, Galea Sandro, Vlahov David, editors: *Cities and the health of the public*, Nashville, TN, 2006, Vanderbilt University Press, pp 61–84.

Knobeloch L, Turyk M, Imm P, et al: Temporal changes in PCB and DDE levels among a cohort of frequent and infrequent consumers of Great Lakes sportfish, *Environ Res* 109:66–72, 2009.

Krieger N, Chen JT, Waterman PD, et al: The inverse hazard law: blood pressure, sexual harassment, racial discrimination, workplace abuse and occupational exposures in US low-income black, white, and Latino workers, *Soc Sci Med* 67:1970–1981, 2008.

Li IC, Chen YC, Hsu LL, et al: The effects of an educational training workshop for community leaders on self-efficacy of program planning skills and partnerships, *J of Adv Nursing* 68(3):600–613, 2011.

Lindland EH, Kendall-Taylor N: *People, polar bears, and the potato salad: mapping the gaps between expert and public understandings of environmental health*, Washington, DC, 2011, FrameWorks Institute.

Martins DC, Burbank PM: Critical interactionism: an upstream-downstream approach to health care reform, *Adv in Nurs Sci* 34(4):315–329, 2011.

Molitor J, Su JG, Molitor NT, et al: Identifying vulnerable populations through an examination of the association between multipollutant profiles and poverty, *Environ Sci Technol* 45(18):7754–7760, 2011. Available from <http://dx.doi.org/10.1021/es104017x>.

National Institute of Health, National Institute of Environmental Health Sciences. GuLF Study. Available from <https://gulfstudy.nih.gov/en/index.html>. Accessed Jan 2014.

Nelson MC, Gordon-Larsen P, Song Y, et al: Built and social environments: associations with adolescent overweight and activity, *Amer J Prev Med* 31(2), 2006.

Northridge ME, et al: Environmental equity and health: understanding completely and moving forward, *Am J Public Health* 93(2):209–213, 2003.

Nweke OC: Achieving environmental justice: perspectives on the path forward through collective action to eliminate health disparities, *Am J Public Health* 101(S1):S6–S8, 2011.

O'Neill MS, Ebi KL: Temperature extremes and health: impacts of climate variability and change in the United States, *Journal of Occupational and Environmental Medicine* 51(1):13–25, 2009.

Pan TC, Kao JJ: Inter-generational equity index for assessing environmental sustainability: an example of global warming, *Ecol Indic* 9(4):725–1721, 2009.

Rauh VA, Landrigan PJ, Claudio L: Housing and health: intersection of poverty and environmental exposures, *Ann N Y Acad Sci* 1136:276–288, 2008.

Renalds A, Smith T, Hale P: A systematic review of built environment and health, *Fam and Comm Health* 33(1):68–78, 2009.

Ron E: Thyroid cancer incidence among people living in areas contaminated by radiation from the Chernobyl accident, *Health Phys* 93(5):502–511, 2007.

Rylander C, Odland JO, Sandanger TM: Climate change and the potential effects on maternal and pregnancy outcomes: an assessment of the most vulnerable—the mother, fetus, and newborn child, *Glob Health Action* 11(6):1–9, 2013.

Sanchez F, Kosson DS: Probabilistic approach for estimating the release of contaminants under field management scenarios, *Waste Manag* 25(4):463–472, 2005.

Sattler B: The greening of health care: environmental policy and advocacy in the health care industry, *Policy Polit Nurs Pract* 4(1):6–13, 2003.

Schrieberg D: Death from a healing machine: radioactive waste goes on Mexican odyssey after sale of medical device, *San Francisco Examiner* 1:12, 1991.

Schwartz J: Air pollution and children's health, *Pediatrics* 113:1037–1046, 2004.

Sheffield PE, Knowlton K, Carr JL, et al: Modeling of regional climate change effects on ground-level ozone and childhood asthma, *Am J Prev Med* 41(3):251–257, 2011.

Schulz A, Mentz G, Johnson-Lawrence V, et al: Independent and joint associations between multiple measures of the built and social environment and physical activity in a multi-ethnic urban community, *J Urban Health*, 2013.

Stevens PE, Hall JM: Applying critical theories to nursing in communities, *Public Health Nurs* 9:2–9, 1992.

Tarr J: Knoxville's pollution rivals that of Los Angeles, Houston and Atlanta, but Green Power might help clear the air, *Metro Pulse* 11(18), 2001.

Thompson B, et al: *Para Ninos Saludables:* a community intervention trial to reduce organophosphate pesticide exposure in children of farmworkers, *Environ Health Perspect* 116(5):687–694, 2008.

Troped PJ, Tamura K, Whitcomb HA, et al: Perceived built environment and physical activity in U.S. women by sprawl and region, *Am J Prev Med* 41(5):473–479, 2011.

U.S. Department of Health and Human Services, Office of Disease Prevention and Health Promotion: *Healthy People 2020*, n.d. Available from <http://www.healthypeople.gov/2020/>. Accessed March 6, 2013.

U.S. Department of Labor, Occupational Safety and Health Administration: *OSHA QUICK-CARD: Hazard communication safety data sheets*, 2013. Available from <http://www.osha.gov/Publications/HazComm_QuickCard_SafetyData.html>.

U.S. Food and Drug Administration: *Food safety for moms-to-be: Medical professionals fast facts*, 2013. Available from <http://www.fda.gov/Food/FoodborneIllnessContaminants/PeopleAtRisk/ucm091671.htm>.

U.S. Geological Survey: *What is ground water?* September, 2005. Available from <http://pubs.usgs.gov/of/1993/ofr93-643/>.

Whitney SL, Maltby HJ, Carr JM: "This food may contain...." What nurses should know about genetically engineered foods, *Nurs Outlook* 52:262–266, 2004.

World Health Organization: *World day for safety and health at work 2005: a background paper*, Geneva, 2005, International Labour Office.

World Health Organization: *Preventing disease through healthy environments*, Geneva, 2006, Author.

World Health Organization: *Influenza A (H1N1) update 46*, 2009a. Available from <http://www.who.int/csr/disease/swineflu/en/index.html>.

World Health Organization: *Ionizing radiation in our environment*, 2009b. Available from <http://www.who.int/ionizing_radiation/env/en/>.

World Health Organization: *Global alert and response (GAR): Severe acute respiratory syndrome (SARS)*, 2013. Available from <www.who.int/csr/sars/guidelines/en/index.html>.

World Health Organization: *Environmental health*, 2013. Available from <http://www.who.int/topics/environmental_health/en/>.

Wu Q, Shi H, Adams CD, et al: Oxidative removal of selected endocrine-disruptors and pharmaceuticals in drinking water treatment systems, and identification of degradation products of triclosan, *Sci Total Environ* 439:18–25, 2012.

CHAPTER

15

Health in the Global Community

Julie Cowan Novak

OBJECTIVES

Upon completion of this chapter, the reader will be able to do the following:

1. Describe globalization and international patterns of health and disease.
2. Discuss the World Health Organization's concepts of "health for all" and primary health care.
3. Identify international health care organizations and how they collaborate to improve global nursing and health care.

4. Describe the role of the community or public health nurse in international health.
5. Discuss key elements and effective models for successful international service learning community health projects, including the International Community Assessment Model and the Furco service learning framework.

KEY TERMS

Bill and Melinda Gates Foundation
Carter Center
Centers for Disease Control and
    Prevention
Declaration of Alma-Ata
globalization
health for all by the year 2000

International Council of Nurses (ICN)
Millennium Development Goals
nongovernmental organizations
Pan American Health Organization
primary care
primary health care
United Nations

United Nations International Children's Emergency Fund (UNICEF)
U.S. Department of Health and Human Services
World Bank
World Health Organization

OUTLINE

Population Characteristics
Environmental Factors
Patterns of Health and Disease
International Agencies and Organizations

International Health Care Delivery Systems
    The Role of the Community Health Nurse in International Health Care
Research in International Health

Health care and health care reform are subjects of critical debate throughout the world. Human health and its influence on every aspect of life are central to the global agenda. Nurses, as first responders, expert care providers, and leaders in international health care assessment, planning, evaluation, and policy development, promote and restore health to individuals, families, and communities across settings and geographic boundaries. Nurses must study models of health promotion, community assessment, community empowerment, and service learning to improve health care access and efficient and effective delivery. Community public health nurses must also be aware of forces that threaten health in the global community. Our global society, the Internet, and reduction in travel time provide access that was unimaginable a decade ago. Globalization—the process of increasing social and economic dependence and integration as capital,

goods, persons, concepts, images, ideas, and values cross state boundaries—is inextricably linked to the benefits and challenges of our time.

This chapter highlights population characteristics; international patterns of health and disease; social, cultural, and economic factors; international health care agencies and organizations; health care providers; health care delivery systems; and the community public health nurse's role as a leader in the global community. The chapter presents an International Community Assessment Model (ICAM; see Case Study 15-1 later in chapter) and the Furco service learning framework (Furco and Billig, 2002) for faculty and student discovery, learning, reflection, engagement, policy, and system design.

Population characteristics, including patterns of growth, demographics, and pandemics, are among the many health issues that merit attention and study because they have global effects that threaten human life. This chapter explores these issues and other environmental factors, including identified stressors and patterns of health and disease.

POPULATION CHARACTERISTICS

More than 1 billion people entered the twenty-first century without benefiting from the health care revolution. Enormous population growth presents a threat to the health and the economy of many nations. The exponential nature of world population growth is evident. In 1804, after 2 to 5 million years of human existence, the world population exceeded 1 billion. Between 1804 and 1927, the population reached 2 billion and, between 1927 and 1960, 3 billion. The population soared to 4 billion between 1960 and 1974 and to 5 billion between 1974 and 1987. In 1999, the world population grew to 6 billion and, in 2006, to 6.6 billion. The population is projected to reach 8 billion by 2025 and 10 to 12 billion by mid-century (United Nations, 2008). Ninety-nine percent of the growth is expected to occur in resource-poor countries (Population Reference Bureau [PRB], 2006).

In any society, large populations create pressure. For example, feeding a population becomes problematic in developing countries when famine, international trade problems, and war occur. Malnutrition, disease, or death may be the outcome. Pressures from population growth are also felt in industrialized nations. Although food may be plentiful, overcrowding leads to pollution, stress, disease, and violence. Each of these challenges represents a major barrier to economic growth. The poor suffer this burden of excess mortality and morbidity disproportionately. Thus, health promotion, effective health care delivery systems, and the enhancement of the environmental infrastructure will address the origins of poverty and ultimately increase productivity and improve quality of life (QOL).

World population distribution is uneven. More than 50% of the population lives in China (1.3 billion), India (1.1 billion), the United States (299 million), and Indonesia (225 million) (PRB, 2006). In 2007, 30% of the world population consisted of children. 8% were over 60 years of age (WHO, 2009). In developed countries life expectancy is increasing; however, in countries severely affected by the human immunodeficiency virus/acquired immunodeficiency syndrome (HIV/AIDS) epidemic, life expectancy has dropped to 35 to 40 years. In these countries the working-age population has dwindled and the birth rate has risen. At today's age-specific mortality rates, a girl born in Zambia can expect to live 43 years, whereas a girl born in Japan can expect to live 86 years. Malcolm Potts (1994), a world-renowned population theorist, predicted that "the world may end up divided not into political or economic groups but by demographic structure," in which countries will be classified into slow-growth or fast-growth countries instead of rich or poor countries. This will eventually further divide the rich and poor.

As the world population grows, a global trend toward urbanization occurs; people live closer together and migrate to urban areas for employment. For example, in 1975, 38.5% of the world's population lived in urban areas. By 1994, the proportion of urban dwellers had swelled to 45%; this proportion is expected to reach 50% by 2015 (United Nations, 2008). With increasingly dense living arrangements and global travel, the health of the general population is threatened by environmental factors and disease, for example, the H1N1 influenza pandemic.

Others say the human population level is OK and can continue to increase because science will meet our needs with new sources of energy and things like that. But even if we sustain 10 billion people, then as it goes, it will be 15 billion, then 20 billion. Impossible! (The Dalai Lama, in a speech given at University of Virginia Nobel Laureates Conference, 1998)

ENVIRONMENTAL FACTORS

The relationship between humans and their environment is an important component of individual, family, and global health. The field of environmental health and sustainable development has exploded since 1990. Environmental stressors are categorized into five types. First, stressors such as lead poisoning and air pollution directly assault human health. Second, stressors such as the effects of air pollution on products and structures damage society's goods and services. Third, stressors such as noise and litter affect QOL. Fourth, stressors such as global warming interfere with the ecological balance. Finally, natural disasters, terrorism, and war affect all of these aspects of life.

Air pollution, water pollution, and land pollution are among the consequences of environmental stressors. For example, 50% of the worldwide air pollution problem is attributable to the chemical pollutant carbon monoxide. Other primary pollutants, such as nitrogen monoxide, sulfur oxides, particulate matter, and hydrocarbons, combine with carbon monoxide to create 90% of the world's pollution. In developing countries, only 75% of the urban population and 50% of the rural population have sanitation facilities, the lack of which is a significant contributing factor to water pollution.

Agricultural, industrial, residential, and commercial wastes increase land pollution. For example, chemical fertilizers have displaced natural fertilizers; synthetic pesticides have displaced natural means of pest control; and petrochemical products, such as detergents, synthetic fiber, and plastics, have replaced soap, cotton, and paper. Disposable goods have replaced reusable goods, resulting in increased waste. Production technologies are contributing to worldwide environmental and ecological stress.

PATTERNS OF HEALTH AND DISEASE

Lifestyles, health and cultural beliefs, infrastructure, economics, and politics affect existing illnesses and society's commitment to prevention. Disease patterns vary throughout the world; therefore primary causes of death differ in developed and developing countries. Racial, ethnic, and access disparities exist within and between countries. Of 57 million deaths worldwide in 1 year, 33 million are from noncommunicable disease, 18 million are from communicable disease, and 5 million are from injuries and violence (Marmot, 2008).

Cardiovascular disease (CVD), cancer, respiratory disease, stroke, violence, and traumatic injury are the primary causes of mortality in *developed countries*. Infections, malnutrition, and violence are the primary causes of mortality in *developing countries*; however, CVDs are becoming more prevalent. Once plagued with high rates of infectious disease, developed countries significantly reduced such rates through improved sanitation, nutrition, immunization, and improved health care. Most developed countries have a more stable economy and a wide range of industrial and technological development. These countries experience an epidemiological transition. For example, the morbidity and mortality profile of a country changes from a lesser developed one to a developed one. Many developed countries experienced an epidemiological transition from having an infectious disease profile to having a chronic disease profile and are now plagued by chronic diseases such as CVD, respiratory disease, and cancer, secondary to air pollution and the tobacco use pandemic. This altered profile has created a demographic transition from traditional societies, in which almost everyone is young, to societies with rapidly growing numbers of middle-aged and elderly people.

Among the infectious diseases that contribute to high rates of mortality in developing countries are AIDS, tuberculosis (TB), endemic malaria, hepatitis B, rheumatic heart disease, parasitic infection, and dengue fever. These diseases claim the lives of millions, yet it is estimated that the diseases could be reduced by up to 50% through effective public health interventions. Many of these diseases will join smallpox as a disease known only to history through the development and implementation of immunization programs or to the twenty-first century through threats of bioterrorism. Immunization is the most powerful and cost-effective strategy at our disposal for many infectious diseases (Centers for Disease Control and Prevention [CDC], 2005). TB recommendations included in the "Commission for Africa" report called for wealthy nations to double their aid to Africa in order to rebuild systems to deliver public health services, provide staff training, develop new medicines, and provide better sexual and reproductive health services. The WHO "two diseases, one patient" strategy should be supported to provide integrated TB and HIV care as the majority of people worldwide who have both HIV and TB are in Africa (WHO, 2005b). The bacille Calmette-Guérin (BCG) vaccine series induces active immunity to TB, but it does not reduce the transmission of infectious types of TB. At least one third of the world's population harbors the TB pathogen, *Mycobacterium tuberculosis*. The WHO programs Roll Back Malaria, Stop TB, HIV/AIDS Control, Tobacco Free Initiative (TFI), Avian Influenza Pandemic Preparedness, and more recently the H1N1 pandemic target key infectious and chronic disease issues of the twenty-first century.

AIDS continues to be a grave global concern. In 2012, more than 25 million adults and children were estimated to be living with AIDS in sub-Saharan Africa, and 35.3 million adults and children to be doing so worldwide. The total number of AIDS deaths from 1981 to 2012 exceeds 30 million (UNAIDS, 2013). Newly infected HIV cases totaled 2.3 million, and there were 1.6 million AIDS deaths in 2008 (UNAIDS, 2013).

Although AIDS is a global epidemic, it varies demographically in different parts of the world. For example, the estimated male-to-female ratio of HIV infections in North America is 5:2, whereas in Africa the ratio is 1:1 (WHO, 2007a). Urbanization and within-country migration play a role in the spread of AIDS. For instance, in Rwanda the HIV seroprevalence is 14 to 20 times higher in urban areas than in rural areas. Annually, HIV threatens more lives as more people migrate to the world's largest cities. In 2010, 50% of the developing world lived in cities. This is an increase from 25% in 1970.

Substantial reductions in HIV seroprevalence occurred after several countries deployed ABC (Abstinence, Be faithful, Condom use) strategies. In 1985, 35% of those infected with HIV were women. By 2004, 50% of infected people worldwide were women (Dworkin and Ehrhardt, 2007).

Malaria is a life-threatening parasitic disease transmitted by mosquitoes. Today approximately 40% of the world's population is at risk for malaria. The disease is found throughout the tropical and subtropical regions of the world and causes more than 300 million acute illnesses and at least 1 million deaths annually. Malaria kills an African child every 30 seconds. Effective low-cost strategies are available for its prevention, treatment, and control, including insecticide-treated nets and new-generation medications, such as artemisinin-based combination therapies (WHO, 2005a). Efforts are ongoing to develop a malaria vaccine.

With 4.9 million deaths annually worldwide due to the use of tobacco, tobacco control is a critical component of the international health care agenda. By 2020, an estimated one in seven deaths will be tobacco related. Since 1990, tobacco control and secondhand smoke policies have been implemented at various political levels in the United States and abroad. The magnitude and consequences of the tobacco pandemic were unexpected. Smoking prevention and cessation programs, state and federal mandates, tobacco taxation, the 1998 Tobacco Master Settlement Agreement, antitobacco media campaigns, strict licensing of tobacco retailers, the elimination of tobacco vending machines and point-of-sale advertising, and the elimination of tobacco sales by pharmacies have had an impact on tobacco sales in the United States. Because of health concerns and cost, many countries from Ireland to New Zealand have developed tobacco-free policies. Although American adults have enrolled in cessation programs, the tobacco industry has targeted youth and dramatically increased international exports. A global commitment to tobacco control can avert millions of premature deaths in the next half century.

In 2003, the first global public health treaty was adopted at the World Framework Convention on Tobacco Control. The treaty was designed to reduce tobacco-related deaths and diseases around the world (WHO, 2007a). In 2005, the WHO Tobacco Free Initiative (TFI) group was convened by the WHO Tobacco Laboratory Network. Proposed activities of the initiative were as follows (WHO, 2009):

- Assess capabilities of each member, and make an inventory.
- Conduct collaborative study on smokeless tobacco.
- Initiate a quality management program that will lead to accreditation in the future.
- Develop and initiate training programs and capacity building.
- Establish a communication channel for network members, including a website and an expert panel for assistance.
- Develop a compendium of global testing methods for tobacco product emissions and contents.
- Participate in international research and standardization activities.
- Define periodic meetings for scientific research and exchange of information and to identify research priorities and agendas.
- Exchange information with policy makers and regulators.

The global approach to tobacco control can guide the development of effective interventions based on best evidence and best practice. Countering potential threats to health resulting from economic crises, unhealthful environments, or risky behavior is critical. Promotion of a healthy lifestyle underpins a proactive strategy for risk reduction, tobacco use prevention and cessation, immunization provision, cleaner air and water, adequate sanitation, healthful diets, fitness and exercise programs, and safe transportation.

INTERNATIONAL AGENCIES AND ORGANIZATIONS

Promoting worldwide health is humankind's greatest challenge. Several global agencies, such as the WHO, the Pan American Health Organization (PAHO), the United Nations, the United Nations International Children's Emergency Fund (UNICEF), the World Bank, the CDC, and nongovernmental organizations play important roles in improving the health of all nations. Founded in 1948, the World Health Organization is an international health agency of the United Nations. With six regional offices in the United States, Congo, Denmark, Egypt, India, and the Philippines, the WHO directs and coordinates international health efforts, producing and disseminating global health standards and guidelines, helping countries to address public health issues, and supporting health research (WHO, 2007a). The WHO goal of "health for all by the year 2000" was framed at the conference in Alma-Ata, the former USSR (now known as Almaty, Kazakhstan), in 1978. The conference defined "health for all" as "the attainment by all citizens of the world by the year 2000 of a level of health that will permit them to lead a socially and economically productive life" (WHO, 1999, p. 65). The target year for achievement was extended to 2010, once again without attainment.

The Alma-Ata conference on primary health care expressed the need for urgent action by all governments. The WHO's statement of beliefs, goals, and objectives is outlined in the Declaration of Alma-Ata, which is presented in Box 15-1. The concept of primary health care stresses health as a fundamental human right for individuals, families, and communities; the unacceptability of the gross inequalities and disparities in health status; the importance of community involvement; and the active role of all sectors. Primary health care seeks to obtain the highest level of health care for all people. The program promotes seven elements of primary health care: health education regarding disease prevention and cure, proper food supply and nutrition, adequate supply of safe drinking water and sanitation, maternal and child health care, immunizations, control of endemic diseases, and the provision of essential drugs. According to the Declaration, a primary health care system should provide the entire population with universal coverage; relevant, acceptable, affordable, and effective services; a spectrum of comprehensive services that provide for primary, secondary, and tertiary care and prevention; active community involvement in the planning and delivery of services; and integration of health services with development activities to ensure that complete nutritional, educational, occupational, environmental, and safe housing needs are met. In 2004, the WHO Global Strategy on Diet, Physical Activity, and Health was adopted (WHO, 2007a).

The Pan American Health Organization (PAHO) is an international public health agency with nearly a century of experience in working to improve the health and living standards of the Americas. It serves as the regional office of WHO and is recognized as part of the United Nations system.

Founded in 1945 after World War II, the United Nations (UN) now comprises 192 nations committed to world peace and security through international cooperation. The UN provides the means to resolve global conflicts and formulates policies that affect all nations. Regardless of size, wealth, or political system, all member nations have an equal vote in the decision-making process. UN decisions reflect world opinion and the moral authority of the community of nations (United Nations, 2008). In 2000, the Millennium Development Goals were developed to coordinate and strengthen global efforts to meet the needs of the poorest of the poor. Governments throughout the world and leading global development agencies agreed on a target date of 2015 for meeting the following goals (United Nations, 2000, 2013):

1. Eradicate extreme hunger and poverty.
2. Achieve universal primary education.
3. Promote gender equality, and empower women.
4. Reduce child mortality.
5. Improve maternal health.
6. Combat HIV/AIDS, malaria, and other infectious diseases.
7. Ensure environmental sustainability.
8. Develop global partnerships.

Collaborating with the UN are nongovernmental organizations (NGOs) such as the Carter Center and the Bill and Melinda Gates Foundation. Founded in 1982, the Carter Center is a nonprofit NGO founded by former President and First Lady Jimmy and Rosalynn Carter and based in Atlanta, Georgia. The Carter Center has three objectives: (1) to prevent and resolve conflicts, (2) to enhance freedom and democracy, and (3) to improve health.

BOX 15-1 DECLARATION OF ALMA-ATA

The International Conference on Primary Health Care, meeting in Alma-Ata this twelfth day of September in the year Nineteen hundred and seventy-eight, expressing the need for urgent action by all governments, all health and development workers, and the world community to protect and promote the health of all the people of the world, hereby makes the following Declaration:

I. The Conference strongly reaffirms that health, which is a state of complete physical, mental, and social well-being and not merely the absence of disease or infirmity, is a fundamental human right and that the attainment of the highest possible level of health is a most important worldwide social goal, whose realization requires the action of many other social and economic sectors in addition to the health sector.

II. The existing gross inequality in the health status of the people, particularly between developed and developing countries and within countries, is politically, socially, and economically unacceptable and is therefore of common concern to all countries.

III. Economic and social development, based on a New International Economic Order, is of basic importance to the fullest attainment of health for all and to the reduction of the gap between the health status of developing and developed countries. The promotion and protection of the health of the people are essential to sustained economic and social development and contribute to a better quality of life and to world peace.

IV. The people have the right and duty to participate individually and collectively in the planning and implementation of their health care.

V. Governments have a responsibility for the health of their people which can be fulfilled only by the provision of adequate health and social measures. In the coming decades, a main social target of governments, international organizations, and the whole world community should be the attainment by all peoples of the world by the year 2000 of a level of health that will permit them to lead a socially and economically productive life. Primary health care is the key to attaining this target as part of development in the spirit of social justice.

VI. Primary health care is essential health care based on practical, scientifically sound, and socially acceptable methods and technology made universally accessible to individuals and families in the community through their full participation and at a cost that the community and country can afford to maintain at every stage of their development in the spirit of self-reliance and self-determination. It forms an integral part both of the country's health system, of which primary health care is the central function and main focus, and of the overall social and economic development of the community. It is the first level of contact for individuals, the family, and the community with the national health system bringing health care as close as possible to where people live and work and it constitutes the first element of a continuing health care process.

VII. Primary health care:

1. reflects and evolves from the economic conditions and socio-cultural and political characteristics of the country and its communities and is based on the application of the relevant results of social, biomedical, and health services research and public health experience;

2. addresses the main health problems in the community, providing promotive, preventive, curative, and rehabilitative services accordingly;

3. includes at least: education concerning prevailing health problems and the methods of preventing and controlling them; promotion of food supply and proper nutrition; an adequate supply of safe water and basic sanitation; maternal and child health care, including family planning; immunization against the major infectious diseases; prevention and control of locally endemic diseases; appropriate treatment of common diseases and injuries; and provision of essential drugs;

4. involves, in addition to health sector, all related sectors and aspects of national and community development, in particular agriculture, animal husbandry, food industry, education, housing, public works, communication, and other sectors; and demands the coordinated efforts of all those sectors;

5. requires and promotes maximum community and individual self-reliance and participation in the planning, organization, operation, and control of primary health care making fullest use of local, national, and other available resources; and to this end, develops through appropriate education the ability of communities to participate;

6. should be sustained by integrated, functional, and mutually supportive systems, leading to the progressive improvement of comprehensive health care for all, and giving priority to those most in need;

7. relies, at local and referral levels, on health workers, including physicians, nurses, midwives, auxiliaries, and community workers, as applicable, and on traditional practitioners as needed, suitably trained socially and technically to work as a health team and to respond to the expressed health needs of the community.

VIII. All governments should formulate national policies, strategies, and plans of action to launch and sustain primary health care as part of a comprehensive national health system and in coordination with other sectors. To this end, it will be necessary to exercise political will, to mobilize the country's resources, and to use available external resources rationally.

IX. All countries should cooperate in a spirit of partnership and service to ensure primary health care for all people because the attainment of health by people in any one country directly concerns and benefits every other country. In this context the joint WHO-UNICEF report on primary health care constitutes a solid basis for the further development and operation of primary health care through the world.

X. An acceptable level of health for all the people of the world by the year 2000 can be attained through a fuller and better use of the world's resources, a considerable part of which is now spent on armaments and military conflicts. A genuine policy of independence, peace, détente, and disarmament could and should release additional resources that could well be devoted to peaceful aims and in particular to the acceleration of social and economic development of which primary health care, as an essential part, should be allotted its proper share.

The International Conference on Primary Health Care calls for urgent and effective national and international action to develop and implement primary health care throughout the world and particularly in developing countries in a spirit of technical cooperation and in keeping with a New International Economic Order. It urges governments, WHO and UNICEF, and other international organizations, and multilateral and bilateral agencies, nongovernmental organizations, funding agencies, all health workers and the whole world community to support national and international commitment to primary health care and to channel increased technical and financial support to it, particularly in developing countries. The Conference calls on all the aforementioned to collaborate in introducing, developing and maintaining primary health care in accordance with the spirit and content of this Declaration.

Reprinted, by permission, from *Alma-Ata 1978: Primary health care, report of the international conference onprimary health care,* Alma Ata, USSR, 6-12 September, 1978. (Health for All Series, 1:2-6.) Geneva, 1978, World Health Organization.
UNICEF, United Nations International Children's Emergency Fund; *WHO,* World Health Organization.

The bond of our common humanity is stronger than the divisiveness of our fears and prejudices. God gives us the capacity for choice. We can choose to alleviate suffering. We can choose to work together for peace. We can make these changes—and we must. (Former U.S. President Jimmy Carter, Carter Center, 2008)

Founded in 2000, the Bill and Melinda Gates Foundation has local, national, and global objectives. Globally, the foundation focuses on reducing extreme poverty, improving health, and increasing public library access. Within Africa, the foundation has had a profound effect on improving access to antiviral medications and prevention and treatment for HIV/AIDS, TB, and malaria.

Created in 1946, the United Nations International Children's Emergency Fund (UNICEF) was founded to assist millions of sick and hungry children in war-ravaged Europe and China. In 1950, the UNICEF mandate was expanded to address the needs of children and women throughout the world. UNICEF works for children's survival, development, and protection by developing and implementing community-based programs with well-documented achievements in child health, nutrition, education, water, sanitation, and women's rights. In 1953 the name was shortened to the UN Children's Fund; however, the UNICEF acronym was retained (WHO, 2007a).

Within a dramatically changing world economy, the major goal of the World Bank is to improve the health status of individuals living in areas that lack economic development. Since 1970, the World Bank has become more focused on health-related initiatives to promote sustainable economic growth (Ruger, 2005). Projects range from alleviation of poverty to safe water to effective sanitation to affordable housing. The Bank has provided financial assistance for the education of health care providers and the improvement of internal infrastructures, and funding for projects related to health status and disease prevention and control. The five largest shareholder countries are France, Germany, Japan, the United Kingdom, and the United States (World Bank, 2007a). Since 1963, the World Bank has provided $31 billion in loans and credits, currently funds 158 educational projects in 83 countries, and commits, on average, $1 billion for health, nutrition, and population projects in new lending annually (World Bank, 2007b).

The Centers for Disease Control and Prevention, located in Atlanta, Georgia, is one of the 13 major operating components of the U.S. Department of Health and Human Services (USDHHS, also called HHS). The principal agency in the U.S. government for protecting the health and safety of all Americans and for providing essential human services, the CDC was founded in 1946 to help control malaria. The agency has remained at the forefront of public health efforts to prevent and control infectious and chronic diseases, injuries, workplace hazards, disabilities, and environmental health threats. Today, the CDC is globally recognized for conducting research and investigations and for its action-oriented approach. The CDC applies research and findings to improve people's daily lives and responds to health emergencies—a feature that distinguishes the CDC from many of its peer agencies. The CDC is committed to achieving evidence-based health improvements. The agency is

defining specific health impact goals to prioritize and focus its work and investments, to measure progress, and to work toward attainment of its National Public Health Performance Standards and accreditation of U.S. public health departments.

Representing 12 million nurses in 129 countries, the International Council of Nurses (ICN) has addressed nursing and health care needs for more than a century. Nursing research, advanced practice nursing, doctoral education, first responders, disaster preparedness, mass casualties, policy, and advocacy have received increased emphasis over the past two decades in ICN and other nursing organizations worldwide. The ICN has five core values: visionary leadership, inclusiveness, flexibility, partnership, and achievement. The ICN Code for Nurses is the foundation for ethical nursing practice throughout the world (ICN, 2008). ICN and WHO are attempting to address the global shortage of nurses and other health care providers.

The U.S. Department of Health and Human Services created a program titled *Healthy People* that serves as the foundation for efforts throughout the HHS to create a healthier Nation. *Healthy People 2020* is based on the accomplishments of the following four previous *Healthy People* initiatives: (1) 1979 Surgeon General's Report, *Healthy People: The Surgeon General's Report on Health Promotion and Disease Prevention*; (2) *Healthy People 1990: Promoting Health/Preventing Disease: Objectives for the Nation*; (3) *Healthy People 2000: National Health Promotion and Disease Prevention Objectives*; and (4) *Healthy People 2010: Objectives for Improving Health*.

Healthy People provides science-based, 10-year national objectives for improving the health of all Americans. *Healthy People 2020* is the result of a multiyear process that reflects input from a diverse group of individuals and organizations. The vision of *Healthy People* is a society in which all people live long healthy lives. The overarching goals of *Healthy People* are to:

- Attain high-quality, longer lives free of preventable disease, disability, injury, and premature death; achieve health equity, eliminate disparities, and improve the health of all groups.
- Create social and physical environments that promote good health for all.
- Promote quality of life, healthy development, and healthy behaviors across all life stages.

Four foundation health measures that serve as an indicator of progress towards achieving these goals are general health status, health-related quality of life and well-being, determinants of health, and disparities.

INTERNATIONAL HEALTH CARE DELIVERY SYSTEMS

In the comparison of health care systems, developed and developing countries can learn much from one another. Although transferring specialized medical technologies from developed to developing countries may not always be appropriate, developing countries are currently learning from health care reform policies and the technological revolution in developed countries. Likewise, developed countries have much to learn about low-technology initiatives, such as oral rehydration therapy for the treatment of diarrhea and the delivery of primary health care as defined by the WHO. Participatory approaches to health care delivery, such as community involvement in health and education, are also essential. This exchange is important given the state of the current health care policy in developed countries, many of which have made health care inaccessible to portions of their general public.

Even in countries with socialized medicine, medical costs rise annually and citizens are faced with paying supplemental medical fees or co-payment. There is a need to expand the knowledge base that made the twentieth-century health care revolution possible. In the twenty-first century, it is critical to provide research and development that are relevant to the infectious diseases that overwhelmingly affect the poor. In addition, it is necessary to systematically generate an information base that countries can use to shape the future of their health care systems (WHO, 2010).

The Lalonde Report (1974), on the health of Canadian citizens, proposed the "health field concept" as a useful way to consider the determinants of health such as biology, lifestyle, environment, and health services. This report emphasized lifestyle and environment as determinants of health outside the traditional medical sphere. It became the basis for rethinking new paradigms for health care delivery. The report signified the early beginnings of a health care paradigm shift from the traditional medical model to a more holistic system–environment perspective (Boothroyd and Eberle, 1990). In the 1980s and 1990s, the rising costs of health care were a major catalyst for change, focusing attention on the need to provide alternative models of care. Over the past three decades, population-based approaches to health promotion and disease prevention have been developed to address system access, cost, efficiency, and effectiveness (Wall, Novak, and Wilkerson, 2005). Day surgery and outpatient services, nurse-managed clinics, ambulatory care, and home care provide alternatives to hospital-based care. In each of these areas, the nurse plays a prominent role and has the potential to bring a needed dimension of health promotion and disease prevention to individuals, families, and communities attempting to navigate a complex health care system.

Nurses must think more broadly about potential collaborators in solving the problems of the health care delivery system. Disciplines such as industrial engineering have much to offer nursing and other health care professionals, because engineering principles are applied to information technology, system design, patient safety, medication administration and reconciliation, simulation, chronic disease management, and hospital and clinic development, design, and renovation. The doctor of nursing practice (DNP) was developed by nursing leaders and endorsed by the American Association of Colleges of Nursing in order to reengineer health care (Wall et al, 2005). More than 100 programs have admitted DNP students, and 200 programs are in the developmental phase.

In 2012, U.S. expenditures for health care were projected to be 17.2 of the gross domestic product (GDP) (Centers for Medicaid and Medicare Services [CMS], 2013) and 46 million Americans were uninsured (Urban Institute, 2014). A market-based, developed country such as the United States treats health care as a market commodity; therefore it focuses on curative medicine rather than preventive medicine because doing so creates more capital. A market-based health care system could lead to a goal opposite that of health for all. Theoretically, the advent of the managed care system in the United States proposed a capitated model to cut health care. The Affordable Care Act was passed in 2010 to address the problem of the large number of uninsured Americans.

Given the two basic health care systems, market-based and population-based, and the fact that countries at different levels of development need to learn from one another, it is evident that a single model of health care delivery is not appropriate for every country. For example, in 1985, Cuba was recognized for reaching WHO's goal of "health for all." Cuba began to demonstrate to the world that health care could be provided as a basic human right rather than a privilege. In addition, Canada developed a universal health care system, and Canadian community health nurses (CHNs) created innovative models for practice. A 1986 report by the Canadian Minister of National Health and Welfare, entitled *Achieving Health for All,* offered a health promotion framework that involves fostering public participation in decisions that affect health, strengthening community health service networks with the disadvantaged communities they serve, and coordinating public health policy efforts (Epp, 1986).

The pressure for change provides the opportunity for reform, and the broad goal of health for all should guide this reform. Effective health care delivery systems must increase access and efficiency; improve health status through health promotion and disease prevention; eliminate health disparities; and protect individuals and families from financial loss due to catastrophic illness. One lesson learned from Canada's experience is that a narrow focus on individual responsibility and biology with acute interventions does not ensure the overall health of a country. Thirty years after the start of the "Health for All" programs, inequity in health in Canada is still linked to socioeconomic rank. This fact suggests that a collective responsibility or population-based focus must be established with less emphasis on the individual. Collective mandates, such as required physical education classes in elementary and middle schools, will be instrumental in changing the social and economic environments in which people live. Preventive health programs are the first line in reducing disease by providing education on healthy living choices (Low, 2008). McKinlay, as cited by Low (2008), argues that treatment of disease is akin to standing downstream and pulling people out of the river after they have fallen in. In contrast, health promotion stresses preventive health care, taking into account how social structure produces ill health and the economic framework of a society shapes lifestyle choices. They are thus analogous to upstream activities by which people are prevented from falling into the river in the first place (Low, 2008).

The Role of the Community Health Nurse in International Health Care

In a rapidly changing health care environment, the nursing role is becoming less traditional and much more diverse. The traditional structure of provider roles is challenged as professional disciplines are recruited to provide expanded and diverse health care services. The nursing role is reciprocal and interdependent with clients and families, physicians, and other health care professionals. The nurse's role expectations and societal expectations influence the formation of behavior patterns specific to the professional nursing role. These expectations provide the basis for the role of the community and public health nurse in international health care.

Florence Nightingale was the first nurse to establish international linkages and networks that became vastly important to her own country and to nursing throughout the world. As the first woman and first nurse inducted into the Royal Statistics Society, she recognized the importance of evidence-based nursing and health care. Every obstacle to health and wellness confronted her. She overcame obstacles systematically, developing the foundation and legacy for modern nursing and for community and public health nursing. Nightingale channeled her energies into all aspects of health from the care of wounded soldiers at Scutari in the Crimea to the broad public policies that affected health in her time.

CHNs seek to ensure the attainment of health for all in a cost-effective, efficient, accessible health care system. They must be involved in research, community assessment, planning, implementation, management, evaluation, health services delivery, disaster preparedness and emergency response, health policy, advocacy, and legislation. Nurses in all countries coordinate their work with other health care personnel as well as with local and global community leaders. Health for all requires attitudes, levels of competence, knowledge, and skills that differ substantially from those required in traditional nursing. The changes in the health environment, such as technological advancements, changes in the morbidity and mortality patterns of the population, and social and political changes, all form the basis for the nursing role.

With the development of the nurse practitioner (NP) role over the past 40 years in the United States and over the past 20 years abroad, nurses with advanced degrees and areas of specialization have strengthened the community-based health care system. The development of the DNP degree in the United States and PhDs in nursing in a variety of countries further elevates the knowledge and skill base for nursing's role in reengineering health care (Wall et al, 2005).

Because primary health care and primary care may be practiced differently in other countries, the NP and the CHN face multiple challenges. Primary health care refers to essential services that support a healthy life. It involves access, availability, service delivery, community participation, and the citizen's right to health care. In contrast, primary care refers to first-line or point-of-access medical and nursing care controlled by providers and focused on the individual.

Primary care may not be the norm, particularly in communities in developing or less-developed countries that have overwhelming needs for basic necessities such as safe drinking water and sanitation. The needs of the group outweigh the needs of the individual.

Nurses can make a difference in helping solve the existing and emerging health problems in countries throughout the world. The advent of technology has enhanced global communication and facilitated travel. It is important that nurses throughout the world understand and learn from one another. Nurses are the most valuable assets of any health care system. Community public health nursing can improve access to care for the most vulnerable and hard-to-reach groups in any country. In its many forms, nursing is relevant and will further expand in the future. The future demands evidence-based learning, engagement, service and growth in information technology, and local and global health policy. Population-based nursing experts are critical to solving the challenges of the fragmented, mismanaged, expensive, ineffective, inefficient health care delivery system that exists in many parts of our global community.

RESEARCH IN INTERNATIONAL HEALTH

Since 1990, international nursing research has focused predominantly on the following three areas: (1) student and faculty educational exchange programs, (2) diverse clinical experiences, and (3) the international development of home care or transition from hospital to home.

WHO collaborating centers in nursing provide a framework for research, education, and service delivery partnerships. Purdue University and the University of Virginia, both affiliates of Case Western Reserve University and the University of Mexico WHO Collaborating Centers, contributed to a partnership for educational programming, clinical practice, and research for graduate students in primary health care nursing and community health. Team Reach Out South Africa, one of the resulting programs, is presented in Case Study 15-2.

Crigger and colleagues (2004) have focused on ethical issues related to introducing antibiotic resistance into the second- and third-world community assessment and clinic development in Honduras, whereas Altman (2009) has immersed her "Spanish for Health Care Professionals" nursing students in orphanages and clinics in Nicaragua.

U.S. models of home health care are developing in many countries. These models provide a variety of services to bridge the gap between the hospital and community-based care. Sources of home care include home visits by nurses from official government public health agencies, nonprofit voluntary agencies, and for-profit home care agencies. Examples of home care services include assistance with activities of daily living, treatment, rehabilitation, transportation, and respite for caregivers. Home care service providers in the United States and abroad face many challenges. Estimating financial implications and calculating potential caseloads are complex factors in the design of effective delivery systems.

HEALTH INITIATIVES TAKING PLACE THROUGHOUT THE WORLD

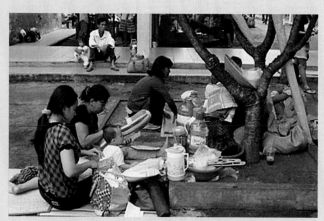

University of Texas Health Science Center at San Antonio Educational Initiative, Ho Chi Minh City, Vietnam. (Courtesy Dr. Kay Avant.)

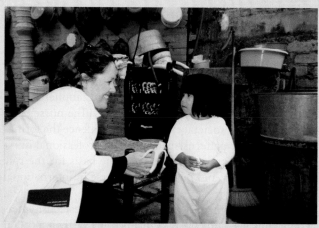

Home health visit, San Luis, Xochimilco, Mexico. (Courtesy Dr. Julie Novak.)

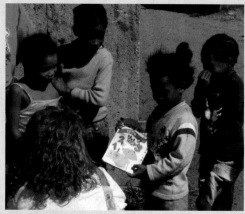

Community home health visits, Cape Town, South Africa. (Courtesy Dr. Julie Novak.)

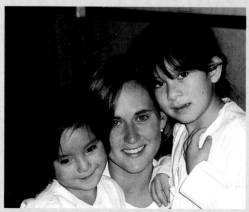

Nurse-managed clinics San Luis, Xochimilco, and Mexico City. (Courtesy Dr. Julie Novak.)

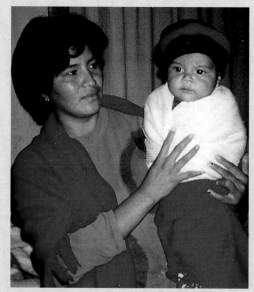

Nurse-managed public health clinic, Universidad Nacional Autonomo de Mexico, San Luis, Xochimilco, Mexico. (Courtesy Dr. Julie Novak.)

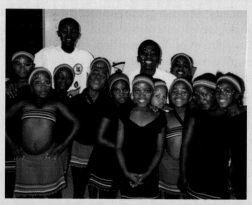

Cape Town, South Africa, school inauguration and health fair. (Courtesy Dr. Julie Novak.)

CASE STUDY 15-1   APPLICATION OF INTERNATIONAL COMMUNITY ASSESSMENT

International Community Assessment Model (ICAM): A Collaborative Model for Community Assessment, Education, and Health Care Delivery

In Mexico and South Africa the provision of equitable health care services to a population that is geographically and educationally disparate is both economically and logistically challenging. Both countries are further challenged by a lack of infrastructure necessary for health promotion, protection, and maintenance. South Africa is challenged by extreme poverty and staggering rates of HIV/AIDS and TB. In planning interventions, nurses need a globally diverse assessment tool and methodology to empower communities in developing countries to achieve health care goals and reduce health care costs. U.S. nursing students gaining international health care experience in a community in rural Mexico and urban South Africa can implement the International Community Assessment Model (ICAM) (Fig. 15-1) before planning targeted programs with local community leaders. The ICAM, tested in rural Mexico and as a component of Team Reach Out South Africa (see Case Study 15-2), is part of an ongoing project. U.S. nursing students compare and contrast practices in various countries using the ICAM and Furco Service Learning Model (Fig. 15-2). Service learning is discipline specific, experiential, and embedded in course objectives and relies heavily on reflection and journaling.

The Model
Community Empowerment
Nurses can collaborate with health and environmental experts in implementing a community empowerment framework. In community empowerment, the community identifies its problems and a plan of action, and environmental experts and nurses remain consultants and team members to assist community members (May, Mendelson, and Ferketich, 1995). This process helps the community to develop interventions that are culturally acceptable, breaking down cultural barriers. In developing countries, health-promotion programs that do not involve community participation and education often fail after the experts leave the community.

Assessment
During the assessment phase, the nurse identifies key influential community members and leaders and encourages them to join a board of community partners with the goal of assessing community health. The community partners may choose to use the ICAM for the purpose of providing a globally diverse assessment framework and for data gathering. Assessment of community culture helps identify potential cultural barriers to nursing interventions. The center of the model assesses the heart of the community's culture by identifying individual, family, and community characteristics, including their history, demographics, values, beliefs, rituals, and the effect of these characteristics on social and economic conditions.

The ICAM assesses the following:

Recreation: Community cardiovascular fitness; stress management; energy renewal; and relaxation through sports, hobbies, and games.

Perceptions: Community perceptions of health, including community members' physical, social, and mental balance and lifestyle choices.

Spirituality: The community's religious beliefs and practices.

Support systems: Family support systems, including parental support of children and adult children, adult children's support of their parents, and support among extended family members. (*Family* is defined as a group of individuals who have common experiences and goals and are often linked together by genetics, marriage, living situation, or a common emotional bond.)

The physical environment encompasses the community's infrastructure, including homes, water sources, waste disposal sites, roadways, buildings for businesses and shops, factories, power lines, and considerations related to occupational health (e.g., nurses must seek new collaborators in solving the complex problems of the health care delivery system). Industrial and biomedical engineering have much to offer nursing and the other health care disciplines, because engineering principles are applied to system design, information technology, patient safety and quality, simulation, and hospital and clinic development, design, and renovation. Throughout the United States advanced practice nursing is evolving to the DNP. This innovation in

FIGURE 15-1 International Community Assessment Model. Courtesy J.C. Novak

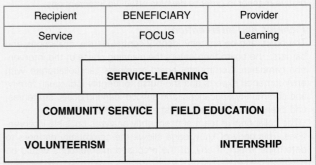

Recipient	BENEFICIARY	Provider
Service	FOCUS	Learning

FIGURE 15-2 Distinction Among Service Programs. (Furco, Andrew. "Service-Learning: A Balanced Approach to Experiential Education." Expanding Boundaries: Service and Learning. Washington DC: Corporation for National Service, 1996. 2-6.)

CASE STUDY 15-1 **APPLICATION OF INTERNATIONAL COMMUNITY ASSESSMENT—cont'd**

nursing will revolutionize health care and improve public health safety and quality (Wall et al, 2005). More than 100 programs have admitted DNP students with 200 programs in developmental phase.

The ICAM also assesses the following:

Education: The concept of education reflects the community's knowledge, skills, level of schooling or training, and literacy rate.

Transportation: Defined as how community members travel from point A to point B.

Safety: Evaluation of the community's safety includes examining both the potential dangers in the community that could lead to injury or death and the safety measures and plans developed by the community to prevent these problems.

Government and politics: How the community is governed or ruled.

Economy: The efficacy of economic resources is analyzed in terms of production, dispersal, and expenditure of resources.

Communication: Communication is evaluated by examining face-to-face and community-wide information exchange through speech, body language, writing, and drawings. Key components of the community's communication are native languages and forms of communication, such as letters, telephone, computer networks, electronic health records, the Internet, fax machines, television, billboards, signs, magazines, newspapers, and telegrams.

Access: Electricity, public sanitation, public water systems, radio, television, technology, computers, the Internet, fax machines, libraries, industrial machinery, and agricultural practices must be examined.

The ICAM allows the board of partners to examine all the public health threats to the community and additional barriers to an effective cultural awareness, sensitivity, proficiency, and humility.

The ICAM also reflects the importance of assessing the country of origin and global effects on the community. When assessing a community, the nurse must consider the external factors affecting the community. For example, the economy depends on vendors and international purchasing of their main exports.

After the community assessment, the collaborative team should develop an educational program that identifies potential challenges to an educational program or intervention. This program should motivate community partners to identify these problems and then search for effective solutions. As partners become further aware of the health care barriers or health hazards, resources should be provided that will aid in their response.

Next, partners should be assisted in completing a survey and offering focus groups related to needs assessment and attitudes.

The nursing team, local experts, key community informants, and partners need to establish the root cause of problems in a collaborative manner in order to develop effective interventions.

Planning and Intervention

The board and community identify central issues, challenges and barriers. The board then enters the planning phase of the intervention campaign. Community board members can collaborate with environmental experts and the nurse to identify individual, family, and community educational and service learning goals, strategies, and interventions based on best evidence and practice.

The collaborative team subsequently analyzes possible interventions. This body of knowledge allows the community partners to determine which, if any, of the proposed interventions would be relevant and appropriate for their community. In addition, they may be able to apply these ideas in creating their own interventions. When the community partners have selected or developed an intervention for their project, they can be encouraged to create strategies to educate the community.

Implementation

Before the project is implemented, the outcome of the community needs assessment must be clarified. The community must be given the opportunity to provide feedback to all collaborators regarding proposed interventions. The partners should be willing to compromise to meet the community's needs. After the community-wide education has occurred and necessary consensus and compromise have been achieved, the project can be implemented. At this point, the community members are trained to maintain the project. Once the implementation is completed, evaluation of the project can begin to ensure that the goals and objectives of the board are met.

Evaluation

The collaborative team should evaluate the project in a formative and summative manner. In addition, the nurse should conduct community surveys to determine whether members continue to recognize the need to maintain the project and to provide feedback related to progress.

Applications

The ICAM was tested in rural Mexico and is being tested in South Africa as part of the ongoing Team Reach Out project. The targeted communities have a high incidence of poverty. As a result, 80% of the communities reside in crowded living conditions. Many factors in the community pose serious health threats, including infectious disease, chronic conditions, tobacco use, secondhand smoke, farm chemicals, and air pollution. Field workers are often powerless and have minimal recourse when exposed to unhealthy environmental contaminants causing increased morbidity and mortality.

In rural Mexico, the top three causes of mortality in the communities are cardiac disorders, diabetes, automobile accidents, and dramatic increases in violence, particularly in urban Mexico and border communities. The leading causes of morbidity are respiratory infections, diabetes, hypertension, and gastrointestinal illnesses. The community's high rate of gastrointestinal illness is related to poor access to potable water. The community historians, community political leaders, key employers, full-time staff at nurse-run clinics, local community health faculty, and the *pasantes* (nursing graduates who have completed 1 year of community service at nurse-run clinics and public health agencies) are critical to the success of the project.

A multidisciplinary team of key influential community members, environmental experts, and nurses will further assess the community using the ICAM model. The goal of this assessment is to assist the community members in further diagnosing the community's health care needs and other issues as they are identified. Nurses collaborate with community partners to develop culturally proficient interventions. After the interventions are developed, the local partners, clinic staff, and *pasantes* continue to evaluate the effectiveness of these interventions, promoting a sense of ownership of the project in the community and helping to ensure improvements in health care long after the multidisciplinary team leaves the community (see Case Study 15-2).

CASE STUDY 15-2   TEAM REACH OUT SOUTH AFRICA

Team Reach Out started as a student-initiated service learning project with the goal of providing ongoing assistance to the victims of Hurricane Katrina. Four years after Hurricane Katrina, Team Reach Out refocused its efforts in Cape Town, South Africa. In 2009, four senior nursing students and one science student integrated their leadership skills with the application of public health knowledge, compassion, and concern as they worked in partnership with several international health agencies. This case reviews the service learning framework (Furco, 1996, 2002), course planning, implementation, and evaluation.

Service learning is a reciprocal partnership that bridges the gap between professional education and society. It is a powerful teaching and learning strategy that engages students in learning while helping communities help themselves (Poirrier, 2001). Service learning provides an experiential, collaborative, discipline-based relationship between students and community members for a reciprocal learning experience and allows an opportunity for reflection. Service learning sets the stage for a lifelong commitment to the development of civic duty, social awareness, and engagement while providing unique learning experiences that focus on building citizenship, cultural diversity, community partnerships, knowledge of community resources, critical thinking skills, and respect for humankind.

Both students and the community benefit from service learning. Students benefit from the exposure to real-life dilemmas and first-hand experience of joint team efforts. Communities benefit from the knowledge and creativity available from academia (Richards et al., 2009).

The faculty team leader/advisor completed an exploratory trip to Johannesburg and Cape Town, South Africa, in March 2008, meeting with prospective community partners. Each of the local health care leaders invited the development of a collaboration. Because of the richness of each setting and the overwhelming need for human and financial resources, the choice was extremely difficult. Cape Town was selected as the city site through a comprehensive assessment using the International Community Assessment Model (ICAM) (Richards, Novak and Davis, 2009; Richards and Novak, 2010). Health care and educational partners within the city were selected in collaboration with the school nurse, faculty, and staff of Christel House Academy of Cape Town. Subsequently, students from the School of Nursing and College of Science were invited to apply through notification in their respective student newsletters. Selection was based on the clarity of the student's goals and understanding of cultural humility and service learning. After selection, each student wrote an additional travel grant application to the university's Office of Engagement. Following is a description of the partners involved in this project and the experiences each provided.

Partners

Christel House International is a 501(c)(3) public charity that operates learning centers in impoverished neighborhoods with the goal of creating sustainable social and educational impact. Between 1999 and 2002, Christel House opened five learning centers in Mexico, India, South Africa, Venezuela, and the United States. Currently, Christel House serves more than 3000 students, their families, and communities. Christel House K-12 Academy in Cape Town helps children around the world break the cycle of poverty, realize their hopes and dreams, and become self-sufficient, contributing members of society (Christel House, 2009). The Academy invited the students to participate in the inaugural celebration of a new school facility and campus. Weekend cultural experiences included a trip to Robben Island, an ecological and historical heritage site where Nelson Mandela was imprisoned from 1963 to 1990; Table Mountain, a protected natural habitat with 1500 plant species; and a game and nature preserve.

The Themba Care Orphanage provides a safe and compassionate environment for approximately 20 children who are HIV positive. In the majority of cases their parents have died of AIDS; however, some children were placed in the setting by their parents to avoid stigma within their respective communities. The orphanage is run by an executive director, two registered nurses/"sisters," a teacher, a staff of five nursing assistants, and local volunteers. Team Reach Out worked with volunteers from three different U.S. universities on site. In addition to one older child, 95% of the children at the orphanage ranged in age from 18 months to 4 years. Students were able to complete Denver Developmental Screenings and health assessments and to work with the sisters in medication dispensation and reconciliation. The majority of the children demonstrated global developmental delay on the screenings. Students played with, fed, and cared for the children in this warm, caring, inviting preschool environment. The students reflected on their difficulty in saying goodbye to the children.

The Gatesville Medical Center is a multispecialty large private Indian hospital located in Cape Town. Team Reach Out students were able to care for pediatric patients and effectively compare and contrast this South African state-of-the-art private hospital with other health care settings. Diagnoses included respiratory syncytial virus, pneumonia, asthma, gastroenteritis/dehydration, and meningitis.

The Tafelsig Community Health Center provides care to approximately 9000 low-income patients each month. Patients receive health promotion visits throughout the lifespan. They are also treated for diseases, upper and lower respiratory tract infections, gastroenteritis, and urinary tract infections being common diagnoses. A minor emergency/urgent care clinic is on site. Tafelsig also has one of the largest TB and HIV/AIDS patient populations in Cape Town. Students were able to complete health assessments and immunize patients under the supervision of South African registered nurse specialty clinic coordinators and their faculty advisor.

The students' week of clinical experiences culminated with a presentation of a health fair at the academy. This health fair focused on school and family health promotion and included the following stations: prenatal and newborn care and parenting; prevention of TB, HIV/AIDS, and malaria; health care careers; science experiments (with premed students); and health screenings, including measurements of height, weight, blood pressure, glucose, and cholesterol. The academy ran special bus routes from the school to and from area shanty towns to bring parents and other community members to the school health fair. The students worked with the World Health Organization, the Centers for Disease Control and Prevention, Johnson & Johnson, and local Cape Town universities to ensure culturally appropriate materials for the health fair. The Christel House Academy Health Fair was attended by 600 children and 200 parents.

Student Responses

Team Reach Out South Africa students provided poignant and insightful reflections about their experiences. Community partners indicated that the students were very professional and were able to provide much-needed support.

Summary

Students felt strongly that service learning enhanced their community public health experience while building relationships with community service organizations. Students reported encountering minimal barriers to the implementation of this project and also were not reluctant to participate in these activities. Students also agreed that they would continue to participate in service-learning activities in the near future. Table 15-1 includes more student reflections on their experiences. Table 15-2 and Box 15-2 highlight students' feelings about service learning in general (Richards and Novak, 2010).

TABLE 15-1	STUDENT REFLECTIONS ON TEAM REACH OUT PROJECTS

Reflections from Team Reach Out Biloxi

"It was a wonderful experience to be able to meet so many interesting people and use our knowledge of health care to provide support to this community."

"Every victim was thinking about their neighbor in terms of their needs."

"Everyone expressed appreciation and hope."

"My most meaningful memory is the incredible impression each Mississippian made on me. It was amazing to me that through all of the tragedy, devastation, and loss, their southern hospitality and gentleness was still very much alive."

Reflections from Team Reach Out South Africa

"We were so fortunate to see the health care extremes, from the poorest of the poor clinics to the private hospitals. It was such a diverse spectrum to work in."

"Traveling to South Africa was an eye-opening experience in so many ways. I'll never forget the striking beauty of the country contrasted with the devastating poverty that runs rampant; I was both impressed and surprised by the resourcefulness of their health care system."

"The trip was incredible. So much poverty and beauty and riches in the same area. The people touched my life and I hope that I did the same for some of them."

BOX 15-2	STUDENT RESPONSES: WHAT IS THE DEFINITION OF SERVICE LEARNING?

Service learning is:

- Providing services to those in need while at the same time learning in your field of interest and having the ability to work with those less fortunate. It is a hands-on learning experience that, for me, was life changing and eye opening.
- Volunteering with doing something that you are in the field of doing or obtaining a degree in.
- A unique way of learning in and about a community and providing services for the betterment of a community. Service projects provide communities with people who are able to use their time, resources, and expertise in order to improve or help the community in which they are serving. At the same time, the people involved in the service project are learning from their experiences with the project.
- A volunteering project that is done to help the community in some positive way while the volunteer has the opportunity to broaden their own horizons by learning something new.
- Utilizing skills and knowledge acquired in the classroom as a means to enhance the community.

Modified from Richards E, Novak J: From Biloxi to Cape Town: Curricular integration of service learning, *J Community Health Nurs* 27(1):46-50, 2010.

TABLE 15-2	STUDENT AND PROVIDER RESPONSES TO SERVICE LEARNING QUESTIONNAIRE

PURDUE UNIVERSITY SCHOOL OF NURSING SERVICE-LEARNING QUESTIONNAIRE: STRONGLY AGREE (5), AGREE (4), UNDECIDED (3), DISAGREE (2), STRONGLY DISAGREE (1)	STUDENT AVERAGE (N = 5)
1. Service learning at Purdue University School of Nursing may be a catalyst for	
a. Assisting societal needs	4.75
b. Student learning	4.8
c. Building relationships with community service organizations	4.6
d. Engagement opportunities	4.8
2. I encountered significant barriers to completing this service-learning activity.	1.8
3. Service learning should only be integrated into senior course leadership.	2.4
4. Service learning enables a positive change through leadership.	4.4
5. I was reluctant to participate in community and civic service-learning activities.	1.2
6. Service learning is a community-building and democracy-building activity.	4
7. I plan to continue service-learning activities in the immediate future.	4.2
8. This experience embraced the concepts of reciprocity between learning and the community being served.	4.2
9. This experience allowed students to engage in activities that addressed community needs.	4.8

Modified from Richards E, Novak J: From Biloxi to Cape Town: Curricular integration of service learning, *J Community Health Nurs* 27(1): 46-50, 2010.

SUMMARY

Community public health nurses face many exciting challenges in health care reform and the design of effective systems of health care delivery. These include being responsive to emerging needs and health issues in the population, developing multidisciplinary practice models that adhere to the principles of primary health care in the context of a reengineered health care system, and mobilizing research dissemination and practice implementation strategies to ensure evidence-based practice as the norm rather than the exception. Using evidence-based models as a framework for local to global community public health partnerships and projects should be tested and evaluated. There is still much to be done to meet the challenge of WHO's goal of "health for all." Studying the progress achieved in other countries is critical; however, success will ultimately depend on societal commitment to addressing complex issues of poverty, disparity, and health care inaccessibility.

LEARNING ACTIVITIES

1. Discuss population characteristics and the threat of population growth to health and health care systems.
2. Compare and contrast the incidence and treatment of people living with AIDS, TB, and malaria. Discuss methods of prevention.

3. Explain the incidence of death from AIDS in Africa, Mexico, and the United States. What might account for the differences?
4. Compare population-focused nursing in a developing country with community health nursing in the community. How are they the same, and how do they differ?
5. Conduct research and compare the rates of life expectancy and infant mortality in Africa, Mexico, and the United States. What factors might account for the similarities and differences in rates between the developing and the developed countries?
6. Describe the key elements of an effective health care delivery system. Will the focus of future health care services reflect downstream thinking, or will the orientation uphold models of prevention and promotion that deal with root causes of health problems?
7. Test the International Community Assessment Model (ICAM) in a community. Evaluate its effectiveness.
8. Describe the Furco Service Learning Model and its potential application in local to global projects in your university.

Ⓔ EVOLVE WEBSITE

http://evolve.elsevier.com/Nies
- NCLEX Review Questions
- Case Studies
- Glossary

REFERENCES

Altman MI: Culture and healthcare delivery in Nicaragua: crossing a cultural divide, *Purdue Nurse* 12, 2009. January.

Boothroyd P, Eberle M: *Healthy communities: what they are, how they're made, CHS Research Bulletin, UBC Centre for Human Settlements,* Vancouver, 1990, University of British Columbia.

Carter Center: *About the center,* 2008. Available from <www.cartercenter.org/about/index.html>.

Centers for Disease Control and Prevention: 2005. Available from <www.cdc.gov>.

Centers for Medicare and Medicaid Services: *Table 1: National health expenditures aggregate,* 2013. Available from <www.cms.gov/nationalhealth ExpendData/downloads/tables.pdf>.

Christel House: *About us,* n.d. Available from <http://www.christelhouse.org/about-us>.

Crigger NJ, Holcomb L, Grogan RL, et al.: A model of antibiotic use in a lay Honduran population, *Int J Nurs Stud* 41(7):745–753, 2004.

Dworkin SL, Ehrhardt AA: Going beyond "ABC" to include "GEM": critical reflections on progress in the HIV/AIDS epidemic, *Am J Public Health* 97(1):128–134, 2007.

Epp J: *Achieving health for all: a framework for health promotion,* Ottawa, 1986, Health and Welfare Canada.

Furco A: Service learning: A balanced approach to experiential education. In Raybuck J, Taylor B, editors: *Expanding boundaries: Serving and learning,* Washington, DC, 1996, Corporation for National Service.

International Council of Nurses: *About ICN,* n.d. Available from <www.icn.ch/abouticn.htm>.

Lalonde M: *A new perspective on the health of Canadians,* Ottawa, 1974, Minister of Supply and Services.

Low J, Theriault L: Health promotion policy in Canada: Lessons forgotten, lessons still to learn, *Health Promot Int* 23(2):200–206, 2008.

Marmot M: *The social determinants of global health and resolving tensions: Readings in global health,* Washington, DC, 2008, American Public Health Association. 3.

May KM, Mendelson C, Ferketich S: Community empowerment in rural healthcare, *Public Health Nurs* 12(1):25–30, 1995.

Poirrier G: *Service learning: curricular applications in nursing,* New York, 2001, National League for Nursing.

Population Reference Bureau: *2006 world population data sheet.* Available from <http://www.prb.org/Publications/Datasheets/2006/2006WorldPopulationDataSheet.aspx >.

Potts M: Common sense prevailing at population conference, *Lancet* 344:809, 1994.

Richards E, Novak J: From Biloxi to Cape Town: Curricular integration of service learning, *J Community Health Nurs* 27(1):46–50, 2010.

Richards E, Novak J, Davis L: Disaster response after Hurricane Katrina: a model for an academic-community partnership in Mississippi, *J Community Health Nurs* 26(3):114–120, 2009.

Ruger JP: The changing role of the World Bank in global health, *Am J Public Health* 95(1):60–70, 2005.

UNAIDS: Global Report: UNAIDS report on the global AIDS epidemic, 2013. <http://www.unaids.org/en/media/unaids/contentassets/documents/epidemiology/2013/gr2013/UNAIDS_Global_Report_2013_en.pdf>.

United Nations: *Resolution adopted by the General Assembly: United Nations Millennium Declaration,* New York, 2000, The Author.

United Nations: *The UN in brief,* 2008. Available from <un.org/Overview/uninbrief/>.

Urban Institute: *The uninsured.* 2014 <http://www.urban.org/health_policy/uninsured/index.cfm>.

Wall B, Novak J, Wilkerson S: The doctor of nursing practice: reengineering healthcare, *J Nurs Educ* 44(9):396–403, 2005.

World Bank: *About us,* 2007a. Available from <http://www.worldbank.org/en/about>.

World Bank: *Ten things you never knew about the World Bank,* Washington, DC, 2007b, Author.

World Health Organization: *Roll back malaria info sheet,* Geneva, 2005a, Author. <www.who.int/malaria/docs/Basicfacts.pdf>.

World Health Organization: *TB recommendations included in the "Commission for Africa" report,* 2005b. Available from <www.who.int/tb/commission_for_africa/en/print.html>.

World Health Organization: *The 3 by 5 initiative,* 2005c. Available from <www.who.int/3by5/about/initiative/en/index.html>.

World Health Organization: *Working for health: an introduction to the World Health Organization,* Geneva, 2007a, WHO Press.

World Health Organization: *Tobacco free initiative,* 2009. Available from <www.who.int/tobacco/global_interaction/en>.

World Health Organization: *Global health atlas database,* 2010, Author.

Child and Adolescent Health

*Susan Rumsey Givens**

Upon completion of this chapter, the reader will be able to do the following:

1. Identify major indicators of child and adolescent health status.
2. Describe social determinants of child and adolescent health.
3. Discuss the individual and societal costs of poor child health status.
4. Discuss public programs and prevention strategies targeted to children's health.
5. Apply knowledge of child and adolescent health needs in planning appropriate, comprehensive care at the individual, family, and community levels.

KEY TERMS

child maltreatment
childhood immunization
Children's Health Insurance Program (CHIP)
Early and Periodic Screening, Diagnosis, and Treatment (EPSDT)
fetal alcohol spectrum disorders (FASD)
infant mortality
late preterm birth
lead poisoning
low birth weight
Medicaid
preconception health
prenatal care
preterm birth
Safe to Sleep
Special Supplemental Nutrition Program for Women, Infants, and Children (WIC)
Teen childbearing
Teen dating violence

OUTLINE

Issues of Pregnancy and Infancy
Infant Mortality
Preterm Birth and Low Birth Weight
Preconception Health
Prenatal Care
Prenatal Substance Use
Breastfeeding
Sudden Unexplained Infant Death
Childhood Health Issues
Accidental Injuries
Unhealthy Weight
Immunization
Environmental Concerns
Child Maltreatment
Children with Special Health Care Needs
Adolescent Health Issues
Sexual Risk Behavior
Violence
Tobacco, Alcohol, and Drug Use
Factors Affecting Child and Adolescent Health
Poverty
Racial and Ethnic Disparities
Health Care Use
Strategies to Improve Child and Adolescent Health
Monitoring and Tracking
Healthy People 2020: Child and Adolescent Health
Health Promotion and Disease Prevention
Public Health Programs Targeted to Children and Adolescents
Health Care Coverage Programs
Direct Health Care Delivery Programs
Sharing Responsibility for Improving Child and Adolescent Health
Parents' Role
Community's Role
Employer's Role
Government's Role
Community Health Nurse's Role
Legal and Ethical Issues in Child and Adolescent Health
Ethical Issues

* The author would like to acknowledge the contribution of Mary Brecht Carpenter, who cowrote this chapter for the previous edition.

A nation's destiny lies with the health, education, and well-being of its children. The United States has made tremendous progress over the past century toward improving children's lives. Advancements in public health measures—such as sanitation, infectious disease control, environmental regulation, health screening, and education—and remarkable strides in medical care have all contributed to the good health status that most children enjoy. However, these improvements have not equally benefited children of all races and ethnic groups, children at all income levels, or children in all geographic areas of the country. For example, significant disparities persist in the health status of white children versus children of color. Children living in suburban areas and most outer urban areas experience access to health care services superior to that of children living in rural areas and inner cities, especially if they are poor.

Although most of the nation's children are healthy and succeed in school, many are not enjoying optimal health and well-being and are not reaching their full potential as contributing members of society. Despite improvements, the mortality and morbidity rates for U.S. children in all age groups are unacceptably high. Consider the following facts:

- Each year, more than 25,000 infants die before reaching their first birthday. Black infants are more than twice as likely to die as white infants.
- Nearly one-half million babies are born prematurely each year. Prematurity is the leading cause of infant death and long-term neurological disabilities.
- Twenty-two percent of children aged 0 to 18 years live in poverty.
- Every day, five children die as the result of child abuse; most are younger than 4 years.
- More than 367,000 girls aged 15 to 19 years give birth each year.
- Seventeen percent of twelfth graders are cigarette smokers. Nearly 23% smoke marijuana.
- Well over half of children currently residing in the United States will be affected by violence, crime, abuse, or psychological trauma this year.

The health of a child has long-term implications. Health habits adopted by children and youth will profoundly influence their potential to lead healthy, productive lives. The physical and emotional health experienced by a child plays a pivotal role in his or her overall development and the well-being of the entire family. Children who go to school sick or hungry, who cannot see well enough to read, who cannot hear the teacher, who have learning disabilities, who are troubled by abusive parents or disruptive living circumstances, or who fear for their safety at home or in school often do not perform on the level of their counterparts who are healthy, well nourished, well cared for at home, and safe and secure in their world. From fetal life onward, the health and well-being of individuals has a substantial impact on their futures.

In 2011 there were 73.9 million United States children younger than 18 years. Children represent about 24% of the

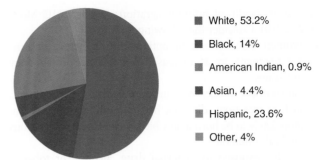

FIGURE 16-1 Percentage distribution of U.S. children by race/ethnicity, 2013. (From Federal Interagency Forum on Child and Family Statistics: *America's children in brief: key national indicators of well-being, 2012.* Retrieved March 8, 2013, from <www.childstats.gov/americaschildren/demo.asp.>.)

country's population, down from a peak of 36% at the end of the mid-1960s baby boom. The birth rate for children of all races has declined in recent years, and the racial and ethnic diversity of children is changing rapidly. For example, by 2050, Hispanic children are expected to account for 39% of the population, up from 24% in 2012. The percentage of children who are Hispanic has increased faster than that of any other racial or ethnic group (Federal Interagency Forum on Child and Family Statistics, 2012) (Figure 16-1).

Children are a dependent population and rely primarily on parents or other adults to protect and promote their health and well-being. Community health nurses can learn more about this important population group and the positive and negative factors that influence their health. Nurses can use this information to help improve the chances that children will grow up to be healthy, both physically and emotionally.

This chapter focuses on the health status of children and adolescents and the medical, socioeconomic, cultural, environmental, educational, safety, and public health factors that community health nurses must address to improve child and adolescent health. The chapter also discusses the individual and societal costs of poor child health, public programs targeted to children's health, and strategies to improve child and adolescent health at the individual, family, and community levels.

ISSUES OF PREGNANCY AND INFANCY

The health of the mother before, during, and after pregnancy has a direct impact on the health and well-being of her child. The conditions that surround a child's fetal development and early years shape his or her life. Adapting healthy lifestyles and obtaining regular medical care before becoming pregnant can help ensure a healthy pregnancy. Unfortunately, many women face barriers to good health throughout their lives, including racism, violence, poverty, and lack of access to health care. A comprehensive approach that helps women identify and treat potential risks and overcome barriers to good health before, between, and beyond their pregnancies will help protect and promote the health of women and children and can help ensure the health of future generations (Moos, 2010; Moos et al., 2010). Consider the following findings:

- Women who are not in optimal health before becoming pregnant are at increased risk for poor pregnancy outcomes.
- Babies whose mothers have uncontrolled medical conditions, such as infections, diabetes, hypertension, and obesity, are more likely to be born at low birth weights and with serious medical conditions.
- A fetus exposed to maternal drug, alcohol, or tobacco exposure or poor nutrition is more likely to have chronic conditions that affect health and well-being.
- Infants exposed to unsafe environmental conditions, such as secondhand smoke and lead-based paint, are more likely to have chronic conditions throughout childhood and, in some cases, through adolescence and adulthood.
- Children who do not receive preventive health care and do not obtain all necessary immunizations are more likely to have preventable diseases or chronic conditions that could have been prevented or minimized and controlled.

Infant Mortality

Infant mortality, the deaths of children during the first year of life, is a critical gauge of children's health status. It is an important marker because it is related to several factors, including maternal health, medical care quality and access, socioeconomic conditions, and public health practices. infant mortality reflects the health and welfare of an entire community and is used as a broad indicator of health care and health status. Box 16-1 lists some terms and definitions associated with infant health and mortality. The five leading causes of infant death are congenital defects; disorders related to short gestation or low birth weight; sudden infant death syndrome (SIDS; see later); maternal complications of pregnancy; and accidents such as suffocation. These five factors account for close to 60% of all infant deaths (Hoyert and Xu, 2012). Box 16-2 lists sources of vital statistics birth data.

Surprisingly, the United States ranks a dismal twenty-seventh in infant mortality, behind most other industrialized nations, including Japan, Sweden, Spain, Hong Kong, Italy, France, and Canada (Table 16-1). Fifty years ago, the United States ranked twelfth (Organisation for Economic Co-operation and Development [OECD], 2012). The gap in infant mortality between the United States and other nations has occurred in spite of the United States' comparatively high per capita spending on health care and technological advancements.

Despite a poor ranking among other nations in the world, the infant mortality rate in the United States has declined every year since 1940 with the exception of 2002 (Figure 16-2). The 2011 figure, 6.05 deaths per 1000 live births (Hoyert and Xu, 2012), was the lowest infant mortality rate ever recorded in this country. This drop can be attributed largely to public health measures and improved standard of living (e.g., better

BOX 16-1 INFANT HEALTH DEFINITIONS

Infant death: Death of an infant before his or her first birthday.
Infant mortality rate: Number of infant deaths per 1000 live births.
Preterm birth: Birth before 37 completed weeks of gestation.
Very preterm birth: Birth before 32 completed weeks of gestation.
Late preterm birth: Birth from 34 to 36 completed weeks of gestation.
Term birth: Birth from 37 to 41 completed weeks of gestation.

From MacDorman MF, Mathews TJ: *Recent trends in infant mortality in the United States* (NCHS Data Brief no. 9), Hyattsville, MD, 2008, National Center for Health Statistics. Retrieved from <http://www.cdc.gov/nchs/data/databriefs/db09.pdf>.

BOX 16-2 SOURCES OF VITAL STATISTICS DATA FOR CHILDREN

In the United States, laws require birth certificates to be completed for all babies born. Information concerning an infant's birth, including the total number of the mother's prenatal care visits, the mother's and father's ages and race, mother's marital status and education, and the infant's weight, gestational age, and birth date, appears on a baby's birth certificate.

Information concerning an infant's death, such as the cause(s), date, and other details, appears on the death certificate. In each state, the vital statistics office in the state health department stores these certificates. This agency collects and regularly reports the aggregated data and forwards them to the National Center for Health Statistics.

The National Center for Health Statistics collects, analyzes, and publishes numerous reports on the health and well-being of the nation's infants. These data sources are very important in tracking the health of infants as well as of other population groups; they help determine necessary interventions from various perspectives (e.g., clinical, public health, public policy, and environmental).

From National Institute of Child Health & Human Development: Safe to sleep public education campaign. 2012.

sanitation, a clean milk supply, immunizations against deadly childhood diseases, the increased availability of nutritious food, and enhanced access to maternal health care). Technological advances in neonatal care, for example, the introduction of synthetic lung surfactant, have also contributed to reductions in infant mortality.

However, declines in infant mortality have stagnated during the past decade, and the gap between black and white infant mortality rates remains stubbornly high, with black infants dying at a rate 2.2 times higher than that of white infants. Identifying and remedying the causes of higher infant mortality rates among certain population subgroups remains a vexing societal problem and one that cannot be ignored (Figure 16-3).

The first year of life is the most hazardous a person faces until he or she reaches 65 years. Therefore, it is particularly important for women to be as healthy as possible before becoming pregnant, and to receive prenatal care and adopt healthy lifestyle choices, and for infants to receive primary health care to maintain health and prevent or minimize serious, long-lasting health problems.

TABLE 16-1	INTERNATIONAL COMPARISONS OF INFANT MORTALITY RATES* FOR SELECTED COUNTRIES AND TERRITORIES (2011)		
WORLD RANK	**COUNTRY**	**1960**	**2011**
1	Iceland	13.0	0.9
2	Sweden	16.6	2.1
3	Japan	30.7	2.3
4	Finland	21.0	2.4
4	Norway	16.0	2.4
6	Czech Republic	20.0	2.7
7	Republic of Korea	–	3.0
8	Portugal	77.5	3.1
9	Spain	43.7	3.2
10	Belgium	31.4	3.3
11	Italy	43.9	3.4
11	Greece	40.1	3.4
13	France	27.7	3.5
13	Israel	–	3.5
13	Ireland	29.3	3.5
16	Germany	35.0	3.6
16	Austria	37.5	3.6
16	Denmark	21.5	3.6
16	Netherlands	16.5	3.6
20	Switzerland	21.1	3.8
20	Australia	20.2	3.8
22	United Kingdom	22.5	4.3
23	Poland	54.8	4.7
24	Slovakia	28.6	4.9
24	Hungary	47.6	4.9
26	New Zealand	22.6	5.5
27	**United States**	**26.0**	**6.1**
28	Chile	120.3	7.4
29	Turkey	189.5	7.7
30	Mexico	92.3	13.6

*infant mortality rate represents infant deaths per 1000 live births.
From Organisation for Economic Co-operation and Development: *Health: Key Tables from OECD, No. 14: infant mortality*, 2013. ISSN 2075-8480. © OECD 2013. Retrieved from <http://www.oecd-ilibrary.org/social-issues-migration-health/infant-mortality_20758480-table9>; Centers for Disease Control and Prevention: Table 20. infant mortality rates and international rankings: organization for economic co-operationand development (OCED countries selected by years 1960-2008. *Health United States 2011*. Retrieved from <http://www.cdc.gov/nchs/hus/contents2011.htm#020>.

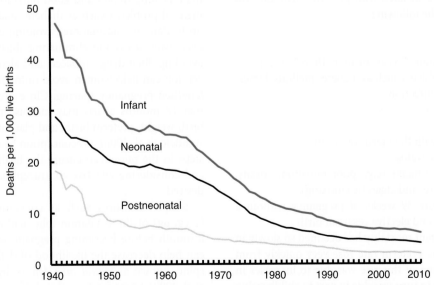

FIGURE 16-2 Infant, neonatal, and postneonatal mortality rates: United States, 1940-2010. (From Murphy SL, Xu J, Kochanek KD: *Deaths: Final data for 2010* [National Vital Statistics Report vol. 61 mo.4], 2013. Retrieved from <http://www.cdc.gov/nchs/data/nvsr/nvsr61/nvsr61_04.pdf>.)

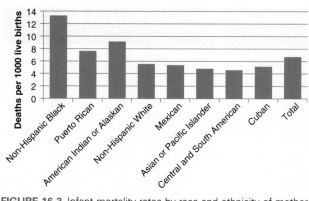

FIGURE 16-3 Infant mortality rates by race and ethnicity of mother, 2011. (Data from MacDorman MF, Mathews TJ. *Understanding racial and ethnic disparities in U.S. infant mortality rates* [NCHS Data Brief no 74], Hyattsville, MD, 2011, National Center for Health Statistics. Retrieved from <http://www.cdc.gov/nchs/data/databriefs/db74.htm>.)

Preterm Birth and Low Birth Weight

Preterm birth (birth before 37 completed weeks of gestation) and low birth weight (weighing less than 5.5 pounds at birth) are the most important predictors of infant health. About 12% of babies in the United States are born prematurely; 8% of babies are born at low birth weight. Black women are about twice as likely as white women to have a preterm birth or babies born at low birth weight (Martin et al, 2012).

Infants born preterm or at a low birth weight have a far greater risk of death as well as of mental and physical disabilities such as cerebral palsy, visual problems such as retinopathy of prematurity, feeding problems, and hearing loss than infants born at term with normal weight. Even babies born late preterm (34-36 completed weeks of gestation) carry a risk for physical problems and developmental delay that is much higher than for babies born at full term. Important growth and development occur even in the last few days of a pregnancy. Factors associated with preterm birth and low birth weight include the following:

- Minority status
- Chronic stress
- Maternal age less than 17 years or more than 35 years
- Chronic health problems such as diabetes mellitus, hypertension, and some infections
- Lack of prenatal care
- Multiple births
- Certain problems with the uterus or cervix
- Low socioeconomic status
- Unhealthy maternal habits (e.g., poor nutrition, obesity, alcohol and drug use, and cigarette smoking)
- Induced labor before 39 weeks of pregnancy without a medical indication and elective cesarean birth

One reason that infant mortality has declined so slowly in recent years is that the preterm rate rose very quickly from 1990 to 2006. A portion of this rise was due to increases in multiple births, which in turn was due in part to childbearing in later years, which increases the likelihood of multiple conceptions. Also there was an increase in the rate of multiples

that resulted from assisted reproductive technology. Yet the rate of preterm births among singleton births also rose during this time. Medical management of pregnancy has increased the numbers of labor inductions and elective cesarean births and has helped push the rate of late preterm births upward (Martin et al, 2012). Success stories of tiny survivors are sensationalized in the news, but the long-term consequences of babies born even a few weeks early are not well publicized. Consequences of preterm and late preterm birth can be long-lasting and costly (Engle and Kominiarek, 2008; Morse et al, 2009; Petrini et al, 2009; Ramachandrappa and Jain, 2009). Because late preterm births account for the majority of preterm births, it is imperative that all possible measures are taken to decrease elective births before 39 weeks of gestation (Oshiro et al, 2009).

Preventing the occurrence of prematurity and low birth weight is a high priority for clinical and public health research and policy. Nurses can play important roles in preventing prematurity, through the provision of evidence-based primary care, research, screening, counseling, education, advocacy, referral, and implementation of interventions to reduce risk among target population groups.

Preconception Health

Developing fetal organ systems are highly vulnerable to the effects of poor maternal nutrition, drugs, alcohol, tobacco, chronic maternal diseases, environmental toxins, and other exposures. The fetus can suffer damage very early in pregnancy (3 days after a missed period), even before a woman knows she is pregnant. Because approximately half of the pregnancies in the United States are unintended (Finer and Zolna, 2011), achieving good health for all women throughout their reproductive years—preconception health—can help ensure optimal fetal health and development should pregnancy occur. Healthy lifestyle measures for women (regardless of their intent to become pregnant) include attaining a healthy weight and good nutrition; tending to chronic medical problems such as diabetes and hypertension; being up-to-date on vaccinations; avoiding environmental toxins; decreasing stress and eliminating abusive relationships; and avoiding illicit drugs, tobacco, and alcohol. Effective contraception can help women avoid unintended pregnancies and lengthen pregnancy spacing. Close pregnancy spacing (less that 18 months apart) may increase the likelihood of low birth weight, preterm birth, and placental problems (Conde-Agudelo et al, 2006). preconception health focuses on taking steps in the present to ensure the health of future children, and considering effective contraception if pregnancy is not desired.

Simple measures such as consuming 400 micrograms (mcg, μg) of the B vitamin folic acid every day for at least a month before becoming pregnant and during pregnancy can help decrease the likelihood of defects of the brain and spine, known as *neural tube defects,* by 50% to 70% (Wolff et al, 2009). Some foods, such as leafy vegetables, bananas and beans, are naturally high in folic acid. Other foods, including breads, cereals, flours, cornmeal, pastas, rice, and select grain products, are enriched with folic acid as required by the U.S. Food and Drug Administration (FDA).

Prenatal Care

Obtaining early and regular prenatal care enhances a woman's chance of delivering a healthy, term baby. Prenatal care includes client education, risk identification, and monitoring and treatment of symptoms. It also includes referral to health, nutrition, childbirth education, and social service programs that can help a woman optimize her chances for a healthy pregnancy. Until the late twentieth century, prenatal care was seen as the best solution for improving birth outcomes. But even with expansions in the Medicaid program to cover health care for increasing numbers of low-income pregnant women and infants, and significant federal, state and local investments, poor pregnancy outcomes have persisted, especially for non-Hispanic black, American Indian, and Puerto Rican women.

Although prenatal care is not the *only* solution to reducing infant mortality, comprehensive prenatal care can improve the identification of specific and treatable causes of infant morbidity and mortality, such as maternal anemia, diabetes, hypertension, urinary tract infections, sexually transmitted infections, and poor nutrition. Comprehensive prenatal care is important for all women, but it is particularly important for low-income women. It can help them obtain other services, such as the Special Supplemental Nutrition Program for Women, Infants, and Children (WIC), food stamps, smoking cessation services, housing, child care, job training, substance abuse treatment, and domestic violence screening and counseling. Health education and counseling can provide women with the information they need to make lifestyle changes to help ensure a healthy pregnancy. Ideally, such counseling and treatment of chronic health conditions should begin before a woman becomes pregnant. Optimal health throughout her life, including treatment of chronic health conditions and the adaptation of a healthy lifestyle, will have far more of an impact on healthy pregnancy than prenatal care alone.

Prenatal Substance Use

Tobacco, alcohol, and illicit drug use are social factors that affect the health of women and their children. During pregnancy, substance use profoundly affects the neurological and physical development of the fetus. The use of these substances, in any combination, is dangerous to a woman's health and worsens infant health and development outcomes.

Tobacco

Smoking tobacco during pregnancy is one of the most preventable causes of infant morbidity and mortality. The adverse health effects of tobacco use during pregnancy are well documented; they include low birth weight, prematurity, stillbirth, intrauterine growth retardation, preterm premature rupture of membranes, placenta previa, placental abruption, neurodevelopmental impairment, and SIDS

(Centers for Disease Control and Prevention [CDC], 2010). Cigarette smoke contains more than 2500 chemicals. The fetal effects of most of these chemicals are unknown. What is known, however, is that when a pregnant woman inhales cigarette smoke, the oxygen supply to her fetus is disrupted by nicotine and carbon monoxide. Nicotine crosses the placenta and becomes concentrated in fetal blood and amniotic fluid. Nicotine concentrations in the fetus of a smoking woman can be as much as 15% higher than maternal levels. Secondhand smoke exposure also is dangerous to the fetus and newborn. It is linked to SIDS, decreased respiratory functioning, and childhood asthma. Pregnant women who are exposed to secondhand smoke have 20% higher odds of giving birth to low-birth-weight babies than women who are not exposed to secondhand smoke during pregnancy (CDC, 2010; Leonardi-Bee et al, 2008).

An estimated 13% of women report smoking during the last 3 months of pregnancy. Teenagers and young women have the highest rates of maternal smoking (CDC, 2010). The elimination of tobacco use among pregnant women would significantly reduce the rates of low-birth-weight infants, preterm delivery, intrauterine growth restriction, and infant mortality. Quitting is very difficult because the nicotine in tobacco is addictive, but quitting is best. Merely reducing cigarette use during pregnancy may not be enough to benefit the fetus because women who cut back tend to inhale more deeply or take more puffs to get an equivalent amount of nicotine.

The need for widespread implementation of smoking cessation programs for women in the childbearing years is clear. Many smoking cessation programs have been developed and implemented by national, state, and local governments and organizations. Because pregnant women who have received even brief smoking cessation counseling are more likely to quit smoking, the nurse should offer evidence-based smoking cessation interventions to the pregnant smoker at the first prenatal visit and throughout the pregnancy (Lumley, et al, 2009; Tong et al, 2008).

Alcohol and Illicit Drugs

The use of alcohol and illicit drugs is a major risk factor for poor infant outcomes. Alcohol exposure during pregnancy can lead to fetal alcohol syndrome (FAS) and other fetal alcohol spectrum disorders (FASDs). FASDs range from mild, subtle learning disabilities to severe learning disabilities. Children with FASDs are at risk for psychiatric problems, criminal behavior, unemployment, and incomplete education. Many children with FASDs also have physical abnormalities, growth deficiencies, and central nervous system disorders. *No level of alcohol intake has been determined to be safe during pregnancy, and there is no safe time to drink during pregnancy.* Women who are pregnant or who may become pregnant should abstain from drinking alcohol (CDC, 2012b).

An estimated 7.6% of pregnant women drink during their pregnancies. Binge drinking, which is defined for women as four or more drinks on an occasion in the past 30 days, is especially harmful to fetal development. About 1.4% of pregnant women report binge drinking (CDC, 2012a). There is a compelling need for research on intervention strategies that can help prevent alcohol-exposed pregnancies.

Like alcohol, illicit drugs can cause permanent harm to an unborn baby. Nearly 5% of pregnant women report using drugs such as marijuana, cocaine, ecstasy and other stimulants, and heroin (Substance Abuse and Mental Health Services Administration [SAMHSA], 2012). Risks to the baby include prematurity, low birth weight, birth defects, newborn withdrawal symptoms, and learning and behavioral problems. Substance use is often a sign of more complex psychosocial problems, such as depression, poverty, abuse, and violence. Illicit drug use often goes hand in hand with other maternal risks including tobacco and alcohol use, poor nutrition, intimate partner violence, and risk of sexually transmitted infections. Surveys now indicate that many pregnant women *do* understand the negative impact of substance use during pregnancy and cut back or stop use but then rapidly resume use after pregnancy. Evidence-based public health measures are needed to further reduce substance use during pregnancy and to prevent postpartum resumption (SAMHSA, 2009).

Because of serious potential risks to the developing fetus, women who are pregnant or who could become pregnant should be asked about substance use and counseled to abstain from alcohol, tobacco, and the use of illicit drugs, through the use of evidence-based practices. For women who already use alcohol, tobacco, and illicit drugs, a comprehensive and long-lasting approach to treatment is required.

Breastfeeding

Breastfeeding is a natural and beneficial source of nutrition and provides the healthiest start for an infant. In addition to the nutritional benefits, breastfeeding promotes a unique and emotional connection between mother and baby. (American Academy of Pediatrics, 2012)

The American Academy of Pediatrics (AAP) recommends exclusive breastfeeding for about the first 6 months of a baby's life, followed by breastfeeding in combination with the introduction of complementary foods until at least 12 months of age, and continuation of breastfeeding for as long as mutually desired by mother and baby. Breastfeeding has many advantages for the mother, for the baby, and for society. The cells, hormones, and antibodies in breast milk protect babies from illness such as infections and lower the childhood risk of asthma, obesity, diabetes, and SIDS. For mothers, breastfeeding is linked to a lower risk of breast and ovarian cancer, postpartum depression, and type 2 diabetes. Breastfeeding can save more than $1500 per year in formula and supplies, and even more in the costs of infant illness (Womenshealth.gov, n.d.).

Initiation of breastfeeding occurs in about 77% of hospital births. Maternity practices that discourage separation of mothers and their babies have helped boost these rates, but more attention is required to meet AAP recommendations.

The breastfeeding initiation rate for Hispanic infants is 80%, compared with 75% for white infants and 60% for black infants. Only about 24% of infants are being breastfed by 12 months. The prevalence is 12% for black infants. Black infants have the lowest rates of breastfeeding initiation and duration (CDC, 2013c). This gap points to the need to understand and act upon barriers to breastfeeding that are unique to black women.

The 2011 *Surgeon General's Call to Action to Support Breastfeeding* suggests actions aimed at increasing societal support for women breastfeeding women. These suggestions call on communities, employers, health care providers, governments, and nonprofit organizations to implement strategies to support breastfeeding (U.S. Department of Health and Human Services [USDHHS], Office of the Surgeon General, 2011). There are many community sources of support for breastfeeding mothers, and nurses can play a key role in linking breastfeeding mothers with help, if it is needed. In addition to nurses, health professionals such as **lactation consultants, childbirth educators,** physicians, trained home visitors and doulas can provide assistance. Peer support groups such as La Leche League and breastfeeding centers can also be helpful. The federally supported WIC program also provides counseling and support for breastfeeding mothers.

Sudden Unexplained Infant Death

Sudden unexplained infant death (SUID) is defined as death in an infant less than 1 year of age that occurs suddenly and unexpectedly, the cause of which is not immediately obvious prior to investigation. About 4500 infants die each year from SUID. Later investigation may reveal death in infants with SUID to be from poisoning, metabolic disorders, hyperthermia or hypothermia, neglect and homicide, and suffocation. About half of the infants who die from SUID die from SIDS (Sudden Infant Death Syndrome), defined as the sudden death of an infant less than 1 year of age that cannot be explained after a thorough investigation is conducted, including a complete autopsy, examination of the death scene, and review of the clinical history. SIDS is the third leading cause of infant mortality. Non-Hispanic black and American Indian/Alaska Native infants are far more likely to die from SIDS than infants of other races (CDC, 2013d).

In 1994, with the recognition that placing infants on their backs for sleep lowered SIDS rates, the federal government along with private entities launched the successful Back to Sleep Campaign to heighten awareness of the safety of positioning infants on their backs for sleep. Since 1994, SIDS deaths have declined by more than 50% (CDC, 2013d) (Box 16-3). More has been learned about other factors that can lower the risk of SIDS. In 2012, the AAP released new guidelines for safe sleeping environments (AAP, 2011). Drawing from the success of Back to Sleep, the **Safe to Sleep** campaign was launched to educate parents, caregivers, and health care providers about ways to reduce the risk of infant death from SIDS as well as death from known sleep-related causes, such as suffocation.

BOX 16-3 "SAFE TO SLEEP" PUBLIC EDUCATION CAMPAIGN

Recommendations to Reduce the Risk of Sudden Infant Death Syndrome (SIDS) and Sleep-Related Causes of Infant Death

- Always place a baby on his or her back to sleep, for naps and at night.
- Use a firm sleep surface, covered by a fitted sheet.
- Your baby should not sleep in an adult bed, on a couch, or on a chair alone, with you, or with anyone else.
- Keep soft objects, toys, and loose bedding out of your baby's sleep area.
- Do not smoke during pregnancy, and do not smoke or allow smoking around your baby.
- Breastfeed your baby.
- Do not let your baby get too hot during sleep.
- Follow health care provider guidance on your baby's vaccines and regular health checkups.
- Avoid products that claim to reduce the risk of SIDS and other sleep-related causes of infant death.
- Get regular health care during pregnancy, and do not smoke, drink alcohol or use illegal drugs during pregnancy or after the baby is born.

From National Institute of Child Health & Human Development: *Safe sleep for your baby* (NIH Pub. No. 12-7040), 2013. Retrieved from <https://www.nichd.nih.gov/publications/pubs/Documents/STS_SafeSleepForYourBaby_General_2013.pdf>.

BOX 16-4 NEWBORN SCREENING

Newborn screening checks for rare but serious health conditions shortly after birth. Often babies with certain health disorders appear healthy at birth; thus all babies are tested for selected conditions that can be treated if they are identified early. Babies can be screened for blood, heart and hearing conditions.

Screening can be conducted in three ways. Blood screening is conducted by collecting a few drops of blood from the newborn's heel. This sample is tested at a laboratory, and parents are notified of abnormalities. Hearing screening requires that a tiny, soft speaker be placed in the baby's ear to see how the baby responds to sound. Heart screening uses pulse oximetry to evaluate the baby for congenital heart disease.

Newborn screening is state-based, and the number of conditions that babies are screened for varies from state to state. All U.S. states and territories currently test for 26 health conditions, including phenylketonuria, galactosemia, congenital hypothyroidism, and sickle cell disease.

Modified from March of Dimes: *Newborn screening*, n.d. Retrieved from <http://www.marchofdimes.com/baby/newborn-screening.aspx>.

CHILDHOOD HEALTH ISSUES

At all ages, appropriate and timely medical care plays an important role in children's health status. However, other factors, including parental influences, nutrition, environment, community safety, and the overall quality of home life, exert even stronger influences over a child's well-being. Childhood is generally a healthy time of life, as evidenced by the improvement in many indicators of child health status over the past century. For example, the incidence of childhood disease has diminished because the majority of children receive a full complement of immunizations during infancy and toddlerhood.

The causes of childhood death vary with age. Parents and the community have important responsibilities in promoting healthy lifestyles, creating safe environments, and ensuring access to medical care. They must take steps to protect children from the leading threats to children's health (i.e., accidental injury and exposure to environmental toxins, abuse, and violence). Box 16-4 discusses the screening of newborns for genetic disorders.

Accidental Injuries

Infants and young children are at great risk for accidental injuries. They are curious and eager to explore their environments, but they often lack the coordination and cognitive abilities to keep themselves safe from harm. Their small size and developing bones and muscles make them especially susceptible to injury. The leading cause of injury death for children younger than 1 year is accidental suffocation due to choking or strangulation. Unintentional injury is the leading cause of death for children ages 1 to 14. For children younger than 5, drowning is the leading cause of death. From 5 to 14 years, motor vehicle–related injuries are the cause of most deaths. Low income and minority children suffer disproportionately from accidental injuries. They are more likely to sustain injuries and more likely to die from their injuries. For example, Native American children are more than twice as likely to experience accidental injury as their white counterparts (Safe Kids USA, 2013).

Many accidents can be avoided by improving that safety of a child's environment. Ensuring a child's safety in a motor vehicle is critical. The most important steps that a parent can take to ensure a child's safety in a motor vehicle is to correctly secure the child into a car seat based on the child's age and size. To maximize safety, children should be in car seats located in the back seat of the car until they are at least 12 years old (National Highway Traffic Safety Administration, 2013). Leaving children unattended in a motor vehicle is another safety concern. In only a few minutes a car can become hot enough to cause heat stroke in a youngster. Children can also become entrapped in a car trunk or locked in a car. They should never be left alone in a car.

Smoke alarms should be installed on every level of the home and in bedroom. Escape plans should be practiced often. Small children can drown in as little as an inch of water. Toilets, buckets, bathtubs, and pools are all potential drowning hazards. Storage of medications and hazardous substances and playground safety are also important safety education topics.

Head injury from cycling and other wheeled sports, such as skateboarding, is a leading cause of child death and disability. Without proper head protection, a fall from as little as 2 feet can cause traumatic brain injury. The use of helmets and proper protective equipment can substantially reduce the risk of injuries.

COMMUNITY HEALTH VISIT

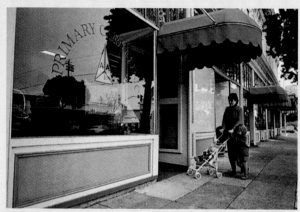

This clinic provides services through the Early and Periodic Screening, Diagnosis, and Treatment (EPSDT) Program, which was developed to provide health care for children in low-income families receiving Medicaid.

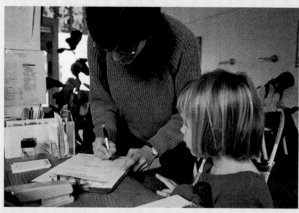

The nurse has an opportunity to observe the client and the family as they register and wait for their appointment. The parent registers the 5-year-old daughter for a school entry health physical examination. Medicaid insurance is verified for the physical.

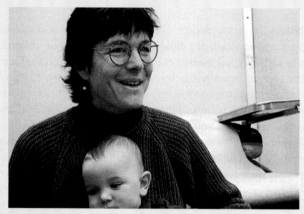

Trust can be established in a short time. The nurse can begin by explaining the steps in the clinic process so that the client knows what is expected. The nurse should always listen to the client attentively and should allow enough time for the client to reflect and respond to questions.

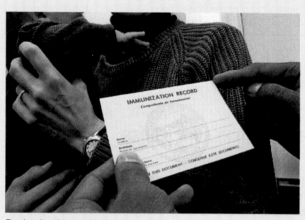

Reviewing immunization records is an important primary prevention role for the community health nurse. This is a teachable opportunity for the nurse to stress the importance of maintaining immunizations for the child. In California parents are provided with a yellow state immunization record for the child, which they should use to record all immunizations and to show proof of immunizations when needed.

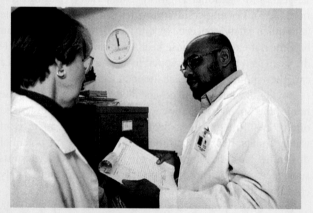

The nurse discusses any concerns about the client with the practitioner before the examination.

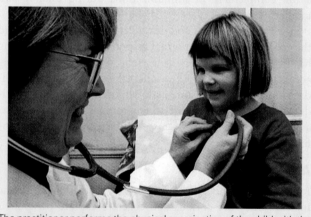

The practitioner performs the physical examination of the child with the help of the parent. The practitioner discusses the result of the vision test with the parent and the need for a follow-up appointment with an ophthalmologist. The child has not undergone a blood lead measurement and requires booster immunizations. The practitioner orders laboratory tests, immunizations, and a referral to an ophthalmologist.

Continued

COMMUNITY HEALTH VISIT—cont'd

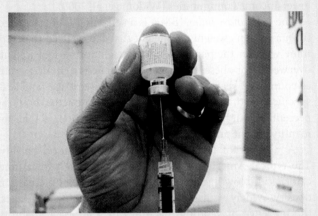

The clinic staff performs the laboratory work: hematocrit, urinary analysis, and lead measurement. The immunization consent forms have been signed by the parent. The nurse administers the immunizations and takes this opportunity to reinforce the importance of immunizations for both children.

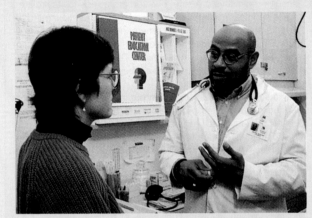

The nurse also offers suggestions to relieve the common side effects of immunizations.

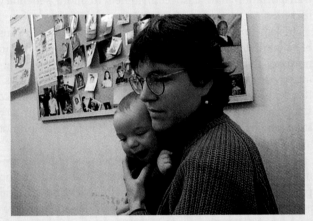

The parent asks about an ophthalmologist who takes Medicaid and about day care facilities in the area for the younger child. The parent also asks about family planning services in the community.

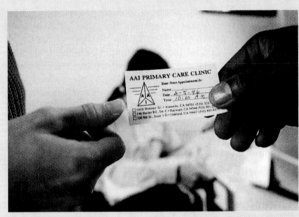

The community health nurse gives the parent a business card with the nurse's name and the agency's address and phone number. The nurse advises the parent to call the nurse if there is anything else that the family may need.

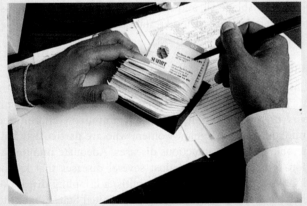

The nurse searches for resources for an ophthalmologist and a family planning clinic that accept Medicaid and a resource for day-care providers. The nurse obtains phone numbers for a couple of ophthalmologists, a family planning clinic, and a day care consortium service.

Story by Leonard Kaku, RN, MSN. Photography by George Draper.

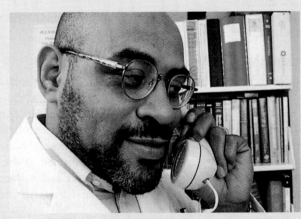

The nurse calls the family with the referrals for an ophthalmologist and a phone number to obtain a list of day care providers.

BOX 16-5   TOY-RELATED INJURIES

Although most toys are safe, children are at risk for toy-related injuries and death. Approximately 168,000 children younger than 14 years are treated in hospital emergency departments for toy-related injuries. Though the majority of toy-related injuries are minor, permanent disability can occur. Riding toys, such as non-motorized scooters and tricycles, are associated with more injuries than any other toy group.

Laws and regulations have been put into place to protect children from toy injuries. An example is the Federal Hazardous Substances Act, which bans children's toys that contain any hazardous substance, such as lead. The Child Safety Protection Act of 1994 was designed to reduce toy-related choking and requires manufacturers to place choking hazard warning labels on balloons, marbles, small balls, and games with small parts intended for use only by children 3 years and older. The act also requires manufacturers, importers, distributors, and retailers to report choking incidents involving such products to the Consumer Product Safety Commission. The U.S. Department of Commerce requires toy guns to be distinguished from real guns. In addition, the toy industry has established voluntary safety standards to minimize risk of injury.

Although regulations and laws are helpful, parents and caretakers must also provide adequate supervision of children and must adopt strategies recommended to prevent toy-related injuries, as follows: use only age-appropriate toys; use Mylar balloons instead of latex (which can cause children to choke or suffocate); purchase a "small parts" tester to determine whether small toys pose choking hazards; check the website of the U.S. Consumer Product Safety Commission (www.cpsc.gov) to obtain information on toy recalls; follow age and safety recommendations on toy labels; and ensure that toys are used in a safe and proper environment.

Data from Safe Kids USA: *Preventing accidental injury: toy safety*. Retrieved March 8, 2013, from <www.safekids.org/>.

Low-income parents may have difficulty affording safety equipment such as safety latches for cabinets, smoke alarms, car seats, and helmets. The grassroots coalition Safe Kids USA can help link parents and professionals to child injury prevention advocacy and events in local communities (Safe Kids USA, 2013).

Box 16-5 discusses how toys can be another threat to small children.

Unhealthy Weight

Childhood obesity has become a health crisis in the United States. The rate of obesity has more than doubled in children and tripled in adolescents over the past 30 years. An estimated one third of children are overweight or obese Ogden et al, 2012). Children who are overweight are more likely to experience cardiovascular disease, diabetes, bone and joint disease, and sleep apnea and to face social discrimination that can lead to poor self-esteem and depression.

Obesity prevalence is higher among non-Hispanic black and Hispanic children and adolescents than among non-Hispanic white youth (Ogden et al, 2012). Minority groups, those with less income, and those with lower education levels are more likely to be overweight. The higher cost and

unavailability of healthy foods, food insecurity, and the lack of access to safe places to exercise contribute to obesity in lower-income communities (Widome et al, 2009).

The *body mass index* (BMI) is a screening tool calculated from a person's weight and height that can be used to determine whether the person is underweight, of normal weight, overweight, or obese. BMI can be calculated in children from as young as 2 years to teen age with the use of age- and sex-specific growth charts. BMI does not calculate actual body fat percentage, but it is an easy and inexpensive method that can identify weight problems (CDC, 2011a).

A number of factors contribute to childhood obesity. The typical American diet, which is both high in fat and calories and low in nutrients, has resulted in an increase in obesity. Widely available fast food, increasing portion sizes, the presence of vending machines in schools, availability of sugar-sweetened drinks, and the eating of fewer meals at home have contributed to the trend. Modern technologies such as electronic games and television, a lack of safe convenient outdoor exercise areas, and readily accessible transportation have also contributed to more sedentary lifestyles.

In some urban neighborhoods, where high concentrations of people living in poverty are prevalent, there may be little to no access to fresh, nutritious, affordable foods, also contributing to obesity. Such neighborhoods are called "food deserts." Residents are limited to obtaining food from convenience stores and fast food restaurants rather than from grocery stores and fresh food markets. Nutritious foods are simply not available.

Nurses can play a leading role in generating public awareness of factors that contribute to obesity and can focus on preventive measures such as healthy lifestyles and physical activity. For example, breastfeeding provides some protection against later obesity. At least 60 minutes of moderately strenuous exercise is recommended for children most days of the week. Nurses can design and implement nutrition, healthy eating, and physical activities policies and standards in schools, take part in initiatives that make fresh, healthy foods available to all, and challenge policymakers and industry leaders such as fast-food restaurants to mobilize resources for good nutrition and fitness.

Immunization

Childhood immunization is a benchmark of child health. Maintaining appropriate immunization protects all members of the community, especially immune-compromised individuals and pregnant women, who are particularly vulnerable to certain infectious diseases. Adequate immunization protects children against several diseases that kill or disable many children. Poliomyelitis, a crippling disease of the past, has been eliminated in the United States thanks to the public health effort that made the polio vaccine accessible and affordable. Over the ensuing decades, new vaccines have been developed, and children can now be protected from more than 14 vaccine-preventable diseases. State laws requiring proof of vaccination before entry to school or child care have helped to ensure high vaccination levels in the population.

Vaccine-preventable disease levels are at or near record lows, but many children and adolescents remain under-immunized. Concerns about the frequency and timing of vaccines and widespread fears that childhood vaccines are linked to autism have prevented some parents from vaccinating their children (Institute of Medicine, 2013). In 2009, however, the U.S. Court of Federal Claims ruled that childhood vaccines do not cause autism. This ruling was consistent with 18 major scientific studies that failed to show a link between vaccines and autism (U.S. Court of Federal Claims, n.d.). Nurses can help to educate community members about the safety of vaccines and recommended vaccination schedules and about the consequences of under-vaccination. The following vaccines are recommended for children and adolescents (CDC, 2013a):

- Tetanus, diphtheria, acellular pertussis
- Inactivated polio
- Rotavirus
- Influenza
- Measles, mumps, and rubella vaccine
- Hepatitis A vaccine
- Hepatitis B vaccine
- Varicella (chickenpox) vaccine
- *Haemophilus influenzae* type b (Hib)
- Pneumococcal conjugate
- Human papillomavirus vaccine (males and females)
- Meningococcal conjugate

Most insurance plans cover the cost of childhood vaccines. The Affordable Care Act requires new insurance plans to eliminate co-pays and deductibles for preventive services such as vaccinations. Another source of assistance is the Vaccines For Children (VFC) program, a federally funded program that provides vaccines at no cost to children who might not otherwise be vaccinated because of inability to pay.

Environmental Concerns

Potential threats to the health of children sometimes exist in their living environments. Threats can be found in the air, in the water, and from toxic exposures to chemicals. For example, air pollution, poor indoor air quality, and second-hand smoke can cause or trigger childhood asthma. Asthma is one of the most common chronic childhood disorders, affecting an estimated 9.3 children every year (CDC, 2011b). Lead, a neurotoxin, that can sometimes be found in drinking water (often from lead pipes and fittings), in old paint dust or chips that crumble from walls on older housing units, and in contaminated soil is a cause of childhood death, cognitive and behavioral problems, decreased growth, and neurological disabilities. The reduction of childhood blood lead levels is among the greatest public health stories of the latter half of the twentieth century, but unfortunately lead is still a threat. Although lead is banned from the manufacture of paint, many millions of housing units in the United States still contain lead-based paint. Most of these units are located in poor, inner-city neighborhoods. Despite dramatic declines in blood lead levels for most U.S. populations, levels remain high among children in low-income families who live in older housing with lead-based paint. Treatment for children with elevated blood lead values is long and difficult and carries risks. Better prevention, elimination of risks in the environment, particularly in older housing units, more efficient tracking, and education of the public are essential to further reduce the menace of lead poisoning.

Exposure to toxic cleaning products, pesticides, medicines, and herbicides is another area of concern. Simple steps can help protect children from accidental exposures, including child-resistant packaging, cabinet safety latches, and careful supervision.

Child Maltreatment

Child maltreatment is another indicator of children's physical and emotional health status. Five children die every day in the United States from abuse and neglect. About 80% of these children are younger than 4 years (USDHHS Administration for Children and Families, 2011). Because of the lack of identification and recognition and because of underreporting, the extent of child maltreatment is probably far greater than these statistics reveal.

Child abuse may be physical, sexual, or emotional. Neglect is by far the most prevalent form of child maltreatment. *Child neglect* is the failure to provide for a child's basic physical, medical, emotional, or educational needs or to protect a child from harm or potential harm. It may include failure to provide affection, warmth, understanding, and supervision adequate for healthy development (Leeb et al, 2008).

Child maltreatment affects children of all races, ages, and ethnicities. Factors that place children at a higher risk for maltreatment include a living in a family that is stressed by drug and alcohol abuse, poverty, chronic health problems, violence in the community or at home, and social isolation (USDHHS Administration for Children and Families, 2011).

There are many long-term effects of child abuse and neglect. The effects may be physical, such as brain damage in shaken baby syndrome; emotional, such as depression and low self-esteem; and behavioral, such as delinquency, promiscuity, eating disorders, poor academic achievement, and drug abuse. Extreme stress caused by abuse and neglect interferes with normal brain development, harming the basic architecture of the brain. Healthy brain development relies on consistent, reciprocal, and appropriate interactions between young children and their caretakers. Chronic deprivation of healthy, reciprocal interactions can lead to the persistent activation of the stress response, leading to poor academic achievement, low self-esteem, depression, promiscuity, drug abuse and chronic health problems (Center on the Developing Child at Harvard University, 2012).

Most often, the perpetrators of maltreatment are parents, who themselves were victims, forming a cycle of abuse. The two dominant characteristics of abusive parents are a history of substance abuse and abuse from their own parents. Often, caretakers do not intend to hurt their children. They may be stressed by poverty, illness, or disability, and they may lack social support systems or coping skills. Young and inexperienced parents may not understand the physical, emotional, and behavioral needs of their children.

Children are never responsible for the harm done to them by others, and yet they may feel guilty for causing it. Many professionals, including nurses, social service workers, and teachers, are required by law to report child abuse. Nurses in the community must understand their ethical and legal obligations to report child maltreatment. They can also help create a climate that supports families and provides parents with alternatives to abusive behavior. Programs for parents can take many different forms. Positive parenting skills are at the core of such programs. Positive parenting skills include responsiveness to the emotional and physical needs of children, good communication, and appropriate discipline. This education may occur in parents' homes, in schools, in medical or mental health clinics, or in other community settings. Nurse home visitors can be key in providing education. The ultimate goal is to prevent child maltreatment before it starts.

Children with Special Health Care Needs

Children and youth with special health care needs are those who have chronic physical, developmental, behavioral, or emotional conditions that necessitate health and related services beyond those required by children generally. These conditions include developmental disorders such as Down syndrome and autism spectrum disorder, mental health disorders such as depression and anxiety, seizures, allergies, asthma, and attention-deficit/hyperactivity disorder (ADHD). Chronic conditions are those expected to last 12 months or more. Often children with special health care needs experience two or more chronic conditions (USDHHS, Health Resources and Services Administration, 2012).

Children with special health care needs frequently have multiple service needs, including public health, physical and mental health care, specialized diagnostic services, social services, and educational, vocational, and sometimes corrective services. Families trying to obtain care for children with special needs face challenges in dealing with differing eligibility criteria, duplication and gaps in services, inflexible funding sources, geographic, cultural, and financial barriers, and poor coordination of care. Children with special needs can benefit from a coordinated, comprehensive, integrated system of care—often called a medical home. A *medical home* is not a place but, rather, an approach to providing care. Having a medical home strengthens the ability of children with multiple service needs to receive comprehensive care for complex conditions (Box 16-6).

The Individuals with Disabilities Education Act (IDEA), enacted by Congress in 1975, is intended to ensure that children with disabilities receive a free, appropriate public education. The law has been amended many times and addresses the needs of babies through school-age children. IDEA is known as the nation's "special education law" and is administered through the U.S. Department of Education (n.d.).

BOX 16-6 THE PATIENT-CENTERED MEDICAL HOME

The American Academy of Family Physicians (AAFP), American Academy of Pediatrics (AAP), American College of Physicians (ACP), and the American Osteopathic Association have long endorsed the concept of a "medical home." This ideal suggests that every child, including special needs children, should have "accessible, continuous, comprehensive, family-centered, coordinated, culturally effective and compassionate" health care (AAP, 1992).

A medical home should be within a community-based system that has coordinated networks designed to promote the healthy development and well-being of children as they move from adolescence to adulthood. Such a system requires appropriate financing to support and sustain quality care, optimal outcomes, family satisfaction, and cost-efficiency (AAP, 1992, n.d.).

ADOLESCENT HEALTH ISSUES

Adolescence is a time of generally good health. It is a period when preteens and teens form lifelong health habits, including dietary and exercise habits and emotional health skills such as problem-solving and coping strategies. Typically, adolescents do not use health services unless they have an underlying chronic condition or an acute illness. They rarely use preventive health services.

In their struggle to gain independence many adolescents engage in risk-taking behaviors, including alcohol and drug abuse, tobacco use, early and unprotected sexual activity, unsafe driving, and participation in delinquent and violent activities that threaten their health. Such behaviors are influenced by peers, the family, and characteristics of communities in which they live. Risk taking among adolescents is greatly influenced by their ability to control their impulses at this stage of brain development. The part of the brain that is responsible for "executive functioning," the prefrontal cortex, is not fully mature until near age 25. Even though a teen may understand that a behavior is risky, he or she may have difficulty "putting on the brakes" because of the immaturity of brain development and connections (USDHHS, Office of Population Affairs, 2013).

Traditional approaches to improving adolescent health have focused on specific risks; however, a collaborative, multipartner approach that centers on the strengths of the whole person in the community, rather than focusing on individual risks, may be more effective in helping adolescents avoid risks and develop social competence. The community health nurse can help parents and communities understand the nonmedical, public health nature of risky behaviors and can assist in the development of community-wide strategies to effectively deal with them. The Youth Risk Behavior Surveillance System (YRBSS), administered by CDC's Division of Adolescent and School Health, monitors health risk behaviors in ninth through twelfth graders that lead to morbidity and mortality (CDC, 2012c).

Sexual Risk Behavior

One of many risk-taking adolescent behaviors is sexual intercourse. Adolescent sexual activity is often unprotected and can result in unintended pregnancy, infection with human immunodeficiency virus (HIV), and other sexually transmitted infections (STIs).

Among students surveyed in 2011, about 47.4% had ever had sexual intercourse. Nearly 34% had engaged in sexual intercourse during the 3 months preceding the survey. Of these, 60.2% reported that either they or their partner had used a condom during last sexual intercourse. Another 23.3% used another form of birth control, such as birth control pills, an injectable form of birth control, a birth control ring, an implant, or an intrauterine device (IUD) to prevent pregnancy. Thirteen percent used no method of birth control during the last sexual intercourse. Twenty-two percent had used alcohol or drugs before last sexual intercourse (CDC, 2012b).

RESEARCH HIGHLIGHTS

Does a Satisfactory Relationship With Her Mother Influence When a 16-Year-Old Female Begins to Have Sex?

A prospective, panel study of more than 1500 female adolescents (not randomly selected) examined whether the dimensions within the mother-daughter relationship during young adolescence influenced sexual initiation prior to age 16 years. Researchers found that three dimensions within the relationship were associated with delayed sexual initiation: positive cohesion, communication, and satisfaction with time spent together. The researchers concluded that efforts in delaying sexual initiation in young adolescents need to be directed toward promoting positive mother-daughter relationships.

Data from Kovar C, Salsberry P: Does a satisfactory relationship with her mother influence when a 16-year-old begins to have sex? *MCN, Am J Maternal/Child Nurs* 37(2):122-129, 2012.

Teen childbearing has been on the decline since the late 1950s, reaching a historic low at 34.3 births per 1000 women aged 15 to 19 years (Ventura and Hamilton, 2011). In recent years, teens seem to be less sexually active, and more of those who are sexually active seem to be using birth control than in previous years (Martinez, Copen, and Abma, 2011). Despite the declines in teen childbearing, the U.S. adolescent birth rate remains one of the highest among industrialized nations (United Nations Statistics Division, 2011). Large disparities exist among racial and ethnic groups. The teen pregnancy rate is lowest among Asian and Pacific Islanders and highest among Hispanic teenagers (Hamilton and Ventura, 2012).

The consequences of early childbearing to mothers, children, and society are significant. Teen childbearing contributes greatly to high school dropout rates. Only half of teen mothers receive a high school diploma by 22 years of age, compared with approximately 90% of girls who did not give birth during adolescence (Perper, Peterson, and Manlove, 2010). For the infant, having a teenage mother poses serious health risks, including death, prematurity, low birth weight, and social risks, including lower school achievement, incarceration, teen pregnancy, and adult unemployment. Children born to teenage parents have lower school achievement and are more likely to drop out of high school. They are more

likely to be incarcerated at some time during adolescence, father children as teenagers, require public assistance, and face unemployment as young adults. According to an analysis by the National Campaign to Prevent Teen Pregnancy, the estimated cost of teen childbearing in the United States for taxpayers (federal, state, and local) is at least $109 billion (National Campaign to Prevent Teen and Unplanned Pregnancy, 2013).

Sexually transmitted infections are another consequence of sexual risk behavior. STIs include human papillomavirus (HPV), *Chlamydia trachomatis*, herpes simplex virus type 2 (HSV-2), human immunodeficiency virus/acquired immunodeficiency syndrome (HIV/AIDS), hepatitis B, gonorrhea, syphilis, and vaginal trichomoniasis. Teenagers are more likely than adults to acquire STIs (CDC, 2011c). For some infections, such as *Chlamydia trachomatis*, the difference may be due to a physiological susceptibility. Barriers to health care such as lack of transportation, concerns about confidentiality, and lack of access to preventive health services also contribute to a higher prevalence of STIs among teens. STIs may be asymptomatic in both males and females. Although many STIs clear on their own, others can persist over time, putting women at high risk for cervical cancer, pelvic inflammatory disease, ectopic pregnancy, and infertility. Not only is a woman's health affected, especially if the infections go untreated, but the infant born to a woman with an STI is at risk of infection and can suffer long-term consequences. Routine counseling and voluntary testing for sexually active teens and pregnant women is recommended. Two vaccines (Cervarix [GlaxoSmithKline] Inc. [Philadelphia, PA] and Gardasil [Merck, Whitehouse Station, NJ]) can protect females against the types of HPV responsible for most cervical cancers, and either is recommended for 11- and 12-year-old girls. Gardasil is also recommended for 11- to 21-year-old boys.

The causes and effects of risky sexual behaviors are complex, and the solutions are multifaceted. A recent survey found that most parents feel that they play an important role in providing guidance to their children about healthy sexual behavior, yet half of children are uncomfortable with these conversations. Parents who were surveyed overwhelmingly support school-based sex education programs including information about birth control (Planned Parenthood, 2012)

Abstinence from vaginal, anal, and oral intercourse is the only 100% effective way to prevent HIV, other STIs, and pregnancy. Primary prevention models are most successful when they are evidence-based and tailored to the community's individual needs. Components of such programs can include the following:

- Abstinence promotion
- Education about contraception and its availability
- Sex education
- Character development
- Problem-solving skill development
- Peer counseling programs
- Strategies for ensuring teenagers' school success
- Job training

Such efforts are more likely to succeed when there are partnerships among parents, adolescents, and agencies for health, education, religion, social service, and government. Nurses working within such organizations can play leadership roles in developing community programs for prevention of adolescent sexual risk behaviors.

Violence

Youth violence can be seen as a reflection of how well parents, schools, and the community are able to supervise and channel youth behavior in positive ways. Children and adolescents can be victims of, aggressors in, or witnesses to violence. For the victims, violence can cause both emotional and physical harm. For too many of the nation's youth, violence is a way of life, a way of coping with challenging and difficult situations, and a significant public health problem.

The rate of serious violent crime against youth ages 12 to 17 years declined 77% between 1994 and 2010. In 2010, male (14.3 victimizations per 1000) and female (13.7 per 1000) youth were equally likely to experience serious violent crime—rape or sexual assault, robbery, and aggravated assault. Black males are the racial group most likely to be victimized (Lauritsen and White, 2012). Homicide is the second leading cause of death for young people ages 15 to 24 years. Of victims in 2010, 82.8% were killed with a firearm (CDC, 2012d). Handguns are readily accessible to America's youth. Federal law prohibits anyone under age 21 years from purchasing a handgun from a licensed dealer, but it does not prohibit anyone under age 21 years from purchasing a handgun from a non-licensed dealer.

Teen dating violence consists of physical, sexual, or psychological/emotional violence (including stalking) within a dating relationship. In the 2011 Youth Risk Behavior Survey, 9.4% of high school students reported having been hit, slapped, or physically hurt on purpose by their boyfriend or girlfriend in the preceding 12 months (CDC, 2012c). Teen dating violence can be emotionally and physically traumatizing and can lead to victimization and unhealthy relationships in the future.

Violence among youth is a multifaceted problem. Social factors, such as unemployment and poverty, strongly influence the risk of exposure to violent behavior. Violence in the home, in the media, and in the community; gun ownership; and child abuse, violence, or severe corporal punishment may socialize youth to viewing violence as an expected and unavoidable part of life.

Teen violence does not have simple remedies. Solutions require community and neighborhood efforts to help young people diffuse anger and frustrations before they escalate; to help parents, religious organizations, and schools assist their youth in managing anger and resolving conflicts; and to work with children and teenagers to assure them that they are loved, appreciated, and accepted for who they are and that help is available. Reducing children's unsupervised exposure to guns, engaging communities in strengthening law enforcement, modifying the design of guns, and limiting the flow of illegal guns to youth are also strategies to reduce youth gun violence (Reich, 2002).

Tobacco, Alcohol, and Drug Use

The use of tobacco, alcohol, and illicit drugs has serious and long-lasting consequences for adolescents and for society. The YRBSS (CDC, 2012c) provides a snapshot of behavioral trends. In 2011, the Survey revealed the following:

- 18.1% of students had smoked cigarettes in the 30 days prior to the survey.
- 44.7% of students had ever tried cigarette smoking.
- 38.7% of students had had at least one drink of alcohol in the 30 days prior to the survey.
- 21.9% of students had had five or more drinks of alcohol in a row, (i.e., within a couple of hours—also known as binge drinking) in the 30 days prior to the survey.
- 70.8% of students had had at least one drink of alcohol on at least 1 day during their lives (i.e., had ever drunk alcohol).
- 20.7% of students had taken prescription drugs (e.g., Oxy-Contin, Percocet, Vicodin, codeine, Adderall, Ritalin, or Xanax) without a doctor's prescription one or more times during their lives (i.e., had ever taken prescription drugs without a doctor's prescription).
- 39.9% of students had used marijuana one or more times during their lives (i.e., had ever used marijuana).
- 23.1% of students had used marijuana one or more times during the 30 days before the survey (i.e., current marijuana use).
- 25.6% of students had been offered, sold, or given an illegal drug by someone on school property during the 12 months before the survey.

Among the findings of the latest YRBSS survey are that smoking rates among teens have declined since peaking in the mid-1990s. In contrast, illicit drug use by youths is constantly evolving as new drugs in new forms are introduced. "Designer drugs" or synthetic cannabinoids (a.k.a. "Spice" or "K2") have been banned in most states, but minor changes to the chemical make-up of these substances result in new substances that are not covered under revised laws (National Conference of State Legislatures, 2012). Also, prescription drugs used outside of medical supervision, for example Oxy-Contin, Ritalin, and steroids, have become more popular. According to the Monitoring the Future Project of the University of Michigan, rumors of the supposed benefits of using a drug usually spread much faster than information about the adverse consequences. It generally takes much longer for evidence of adverse consequences, such as death, disease, overdose, and addictive potential, to become widely known, thus contributing to the widespread use of both legal and illegal drugs (Johnston et al, 2009).

Adolescence is a critical time to prevent substance addiction. Drugs change brains, and early use of drugs increases a person's chances of more serious drug abuse and addiction (National Institute on Drug Abuse, 2010). Broad evidence-based prevention efforts, including addressing the issues of housing, poverty, and crime, are needed.

FACTORS AFFECTING CHILD AND ADOLESCENT HEALTH

As in other age groups, social, nonmedical factors largely determine children's health. Children depend on their families or caregivers for their health and well-being; therefore the following factors significantly impact children's physical health, mental health, and overall well-being:

- Parents' or caregivers' income, education, and stability
- Security and safety of the home
- Nutritional and environmental issues
- Health care access and use

Poverty

Poverty is the greatest threat to child health. Child poverty in the United States is higher than in most other industrialized countries, and the rate is rising (National Center for Children in Poverty, 2013). About 16 million (22%) of the nation's children live below the federal poverty level. The official poverty level is calculated by using poverty thresholds that are issued each year by the U.S. Census Bureau. The thresholds represent the annual amount of cash income minimally required to support families of various sizes. The 2014 poverty guideline for a family of three in the 48 contiguous states and the District of Columbia was $23,850 (USDHHS, 2012). Many more children (about 44%) live in low-income families that are close to the poverty level and unable to meet basic living expenses. Children are far more likely than adults to live in poverty. Poverty rates are highest for black, Hispanic, and American Indian children.

Factors associated with poverty include parental education, employment, and single parenting. Eighty-five percent of children whose parents do not have a high school education live in low-income families. Even if parents have full-time employment, low education levels make their children susceptible to poverty. Likewise, children in households headed by a single parent (usually the mother) are far more likely to live in poverty and thus to have more health risks; 69% of all children with single parents live in low-income families (National Center for Children in Poverty, 2013).

Poverty by itself does not always put a child at risk; however, poor children face the following health and socioeconomic risks that can compound the burdensome influence of poverty (Federal Interagency Forum on Child and Family Statistics, 2013):

- Children in poverty have less access to nutritious food, shelter, and health care.
- Poor children are often deprived of advantages such as good schools, libraries, and other community resources.
- Deaths from unintended injuries, child maltreatment, homicide, STIs, and infectious diseases (including AIDS) are more common among poor children.
- Many poor children live in substandard housing, have stressful home lives, may live surrounded by drugs and crime, and lack positive and nurturing adult role models.
- Poor children may feel hopeless about the future.

- Poor children often suffer from low birth weight, asthma, dental decay, high blood lead levels, learning disabilities, and teenage unmarried childbearing.
- Poor children are more likely to move frequently. Residential instability and extreme living conditions of poor children who are homeless or migrants usually compound their health problems.

These social and economic burdens can be overwhelming to parents or caregivers and may cause them to neglect other matters, such as providing a nutritious breakfast before school, taking a child for a well-child appointment, and getting his or her immunizations completed on schedule. They can create a sense of despair and hopelessness among parents and children, which greatly hinders healthy behavior. These factors clearly increase a child's physical and emotional health risks.

Racial and Ethnic Disparities

Although children in the United States are healthier now than in any other time in our nation's history, overall improvements in health mask the poor health of some racial and ethnic subgroups (Figure 16-4). For example, as mentioned previously, the infant mortality rate has plunged over the past century, yet infants born to non-Hispanic black women are two-and-one-half times more likely to die in the first year of life than babies born to non-Hispanic white mothers. Native Americans and African Americans account for a disproportionate share of disabilities and deaths due to fetal alcohol exposure. African American youth are at higher risk for gun violence than white youth and are more than four times as likely to die from asthma as non-Hispanic White children. Childhood obesity affects racial and ethnic minority children at much higher rates than non-Hispanic Whites, driving up rates of associated diabetes.

Eliminating health disparities is an important national health priority. *Healthy People 2020* (USDHHS, 2013; see later) targets persistent differences in health among children of varying racial and ethnic groups and calls for the elimination of disparities in health. Social determinants of health—the circumstances into which children are born—exert a strong and persistent influence over their lifelong health. A child's ability to be healthy and productive in life is negatively impacted by poverty, violence, and a family history of poor health along with systemic inequities such as limited access to quality health care, education, and job opportunities.

Community health nurses can develop an understanding of differences in health based on race, ethnicity and economic circumstances. They can translate experiences in the field into evidence-based intervention strategies that incorporate social programs such as education, employment, and housing into solutions for addressing health disparities.

Health Care Use

Children grow and develop rapidly between infancy and adolescence; therefore they are extremely vulnerable to the effects of illness and of environmental factors that influence physical and emotional health. Preventive health and dental care

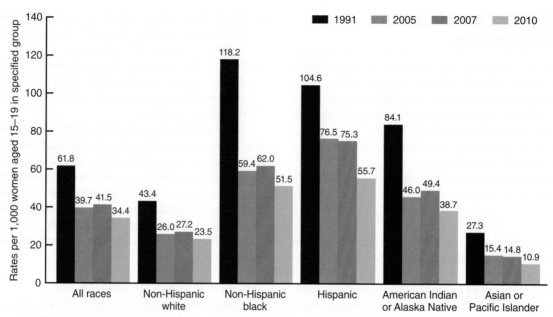

FIGURE 16-4 Birth rates for women aged 15 to 19 years, by race and Hispanic origin: United States, 1991, 2005, 2007, and 2010. (From Hamilton BE, Ventura SJ: *Birth rates for U.S. teenagers reach historic lows for all age and ethnic groups* [NCHS Data Brief no 89], Hyattsville, MD, 2012, National Center for Health Statistics. Retrieved from <http://www.cdc.gov/nchs/data/databriefs/db89.pdf>.)

offer children and parents a chance to periodically meet with a health care provider to do the following:

- Discuss the child's physical and emotional growth and development.
- Learn about good nutrition.
- Address safety issues, such as the use of car seats and seatbelts.
- Receive immunizations and vision and hearing screening.
- Learn about potential environmental threats to the child's health.
- Begin prompt treatment for a condition discovered during the examination.
- Ask other questions or obtain a referral if necessary.

Access to a regular health care source can facilitate prompt attention to acute medical problems, which can help prevent chronic, disabling conditions. For example, untreated ear infections can cause hearing loss, which can lead to learning disabilities, school problems, and even school dropout. Resulting low self-esteem can increase the likelihood of depression, behavior problems, early sexual activity, STIs, and unplanned pregnancy. Comprehensive, regular health care helps all children achieve their potential.

STRATEGIES TO IMPROVE CHILD AND ADOLESCENT HEALTH

One of the most important ways to ensure the success and well-being of future generations is for each child to start life healthy and maintain his or her physical and emotional health status throughout childhood and adolescence. Since the beginning of the twentieth century, the nation has made remarkable progress in many areas of child and adolescent

BOX 16-7 RESOURCES: MONITORING THE HEALTH AND WELL-BEING OF CHILDREN

Centers for Disease Control and Prevention (CDC): Monitors many health and disease prevention efforts, including the Youth Risk Behavior Surveillance System, which monitors youth tobacco, alcohol, and drug use; dietary behaviors; and sexual behaviors contributing to unintended pregnancy and sexually transmitted infections. (www.cdc.gov.)

Federal Interagency Forum on Child and Family Statistics: On an annual basis, produces *America's Children: Key National Indicators of Well-Being,* a report containing detailed information on a set of key indicators of child well-being. (www.childstats.gov.)

National Center for Education Statistics (NCES): The primary federal agency for collecting and analyzing data related to education in the United States. (www.nces.ed.gov.)

National Center for Health Statistics (NCHS): Provides birth and death data, including birth certificate information. (www.cdc.gov/nchs.)

U.S. Bureau of Justice Statistics: Collects information about juvenile offenders. (www.ojp.usdoj.gov/bjs.)

U.S. Bureau of Labor Statistics: Provides a variety of employment data. (http://www.bls.gov/)

U.S. Census Bureau: Provides current census figures and analysis. (www.census.gov.)

U.S. Department of Health and Human Services (USDHHS): Program *Healthy People 2020* is a framework of goals and objectives for the nation's health. (www.healthypeople.gov.)

health, but the results are mixed. Fortunately, scientific, medical, environmental, parenting, and other knowledge can lessen or eliminate many of the problems. It is a matter of making these concerns a priority and taking the necessary steps to elicit change. Box 16-7 lists several resources for monitoring the health and well-being of children.

Monitoring and Tracking

Federal, state, and local governments and many national organizations collect and analyze data to track the well-being of children and adolescents. For example, the Maternal and Child Health Bureau of the USDHHS (2012) generates a yearly report, *Child Health USA*, on child population characteristics, health status, and health care utilization. Such data are readily accessible online to citizens, health professionals, policymakers, and the media. A number of key indicators are tracked on a regular basis by the federal statistical system so that trends are revealed. State and local data also are used to track the well-being of children.

Healthy People 2020: Child and Adolescent Health

Many professions establish goals and set measurable objectives. Educators use these techniques to organize their teaching materials, measure their students' progress, and evaluate the effectiveness of their teaching strategies and plans. Health care professionals use them for similar purposes in client care. The individual community health nurse uses them in working with a family to ensure that the nurse and family are organized and are guided by common purposes. Goals and objectives help the nurse and family evaluate progress and make necessary midcourse corrections.

These strategies are also important at the macro level and the programmatic level, where multiple players must collaborate to address complicated statewide or nationwide problems. In 1979, the Surgeon General of the United States embarked on an ambitious task of convening hundreds of public health experts, health care researchers, health professional organizations, and others to develop the first health goals and objectives for the nation. At each of the intervening decades, these groups have developed a new set of goals and objectives to help bring clear focus to the health concerns of the nation and to set measurable and attainable goals for different age-groups and issues across the country.

Healthy People 2020 (USDHHS, 2013) sets broad national health goals for the first decade of the twenty-first century. This initiative, like its predecessors, helps define the nation's health agenda and guides policy development. *Healthy People 2020* addresses many challenges facing the country and helps the public and private sectors understand the nation's leading health problems, helps the two sectors develop strategic plans for addressing them, and collaborates to reach common goals. The *Healthy People* table lists selected objectives from *Healthy People 2020* related to child and adolescent health.

Since the inception of the *Healthy People* initiative in 1979, child and adolescent health has improved. For instance, there have been improvements in infant, child, and adolescent mortality, adolescent smoking, pregnancy, and violence.

Health Promotion and Disease Prevention

Health promotion and disease prevention are more significant and cost-effective for children than for any other age group. Primary health care and early intervention for children and

❤ HEALTHY PEOPLE 2020

Selected Objectives for Child and Adolescent Health

AH 2020-1: Increase the proportion of adolescents who have had a wellness checkup in the past 12 months.

AH HP2020–2: Increase the percentage of adolescents who participate in extracurricular and out-of-school activities.

EMC HP2020–1: (Developmental) Increase the proportion of children who are ready for school in all five domains of healthy development: physical development, social-emotional development, approaches to learning, language, and cognitive development.

EMC HP2020–3: Increase the proportion of elementary, middle, and senior high schools that require school health education.

EH HP2020-3: Reduce air toxic emissions to decrease the risk of adverse health effects caused by mobile, area, and major sources of airborne toxics.

FP HP2020–8: Reduce pregnancies among adolescent females.

FP HP2020–12: Increase the proportion of adolescents who received formal instruction on reproductive health topics before they were 18 years old.

NWS HP2020-10: Reduce the proportion of children and adolescents who are considered obese.

IID HP2020–1: Reduce chronic hepatitis B virus infections in infants and young children (perinatal infections).

IID HP2020–14: Reduce or eliminate or maintain elimination of cases of vaccine-preventable disease.

IVP HP2020–16: Increase age-appropriate vehicle restraint system use in children.

IVP HP2020–28: Increase the proportion of public and private schools that require students to wear appropriate protective gear when engaged in school-sponsored physical activities.

MICH HP2020–1: Reduce the rate of child deaths.

MICH HP2020– 9: Reduce preterm birth.

MICH-HP2020-16: Increase the proportion of women delivering a live birth who received preconception care services and practiced key recommended preconception health behaviors.

OH HP2020–4: Increase the proportion of low-income children and adolescents who received any preventive dental service during the past year.

PA HP2020–8: Increase the proportion of children and adolescents who do not exceed recommended limits for screen time.

SA HP2020–3: Increase the proportion of adolescents who disapprove of substance abuse.

TU HP2020–3: Reduce the initiation of tobacco use among children, adolescents, and young adults.

From U.S. Department of Health and Human Services: *Healthy People 2020,* Washington, DC, 2010, U.S. Government Printing Office. Retrieved from <http://www.healthypeople.gov/2020/default.asp>.

families can help prevent costly problems, suffering, and lost human potential. The following examples illustrate this point:

- Preterm birth, the leading cause of infant death and long-term neurological disabilities in children, costs the U.S. health care system more than $26 billion each year (CDC, 2013b).
- Preventing pregnancy among teenagers can reduce the rates of school dropout, welfare dependency, low birth weight, and infant mortality. It has been estimated that teen childbearing costs taxpayers at least $10.9 billion every year in expenses associated with health and foster care, criminal justice, and public assistance (National Campaign to Prevent Teen and Unplanned Pregnancy, 2013).

Health promotion and disease prevention strategies for improving child and adolescent health come in many forms and originate in research institutions, public agencies, private businesses, and community-based organizations. They can include the following:

- Clinical interventions
- Public health efforts that identify trends and develop population-based, community-wide, or individual strategies to affect them
- Philanthropic endeavors that fund initiatives at the community, state, and regional levels
- Public policy initiatives that create or improve public programs or provide incentives for nongovernmental entities to address identified problems

PUBLIC HEALTH PROGRAMS TARGETED TO CHILDREN AND ADOLESCENTS

A number of public programs address the health needs of children, and many target medically underserved or low-income individuals and families. In addition, local and state public health and social service agencies aim to protect the health of an entire community or state through programs such as water fluoridation, sanitation, and infectious disease control. Furthermore, broad-based strategies such as lead-based paint elimination, mandatory child safety seats in automobiles, bicycle helmet laws, teen pregnancy prevention programs, comprehensive school health clinics, and drug and violence prevention programs serve to improve the health of children using community-wide approaches.

Health Care Coverage Programs

Approximately 9.4% of American children under 18 years of age do not have health insurance. Hispanic children are far more likely than children of other races to be uninsured (DeNavas-Walt, Proctor, and Smith, 2012) (Figure 16-5). Those who do not have health insurance are more likely to lack a source of health care, to have unmet health needs, and to experience worse health outcomes than children with insurance. Efforts to expand health care coverage for pregnant women and children have been successful, and provisions of the Affordable Care Act promise to further ensure affordable preventive services and health care coverage for all Americans.

Affordable Care Act

The Affordable Care Act (ACA), signed into law by the President on March 23, 2010, and upheld by the U.S. Supreme Court on June 28, 2012, puts into place health care reforms set to roll out through 2014 and beyond. Among other features, the ACA lowers premium costs for millions of working families and small businesses by providing hundreds of billions of dollars in tax relief—the largest middle class tax cut for health care in history. It also reduces what families will have to pay for health care by capping out-of-pocket expenses and requiring preventive care to be fully covered without any out-of-pocket expense (USDHHS, n.d.).

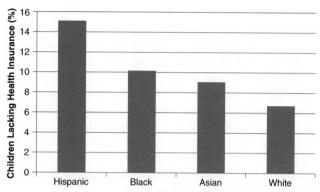

FIGURE 16-5 Children less than 18 years of age and lacking health insurance by race, 2011. (Data from DeNavas-Walt C, Proctor D, Smith J: *Income, poverty, and health insurance coverage in the United States: 2011* [U.S. Census Bureau Current Population Reports], 2012. Retrieved from <http://www.census.gov/prod/2012pubs/p60-243.pdf>.)

For pregnant women, the ACA expands options for health care insurance and makes them more affordable. Job-based health plans and new insurance plans are not allowed to deny or exclude coverage for pregnant women or children on the basis of a pre-existing condition, including a disability. The ACA mandates certain preventive services at no cost, such as vaccinations for children and breastfeeding support. Teens and adults younger than 26 years can stay insured under their parent's insurance plan if the plan allows dependent coverage.

Medicaid and the Children's Health Insurance Program

The ability to pay for health care greatly influences whether a parent takes a child to see a health care provider. Medicaid (Title XIX of the Social Security Act) is a health insurance program for poor and low-income people. It is a federal/state entitlement program that plays an important role in providing health coverage for low-income women and children. The federal government sets the minimum guidelines for Medicaid eligibility, and states can chose to expand eligibility through the Children's Health Insurance Program (CHIP). The average CHIP income eligibility level for children is 241% of the federal poverty level (FPL). Together, Medicaid and CHIP serve about half of low-income children (Centers for Medicare and Medicaid Services, n.d.).

Within broad national guidelines, each state establishes eligibility standards based on a family's income in comparison with the federal poverty level, determines the type and scope of services, and administers its own Medicaid and CHIP programs. States have some discretion in determining which population groups their programs will cover. Thus, a pregnant woman or child who is eligible for the program in one state may not be eligible in another.

Through the Early and Periodic Screening, Diagnosis, and Treatment (EPSDT) program, a child covered by Medicaid can receive a range of health and health-related services beginning in infancy. The program is designed to assure availability and accessibility of health care resources and to help

Medicaid recipients and their parents effectively use them. The program's services far exceed those usually covered by private insurance and include the following:

- Health, developmental, and nutritional screening
- Physical examinations
- Immunizations
- Vision and hearing screening
- Certain laboratory tests
- Dental services

Expansions in public health care insurance programs have helped many children achieve insurance coverage, but many children still lack insurance or other health care coverage like Medicaid or CHIP for many reasons, some of which are as follows:

- Insurance is too expensive.
- Medicaid has a welfare stigma, and parents do not want to be associated with it.
- Medicaid application forms and processes can be complex and burdensome and can intrude on a family's privacy.
- Parents may be concerned that their illegal immigration status may be revealed.
- Parents may not consider the importance of health insurance.
- Parents may not know their child is eligible for programs such as Medicaid and CHIP.
- Applications and other information may not be available in the family's language.

Although insurance gives a child financial access to health care, some children may not obtain the health care they need for other reasons. Numerous health care or family barriers can still stand in the way. They include the following:

- Lack of transportation
- Language barriers
- Misunderstanding or denial of the child's health problem
- Clinic or office hours that conflict with work or school schedules
- Overcrowded clinics with long delays in the waiting room (and parents often have more than one child in tow)
- Competing family or personal priorities that reduce the importance of obtaining care
- Some doctors' unwillingness to see Medicaid or low-income clients
- Parents' concerns that care providers are either unresponsive to their medical needs or interpersonally disrespectful
- Cost of deductibles or co-payments

To successfully meet the health needs of children and adolescents, especially those with known risk factors, the community health nurse must be cognizant of health care access issues, family and neighborhood influences, and other social concerns in a child's life. The nurse must be prepared to help the family solve problems, to be their health care system advocate, and to address the child's health needs in a culturally competent manner.

Direct Health Care Delivery Programs

Although Medicaid and CHIP finance health care for their enrollees like private insurance, several other public programs deliver health care services directly to underserved populations. Most underserved aggregates live in inner cities or rural areas with few health care providers and facilities. Some have Medicaid, CHIP, or other insurance coverage, but many are uninsured.

Maternal and Child Health Block Grant

The Maternal and Child Health (MCH) Block Grant program (also called Title V, because it is the fifth section, or title, of the Social Security Act) allocates federal funds to the states, and the states must contribute their own funds for maternal and child health services. It is administered by the Maternal and Child Health Bureau as a part of the USDHHS's Health Resources and Services Administration. Established in 1935, the Title V MCH Block Grant has provided a foundation of health care services for mothers, children, including those with special health care needs, and families over the years. States must match every four dollars of federal Title V money with three dollars of state and or local funding to help ensure the delivery of basic health care to pregnant women and children and help deliver additional services to children with special health care needs. Agencies in state health departments also monitor the health status of mothers and children throughout their respective states and work with other state agencies to develop programs to improve the health of this population.

The Consolidated Health Centers Program, managed by the Health Services Administration (HRSA) within the Department of Health and Human Services (HHS), provides funding to more than 9000 primary health care clinics (Health Care Clinics) in geographically isolated and economically distressed areas.

These health centers provide comprehensive, culturally competent, primary and preventive health care to a diverse population including individuals who are low income, uninsured and experiencing homelessness. Two thirds of those served are members of ethnic and minority groups, 36% percent are uninsured and more than one third are children. One out of every people living in the United States relies on a HRSA funded health clinic. This successful program provides primary care services including health, dental, mental health, pharmacy as well as services that promote access to health care such as language interpretation, case management, and transportation. Health Care clinics will play a key role in the implementation of the Affordable Care Act (USDHHS, n.d.)

School-Based Health Centers

Adolescents are the least likely aggregate to use health care services, especially preventive services. Their adolescent health care needs are different from their childhood needs, and they may be uncomfortable seeing a pediatrician or their childhood provider. Furthermore, they may or may not be able to discuss sensitive topics such as sexuality, substance use, and peer relationships with their parents. Some may not want their parents to know they have a health problem; therefore they may not want to see the family's health care provider out of concern about privacy and confidentiality. Therefore their health care needs may go unmet.

School-based health centers typically provide a combination of screening and preventive services, primary care, mental health and substance abuse counseling, dental health, nutrition education, and other health promotion activities. State dollars, mostly from general funds and the MCH Block Grant, are the primary sources of funding for school-based health care. A growing number of health centers participate in the Medicaid and CHIP programs, and some provide services within a managed care network. Expansion of school-based health centers has been made possible under the Affordable Care Act.

Special Supplemental Nutrition Program for Women, Infants, and Children (WIC)

Although it is not a health program exclusively, WIC gives federal grants to states for the purpose of serving nutritionally at-risk, low-income, pregnant and postpartum women and their children up to 5 years of age. WIC programs provide highly nutritious foods, nutrition education and counseling, and screening and referral to needed services. To be eligible, women and children must meet income guidelines established by each state, and a health professional must determine they are at "nutritional risk." Women and children who participate in Medicaid, the Food Stamp program, or the Temporary Assistance for Needy Families program are automatically income eligible for WIC. Fifty-three percent of all infants born in the United States are served by WIC (U.S. Department of Agriculture Food and Nutrition Service, 2013).

WIC clinics operate in a number of sites, including health clinics, hospitals, schools, public housing sites, and mobile clinics. Women participating in the program are encouraged to obtain prenatal care if they are pregnant. They are also encouraged to maintain healthy diets and obtain preventive health care for themselves and their children, including childhood immunizations. WIC participants receive checks or vouchers to purchase specific, nutritious foods. Most grocery stores and supermarkets participate in WIC and carry the foods designated by the program.

Established in 1972, WIC is one of the most successful, popular, and cost-effective public health programs. Some of the many benefits attributed to WIC include the following:

- Improvements in birth outcomes and health care cost savings
- Improved infant feeding practices, better low-birth-weight rate, and more regular primary care
- Lower rates of childhood obesity

SHARING RESPONSIBILITY FOR IMPROVING CHILD AND ADOLESCENT HEALTH

Most children in the United States are born healthy and remain healthy throughout childhood. However, the protective factors operating in the lives of healthy children and the interventions they receive are not available to all children. Although public sector programs have attempted to provide a "safety net" for children, these interventions cannot address all the needs of children. For example, the health care system

---

BOX 16-8   BREASTFEEDING: THE FEEDING METHOD OF CHOICE

Breastfeeding is uniquely superior for infant feeding. The practice imparts many health benefits for mothers and babies.
  Benefits for children include the following:
- Decreased incidence and severity of a wide range of infectious diseases
- Decreased infant mortality
- Decreased risk of Sudden Infant Death Syndrome
- Reduction in the incidence of diabetes, respiratory infections, and some cancers
- Lower risk of overweight and obesity
- Enhanced cognitive development
  Benefits of breastfeeding for mothers include the following:
- Decreased postpartum bleeding
- Earlier return to prepregnancy weight
- Decreased risk of breast and ovarian cancer

  The American Academy of Pediatrics (AAP) and many other health organizations recommend exclusive breastfeeding for the first 6 months of life with continuation of breastfeeding for 1 year or longer as mutually desired by mother and infant (AAP, 2012).

---

may provide emergency care to a 9-year-old child injured by gunfire in a drive-by shooting, but it cannot address the community conditions that perpetuate violence.

Child health is affected by many factors; therefore, the responsibility for improving children's health rests with the entire community. This responsibility begins with parents and includes health care professionals, community groups, businesses, and the public sector. When a child is older, he or she can be responsible for practicing healthy behaviors and obtaining proper health care.

Parents' Role

Even before conception, a woman can help ensure the health of her fetus by practicing healthy behaviors herself. Reproductive life planning can help a woman set personal goals and priorities and design strategies to meet these goals. This planning may entail avoiding unwanted pregnancy and/or learning about specific actions she can take to increase her chances for having a healthy baby should she desire a child in the future. If pregnancy is desired, a woman can learn to manage chronic health conditions and to develop healthy behaviors, including proper nutrition with folic acid supplementation, avoidance of tobacco, alcohol, drugs, and other behaviors that could harm a developing baby. It is also important for the mother to receive prenatal care early in pregnancy.

Starting with breastfeeding, parents must give their children nutritious food and ensure that they are immunized, receive needed health care services, and acquire healthful lifestyles. Breastfeeding provides many health benefits for mothers and their children (Box 16-8).

Another important task for parents is to ensure that their children have a safe environment at home, in the neighborhood, and at school. They must protect their children from injury, violence, abuse, and neglect. Parents must learn how to nurture, guide, and protect their children effectively through the developmental stages of childhood and adolescence.

Community's Role

Families need support from their community and society to fulfill their roles and responsibilities. This is particularly true for families who live in poverty and for parents who are isolated and disenfranchised. Ensuring access to health care is an important community role, but communities are also responsible for promoting well-being, which goes far beyond the provision of traditional medical care.

Communities should work to create safe neighborhoods and support the development of community-based comprehensive health, education, housing, and social service programs. Collaborative, multi-partner approaches that concentrate on helping children and adolescents avoid risks and develop social competence are more likely to be effective than fragmented programs focusing on individual risks, such as teen drug use. Communities are well situated to facilitate the integration of health, education, and social services; to eliminate fragmentation and duplication of services; to provide culturally competent care; and to better organize more comprehensive and streamlined systems of care. Although many health and social service programs exist, they can be poorly coordinated with one another, with little collaboration among the professional disciplines.

The media are part of the community at large and should be involved in promoting child and adolescent health. The media significantly influence children's lives, their perceptions of the world, and their self-images. From developing informational campaigns about prenatal care and immunizations to discouraging violence and explicit sex in advertising and popular television programs, the media can have a profound effect on improving children's health and well-being.

Employer's Role

Business and industry have an enormous stake in the health of the nation's children. A strong, productive workforce is ensured only when the health, social, and educational needs of the next generation of workers are met. Furthermore, health risks cost employers in lost productivity and increased health care costs.

The private sector can play a role in improving the health of individual children or the community in general. An employer can make health care more accessible to families with children by offering affordable health insurance that covers employees and dependents. The provision of insurance plans that offers full pregnancy and well-child health care benefits is essential to employee health promotion. Employers can meet the requirements of the U.S. Department of Labor (2013) by supporting nursing mothers in the workplace. This includes providing reasonable break time to express milk and a private space other than a bathroom in which to do so.

Maintaining a workplace that allows flexible leave for prenatal and pediatric health care and allows time off to care for newborn and sick children can also contribute to child health improvements. In 1993, the Family and Medical Leave Act mandated that employers with 50 or more employees must allow a total of 12 work weeks of unpaid leave during any 12-month period for the birth, adoption, or foster care of a child or for the care of a seriously ill family member or the employee himself or herself (U.S. Department of Labor, n.d.).

In addition, employers can sponsor education opportunities for employees about topics such as healthy diets, healthy pregnancies, substance abuse, and stress management. Businesses can also offer on-site child care and can work with community leaders and public officials to initiate community-wide health promotion projects targeted to children. Finally, employers can be catalysts in their communities for linking health, education, and social services for children.

Government's Role

In the United States, government's role in promoting or ensuring children's health is more limited than in many other countries. Other countries often have defined policies on children's health; the United States does not. Such policies not only indicate that children are a priority of the citizenry but also help shape the operation of programs and their funding.

As discussed earlier, U.S. state and federal governments have several public health programs that provide assistance to children, especially to those at risk from poverty or other disadvantages. Monitoring the health of children is also a governmental role. Although these programs are not a substitute for a family or caregiver's care and concern, they are important in protecting and promoting health and delivering services to those who would otherwise go without. Programs with significant funding exist, but many children with health problems do not receive the services they need for reasons previously discussed.

Managers and front-line workers (e.g., community health nurses, social workers, physicians, and caseworkers) in effective community programs should be encouraged to collaborate and thereby assist children with problems that adversely impact their health. "One-stop shopping" (i.e., user-friendly, accessible services for children and families) is an important concept for public and community programs to embrace to ensure that children easily receive needed services. Outreach and referral efforts should be an integral part of health initiatives to provide children with the services they require. Community health nurses are often an essential part of these efforts.

Community Health Nurse's Role

Public health nurses have always played pivotal roles in improving the health status of pregnant women, children, and adolescents. Within the community, the community health nurse is often most aware of children's health status, any barriers that prevent children from receiving necessary care, and other factors that may adversely affect their health. Armed with this information and knowledge about available health resources in the community, the community health nurse is:

- An advocate for improved individual and community responses to children's needs
- A researcher for effective strategies to serve women and children
- A participant in publicly funded programs

- A promoter of social interventions that enhance the living situations of high-risk families
- A partner with other professionals to improve service collaboration and coordination

One important role of the community health nurse is to help link local health and social services with the school system. Children must be healthy to learn; however, children may come to school with vision, hearing, and other health problems that appropriate education, screening, and treatment could have prevented or alleviated. When children pass the preschool years, the school health nurse is sometimes their only connection to the health care system. School health nurses can be important sources of primary health care and health information for students and their families.

Community health nurses can alert the health professional community, business leaders, religious groups, and voluntary organizations to children's and adolescents' needs and to the strategies that can improve their health. Community health nurses can influence the planning and implementation of necessary changes in the health care system to ensure improved children's health and to achieve the national health goals for the year 2020. Also, they can promote commitment within their own institutions for comprehensive, culturally competent care.

Home visiting is a promising strategy that connects community health nurses, paraprofessionals or lay home visitors to families in order to provide education, support, and referrals (Olds et al, 2010). One home visiting model, administered through Nurse-Family Partnership, partners low-income, first-time mothers with maternal and child health nurses. Pregnant women develop trusting relationships with their nurse home visitors and receive the care and support needed for healthy pregnancy and parenting. Financial self-sufficiency is encouraged (http://www.nursefamily partnership.org/).

LEGAL AND ETHICAL ISSUES IN CHILD AND ADOLESCENT HEALTH

Every day, community health nurses are involved in making decisions. In each encounter with a client, the nurse's decisions or the family's choices have the potential to influence the health and well-being of the family or the community at large for better or for worse.

People often assume that health care professionals, particularly nurses, are by nature attuned to the ethical implications of their decisions. In addition, the community trusts that nurses are aware of the legal ramifications of their actions and decisions, of their clients' decisions, and of the health care and legal systems' decisions. In reality, the ever-changing pressures of serving the community's health care needs leave little time to reflect on the ethical and moral implications of a given situation. In some cases, it may seem easier to avoid tough decisions. An ethical approach to decision making allows the community health nurse to evaluate a client's or a population's needs more honestly and completely and take appropriate action. Understanding the legal environment will help the nurse make informed decisions and effectively assist clients with their decision-making processes.

Ethical Issues

The complex nature of public health and health care delivery environments often sets the stage for conflicts of interest and values. Meanwhile, nurses and other health professionals must work within the system to improve child and adolescent health in a country of great differences. Such differences exist between races and cultures, and there are great dichotomies, such as the affluence of some and the poverty of many others. For the perinatal nurse, for example, ethical dilemmas may arise because she is an advocate for two clients: the pregnant woman and her fetus. The scope of ethical and legal dilemmas is broad. The Ethical Insights box lists specific ethical issues related to child and adolescent health.

⚖ ETHICAL INSIGHTS

Ethical Issues Related to Child and Adolescent Health

Allocation decisions: Given limited time and resources, what level of care should a nurse offer a child and his or her family?

Maternal-fetal conflict: Sometimes there are opposing ethical concerns for the pregnant woman and her fetus—for example, whether the benefits of prolonging a pregnancy justify the risk of complications for a pregnant woman or whether court-ordered treatment for a substance-abusing pregnant woman overrides the right to autonomy for a pregnant woman.

Client autonomy: In each specific case, who should make health care decisions for a young client, especially when opposing opinions arise? The client? The parents or guardian? The nurse or other health care professional? At what age does a child become mature enough to participate in such decision making? What laws does any given state have that affect adolescent client autonomy? What should the community health nurse do if he or she believes the client's or parent's decisions are not in the best interest of the client?

Privacy and confidentiality: Is an intervention appropriate if the community health nurse identifies gross noncompliance, neglect, or abuse? Is an intervention appropriate if in making it the nurse must break confidentiality? When and how should the nurse take action?

"Gaming the system": When the health care system's rules appear to impede the nurse's ability to serve the client's best interest, is it acceptable to circumvent the system? If so, what are the moral and legal costs?

Cultural competence: The United States will continue to experience huge demographic changes and greater diversity; nurses will face different cultural definitions of what is and what is not acceptable or ethical. How should the community health nurse respond to a client or population group that does not share the same cultural outlook on health? What is the nurse's legal justification, if any, for responding in a certain way?

Health disparities and access to care: What are the nurses' responsibilities in ensuring that women and children have access to health care? How can nurses influence policy decisions that impact community health care?

Prenatal diagnosis and newborn screening: What are potential long-term consequences of identifying genetic conditions? Are parents fully informed of negative consequences of genetic diagnoses, including stigmatization, discrimination, and psychological effects?

These issues invariably involve value judgments and challenge a nurse's bounds of professional and personal duty. They also require the community health nurse to stay abreast of legislative changes at the local, state, and national levels and participate in professional activities that can help him or her stay current in these important matters. By recognizing the ethical implications of the care and advice they give or the actions they take, nurses can embrace their duty to promote the health and well-being of individual clients and the community more completely, protect their clients from harm, and strive for health care fairness and justice for all clients.

Recognizing the value of engaging in a shared dialogue with colleagues regarding ethical decision-making issues and understanding the possible legal implications of their decisions are equally important. The choices can be complex; therefore receiving the guidance of an ethics board or gaining a second opinion can be critical to making the right choices. On a broader scale, a community health nurse's ethical perspective can enhance any discussion about individual client care and overall community health and also can affect the direction of the country's public health policy.

CASE STUDY APPLICATION OF THE NURSING PROCESS

By applying the principles of the nursing process to the individual, family, and community, the community health nurse can provide services to children and adolescents more systematically and effectively. Most communities offer a range of preventive services and other important programs that children need. The community health nurse must thoroughly understand the needs of the individual child and family and must be aware of available community resources to help meet the child's health needs, as this case study illustrates.

Maria Martinez, a community health nurse working for the county health department, received a call from the high school nurse informing her that a 16-year-old high school student named Kaylah M. would come in that afternoon for a pregnancy test. Kaylah had already missed three menstrual periods and was afraid to talk about it with her family. She had a long discussion with the school nurse and asked her boyfriend, also aged 16, to take her to the health department clinic after school for the pregnancy test.

Assessment

Kaylah's pregnancy test result was positive, and she was an estimated 3 months pregnant. She was upset and would not speak with Maria at the health department. With agreement from Kaylah, Maria arranged to make a home visit the next afternoon.

Knowing that she needed to address a number of issues at the first home visit, Maria prepared by developing a list of possible assessment areas that covered individual, family, and community concerns, as follows:

Individual
- Medical risk factors
- Emotional well-being, including concerns about community safety, domestic violence, and sexual abuse
- Cultural beliefs and attitudes toward pregnancy and medical care
- Barriers to communication with providers, such as language, hearing, and sight
- Understanding and acceptance of pregnancy
- Health-promoting and risk-taking behaviors
- Understanding the importance of obtaining preventive care services
- Health insurance status
- Access to transportation

Family
- Adequacy of housing structure
- Safety of neighborhood
- Ability of family members to provide emotional support
- Ability of family to provide financial support
- Ability and willingness of the father of the baby to provide support

Community
- Availability of affordable and culturally sensitive prenatal and pediatric care
- Health and social services coordination
- Emotional guidance and counseling

- Educational opportunities for pregnant and parenting teenagers
- Job training
- Nutrition services such as WIC and food stamps
- Pregnancy and parenting education
- Child care availability

Assessment Data
Individual
- Kaylah was already in the early second trimester of pregnancy and had not received prenatal care. She also engaged in risk-taking behaviors (i.e., smoking, alcohol use, unprotected sex, and poor eating habits) potentially detrimental to her baby.
- During the interview, Kaylah seemed quiet and reserved. She said she was excited to have a baby but feared labor and delivery.
- Her boyfriend wanted her to keep the baby but was not committed to supporting Kaylah or the baby. He did not want to involve his own parents.
- She said she did not think about prenatal care much but would probably visit a health clinic sometime before her delivery. Her family did not have health insurance, and she said they could not afford prenatal care.
- She wanted to keep the baby and remain in school, yet she did not have a realistic understanding of parental responsibilities.

Family
- When Kaylah told her parents she was pregnant, they expressed disappointment. Her mother voiced a willingness to provide emotional support, but her seemingly emotionally distant father expressed anger.
- Both parents expressed concern about how the family would manage financially.
- After a brief review of the family's financial situation, it appeared that Kaylah was eligible for Medicaid and WIC.
- Her parents wanted her to have no further contact with her boyfriend.

Community
- Maria determined that prenatal services were available, but only during school hours. Although the only clinic that accepted Medicaid clients was on the other side of town, a nearby obstetrical practice with a certified nurse-midwife on staff accepted clients with Medicaid coverage. However, their primary clientele consisted of middle-class, married women.
- Applying for Medicaid and the WIC program required Kaylah to go to the welfare office and apply during school hours. However, the hospital outpatient department could make a preliminary Medicaid eligibility determination, which might be more convenient.
- Although Medicaid would pay for some prenatal classes, those nearby were geared to older, married couples.
- Kaylah's school encouraged her to remain in regular classes until her delivery date and participate in home study for a limited time thereafter.

- No parenting classes geared toward adolescents were available.
- Child care was not available at the high school, making a return to school more difficult for Kaylah.
- Although the community has a lay home visitor program that matches mentors with pregnant and parenting teens and provides health information and encouragement, the project does not serve Kaylah's neighborhood.

Diagnosis

Individual

- Unhealthy lifestyle choices related to the lack of prenatal care and the effect of poor nutrition, smoking, and alcohol use on fetal development
- Parenting issues related to unrealistic expectations about parenting responsibilities
- Lack of knowledge related to infant and child safety issues, such as the use of child safety seats, advantages of breastfeeding, safe sleep for infants, and use of preventive health care, including immunizations

Family

- Disrupted family dynamics related to anger and disappointment over daughter's pregnancy
- Altered financial status resulting from the addition of another dependent to the family

Community

- Lack of coordinated, culturally sensitive, accessible prenatal and parenting services for adolescents
- Existing lay home visitor program not available

Planning

To ensure the action plan is complete, realistic, and successfully implemented, Maria must thoroughly identify the factors affecting Kaylah's health and well-being. In addition, Kaylah, her family, and Maria must set mutual goals.

Individual

Long-Term Goals

- Pregnancy outcome will be healthy for mother and infant.
- Kaylah will demonstrate successful parenting behaviors.
- Kaylah will complete high school.

Short-Term Goals

- Kaylah will obtain prenatal care.
- Kaylah will understand the reasons to change nutrition and substance use habits.
- Kaylah and the nurse will plan actions to change poor health habits.
- Kaylah will remain in school throughout her pregnancy and will use the home study program until she returns to school after her baby is born.
- Kaylah will enroll in parenting class. If classes are not available, she will use age-appropriate reading materials, films, CDs, Internet resources, opportunities for group discussion with other teens, or visits with experienced parents.
- Kaylah will breastfeed her baby.
- Kaylah will speak with the community health educator to determine methods to protect the health and safety of her newborn.

Family

Long-Term Goal

- The family's ability to handle crises will improve with their ability to discuss problems and engage in mutual problem solving.

Short-Term Goal

- Kaylah's parents will display supportive behaviors, such as accompanying her to prenatal care appointments, helping her engage in healthy behaviors, and helping her arrange child care so she can remain in school.

Community

Long-Term Goal

- Accessible, comprehensive, culturally sensitive prenatal and other health care services will be established, including home visiting and parenting classes targeted to adolescents.

Short-Term Goals

- The health department clinic will extend evening hours to accommodate students and working families.
- A child care facility will open in or near the high school.

Intervention

The nurse, family, and individual must address their immediate, mutual goals to help Kaylah achieve a healthy birth outcome and begin successful parenting. Interdisciplinary planning among Kaylah's school health nurse, caseworker, community health nurse, primary pregnancy care provider, childbirth educator, and family planning nurse is critical. In addition, Maria must be an advocate for community-wide change to ensure that the community is meeting individuals' needs.

Individual

Maria worked with the school nurse and other health professionals to help Kaylah obtain Medicaid and WIC; she was referred to an obstetrician who saw her regularly. Kaylah's pregnancy was also monitored by the school nurse, who had her come to the clinic on a weekly basis to check her weight and blood pressure and to talk with her about pregnancy-related issues.

Working with the school nurse, Maria provided Kaylah with information on childbirth classes and nutrition as well as booklets detailing how to promote a healthy pregnancy. She was counseled to avoid tobacco, alcohol, and all drugs. Near the end of the pregnancy, Kaylah was encouraged to attend parenting classes with her boyfriend.

Family

Maria and the social worker referred Kaylah's parents to other social service agencies that might be able to help financially. In particular, they focused on providers who could assist with utilities, job placement, and child care. The family was also referred to a family counselor who specialized in working with families with adolescent children.

Community

Maria worked with the maternal-child health division of the county health department to help facilitate offering parenting classes at an area high school, targeting the learning needs of pregnant teens. She and the school nurse also met with school district officials and community leaders to stimulate dialogue about the consequences of dropping out of high school and to facilitate action in policies such as child care for parenting teenagers to help them remain in school.

Evaluation

Evaluation strategies must involve both process and outcome measures on the individual, family, and community levels.

Individual

The school nurse was able to monitor Kaylah throughout her pregnancy and was aware that she finished classes for the term. Kaylah's pregnancy was unremarkable, and she delivered a healthy boy. Their health care expenses were covered by Medicaid, and the baby was determined to also be eligible for CHIP. A home-based teacher was assigned to work with Kaylah for 1 month after delivery

Continued

CASE STUDY   APPLICATION OF THE NURSING PROCESS—cont'd

to ensure that she was able to keep up with her coursework. With the assistance of the social worker, Kaylah was able to place the baby in a subsidized day care facility, allowing her to finish school.

Family

Family counseling helped the family resolve some of their issues. Maria observed that Kaylah's parents were proud of their grandson and eager to help with his care.

Community

With the help of the school nurse and other interested parties, Maria was able to initiate a collaborative program in which health department nurses and developmental specialists offered parenting classes in high schools on a regular basis. They were also planning on writing for a Maternal Child Health Block Grant to implement a school-based clinic focusing on the needs of pregnant teens and their infants.

Levels of Prevention

Primary

- Primary prevention depends largely on the child's age. For the youngest children, strategies include encouraging healthy behaviors by girls and women.

- Primary prevention also includes the prevention of unwanted pregnancy, which is especially important for adolescents.

Secondary

- Once pregnant, the woman must receive early and adequate prenatal care, practice healthy behaviors, obtain necessary social and supportive services, and prepare herself for becoming a parent.
- It is incumbent on the community to ensure that adequate preventive health services, such as prenatal care, nutrition and dietary counseling, pregnancy and parent education, and social services, are available.

Tertiary

- Initiate programs and services that prevent future unwanted pregnancy among teenagers and help the parenting teenager provide the best possible care to the child.
- Establish programs such as parenting classes; support services to help adolescents complete their education; coordination of health and social services for the mother and her child; and well-child care, immunizations, and nutrition services.

SUMMARY

Child and adolescent health status remains an important indicator of the nation's health. The health of a child sets the foundation for school readiness and future success. Child and adolescent health problems are reflections of rapidly changing social conditions, not isolated events. Despite generally improving trends in health for most children, community health nurses must address discrepancies that exist between racial and ethnic groups. Poverty is the basis for many continuing health problems among children in this country, and nurses must recognize and treat it as such.

The best way to ensure the success and well-being of future generations is for each child to begin life healthy and maintain that health status throughout childhood. Any health problem (e.g., hunger and poor nutrition, asthma, poor vision or hearing, anemia, dental caries, mental health problems, illicit drug use, or teen pregnancy) can interfere with school attendance, academic success, normal growth and development, learning ability, and life success.

The prevention of health problems is most significant and cost-effective for children. Each dollar spent on the prevention of physical and emotional problems in children is a sound investment. Primary health care and early intervention for children and families can help prevent costly problems, suffering, and the loss of human potential. Community health nurses can use their experience and "inside knowledge" of barriers to child health to educate others. Rather than limiting their approach to caring for the individual and family only, community health nurses can maximize their roles to collaborate and forge necessary alliances to solve children's health problems. Nurses are authority figures in the least expected places. Working on health care's front line is

a powerful and very real position to members of Congress, state legislators, mayors, and other leaders. By creatively using this kind of power, community health nurses can contribute greatly to improving the health and well-being of all children.

LEARNING ACTIVITIES

1. Examine infant mortality statistics in the community, and compare the rates with state and national averages. Is infant mortality higher for any particular racial or ethnic group within the community?
2. Determine how a non–English-speaking immigrant without finances or available transportation would obtain prenatal care.
3. Accompany a pregnant woman to a local department of social services, and observe as she tries to establish Medicaid eligibility for herself and her unborn child.
4. Develop strategies to inform parents whose children are uninsured about the availability of CHIP.
5. Spend a day with a school health nurse, and analyze what could help prevent or address the health problems and issues he or she encountered throughout the day.
6. Survey businesses in the community to determine whether they offer maternity health insurance benefits, paid or unpaid maternity or paternity leave, and leave for prenatal care appointments. Is there a location within each worksite where women can pump breast milk? Use this information to develop a strategy to encourage family-friendly policies and practices in the business community.
7. If the community has a lay home visitor program, meet with a home visitor and, if possible, accompany him or her during home visits.

8. Communicate with those in policy-making positions by writing letters or holding meetings about children's needs.
9. Identify the public health and advocacy organizations in the community that are working to address children's health needs, and identify their strategies for promoting child health within the community.

ⓔ **EVOLVE WEBSITE**

http://evolve.elsevier.com/Nies
- NCLEX Review Questions
- Case Studies
- Glossary

REFERENCES

American Academy of Pediatrics: Ad Hoc Task Force on Definition of the Medical Home: The medical home, *Pediatrics* 90(5):774, 1992. Also available from <http://pediatrics.aappublications.org/content/90/5/774.abstract?sid=655ecdcd-5e4f-47ab-9dad-59ab0865762a>.

American Academy of Pediatrics: Section on Breastfeeding: Breastfeeding and the use of human milk, *Pediatrics* 129(3):e827–e841, 2012. Also available from <http://pediatrics.aappublications.org/content/early/2012/02/22/peds.2011-3552>.

American Academy of Pediatrics National Center for Medical Home Implementation: *National initiatives overview*, n.d. Available from <http://www.medicalhomeinfo.org/national/>.

American Academy of Pediatrics: Task Force on Sudden Infant Death Syndrome: SIDS and other sleep-related infant deaths: expansion of recommendations for a safe infant sleeping environment, *Pediatrics* 128(5):e1341–e1367, 2011. Also available from http://pediatrics.aappublications.org/content/128/5/e1341.full?sid=bd9574fb-4575-4d35-a46e-a63394e68331.

Center on the Developing Child at Harvard University: *The Science of neglect: The persistent absence of responsive care disrupts the developing brain: working paper 12*, 2012. Available from <www.developingchild.harvard.edu>.

Centers for Disease Control and Prevention: *How tobacco smoke causes disease: A report of the surgeon general*, Atlanta, 2010, U.S. Department of Health and Human Services. >.

Centers for Disease Control and Prevention: *About BMI for children and teens*, 2011a. Available from <http://www.cdc.gov/healthyweight/assessing/bmi/childrens_bmi/about_childrens_bmi.htm>.

Centers for Disease Control and Prevention: Health disparities and inequalities report—United States, 2011, *Morb Mortal Wkly Rep* 60(Suppl):1–114, 2011b. Also available from <http://www.cdc.gov/mmwr/pdf/other/su6001.pdf>.

Centers for Disease Control and Prevention: *Sexually transmitted disease surveillance*, 2011c. Available from <http://www.cdc.gov/std/stats11/Surv2011.pdf>.

Centers for Disease Control and Prevention: Alcohol use and binge drinking among women of childbearing age —United States, 2006–2010, *MMWR Morb Mortal Wkly Rep.* 61(28):534–538, 2012a. Also available from <www.cdc.gov/mmwr/preview/mmwrhtml/mm6128a4.htm?s_cid=mm6128a4_e%0D%0A>.

Centers for Disease Control and Prevention: *fetal alcohol spectrum disorders: Preventing alcohol use during pregnancy*, 2012b. Available from <http://www.cdc.gov/ncbddd/fasd/research-preventing.html>.

Centers for Disease Control and Prevention: Youth risk behavior surveillance—United States, 2011, *MMWR Morb Mortal Wkly Rep 2012* 61(SS-4), 2012c.

Centers for Disease Control and Prevention: *Youth violence: Facts at a glance*, 2012d. Available from <http://www.cdc.gov/ViolencePrevention/pub/YV_DataSheet.html>.

Centers for Disease Control and Prevention: *Immunization schedules*, 2013a. Available from <http://www.cdc.gov/vaccines/schedules/>.

Centers for Disease Control and Prevention: *preterm birth*, 2103b. Available from <http://www.cdc.gov/reproductivehealth/maternalinfanthealth/PretermBirth.htm>.

Centers for Disease Control and Prevention: Progress in increasing breastfeeding and reducing racial/ethnic differences—United States, 2000–2008 births, *Morb Mortal Wkly Rep* 62(05):77–80, 2013c. Also available from <http://www.cdc.gov/mmwr/preview/mmwrhtml/mm6205a1.htm?s_cid=govD_dnpao_260>.

Centers for Disease Control and Prevention: *Sudden unexpected infant death (SUID)*, 2013d. Available from <http://www.cdc.gov/sids/>.

Centers for Medicare and Medicaid Services: *Medicare.gov: Children*, n.d. Available from <http://www.medicaid.gov/Medicaid-CHIP-Program-Information/By-Population/Children/Children.html>.

Conde-Agudelo A, Rosas-Bermúdez A, Kafury-Goeta A: Birth spacing and risk of adverse perinatal outcomes: A meta-analysis, *JAMA* 295(15):1809–1823, 2006, http://dx.doi.org/10.1001/jama.295.15.1809.

DeNavas-Walt C, Proctor D, Smith J: *Income, poverty, and health insurance coverage in the United States: 2011* (U.S. Census Bureau Current Population Reports), 2012. Available from <http://www.census.gov/prod/2012pubs/p60-243.pdf>.

Engle WA, Kominiarek MA: Late preterm infants, early term infants and timing of elective deliveries, *Clin Perinatol* 35(2):325–341, 2008.

Federal Interagency Forum on Child and Family Statistics: *America's children in brief: key indicators of wellbeing*, 2013. Available from <www.childstats.gov/americaschildren/demo.asp>.

Finer LB, Zolna MR: Unintended pregnancy in the United States: incidence and disparities, 2006, *Contraception* 84(5):478–485, 2011.

Hamilton BE, Ventura SJ: *Birth rates for U.S. teenagers reach historic lows for all age and ethnic groups (NCHS Data Brief no 89)*, Hyattsville, MD, 2012, National Center for Health Statistics. Also available from <http://www.cdc.gov/nchs/data/databriefs/db89.pdf>.

Hoyert DL, Xu JQ: *Deaths: Preliminary data for 2011 (National Vital Statistics Reports vol. 61, no. 6)*, Hyattsville, MD, 2012, National Center for Health Statistics.

Institute of Medicine: *The childhood immunization schedule and safety: Stakeholder concerns, scientific evidence, and future studies*, Washington, DC, 2013, National Academies Press. Also available from <http://www.iom.edu/Reports/2013/The-Childhood-Immunization-Schedule-and-Safety.aspx>.

Johnston LD, O'Malley PM, Bachman JG, et al.: *Monitoring the future national results on adolescent drug use: overview of key findings, 2008 (NIH Publication no. 09–7401)*, Bethesda, MD, 2009, National Institute on Drug Abuse.

Kovar C, Salsberry P: Does a satisfactory relationship with her mother influence when a 16-year-old begins to have sex? MCN, *The American Journal of Maternal/Child Nursing* 37(2):122–129, 2012.

Lauritsen J, White N: *Violent crime against youth, 1994-2010*, Office of Justice Programs, Bureau of Justice Statistics, U.S. Department of Justice, 2012. Available from <http://bjs.ojp.usdoj.gov/index.cfm?ty=pbdetail&iid=4575>.

Leeb RT, Paulozzi L, Melanson C, et al.: *Child maltreatment surveillance: uniform definitions for public health and recommended data elements, version 1.0*, Atlanta, 2008, Centers for Disease Control and Prevention, National Center for Injury Prevention and Control.

Leonardi-Bee J, Smyth A, Britton J, et al.: Environmental tobacco smoke and fetal health: systematic review and meta-analysis, *Arch Dis Child Fetal Neonatal Ed* 93:F351–F361, 2008.

Lumley J, Chamberlain C, Dowswell T, et al.: Interventions for promoting smoking cessation during pregnancy, *Cochrane Database of Systematic Reviews* (3):CD001055, 2009, http://dx.doi.org/10.1002/14651858.CD001055.pub3.

MacDorman MF, Mathews TJ: *Recent trends in infant mortality in the United States (NCHS Data Brief no. 9)*, Hyattsville, MD, 2008, National Center for Health Statistics.

MacDorman MF, Mathews TJ: *Understanding racial and ethnic disparities in U.S. infant mortality rates (NCHS Data Brief no 74)*, Hyattsville, MD, 2011, National Center for Health Statistics. Also available from <http://www.cdc.gov/nchs/data/databriefs/db74.htm>.

Martin JA, Hamilton BE, Ventura SJ, et al: *Births: Final data for 2010, (National Vital Statistics Reports vol. 61 no. 1),* Hyattsville, MD, 2012, National Center for Health Statistics.

Martinez G, Copen CE, Abma JC: Teenagers in the United States: Sexual activity, contraceptive use, and childbearing, 2006–2010, national survey of family growth, *Vital Health Stat* 23(31):1–35, 2011.

Moos M-K: From concept to practice: Reflections on the preconception health agenda, *Journal of Women's Health* 19(3):561–567, 2010.

Moos M-K, Badura M, Posner S, et al.: Quality improvement opportunities in preconception and interconception care. In *March of Dimes: Toward improving the outcome of pregnancy, III,* White Plains, NY, 2010, March of Dimes Foundation.

Morse SB, Zheng H, Tang Y, et al: Early school-age outcomes of late preterm infants, *Pediatrics* 123(4):e622–e629, 2009.

National Campaign to Prevent Teen and Unplanned Pregnancy: *Counting it up: the public costs of Teen childbearing.* Available from <http://www.thenationalcampaign. org/costs/ciu/counting-it-up-2013.pdf >. Accessed March 7, 2013.

National Center for Children in Poverty: *Child poverty,* 2013. Available from <http://www. nccp.org/topics/childpoverty.html>.

National Conference of State Legislatures: *Synthetic drug threats,* 2012. Available from <http://www.ncsl.org/issues-research/justice/synthetic-drug-threats.aspx>.

National Highway Traffic Safety Administration: *Child safety: Is your child in the right car seat?* 2013. Available from <http://www. nhtsa.gov/Safety/CPS>.

National Institute on Drug Abuse: *Preventing drug abuse: The best strategy,* 2010. Available from <http://www.drugabuse.gov/publica tions/science-addiction/preventing-drug-abuse-best-strategy>.

Olds DL, Kitzman HJ, Cole RE, et al: Enduring effects of prenatal and infancy home visiting by nurses on maternal life course and government spending: follow-up of a randomized trial among children at age 12 years, *Arch Pediatr Adolesc Med* 164(5):419–424, 2010.

Ogden CL, Carroll MD, Kit BK, et al: Prevalence of obesity and trends in body mass index among US children and adolescents, 1999-2010, *JAMA* 307(5):483–490, 2012.

Organisation for Economic Co-operation and Development: *Health: Key Tables from OECD, No. 14: Infant mortality,* 2013. Available from < http://www.oecd-ilibrary.org/social-issues-migration-health/infant-mortality_20758480-table9>.

Oshiro BT, Henry E, Wilson J, et al: Decreasing elective deliveries before 39 weeks of gestation in an integrated health care system, *Obstet Gynecol* 113:804–811, 2009.

Perper K, Peterson K, Manlove J: *Diploma attainment among teen mothers (Child Trends, Fact Sheet Publication #2010-01,* Washington, DC, 2010, Child Trends.

Petrini JR, Dias T, McCormick MC, et al: Increased risk of adverse neurological development for late preterm infants, *J Pediatr* 154:169–176, 2009.

Planned Parenthood. Parents and teens talk about sexuality: A national survey 2012. Survey conducted by GfK Custom Research, LLC on behalf of Planned Parenthood, Family Circle magazine, and CLAFH. Available at http://www.plannedparenthood.org/imag es/LT_2012_Poll_Fact_Sheet_final(2).pdf

Ramachandrappa A, Jain L: Health issues of the late preterm infant, *Pediatr Clin North Am* 56(3):565–577, 2009.

Reich K, editor: *Children, youth, and gun violence,* Future Child 12(2):1–173, 2002. Available from <www.futureofchildren.org/pubs-info2825/ pubs-info_show.htm? doc_id=154414>.

Safe Kids USA: Preventing injuries: at home, at play, and on the way, 2013. Available from <http://www.safekids.org/search?search_api_vi ews_fulltext=preventing+injuries h>.Accessed February 22, 2013.

Substance Abuse and Mental Health Services Administration: *Results from the 2011 national survey on drug use and health: summary of national findings (NSDUH Series H-44, HHS Publication No. [SMA] 12–4713),* Rockville, MD, 2012, Author. Also available from <http://www.samhsa.gov/data/NSDU H/2k11Results/NSDUHresults2011.htm>.

Substance Abuse and Mental Health Services Administration, *Office of Applied Studies: The NSDUH report: Substance use among women during pregnancy and following childbirth,* 2009. Available from <http://oas.samh sa.gov/2k9/135/PregWoSubUseHTML.pdf>.

Tong VT, England LJ, Dietz PM, et al: Smoking patterns and use of cessation interventions during pregnancy, *Am J Prev Med* 35(4):327–333, 2008.

U.S. Court of Federal Claims: *Autism decisions and background information,* n.d. Available from <http://www.uscfc.uscourts.gov/omni bus-autism-proceeding>

U.S. Department of Agriculture Food and Nutrition Service: *Women, infants, and children (WIC),* 2013. Available from <http://www.fns.usda.gov /wic//women-infants-and-children-wic>.

U.S. Department of Education: *Building the legacy: IDEA 2004,* n.d.. Available from <http://idea.ed.gov/explore/home>.

U.S. Department of Health and Human Services: *About the law,* n.d. Available from <http://www.healthcare.gov/law/>.

U.S. Department of Health and Human Services: *Healthy People 2020,* Washington, DC, 2013, U.S. Government Printing Office. Also available from <http://www.healthypeople. gov/2020/default.asp>.

US. Department of Health and Human Services: Primary care: the health center program, n.d available from http://bphc.hrsa.gov/healthce nterdatastatistics/index.html

U.S. Department of Health and Human Services: *2012 poverty guidelines.* Federal Register 77(17):4034–4035, 2014. Also available from <http://aspe.hhs.gov/poverty/14poverty.cfm>.

U.S. Department of Health and Human Services, Administration for Children and Families, Administration on Children, Youth and Families, Children's Bureau: *Child maltreatment 2010,* 2011. Available from <http://www.acf.hhs.gov/programs/cb/ resource/child-maltreatment-2010>.

U.S. Department of Health and Human Services, Office of Population Affairs: *Title X family Planning Annual Report: 2012 National Summary,* 2013 http://www. hhs.gov/opa/pdfs/fpar-national-summary-2012.pdf

U.S. Department of Health and Human Services, Health Resources and Services Administration, Maternal and Child Health Bureau: *Child health USA,* Rockville, MD, 2012, Author. Also available from < http://mchb.hrsa.gov/chusa12/>.

U.S. Department of Health and Human Services, Office of the Surgeon General: *The surgeon general's call to action to support breastfeeding,* Washington, DC, 2011, Author. Available from <http://www.surge ongeneral.gov/library/calls/breastfeeding/ index.htm>.

U.S. Department of Labor, Wage and Hour Division: *Fact sheet #73: Break time for nursing mothers under the FLSA,* revised December 2013. Available from <http://www.dol.gov/ whd/regs/compliance/whdfs73.htm>.

U.S. Department of Labor, Wage and Hour Division: *Family and medical leave act,* n.d. http://www.dol.gov/whd/fmla/. Accessed March 8, 2013.

Ventura SJ, Hamilton BE: *U.S. teenage birth rate resumes decline (NCHS Data Brief no. 58),* Hyattsville, MD, 2011, National Center for Health Statistics. Also available from <http://w ww.cdc.gov/nchs/data/databriefs/db58.htm>.

Widome R, Neumark-Sztainer D, Hannan PJ, et al: Eating when there is not enough to eat: eating behaviors and perceptions of food among food-insecure youths, *Am J Public Health* 99:822–828, 2009.

Wolff T, Witkop CT, Miller T, et al: Folic acid supplementation for the prevention of neural tube defects: an update of the evidence for the United States Preventive Services Task Force, *Ann Intern Med* 150:632–639, 2009.

Womenshealth.gov: *Breastfeeding,* n.d. Available from <http://www.womenshealth.gov/breast feeding/index.html>.

CHAPTER

17

Women's Health

Lori Glenn

OBJECTIVES

Upon completion of this chapter, the reader will be able to do the following:

1. Identify the major indicators of women's health.
2. Examine prominent health problems among women of all age-groups (i.e., from adolescence to old age).
3. Identify barriers to adequate health care for women.
4. Discuss issues related to reproductive health.
5. Explain the influence of public policy on women's health.
6. Discuss issues and needs for increased research efforts focused on women's health.
7. Apply the nursing process to women's health concerns across all levels of prevention.

KEY TERMS

breast cancer
Cesarean section
Civil Rights Act
cardiovascular disease
domestic violence

ectopic pregnancy
Family and Medical Leave Act
hypertension
life expectancy
maternal mortality

multiple family configurations
osteoporosis
pelvic inflammatory disease
sexual harassment

OUTLINE

Major Indicators of Health
 Life Expectancy
 Mortality Rate
 Morbidity Rate
Social Factors Affecting Women's Health
 Health Care Access
 Education and Work
 Employment and Wages
 Working Women and Home Life
 Family Configuration and Marital Status
Health Promotion Strategies for Women
 Chronic Illness
 Reproductive Health
 Other Issues in Women's Health
Major Legislation Affecting Women's Health
 Public Health Service Act
 Civil Rights Act

 Social Security Act
 Occupational Safety and Health Act
 Family and Medical Leave Act
Health and Social Services to Promote the Health of Women
 Women's Health Services
 Other Community Voluntary Services
Levels of Prevention and Women's Health
 Primary Prevention
 Secondary Prevention
 Tertiary Prevention
Roles of the Community Health Nurse
 Direct Care
 Educator
 Counselor
Research in Women's Health

To achieve "health for all" in the twenty-first century, health care services must be affordable and available to all. Although adequate health care for women is a key to realizing this goal, a significant number of women and their families face tremendous barriers to health care access. Additionally, knowledge deficits related to health promotion and disease prevention activities prevent women of all educational and socioeconomic levels from assuming responsibility for their own health and well-being.

Beginning in the 1970s, the women's movement called for the reform of systems affecting women's health. Women were encouraged to become involved as consumers of health services and as establishers of health policy. More women entered health professions in which they were previously underrepresented, and those in traditionally female-dominated professions, such as nursing and teaching, became more assertive in their demands to gain recognition for their contributions to society. Health care for women has evolved from a focus on the pelvic area and breast to viewing the woman as a holistic being with specialized needs.

In "Preamble to a New Paradigm for Women's Health," Choi (1985) declared that collaboration and an interdisciplinary approach are necessary to meet the health care needs of women. She further stated, "essential to the development of health care for women are the concepts of health promotion, disease and accident prevention, education for self-care and responsibility, health risk identification and coordination for illness care when needed" (p. 14). To realize this paradigm, community-based health care focuses on health beyond the biophysical, disease-focused approach. Health from a social perspective considers the interaction of individual physiology along with work environment, living conditions, lifestyle choices, and health habits (Ruzek et al, 1997). Community health nurses must work with other health care professionals to formulate upstream strategies that modify the factors affecting women's health. Many *Healthy*

People 2020 objectives address health problems pertaining to women and include specific targets and strategies to improve the health of this aggregate. The *Healthy People 2020* boxes in this chapter present a small selection of these objectives. This chapter examines the health of women from adolescence to old age. It explores the major indicators of health, including specific health problems and the socioeconomic, sociocultural, and health policy issues surrounding women's health. The chapter also discusses identification of current and future research aimed at improving the health of women. An understanding of these points will enable community health nurses to appropriately apply this expertise in a community setting to help improve women's health.

MAJOR INDICATORS OF HEALTH

In the United States, data collected on major causes of death and illness appraise the health status of aggregates. These data are typically presented in terms of gender, age, or ethnicity and can help us interpret the levels of health in different groups. The primary indicators of health this chapter covers are life expectancy, mortality (i.e., death) rate, and morbidity (i.e., acute and chronic illness) rate.

♥ HEALTHY PEOPLE 2020

Selected Objectives for Women's Health

Objective	Baseline (Year)	Target (2010)	Final (Year)	Target (2020)
3-3: Reduce breast cancer death rate.	26.6 deaths per 100,000 (1999)	21.3 deaths per 100,000	22.9 deaths per 100,000 (2007)	20.6 deaths per 100,000
3-4: Reduce death rate from cervical cancer.	2.8 deaths per 100,000 (1999)	2.0 deaths per 100,000	2.4 deaths per 100,000 (2008)	2.2 deaths per 100,000
3-11b: Increase the proportion of women 21 years of age and older who have received a Papanicolaou smear test within the preceding 3 years.	79%* (1998)	90%	84.5%* (2008)	93%
3-13: Increase the proportion of women who have received breast cancer screening based on most recent guidelines in 2008.	67%† (1998)	70%	67%† (2008)	81.1%
16-4: Reduce maternal deaths.	9.9 deaths per 100,000 live births (1998)	4.3 deaths per 100,000 live births	12.7 deaths per 100,000 live births (2007)	11.4 deaths per 100,000 live births
16-5a: Reduce maternal complications during labor and delivery.	31.2% (1998)	24%	31.1% (2007)	28%
16-6a: Increase the proportion of pregnant women who receive early and adequate prenatal care beginning in the first trimester.	83% (1998)	90%	70.8% (2007)	77.9%
16-15: Reduce the occurrence of neural tube defects (spina bifida and anencephaly).	60 cases per 100,000 live births (1996)	50 cases per 100,000 live births	60 cases per 100,000 live births (2007)	52 cases per 100,000 live births
25-1a: Reduce the proportion of females 15 to 24 years of age attending Sexually Transmitted Disease clinics with *Chlamydia* infections.	5% (1997)	3%	7.4% (2008)	6.7%
25-6: Reduce the proportion of females 15 to 44 years of age who have required treatment for pelvic inflammatory disease.	8% (1995)	5%	4.2% (2006-2010)	3.8%

*Reflects a change in practice guidelines: Through 2008, women >18 years old were recommended for routine Pap smear screening, but guidelines changed the age to 21 years old in 2008.
†Reflects a change in practice guidelines. Prior to 2008, the measurement was mammograms within the past 2 years for women older than 40 years.
Data from U.S. Department of Health and Human Services: *Healthy People 2020,* ed 3, Washington, DC, 2010, Author; and National Center for Health Statistics: *Healthy People 2010 final review,* 2012. Available from <http://www.cdc.gov/nchs/data/hpdata2010/hp2010_final_review.pdf>.

There are 156.9 million women in the United States (Howden, 2010). Of these women, 11% are considered in fair to poor health, a 12% have conditions that impair their daily functioning (Adams et al, 2011). Many factors that lead to death and illness among women are preventable or avoidable (see Veteran's Health box). If certain conditions receive early detection and treatment, a significant positive influence on longevity and the quality of life could ensue. Recognition of patterns demonstrated by these indicators can address problems preventively. This section presents an overview of these major indicators of health among women.

VETERANS' HEALTH

Women in the Military

Women veterans are a growing segment of the veteran population, as indicated by the following findings:
- There were an estimated 1.8 million women serving in the military in 2010
- 49% have a bachelor's degree
- 61.5% are from the post-Vietnam era
- The average age of women veterans is 48 years, compared with 63 years for men
- 240,000 sought care at Veterans Administration (VA) facilities
- Top diagnoses were postttaumatic stress disorder, hypertension, and depression
- 1 in 5 women responded "yes" when screened by the VA for military sexual truama (MST)

Health care professionals must recognize that this special cohort may have health concerns related to their service. Public health nures should be prepared to counsel women verterans and to be aware of community resources for referrals to meet health needs of this special group of women.

Modified from a presentation created by Bridgette Crotwell Pullis, PhD, RN, CHPN.

Life Expectancy

Except in a few countries, such as Bangladesh, Malawi, Niger, Pakistan, Qatar, and Zimbabwe, women typically experience greater longevity than their male counterparts (World Health Organization [WHO], 2013). For example, women born in the 1970s in the United States have an average life expectancy of 74.7 years, or 7.6 years longer than men born in the same year.

Life expectancy for Americans is at an all-time high, but the discrepancy between males and females remains. Males born in 2011 have a life expectancy of 76 years, compared with 81 years for females. This suggests a trend toward narrowing the gap between male and female life expectancies. Ethnic/racial disparities in life expectancy unfortunately continued into the twenty-first century, as there is considerable variation among races. For example, black females gained an additional 7.1 years, from 69.4 years for those born in 1970 to 78 years for those born in 2005. Although that is a significant gain, it falls behind the 81 years of life expectancy for white females born in 2005 (Hoyert & Xu, 2012).

Mortality Rate

Table 17-1 lists the six major causes of death among American women in 2009 by age-group (Centers for Disease Control

and Prevention [CDC], 2009d). As age increases, the leading causes of death change. In the adolescent to early adulthood years, the leading cause is unintentional injuries (i.e., motor vehicle accidents, drug overdose). Changes since 1999 include (1) human immunodeficiency virus (HIV) as a cause of death is no longer in the top six causes for the 25- to 44-year group and (2) death from pregnancy complications is higher in the list for the 20- to 34-year group. As middle age approaches, cancer becomes the number one cause for women aged 35 to 74 years. Finally after age 75, cardiovascular disease is the most common cause of death.

RESEARCH HIGHLIGHTS

Nurse Researchers Study the Inclusion of Women in Research

A group of nurse researchers (Crane et al, 2004) examined more than 1000 articles published in nursing journals between 1995 and 2001 to determine whether women had been included in research studies focusing on the leading causes of mortality. They found that 87% of the studies did include women participants. They also noted that there appeared to be a slight increase in inclusion of women from the earlier years to the later years.

Cardiovascular Disease

About one in four Americans has one or more forms of cardiovascular disease (CVD) (e.g., high blood pressure, coronary heart disease, stroke, congenital defects, or rheumatic heart disease). CVD accounts for about 35.3% of all deaths in the United States, or about 1 out of every 2.8 deaths. One in ten women under age 60 has some form of CVD; the ratio increases to one in three after age 65. Black women are more likely to die from CVD than white women. In 2005, the CVD death rate among white women was 230.4 per 100,000, compared with 319.7 per 100,000 for black women. Black women are also more likely to die from stroke than white women (60.7 per 100,000 and 44 per 100,000, respectively) (American Heart Association, 2013).

Cardiovascular disease continues to be the number one overall killer of women. One out of every 3 deaths is from CVD, whereas one out of every 29 deaths is from breast cancer. Since 1984, CVD caused more deaths among females than males. In 2010, 386,436 men and 401,4950 women died from CVD (AHA, 2013). The overall number of deaths due to CVD decreased dramatically from 424.2 per 100,000 in 1950 to 236 per 100,000 in 2010, with significant differences between white women (190.4 per 100,000) and black women (267.9 per 100,000).

Disparities continue in relation to prevention, diagnosis, and management of heart disease in women, although research has focused more on the unique aspects of women and heart disease. After age 65, women are twice as likely as men to die from heart disease (Vaccarino et al, 2003). Women have higher rates of complications after revascularization procedures (Jacobs, 2003) and higher rates of death after myocardial infarction (Wenger, 2004). This phenomenon

TABLE 17-1   SIX LEADING CAUSES OF DEATH AMONG AMERICAN WOMEN FOR ALL RACES BY AGE-GROUPS IN 2009

AGE-GROUP (YEARS)	CAUSE OF DEATH (IN RANK ORDER)
15 to 19	Unintentional injury or accidents (43.9%) Suicide (9.1%) Homicide (8.1%) Cancer (8.1%) Heart disease (3.4%) Birth defects (3.1%)
20 to 24	Unintentional injury or accidents (36.8%) Suicide (9.1%) Homicide (8.1%) Cancer (7.8%) Heart disease (4.9%) Pregnancy complications (3.6%)
25 to 34	Unintentional injury or accidents (26.5%) Cancer (13.9%) Suicide (7.7%) Heart disease (7.6%) Homicide (5.6%) Pregnancy complications (3.0%)
35 to 44	Cancer (25.3%) Unintentional injuries (15.8%) Heart disease (11.9%) Suicide (5.5%) Stroke (3.1%) Chronic liver disease (3.0%)
45 to 54	Cancer (34.6%) Heart disease (14.4%) Unintentional injuries (9.0%) Stroke (3.8%) Chronic liver disease (3.6%) Chronic lower respiratory disease (3.3%)
55 to 64	Cancer (40.1%) Heart disease (26.6%) Chronic lower respiratory disease (5.7%) Stroke (3.8%) Diabetes mellitus (3.8%) Unintentional injuries (2.9%)
65 to 74	Cancer (36.5%) Heart disease (19.1%) Chronic obstructive pulmonary disease (8.9%) Stroke (4.7%) Diabetes mellitus (3.7%) Kidney disease (2.2%)
75 to 84	Heart disease (23.8%) Cancer (23.5%) Chronic obstructive pulmonary disease (8.0%) Stroke (7.0%) Alzheimer's disease (4.6%) Diabetes mellitus (3.1%)
85+	Heart disease (31.1%) Cancer (10.5%) Stroke (8.0%) Alzheimer's disease (8.0%) Chronic obstructive pulmonary disease (4.6%) Influenza and pneumonia (3.0%)

Data from Centers for Disease Control and Prevention: *Leading cause of death by age group, all females-United States, 2009.* Available from <http://www.cdc.gov/women/lcod/2009/index.htm>.

exists because women display different symptoms of heart disease and are managed differently from men (Chang et al, 2003; Martin et al, 2004; Schulman et al, 1999). Women have smaller arteries and higher rates of metabolic syndrome, diabetes, heart failure, and other comorbidities. They tend to be older at their first cardiovascular event, with more urgent and emergency presentations (Jacobs, 2003). These differences result in fewer preventive interventions, such as cholesterol screening and the use of aspirin and other fibrinolytic therapy and of statin drugs to lower cholesterol (Downs, Clearfield, and Weis, 1998).

Rates of CVD among women can decline further when individuals become more aware of risk factors and accept responsibility for managing their own health and well-being (Kuehn, McMahon, and Creekmore, 1999). Concerned and motivated providers must encourage women to practice heart-healthy behaviors. In 2002, the American Heart Association launched the "Go Red" campaign for women and "The Heart Truth" program for health care providers, which were designed to educate both groups about the unique features of women and heart disease.

Cancer

Cancer is the second leading cause of death in the United States. One out of 4 deaths in the United States is due to cancer (Siegel et al, 2014). Cancer rates rose through the early 1990s for a number of reasons, including lifestyle choices (smoking, diet, sun exposure), increasing exposure to environmental carcinogens, and, probably most important, greater life expectancy. Because of improvements in early detection, screening, and treatment of the major cancers, incidence rates have leveled off and in some cases decreased (ACS, 2009). To illustrate, death rates from cancer among women have increased from 136 per 100,000 women in 1960 to 167.3 per 100,000 women in 2000 (CDC, 2004). Yet there was a decline in the cancer death rate from 2002 to 2004, about 2% per year, which was "large enough to overcome the impact of the growth and aging of the population" (ACS, 2013b). The ACS (2013a) estimates that 273,430 deaths will have occurred among women as a result of cancer in 2013.

In 1987, lung cancer surpassed breast cancer as the leading cause of cancer deaths in women, and death rates from lung cancer increased sharply until about 1990. Lung cancer deaths leveled off in 2005, when 26% of cancer deaths in American women were attributed to lung cancer. Breast cancer was the second most common cause, accounting for 15% of all cancer deaths (ACS, 2013a). Colorectal cancer, the third most frequent cause of cancer deaths, accounts for 9% of all cancer deaths and claims the lives of some 28,000 women annually.

Other female-specific cancers include ovarian cancer (fifth most common cancer), uterine cancer (sixth most common cancer), and cervical cancer. Cervical cancer, in particular, has received considerable attention of late because it has been determined that 90% of women with cervical cancer have evidence of cervical infection with human papillomavirus (HPV) (ACS, 2013c). In June 2006, the U.S. Food and Drug Administration (FDA) licensed Gardasil (Merck and

Co, Inc.), the first vaccine to prevent HPV infection (CDC, 2012a; CDC 2012b). Through March of 2013, 57 million doses have been given (CDC, 2014). Gardasil has been shown to be highly effective in preventing the most common types of HPV infection and was approved for use in females between 9 and 26 years of age. For additional information, consult the CDC's website (http://www.cdc.gov/vaccinesafety/vaccines/HPV/Index.html).

The good news is that healthy lifestyle changes and early detection and intervention have contributed to the decreases in mortality rates from some cancers. For example, the death rate for colorectal cancer has been dropping since the mid-1980s as a result of early detection and treatment (ACS, 2011). Lung cancer deaths are beginning to show a slight decline that parallels a lower incidence of smoking by women older than 18 years (ACS, 2008).

Five-year survival rates vary according to the type of cancer and stage at diagnosis. For instance, the 5-year survival rate for all clients with lung cancer is only 18%. For those with localized breast cancer, it is 98%, decreasing to 23% for those diagnosed with distant metastases. Of cancers related to the reproductive tract, ovarian cancer has the lowest survival rate, as only around 46% of women survive for 5 years. With diagnosis at an early stage, the 5-year survival rate is 91% for women with colon cancer and 89% for those with rectal cancer (NCI, 2013d; 2013e).

Early diagnosis and prompt treatment are major factors in surviving many types of cancer. According to the ACS (2008), this approach includes routine cervical cancer screening with Papanicolaou (Pap) smear and HPV tests beginning 3 years after the onset of intercourse and continuing annually. After age 30, women with who have three negative annual Pap smear results can be screened every 3 years. Breast cancer screenings include regular breast self-examination and annual clinical breast examination, with the addition of mammography after age 40, or sooner in those with increased risk of hereditary breast cancer. Colorectal cancer screenings include annual fecal occult blood tests along with sigmoidoscopy every 5 years or colonoscopy every 10 years (ACS, 2008).

Certain health choices may reduce an individual's risk of cancer. Women reduce their risk for cancer by never smoking or by quitting if they already use tobacco products. Eating a nutritious, plant-focused, high-fiber diet along with adopting a physically active lifestyle and maintaining a healthy body weight protects against both heart disease and many cancers. Nutrition guidelines include avoiding salt-cured, smoked, nitrite-containing, and charred foods, high-fat foods, and excessive alcohol (Rhodes, 2002; Vogel, 2003). Obesity has been associated with an increased risk for cancers of the colon and rectum, endometrium, and breast (ACS, 2008). Finally, the practice of safe sex has been shown to reduce the spread of cancer associated with sexually transmitted diseases such as HPV, hepatitis B and C, and HIV.

Community health nurses must encourage all females (i.e., from childhood to old age) to adopt these healthy lifestyle choices and pursue early cancer detection. Community health nurses play a major role in providing cancer control

services that should be culturally sensitive and appropriate to the targeted aggregate. If providers and clients applied everything known about cancer prevention, approximately two thirds of cancer cases would not occur.

Diabetes

In 2008, the number of diabetics in the United States reached 24 million, 8% of the population, with 25% of the population over age 60 being affected (CDC, 2008a). From 2003 to 2006, the number of diagnosed diabetics rose by 7.8%, especially among women (Cheung, Ong, and Cherny, 2009).

Diabetes mellitus is a chronic disease that causes the premature death of many women and overall ranks sixth in mortality among that group, being highest after the age 45. Diabetes ranks fourth as the cause of death among several aggregates, including Native Americans, blacks, and Asians, and is fifth among Hispanics (National Center for Health Statistics, 2013).

In addition to being a serious illness in itself, diabetes is a risk factor for the development of CVD; furthermore, it dramatically influences the severity and course of the CVD. In death certificates from 2004 on which the cause of death was related to diabetes, 68% also listed CVD and 16 % also listed stroke (CDC, 2008a). When comparing men and women with diabetes, of those who suffer myocardial infarction before age 65, women are more likely to die and suffer long term health problems (Norhammar, Stenestrand, Lindbäck, and Wallentin, 2008). The good news is that the number of women hospitalized for diabetes has dropped, indicating that better management with tighter control of blood glucose has decreased complications (CDC, 2008a). The community health nurse is an important resource for supporting the tight control of diabetes to prevent its complications. An upstream approach to this problem includes helping women maintain a desirable weight throughout life in an effort to avoid nutrition-related causes of death such as diabetes and CVD.

Maternal Mortality

According to the WHO (2012), 800 women die every day from complications of pregnancy and childbirth, which are the leading cause of disability and death among women worldwide between the ages of 14 and 49 years. Maternal mortality in developing countries is 240 per 100,000 live births, whereas it is 16 per 100,000 in developed countries. Forty percent of women experience complications during pregnancy, childbirth, and the postpartum period, 15% of which are life-threatening.

Before 2003, in the United States, maternal mortality was defined as the deaths of women while pregnant or within 42 days after termination of pregnancy. The U.S. Standard Certificate of Death and the tenth revision of WHO's *International Statistical Classification of Diseases and Related Health Problems* (ICD-10) revised this definition in 2003 to include late causes of maternal death, defined as occurring more than 42 days but less than 1 year after the end of the pregnancy (Hoyert and Xu, 2012 WHO, 2007). The duration and the site of the pregnancy are irrelevant, and causes are defined as related to or aggravated by the pregnancy or its management but not to accidental or incidental causes.

The United States ranks seventeenth in maternal mortality among all nations. In 2012 the rate of maternal death was 12.1 per 100,000 pregnancies (WHO, 2012). Reduction of maternal mortality is one of the *Healthy People 2020* objectives for the United States. See Box 17-1 for information on a group approach to prenatal care.

Beginning in the 1950s, maternal mortality rates began to decline in the United States owing to the use of blood transfusions, the availability of antimicrobial drugs, and the maintenance of fluid and electrolyte balance during serious complications of pregnancy and birth. The development of obstetrical training programs and obstetrical anesthesia programs was also important.

Racial discrepancy persists, however, in maternal mortality rates as in life expectancy. Table 17-2 illustrates how nonwhite women have a significantly higher incidence of death during pregnancy than white women. The gap in maternal mortality rates between black and white women has widened over the past several decades. Early in the twentieth century, black women were two times more likely to die of pregnancy-related complications than white women. Currently, black women are nearly four times more likely to die (CDC, 2009). Major risk factors for maternal death include lack of antepartum care and family planning services, inadequate health education, and poor nutrition. An additional risk factor, regardless of race, is advancing age. Women 40 years and older have more than three times the risk of dying from a pregnancy-related cause as women aged 30 to 39 years (National Center for Health Statistics, 2008). Intrinsic maternal factors, such as higher frequency of hypertension and

greater likelihood of uterine hemorrhage, help explain this increase in the mortality rate among older mothers.

In 2005, maternal mortality in the United States was 17 per 100,000 live births, up from 12 births in 1990 (Hogan et al, 2010). Historically, the leading cause of maternal death is pulmonary embolism (17%), followed by pregnancy-induced hypertension, ectopic pregnancy, hemorrhage, stroke, and anesthesia (Cunningham et al, 2010). Of growing concern are the increasing cesarean section rate, the rising incidence of maternal obesity, and the greater age of mothers, all of which may be contributing to the rise in this rate (Kaiser Daily, 2009). Death associated with legal surgical abortion is rare in the United States, with 12 cases reported in 2008 (CDC, 2012). Complications that result in death from legal abortion relate to the woman's age, the type of procedure, the gestational age of the fetus, and general health problems at the time of the abortion (Cates, Ellertson, and Stewart, 2004).

A medical, or induced, method of abortion using mifepristone (i.e., RU-486), an antiprogestin medication, together with prostaglandins has been used in the United States since September 2000. This method is as effective as surgical abortion and is considered a safe alternative to surgical abortion in pregnancies of less than 49 days (7 weeks). In 2005, 9.9% of the 820,151 legal abortions in the United States employed this method. Curettage as an abortion procedure is still the most widely used (Gamble et al, 2008).

Abortion is a controversial issue for providers and for the women in their care. Adequate access to affordable family planning services are key to decreasing the need for elective abortions. Consider statement by Dr. Jocelyn Elders (2009): "I never knew a woman who needed an abortion who wasn't already pregnant." Nurses must continue to keep abreast of all available pregnancy prevention and termination options to provide the best counsel for women.

Ectopic pregnancy is the leading cause of maternal death in the first trimester. Since the 1980s, the incidence of ectopic pregnancy has decreased from 1.15 to 0.50 per 100,000 live births, the cause of death being hemorrhage in 67% of cases. Racial discrepancy is evident, with rates 6.8 times higher in African Americans. Rates are also 3.5 times higher in women older than than 35 years than in those younger than 25 years. The rates are possibly higher because sexually transmitted diseases (STDs) are diagnosed more frequently in this older population and may cause damage and scarring of fallopian tubes, raising the risk of ectopic pregnancy (CDC, 2012d; Creanga et al, 2011).

The most significant risk for ectopic pregnancy is previous pelvic inflammatory disease (PID) or salpingitis. Early diagnosis and treatment greatly lower the mortality rate. Prevention interventions for women at risk for acquiring STDs are critical in reducing a woman's risk for an ectopic pregnancy. An important task of health care providers is to educate women and men about methods to reduce sexual health risk-taking behaviors. Additional risk factors for ectopic pregnancy include tubal pathology, previous ectopic pregnancy, tubal surgery, and the use of intrauterine contraceptive devices.

BOX 17-1   CENTERING PREGNANCY: MODEL FOR PRENATAL CARE

Developed in 1993, the Centering Pregnancy model uses a group approach to prenatal care. The prenatal visit occurs with women of similar gestational ages and includes an assessment with the provider along with group learning, facilitated discussion, and support among women. The group dynamic contributes to health-promoting behaviors and to normalizing attitudes to pregnancy. Women report high satisfaction with the care and go onto have fewer preterm births and babies of optimal weight (Centering Health Care, 2013; Manant and Dodgson, 2011).

TABLE 17-2   MATERNAL MORTALITY RATE PER 100,000 LIVE BIRTHS—SELECTED YEARS

YEAR	TOTAL	WHITES	BLACKS	OTHER (NON-WHITE)
1992	7.8	5.0	20.8	18.2
1999	13.2	9.5	32.2	14.5
2001	14.7	10.2	36.8	9.9
2003	16.8	11.7	43.5	18.9
2005	15.4	10.7	38.7	15.9

Data from Berg CJ, Callaghan WM, Syverson C, Henderson Z: Pregnancy-related mortality in the United States, 1998 to 2005, *Obstet Gynecol* 116(6):1302-1309, 2010.

Morbidity Rate
Hospitalizations

The 2007 National Hospital Discharge Survey reported that more women than men are hospitalized each year in the United States (Hall, et al, 2010). Pneumonia resulted in an average hospital stay of 5.0 days, which occurred most frequently among women aged 65 or older. Fractures accounted for an average 5.1 days, malignant neoplasms for an average 6.5 days, and diseases of the heart for an average 4.4 days. The primary reason for hospitalization was childbirth, followed by circulatory, digestive, and respiratory diseases, and finally injury or poisoning (DeFrances et al, 2008).

The prospective payment system for hospitalization resulted in a greater demand for skilled nursing services in the home. After community members have been hospitalized for any of several of these conditions, community health nurses may provide ongoing nursing care in the home by referral. Nurses practicing in home environments must be prepared to deliver "high-tech" and "high-touch" services. Chapter 33 discusses home health care in detail.

Chronic Conditions and Limitations

Women are more likely than men to be disabled by chronic conditions. Arthritis and rheumatism, hypertension, and impairment of the back or spine decrease women's activity level more often than they affect their male counterparts. In fact, twice as many women (24.3%) as men (11.5%) are limited in activity from arthritis and rheumatism. Women are more likely than men to have difficulty performing activities such as walking, bathing or showering, preparing meals, and doing housework (CDC, 2009f).

Functional limitations may require home health care that community health nurses supervise and deliver. Nurses plan and implement interventions on the basis of functional assessments. Each care plan facilitates optimal resumption of the individual's independence in personal care activities.

Surgery

Women are more likely than men to have surgery. Hysterectomy is the second most frequently performed major surgical procedure among women of reproductive age after cesarean section. Approximately 600,000 hysterectomies are performed each year (CDC, 2008). Hysterectomy rates for women in the south are slightly higher than those in the northeast (6.3 and 4.9 per 1000 women, respectively). Overall, rates of hysterectomy decreased from 5.4 to 5.1 per 1000 in the years 2000 through 2004 (Whiteman, Hillis, and Jameson, 2008).

The most common reason for hysterectomy is uterine fibroids or leiomyoma, which contributes to more than one third of all such surgeries, but considerably more in blacks (68%) than in whites (33%) (CDC, 2007). White women are more often diagnosed with endometriosis and uterine prolapse, which are the second and third most common reasons for hysterectomy. Hysterectomy rates are the highest in women aged 40 to 44 years (CDC, 2008c).

Optional procedures are becoming available to women. Myomectomy—removal of only the tumors with repair of the uterus—uterine artery ablation, and the use of a gonadotropin-releasing hormone to shrink the tumors can decrease the need for hysterectomy, but women may not know about these alternatives. Community health nurses function as advocates for women and can provide health education programs related to alternatives to hysterectomy, indications for hysterectomy and oophorectomy (i.e., removal of ovaries), and information regarding the type of surgical approach and the purpose of a second opinion. Second opinions and higher levels of education tend to lower the rate of hysterectomies (Finkel and Finkel, 1990).

Birth by cesarean section is the most prevalent surgical procedure experienced by women in the United States and accounts for 32% of births. This rate has gone up more than 50% since 1996 (Martin, Hamilton, and Ventura, 2011). Several factors contribute to the high rates of C-section, including physician fear of malpractice suits, routine use of early induction of labor, and epidural anesthesia. The technology of fetal monitoring has been shown to increase the C-section rate without improving neonatal outcomes.

Mental Health

The most frequently occurring interruption in women's mental health relates to depression. Well-controlled epidemiological studies consistently demonstrate that women experience depression at two to three times the rate of men (American Psychological Association, 2005). Symptoms of depression include depressed mood, apathy, anxiety, irritability, and thoughts of death and suicide (Evans et al, 1999). Unique to women are atypical symptoms including anxiety, increased appetite, weight gain, and somatic complaints along with increased rates of comorbid conditions. Women are more likely to attempt suicide but less likely to be successful (Urbanic, 2009). Women with socioeconomic barriers, such as lower income and lower educational levels, racial/ethnic discrimination, unemployment, poor health, single parenthood, and high-stress jobs, are at greater risk for depression than women with higher educational levels or higher economic status. Other risk factors are childhood negligence and abuse, parental death, negligence, and alcoholism (Urbanic, 2009).

Nurses practicing in community health settings should be aware of the signs and symptoms of depression and should identify referral sources for professional help within the community. The community health nurse plays a vital role in identifying mothers who suffer from postpartum depression. The CDC (2008d) reports that up to 12% of women suffer postpartum depression that interferes with a woman's ability to care for her self, baby, and family. The nurse needs to also be aware of the impact a mother's depression may have on her child's development and family functioning. A woman experiencing depression displays a variety of symptoms, including depressed mood, weight changes, sleep disturbances, and fatigue among others which and be found in the Diagnostic and Statistical Manual of Mental Disorders (APA, 2013).

SOCIAL FACTORS AFFECTING WOMEN'S HEALTH

Health Care Access

In 2012, 18.2% of the U.S. population, or 48.2 million U.S. citizens, lacked health insurance coverage, (CDC, 2012e). Owing to the nature of their employment, women frequently lack health insurance but may not be eligible for Medicaid benefits because their income is too high. Young adults (i.e., those between ages 16 and 24 years) make up approximately 50% of individuals without health insurance. Lacking economic means for meeting the costs of health care, these women are not likely to seek health care until they or a family member is in acute distress. Others may rely on home remedies, over-the-counter drugs, or folk healers for health care. Older women on fixed incomes may have difficulty meeting co-payments required by Medicare and paying for prescription medications. Many senior citizens have paid hospitalization insurance premiums for policies that fail to meet the gap.

Education and Work

In the workplace, women traditionally predominated as secretaries, administrative assistants, registered nurses, teachers, cashiers, and retail sales people. However, in the 1980s, more women began to enter professions traditionally held by men (e.g., lawyers, physicians, and dentists), and in 2008, more than half (51%) of young professionals were women (U.S. Department of Labor, 2008). In 1970, 55.4% of all women aged 25 or older were high school graduates, compared with 81.6% in 1995 and 85% in 2003. Of this same age-group in 2003, 25.7% had completed college, which was more than three times the 1970 rate of 8.1% (U.S. Census Bureau, 2005). A growing number of women have earned degrees in traditionally male-dominated professions. Table 17-3 reflects the changes occurring in percentages of women receiving degrees in medicine, dentistry, law, and theology.

Employment and Wages

In 2008, 46.5% of the workforce were women. In addition, more than half (62%) of women with young children (younger than 6 years) were working outside the home (U.S. Department of Labor, 2005). In 1950, only 12% of women were combining these roles (Chadwick and Heaton, 1992).

Several questions concern women's health and well-being relate to employment issues. A review of female-dominated versus male-dominated jobs discloses inequalities in wage and salary scales; despite the diminishing gap between women's and men's incomes, there is still much room for improvement. Table 17-4 depicts median annual income by sex and ethnicity for both men and women (DeNavas-Walt, Proctor, and Smith, 2011). Disparities in income, based on sex and ethnicity, are clear.

Women heads of households and their children are the poorest aggregate in the United States (Table 17-5). This phenomenon is labeled "the feminization of poverty." In 2005, the poverty rate for single female heads of household was 36.9%, compared with 17.6% for single male heads of households (Thibos, Lavin-Loucks, and Martin, 2007). The nurse working with impoverished families should be aware of social services, child care programs, emergency services, and other resources for families in need. The community health nurse often needs to act as case manager and advocate for families with social service agencies and other public entities.

Working Women and Home Life

Added to inequalities outside the home are inequalities within the home. A working woman is less likely to have a spouse or partner help with the home and children. Even when a spouse or partner is present, the burdens of housework and child care usually fall more heavily on the woman, regardless of ethnicity. Mothers generally spend more time than fathers preparing meals and training and disciplining their children. These multiple-role demands and conflicting expectations contribute to stress (American Academy of Pediatrics, 2005; Matthews and Power, 2002).

However, changes are occurring, as both younger and older men now report spending more time in family activities than middle-aged men. Black and Hispanic men tend to spend a little more time working at family tasks than white men. Books and articles encourage wives and husbands to make their needs known, encouraging greater communication

TABLE 17-3	PERCENTAGES OF DEGREES RECEIVED BY WOMEN					
DEGREE	1970	1980	1988	1996	2002	2007
Medicine (MD)	8.4	23.4	33.3	40.9	44.4	49.2
Dentistry (DDS or DMD)	0.9	13.3	26.7	35.8	38.5	44.5
Law (LLB or JD)	5.4	30.2	40.8	43.4	48.0	47.6
Theology (BD, MDiv, or MHL)	2.3	13.8	19.3	23.3	33.2	33.2

From U.S. Department of Education: *Digest of education statistics*, Washington, DC, 2008, Author.

TABLE 17-4	MEDIAN ANNUAL EARNINGS BY TYPE OF HOUSEHOLD IN 7 YEARS BETWEEN 1969 AND 2011						
HOUSEHOLD TYPE	1969	1979	1989	1999	2003	2007	2011
Married couple with children	41,453	47,793	50,613	56,827	62,405	72,785	74,130
Female householder with children	16,327	18,468	17,651	26,164	29,307	33,370	33,637
Male householder with children	33,749	36,619	34,646	41,830	41,959	49,839	49,567

From DeNavas-Walt C, Proctor D, Smith J: *Income, poverty, and health insurance coverage in the United States: 2011* (U.S. Census Bureau Current Population Reports), 2012. Retrieved from <http://www.census.gov/prod/2008pubs/p60-243.pdf>.

TABLE 17-5	CHARACTERISTICS OF BLACK, WHITE, AND HISPANIC FEMALE-HEADED HOUSEHOLDS: 2009		
CHARACTERISTIC	**BLACK**	**WHITE**	**HISPANIC**
Never married	51.5	27.4	39.7
Married and spouse absent	12.1	11.3	17.8
Widowed	11.1	16.9	9.6
Divorced	21.7	40.6	26.4
Number of children per female-headed household	1.87	1.65	1.82

Modified from U.S. Census Bureau: *Current population reports* and *America's families and living arrangements: 2007.* Available from <http://www.census.gov/population/www/socdemo/hh-fam/cps2007.html>.

between partners. Marriage enrichment programs, often offered through churches and synagogues, teach couples how to communicate more effectively with each other, fostering equality between partners.

Family Configuration and Marital Status

Women are members of multiple family configurations (e.g., nuclear families, extended family units, single-parent units, families of group marriages, blended family units, adoptive family units, non-legal heterosexual unions, and lesbian family units). This diversity causes changes in women's roles within families. Whether or not they function in a traditional role, most women do whatever is necessary to maintain the integrity of their families. Early assessment of the strengths of family units by the community health nurse provides a database for positive nursing interventions established on upstream strategies to enhance each family's level of health and well-being.

Many women are delaying marriage, and an increasing number are not marrying. Overall, marriage rates have remained stable, perhaps because the increasing number of remarriages balances the declining rate of first marriages. When a relationship ends in divorce or separation, more women than men have the responsibility of providing for themselves and their children. According to the U.S. Census Bureau (2007), single-parent households in 2006 represented 9% of all households with children, and a third of all children lived with a single parent. Single mothers are most often the head of a single-parent family. Even in the face of changing lifestyles, divorce, and increased mobility, which leads to long-distance relationships, most Americans report that they remain connected to their extended families through parents, grandparents, siblings, aunts, and uncles.

One contemporary family configuration involves single women with one or more adopted children. Single-parent adoptions are legal, and a growing number of single women are becoming adoptive parents. An often-ignored family structure is one headed by a lesbian parent. Lesbians who become parents have needs similar to those of all mothers. Many cities have lesbian-gay parent groups that provide support, anticipatory guidance, and strategies for coping in society. However, lesbian women often neglect their own health.

This self-neglect may be traced to hostile and rejecting attitudes of health care providers (Zeidenstein, 2004). However, the parents or guardians must remain healthy to ensure the child's well-being.

HEALTH PROMOTION STRATEGIES FOR WOMEN

A woman's ability to carry out her important roles can affect her entire family; therefore women should receive services that promote health and detect disease at an early stage. Early detection and improved treatments for disease allow women to return to work or remain working throughout the course of an illness. Although work is essential to the economic and social well-being of many women's families, the workplace itself creates physical and social stress. As more women enter the workforce and face many of the same risks and stressors as men, it is not surprising that their formerly favorable mortality and morbidity rates have been declining.

Many women seek information that will allow them to be in control of their own health. Since the early 1970s, women have met in self-help groups to develop a better understanding of their own health needs. Some of the health behaviors that women learn in self-help groups are the importance of nutrition and exercise, breast self-examination (BSE), pregnancy testing and contraceptive awareness; recognition of the early signs of vaginal infections and STDs; and awareness of the variations in female anatomy and physiology.

For women who desire to become more knowledgeable about their own health, there are books available in bookstores, in public libraries, and among the holdings of traditional women's groups such as sororities and federated women's clubs. An excellent resource for women is the FDA Consumer (http://www.fda.gov/fdac/), the official consumer site of the FDA, which reports on studies that cover a variety of women's health issues, such as mammography standards, menopause, treatment for STDs, eating disorders, infertility, cosmetic safety, silicone breast implants, and osteoporosis. Another resource is the U.S. Department of Health and Human Services' Office on Women's Health (www.WomensHealth.gov) which highlights positive health behaviors for women and girls. The community health nurse can use models such as Pender's Health Promotion Model in teaching health behaviors that lead to general health promotion among women. Pender notes that health-promoting behaviors are directed toward sustaining or increasing the level of well-being, self-actualization, and fulfillment of a given individual or group (Pender, Murdaugh, and Parsons, 2006). However, because many models were developed for the middle class, they may not be useful to community health nurses working with low-income families.

Knowledge deficits related to body awareness prevail among all women, regardless of socioeconomic or educational level. For example, a woman may ask whether she will menstruate after a hysterectomy, whether she should perform a BSE, or what she can do to prevent recurrent episodes of vaginitis. Nurses can play an instrumental role in helping women develop a greater sense of self-awareness.

Furthermore, community health nurses can remove the mystery surrounding the woman's body and encourage clients to ask previously unmentionable questions.

Chronic Illness

Included among chronic diseases that may affect a woman during her life span are coronary vascular disease and metabolic syndrome, hypertension, diabetes, arthritis, osteoporosis, and cancer.

Coronary Vascular Disease and Metabolic Syndrome

Evidence suggests that cardiovascular disease (CVD) and metabolic syndrome in most women are preventable. CVD is caused by atherosclerosis, which results in buildup of plaque that in turn narrows arteries, decreasing blood flow to the heart muscle. Metabolic syndrome is a group of risk factors that have been linked to an increased risk of cardiovascular events. These factors are abdominal obesity (waist circumference more than 35 inches in women), dyslipidemia (elevated triglyceride and low high-density lipoprotein cholesterol values), insulin resistance, and elevated blood pressure. The underlying etiology of metabolic syndrome is related to the combination of inactivity, obesity, and genetics.

At-risk women have nonmodifiable risk factors such as increasing age, race, gender, or family history of CVD and diabetes. Where the greatest impact can be made is with the modifiable risk factors, which are as follows (AHA, 2013):

- Cigarette smoking
- Obesity
- Diet high in calories, total fats, cholesterol, refined carbohydrates, and sodium
- Glucose intolerance
- Elevated serum lipid values
- Sedentary lifestyle
- Personality type
- Hypertension
- Stress
- Alcohol use

Education by community nurses can assist women in identifying their risk of CVD and metabolic syndrome along with health behaviors that decrease modifiable risk factors. Also important are evidence-based recommendations for high-risk women with existing CVD, including aspirin therapy and omega-3 fatty acid supplementation (Mosca, 2007).

Hypertension

The latest report of the Joint National Committee on Prevention, Detection, Evaluation, and Treatment of High Blood Pressure defines **hypertension** as blood pressure of 140 mm Hg or greater systolic and 90 mm Hg or greater diastolic. The guidelines include the category "prehypertension," which refers to systolic pressure 120 to 139 mm Hg and/or diastolic pressure 80 to 89 mm Hg. Clients with prehypertension are at increased risk for progression to hypertension and require lifestyle modifications to prevent CVD (Chobanian et al, 2003). Essential hypertension is the most common type of chronic hypertensive disorder in women of childbearing age, accounting for 85% of such cases. It is also responsible for approximately one third of all hypertension cases during pregnancy. Hypertension is more common in women than in men and affects more blacks than whites. Additional factors associated with primary hypertension are age (older than 35 years), family history of hypertension, obesity, cigarette smoking, and diabetes mellitus (AHA, 2012). Hypertension usually starts with an asymptomatic phase; therefore, every woman should be screened on an average of every 2 years beginning in her teenage years. Diagnosis is crucial to prevent or modify possible complications of this disease.

Diabetes

According to the U.S. Department of Health and Human Services (2011), 25.8 million people (8.3% of the population) have diabetes in the United States, and the number is growing every year. Furthermore, although an estimated 18.8 million have been diagnosed, some 7.0 million people are not aware they have the disease. In previous years, community health nurses have worked to educate women to assume responsibility in their management of diabetes mellitus. More recently, community health nurses have been actively involved in education and screening programs for groups at high risk. Included in these groups are individuals who have a family history of diabetes, those who are obese, and older adults. Nurses who design education programs need to be aware of the ethnic differences in the prevalence of diabetes. African American, Hispanic, American Indian, and Asian women are two to four times more likely to have diabetes than their non-Latino white counterparts (USHHS, 2011).

According to Cunningham and colleagues (2010), pregnancy is potentially diabetogenic. Pregnancy may aggravate the condition, and clinical diabetes may appear in some women only during pregnancy. Consequently, screening for diabetes is routine in pregnancy.

Controversy surrounds the most effective method of screening for diabetes, but regardless of the selected method, the nurse is involved in explaining the purpose of the screening and how to prepare for the tests. In most public health settings, the nurse is responsible for explaining the results.

Arthritis

In 2009, 50 million people in the United States, nearly one in five adults, were afflicted with arthritis.

The incidence of arthritis is higher in women than in men: approximately 25.9 million women have the condition, compared with 18.3 million men (CDC, 2010).

Osteoarthritis (OA) is the most common form of the disease. It is characterized by degeneration of the joints and is more common with increasing age and in women. OA of the knee is the leading cause of disability in the U.S. Modifiable risk factors for OA include excess body mass, joint injury, occupation, and estrogen deficiency (CDC, 2008b).

Rheumatoid arthritis (RA) can affect anyone, but for every man affected, 2.5 women have the disease. Onset usually occurs between 30 and 50 years of age. RA often goes into remission in a pregnant woman, although symptoms tend to increase in intensity after the baby is born, and RA develops more often than expected the year after giving birth. Although women are two to three times more likely to have RA than men, men tend to be more severely affected when they do have it (Arthritis Foundation, 2014).

Arthritis is the leading cause of disability in the United States (CDC, 2007b). Nursing interventions focus on prevention of joint deformity and modification of lifestyle if necessary.

Osteoporosis

Osteoporosis is a major disorder affecting women, occurring in 25% to 50% of postmenopausal women. Although men may experience osteoporosis, it is four times more common among women. The National Osteoporosis Foundation (2014) estimates that of the 10 million Americans who have osteoporosis, 8 million are women and 2 million are men. An additional 34 million Americans have osteopenia. Half of all non-Hispanic white women in the United States will experience an osteoporosis-related fracture during their lifetimes. The most serious complication of osteoporosis is hip fracture, which is experienced by 280,000 Americans annually. Approximately 24% die within a year from complications of hip fracture (U.S. Department of Health and Human Services [USDHHS], 2000).

Postmenopausal white women are at highest risk for osteoporosis. Loss of bone begins at an earlier age in women and proceeds twice as rapidly as in men. Guidelines issued by the National Osteoporosis Foundation recommend bone mineral density tests for selected postmenopausal women and the use of oral bisphosphonates as the first-line pharmacological treatment of osteoporosis. In light of the results of the Women's Health Initiative Study showing that non-estrogen therapies fail or cause intolerance to side effects, hormone replacement therapy is currently considered second-line therapy for the disease (Wei et al, 2003). Osteoporosis has no cure; therefore prevention is especially important early in life. Prevention involves an awareness of dietary practices such as maintaining a correct balance of calcium, vitamin D, and protein throughout life, in addition to regular weight-bearing, muscle-strengthening, and aerobic exercise.

Nurses in ambulatory health practices should encourage women to become more knowledgeable of the strategies to prevent osteoporosis. For women diagnosed with osteoporosis, nurses can assist in various aspects of management (e.g., education regarding prescribed medication, follow-up care, avoidance of complications, and dietary modifications as needed).

Breast Cancer

The incidence of breast cancer has been rising since the 1950s. Currently, one of every eight women will have breast cancer sometime in her life. The chance of dying from breast cancer is about 1 in 35. The National Cancer Institute (NCI) (2013c) estimated that 226,870 women in the United States will have been found to have invasive breast cancer in 2013 and that 39,510 will die from it. Risk factors include aging, personal or family history (especially mother or sister) of breast cancer, early age at menarche, late age at menopause, never having children, and having a first child after age 30. Female gender and aging are the most significant risk factors for breast cancer (ACS, 2008). An additional risk is a genetic mutation of tumor suppressor genes, known as *BRCA1* and *BRCA2*. The lifetime risk for women with this mutation to be diagnosed with breast cancer is 60%, compared with 12% for the general population. Additional risks are for ovarian cancer, with a 40% lifetime risk for those who inherit the gene, compared with 1.4% for the general population (NCI, 2013a). Genetic testing is available, and the rights of those tested is protected legally, so insurers and employers cannot use this information to discriminate against those testing positive (Genetic Information Nondiscrimination Act, 2008, NCI, 2013a & 2013d).

In 2009 the United States Preventive Services Task Force (2009) published recommendations based on review of scientific evidence that women should not have routine mammography screening between ages 40 and 49 years but should have biennial screenings between the ages 50 and 74 years. This was a major shift from the recommendation of annual screening mammograms for women older than 40 years. The researchers cited the reason for this recommended change as improvements in mammography screening films that lead to more accurate diagnosing. They also cited the high cost and harmful psychologic effect of screening on women related to unnecessary diagnostic testing resulting from the high number of false-positive results. Despite that recommendation, the America Cancer Society (2012) continues to recommend annual mammograms after age 40, whereas the NCI (2013c) recommends screening every 1 to 2 years, except in women at higher risk, who should begin prior to age 40. Key to mammogram screening is a woman's informed choice based on individual risk factors for development of breast cancer as well as the benefits (early detection and improved survival) and potential harms (false-positive results or missed cancer).

The current position of the U.S. Preventive Services Task Force is that there is insufficient evidence to recommend for or against the teaching of BSE (Thomas et al, 2002). Studies support the contention that BSE contributes to awareness, helping women be alert to changes in their breasts. However, for women 40 years and older, the greatest potential to save lives from breast cancer is through early detection with clinical breast examination and mammography (ACS, 2012).

The ACS (2012) recommendations for BSE are as follows:
- BSE's benefits and limitations should be taught to women beginning their 20s.
- The correct technique for BSE should be taught to improve detection of abnormalities.
- Recommendations for the frequency of BSE are no longer specified.
- It is acceptable for women to choose to perform BSE, and this practice should not be discouraged.
- It is acceptable for women to choose not to perform BSE.
- There may be an added benefit for the woman at higher risk of breast cancer to perform regular BSE.

In addition to annual mammography and clinical breast examinations, breast cancer detection may involve ultrasound, magnetic resonance imaging, positron emission tomography, and genetic testing for *BRCA1* and *BRCA2* (NCI, 2013a). Box 17-2 lists resources that provide information about breast cancer and early detection.

RESEARCH HIGHLIGHTS

Breast Cancer Study

A study of the data collected in the U.S. National Cancer Institute's Surveillance, Epidemiology, and End Results (SEER) program demonstrated an increase in the incidence of breast cancer with distant involvement in younger women. From 1976 to 2009 there was a 2.07% average compounded increase in this diagnosis in women 25 to 39 years old but not in older women. This increase was highest in Hispanic and African American women (Johnson, Chien, and Bleyer, 2013).

The Centers for Disease Control looked at data from United States Cancer Statistics (USCS) to determine whether race impacted breast cancer outcomes. Black women had a lower incidence of breast cancer diagnosis than white women, yet cancers were diagnosed at more advanced stages and the death rate was 41% higher in the former group from 2005 through 2009 in the United States. Self-reports of mammogram frequency did not differ in the two groups. However, research shows that in black women, differences do exist in breast cancer screening, follow-up, and treatment after diagnosis, leading to greater mortality (Cronin et al, 2012).

Lung Cancer

Although breast cancer is the most common cancer among women after skin cancer, cancer of the lung and bronchus is responsible for more cancer deaths. The NCI (2013d) predicted that in 2013, 109,690 women will have been diagnosed with lung cancer. Lung cancer is responsible for more deaths yearly in U.S. women than breast cancer. From 2005 to 2009, 39.6 of every 100,000 women died from lung cancer, compared with 23 per 100,000 from breast cancer. In fact, lung cancer kills more women annually than breast, ovarian, and uterine cancers combined (ACS, 2008). Between 1990 and 2003, there was a 60% increase in the number of new cases of lung cancer in American women, whereas the number of men diagnosed with lung cancer remained stable (Patel, 2005). The rise in the incidence of lung cancer in women is due primarily to an increase in their tobacco use: 85% to 90% of all clients who have lung cancer have a history of cigarette smoking. Yet lung cancer develops in only 20% of cigarette smokers, suggesting that the cause of lung cancer is multifactorial.

Widely accepted risk factors for lung cancer include exposure to environmental tobacco smoke, certain occupational exposures (especially asbestos), genetic predisposition, sex, gender, diet, chronic lung disease, and a history of tobacco-related cancer (Rivera and Stover, 2004). Studies have shown that the risks for development of lung cancer are different in women and men and that lung cancer appears to be a biologically different disease in women. Women smokers are more likely than men to have adenocarcinoma of the lung, and women who have never smoked are more likely to have lung cancer than men who have never smoked. These differences are due to hormonal, genetic, and metabolic differences between the sexes (Patel, 2005).

Although medical treatment may be similar for men and women, the symptom distress, quality of life, and demands of illness experienced by women may be different from those in men because the competing household, child care, and other role-related demands take a toll on many women (Sarna and McCorkle, 1996). Further, women with advanced lung cancer

BOX 17-2 RESOURCE MATERIALS FOR BREAST CANCER

BCCCP (Breast and Cervical Cancer Control Program)
Federally funded free breast and cervical cancer screening through state departments of community health

American Cancer Society
Website
   Breast Cancer: Early Detection (available from http://www.cancer.org/acs/groups/cid/documents/webcontent/003165-pdf.pdf)

Publications
   Breast Cancer Awareness Information Packet*
   ABC's of Breast Health*
   The Older you Get, the More you Need a Mammogram* (pamphlet)
   Breast Health(card)
   How to Check your Breasts* (pamphlet)
   Let's Talk about Mammograms (pamphlet)
   For copies, call (800) ACS-2345. For more information, visit http://www.cancer.org/acs/groups/cid/documents/webcontent/003165-pdf.pdf.

National Cancer Institute
Website
   General Information About Breast Cancer (available from http://www.cancer.gov/cancertopics/pdq/screening/breast/Patient/page2)

Publications and Videos
   A Mammogram Once a Year . . . For a Lifetime (video)
   Smart Advice for Women 40 and Over: Have a Mammogram (pamphlet)
   Guidelines for Screening Mammography (pamphlet)
   A Mammogram Could Save Your Life*
   Take Care of Your Breasts*
   For copies, call (800) 4-CANCER. For more information, visit http://www.cancer.gov/cancertopics/pdq/screening/breast/Patient/page2.

U.S. Department of Health and Human Services, and Health Care Financing Administration
   Get a Mammogram: A Picture That Can Save Your Life (pamphlet)
   Medicare Covers Mammograms (pamphlet)
   For copies and more information, call (800) 4-CANCER (breast cancer and mammograms) or (800) MEDICARE (Medicare coverage).

*Specifically designed for low-literacy audiences; some resources are available in Spanish and English.

report more psychological symptoms than men (Hopwood and Stephens, 1995).

Lung cancer is often a fatal illness because it is diagnosed most commonly at an advanced stage; early detection is difficult, and treatment for advanced disease is not as effective. Women appear to have a slight survival advantage over men: the 5-year survival rate is 15.6% for women with lung cancer, and 12.4% for men (Patel, 2005).

The primary factor in preventing lung cancer is for individuals either to never start smoking or to quit smoking. Nurses must work with other health care providers to reverse the morbidity and mortality rates related to this disease. The

Agency for Healthcare Research and Quality has developed a useful guideline for health care professionals to assist women and their families in smoking cessation efforts plus summaries of more than 400 guidelines on a wide variety of topics, which can be found on their website (http://www.ahrq.gov).

Gynecological Cancers

About 20% of all malignant diseases in women occur in the genital tract. The incidence of invasive cervical cancer has declined dramatically as a result of regular Pap smears, which allow for identification of precancerous conditions. However, 3909 women died from the disease in 2009 (CDC, 2013a). Cervical cancer used to be the leading cause of cancer death, but the use of cytological screening has decreased the mortality rate. One major risk factor is infection with HPV, which is linked to 65% of cervical cancer cases. Other risk factors include coitus at an early age, multiple sexual partners, cigarette smoking, history of *Chlamydia* infection, long-term oral contraceptive use, multiple pregnancies, HIV, family history, and low socioeconomic status (ACS, 2013c). It is most commonly diagnosed in women between the ages of 30 and 50 years because the cellular changes that lead to cancer are caused by chronic infection and inflammation. It is uncommon for women who undergo regular screening to be diagnosed with cervical cancer.

Current guidelines recommend cervical cancer screening to begin approximately 3 years after a woman begins having vaginal intercourse, but no later than 21 years of age. Screening should then be performed every 3 years until the age 65 using regular or liquid-based Pap smear tests, or every 5 years with a co-test for HPV DNA (CDC, 2013a). HPV DNA testing is not recommended for routine screening in adolescent women, because the prevalence of HPV is 60% to 80% at this age, and more 90% of those who test positive will clear the HPV within 1 to 2 years of their sexual debuts (Wright et al, 2006). HPV infection is linked to 5% of cancers worldwide, 85% affect the anus and at least half of those in the vagina, vulva, and throat (NCI, 2013b). Current recommendations are that girls and boys be vaccinated for HPV beginning at the age of 11 or 12 years. As of June 2012, more than 46 million doses of HPV vaccine had been administered without serious safety concerns. Because of the Affordable Care Act, vaccinations are covered by private insurers and through the Vaccines for Children Program for eligible children who would otherwise not have access (CDC, 2012).

According to the ACS (2013a), the incidence of carcinoma of the endometrium has increased lightly for black women from 2005-2009, but remained stable for white women. This drop has been attributed to the decline in the use of unopposed exogenous estrogen to control menopausal symptoms. This cancer is commonly found in women during their sixth and seventh decades of life (i.e., 80% of women with this condition are postmenopausal). Approximately 7,470 women in the United States died from endometrial cancer in 2009. The incidence of endometrial cancer is highest among white women, but mortality is higher among black women, suggesting disparity in diagnosis and/or treatment. Factors related to its occurrence are obesity, low parity, diabetes mellitus, and conditions in which high circulating estrogen levels are not countered by adequate progesterone levels. The most common sign of endometrial cancer, occurring in 90% of women, is abnormal vaginal bleeding. Postmenopausal women experiencing vaginal bleeding should seek immediate gynecological evaluation.

Cancer of the ovary causes more deaths than any other pelvic malignancy. According to the NCI (2013e), the lifetime risk of ovarian cancer is 1.38%. The incidence increases with age, peaking in women 75 to 79 years old at 56.7 per 100,000. Risk factors include increasing age, nulliparity, never having breastfed, a history of breast cancer, postmenopausal use of hormone replacement therapy, obesity, a family history of breast and ovarian cancer, as well testing positive for the *BRCA* mutation. Protective factors against ovarian cancer include use of oral contraceptives, having and breastfeeding children, tubal sterilization, hysterectomy, and prophylactic oophorectomy (NCI, 2013e).

Ovarian cancer is a silent cancer. Early-stage detection of ovarian cancer is difficult; therefore it has usually reached an advanced stage when discovered. The health professional should be alert to ovarian enlargement on pelvic examination with suspicion that ovarian malignancy may be present, especially in a postmenopausal woman. The most common sign a woman experiences is abdominal enlargement. She may complain that her skirts and slacks are getting tighter in the waist. Any woman older than 40 years who experiences vague digestive complaints that persist and are not explained by another cause must have a thorough evaluation for ovarian cancer. According to the ACS (2008), transvaginal ultrasound and a blood test for tumor marker CA-125 may assist in the diagnosis of ovarian cancer. These tests are not recommended for routine screening of all women but are recommended for those with risk factors related to family history (strong family history of ovarian and breast cancer, positive for genetic mutations *BRCA1* and *BRCA2*).

Mental Disorders and Stress

Various circumstances and conditions influence the mental health of women. Women face stressful decisions about career and family, and many express anxieties about these decisions. A woman may feel pressured to make decisions regarding childbearing before she has fulfilled her career goals. Deciding to focus on a career may mean decreased authority and the suffering of stress in the workplace. More women are occupying middle-management positions, which are known for creating stress-related illnesses associated with high demands and little or no power. Women combining motherhood and a career have additional decisions, such as whether to work during pregnancy and choice of child care.

A woman's emotional state can be influenced by ovarian function from the onset of menstruation to the cessation of menstrual periods. Depression may be triggered or worsened by premenstrual hormonal changes. Women with a history of depression are also at increased risk for a recurrent episode of depression during the postpartum period, and they also are at risk for depression during the perimenopausal transition (Blehar, 2003). Depression is more prevalent among women than among men. In all age-groups from adolescents through the elderly, approximately two thirds of those affected with depression are women. According to Bhatia and Bhatia (1999), the higher prevalence of depression in women is most likely due to a combination of gender-related differences in cognitive styles, certain biological factors, and a higher incidence of psychosocial and economic stressors.

Mental disorders often go undiagnosed and untreated or undertreated despite the availability of effective treatments. Women may not recognize or correctly identify their symptoms, and even when they do, they may be reluctant to seek care because of stigma associated with mental illness (Blehar, 2003). Community health nurses are in a good position to assess women's moods in diverse aggregates. Being familiar with the symptoms of common mental disorders, nurses can identify these problems and can help women in seek and maintain continuity of care.

Reproductive Health

Community health nurses provide a variety of services in the area of women's reproductive health from menarche through postmenopause. Nurses, in collaboration with other health care professionals, have identified a persistent group of preventable and correctable problems related to maternal-child health. *Healthy People 2020* (USDHHS, 2000b) provides numerous recommendations for improving maternal and infant health, including reduction of cigarette smoking, reduction of alcohol and other drug use, optimal nutrition, improved socioeconomic opportunities (including education), and decreased environmental hazards.

For the *Healthy People 2020* initiative, some of the family planning objectives demonstrated progress. Adolescent pregnancy rates decreased until the year 2005, but a 5% increase occurred between 2005 and 2007 (CDC, 2009b). There were also improvements in rates of adolescent abstinence, contraceptive failure, and condom use. However, health disparities remain an issue for Hispanic and black populations. With *Healthy People 2020* family planning objectives, the focus is on the positive that "all pregnancies should be intended." Examples of *Healthy People 2020* objectives related to family planning are shown in the *Healthy People 2020* box (National Center for Health Statistics, 2012).

Dysmenorrhea is another reproductive health problem affecting approximately 50% to 80% of the female population between ages 15 and 24 years (Nelson, 2004). At least 10% to 20% of women with dysmenorrhea are incapacitated for 1 to 3 days each month. Dysmenorrhea is the greatest single cause of absenteeism

from school and work among young women and causes the loss of approximately 140 million working hours annually; therefore the economic influence of this condition is significant.

⚖ ETHICAL INSIGHTS

Working With Women's Health

Community health nurses working in the field of women's health will be exposed to ethical dilemmas during their careers. For this reason, nurses must have a working knowledge of the principles of health care ethics. The commonly accepted principles include the following:

- Respect for autonomy
- Beneficence
- Non-maleficence
- Justice

Nursing care revolves around moral values such as compassion, empathy, honesty, trust, and respect. Most encounters will be nonproblematic. Occasionally, nurses may be exposed to clinical situations that challenge their values and beliefs. Clients and family members may, at times, also disagree with the nurse's professional advice/plan. It is important for the nurse to keep his or her personal philosophy, politics, religion, and moral values out of clinical work with individuals and families.

Examples of potential ethical dilemmas related to women's health care are emergency contraception, abortion, assisted reproductive technology, and end-of-life issues.

The average age of menopause in the United States is 51 years. *Menopause* is defined as the cessation of menses for at least one full year, but it is characterized by several years of symptoms as the hormonal shifts occur, called perimenopause (Schuiling and Likis, 2013). At this stage, women's health concerns become focused on the symptoms associated with this transition. The most common complaints are related to vasomotor changes causing hot flushes, increased heart rate, insomnia and night sweats, urogenital atrophy causing incontinence, vaginal dryness and dyspareunia, and mood alterations including irritability, depression, and anxiety (North American Menopause Society, 2012; PubMed Health, 2011). Community health nurses can play a key role in helping women find resources to deal with symptoms and develop an understanding of the normal processes associated with menopause. Also, women in menopause need guidance in promoting a healthy lifestyle because they have an increased risk for development of chronic conditions such as osteoporosis, coronary heart disease, hypertension, and type 2 diabetes.

♥ HEALTHY PEOPLE 2020

Selected Objectives for Family Planning

Objective	Baseline (Year)	Target (2010)	Final (Year)	Target 2020
9-1: Increase the proportion of pregnancies that are intended.	52% (2002)	70%	51% (2002)	56%
9-7: Reduce pregnancies among adolescent females (pregnancies per 1000 females 15 to 17 years of age).	63 (1996)	39	40.2 (2005)	36.2
9-11: Increase the proportion of women who have received formal instruction on birth control methods before turning 18 years of age.	70% (2002)	73%	70.5% (2006-10)	77.6%
9-12: Reduce the proportion of married couples whose ability to conceive or maintain a pregnancy is impaired.	13% (1995)	10%	11% (2006-2008)	10.8%

Data from U.S. Department of Health and Human Services: *Healthy people 2020*, ed 3, Washington, DC, 2010, Author.

Nutrition

One of the most important factors in a woman's reproductive health is her total life nutritional experience from infancy through childhood and adolescence. Obesity has become a major public health concern. The community health nurse is in an advantageous position to provide nutritional counseling. The U.S. Department of Agriculture updates the dietary recommendations every 5 years on the basis of current scientific information. In 2011, the "My Plate" approach to health eating was unveiled. This approach is intended to encourage persons to be mindful of the foods they eat in terms of both portion size and proportion to other foods. One half of the plate should consist of fruits and vegetables, one quarter each for meats/proteins and grains, preferably whole grains. Recommendations also include eating less sodium and fewer sugary foods (U.S. Department of Agriculture, 2013).

Pregnancy may provide a motivational factor for developing an awareness of proper nutrition. During the nutritional assessment of a prenatal client, the community health nurse can take the opportunity to determine dietary habits and initiate a referral to the Special Supplemental Food Program for Women, Infants, and Children (WIC). This program provides food vouchers for pregnant or breastfeeding women, infants, and children who are at nutritional risk.

Good nutrition must include factors other than kinds and amounts of foods. Elements to consider include age, lifestyle, economic status, and culture. For example, when counseling an pregnant adolescent, the nurse can include the primary person responsible for meal preparation. The nurse should include the adolescent in the planning of her diet, asking her to identify foods that she likes from those recommended. The nurse should make the adolescent aware of the influence of her nutrition on fetal growth and development. This information must be balanced with the young woman's individual needs.

Sexually Transmitted Diseases

STDs are commonly found among U.S. women. Community health nurses and other health providers, including physicians, nurse practitioners (NPs), nurse midwives, and social workers, must be prepared to provide age-appropriate STD prevention, education, and counseling.

In 2007, the CDC reported the most common sexually transmitted disease was infection with *Chlamydia trachomatis* (1,108,374 cases), followed by *Neisseria gonorrhea* (355,991 cases). This was the largest number of *Chlamydia* cases ever reported. *Chlamydia* infection is diagnosed three times more in women than men, most likely because of the CDC's recommendation for routine screening of any sexually active woman of childbearing age to prevent infertility. Gonorrhea is also diagnosed more often in women, but particularly in black women, who are diagnosed 15 times more often than white women. The Gonococcal Isolate Surveillance Project (GISP) demonstrated that gonorrhea was becoming resistant to treatment with CDC-recommended fluoroquinolone drugs in 2007, prompting the CDC to revise treatment guidelines (CDC, 2007).

When rates of syphilis, another STD, dropped nearly 90% between 1990 and 2000, the CDC initiated the National Plan to Eliminate Syphilis. However, rates have increased yearly since 2001. Racial disparity in cases of syphilis has improved from 1999, when 29 times more blacks than whites were diagnosed, down to a rate that is now 7 times higher. The major increase in syphilis between 2001 and 2007 has been in men, especially men having sex with men, and less in women (CDC, 2007).

Treatments of STDs are outlined in the CDC guidelines, which are updated regularly and available online (http://www.cdc.gov/std/treatment/2010/default.htm). A vital role of the community health nurse is to follow up with the woman's sex partner(s) who require(s) evaluation and treatment. Partner notification and expedited treatment, along with avoidance of sexual activity until treatment/cure, are key to stopping the spread of STDs. In addition to medications, women and their partners need individualized counseling on reducing risky sexual behaviors.

Human Immunodeficiency Virus and Acquired Immunodeficiency Syndrome. Today, the HIV/acquired immunodeficiency syndrome (AIDS) epidemic represents a growing and persistent health threat to women in the United States, especially young women and women of color. According to the CDC (2009c), in 2005, HIV infection was the third leading cause of death for African-American women aged 25 to 44 years and was the fourth leading cause for those aged 45 to 54 years. Among women diagnosed with HIV/AIDS, 64% are black, yet black women make up only 13% of the general U.S. population. The majority of infants born with HIV are black. For all ethnicities, primary transmission in men occurs through sexual contact with other men, whereas in women, the route is high-risk heterosexual contact. In 2005, HIV disease was the fifth leading cause of death among Hispanic women aged 25 to 44 years. Worldwide, AIDS is a leading cause of death among young women (WHO, 2004).

According to the CDC (2009c), risk factors for and barriers to prevention of HIV/AIDS for women include the following:

- Young age at sexual initiation
- Lack of awareness regarding disease and condom use
- Sexual inequality in relationships
- Biological vulnerability to sexually transmitted infections
- Substance abuse
- Poverty; dropping out of school
- Stigma surrounding testing and treatment
- Working in the sex trade
- Participants in unprotected sex

In November 2008, the USDHHS released the updated *Guidelines for the Use of Antiretroviral Agents in HIV-1 Infected Adults and Adolescents* (USDHHS, 2013). Treatment guidelines continually evolve with new research and experience. The use of antiretroviral drugs has reduced the rate of death for HIV disease in women, which peaked in 1993-1994 at 6 per 100,000, down to 2.5 per 100,000 (CDC, 2009c). It is imperative that the community health nurse working with this population stays abreast of the current trends for both counseling and treatment options. Community health nurses also must target at-risk populations and campaign for the use of safer sex practices and routine HIV testing for those at risk.

Other Issues in Women's Health
Unintentional Injury or Accidents and Domestic Violence

Although unintentional injury affects women less commonly than men, several areas of concern still exist for women. For example, older women are at increased risk for accidents such as falls. Falls account for the majority of serious unintentional injuries and lead to 40% of all deaths from injury in people older than 75 years (Stevens, 2005). Factors that may be responsible for this major cause of injury among older adults are an unsteady gait, reduced vision, and a hazardous environment. Older women experience an increasing number of falls; therefore the nurse must identify the preventable factors. Whether working with older adults in the home or in institutional settings, nurses must be knowledgeable about hazards that may be corrected to decrease the incidence of falls.

Domestic violence is the single largest cause of injury to women between the ages of 15 and 44 in the United States— more common than muggings, car accidents, and rapes combined. Each year 4.8 million women are battered. In 2004, 1,158 of these women died from their injuries. Two thirds of women are abused by a current or former intimate partner (CDC, National Center for Injury Prevention and Control, 2006).

Abuse in women is often explained as accidental injury. Approximately 6% of visits made by women to emergency departments are for injuries that result from physical battering by their husbands, former husbands, boyfriends, or lovers. Domestic violence includes physical, sexual, and psychological attacks and economic coercion (Warshaw, Ganley, and Salber, 1995). Reports of teen dating abuse indicate that one in five teens reports some sort of abuse and one in four girls report being sexually coerced. (CDC, 2013b).

Nurses employed in community health settings need to know how to make assessments, provide support, and make referrals to agencies dealing with domestic violence (see Boxes 17-3 through 17-5). Understanding the state laws related to reporting known or suspected domestic violence is important. The American Medical Association and American Nurses Association advocate that all women should be assessed for intimate partner violence. Questions should be posed privately, in nonjudgmental but specific terms (i.e., "Do you feel safe?" "Have you ever been hit, punched, slapped, or kicked?") with follow-up questions if the woman responds "yes" (Kovach, 2004). Many nurses are past or current victims of abuse; assessing abuse with clients can evoke painful emotions that the nurse may not be ready to confront. Chapter 27 contains additional information about domestic violence.

Disability

More women than men have disabilities resulting from acute conditions, but women experience fewer disabilities resulting from chronic conditions because they report their symptoms earlier and receive necessary treatment. There are 56.7 million disabled persons, which is 18.7% of the population and 19.8% are women (Brault, 2012). Women report proportionately more days of restricted activity than men.

> **BOX 17-3   DOMESTIC VIOLENCE STRATEGIES FOR NURSES**
>
> It is important not to re-victimize the woman who admits to intimate partner violence. Avoid asking the woman "why" or talking negatively about the abuser. Sit down with her, give her time to talk, listen actively. Provide her with privacy and confidentiality as much as you can. Useful statements include:
> "I believe what you are telling me."
> "I am here for you."
> "This will only get worse."
> "You deserve better."
> "I am afraid for you safety."
> "You deserve to be treated with respect."
> "It is a crime."
> This approach will empower the victim. Episodes of imminent danger must be reported to the police. An emergency plan should be formulated with the woman. Resources including phone numbers for hotlines and the local women's shelter should be provided in a format that is easy to conceal (such as on a business card).

Adapted from Perry SE, Hockenberry MJ, Lowermilk DL, Wilson D: *Maternal child nursing care*, Maryland Heights, MI, 2010, Mosby, p. 62.

> **BOX 17-4   SIGNS OF INTIMATE PARTNER VIOLENCE**
>
> - Overuse of health services
> - Nonspecific, vague complaints
> - Missed appointments
> - Injuries without legitimate explanation
> - Injuries not matching reported cause
> - Untreated serious injuries
> - Intimate partner describing the cause of injuries
> - Intimate partner refusing to leave the woman's room

Adapted from Krieger CL: Intimate partner violence: a review for nurses, *Nursing Women's Health* 12(3):224-334, 2008.

> **BOX 17-5   RESOURCES FOR VICTIMS OF DOMESTIC VIOLENCE**
>
> National Domestic Violence Hotline: 1-800-799-SAFE (7233) and http://www.thehotline.org
> Dating Violence on Women's Health.gov: http://womenshealth.gov/violence-against-women/
> National Coalition Against Domestic Violence: http://www.ncadv.org
> Office on Violence Against Women: http://www.ovw.usdoj.gov

Disabling conditions limit the physical functional abilities of many women, but the health care delivery system has often overlooked the unique needs of this aggregate. In planning care for disabled women, community health nurses should focus attention on enabling women to strengthen their capabilities. In addition, nurses should be sensitive to barriers in the clinical setting that affect the access of disabled women to health care services. Chapter 21 discusses the needs of disabled people in greater detail.

MAJOR LEGISLATION AFFECTING WOMEN'S HEALTH

Several legislative acts have direct or indirect influence on the health of women. Many changes have been made in the past five decades that have the potential for improving the health and welfare of all women.

Public Health Service Act

The Public Health Service (PHS) Act, passed in 1944, provides for biomedical and health services research, information dissemination, resource development, technical assistance, and service delivery. In the area of women's health, the PHS Act supports activities related to general health issues, reproductive health, social and behavioral issues, and mental health. Aggregates of women targeted by the PHS Act include those disabled by specific diseases, victims of sexual abuse and domestic violence, recent immigrants, and occupational groups.

Title X of the PHS Act is the Family Planning Public Service Act, which helped 5 million women obtain family planning services in 2008. Since 1970, federally subsidized family planning funds have been available to clinics and health departments throughout the country. These facilities provide access not only to contraception but also to routine preventive health services, education, and counseling. The program is an important part of the public effort to prevent low birth weight through addressing the relationship between lack of family planning and women at greatest risk for low-birth-weight infants (women who are adolescents, single, and/or low-income) (Fowler, 2010).

Civil Rights Act

Title VII of the Civil Rights Act of 1964 prohibits discrimination based on sex, race, color, religion, or national origin in determining employment eligibility or termination, wages, and fringe benefits. The Act has been amended to prohibit discrimination against pregnant women and conditions involving childbirth or pregnancy. This landmark legislation makes it unlawful for employers to refuse to hire, employ, or promote a woman because she is pregnant. In addition, employee benefit plans that continue health insurance, income maintenance during disability or illness, or any other income support program for disabled workers must include disabilities resulting from pregnancy, childbirth, and other related conditions. If employers allow disabled employees to assume lighter or medically restricted assignments, the same considerations must extend to pregnant women.

Sexual harassment is a violation of the Civil Rights Act. Sexual harassment is "conduct of a sexual nature ... unwelcome by the target .. severe or pervasive enough to create an intimidating work environment" (Women Employed Institute, 1994). Female and male workers may face unwelcome sexual advances or requests for sexual favors or other verbal or physical conduct of a sexual nature. Awareness of sexual harassment in the workplace has increased dramatically over the past decade, but sexual harassment has not been eliminated.

Social Security Act

The Social Security Act provides monthly retirement and disability benefits to workers and survivor benefits to families of workers covered by Social Security. Full retirement benefits are available after 10 years of covered employment, and workers can collect partial benefits beginning at age 62 and full benefits after age 67.

The Social Security Act permits a divorced person to receive benefits based on a former spouse's earning record when that spouse retires, becomes disabled, or dies if the marriage lasted at least 10 years. Since January 1985, a woman who has been divorced for at least 2 years can receive spousal benefits at age 62, if her former husband is eligible for benefits, regardless of whether he is actually receiving them.

Medicare and Medicaid also resulted from the Social Security Act. Medicare is the insurance plan that covers the majority of the health care expenses of older adults, including payments for hospital care, physicians, home health care, and other services and supplies after co-payments and deductibles. Medicaid covers health care for indigent and eligible children and includes family planning, obstetrical care, and preventive cancer screening for women, such as mammography and Pap smears. Chapters 10 and 12 describe Medicare and Medicaid in detail, and it is further discussed later in this chapter.

Occupational Safety and Health Act

The Occupational Safety and Health Act, enacted in 1970, helps ensure safe and healthful working conditions for workers throughout the United States. Although there is a growing emphasis on the study of the health of women workers, gaps in knowledge exist. For example, little is known about women who work in cottage industries, as domestic workers, as prostitutes, in agriculture, and in the garment industry. In addition, the work of some women is classified as "women's work" and includes such things as housework, child care, caregiver of the sick, and farming (Misner, Beauchamp-Hewitt, and Fox-Levin, 1995). These women experience physical demands and hazards, yet government economic reports have not recognized them as workers. Investigations of factors that influence the health of these women workers are needed. Table 17-6 lists specific positions in which a large number of women are employed and the potential for health hazards within these positions.

Community health nurses, occupational health nurses, and NPs need to be cognizant of environmental hazards wherever they find women at work. In taking a health history, the nurse should collect data regarding the client's occupational environment to assess the potential risk to emotional, general, and reproductive health. In addition, nurses must work individually and as an aggregate with their legislatures to maintain strong worker health and safety programs to protect the health of all women.

Family and Medical Leave Act

Enacted in 1993, the Family and Medical Leave Act (FMLA) allows an employee a minimum provision of 12 weeks unpaid leave each year for family and medical reasons such as personal illness; an ill child, parent, or spouse; and the birth or adoption of a child. In 2008, the FMLA was updated to include family providing care to members of the Armed Forces injured in the line of duty. This act guarantees the employee the same or an equivalent job with the same pay and benefits upon the employee's return to work. In addition, health benefits must continue throughout the

TABLE 17-6	HAZARDOUS OCCUPATIONS IN WHICH WOMEN ARE EMPLOYED
OCCUPATION	**HEALTH HAZARD**
Clerical workers	Organic solvents in stencil machines, correction fluids, and ozone from copying machines
Textile and apparel workers	Cotton dust, skin irritants, and chemicals
Hairdressers and beauticians	Hair, nail, and skin beauty preparations
Launderers and dry cleaners	Heat, heavy lifting, and chemicals
Electronics workers	Solvents and acids
Hospital and other health care workers	Infectious diseases, heavy lifting, radiation, skin disorders, and anesthetic gases
Firefighters	Exposure to hazardous materials and rescue environments
Laboratory workers	Biological agents; flammable, explosive, toxic, or carcinogenic substances; exposure to radiation; and bites from and allergic reactions to research animals
Construction workers	Exposure to hazardous materials, dangerous environments
Military personnel	Exposure to hostile persons, hazardous materials, harsh environments and sexual assault.

Data from Centers for Disease Control, National Institute for Occupational Safety and Health: *Workplace safety and health topics: Industries & occupations,* 2013. Available from <http://www.cdc.gov/niosh/topics/industries.html>.

leave. In 2011, 14 million people utilized FMLA. Of these 56% were women, 40% took less than 10 days, and those with a new child took and took an average of 22 days (NPF, 2012).

The FMLA is particularly important to female workers because they are more likely to use leave to care for seriously ill family members, whereas male workers more often use leave for personal illness (Gilinson, 1999). Employees who must be away from work for family and medical reasons lose income, with the most significant impact on those without job-protected leave. The FMLA is an important step toward equitable leave policies, but more change is needed.

HEALTH AND SOCIAL SERVICES TO PROMOTE THE HEALTH OF WOMEN

Major changes for women came with the signing of the Affordable Health Care Act (ACA) of 2010 (HHS, 2012). Particular to women are protections from being denied coverage by insurance companies and from being charged more for health care services because of gender. As of August 1, 2012, 47 million women gained access to preventive care without co-pays. Services include well-woman visits along with screening and counseling for gestational diabetes, HPV, STDs including HIV, contraception, and domestic violence. Also included are breastfeeding counseling, support, and supplies. The ACA mandates an expansion of Medicaid to include persons younger than 65 years with income below 133% of the Federal poverty level;

estimates are that an additional 22 million would have coverage by 2022 (Holahan et al, 2012; Medicaid.gov, 2012). Medicaid is a health insurance program that was instituted in 1965 for the poor and is funded jointly by the federal and state governments but is administered by individual states. Medicaid is the largest source of funding for medical and health-related services for people with limited income regardless of age eligibility. Medicaid is classified into five broad coverage groups: children, pregnant women, adults in families with dependent children, individuals with disabilities, and individuals 65 years or older.

Pregnant women who are eligible for Medicaid are at high risk for poor pregnancy outcome, including low birth weight. Ideally, a maternity care provider should examine women with high maternal risk immediately after conception. However, too often these women seek prenatal care late in pregnancy or arrive at the emergency department when delivery is imminent without having previously received prenatal care. Barriers limit access to prenatal care for those most in need. Medicaid allows some access to care. Greater public awareness of facilities and maternity care providers who accept Medicaid are necessary.

Clinical Example

Anita Rogers, a 16-year-old unemployed single woman, arrived at the Family Services Health Center seeking initial prenatal care at 36 weeks of gestation. She stated that for a few days she noted some brown discharge from her vagina. She told the nurse she knew she should have begun prenatal care earlier, but when she called several physicians' offices, the receptionists told her she should bring $1000 for her first visit. She said that neither she nor her parents had that much money. Her father was unemployed, and her mother worked at a cafe as a waitress. She also had difficulty with transportation. Anita was sent to the hospital immediately for an ultrasound examination. The sonogram revealed triplets, but two of them had died in utero. Anita was hospitalized and began to hemorrhage. She delivered a 3-lb infant.

Women's Health Services

Since the mid-1970s, women have sought health services beyond the conventional mode of care delivery. Women desire a participatory role in their health and have become more assertive. Health care facilities have recognized the importance of meeting women's health needs. A notable evolution has occurred in maternity care, in which the demands of women as consumers lead to the emergence of freestanding and hospital-based birth centers and family- and sibling-attended births.

The National Women's Health Network (NWHN) has been a strong advocate for women's concerns and has provided testimony at congressional hearings dealing with women's issues. This organization is concerned with women's rights, environmental safety, reproductive rights, warnings about the effects of alcohol and drugs on the developing fetus, safety in relation to medical devices, and to drugs, especially those that may have teratogenic or carcinogenic effects. Examples of the organization's work include recall of the Dalkon Shield intrauterine device, identification of women who may have been exposed to diethylstilbestrol (DES) in utero, and promotion of well-woman health care.

Other Community Voluntary Services

Networking, the exchange of information among interconnected or cooperating individuals, has been one of the major movements during the past two decades. It is a means by which women seek to advance their careers, improve their lifestyles, and increase their income while helping other women become successful. Networking in business, professional support, politics and labor, arts, sports, and health is established throughout the United States enabling women to develop and become empowered to achieve mutual goals.

Many private voluntary organizations spend money, time, and energy in attempting to increase health awareness among its members and provide direct services to the public. Most urban areas have crisis hotline services in which women volunteer to provide counseling to battered women, battering parents, rape victims, those considering suicide, and those with multiple needs. One of the most effective, low-cost, voluntary efforts to assist abused women involves shelters and safe houses scattered throughout the United States. One of the goals of *Healthy People 2020* relates to this issue, as many women needing shelter are often denied emergency housing.

Women's organizations have a long history of voluntary involvement with the community. An increasing number have added activities to their agendas to improve pregnancy outcomes, prevent teen pregnancy, and support older women's rights. Organizations such as the Older Women's League, United Methodist Women, women's groups of other religious denominations, Urban League, sororities, Junior League, Young Womens' Christian Association, and the National Association of Colored Women's Clubs, have made women's health a major item on their agendas.

LEVELS OF PREVENTION AND WOMEN'S HEALTH

Primary Prevention

The focus of primary prevention is preventing disease from occurring. Women should recognize the risk of disease and target their health care behaviors accordingly. Types of primary prevention include never smoking, following a nutritious diet, practicing safe sex, avoiding drugs, limiting alcohol consumption, and staying physically active.

Consider Jackie, a 39-year-old woman with three first-order relatives diagnosed with breast and/or ovarian cancer. She is at risk for hereditary cancer and should seek genetic counseling and possibly testing. If genetic test results are positive, she should be given information on measures that could prevent cancer from occurring, a process that constitutes primary prevention. These measures include lifestyle choices (early childbearing/breastfeeding); prophylactic surgical procedures (oophorectomy/mastectomy); and medical treatment (contraceptive pills, tamoxifen). Vigilant screenings (pelvic ultrasound with Ca-125 measurement or breast magnetic resonance imaging) to detect cancer early would be considered secondary prevention.

Secondary Prevention

The focus of secondary prevention is detecting the disease once it has begun but before it appears clinically. Examples of this level of prevention are routine screening for cervical cancer through Pap smears, for chlamydial infections through nucleic acid amplification tests on either urine or cervical specimens, and clinical breast examination and mammogram.

Tertiary Prevention

Tertiary prevention seeks to stop further complications after a disease has become clinically evident. For example, Sandra Smith, a 55-year-old Native American, has had diabetes mellitus for the past 3 years. She attended an urban clinic for monitoring of the diabetes. After the physician examined her, he suggested that she have her annual pelvic examination. She was overdue for one and agreed to be seen by the women's health care NP. Ms. Smith described symptoms of a yeast infection (e.g., increase in vaginal discharge and itching) to the nurse. Her examination and a wet mount examination confirmed the diagnosis of *Candida albicans* infection, a common problem among diabetic women. Sandra then learned about the nature of, predisposing factors for, and treatment of the infection.

CASE STUDY   APPLICATION OF THE NURSING PROCESS

John Lawrence, an educator at the state women's correctional center, contacted Donna Williams, a women's health care nurse practitioner and faculty member at the College of Nursing, and expressed concern for the health of an inmate, Lela Marvin. According to Mr. Lawrence, Lela, a 19-year-old pregnant primigravida, was being seen at the state-supported hospital for antepartal care; however, she was not permitted to attend perinatal education classes. He stated that other pregnant women in the facility could benefit from perinatal education. In fact, approximately 6.1% of female state prison inmates are pregnant when admitted to prison and could benefit from perinatal education (Snell, 1994).

Lawrence's call was followed by a call from Herman Martin, an RN who also expressed concern for the other women's needs for information regarding their personal hygiene. Although an RN, Mr. Martin was not knowledgeable of women's health because his primary clinical focus was emergency and trauma care. He indicated that many of the women were overweight, cared little about themselves, and lacked a general knowledge of how to maintain their health.

Assessment

After gaining clearance from the prison officials, Ms. Williams made an assessment of health care information needs and started offering classes for the inmates. The immediate need was for perinatal education for women in the last weeks of pregnancy. Lela said she wanted to learn about labor because she had heard only horror stories from other women. Ms. Williams noted that three other women were close to term and they also seemed eager to learn. She knew that students' readiness to learn was key to the course's success. Success of this course would be crucial to future course offerings.

The traditional perinatal education course was designed to promote healthy birth outcomes and an emotionally satisfying birth experience. These goals are also important to pregnant women in a

CASE STUDY APPLICATION OF THE NURSING PROCESS—cont'd

correctional facility; however, perinatal education would have to be modified to meet this group's special needs. For example, information on newborn care is not appropriate because the infant born to an inmate is usually placed with the mother's family or in foster care.

Assessment of nonpregnant women provided opportunities for other health education classes. The next spring and each spring thereafter, junior nursing students under Ms. Williams's guidance were assigned to develop and carry out 1-hour weekly health education and awareness sessions at the correctional facility. Although each student expressed some initial anxiety about the experience, each evaluated it as being worthwhile.

Diagnosis
After assessment, the community health nurse developed community and aggregate diagnoses, which served as the basis for the care plan.

Individual
- Inadequate preparation for childbirth related to lack of resources in prison (Lela)
- Lack of family support related to separation secondary to incarceration (Lela)
- Potential for feelings of loss related to separation from infant after birth (Lela)

Family
- Lela's family visits were rare; therefore she looked for others to provide support during her pregnancy. Lela told Ms. Williams that her cellmate, Julieanna, offered to be her labor support person.
- Lack of knowledge of her role as a labor support person (Julieanna).

Community
- Lack of adequate health-seeking behaviors of women in the correctional facility (i.e., pregnant and nonpregnant women)
- Lack of programs to promote health and prevent diseases among women prisoners

Planning
After the nursing diagnosis was validated with the individual, family, or community, the plan of care was developed. Examples of long- and short-term goals follow.

Individual
Long-Term Goal
- Individual family members will have a positive birth experience (Lela).

Short-Term Goal
- Family member or friends will help Lela use relaxation techniques to cope with the discomforts of labor.

Family
Long-Term Goal
- The family members will be strengthened through their newly acquired knowledge and skills.

Short-Term Goal
- The family members will demonstrate increased ability to perform their role as labor support people.

Community
Long-Term Goal
- The health and well-being of incarcerated women (i.e., pregnant and nonpregnant) will improve.

Short-Term Goal
- Health education programs will be instituted for individuals, families, and aggregates in the correctional facility.

Intervention
The community health nurse worked with the individual, family, or community to achieve mutually established goals. Intervention was aimed at empowering individuals and groups to take responsibility for themselves and to form links with others to accomplish goals.

Individual
Providing a perinatal education program for Lela was Ms. Williams's first priority. In addition, counseling related to feelings of loss after birth might be appropriate. Referral to a counselor might be necessary, and Ms. Williams had to become familiar with available resources.

Family
Teaching the family the roles and responsibilities of a labor support person was an important intervention. In the correctional facility, interventions must ensure that Lela has a labor support person with whom to practice her relaxation techniques and to be available. In this case, Lela's cellmate, Julieanna, was willing to act in this role, and the nurse had to negotiate with prison officials to allow this arrangement.

Community
Specific interventions with a group of pregnant women in the correctional facility were based on the specific needs of the group. The community health nurse had to identify prison officials who were supportive of health education programs and request their input as to which women should be targeted for such programs. Then the nurse met with targeted women to assess their level of knowledge and skills regarding women's health. For example, the nurse surveyed what each woman perceived as learning needs (e.g., well-woman care, women's anatomy and physiology, self-care in health promotion, health protection, and disease prevention). Then the nurse tailored an intervention that was compatible with the community. Ms. Williams asked each nursing student to select a topic the basis of the survey and to develop a teaching plan for presentation to female prisoners (i.e., pregnant and nonpregnant) at least once during the spring semester.

Evaluation
The community health nurse compared the actual and predicted outcomes to determine the efficacy of the plan of care and make revisions.

Individual
For example, Lela learned necessary relaxation techniques that were useful to her in labor and helped make the birth experience positive. Follow-up of Lela's psychosocial concerns in postpartum was also important.

Family
Evaluation of this nontraditional family would include their level of satisfaction with their role in the birth experience. Evaluation would also include learning how this interaction between family members (i.e., Lela and Julieanna) prepared them for other situations.

Community
The aggregate evaluation focuses on the community. For example, in health education programs designed for pregnant and

Continued

nonpregnant women in the correctional facility, it was important to do the following:

- Maintain attendance records.
- Seek feedback from women, the referring nurse-educator, and prison officials regarding changes in self-care behavior regarding health.
- Obtain student response to learning experience.
- Make changes in health education programs on the basis of evaluation.

Levels of Prevention

The following are examples of the three levels of prevention as applied to the individual, family, and community.

Primary

- Assessment and teaching perinatal education course to pregnant inmates

- Assessment and teaching health education classes to nonpregnant inmates
- Teaching the family the roles and responsibilities of a labor support person

Secondary

- Screening at the community level (correctional facility) of what is perceived as learning needs
- Educating the family and community of the signs of postpartum depression

Tertiary

- Educating HIV-positive pregnant inmates on the need for antiviral treatment and delivery by cesarean section
- Educating family members and foster parents about the need for neonatal follow-up with regard to HIV status
- Assessing available community resources for counseling and treatment of postpartum depression

ROLES OF THE COMMUNITY HEALTH NURSE

Direct Care

The community health nurse provides direct care in a variety of settings. Often, this care is considered the "hands-on" nursing care given to a client in the home or a clinic.

Educator

The nurse encounters many opportunities for teaching. To be successful with health education, the nurse must attempt to gain the client's trust and must be sensitive to any cultural issues present. The nurse must also be aware of the emotional and physical state of the client. If the client is anxious or in pain, teaching may be ineffective.

Counselor

The counseling role of the nurse occurs in almost every interaction in the area of women's health. Before counseling in the area of reproductive health is begun, it is essential for effective intervention that the nurse become aware of his or her value system, including how biases and beliefs about human sexual behavior affect the counseling role.

RESEARCH IN WOMEN'S HEALTH

Women have long been the major users of the health care system. Research involving women is beginning to provide information enabling prediction, explanation, or description of phenomena affecting health. In the past, medical treatment for women was based on findings of research performed with male subjects exclusively, even in conditions that caused more deaths in women. Since the federal mandate regarding women and research was instituted, research efforts to include women in studies have grown. If women are not included in a research project, a rationale must be given for their exclusion.

The National Institutes of Health established the Office of Research on Women's Health (ORWH) in 1990. Through

a special task force, recommendations were made for the research agenda for women's health. In addition, nurse researchers are encouraged to test interventions and question rituals in nursing by conducting research. Following are some of the areas for exploration and research among women:

- Alcohol, tobacco and other drug use
- Domestic violence
- Heart disease
- Health behaviors
- Genetic screening and breast cancer
- Bone and musculoskeletal disorders
- Cancer prevention, screening, diagnosis, and treatment
- Health education at various literacy levels
- Wellness throughout the life cycle
- Differences among women experiencing menopausal symptoms
- Dysmenorrhea
- Safe and effective contraception
- Promotion of breastfeeding
- Infertility
- Coping with chronic illness, such as systemic lupus erythematosus or arthritis
- Discomforts of pregnancy, including morning sickness
- Strengths of single, female heads of households
- Adolescent sexuality
- Multiple-role adaptation
- Menstrual cycle variations
- Control of obesity
- Substance abuse and its effect on pregnancy
- HIV infection and pregnancy
- Influence of diet on osteoporosis
- Effect of socialization on role
- Gender differences in pharmacology

Currently, research on the financing and delivery of health services for women has been supported. The American Recovery and Reinvestment Act of 2009 provided funding to the National Institutes of Health to support research in women's health by the ORWH. Overarching themes in women's health research identified by the ORWH include:

- Effects of developmental, psychological, spiritual, and physiological factors on lifespan
- Effects of female determinants, such as genetics and gender expectations, on health
- Health disparities and diversity
- Diseases and conditions affecting women
- Career development and advancement of women in the sciences

With the increased emphasis on community health, community health nurses can make significant contributions to the improvement of women's health through scholarly research, either as principal investigators or through data gathering. Furthermore, they can become consumers of research and develop nursing interventions based on sound research and recommendations.

SUMMARY

Women's health care has multiple facets, with many areas for community health nursing intervention. Nurses are advocates and activists for women's health through their involvement in health policy making as a profession. Along with other multidisciplinary and consumer groups, professional nurses are in the forefront of making changes in the health care delivery system that will promote an overall quality and research-based health plan for women. Women are at the center of the health of the United States; therefore, if better models are developed for improving the health of women, the health of the entire nation will benefit.

LEARNING ACTIVITIES

1. Identify examples from everyday life that support or encourage violence against women (e.g., magazines, books, and television advertisements). Share findings with classmates.
2. Survey lay magazine advertisements and estimate the percentage of total pages that use a woman's image, including aging, menopause, overweight and obesity, and sexuality, to sell products. Share these with classmates.
3. Discuss the need for cancer screening with female relatives; refer to the ACS guidelines.
4. Discuss with female relatives the need for a heart-healthy nutritional plan based on AHA guidelines.
5. Identify resources for mammograms and Pap smears for low-income women.
6. Visit with a women's group in the community (e.g., business, church, sorority, Parents Without Partners, Red Hat Society) to discuss members' health care needs and concerns. From these data, develop research questions.
7. Call a family planning clinic and determine the population served (i.e., eligibility), available services, and costs.
8. Review county or state health department statistics for leading causes of death among women of varying ethnic or racial groups.

ⓔ **EVOLVE WEBSITE**

http://evolve.elsevier.com/Nies

- NCLEX Review Questions
- Case Studies
- Glossary

REFERENCES

Adams PF, Martinez ME, Vickerie JL, et al: Summary health statistics for the US Population: National Health Interview Survey, 2010. *National Center for Health Statistics, Vital Health Stat* 10(251):1–117, 2011.

American Academy of Pediatrics: *Family pediatrics: report of the task force on the family, 2003,* Elk Grove Village, Ill, 2005, Author.

American Cancer Society: *American Cancer Society recommendations for early breast cancer detection in women without breast symptoms,* 2012. Available from <http://www.cancer.org /cancer/breastcancer/moreinformation/bre astcancerearlydetection/breast-cancer-early -detection-acs-recs>.

American Cancer Society: *Cancer facts and figures 2013,* 2013a. Available from <http://www.cancer. org/acs/groups/content/@epidemiologysurveilance /documents/document/acspc-036845.pdf>.

American Cancer Society: *Colorectal facts & figures 2011-2013,* Atlanta, 2011, American Cancer Society. Available from <http://www.cancer.org /acs/groups/content/@epidemiologysurveilanc e/documents/document/acspc-028323.pdf.>

American Cancer Society: *Guidelines for the early detection of cancer,* 2013b. Available from <http://www.cancer.org/healthy/ findcancerearly/cancerscreeningguidelines/am erican-cancer-society-guidelines-for-the-early- detection-of-cancer.>

American Cancer Society. *What are the risk factors for cervical cancer?* 2013c. Available from <http://www.cancer.org/cancer/cervicalcancer/ detailedguide/cervical-cancer-risk-factors>.

American Diabetes Association: *All about diabetes: Total prevalence of diabetes and pre-diabetes,* 2009. Available from <http://www.diabetes.org/diabetes-statistics/pre valence.jsp. Accessed May 22, 2009.

American Heart Association. *Understand your risk for high blood pressure.* 2012 <http://www- .heart.org/HEARTORG/Conditions/HighBlo odPressure/UnderstandYourRiskforHighBlo odPressure/Understand-Your-Risk-for-High- Blood-Pressure_UCM_002052_Article.jsp.>

American Heart Association: *Statistical fact sheet, 2013 update: Women and cardiovascular disease,* 2013. Available from <http://www.heart.org/idc /groups/heart-public/@wcm/@sop/@smd/docu ments/downloadable/ucm_319576.pdf>.

American Psychological Association: *Diagnostic and statistical manual of mental disorders,* ed 5, Washington, D.C, 2013, Author.

American Psychological Association: *Women and depression,* 2005. Available from <http://www.apa. org.ppo/issues/pwomenanddepress.html>.

Arthritis Foundation. Learn about arthritis Arthritis is Women. 2014. Available from <http://www.arthritis.org/conditi ons-treatments/disease-center/women/.>

Berg CJ, Callaghan WM, Syverson C, et al: Pregnancy-related mortality in the United States, 1998 to 2005, *Obstetrics and Gynecology* 116(6):1302–1309, 2010. 2010.

Bhatia SC, Bhatia SK: Depression in women: diagnostic and treatment considerations, *Am Fam Physician* 60(1):225, 1999.

Blair T: Domestic abuse: What is the Ob/Gyn nurse's role? *Ob Gyn Nurse Forum* 7(2):1, 1999.

Blehar M: Public health context of women's mental health research, *Psychiatric Clinics of North America* 26:781–799, 2003.

Brault Matthew W: *"Americans With Disabilities: 2010," Current Population Reports,* Washington, DC, 2012, U.S. Census Bureau. Available at <http: //www.census.gov/prod/2012pubs/p70-131.pdf.>

Cates W, Ellertson C, Stewart F: Abortion. In Hatcher RA, Trussell J, Stewart F, et al: *Contraceptive technology*, ed 18, New York, 2004, Ardent Media.

Centering Health Care: *Centering pregnancy overview*, 2013. Available from <http://www.centeringhealthcare.org/pages/centering-model/pregnancy-overview.php>.

Centers for Disease Control and Prevention: *National diabetes fact sheet: general information and national estimates on diabetes in the United States*, 2007a. Available from <http://www.cdc.gov/diabetes/pubs/pdf/ndfs_2007.pdf>.

Centers for Disease Control and Prevention: *Newest estimates for specific forms of arthritis*, 2007b. Available from <http://www.cdc.gov/arthritis/resources/spotlights/dsarthritis.htm>.

Centers for Disease Control and Prevention: *Age-adjusted hospital discharge rates for diabetes as any-listed diagnosis per 1,000 diabetic population, by sex, United States, 1980-2005*, 2008a. Available from <http://www.cdc.gov/diabetes/statistics/dmany/fig5.htm>.

Centers for Disease Control: *Arthritis types*, 2008b. Available from <http://www.cdc.gov/arthritis/basics/types.htm>.

Centers for Disease Control and Prevention: Birth rates for teens aged 15-19 years, by age group—United States, 1985-2007, *Morbid Mortal Wkly Report* 58(12):313, 2009b. Also available from <http://www.cdc.gov/mmwr/preview/mmwrhtml/mm5812a5.htm>.

Centers for Disease Control and Prevention: Cancer mortality surveillance United States, 1990-2000. *MMWR*, 53(3): 1-108, 2004.

Centers for Disease Control and Prevention: *Cervical cancer screening guidelines for average-risk women*, 2012a. Available from <http://www.cdc.gov/cancer/cervical/pdf/guidelines.pdf >.

Centers for Disease Control and Prevention: *Cervical cancer statistics*, 2013a. Available from <http://www.cdc.gov/cancer/cervical/statistics/#2>.

Centers for Disease Control and Prevention. *Faststats: Health insurance coverage*. 2012e. Available from <http://www.cdc.gov/nchs/fastats/hinsure.htm>.

Centers for Disease Control and Prevention: *HPV-associated cervical cancer rates by race and ethnicity*, 2012b. Available from <http://www.cdc.gov/cancer/hpv/statistics/cervicalhtm>.

Centers for Disease Control and Prevention: *HPV vaccine information for clinicians—fact sheet*, 2012. Available from <http://www.cdc.gov/std/HPV/STDFact-HPV-vaccine-hcp.htm>.

Centers for Disease Control and Prevention: Pregnancy related mortality in the United States, 2012c. Available from <http://www.cdc.gov/reproductivehealth/MaternalInfantHealth/Pregnancy-relatedMortality.htm>.

Centers for Disease Control and Prevention: Death rates* for human immunodeficiency virus (HIV) disease among women, by race and age group United States, 1987-2005, *Morbid Mortal Wkly Report* 58(11):286, 2009c. Also available from <http://www.cdc.gov/mmwr/preview/mmwrhtml/mm5811a4.htm>.

Centers for Disease Control and Prevention: *Leading cause of death by age group, all females—United States, 2009d*. Available from <http://www.cdc.gov/women/lcod/2009/09_all_women.pdf.>

Centers for Disease Control and Prevention: Prevalence of doctor-diagnosed arthritis and arthritis-attributable activity limitation United States, 2007-2009, *Morbidity And Mortality Report.*, 2010.

Centers for Disease Control and Prevention: *Prevalence of Self-Reported Postpartum Depressive Symptoms in 17 states, 2004-2005*. 2008d. Available from <http://www.cdc.gov/mmwr/preview/mmwrhtml/ss5610a1.htm.>

Centers for Disease Control and Prevention: Prevalence and most common causes of disability among adults—United States, 2005, *Morbid Mortal Wkly Rep* 58(16):421–426, 2009f. Also available from <http://www.cdc.gov/mmwr/preview/mmwrhtml/mm5816a2.htm#tab1>.

Centers for Disease Control and Prevention. *STDs in Women & infants*. 2012d. Available from <http://www.cdc.gov/std/stats11/womenandinf.htm#foot22>

Centers for Disease Control and Prevention: Teen Dating Violence. 2013b. Available from <http://www.cdc.gov/violenceprevention/intimatepartnerviolence/teen_dating_violence.html.>

Centers for Disease Control and Prevention. *Vaccine safety: human papilloma virus*. 2014. Available from <http://www.cdc.gov/vaccinesafety/Vaccines/HPV/index.html>.

Centers for Disease Control and Prevention. *Women's reproductive health: Hysterectomy*. 2008c. Accessed at <http://www.cdc.gov/reproductivehealth/WomensRH/Hysterectomy.htm.>

Centers for Disease Control and Prevention: Abortion Surveillance, United States, 2009; MMWR 61(SS08), 1-44, 2012. http://www.cdc.gov//mmwr/preview/mmwrhtml/ss6108a1.htm?s_cid=ss6108a1_w.

Centers for Disease Control and Prevention, National Institute for Occupational Safety and Health: *Workplace safety and health topics: Industries & occupations*, 2013. Available from <http://www.cdc.gov/niosh/topics/industries.html>.

Chadwick BA, Heaton TB, editors: *Statistical handbook on the American family*, Phoenix, 1992, Oryx Press.

Chang WC, Kaul P, Westerhout CM, et al: Impact of sex on long-term mortality from acute myocardial infarction vs. unstable angina, *Arch Intern Med* 163:2476–2484, 2003.

Cheung BM, Ong KL, Cherny SS: Diabetes prevalence and therapeutic target achievement in the United States, 1999 to 2006, *American Journal of Medicine* 122(5):443–453, 2009.

Chobanian AV, et al: The seventh report of the joint national committee on prevention, detection, evaluation, and treatment of high blood pressure, *JAMA* 289(19), 2003.

Choi M: Preamble to a new paradigm for women's health, *Image* 17:14, 1985.

Crane PB, Letvak S, Lewallen L, et al: Inclusion of women in nursing research: 1995-2001, *Nurs Res* 53(4):237–242, 2004.

Creanga AA, Shapiro-Mendoza CK, Bish CL, et al: Trends in ectopic pregnancy mortality in the United States: 1980-2007, *Obstetrics and Gynecology* 117(4):837–843, 2011.

Cronin KA, Richardson LC, Henley SJ, et al: Vital signs: Racial disparities in breast cancer severity—United States, 2005–2009, *Morbid Mortal Wkly Rep* 61(45):922–926, 2012. Also available from <http://www.cdc.gov/mmwr/preview/mmwrhtml/mm6145a5.htm?s_cid=mm6145a5_w>.

Cunningham FG, Gant NF, Wenstrom K, et al: *Williams' obstetrics*, ed 23, Norwalk, CT, 2010, Appleton and Lange.

DeFrances C, Lucas C, Buie V, et al: 2006 National Hospital Discharge Survey, *National Health Statistics Report* 30(5):1–20, 2008.

DeNavas-Walt C, Proctor D, Smith J: *Income, poverty, and health insurance coverage in the United States: 2011* (U.S. Census Bureau Current Population Reports), 2012. Available from <http://www.census.gov/prod/2008pubs/p60-243.pdf>.235.pdf.>

Downs J, Clearfield M, Weis S: Primary prevention of acute coronary events with lovastatin in men and women with average cholesterol levels: results of AFCAPS, *JAMA*(279)1615–1622, 1998.

Elders J: *Speech given at 2009 Public Health Practice Symposium: Public Health Leadership to Improve the Health of Young People*, Ann Arbor, January 27, 2009, Michigan.

Evans DL, et al: Depression in the medical setting: biopsychological interactions and treatment considerations, *J Clin Psychiatry* 60(suppl 4):40, 1999.

Finkel ML, Finkel DJ: The effect of a second opinion program on hysterectomy performance, *Med Care* 28:776, 1990.

Fowler CI, Gable J, Wang J, et al: *Family planning annual report: 2009 National summary*, Research Triangle Park, NC, 2010, RTI International Available from <http://www.hhs.gov/opa/pdfs/fpar-2009-national-summary.pdf.>

Gamble SB, Strauss LT, Parkere WY, et al: Abortion Surveillance, United States, 2005, *Morbid Mortal Wkly Report* 57(SS13):1–32, 2008. Also available from <http://www.cdc.gov/mmwr/preview/mmwrhtml/ss5713a1.htm>.

Genetic Information Nondiscrimination Act of 2008, 493 H.R., § 110 (2008).

Gilinson T: Know family, medical leave rights for yourself, your patients. Am Nurse 31(14): 1484-1486, 1999.

Hall MJ, DeFrances CJ, Williams SN, et al: National Hospital Discharge Survey: 2007 summary, *Natl Health Stat Report* 26(29):1–20, 2010. 24.

Health & Human Services. *Health Care: Improvements for Women*. 2012. Available at <http://www.hhs.gov/healthcare/prevention/women/index.html>

Hogan MC, Foreman KJ, Naghavi M, et al: Maternal mortality for 181 countries, 1980–2008: A systematic analysis of progress towards Millennium Development Goal 5, *The Lancet*. 375(9726):1609–1623, 2010.

Holahan J, Buttgens M, Caroll C, et al: Kaiser Commission on Medicaid and the Uninsured: *The cost and coverage implications of the ACA Medicaid expansion: National and state-by-state analysis, 2012.* Available from <http://kaiserfamilyfoundation.files.wordpress.com/2013/01/8384.pdf>.

Hopwood P, Stephens RJ: Medical Research Council (MRC) Lung Cancer Working Party: Symptoms at presentation for treatment in patients with lung cancer: implications for the evaluation of palliative treatment, *Br J Cancer* 71:633, 1995.

Hoyert DL, Xu JQ. Deaths: Preliminary data for 2011. *National vital statistics reports*; 61:6. Hyattsville, MD: National Center for Health Statistics. 2012.

Jacobs A: Coronary revascularization in women in 2003: sex revisited, *Circulation* 107:375–377, 2003.

Johnson RH, Chien FL, Bleyer A: Incidence of breast cancer with distant involvement among women in the United States, 1976 to 2009, *Journal of the American Medical Association.* 27(309):1229, 2013.

Kaiser Daily: *Women's health policy*, 2009. Available from <http://www.kaisernetwork.org/daily_reports/rep_index.cfm?hint=2&DR_ID=47116>. Accessed May 4, 2009.

Kovach K: Trauma nursing: intimate partner violence, *RN* 67:38, 2004.

Krieger Carol L: Intimate partner violence: A review for nurses, *Nursing for Women's Health* 12(3):224–334, 2008.

Kuehn J, McMahon P, Creekmore S: Stopping a silent killer. Preventing heart disease in women, *AWHONN Lifelines* 3(2):31–35, 1999.

Johnson RH, Chien FL, Bleyer A: Incidence of breast cancer with distant involvement among women in the United States, 1976 to 2009, *Journal of the American Medical Association* 309(8):800–805, 2013.

Manant A, Dodgson JE: Centering pregnancy: An integrative literature review, *Journal of Midwifery and Women's Health* 56:94–102, 2011.

Martin JA, Hamilton BE, Ventura SJ, et al *Births: Final data for 2009.* National Vital Statistics Reports; 60(1). Hyattsville, MD: National Center for Health Statistics. 2011. Accessed from <http://www.cdc.gov/nchs/data/nvsr/nvsr60/nvsr60_01.pdf.>

Martin R, et al: Gender disparities in common sense models of illness among myocardial infarction victims, *Health Psychol* 23:345–353, 2004.

Matthews S, Power C: Socio-economic gradients in psychological distress: A focus on women, social roles and work-home characteristics, *Soc Sci Med* 54:799–810, 2002.

Medicaid.gov. (2013). *Affordable Care Act: Eligibility*, n.d. Available from <http://www.medicaid.gov/AffordableCareAct/Provisions/Eligibility.html>.

Misner ST, Beauchamp-Hewitt JB, Fox-Levin P: Occupational issues in women's health. National League for Nursing.19:2546, 29–35.

Mosca CL: Evidence-based guidelines for cardiovascular disease prevention in women: 2007 Update, *Circulation* 115:1481–1501, 2007.

National Cancer Institute: *BRCA1 and BRCA2: Cancer risk and genetic testing*, 2013a. Available from <http://www.cancer.gov/cancertopics/factsheet/Risk/BRCA>.

National Cancer Institute: *HPV and cancer*, 2013b. Available from <http://cancer.gov/cancertopics/factsheet/Risk/HPV>.

National Cancer Institute: *Mammograms*, 2013c. Available from <http://www.cancer.gov/cancertopics/factsheet/detection/mammograms>.

National Cancer Institute, Surveillance, Epidemiology, and End Results Program: *SEER Stat fact sheets: Breast, surveillance epidemiology & end results*, 2013d. Available from <http://seer.cancer.gov/statfacts/html/breast.html>.

National Cancer Institute, Surveillance, Epidemiology, and End Results Program: *SEER Stat fact sheets: Ovary cancer*, 2013e. Available from <http://seer.cancer.gov/statfacts/html/ovary.html>

National Center for Health Statistics. *Health, United States, 2007 with chartbook on trends in the health of Americans*, 2008. Available from <http://www.cdc.gov/nchs/hus.htm>.

National Center for Health Statistics. *Health, United States, 2012: with special feature on emergency care.* Hyattsville, MD. 2013. 88–90. Available from <http://www.cdc.gov/nchs/data/hus/hus12.pdf#045>.

National Center for Health Statistics. *Healthy People 2010 Final Review*, 2012. Available from <http://www.cdc.gov/nchs/data/hpdata2010/hp2010_final_review.pdf>.

National Partnership for Women & Families. A look at the U.S. Department of Labor's 2012 family and medical leave act employee and worksite surveys. 2013. Available at <http://go.nationalpartnership.org/site/DocServer/DOL_FMLA_Survey_2012_Key_Findings.pdf?docID=11862.>

National Osteoporosis Foundation: What women need to know. 2014. Available at <http://www.nof.org/235.>

Nelson AL: Menstrual problems and common gynecologic concerns. In Hatcher RA, Trussell J, Stewart F, et al: *Contraceptive Technology*, ed 18, New York, 2004, Ardent Media.

Norhammar A, Stenestrand UJ, Lindbäck J, et al: Women younger than 65 years with diabetes mellitus are a high-risk group after myocardial infarction: a report from the Swedish Register of Information and Knowledge about Swedish Heart Intensive Care Admission (RIKS-HIA), *Heart* 94:1565–1570, 2009.

North American Menopause Society: The 2012 hormone therapy position statement of the North American Menopause Society, *Menopause* 19(3):265, 2012. Available from <http://dx.doi.org/10.1097/gme. 0b013e31824b970a.>

Patel JD: Lung cancer in women, *J Clin Oncol* 23(14):3212–3218, 2005.

Pender NJ, Murdaugh CL, Parsons MA: *Health promotion in nursing practice*, ed 4, Upper Saddle River, NJ, 2006, Prentice Hall.

Rhodes DJ: Identifying and counseling women at increased risk for breast cancer, *Mayo Clinic Proceedings* 77:355–361, 2002.

Rivera MP, Stover DE: Gender and lung cancer, *Clinical Chest Med* 25(2):391–400, 2004.

Ruzek S, Olsen V, Clark A: *Social, biomedical, and feminist models of women's health. Women's health: Complexities and differences*, Columbus, OH, 1997, Ohio State University Press.

Sarna L, McCorkle R: Burden of care and lung cancer, *Cancer Pract* 4:245, 1996.

Schuiling KD, Likis FE: *Women's gynecologic health*, Sudbury, MA, 2013, Jones and Bartlett.

Schulman KA, Berlin JA, Harless W, et al: The effect of race and sex on physicians' recommendations for cardiac catheterization, *New England Journal of Medicine* 340(8):618–626, 1999.

Siegel R, Ma J, Zou Z, et al: Cancer statisitcs, 2014. CA, *A cancer journal for clinicians* 64(1):9–29, 2014.

Snell T: *Survey of state prison inmates: 1991—women in prison (U.S. Department of Justice, Bureau of Justice Statistics Special Report)*, Washington, DC, 1994, US Government Printing Office.

Stevens JA: Falls among older adults–risk factors and prevention strategies, *Journal of Safety Research* 36(4):409–411, 2005.

Thibos M, Lavin-Loucks D, Martin M: *The feminization of poverty*, Dallas, TX, 2007, The J. McDonald Williams Institute and the YWCA.

Thomas B, et al: Randomized trial of breast self-examination in Shanghai: final results, *J Natl Cancer Inst* 94(19), Oct 2002.

U.S. Census Bureau: *Newsroom: News release: Single-parent households showed little variation since 1994, Census Bureau Reports*, Washington, DC, 2007, U.S. Department of Commerce, Public Information Office.

U.S. Department of Agriculture: *Choose my plate*, 2013. Available from <http://www.choosemyplate.gov/weight management-calories.html>.

U.S. Department of Education: *Digest of education statistics*, Washington, DC, 2008, Author.

U.S. Department of Health and Human Services: National Diabetes Statisitcs, 2011. *National Diabetes Clearinghouse.* Available at <http://diabetes.niddk.nih.gov/dm/pubs/statistics/#fast.>

U.S. Department of Health and Human Services: Panel on Antiretroviral Guidelines for Adults and Adolescents. Guidelines for the use of antiretroviral agents in HIV-1-infected adults and adolescents. 2013. Department of Health and Human Services. Available at <http://aidsinfo.nih.gov/ContentFiles/AdultandAdolescentGL.pdf.>

U.S. Department of Labor: *Women in the labor force: a databook*, Washington, DC, 2005, Author.

U.S. Department of Labor, Women's Bureau: *Quick stats on women workers*, 2008. Available from <http://www.dol.gov/wb/stats/main.htm>.

Urbanic JC: Depressive disorders. In Urbanic JC, Groh CJ, editors: *Women's mental health: a clinical guide for primary care providers*, Philadelphia, 2009, Wolters Kluwer.

Vaccarino V, Lin ZQ, Kasl S, et al: Sex differences in health status after coronary artery bypass surgery, *Circulation* 108(143):2642–2647, 2003.

Vogel WH: The advance practice nursing role in a high-risk breast cancer clinic, *Oncol Nurs Forum* 30:115–122, 2003.

Warshaw C, Ganley AL, Salber PR: *Improving the health care response to domestic violence: a resource manual for health care providers*, San Francisco, 1995, Family Violence Prevention Fund.

Wei G, Jackson JL, Hatzigeorgiou C, et al: Osteoporosis management in the new millennium, *Prim Care* 30(4):711–741, 2003.

Wenger NK: You've come a long way, baby*: cardiovascular health and disease in women: problems and prospects, *Circulation* 109: 558–560, 2004.

Whiteman MK, Hillis SD, Jamieson DJ, et al: Inpatient hysterectomy surveillance in the United States, 2000–2004, *American Journal of Obstetrics and Gynecology* 198(1):1–7, 2008.

Women Employed Institute: *Sexual harassment: the problem that isn't going away*, Chicago, 1994, Author.

World Health Organization. (2007*). International Statistical Classification of Diseases and Related Health Problems, 10th revision*, 2007. Available from <http://apps.who.int/classifications/apps/icd/icd10online/>.

World Health Organization: *Maternal mortality* (Fact Sheet No. 348), 2012. Available from <http://www.who.int/mediacentre/factsheets/fs348/en/>.

World Health Organization: *Life expectancy by country*, 2013. Available from <http://apps.who.int/gho/data/node.main.688>.

World Health Organization: *Department of Reproductive Health and Research: Maternal mortality 1990-2010*. estimates developed by WHO, UNICEF, UNFPA, and the World Bank. Geneva, 2012, Author.

World Health Organization: *World Health Report: 2004*, Geneva, 2004, The Author Available from <http://www.who.int/whr/2004/en/index.html.>

Wright Jr T, Massad L, Dunton, et al: 2006 consensus guidelines for the management of women with abnormal cervical cancer screening tests, *American Journal of Obstetrics and Gynecology* 197(4):346–355, 2006.

Zeidenstein L: Health issues of lesbian and bisexual women. In Varney H, editor: *Varney's midwifery*, ed 4, Sudbury, MA, 2004, Jones and Bartlett.

Men's Health

Jené Hurlbut*

OBJECTIVES

Upon completion of this chapter, the reader will be able to do the following:

1. Identify the major indicators of men's health status.
2. Describe physiological and psychosocial factors that have an impact on men's health status.
3. Discuss barriers to improving men's health.
4. Discuss factors that promote men's health.
5. Describe men's health needs.
6. Apply knowledge of men's health needs in planning gender-appropriate nursing care for men at the individual, family, and community levels.

KEY TERMS

androgen
chronic condition
illness orientation

life expectancy
medical care

morbidity
mortality

OUTLINE

Men's Health Status
  Longevity and Mortality
  Morbidity
Use of Medical Care
  Use of Ambulatory Care
  Use of Hospital Care
  Use of Preventive Care
  Use of Other Health Services
Theories that Explain Men's Health
  Biological Factors
  Socialization
  Orientation Toward Illness and Prevention
  Reporting of Health Behavior
  Discussion of the Theories of Men's Health
Factors that Impede Men's Health
  Medical Care Patterns
  Access to Care
  Lack of Health Promotion

Men's Health Care Needs
Primary Preventive Measures
  Health Education
  Interest Groups for Men and Men's Health
  Men's Growing Interest in Physical Fitness and Lifestyle
  Policy Related to Men's Health
Secondary Preventive Measures
  Health Services for Men
  Screening Services for Men
Tertiary Preventive Measures
  Sex-Role and Lifestyle Rehabilitation
  New Concepts of Community Care

*The author would like to acknowledge the contribution of Carrie Morgan, who wrote this chapter for the previous edition.

It is common knowledge that women live longer than men and that health care use is greater among women than men. Death rates for men are higher than for women in the major causes of death. Although the overall interest in health promotion and illness prevention has increased, men's health issues remain largely unaddressed (Baerlocher and Verma, 2008). Women's health has become a specialty practice with courses and programs available in many colleges of nursing. A specialty in men's health has not yet been established.

This chapter focuses on exploring the health needs of men and the implications for community health nursing. Specific areas that are discussed include the current health status of men, physiological and psychological theories that attempt to explain men's health, factors that impede men's health, factors that promote men's health, men's health needs, and planning gender-appropriate care for men at the individual, family, and community levels.

MEN'S HEALTH STATUS

Traditional indicators of health for all persons include rates of longevity, mortality, and morbidity. Reviewing these rates gives nursing students a better understanding of the community aggregate.

Longevity and Mortality

Major gender differences in longevity and mortality rates reveal that men remain disadvantaged despite advances in technology. Although women are more likely to use health services

STANDARDIZED TERMINOLOGY

In the fields of demography and sociology, the following terms are standardized:

People of all ages: Males and females
Children younger than 18 years: Boys and girls
Adults 18 years of age or older: Men and women
Sex: The biological distinction between males and females
Gender: The attitudes and behavior of men and women that are shaped by socialization and have a potential to be changed
Role: The part one plays in society

Modified from Skelton R: Man's role in society and its effect on health, *Nursing* 26:953, 1988; and Verbrugge LM, Wingard DL: Sex differentials in health and mortality, *Womens Health* 12:103, 1987.

and have higher morbidity rates, mortality rates for men remain higher. Gender differences are generally associated with both physiological and behavioral factors, which place men at greater risk of death. These behavioral factors, together with men's reluctance to seek preventive and health services, have marked implications for community health nursing.

Longevity

Rates of longevity are increasing for both men and women. People can now expect to live more than 20 years longer than their forefathers and foremothers lived at the turn of the nineteenth century. Infants born in the United States in 1996 can expect to live 77 years, whereas those born in 1900, when the death rate was highest, lived an average of 47.3 years. Life expectancy for both males and females has increased; however, since the 1970s this gender gap in longevity has decreased (Table 18-1). Between 2007 and 2008, men and women gained 0.2 year of longevity (Arias, 2012). This change in male longevity may be attributed to the advances in treatment of heart disease and cancer, which have been the major causes of death in U.S. males (Table 18-2).

Factors that influence the incongruencies between males and females are race or ethnic origin, socioecomic status, and education. When reported by race, gender mortality rates show that less advantaged populations in the United States, especially minorities, live significantly fewer years. African American males live 6 years less than white males (Arias, 2012). Hispanics have a life expectancy comparable with that of their white counterparts.

Mortality

The United States lags behind several other countries in premature mortality rates for males. In 2011 only six countries had premature mortality rates higher than that of the United States: Russian Federation, Mexico, Hungary, Estonia, Poland, and Slovak Republic (Organisation for Economic Co-operation and Development [OECD], 2011). In the United States, as in most industrialized countries, males lead females in mortality rates in each leading cause of death. Although males were the primary source of medical data before the 1970s, and most of the treatment advances have been developed from these data, gender-related disparity in death rates continues. Other factors also account for this mortality gender gap.

TABLE 18-1	LIFE EXPECTANCY AT BIRTH ACCORDING TO SEX AND RACE, UNITED STATES: 1900, 1950, 2000, 2005, 2007, AND 2008								
	ALL RACES			WHITE			BLACK		
YR	BOTH SEXES	MALE	FEMALE	BOTH SEXES	MALE	FEMALE	BOTH SEXES	MALE	FEMALE
1900	47.3	46.3	48.3	47.6	46.6	48.7	33.0	32.5	33.5
1950	68.2	65.6	71.1	69.1	66.5	72.2	60.8	59.1	62.9
2000	76.8	74.1	79.3	77.3	74.7	79.9	71.8	68.2	75.1
2005	77.4	74.9	79.9	77.9	75.4	80.4	72.8	69.3	76.1
2007	77.9	75.4	80.4	78.4	75.9	80.8	73.6	70.0	76.8
2008	78.1	75.6	80.6	78.5	76.1	80.9	74.0	70.6	77.2

Data from Arias E: *United States life tables, 2008* (National Vital Statistics Reports vol. 61, no. 3), Washington, DC, 2012, National Center for Health Statistics.

TABLE 18-2 LEADING CAUSES OF DEATH IN MALES, UNITED STATES, 2009

	PERCENTAGE
All Males, All Ages	
1. Heart disease	25.2
2. Cancer	24.4
3. Unintentional injuries	6.2
4. Chronic lower respiratory diseases	5.3
5. Stroke	4.3
6. Diabetes	2.9
7. Suicide	2.4
8. Influenza and pneumonia	2.1
9. Kidney disease	2.0
10. Alzheimer's disease	2.0
White Males, All Ages	
1. Heart disease	25.4
2. Cancer	24.6
3. Unintentional injuries	6.2
4. Chronic lower respiratory diseases	5.7
5. Stroke	4.2
6. Diabetes	2.7
7. Suicide	2.5
8. Alzheimer's disease	2.1
9. Influenza & pneumonia	2.1
10. Kidney disease	1.9
Black Males, All Ages	
1. Heart disease	24.2
2. Cancer	22.9
3. Unintentional injuries	5.5
4. Stroke	4.8
5. Homicide	4.6
6. Diabetes	3.8
7. Chronic lower respiratory diseases	3.1
8. Kidney disease	2.7
9. HIV	2.4
10. Septicemia	1.9
Asian or Pacific Islander Males, All Ages	
1. Cancer	27.0
2. Heart disease	24.4
3. Stroke	6.5
4. Unintentional injuries	5.0
5. Diabetes	3.7
6. Chronic lower respiratory diseases	3.4
7. Influenza and pneumonia	3.2
8. Suicide	2.6
9. Kidney disease	2.0
10. Alzheimer's disease	1.2
Hispanic Males, All Ages	
1. Heart disease	20.9
2. Cancer	20.2
3. Unintentional injuries	10.0
4. Stroke	4.2
5. Diabetes	4.1
6. Chronic liver disease	3.8
7. Homicide	3.4
8. Suicide	2.7
9. Chronic lower respiratory diseases	2.6
10. Influenza & pneumonia	2.4

From Centers for Disease Control and Prevention: *Men's health: leading causes of death in males United States 2009,* 2009. Retrieved from <http://www.cdc.gov/men/lcod/>.

The gender disparity for disease-related deaths has narrowed. Heart disease remains the leading cause of death, but the ratio of death for heart disease decreased by 2.8 between 2005 and 2006. During this same period, the ratio of male deaths to female deaths increased by 1.4. Since the 1990s, cancer-related deaths in women have declined at a slower rate than those in men. Lifetime risk for lung cancer is estimated to be 9.8% among males and 3.8% among females (Lynch, 2008). The death rate for chronic lower respiratory tract disease among females has increased from 14.9 deaths per 100,000 population in 1980 to 39.1 in 2008, and among males from 49.9 in 1980 to 51.4 in 2008 (NCHS, 2012). These rises may be associated with the increase in incidence of lower respiratory disease among the elderly (Lynch, 2008). Unintentional injury deaths for the whole population have decreased 1.2 per 100,000 from 2007 to 2008 (NCHS, 2011). Males continue to be at risk for death due to unintentional injury. Males aged 15 to 64 years are two to three times more likely to die as a result of unintentional injury than females of the same age. Men are three to four times more likely to commit suicide. Males older than 85 years are eleven times more likely than females of the same age to commit suicide (NCHS, 2011).

Race and ethnic background also are factors to be considered in the evaluation of male mortality rates. Black men between ages 45 and 64 years are more than eight times as likely to die of human immunodeficiency virus (HIV) infection as white males. Among males aged 15 to 24 years, African American males are more likely to die of vehicle accidents and seven times more likely to die of homicide (NCHS, 2011). Hispanic males fare somewhat better but are twice as likely as white males to die as a result of homicide.

Morbidity

Despite the differences in mortality rates, men tend to perceive themselves to be in better health than women do (Brown and Bond, 2008). In the National Health Interview Survey (NHIS) of 2010, which asked people to rate their health status, men were more likely to rate their health as excellent or very good as opposed to fair or poor (Schiller et al, 2012). Morbidity rates, or rates of illness, are difficult to obtain and have been available usually only in Western industrialized countries. For example, in the United States, reports of analyses of morbidity rates by gender lag several years behind those of analyses of mortality rates by gender. Gender differences in morbidity rates reflect the latest available reports. The following are common indicators of morbidity rate:

- Incidence of acute illness
- Prevalence of chronic conditions
- Use of medical care

Although variations exist, women are more likely to be ill, whereas men are at greater risk for death.

Chronic Conditions

A chronic condition is a condition that persists for at least 3 months or belongs to a group of conditions classified as chronic regardless of time of onset, such as tuberculosis, neoplasm, and arthritis. In general, women have higher morbidity rates than men. Women are more likely than men to have a higher prevalence of chronic diseases that cause disability and limitation of activities but do not lead to death. However, men have higher morbidity and mortality rates for conditions that are the leading causes of death.

SOURCES OF DATA

Health, United States: Submitted by the Secretary of the Department of Health and Human Services, *Health, United States* is an annual report on the health status of the nation. The data are compiled by the National Center for Health Statistics and the Centers for Disease Control and Prevention. The National Committee on Health and Vital Statistics reviews the report (http://www.cdc.gov/nchs/hus.htm).

National Center for Health Statistics (NCHS): Through the National Vital Statistics System, the NCHS collects data from each state, New York City, the District of Columbia, the U.S. Virgin Islands, Guam, and Puerto Rico on births, deaths, marriages, and divorces in the United States (http://www.cdc.gov/nchs/).

National Health Interview Survey: Directed by the National Center for Health Statistics, the National Health Interview Survey is an annual and continuing, nationwide sample survey in which data are collected by personal interviews about household members' illnesses, injuries, chronic conditions, disabilities, and use of health services (www.cdc.gov/nchs/nhis.htm).

USE OF MEDICAL CARE

The use of medical care—the use of ambulatory care, hospital care, preventive care, or other health services—in the United States also illustrates the different gender patterns.

Use of Ambulatory Care

Men seek ambulatory care less often than women. According to the 2010 NHIS (Schiller et al, 2012), the physician's office is the primary setting for ambulatory care for both men and women. Responses to the survey indicated that men visited physician offices and clinics or health centers less often than women and emergency rooms more frequently. Additionally, 27% of men, compared with 14% women, had made no office visits to a health care provider in the past 12 months. Men were likely to visit a physician only if they experienced a specific health-related symptom (Brown and Bond, 2008). Injury-related visits to hospital emergency departments are higher for males than females. Males aged 18 to 24 years are twice as likely to visit hospital emergency departments for unintentional injuries as females in the same age range. Even though gender differences in ambulatory care utilization are lessening, males continue to delay medical treatment, so they are sicker when they do seek health care and therefore require more intensive medical care.

Use of Hospital Care

The literature indicates that hospitalization rates also vary by sex. In 2008 to 2009, rates of discharges from short-stay hospitals were lower for males (1000.9 per 10,000) than for females (1307.6 per 10,000). However, males had a longer length of stay in the hospital than females (5.4 vs. 4.4 days, respectively). Discharge rates increase for both men and women after 45 years of age; however, rates for men increase more rapidly. After 65 years of age, men's discharge rates continue to be higher than women's rates (NCHS, 2012).

Use of Preventive Care

Preventive examinations and appropriate health-protective behavior are necessary for health promotion and early diagnosis of health problems. Men do not engage in these health-protective behaviors at the same frequency as females (Brown and Bond, 2008). Most men do not have routine checkups. National health surveys indicate that women overall are more likely than men to have visits to various health care providers (NCHS, 2012). Men are twice as likely to report no usual source of care, although eligibility for primary care in males exceeds that in females (Lynch, 2008).

Use of Other Health Services

Overall, the number of visits to health care provider offices and outpatient sites is lower for men aged 18 to 74 than for women in the same age span. Men tend to have fewer dental health care visits (56.2) than women (58.9), percent of persons with a dental visit in the past year for 2010 (NCHS, 2012). In a research study conducted by Frisbee and colleagues (2010), findings supported the importance of oral hygiene as it relates to the overall health of the individual. Additionally, men have lower rates of use of colorectal testing and procedures (men, 54.7; women, 55.1, percent of adults aged 50-75) (NCHS, 2012).

THEORIES THAT EXPLAIN MEN'S HEALTH

As discussed previously, a gender gap exists in health. The data reviewed raise many questions for community health nurses to explore regarding gender differences in health and illness. Although men have shorter life expectancies and higher rates of mortality for all leading causes of death, women have higher rates of morbidity, including rates of acute illness and chronic disease and use of medical and preventive care services. Verbrugge and Wingard (1987) asked why "females are sicker, but males die sooner." Several explanations exist for this paradox.

Nurses traditionally use developmental theories to explain individual behavior. Erickson's model was not gender specific; Levinson focused somewhat on male development. There remains a need for literature detailing the factors and combinations of factors that influence gender differences in the health and illness of populations.

The following explanations proposed by Waldron (1995-e) and Verbrugge and Wingard (1987) attempt to account for gender differences in this important area:

- Biological factors, including genetics, effects of sex hormones, and physiological differences, which may be influenced by genetics, hormones, and environment
- Socialization
- Orientations toward illness and prevention
- Data collection of health behavior

Biological Factors

Several biological factors influence sex differences in mortality and morbidity rates, including genetics, effects of sex hormones, and physiological differences, which may be influenced by genetics, hormones, and environmental factors (Waldron, 1995a-e). The embryo is unisexual until the seventh week of gestation. Androgen, a hormone from the Y chromosome coupled with the maternal androgen sources, results in the development of the male sex. More male births occur than female births. In 2008, 1048 male births occurred for every 1000 female births (Martin, Hamilton, and Sutton, 2010). However, during this period, infant mortality rates for males were 21% higher than for females, thus reducing this ratio (Mathews and MacDorman, 2012). Sex ratios at birth appear to be lower for births to American Indian and black fathers (Martin, Hamilton, and Sutton, 2010).

Whether sex ratios at birth are influenced by sex ratios at conception or sex differentials in mortality rates before birth is unknown. Current evidence suggests that more than two of every three prenatal deaths occur before clinical recognition of the pregnancy. Embryonic research shows excess male fetuses in early pregnancy and fewer males delivered at term. Males' experience of higher mortality rates for perinatal conditions is attributed to biological disadvantages such as males' greater risk of premature birth, higher rates of respiratory distress syndrome, and higher rates of infectious disease in infancy resulting from the influence of male hormones on the developing lungs, brain, and possibly the immune system of the male fetus (Heron et al, 2009). Sex chromosome–linked diseases, such as hemophilia and certain types of muscular dystrophy, are more common among males than females (Waldron, 1995d).

Biological advantages for females may also exist later in life because of the estrogen-related mechanism that protects against heart disease. Some evidence supports the hypothesis that men's higher testosterone levels contribute to their lower high-density lipoprotein cholesterol levels. Body fat distribution, specifically the tendency for men in Western countries to accumulate abdominal body fat versus the tendency for women to accumulate fat on the buttocks and thighs, may also contribute to sex differences in the development of metabolic syndrome (Kirby et al, 2006). Men's higher levels of stored iron also may contribute to risk for ischemic heart disease. Additional physiological gender differences are as follows (Tanne, 1997):

- During the process of aging, men's brain cells die faster than women's brain cells. This finding may explain why men are more often hospitalized for serious mental disease.
- Male immune systems are weaker than women's.

Socialization

A second theory for explaining sex differences in health is socialization, especially in the area of masculinity. Society emphasizes assertiveness, restricted emotional display, concern for power, and reckless behavior in males. Pursuit of these attributes results in higher risks in work, leisure, and lifestyle. Internalization of these norms of masculinity reduces the likelihood of engaging in health promotion behaviors for fear these behaviors might be interpreted as a sign of weakness. Gender-role socialization may influence these differences. Peer pressure plays an important role in the adherence to masculine norms. Many men enculturate their sons to believe that risking personal injury demonstrates masculinity (Brown and Bond, 2008).

According to the National Institute for Occupational Safety and Health's *NIOSH Workers Health Chartbook* (2004), 53.4% of U.S. workers are males. Male workers account for 66.1% of the reported occupational injuries and for 92% of work-related fatalities. Men's higher exposure to carcinogens at the worksite is associated with high rates of mesothelioma and coal worker's pneumoconiosis. In the United States, men score higher than women on measures of hostility and lack of trust of others, which may place them at higher risk of ischemic heart disease. Although occupational hazards to women's health are being identified, evidence indicates that, unlike for men, employment outside the home has a positive effect for U.S. women.

Popular male leisure, sports, and play activities place men at high risk for injury. Males between the ages of 18 and 24 years are twice as likely as women to visit a hospital emergency department because of unintentional injuries, cuts, or piercings or intentional injury (NCHS, 2012). Statistics show that men drive faster than women, receive more traffic violations, and are less likely to wear seat belts, all of which contribute to a greater number of motor vehicle fatalities. Although prevalence of smoking is decreasing, 25.3% of males smoke (NCHS, 2012); 57.6% of men consume alcohol, and men are five times more likely than women to drink heavily. Addtionally, males overall have a greater use of illegal substances and greater nonmedical use of psychotherapeutic drugs (NCHS, 2012).

Men are more likely to be involved in violent crimes, and violence is a typical precursor to homicide. Men are victims in four out of five homicides. For black males, the fifth leading cause of death is homicide. However, for white males, homicide is not one of the top ten causes of death (NCHS, 2012).

Many barriers exist that prohibit positive changes in male health behavior, but female family members were seen as facilitators. Cheatham and colleagues (2008) reported that several studies show males to be more likely to change health behaviors when these changes are suggested and supported by female family members that the males thought were concerned about their well-being.

FOUR DIMENSIONS OF STEREOTYPED MALE GENDER-ROLE BEHAVIOR

No sissy stuff: the need to be different from women
The big wheel: the need to be superior to others
The sturdy oak: the need to be independent and self-reliant
Give 'em hell: The need to be more powerful than others, through violence if necessary

Modified from David DS, Brannon R: The male sex role: our culture's blueprint of manhood, and what it's done for us lately. In David DS, Brannon R, editors: *The forty-nine percent majority: the male sex role*, Reading, MA, 1976, Addison-Wesley.

Orientation Toward Illness and Prevention

Illness orientation, or the ability to note symptoms and take appropriate action, also may differ between the sexes. Most diseases, injuries, and deaths prevalent among men are preventable. However, the stereotypical view of men as strong and invulnerable is incongruent with health promotion. Boys are socialized to ignore symptoms and "toughen up." Surveys done by the magazine *Men's Health* reveal that 9 million men have not seen a health care provider in 5 years. Men may be aware of being ill, but they make a conscious decision not to seek health care to avoid being labeled as "sick." Brown and Bond (2008) suggest that men lack the somatic awareness and are less likely to interpret symptoms as indicators of illness. A desire to rationalize symptoms and denial of susceptibility to disease may contribute to the delay in treatment (Brown and Bond, 2008).

Health-protective behavior, or the ability to take action to prevent disease or injury, also may vary between the sexes. Perhaps as a result of the contraceptive developments of the 1970s, women are more likely to seek preventive examinations. Routine reproductive health screening (e.g., the Papanicolaou smear test and breast examination) has been expanded to include some general screening, such as testing of blood pressure, urine, and blood for signs of chronic problems. Men do not have routine reproductive health checkups that include screening, which would detect other health problems at an early stage. Among respondents to the NHIS, more women than men reported contacting a dentist and a health care provider within the previous 6 months, and 22% of men were without a usual place of health care, compared with 13% of women (Schiller et al, 2012). Men reported spending more time in leisure activities and muscle strengthening activities that met the federal physical activity guidelines. However, 41% of men were considered overweight, compared with 28% of women (Schiller et al, 2012).

Gender differences in preventive health behavior are a fertile ground for continued research. Meryn (2009) reported that 21% of research was devoted to men's health, compared with 53% for female health. He suggests that large-scale research in this area would add to the small evidence bases of health promotion behaviors among men. Specific national health objectives have only recently addressed the health care needs of this aggregate. Uniformly recognized preventive screening programs for males have only recently been developed. With the advent of managed care and initiatives for health care reform, men who are eligible for health care coverage will have access to these routine health screenings. For men coverage would be available for immunizations, colonoscopies, nutritional education, obesity screenings, cholesterol and blood pressure screenings, screenings for HIV, depression screenings, and tobacco counseling (Sommers and Wilson 2012). However, whether men will take advantage of these programs is undetermined. Box 18-1 discusses matters related to men's reproductive health needs.

Reporting of Health Behavior

Data regarding health behaviors are collected from a variety of sources, such as interviews, surveys, questionnaires, and reports. Data from these sources may not be accurate because males are less likely than females to participate in such a data collection process. Men may be less willing to talk, may not recall health problems, and may lack a health vocabulary. Men may be more hesitant to talk about their illnesses. Not only do women participate more in the data collection process but also they are often solicited in health surveys to report the health behavior of men. In this manner, women are proxies, and proxies have a tendency to underreport behavior. The accuracy of the data does increase with male participation, but men may not want to participate in the socialization of sickness and tend to make light of health problems. Males with an extreme conception of masculinity are less likely to admit their health problems and may conceal or suppress pain in an effort to appear strong (Naslindh-Ylispanger, Sihvonen, and Kekki, 2008). Men are far less likely than women to seek counseling. Male socialization to suppress expressiveness may represent the explanation for gender differences in reporting health behaviors.

Discussion of the Theories of Men's Health
Interpreting the Data

Community health nurses should be aware of gender disparity when collecting and interpreting data. To avoid bias, the community health nurse should consider the following issues:

- Gender-specific interview techniques may be necessary to obtain the most accurate health history. Men respond better to direct questions than to open-ended questions.
- How do data obtained by male nurses differ from those obtained by female nurses? Is there personal gender bias in data collection?
- The accuracy of secondary sources of information is skewed toward the interpretation of the source. How do the data provided by women about male health behavior compare with the data collected from men regarding these same behaviors?
- Men are not enculturated to be caregivers. They need assistance to learn how to provide support to a caregiver or to develop a caregiver role.

In response to the question why "females are sicker, but males die sooner," several reasons can be provided. Conditions that affect morbidity rates (e.g., arthritis and gout) do not significantly affect mortality rates. Conditions that affect mortality rates may not significantly affect day-to-day activity until the conditions are advanced. Men tend to delay seeking health care until their conditions are advanced. Although mortality rates are, in large part, the outcome of inherited or acquired risks, gender differences in illness and health promotion behaviors, as well as in the reporting of health behaviors, suggest that social and psychological factors also affect morbidity rates. Although males have higher prevalence and death rates for "killer" chronic diseases, injuries, and accidents, females have higher prevalence rates for a greater number of nonfatal chronic conditions.

BOX 18-1   MEN'S REPRODUCTIVE HEALTH NEEDS

Reproductive health needs are beginning to be recognized as important to both men's health and women's health. Usually the term reproductive health is applied to women of childbearing age. Used here, the term applies to the health of reproductive organs, which develop in utero and with which a person is born, either males or female, regardless of whether he or she has sex or reproduces. Males may have reproductive health needs whether child or adult, straight or gay, or virgin or sexually experienced.

Many sexually transmitted diseases (STDs) are at epidemic proportions in the United States and are a major health hazard for many men and women. Acquired immunodeficiency syndrome (AIDS) in the United States is twice as likely to occur in males as in females. In 2008, death due to HIV in males was 4.8 per 100,000, and for females it was 1.9 per 100,000 (National Center for Health Statistics [NCHS], 2012). Less well known, perhaps, is that many STDs are considered intrinsically "sexist" because clinical evidence, more overt in men, is more likely to facilitate a correct diagnosis in men than in women. These STDs are easier to detect in men because men are more likely to be symptomatic; laboratory tests are more reliable in men; efficiency of transmission is greater from male to female; and men are more likely to seek care for STDs that are symptomatic. For example, the overall incidence rate for *Chlamydia* infection in 2010-2011 for males was 256.9 per 100,000; for females, the rate was 648.9 per 100,000. The rate of gonorrhea was slightly lower among men (98.7 per 100,000 population) than among women (108.9 per 100,000 population). Only syphilis was more common in men than in women (8.2 per 100,000 males; 1.0 per 100,000 females) (National Center for Health Statistics, 2012).

Testicular cancer represents only 1% of cancers in males and is the most common cancer to affect young men between ages 15 and 35 years. Cancer of the prostate is a leading cause of death from cancer in men, was estimated to account for 22.3 deaths per 100,000 population in 2008, and remains twice as common in African American males as in white males (NCHS, 2012). The increase in the incidence of prostate cancer has been attributed to factors such as improved methods of detection and greater exposure to environmental carcinogens.

Mortality rates for all cancers remain high, especially in males older than 75 years. Men older than 85 years are twice as likely to die of cancer as those aged 75 to 84 years (NCHS, 2012).

Many occupational and environmental agents associated with adverse sexual and reproductive outcomes in men have been identified, including pesticides, anesthetic gases in the operating room and dental office, inorganic lead from smelters, paint, printing materials, carbon disulfide from vulcanization of rubber, inorganic mercury manufacturing and dental work, and ionizing radiation from x-rays (Whorton, 1984). Nonchemical agents have also been identified as hazardous in men; for example, hyperthermia experienced by firefighters has been linked to male infertility.

Many pharmacological agents, including prescription, over-the-counter, and recreational drugs, have been found to affect the reproductive outcomes or sexual functioning of men. Examples are drugs from the following categories: antihypertensives, antipsychotics, antidepressants, hormones, sedatives, hypnotics, stimulants, chemotherapy agents used in cancer treatment, amphetamines, opiates, alcohol, marijuana, cocaine, barbiturates, and lysergic acid diethylamide (LSD). Erectile dysfunction has become a "socially acceptable" topic of discussion since many high-profile men, such as U.S. Senator Bob Dole, former National Football League coach Mike Ditka, and retired General Norman Schwarzkopf have openly discussed their problem. Pharmaceutical companies market their products for treatment of this disorder via mass media. Controversy has arisen as to the use of public funding for these products.

A focus on homosexual men's health has come about largely through the advent of AIDS. Today, homosexuality encompasses not only the male but also the entire family. The community health nurse should develop nonjudgmental assessment skills that foster honest and open expression for all members of the community. Nurses may need specialized skills to work with these individuals.

Gender-Linked Behavior

The largest gender differences in mortality rates occur for causes of death associated with gender-linked behavior and suggest that gender-linked behavior, which is more prevalent and encouraged in men, correlates with the following major categories of death:

Tobacco use: Lung cancer, bronchitis, emphysema, and asthma
Substance abuse: Cirrhosis, accidents, and homicide
Poor preventive health habits and stress: Heart disease
Lack of other emotional channels: Cirrhosis, suicide, homicide, and accidents

Physical conditions can be seriously affected by social and environmental conditions, such as occupational hazards (e.g., carcinogens and stress), unemployment, and massive advertising campaigns that use gender and gender roles to sell alcohol and tobacco. These lifestyle factors are compounded by men's lack of willingness to seek preventive care such as screening and to seek health care when a symptom arises. To counter these types of factors, research is needed to determine gender-specific methods of data collection, education, and practice that are aimed at health promotion, illness prevention, and political processes for males.

RESEARCH HIGHLIGHTS

Health Education and Health Screening in a Sample of Older Men: A Descriptive Survey

Two nurse researchers (Dallas and Neville, 2012), conducted a study to describe the health education and health screening practices of older men living in an area of New Zealand and the perceived barriers to and benefits of healthy lifestyle choices. Data were collected using a self-reported instrument. The sample consisted of 59 men ranging in age from 65 to 91 years. The majority of the men in this sample (66%) reported no barriers to making a healthy lifestyle choice. However, of those men who did report barriers, the most common reason was lack of motivation (12%), followed by lack of knowledge related to availability of programs and screenings (8%). Reported external barriers included: lack of programs, associated costs, and transportation challenges. The most common reported benefits of a healthy lifestyle choice were: getting to be with other people (62%), having fun (56%), feeling healthier (54%), and feeling better about self (52%). The majority of the men reported their health as good (67%), and healthy lifestyle as always (43%) or frequently healthy (43%). Dallas and Neville (2012) contend that nurses can have a pivotal role in conducting future research endeavors aimed at understanding the health needs of older men that will ultimately improve their health outcomes.

Data from Dallas J, Neville S: Health education and health screening in a sample of older men: a descriptive survey, *Nurs Prax N Z* 28(1):6-16, 2012.

FACTORS THAT IMPEDE MEN'S HEALTH

There are many factors that function as barriers to men's health, including their risk-taking behaviors and infrequent use of the health care system. In addition, gaps in preventive health behavior and differences in illness and health orientations and reporting of health behavior all contribute to a diminished health status for men. Several other barriers have been proposed, including the patterns of medical care provided in the United States, access to care, and lack of health promotion.

Medical Care Patterns

Although the data that serve as a foundation for medical treatment were collected from males, the concept of a health care provider that specializes in men's health is a relatively new phenomenon. Many health professionals provide care for men with complex health needs in a wide variety of settings. A specialist to which a male could go to for care that "feels right" for him has not been developed. Little effort has been made to create a male-specific health care climate (Haines and Wender, 2006). Urologists, who may see men for genital abnormalities or diseases of the prostate, became the proxy "male health specialists." The medical specialty andrology, which originated in Europe to treat problems of fertility and sterility, is considered too narrow in focus to treat "the whole man." Without a primary care specialty that focuses specifically on men's needs and gender-role influences on health and lifestyle, the gender disparity will continue. Currently, male health concerns are addressed by specialists and generalists who have not received gender-specific training that would enable them to focus on men's health needs. In the current era of managed care and health care reform, men will still be left without gender-specific primary care providers who have training focused specifically on men's needs.

Access to Care
Mission Orientation

Historically, society's interest in men's health has focused on efforts necessary to maintain an effective workforce. Men are socialized to view health as a commodity or resource that enables the body to work. Mission-oriented health care is a priority for large industries and organized sports. Industries provide workers with preventive health care to maintain workplace productivity. Mission-oriented health care in the sports arena has given birth to the specialty of sports medicine. Insurance programs such as health maintenance organizations (HMOs) may provide more comprehensive health care to men. Perhaps the most complete care is currently offered by the military; however, marked deficiencies exist there in the lack of a focus on prevention and health promotion at the individual and aggregate levels and inattention to policy regarding environmental hazards.

Financial Considerations

Another barrier to health care for men is financial ability. A man may receive an annual physical examination if he belongs to a health maintenance organization or if he is an executive or an airline pilot, but many private insurance companies reimburse more fully for a diagnosed condition (e.g., for pathology) and less fully for preventive care. A man is more likely to be insured for acute or chronic illness conditions than for health education, counseling, or other types of preventive health care. Women have annual gynecological examinations that include screening for other conditions and allow a woman to express other physical or psychological needs; however, men have lacked entrance into the health care system for a physical examination on a routine basis. With the advent of managed care and societal interest in preventive health focus, gender differences in routine physical examinations for preventive reasons have narrowed. However, socialization has a marked influence on behavior, and current trends may prevail despite attitudinal changes in health care delivery. Men must become advocates for programs that meet their own health care needs (Porche, 2009).

Time Factors

Historically, medical care could be accessed between the hours of 9:00 AM and 5:00 PM Monday through Friday. Men were reluctant to take time from work for a medical visit, especially for reasons other than illness. Fear of loss of income or the stigmatization of being "weak," "ill," or "less of a man" inhibited medical care access for males. Men in the lower socioeconomic group may be too exhausted from working to access health care, especially preventive health care (Haines and Wender, 2006). Variety in the times and locations of care delivery clinics should improve male access. More walk-in primary care clinics that provide evening and weekend appointments have appeared. These clinics may be housed in occupational settings, malls, and even grocery stores. Data must be collected regarding male utilization of these additional health care sites.

Lack of Health Promotion

Limiting the concept of health to being merely absence of disease eliminates health promotion. Using traditional mortality and morbidity rates as reflective of the state of "health" of a population represents only a biological basis of health. To provide the community health nurse with a clearer picture of male health, the presence of behavioral risk factors such as smoking, alcohol consumption, obesity, and sedentary lifestyle should be considered. When asked, men describe "healthy" people as those with proportional body weight and height who do not engage excessively in behaviors detrimental to health. Physical recovery after impairment, illness, or injury is also considered a factor in men's definition of "healthy." Disease prevention and health promotion are not often reflected in a man's perception of health. Addressing and limiting the precursors of death is a recent health care phenomenon (Box 18-2). Interventions by many disciplines are needed to prevent current health problems. Nursing can play a pivotal role in the contribution to practice and research in this area of concern.

The continued focus on disease cure in the present health care system reinforces men's perception of health. Coronary heart disease, cancer, and stroke are three conditions that

The following precursors of death are frequently unaddressed by the present health care system:
- Heart disease and stroke
- Hypercholesterolemia
- Hypertension
- Diabetes mellitus
- Obesity
- Type A personality
- Family history
- Lack of exercise
- Cigarette smoking
- Cancer
- Sunlight
- Radiation
- Occupational hazards
- Water pollution
- Air pollution
- Dietary patterns
- Alcohol
- Heredity

account for two thirds of all deaths and require the greatest use of health care resources. The increase in life expectancy exhibits the effect these medical advances have had on mortality rates from these diseases. These advances have resulted in an increase in years of disability, which may account for the rise in suicide among men older than 65 years (NCHS, 2012). An increase in health care costs has also resulted.

SOCIAL DEMOGRAPHY AND SOCIAL EPIDEMIOLOGY

Epidemiology is the method of research used to determine the nature and distribution of a health problem in a community. Social demographers and social epidemiologists study social and psychological factors that affect the distribution of health problems in a community. Factors associated with the occurrence of the problems can be identified, and resources can be focused on prevention. Social epidemiologists have identified men as a population at risk for premature death. Concentrated efforts can improve men's health.

ETHICAL INSIGHTS

Social Justice versus Market Justice Ethics

Community health nurses should be involved in political activities that develop health policies that will make a difference in the health of males and the entire population. Such activities are congruent with the philosophy of public health as "health for all" and a commitment to a social justice ethic of health care rather than a market justice ethic of health care. Examining men's health gives the community health nurse an opportunity to observe the market justice ethic of health care's influence on men's health in the United States and how this impacts their traditional roles in the family and within the community. The community health nurse can play a vital role in contributing to a social justice ethic of health care, particularly in relation to promoting men's health. Nurses must focus on health promotion and prevention at the aggregate and population levels rather than on treatment and cure.

Financial resources are invested in traditional disease-curative care rather than health promotion action. An inordinate amount of funding is poured into the health care system each year, with only minimal amounts allotted to public health promotion, as discussed in earlier chapters. In 2009, total health expenditures accounted for 17.4% of the gross domestic product (NCHS, 2012). Of every dollar spent on health care in 2009, more than half went to hospital care and physician services, which are in large part curative in focus. The current health care system is making limited advances in addressing the precursors of death. It is questionable whether medical care, or another medical specialty, is the answer to men's health needs when social, occupational, environmental, and lifestyle factors continue to place men at risk.

Healthy lifestyles are not a matter of free choice but rather a result of opportunities that are not always equally available to people. Although available, prevention and health promotion are not uniformly applied at the aggregate and population levels. Health policies shape these opportunities for a healthy lifestyle for individuals and aggregates. Policies related to environmental and occupational changes beyond an individual's control are required to significantly impact the health of the population (Meryn, 2009).

MEN'S HEALTH CARE NEEDS

DeHoff and Forrest (1984) delineated men's health care needs that draw from the biological and psychosocial causes of men's distinctive health situation, and these health care needs continue today. According to these writers, men need the following:
- Permission to have concerns about health and talk openly to others about their concerns
- Support for the consideration of gender-role and lifestyle influences on their physical and mental health
- Attention from professionals regarding factors that may result in illness or influence a man's expression of illness, including such things as occupational factors, leisure patterns, and interpersonal relationships
- Information about how their bodies function, what is normal, what is abnormal, what action to take, and the contributions of proper nutrition and exercise
- Self-care instruction, including testicular and genital self-examination
- Physical examination and history taking that include sexual and reproductive health and illness throughout the lifespan
- Treatment for problems of couples, including interpersonal problems, infertility, family planning, sexual concerns, and sexually transmitted diseases (STDs)
- Help with fathering (i.e., being included as a parent in child care)
- Help with fathering as a single parent, in particular with a child of the opposite sex, in addressing the child's sexual development and concerns
- Recognition that feelings of confusion and uncertainty in a time of rapid social change are normal and that they may mark the onset of healthy adaptation to change

- Adjustment of the health care system to men's occupational constraints regarding time and location of health care sources
- Financial ways to obtain these goals

Additional health care needs of men are for primary prevention, and for secondary and tertiary prevention at the individual, family, and community levels, to address the precursors of death that influence males so greatly. Men are less likely than women to be consumers in the health care system; therefore alternative approaches must be developed that address their health needs. The most significant approaches in the future will be those that reach men in the community, schools, the workplace, and public settings. These approaches call for political processes that set policy, for health marketing techniques, and for advocacy (Meryn, 2009).

COMMUNITY HEALTH NURSING SERVICES FOR MEN

A male can be seen by a community health nurse in a well-baby clinic, by a school nurse, by an occupational health nurse, and by a community health nurse or home health nurse on a home visit for follow-up of a chronic disease. However, men are less likely than women to be seen by a community health nurse. Not only is maternal and child health a major focus of many health departments, but neither a medical nor a nursing specialty within a health department routinely exists to specifically address men's health. Preventive reproductive health care (e.g., family planning, prenatal care, and cancer screening) and associated general screening are not routinely available for men. The community health nurse's commitment to health for all requires an increased awareness of men's health issues in their social and cultural context as well as individual and group actions that will improve men's physical, psychological, and social well-being.

Meeting men's health care needs can be viewed in a traditional public fashion. By viewing the problem from a primary, secondary, and tertiary intervention method, the nurse can look at the problem in a holistic manner. Factors that promote men's health are in the community, including interest groups in men and men's health, men's growing interest in physical fitness and lifestyle, policy related to men's health, and health services for men.

GAINING SKILLS NECESSARY TO ADDRESS MEN'S HEALTH NEEDS

Assessment skills necessary to carry out screening activities with men to detect reproductive health needs may be lacking in nursing education. One community health nurse who worked in a rural health department felt unqualified to respond to male partners' requests for genital examinations when couples came to seek family planning services. This community health nurse requested to work for specified periods of time with a urologist and in a sexually transmitted disease clinic in a large urban area to gain the necessary skills. On return to the rural health department, she felt comfortable with male patients and taught the skills she had learned to nurse colleagues. Cheatham and colleagues (2008) suggest that providers make efforts to establish a positive patient-provider relationship using nonjudgmental verbal and nonverbal communication techniques. The nurse should engage the male and the female significant other in a manner that is easily understood.

PRIMARY PREVENTIVE MEASURES

Health Education

Health care professionals, including the community health nurse, find that health education is the cornerstone of prevention. Although criticized by some as too narrow, health education can be a means of empowerment that helps individuals make behavioral changes. Education about male health issues should begin early. At school, boys should learn the anatomical and physiological aspects of their bodies and the social aspects of taking responsibility for their health. Coeducational discussion classes that cover a variety of social and personal topics can be a venue to encourage boys to talk about their bodies and their feelings. Adolescent males are shown to lack the use of language in comparison with their female counterparts. This may lead to a less self-conscious attitude to health seeking when boys reach adulthood.

Access to health education should follow males into the workplace. Many employers have experienced benefits such as lower health care costs when their employees receive health education programs coupled with health screening. Government and private insurance incentives given to employers who provide such programs would provide further impetus. Men who are not in the workplace can access health education in other areas, such as shopping malls, barbershops, and local senior centers. Some health care professionals are concerned about such informal dispersion of health literature, citing possible issues with the literacy level of the population. Government benefits programs can function as a medium for health education by including it in their benefit mailings. More control over the readability and the information included can be exerted over this material. Educational material should be written in the context of male interests and should focus on making healthy living relevant to the male (Cheatham et al, 2008).

Interest Groups for Men and Men's Health

The consumer movement that occurred on behalf of women's health in the 1960s and early 1970s has no counterpart for advocation of men's health. However, a viable men's consumer movement is forming. The National Organization for Men Against Sexism is interested in redefining the male role, particularly those aspects of it that are detrimental to health and growth. The American Assembly for Men in Nursing sponsors annual meetings that address issues such as men's health, men's work environments, research on men's health, and networking and support among male nurses. Researchers are beginning to define and study men's health beyond men's occupational role (e.g., reproductive health). Marketing has changed to include male health promotion public service announcements. Peer-reviewed journals such as *International Journal of Men's Health* and *American Journal of Men's Health* are providing scholars with avenues to disseminate men's health concerns.

Men's Growing Interest in Physical Fitness and Lifestyle

Although cardiovascular diseases (CVDs) are a major health hazard for men, research on the validity and usefulness of preventive and treatment modalities is an issue of considerable debate (*Harvard Men's Health Watch*, 2009). Men's interest in altering behavior that places them at risk for cardiovascular and other major diseases is increasing, especially among older males (Shapiro and Yarborough-Hayes, 2008). For example, men's smoking behavior has changed dramatically. In 1965, more than 50% of males smoked compared with 21% in 2010. Today, 52.1% of men report engaging in aerobic activity three times a week or more, compared with 42.7% of females (Schiller et al, 2012).

However, those health behaviors that have shown the greatest change in a positive direction have been those most influenced by legislative action (e.g., seat belt use, use of smoke detectors, and drunk driving). Even with these legislative actions, males remain three times less likely to use seat belts as females of the same age. In the Southeast, use of seat belts in pickup trucks was 25%, compared with more than 75% in other vehicles. The states of Alabama, Florida, Georgia, Kentucky, Mississippi, North Carolina, South Carolina, and Tennessee have engaged in a campaign called "Buckle Up in Your Truck." The campaign's centerpiece is the use of targeted television and radio advertisements to encourage seat belt use. Intensive enforcement mobilizations in the form of Selective Traffic Enforcement Programs (STEPs), like Click It or Ticket, have followed periods of pickup truck advertisements. According to Tison and Williams (2010), the Click It or Ticket program has been an important factor in the improved usage of seat belts across the nation. On the basis of data from this report, seat belt use has increased by 20 percentage points from 1991 through 2007.

Policy Related to Men's Health

Policies related to any group of people should include the opinions and perceptions of those directly affected. Policy related to men's health should include the male perception of health. Community health nurses can encourage and help males to be advocates for policies regarding their health care. Male nurses can be extremely instrumental in this endeavor. Liaisons between male consumers and policy planners should be formed.

SECONDARY PREVENTIVE MEASURES

Health Services for Men

Fewer health care clinics are tailored to men's special needs than to women's special needs. The "well-man clinics" set up in the 1980s were designed to identify lifestyle risk factors, not to provide screening clinics like the women's clinics. Once they are identified, a method or resolution for these lifestyle risk factors is formulated. Although many well-man clinics exist in the United Kingdom, male use of these clinics is far below female use of women's clinics (Roberts and Gerber, 2003). Although not based on the medical model, the Men's Shed movement in Australia has provided men with the socialization needed to make positive health behavior changes. Male screening methods typically have been limited to detecting high blood cholesterol levels and cancers such as prostate cancer, skin cancer, and testicular lumps. The era of managed care and health care reform may not encourage the concept of gender-specific care, as men and women receive primary care from the same health services.

Screening Services for Men

The U.S. Preventive Services Task Force (2004) outlines the kinds of screening tests the population should receive. According to the Task Force, healthy men younger than 50 years should have the following evaluation schedule:

- Dental examination: Yearly
- Eye examination: Every 3 to 5 years
- Blood pressure check: Every 2 years
- Blood cholesterol check for men aged 53 years and older: Yearly
- Prostate examination: Every year after age 50 years; blacks every year after age 40 years
- Colorectal screening: Every 3 to 5 years
- Tobacco use and cessation information every year
- One-time screening for abdominal aortic aneurysm for any man 65 years old who has smoked

Community health nurses should be familiar with these recommended screening test frequencies and should take every opportunity to encourage men to have these screenings. Through the institution of male health care fairs and other organized screenings, nurses are able to work with other health care providers to ensure that such routine screenings are performed.

TERTIARY PREVENTIVE MEASURES

Sex-Role and Lifestyle Rehabilitation

Traditional health services for males are available in both private and governmental arenas. The emphasis of these services is on diagnosis and treatment. The traditional male role may change dramatically from treatment modalities. Rehabilitation services for males must include counseling on lifestyle, role changes, and job retraining. Men must be given permission to express their emotions, such as fear and anxiety, over the resultant change (Cheatham et al, 2008).

Goal setting and possible methods for achievement must be acceptable to the man. For example, after a heart attack, a man may be told to stop smoking and begin an exercise program. For the plan to be successful, the male must be an active partner in its formation. (He may be able to exercise, for example, by walking to the nearest automotive shop to talk with friends rather than spending time on a stationary bicycle at a local gym.)

Time taken away from work because of occupational injuries should be kept to a minimum. Males should be encouraged to return to work in an altered capacity rather than remaining away from work until injuries are completely healed. Occupational accommodation for the treatment regimen will help ensure compliance. Provision of medical care, supportive physical and occupational therapies, and "light-duty" jobs at the worksite help preserve the masculine persona.

DOOR OPENERS: WAYS TO ADDRESS MEN ABOUT HEALTH CONCERNS

Strategies to address men about health concerns include the following:

- Ask a man to talk about the last time he had a physical examination, what was done, why it was done, where it was done, and what the recommendations were.
- Ask a man how he feels about his health insurance coverage. If he lacks health insurance, ask about the resources he used to obtain medical care for himself and for his family.
- Ask a man about how he spends his leisure time, what he is doing to take care of himself, and what his usual physical activities are.
- Observe a man for signs of stress such as moist palms, nail biting, posture (e.g., stooped with lack of eye contact), and nervous movements. If signs of stress are present, ask about how he is coping with an identified health problem, family problem, or being unemployed.
- Observe a man for difficulty clearing the airway (e.g., from smoking) and flushing of the face (e.g., from alcohol). Inquire as to habits of smoking and drinking and whether these habits have increased since the occurrence of the particular health or social problem.
- Involve the man in decision making about health care to instill a sense of control over events.

New Concepts of Community Care

Specific services for men within health departments continue to be lacking in the United States. With the exception of STD clinics and selected family planning service models, male health concerns remain unaddressed. Two male health visitors (the British term for public health nurses) from the National Health Service (NHS) started an innovative public health nursing program directed at men in Glasgow, Scotland. Health visitors Bill Deans and Bob Hoskins established a nurse-run well-man clinic with the help of the NHS and the Scottish Council for Health Education. During home visits with mothers and infants, Deans and Hoskins observed that fathers excused themselves and went to the local pub when they arrived.

Any intervention regarding men's health needs must include men as willing participants (Lynch, 2008). Noting the characteristics of the male population in their community (e.g., overweight, heavy smoking, drinking, and high unemployment), Deans and Hoskins decided to modify their practice to serve their clients' needs. One afternoon per week, the clinic, which is based on a nursing model rather than a medical model, offers health screening, health education, and primary prevention to men. Marketing is important, and men are referred from general practitioners' and specialists' practices and recruited through newspaper advertisements. Clients with clinical signs and symptoms are referred back to their physicians. Lifestyle counseling and education are offered in areas such as fat and fiber content in diet, smoking, alcohol use, and exercise.

Deans and Hoskins consider the clinic a way to extend the health visitor's role in the NHS's efforts in health education with an aim to "nip potential digseases in the bud." Deans and Hoskins are concerned that the NHS does not provide male

services and are clear that "the unemployed chain-smoking husband needs as much care and health education from the health visitor as do his wife and baby" (Sadler, 1979, p. 18). The well-man clinic and well-woman clinic models can now be found in several communities throughout Great Britain and have been expanded to serve inmates in prison (Ballinger, Talbot, and Verringer, 2009; Woodland and Hunt, 1994). After 10 years in existence, the well-man clinics in Great Britain are only sporadically used by males. Even when the services were expanded to the home, nurses found that men were purposely absent at the appointment time. Usage was highest with informal evening clinics directed by male nurses (Roberts and Gerber, 2003). An attempt to evaluate these nationally funded clinics was undertaken in 2003. It was suggested from the data that a collaborative approach to these interventions is a slow process and that adequate time should be provided prior to evaluation (Reid et al, 2009).

In Australia, Men's Shed is a community-based health promotion initiative in men's health. Based on the social rather than medical model, the sheds promote well-being among older males by providing them with accepted and respected activities as well as a male-friendly space for socialization. Ballinger and colleagues (2009) found that participants in these activities reported an increase in recognition of the importance of health determinants and a sense of well-being.

Public health nurses working in the Benton County Health Department in Corvallis, Oregon, responded to the challenge of teen pregnancy in the 1970s by launching a community-wide effort that included developing a men's health clinic and marketing reproductive health services directly to teenage boys and men. An early effort established an advisory committee that included people from churches, schools, and health care facilities. A public health nurse health educator launched an extensive education program in the high school, which focused on decision-making processes and services available in the community. Later efforts involved the establishment of a clinic for men. Teenage boys were members of a consumer advisory committee established by the nurses that recommended the wording and format for advertisements about the clinic that ran in the high school newspaper. The advisory committee also recommended a flyer format that would be attractive to males. Specifically, they requested a card with information about the clinic and how to use condoms that would discreetly fit into their wallets and be available to share with peers.

The nurses have expanded their focus to create inclusive service environments in which teenage girls and boys and adult men and women will feel accepted and comfortable. Particular attention is given to the clinic decor and advertising, reading materials, and posters to transmit a message that includes offering health care for males and females. Clinic staff will see males or females at any time; however, a room in which staff members see men has decor geared toward men (e.g., no gynecological stirrups on the examining table) and pamphlets available for men on topics such as testicular cancer and chewing tobacco. Integrated services exist in the areas of family planning, STDs, and HIV counseling and testing.

CASE STUDY APPLICATION OF THE NURSING PROCESS

Community health nurses are in an ideal position to address the health needs of men at individual, family, and community levels. The community health nurse may promote self-care in male members of the family, facilitate men's health by addressing needed changes at the family level, buttress women's roles as caregivers of the family's health, and bring about change that influences policies that affect men at the community level.

Planning gender-appropriate care for males is outlined in the following case study, which is an application of the nursing process at the individual, family, and aggregate levels initiated in a home visit, and applies the previous discussions about the levels of prevention, roles of the community health nurse, research, and men's health.

Application of the nursing process to aggregates is facilitated by the use of systems theory, in which the nurse identifies the system and subsystems involved. The nurse may use a deductive or an inductive approach. A deductive approach would involve carrying out a community assessment and identifying an area or areas, such as a program needed by the community. Planning, implementation, and evaluation of the program would be carried out at the family or group level. An inductive approach would involve entering the community system through a person or client via a referral about a problem or concern. Assessment of the individual would be followed by identification of those groups to which the client belongs, such as family and community, and assessment of those groups.

Beth Lockwood, a community health nursing student at a health department, received a referral from the high school nurse to visit the Connors family to assess Richard Connors' mental health status. Richard was a 16-year-old sophomore whose academic work in school had declined rapidly after the premature death of his 46-year-old father. The father had died of a myocardial infarction, which he had while cleaning the garage with Richard one evening after school. Richard and the neighbors failed to revive Mr. Connors, and Richard carries feelings of guilt. Household members include Mrs. Connors, age 44 years, and Richard's sister Yvonne, age 12 years.

Assessment

The referral to assess the Connors family called for an inductive approach to assessment. Beth used a deductive approach later, when her experience with the Connors family piqued her concern about the status of men's health in her community. Beth assessed Richard, his mother, and his sister as household members of the family. However, she could not stop with the immediate family; she had to continue to identify the other groups within the community to which each individual family member belonged. Viewing the community as a system and focusing on systems and subsystems helped Beth organize the data she collected during assessment. Knowing that "the whole is greater than the sum of its parts," Beth prepared for her visit by reviewing adolescent theories of development and family theory. Beyond individual assessment, she noted factors related to the development of sex role–related behavior that may influence health. Examples of assessment areas include the following:

- Family configuration, traditional or nontraditional
- Sex role–related behavior of parents, including work patterns in and out of the home, division of household labor, and decision-making patterns
- Patterns of parenting: mothering, fathering, and substitute father figure(s)
- Ability of male children to disclose feelings to family members and others
- Degree of assertiveness in female children
- Ability of family members to give emotional and physical support during crises and noncrises

- Ability of family members to trade off role-related behavior during crises and noncrises
- Risk-taking health behaviors
- Processing of stress and grief
- Communal lifestyle patterns that place the individual or family at risk (e.g., lack of exercise, poor diet, smoking, and drinking)
- Family history of death and illness
- Health care–taking patterns of family members
- Preventive health behaviors
- Leisure activities

Assessment of other groups includes neighborhood and other peer groups, school environments, sports, and church and civic activities.

Diagnosis

Through induction, the nurse makes a diagnosis for each individual and each system component, including family and the community. The following are examples of diagnoses.

Individual

- Loss of interest or involvement in an activity, related to conflicting stages of grief process secondary to premature death of father (Richard)
- Expressed dissatisfaction with parenting role, related to feelings of helplessness and sadness secondary to premature death of husband (Mrs. Connors)
- Risk of interpersonal conflict, resulting from prolonged, unrelieved family stress secondary to premature death of father (Yvonne)

Family

- Decreased ability to communicate, related to family stress secondary to premature death of father
- Risk of family crisis, related to disequilibrium

Community

- Inadequate systematic programs for linking families in crisis to community resources
- Inadequate systematic programs for populations at risk of premature death, related to inadequate planning among community systems

Planning

Planning involves contracting and mutual goal setting and is an outcome of mutually derived assessment and diagnosis. A contract with the family alone is shortsighted and may provide little community benefit over time. The following are examples of other aggregates with which a contract may be established:

- The school subsystem that does not provide ongoing counseling but will meet periodically with family members to evaluate pupil progression
- The school subsystem that provides physical education in football, basketball, and baseball (i.e., nonaerobic, non-lifetime sports) but offers extramural aerobic, lifetime sports such as swimming, tennis, golf, and track after school hours
- The American Red Cross, which does not offer cardiovascular pulmonary resuscitation (CPR) courses on evenings or weekends but offers to consider doing so for a defined minimum-size community

Mutual goal setting requires collaboration regarding long- and short-term goals. Again, mutually defined needs and diagnoses are important to this process. Regardless of the diagnosis, each individual in the family and the subsystem must participate in development of a care plan. The following are examples of goals.

Continued

CASE STUDY   APPLICATION OF THE NURSING PROCESS—cont'd

Individual

Long-Term Goal
* Individual family members will be able to trade off role-related behavior.

Short-Term Goal
* Individual family members will express feelings related to abandonment and loss.

Family

Long-Term Goal
* The family will exhibit an increased ability to handle crisis, as evidenced by ability to discuss roles and interdependencies.

Short-Term Goal
* The family will identify specific ways to recognize and use support services.

Community

Long-Term Goal
* Systematic programs, with ongoing program evaluation, will be established for populations at risk of premature death from coronary heart disease, as evidenced by local planning bodies.

Short-Term Goals
* Information is disseminated to individuals, families, groups, and planning bodies in the community about the incidence of coronary heart disease.
* Existing programs are identified that address coronary heart disease.
* Existing programs are coordinated to bridge gaps and avoid duplication of effort.

Intervention

The nurse, family, and other aggregates carry out interventions contracted during the planning phase to meet the mutually derived goals. Most important, the nurse empowers the family and community to develop the networks and linkages necessary to care for themselves.

Individual

Individual counseling regarding loss and grief may be beneficial to each family member, but options may need to be explored and referrals may need to be reevaluated for members of the rural family. Education regarding preventive measures that combat risk factors for heart disease include those aimed at individual family members and those that address areas such as diet, exercise, smoking, alcohol use, and stress management.

Family

Examples of interventions with the family include counseling, education, and referral aimed at family self-care promotion. For example, Beth's interventions with the Connors family depended on the family's ability to solve problems, investigate community resources, and create linkages between the family and resources. Periodic family conferences at school and more inclusive family therapy may enable the family to work through the death of Mr. Connors; this process results in the development of new roles and the communication necessary to maintain family equilibrium. Education regarding preventive measures to combat risk factors for heart disease may need discussion at the family and individual levels (e.g., diet, exercise, smoking, alcohol use, and stress management).

Community

The nurse must also carry out interventions with other aggregates. These may involve activities such as educating, facilitating program expansion, and tailoring programs to meet community needs. Intervention at the aggregate level calls for group and community work. The nurse carries out interventions at this level in several ways (e.g., by communicating community statistics from a community analysis, relating anecdotes from families served, or linking family experience to program needs by acting as an advocate and bringing family members to board meetings or hearings on community health issues).

Education regarding preventive measures to combat risk factors for heart disease also includes those interventions aimed at the community. A rationale for the development of lifetime aerobic sports is needed not only by Richard but also by school districts. Exploration of options with the school nurse and review of the school district health education curriculum would be beneficial. A community assessment of heart disease awareness, including determination of the availability of resources such as emergency response and CPR courses, is an aggregate intervention. Taking the outcome of the assessment in the form of statistics and the anonymous anecdotal story of the Connors family to planning bodies in the community is also intervention at the aggregate level. Creative programs other communities used (e.g., teaching CPR within the school system) should be investigated and proposed.

Evaluation

Evaluation is multidimensional and ongoing. Using a systems approach to evaluation, the nurse evaluates each component of the system, from individual family member to family and community, in terms of goal achievement. Evaluation consists of noting degrees of equilibrium established, extent of change, how the system handles change, whether the system is open or closed, and patterns of networking. Ongoing evaluation includes noting referrals and follow-up of the individual, the family, and other aggregates in resource use.

Individual

Use of resources such as support groups by the individual family member may be noted. These resources may include a teen support group, a women's support group, support groups for those experiencing the loss of a spouse or other family member, reentry programs for women at a local junior college or university, and Parents Without Partners.

Family

Evaluation of the Connors family would include follow-up of their use of support services specifically for the family, such as counseling options for the family as a unit. Evaluation would also focus on the family's ability to handle crises in the future.

Community

Aggregate evaluation would focus on the community. For example, to what extent do school programs encourage sports options that promote lifetime aerobic activities and prevent premature death from heart disease? Are programs systematically planned in the community for populations that are at risk of premature death from heart disease?

Levels of Prevention

Society's expectations of men and women are in transition. Application of levels of prevention by the community health nurse must take into account men's health status, men's socialization, men's use of health care services, men's primary needs for prevention and health promotion, and the role of women as caregivers in family health.

Primary

Men are more likely to engage in risk-taking behavior than women and are less likely to engage in preventive behaviors; therefore, primary prevention must be marketed specifically to men. Examples of primary prevention for the Connors family are applied at the following individual, family, and community levels:

CASE STUDY   APPLICATION OF THE NURSING PROCESS—cont'd

Individual

- Assessment, teaching, and referral related to diet and exercise behaviors

Family

- Assessment and teaching related to food selection and preparation at home and food selection at fast-food restaurants
- Teaching and role-modeling gender roles that allow male members of the family to use alternative expressions of emotion

Community

- Provision of CPR courses for members of the community; consultation with schools regarding need for aerobic activities in physical education and sports programs
- The nurse must pull men from the family, workplace, or other aggregates into involvement with family planning, education, antepartum and postpartum care, parenting, dental prophylaxis, and accident prevention. In addition, assessment of need for immunizations and classes (e.g., retirement preparation) is considered action aimed at primary prevention.

Secondary

Men have higher mortality, morbidity, and health care use rates for many of the leading causes of death, but they are second to women in overall use of health care services, including preventive physical examinations and screening; therefore, early diagnosis and prompt intervention must also meet men's needs. Examples of secondary prevention regarding the Connors family include the following:

Individual

- Screen for risk factors related to CVD in the individual, such as how the individual handles stress.

Family

- Screen for risk factors related to CVD in the family, such as how the family processes stress.

Community

- Organize screening programs for the community, such as health fairs.
- The nurse must screen individuals and aggregates of men according to lifestyle risk factors, mortality rates at different age levels, morbidity rates, and occupational health risks.

Tertiary

Activities that rehabilitate individuals and aggregates and restore them to their highest level of functioning are aimed at tertiary prevention. The nurse in the community is ideally situated to locate people in need of rehabilitation services. The nurse may provide evaluation and physical, mental, and social restoration services. Men in need of rehabilitation may have special needs because their disabilities influence them, their families, and ultimately their communities. Financial assistance and vocational counseling, training, and placement may be priorities for the well-being of the family. Socialization causes men to have difficulty admitting they need help. Community health nurses who teach men with chronic disease to rest at specified periods during the day or to continue with medical regimens or speech or occupational therapy are providing tertiary prevention. Working with couples as a unit is also important because caregiving patterns may shift as a result of chronic disease and disability. Encouraging men to express their concerns about their health, families, and jobs and their frustration with themselves is important. The following are examples of tertiary prevention with the Connors family.

Individual

- Assist individual family members in dealing with grief from the loss of the father and husband.

Family

- Assist family in dealing with grief and assuming alternative roles.

Community

- Assist the community in dealing with loss of a fully functioning family by providing grief support services that include males or target males and females.

SUMMARY

As the information within this chapter shows, women do get sick and men die. There is gender disparity in all areas of disease and all health entities. Health initiatives and programs are changing as more and more attention is given to the health care of men.

LEARNING ACTIVITIES

1. Examine the vital statistics in the community and compare the gender-specific differences in mortality rates.
2. During a 1-week period, determine the frequency of newspaper articles in the local major newspaper that identify the top 12 causes of death for men.
3. Survey the billboards in the community and determine the frequency of those that depict gender-linked behaviors of men that are associated with risk taking.
4. Survey local businesses and industries in the community to determine what health promotion and prevention programs are available and used by men and women.
5. Select a family that has a man in the household who is accessible. Select two "door openers" appropriate to initiate discussion of health concerns with this man. Devise a gender-appropriate nursing care plan that includes primary, secondary, and tertiary prevention for this man as an individual, for his family, and for his community.
6. Select a family that has a man in the household who is not readily accessible. Interview the female caregiver in the household and obtain information by proxy about the man's health. If possible, arrange to meet the man for lunch, at work, or after work and obtain information about his health. Compare the information obtained by proxy with that obtained from the client.
7. Review major nursing texts (e.g., medical-surgical); examine the tables of contents and the indexes for content on men's health versus women's health.

ⓔ EVOLVE WEBSITE

http://evolve.elsevier.com/Nies

- NCLEX Review Questions
- Case Studies
- Glossary

REFERENCES

Arias E: *United States life tables, 2008 (National Vital Statistics Reports vol. 61, no. 3)*, Washington, DC, 2012, National Center for Health Statistics. Available from <http://www.cdc.gov/nchs/fastats/lifexpec.htm.>

Baerolcher MO, Verma S: Men's health research: under researched and under appreciated, *Meidal Schience Monitor* 14(Part 3), 2008.

Ballinger M, Talbot L, Verrinder G: More than a place to do woodwork: a case study of a community-based Men's Shed, *J Men's Health* 6(1):20–27, 2009.

Brown L, Bond M: An examination of influences on health protective behaviors among Australian men, *Int J Men's Health* 3(7):274–287, 2008.

Centers for Disease Control and Prevention: *Men's health: Leading causes of death in males United States 2009*, 2009. Available from <http://www.cdc.gov/men/lcod/>.

Centers for Disease Control and Prevention. Sexually Transmitted Disease Surveillance 2011. Atlanta: U.S. Department of health and Human Services: 2012.

Cheatham C, Barksdale D, Rodgers S: Barriers to health care and health seeking behaviors faced by black men, *J Am Acad Nurse Pract* 20:555–562, 2008.

Frisbee S, Chambers C, Frisbee J, et al: Associations between dental hygiene, cardiovascular disease risk factors and systemic inflammation in rural adults, *The Journal of Dental Hygiene* 84(4):177–184, 2010.

Haines C, Wender R: Men's health, *Prim Care* 33(1):xiii–xv, 2006.

Harvard Men's Health Watch, Volume 13:8, 2009.

Heron M, Hoyert DL, Murphy SL, et al: *Deaths: final data for 2006*(National Vital Statistics Reports vol. 57, no. 14) Washington, DC, 2009, National Center for Vital Statistics. Also available from <http://cdc.gov/nchs/ data/hus/hus08.pdf>.

Kirby R, Kirby M, Aoroso P, et al: Steps by which better overall health for men could be achieved, *BJU Int* 98(2):285–288, 2006. Also available from <www.bjui.org/ContentFullItem. aspx?id= 81&SectionType=5>.

Lynch L: Men's Health, *Ir Med J* 101(1):5–6, 2008.

Martin JA, Hamilton BE, Sutton PD, et al: *Births: Final data for 2008 (National Vital Statistics Reports vol. 59 no. 1)*, Hyattsville, MD, 2010, National Center for Health Statistics.

Mathews TJ, MacDorman MF: *Infant mortality statistics from the 2008 period linked birth/infant death data set (National Vital Statistics Reports vol. 60, no. 5)*, Hyattsville, MD, 2012, National Center for Health Statistics.

Meryn S: Global man and health, *J Men's Health* 6(1):2–3, 2009.

Naslindh-Ylispangar A, Sihvonen M, Kekki P: Health, utilization of health services, "core" information and reasons for non-participation: a triangulation study among non-respondents, *J Clin Nurs* 17:2972–2978, 2008.

National Center for Health Statistics: *Health, United States, 2011: With special feature on socioeconomic status and health*, Hyattsville, MD, 2012, Author. Also available from.

National Institute for Occupational Safety and Health: *NIOSH workers health chartbook* (NIOSH publ 2004–146), 2004. Available from <www.chc.gov/niosh/doc./chartbook>.

Organisation for Economic Co-operation and Development [OECD]: *Health at a glance*, 2011. Available from <http://www.oecd.org/health/hea lth-systems/healthataglance2011.htm>.

Porche D: Men's health: building the science, *Am J Men's Health* 3(2):92, 2009.

Reid G, van Teijlingen E, Douglas F, et al: The reality of partnership working when undertaking an evaluation of national well men's service, *J Men's Health* 1(6):36–49, 2009.

Roberts A, Gerber L: *Nursing perspective on public health programming in Nunavut, Iqaluit*, Nunavut, Canada, 2003, Department of Health and Social Services. Available from <www.gov.nu.ca/health/Report% 20on%20Nursing% 20Perspectives%20on%2 0Public%20Heatlh%20Programming%20in% 20Nunavut.pdf>.

Sadler C: DIY male maintenance, *Nurs Mirror* 160:16, 1979.

Schiller JS, Lucas JW, Ward BW, et al: Summary health statistics for U.S. adults: National Health Interview Survey, 2010, *Vital Health Stat* 10(252):1–217, 2012.

Shapiro A, Yarborough-Hayes R: Retirement and older men's health, *Generations, Journal of the American Society on Aging* 32(1):49–53, 2008.

Skelton R: Man's role in society and its effect on health, *Nursing* 26:953, 1988.

Sommers B, Wilson L: *Fifty-four million additional Americans are receiving preventive services coverage without cost-sharing under the Affordable Care Act*, 2012. Available from <http://aspe.hhs.gov/he alth/reports/2012/PreventiveServices/ib.shtml>.

Tanne JH: Medicine's new motto: one sex does not fit all, *American Health for Women* 16(5):54–58, 1997.

Tison, J, & Williams, A: *Analyzing the first years of the Ticket or Click It mobilizations* (DOT HS 811 232), 2010. Available from <www.nhtsa.go v/staticfiles/nti/pdf/811232.pdf>.

U.S. Preventive Services Task Force: Men: Stay healthy at 50+: *Checklists for your health*, 2004. Available from <http://www.ahrq.gov/patients-consumers/patient-involvement/healthy-men/men-over-50.html>.

Verbrugge LM, Wingard DL: Sex differentials in health and mortality, *Women's health* 12:103, 1987.

Waldron I: Changing gender roles and gender differences in health behavior. In Gochman DS, editor: *Handbook of health behavior research*, New York, 1995a, Plenum.

Waldron I: Contributions of changing gender differences in behavior and social roles to changing gender differences in mortality. In Sabo D, Gordon DF, editors: *Men's health and illness: gender, power and the body*, Thousand Oaks, CA, 1995b, Sage.

Waldron I: Contributions of biological and behavioral factors in changing sex differences in ischaemic heart disease mortality. In Lopez A, Caselli G, Valkonen T, editors: *Adult mortality in developed countries: from description to explanation*, New York, 1995c, Oxford University Press.

Waldron I: Contributions of changing gender differences in behavior and social roles to changing gender differences in mortality. In Sabo D, Gordon DF, editors: *Men's health and illness: gender, power, and the body*, Thousand Oaks, CA, 1995d, Sage.

Waldron I: Factors determining the sex ratio at birth. In *Sex differentials in infant and child mortality*, New York, 1995e, United Nations.

Whorton MD: Environmental and occupational reproductive hazards. In Swanson J, Forrest K, editors: *Men's reproductive health*, New York, 1984, Springer.

Woodland A, Hunt C: Healthy convictions … well-man clinic for the inmates of Lindholme prison, *Nurs Times* 90:32, 1994.

Senior Health

Mary Ellen Trail Ross and Edith B. Summerlin

OBJECTIVES

Upon completion of this chapter, the reader will be able to do the following:

1. Discuss the aging process.
2. Discuss the demographic characteristics of the elderly population.
3. Describe psychosocial issues related to aging.
4. Describe physiological changes due to aging.
5. Recognize *Healthy People 2020* wellness goals and objectives for older adults.
6. Describe health/illness concerns common to the elderly population.
7. Identify nursing actions that address the needs of older adults.
8. Identify resources available to older adults.

KEY TERMS

advance directives
aging
alternative housing options
Alzheimer's disease
anxiety disorder
crime

depression
elder abuse
falls
glaucoma
guardianship
macular degeneration

Medicaid
Medicare
Social Security
suicide

OUTLINE

Concept of Aging
Theories of Aging
Demographic Characteristics
 Population
 Racial and Ethnic Composition
 Geographic Location
 Gender
 Marital Status
 Education
 Living Arrangements
 Sources of Income
 Poverty and Health Education
Psychosocial Issues
Physiological Changes
Wellness and Health Promotion
 Healthy People 2020
 Recommended Health Care Screenings and Examinations
 Physical Activity and Fitness
 Nutrition
Common Health Concerns
 Chronic Illness
 Medication Use by Elders

Additional Health Concerns
 Sensory Impairment
 Hearing Loss
 Dental Concerns
 Incontinence
Elder Safety and Security Needs
 Falls
 Driver Safety
 Residential Fire–Related Injuries
 Cold and Heat Stress
 Elder Abuse
 Crime
Psychosocial Disorders
 Anxiety Disorders
 Depression
 Substance Abuse
 Suicide
 Alzheimer's Disease
Spirituality
End-of-Life Issues
 Advance Directives
 The Nurse's Role in End-of-Life Issues

In America, the number of individuals aged 65 years or older grew from 3 million in 1900 to 40 million in 2010 (Federal Interagency Forum on Aging-Related Statistics [FIFARS], 2012). Life expectancy is increasing; thus, larger numbers of people are reaching 65 years and beyond. In view of the increasing number of seniors who potentially will remain living in the community, the role of the nurse becomes very important in helping these seniors to continue to live independently and to increase their years of healthy life. For nurses to assist older adults, they must be familiar with the characteristics of seniors, their socioeconomic situations, their health behaviors, health status, health risks, and available community resources. This chapter discusses these issues and gives suggestions as to how nurses might address them.

CONCEPT OF AGING

Aging is a natural process that affects all living organisms. The concept of aging is most often defined chronologically. *Chronological age* refers to the number of years a person has lived. In the United States, an older adult is generally defined as one who is 65 years or older. However, it is important to remember that older adults cannot be grouped collectively as just one segment of the population. The older adult population is a heterogeneous group. The young-old (aged 65 to 74 years), the middle-old (aged 75 to 84 years), the old-old (aged 85 to 99 years), and the elite-old (more than 100 years old) are four distinct cohort groups (Touhy and Jett, 2012).

Functional age, on the other hand, refers to functioning and the ability to perform activities of daily living (ADLs), such as bathing and grooming, and instrumental activities of daily living (IADLs), such as cooking and shopping. This definition of aging is a better measure of age than chronological age. After all, most older adults are more concerned with their functional ability than their chronological age. Helping older adults remain independent and functional is a major focus of nursing care.

THEORIES OF AGING

Since early times, scientists have attempted to explain why humans age. There are many biological and psychosocial theories of aging. Biological theories of aging answer questions such as "How do cells age?" and "What triggers the actual aging process?" (Miller, 2012). The biological theories can be subdivided into two main divisions: stochastic and nonstochastic. Stochastic theories explain aging as events that occur randomly and accumulate over time, whereas nonstochastic theories view aging as predetermined. Some of the popular biological theories are summarized in Box 19-1.

The three classic psychosocial theories of aging are behavioristic and examine how humans experience late life. The disengagement theory, proposed by Cumming and Henry (1961), asserts that aging is inevitable, with mutual withdrawal or disengagement from society and decreased interaction between the aging person and others. The activity theory posits that remaining active and involved is necessary

---

| BOX 19-1 | **BIOLOGICAL THEORIES OF AGING** |

Stochastic Theories

Error Theory

The error theory proposes that an accumulation of errors in protein synthesis occurs over time, resulting in impairment of cellular function. Defective cells are produced, which eventually interfere with biological function (Orgel, 1963).

Somatic Mutation Theory

Similar to the error theory, somatic mutation theory also suggests that when cells are exposed to x-ray irradiation or chemicals, alteration of DNA occurs, increasing the incidence of chromosomal abnormalities and decreasing cellular and organ function. The deleterious effects appear in later life (Morley, 1995).

Free Radical Theory

Free radicals are highly reactive molecules that possess an extra electric charge (free electron) that can damage protein membranes, enzymes, and DNA. The body produces antioxidants that scavenge the free radicals (Hayflick, 1996).

Cross-Linkage Theory

The cross-linkage theory posits that aging causes body chemicals (proteins, lipids, nucleic acid, and carbohydrates) to become cross-linked. The cross-linking causes abnormal metabolic activity and waste products to accumulate in the cells. The result is poor functioning of body tissues and structures (Hayflick, 1996).

Wear-and-Tear Theory

Cells and organs wear out after years of use. Proponents of the wear-and-tear theory view the human body as similar to a machine that eventually wears out because of decline in cellular function, death of cells, and mechanical injury and use (Hayflick, 1996).

Nonstochastic Theories

Programmed Theory

The programmed theory postulates that normal cells divide a specific number of times. The number of cell divisions is proportional to the lifespan of the species. Human cells double 40 to 60 times before the ability to replicate is lost and cellular death occurs (Hayflick, 1996).

Immunological Theory

According to immunological theory, alteration of the B and T cells causes a loss of a self-regulatory pattern between the body and the cells. Autoaggression occurs when cells normal to the body are misidentified as alien and are attacked by the body's immune system (Miller, 1996).

Neuroendocrine Control or Pacemaker Theory

Aging is described in neuroendocrine control theory or pacemaker theory as a programmed decline in the functioning of the nervous, endocrine, and immune systems. Cells lose their ability to reproduce, a process known as replicative senescence (De la Fuente, 2008).

---

to maintain life satisfaction (Havighurst, Neugarten, and Tobin, 1963). The continuity theory suggests that a person continues through life in a similar fashion as in previous years (Havighurst et al, 1968).

Concepts gleaned from the various theories are useful to nurses as they care for older adults. For example, knowledge that the immune system is affected by aging implies the need for nurses to be vigilant about preventing infections (Miller, 2012). Psychosocial theories of aging point out the uniqueness of older individuals as they age and make life adjustments. Knowledge of these theories may help nurses to dispel common myths of aging.

DEMOGRAPHIC CHARACTERISTICS

Population

Americans are living longer than ever before, and it is expected that the older population will continue to grow. Currently, people who survive to age 65 years can expect to live an average of nearly 18 more years. The life expectancy of people who survive to age 85 years today is about 7 more years for women and 6 more years for men. Life expectancy varies by race, but the difference decreases with age. In 1900, people aged 65 years and older made up 4% of the population. In 2010, nearly 40 million people aged 65 years and over lived in the United States, accounting for just over 13% of the total population. The oldest-old population (those 85 years and older) grew from just over 100,000 in 1900 to 5.5 million in 2010 (FIFARS, 2012). In 2010, there were 53,364 centenarians in the United States (U.S. Census Bureau, 2012).

The baby boomers (individuals born between 1946 and 1964) started turning 65 years old in 2011, and the number of older adults will increase dramatically. By 2030, the number of Americans aged 65 years and older is expected to be twice as large as that of their counterparts in 2000, growing from 35 million to 72 million, and will represent nearly 20% of the total U.S. population. The greatest growth will occur in the population aged 85 years and older, whose numbers are projected to grow from 5.5 million in 2010 to nearly 19 million by 2050 (FIFARS, 2012).

Racial and Ethnic Composition

In addition to growing larger, the older population is becoming more diverse, as is the rest of the population. In 2010, non-Hispanic whites accounted for nearly 80% of the U.S. older population. Blacks made up 9%, Asians made up 3%, and Hispanics (of any race) accounted for 7%. The older population will grow among all racial and ethnic groups; however, the older Hispanic population is projected to grow the fastest (FIFARS, 2012).

Geographic Location

The proportion of the population aged 65 years and over varies by state. In 2010, Florida had the highest proportion of people aged 65 years and over (17%). Maine, Pennsylvania, and West Virginia also had high proportions, each more than 15% (FIFARS, 2012). More than half (56.5%) of persons 65 years or older lived in 11 states: California, Florida, New York, Texas, Pennsylvania, Ohio, Illinois, Michigan, North Carolina, New Jersey, and Georgia (Administration on Aging, 2011).

Gender

Older women outnumber older men in the United States. In 2010, women accounted for 57% of the population 65 years and older and 67% of the population 85 years and older (FIFARS, 2012).

Marital Status

Older men are more likely than older women to be married. In 2010, more than three quarters (78%) of men aged 65 to 74 years were married, compared with more than one half (56%) of women in the same age-group. The proportion married is lower at older ages: 38% of women aged 75 to 84 and 18% of women 85 years and older were married. Widowhood is more common among older women than older men. Women aged 65 years and over were three times as likely as men of the same age to be widowed: 40% compared with 13%. In 2010, nearly 73% of women aged 85 years and over were widowed, compared with 35% of men. Relatively small proportions of older men (9%) and women (11%) were divorced in 2010, and a small proportion of the older population has never married (FIFARS, 2012).

Education

Educational attainment has increased among older adults. In 2010, 80% of older adults were high school graduates (compared with 24% in 1965). Older blacks and Hispanics aged 65 years and older completed high school at lower rates than their white and Asian counterparts (65% and 47%, compared with 84% and 74%, respectively). In 2010, 23% of older adults had a bachelor's degree or higher (compared with 5% in 1965). Older Asians had the highest proportion with a bachelor's degree or higher, at 35%, compared with 24% for non-Hispanic whites, 15% for blacks, and 10% for Hispanics. Older men had attained a bachelor's degree more often than older women (28% compared with 18%); however, the gender gap in completion of a college education is narrowing (FIFARS, 2012).

Living Arrangements

As age increases and widowhood rates rise, the percentage of the population living alone increases accordingly. In 2010, 72% of older men lived with their spouses, whereas less than half (42%) of older women did. In contrast, older women were twice as likely as older men to live alone (37% and 19%, respectively). Older Hispanic (36%), black (35%), and Asian (33%) women were more likely than white women (13%) to live with relatives other than a spouse. Older white and black women were more likely than women of other races to live alone (approximately 39% each, compared with about 21% for Asian and 23% for Hispanic women). Older black men (28%) lived alone more than twice as often as older Asian men (12%). Older Hispanic men were more likely than men of other races and ethnicities to live with relatives other than a spouse (FIFARS, 2012).

Housing and Residential Services

Older adults typically prefer to "age in place" or live in their own homes for as long as possible. In 2009, 93% of Medicare enrollees aged 65 years and over resided in traditional community settings. Three percent of the Medicare population aged 65 years and over resided in community housing with at least one service available, such as meal preparation, housekeeping, laundry, and assistance with medication. Approximately 4% resided in long-term care facilities. The percentage of people residing in community housing with services and in long-term care facilities was higher for the older age-groups. For example, among older adults 85 years and older, 78% resided in traditional housing, whereas 8% resided in community housing with services and 14% resided in long-term care facilities (FIFARS, 2012). It's important to make services needed for independent living, such as meal preparation, medication assistance, and housekeeping, accessible to older adults who prefer this type of living arrangement.

Alternative Housing Options for Older Adults

The significant majority (93%) of older adults aged 65 years and older reside in the traditional, single-family home; however, some choose to downsize to smaller housing, such as townhouses or condominiums, where maintenance needs are eliminated or minimized. As mentioned, in 2009, only about 2.7% of elders aged 65 years and over resided in community housing with at least one service available. The types of alternative housing options included retirement communities or apartments, continuing care retirement facilities, assisted-living facilities, and board and care homes. Services at these facilities include meal preparation, housekeeping, laundry, and medication administration. Approximately 4.2% of older adults reside in long-term care facilities that provide personal and/or skilled care 24 hours a day, 7 days a week. The percentage of people residing in community housing with services and in long-term care facilities is higher for individuals 85 years and older. These older adults generally have more functional limitations (FIFARS, 2012). It is important to note that many older adults who would like to change current living arrangements find that organized senior housing is too expensive for middle-class and lower-middle-class citizens. On the other hand, these individuals often have too many assets to qualify for subsidized housing.

Although not considered a housing option, adult day care provides a safe and supportive environment during the day for adults who cannot or choose not to stay alone. This service is often needed for caregivers who work during regular hours or need respite. Socialization, recreational activities, medication supervision, and meals are provided on-site. Often transportation to and from the facility is provided.

Sources of Income

In 2010, the median household income of older adults was $31,410. Aggregate income for the population aged 65 years and over came largely from four sources: Social Security provided 37%, earnings accounted for 30%, pensions provided 19%, and asset income accounted for 11%. Among older Americans in the lowest fifth of the income distribution, Social Security accounts for 84% of aggregate income, and public assistance accounts for another 7%. For those whose income is in the highest income category, Social Security, pensions, and asset income each account for almost one fifth

of aggregate income, and earnings account for the remaining two fifths (FIFARS, 2012).

With aging, a good percentage of income is spent on health care. Most older adults have Medicare, which provides health insurance for those who are 65 years or older, are disabled, or have end-stage renal disease. Medicare is funded, in part, by Social Security contributions from employers, employees, and the self-employed. Medicare Part A is a hospital insurance plan that covers acute care, short-term rehabilitative care, and some costs associated with hospice and home health care. For 2013, the Part A deductible for acute care was $1184 for the first 60 days of a hospital stay per benefit period. This amount increases for longer hospital stays. Rehabilitative care generally provided in skilled nursing facilities is covered only if it occurs after a 3-day hospital stay and requires "skilled care" provided by a licensed nurse or by a physical or occupational therapist. Medicare Part A will pay 100% of the first 20 days of a nursing home stay, with a daily co-pay for days 21 to 100 and no coverage after that (U.S. Department of Health and Human Services [USDHHS]/Centers for Medicare and Medicaid Services [CMS], 2013).

Medicare Part B covers the costs for physician and nurse practitioner services; outpatient services, such as diagnostic procedures (e.g., laboratory and x-ray); qualified physical, speech, and occupational therapy; ambulance services; durable medical equipment; and some home health care services. Charges are paid by Medicare at a rate of 80% of what Medicare considers an "allowable charge." The client is responsible for the remaining 20% of the charge. In addition, the client is responsible for an annual Part B deductible ($147.00 in 2013) and a monthly premium of $104.90. This amount is generally deducted directly from the monthly Social Security check. Most Medicare enrollees have a supplemental insurance (Medigap) policy to pay for services not covered by Medicare. A Medicare Advantage Plan (sometimes called Part C) is another Medicare health plan choice. This plan is offered by private companies approved by Medicare. In addition to the Part B premium, there is usually an additional monthly premium for the Medicare Advantage Plan (USDHHS/CMS, 2013).

The newest component of Medicare is the prescription drug coverage that became available in January 2006. The prescription drug plan is designed to help lower prescription drug costs. The individual chooses the drug plan and pays a monthly premium and most have an annual deductible. Most Medicare prescription drug plans have a coverage gap (also called the "donut hole"). This refers to a temporary limit on what the drug plan will cover. In 2013, once a member and his/her plan have spent $2970 on covered drugs (the combined amount plus the deductible), the member is in the coverage gap and will receive a 52.5% manufacture-paid discount on covered brand-name drugs (www.medicare.gov/part-d/costs/coverage-gap/part-d-coverage-gap.html) (USDHHS/CMS, 2013).

For older adults with low incomes, Medicaid may be available to offset the Medicare deductibles and co-pays and to provide additional health benefits. Each state establishes its own eligibility criteria within the broad guidelines established by the federal government. Medicaid generally covers more services than Medicare, including custodial care in nursing homes, without deductibles or co-pays.

Poverty and Health Education

To determine who is considered poor, the U.S. Census Bureau compares family income (or an unrelated individual's income) with a set of poverty thresholds that vary by family size and composition and are updated annually for inflation. By 2010, the proportion of the older population (65 years and older) living in poverty had decreased dramatically to 9%, compared with 35% in 1959. Older women (11%) were more likely than older men (7%) to live in poverty. Older people who live alone have higher rates of poverty than those who are married. Race and ethnicity are also related to poverty among the older population. In 2010, older whites were less likely than older blacks and Hispanics to be living in poverty (FIFARS, 2012).

Community nurses will be increasingly called upon to care for older adults of diverse backgrounds who have various living arrangements. Although educational attainment has increased among the elderly population, many older adults have less than a high school education; therefore nurses must be sensitive and creative when providing instruction and teaching. Nurses cannot assume that an older adult has had a formal education. In addition, instructions may need to be given at a slower pace. It may also be imperative to include family or significant others when providing instruction. Also, written information may be sent home for further reference.

On the other hand, increased educational levels of current and future elders also provide a challenge for the community health nurse. These elders are, and will be, more informed and will make greater demands for current and scientifically based information, thus requiring the nurse to be knowledgeable about the latest developments in health care.

PSYCHOSOCIAL ISSUES

In addition to adjusting to physiological changes related to aging and health concerns (discussed later in this chapter), older adults must cope with psychosocial and role changes such as retirement, relocation, widowhood, loss of family and friends, and possibly raising their grandchildren. Retirement may be a happy occasion when voluntary; however, the opposite may be true if it is involuntary. When older adults retire, they inevitably must cope with a change in social status and possibly income level; this may be especially difficult for people whose self-concept is related to job status. For retirees who are married, the spouse must also adjust to the changes related to retirement. Indeed, the adjustment may be more difficult for the spouse than the retiree as the retiree's leisure time will be increased. For elders who have no hobbies or interests, this extra leisure time may be a source of boredom. Nurses should encourage older retirees to pursue old hobbies and interests or establish new ones.

Relocation is another psychosocial issue that many older adults must manage. Often, relocation occurs as a result of

health and functional impairment, lack of ability to maintain one's home, unsafe neighborhoods, and lack of assistance with ADLs or IADLs. The relocation may be prompted by the older adult's desire to be closer to family or medical care, or interest in moving to a new location or more supportive housing (as discussed in the section Alternative Housing Options for Seniors).

RESEARCH HIGHLIGHTS

Recognizing the Needs of the Elderly

Tsai (2005) examined factors that predicted distress and depression among elders with arthritis. Performing secondary analysis of data from 234 people aged 65 years and older (mean age 74.1 years), she determined that elders with higher levels of disability, more financial hardship, less social support, and younger age were more likely to have higher levels of distress than those who did not share these characteristics. Furthermore, distress, along with pain and disability, significantly predicted depression. She concluded that nurses should recognize the needs of elders with arthritis, considering a number of both physical (e.g., pain, level of disability) and psychosocial (e.g., social support, financial hardship) factors that might lead to depression, and should intervene where appropriate and feasible.

Data from Tsai P: Predictors of distress and depression in elders with arthritic pain, *J Adv Nurs* 51:158-165, 2005.

Widowhood is an event experienced by most older adults, especially elderly women. According to Miller (2012), common consequences of widowhood are loss of companionship and intimacy; loss of one's sexual partner; feelings of grief, loneliness, and emptiness; increased responsibilities and dependency on others; loss of income and less efficient financial management; and changes in relationships with children, married friends, and other family members. Widowhood may be especially traumatic for elders who have been married for many decades. In addition to the loss of a spouse, older adults must also cope with loss of family members (sometimes their own children) and friends.

On the other hand, many older adults are faced with the responsibility of raising their grandchildren. Substantial increases have occurred in the number of children under age 18 years living in households maintained by their grandparents, often without the presence of the grandchildren's parents. Antecedents to children being raised by grandparents include neglect related to parental substance abuse, abandonment, emotional and physical abuse, parental death, mental and physical illness, incarceration, teen pregnancy, and grandparents assisting adult children who work or attend school. Although there may be rewards to raising grandchildren, such as satisfaction for keeping the family together, sense of purpose in life, and the opportunity to have a close relationship with one's grandchildren, this arrangement may contribute to both physical and psychological problems, such as stress, depression, and poorer health (Musil and Ahmad, 2002; Ross and Aday, 2006; Rubin, 2013; Williams, 2011).

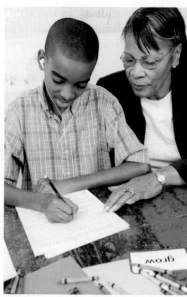

A custodial grandmother doing homework with her grandson. (© 2013 Photos.com, a division of Getty Images. All rights reserved. Image # 86535689.)

Clinical example

Ms. Thomas, age 62, is divorced and has been raising her three grandchildren, ages 11 to 13, for the past 10 years. She was forced to retire from full time teaching to assume this role. Her daughter, the children's mother, is bipolar and schizophrenic, and has tested positive for human immunodeficiency virus (HIV). All of the grandchildren have medical problems and/or special needs, including asthma, attention deficit hyperactivity disorder, and emotional/behavioral concerns. Ms. Thomas is very organized and keeps track of their many medications via a written schedule containing the name of each medication, dose, and time of administration. Ms. Thomas expressed increased stress, tension, and anxiety as a result of caregiving responsibilities and neglect of her own needs. She has hypertension, a "thyroid condition," asthma, gastroesophageal reflux disease, and allergies. She admits to occasionally forgetting to take her own medications because of her busy schedule. She rates her health as "fair" overall and "somewhat worse" in comparison with that of other people her age. She reports significantly less time for herself and leisure activities. Nonetheless, Ms. Thomas is determined to raise her grandchildren as well as possible. Despite her circumstances, she is very positive and optimistic that her grandchildren will grow up to be successful and respectable citizens.

The role of the nurse is to identify, support, and assist older adults experiencing various psychosocial changes and role adjustments. In addition, the nurse should provide information about various community resources and make referrals to agencies that might be helpful.

PHYSIOLOGICAL CHANGES

Normal physiological aging changes occur in all body systems. However, it is important to note that the rate and degree of these changes are highly individualized. These changes are influenced by genetic factors, diet, exercise, the environment, health status, stress, lifestyle choices, and many other elements. Table 19-1 depicts common physiological changes that occur with aging.

WELLNESS AND HEALTH PROMOTION

Wellness is different from "good health." Wellness exists at one end of a continuum with illness at the other end. Health promotion programs focus on helping individuals to maintain their wellness, prevent illness, and manage any chronic illnesses that they may have. Preventive health services are valuable in improving the health status of individuals to their maximum wellness potential.

Healthy People 2020

The USDHHS's program *Healthy People 2020* establishes national objectives for health promotion and disease prevention. High-priority objectives are listed in the Leading Health Indicators section of the *Healthy People* documentation and website. A primary goal is to increase the quality and years of healthy life. Although people are living longer, many older adults have two or more chronic illnesses that interfere with their quality of life. *Healthy People 2020* has incorporated specific objectives related to older adults that are designed to promote healthy outcomes for this population.

❤ HEALTHY PEOPLE 2020
Summary of Objectives for Older Adults

Prevention

OA–1: Increase the proportion of older adults who use the Welcome to Medicare benefit. Target: 8.0 percent.

OA–2: Increase the proportion of older adults who are up to date on a core set of clinical preventive services.

OA–3: (Developmental) Increase the proportion of older adults with one or more chronic health conditions who report confidence in managing their conditions.

OA–4: Increase the proportion of older adults who receive Diabetes Self-Management Benefits.

OA–5: Reduce the proportion of older adults who have moderate to severe functional limitations. Target: 25.5 percent.

OA–6: Increase the proportion of older adults with reduced physical or cognitive function who engage in light, moderate, or vigorous leisure-time physical activities.

OA–7: Increase the proportion of the health care workforce (physicians, psychiatrists, registered nurses, dentists, physical therapists, registered dieticians) with geriatric certification.

Long-Term Services and Supports

OA–8: (Developmental) Reduce the proportion of noninstitutionalized older adults with disabilities who have an unmet need for long-term services and supports.

OA–9: (Developmental) Reduce the proportion of unpaid caregivers of older adults who report an unmet need for caregiver support services.

OA–10: Reduce the rate of pressure ulcer–related hospitalizations among older adults.

OA–11: Reduce the rate of emergency department (ED) visits due to falls among older adults.

OA–12: Increase the number of States, the District of Columbia, and Tribes that collect and make publicly available information on the characteristics of victims, perpetrators, and cases of elder abuse, neglect, and exploitation.

From U.S. Department of Helath and Human Services: *Healthy People 2020 summary of objectives: Older adults,* n.d.. Retrieved from <http://healthypeople.gov/2020/topicsobjectives2020/pdfs/OlderAdults.pdf>.

TABLE 19-1   NORMAL PHYSIOLOGICAL CHANGES ASSOCIATED WITH AGING

PHYSIOLOGICAL CHANGES	NURSING INTERVENTION(S) AND PATIENT INSTRUCTIONS
Sensory Changes	
Vision	
Decreased visual acuity	Use large print for teaching
Decreased visual accommodation	Encourage adequate lighting
Increased opacities	Encourage use of corrective lenses as prescribed
Hearing	
Decreased ability to hear – presbycusis	Decrease extraneous sounds
Decreased ability to hear consonants with high-frequency sounds	Use concise sentences and speak slowly and distinctly in a low-pitched voice
	Encourage hearing examination and use of hearing aids, if needed
Taste	
Diminished taste sensation	Encourage well balanced meals
Decreased saliva production	Advise to drink plenty of fluids
Decreased sensitivity to sweetness and saltiness	Observe for overconsumption of sweets and salt
	Give options for seasoning other than salt
Smell	
Decreased smell acuity	Advise to use other senses and other people to assist with monitoring the environment for safety (e.g., spoiled food and gas fumes)
Touch	
Decreased sensitivity to touch	Monitor for extreme temperature changes in the environment (e.g., water temperature)
	Maintain adequate room temperature
Nervous System	
Reduction in neurons and cerebral blood flow	Assess neurological status
	Ensure frequent position changes
Slower autonomic and voluntary reflexes	Assess for pain and unique responses to pain
Reduced capacity to sense pain and pressure	
Increase in amount of senile plaque and neurofibrillary tangles	
Cognitive Changes and Changes in Balance	
Slower reaction time	Allow adequate time for response; teach fall precautions
Slower learning time	Break instructions into small units
Memory: long-term memory better than short-term memory	Use shorter teaching sessions; use cues and gestures
Personality consistent with earlier years	Relate education to prior experience
	Allow adequate time for completing tasks
Sleep	
Decrease in Stages 3 and 4 sleep pattern	Allow naps as needed
Increase in arousals during the night	Avoid sleep medication use if possible
Slight reduction in total sleep time	Avoid stimulants and caffeine
	Assess quantity and quality of sleep
Cardiovascular System	
Decrease in tone and elasticity of aorta and great vessels	Pace activities
Thicker and stiffer heart valves	Allow rest periods
Slowing down of heart's conduction system	Encourage use of ambulation aids when appropriate
Slower recovery of myocardial contractility and irritability	Monitor for activity intolerance
Decreased cardiac reserve and output	Prevent or eliminate stressors
Decreased ability to increase heart rate when stress occurs	Monitor heart rate and blood pressure
Increased systolic blood pressure	Encourage regular exercise program
Respiratory System	
Reduced size of lungs, lung expansion, activity, and recoil	Encourage influenza and pneumococcal vaccinations
Increased rigidity of lungs and thoracic cage	Encourage regular exercise
Decreased cough response	Encourage adequate fluid intake
Decreased number of alveoli and gas exchange	Monitor oxygen administration

Continued

TABLE 19-1	**NORMAL PHYSIOLOGICAL CHANGES ASSOCIATED WITH AGING**—cont'd	
PHYSIOLOGICAL CHANGES	**NURSING INTERVENTION(S) AND PATIENT INSTRUCTIONS**
Musculoskeletal System	
Atrophy and decrease in muscle fibers	Prevent immobility
Decreased muscle mass and strength	Encourage regular exercise program
Reduced bone minerals and mass, causing porous and brittle bones	Teach safety precautions to prevent falls
Shortening of vertebra	Encourage adequate calcium and vitamin D intake
Gastrointestinal System	
More brittle teeth	Encourage good dental health
Decreased esophageal/colonic peristalsis	Encourage diet that is well balanced and has adequate protein
Decreased stomach motility	and vitamins
Decreased production of saliva, HCl, and digestive enzymes	Encourage adequate fluids
Decreased absorption of fat and vitamins B1 and B12	Encourage fiber in the diet
Decrease in thirst response	Monitor diet for deficiencies
Renal System	
Decreased size of kidneys	Monitor drugs—smaller doses may be needed
Decreased number of nephrons	Observe for adverse responses to drugs
Reduced renal blood flow and tubular function	Monitor electrolytes and laboratory values
Decreased glomerular filtration rate	Prevent dehydration
Genitourinary System	
Weakening of bladder muscle, causing increased urinary frequency, urgency, and nocturia	Assess bladder function and assist with frequent toileting
Decreased bladder capacity	Encourage bladder training program, exercises, and medication when needed
Increased retention	Observe for signs of urinary tract infection
Increased nocturia	
Reproductive System	
Women	
Atrophy of vulva and flattening of labia	Differentiate between changes due to normal aging and those
Vaginal drying	due to disease or medications
Atrophy of cervix, ovaries, and uterus	Advise about use of lubricants for comfort during intercourse
Decreased amount and elasticity of breast tissue	Recommend breast examinations and mammograms
Men	
Decreased elasticity of scrotal skin	Differentiate between changes due to normal aging and those
Prostatic enlargement	due to disease or medications
Erection takes longer to achieve but is maintained longer	Recommend prostate examination
Endocrine System	
Increased fibrosis and nodularity of thyroid gland	Recommend pneumococcal, influenza, and tetanus vaccinations
Shrinkage of thymus and pituitary glands	Monitor electrolytes and glucose
Decrease in adrenal gland secretion of glucocorticoid	Prevent infection
Decreased levels of aldosterone	Encourage good nutrition
Delayed insulin release	Observe for hypoglycemia or hyperglycemia
Reduced ability to metabolize glucose	
Decrease in testosterone, estrogen, and progesterone	
Integumentary System	
Decreased skin elasticity	Encourage frequent position changes and inspect skin
Generalized thinning and dryness	Be careful of skin tears, bruising, and pressure ulcers
Atrophy of sweat glands and diminished sweating	Assess body and environmental temperatures to prevent
Altered thermoregulation	hypothermia and hyperthermia
Variation in pigmentation (age spots)	Ensure adequate clothing and comfortable room temperature

Adapted from Eliopoulos C: *Gerontological nursing,* ed 8, Philadelphia, 2014, Lippincott Williams & Wilkins.

Recommended Health Care Screenings and Examinations

Many organizations, such as the American Cancer Society, the American Heart Association, the U.S. Preventive Services Task Force, and the Agency for Healthcare Research & Quality, have established guidelines for health promotion screenings and examinations. Box 19-2 depicts some of the more widely agreed-on screenings and examinations for older adults. These established recommendations might be very useful to community nurses educating older adults about the benefits of screening and early detection of disease. Frequently, earlier detection of disease allows

BOX 19-2 RECOMMENDED SCREENINGS AND EXAMINATIONS FOR HEALTH PROMOTION AND DISEASE PREVENTION IN OLDER ADULTS

Examinations and Tests

For All Older Adults

Complete physical: Annually

Blood pressure: Annually; more frequently if hypertensive or at risk

Blood glucose: Annually; more frequently if diabetic or at risk

Serum cholesterol: Every 5 years; more frequently if at high risk

Fecal occult blood test: Annually

Sigmoidoscopy: Every 5 years

OR

Colonoscopy: Every 10 years; more frequently if at high risk

Visual acuity and glaucoma screening: Annually

Dental examination: Annually for those with teeth with cleaning every 6 months; cleaning every 2 years for denture wearers

Hearing test: Every 2 to 5 years

For Women

Breast self-examination: Monthly

Clinical breast examination: Annually

Mammogram: Every 1 to 2 years if aged 40 years or older; check with health care provider if 74 years or older

Pelvic examination and Papanicolaou smear: Annually; may check with health care provider about discontinuation at 65 or 70 years after three consecutive negative exam results and no abnormal results in previous 10 years and not otherwise at risk

Digital rectal examination: Annually with pelvic examination

Bone density: Once after menopause and more frequently if at risk

For Men

Digital rectal examination and prostate examination: Annually

Prostate-specific antigen (PSA) blood test: Annually

Immunizations for All Older Adults

Tetanus, diphtheria, pertussis: Every 10 years

Influenza/flu vaccine: Annually

Pneumonia vaccine: Once after age 65 years; ask physician about booster every 5 years

Hepatitis A and B: For those at risk

Herpes zoster (shingles): One-time dose

Varicella: If evidence of lack of immunity and significant risk for exposure

Data from American Cancer Society: *Cancer facts & figures*, Atlanta, 2013, Author; and Centers for Disease Control and Prevention: *Recommended adult immunization schedule, U.S., 2013*, 2013. Available from <http://www.cdc.gov/vaccines/schedules/downloads/adult/mmwr-adult-schedule.pdf>.

better treatment, lower health care costs, and the possibility of cure.

Physical Activity and Fitness

Physical activity is beneficial for the health of people of all ages, including older adults. Although there are various types of exercises, walking is one of the best forms of exercise, and it is free. Many older adults engage in walking, swimming, dancing, yoga, and tai chi for exercise. Regular exercise improves functional status, reduces blood pressure and serum cholesterol level, decreases insulin resistance, prevents obesity, strengthens bones, and reduces falls. Barriers to exercising that have been identified by older adults include lack of access to safe areas to exercise, pain, fatigue, and impairment in sensory function and mobility (Mauk, 2014).

Objective OA-6 of *Healthy People 2020* reads "increase the proportion of older adults with reduced physical or cognitive function who engage in light, moderate, or vigorous leisure-time physical activities" (USDHHS, Office of Disease Prevention and Health Promotion, 2012). Nurses may help older adults accomplish this goal by assessing their understanding of the beneficial effects of exercise and identifying barriers that prevent exercise. Nurses should also educate, encourage, and assist older adults with exercise. When applicable, anti-inflammatory medications may be administered before physical activity to address accompanying pain.

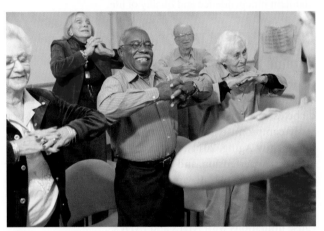

Older adults participate in an exercise class. (© 2013 Photos.com, a division of Getty Images. All rights reserved. Image # 125557433.)

Nutrition

In the 2010 Dietary Guidelines for Americans, the U.S. Department of Agriculture (USDA) and USDHHS provide authoritative advice on what constitutes a healthy diet. A graphic model, MyPyramid, was developed in 1992 to show what foods and in what proportion foods should be eaten. In 2010, MyPyramid was changed to MyPlate (U.S. Department of Agriculture, 2012). The plate picture helps an individual make smart choices from every food group, find balance between food and physical activity, get the most nutrition out of calories, and stay within caloric needs (see Figure 4-9). Food groups emphasized are fruits, vegetables, grains, protein foods, dairy, oils, and empty calories.

In *Healthy People 2020*, nutrition was identified as a priority area of health promotion for people of all ages. Similar to patterns among other age groups, poor nutrition in the elderly population is common. Obesity has been increasing in adults 70 years and older (FIFARS, 2012). Researchers at Tufts University's Gerald J. and Dorothy R. Friedman School of Nutrition Science and Policy have developed a food plate specifically for older adults. The researchers state that the elderly still require the same or higher levels of nutrients for optimal health outcomes. Poor diet quality is associated with cardiovascular disease, hypertension, type 2 diabetes, osteoporosis, and some types of cancer (Lichtenstein et al, 2008). Also, an inappropriate diet is related to constipation, dental disease, physical inactivity, and depression. Normal physiological changes such as a diminished sense of smell may reduce the enjoyment of eating. Gastrointestinal changes can interfere with absorption of vitamin B12 and folic acid, leading to anemia. A diminished thirst sensation may lead to dehydration. Other factors that can affect the nutritional status of the elderly are income, functional status, taking multiple medications, social isolation, lack of transportation, and dependence on others for grocery shopping and cooking. The nutrition checklist presented in Table 19-2 lists warning signs of and risk factors for poor nutritional health described by the mnemonic DETERMINE. The nurse should use this tool to identify the elderly who need help with their dietary intake. The benefits of good nutrition are an important factor in helping to maintain independence and quality of life.

COMMON HEALTH CONCERNS

Chronic Illness

About 91% of older adults have at least one chronic condition, and 73% have at least two chronic conditions, such as diabetes, arthritis, hypertension, and lung disease, that seriously compromise the quality of life of older adults (Center for Healthy Aging, 2011). The most common conditions are arthritis, hypertension, and diabetes. Chronic diseases are the leading causes of death among persons 65 years and older (Table 19-3). The prevalence of chronic diseases rises with age. Chronic illnesses are a major cause of disability and may cause limitations with ADLs and IADLs.

Medication Use by Elders

The high prevalence of chronic diseases in the elderly population causes this group to use a large number of medications. Older adults consume nearly one third of all prescription drugs dispensed and spend billions annually on medications (Vincent and Velkoff, 2010). Older adults also consume many over-the-counter medications as well as "folk" or herbal remedies.

The elderly population is vulnerable to the effects of drugs because of normal aging changes (see Table 19-1) and age-related differences in pharmacokinetics and pharmacodynamics (NIHSeniorhealth.gov, 2011). Polypharmacy may also make older adults vulnerable to drug interactions and dangerous adverse reactions. Budnitz and colleagues (2011) used adverse-event data from the National Electronic Injury Surveillance System–Cooperative Adverse Drug Event Surveillance project (2007-2009) to estimate the frequency and rate of hospitalizations due to emergency department visits for adverse drug events in older adults. The researchers estimated that 99,628 emergency hospitalizations for adverse drug events in U.S. adults 65 years of age or older occurred each year from 2007 to 2009. Nearly half of the hospitalizations were among adults 80 years of age or older. Nearly two thirds of hospitalizations were due to unintentional overdoses. Four medications or medication classes—warfarin (33.3%), insulin (13.9%), oral antiplatelet agents (13.3%), and oral hypoglycemic agents (10.7%)—were implicated alone or in combination in 67% of hospitalizations.

TABLE 19-2	NUTRITION CHECKLIST FOR OLDER ADULTS: WARNING SIGNS OF POOR NUTRITIONAL HEALTH

POSSIBLE PROBLEM	QUESTION TO ANSWER	SCORE FOR "YES" ANSWER (CIRCLE IF "YES")
Disease	Do you have an illness or condition that makes you change the kind and/or amount of food you eat?	2
Eating poorly	Do you eat fewer than two meals per day?	3
	Do you eat few fruits, vegetables, or milk products?	2
	Do you have three or more drinks of beer, liquor, or wine almost every day?	2
Tooth loss/ mouth pain	Do you have tooth or mouth problems that make it hard for you to eat?	2
Economic hardship	Do you sometimes have trouble affording the food you need?	4
Reduced social contact	Do you eat alone most of the time?	1
Multiple medications	Do you take three or more prescribed or over-the-counter drugs a day?	1
Involuntary weight loss/ gain	Have you lost or gained 10 lbs in the last 6 months without trying?	2
Needs assistance in self-care	Are you sometimes physically not able to shop, cook, or feed yourself?	1
Elder years >80 yr	Are you over 80 years old?	1
	TOTAL:	_____

Scoring:
0-2: Good! Recheck your nutritional score in 6 months.
3-5: You are at moderate nutritional risk. See what can be done to improve your eating habits and lifestyle. Your office on aging, senior nutrition program (e.g., Meals on Wheels), senior center, or health department can help. Recheck your nutritional score in 3 months.
6 or more: You are at high nutritional risk. Bring this checklist the next time you see your physician/nurse practitioner, dietitian, or other qualified health or social service professional. Talk with them about any problems you may have. Ask for help to improve your nutritional health.

From The Nutrition Screening Initiative: *Determine your nutritional health,* n.d. Retrieved from <http://www.cdaaa.org/images/Nutritional_Checklist.pdf>.

The researchers concluded that most emergency hospitalizations for adverse drug events in older adults were caused by a few commonly used medications and that relatively few resulted from medications designated as high-risk or inappropriate.

The Beers Criteria catalogues medications that cause adverse drug events in older adults because of the drugs' pharmacological properties and the physiological changes of aging. An updated version of the Beers Criteria for potentially inappropriate medications in older adults has been published

TABLE 19-3	LEADING CAUSES OF DEATH FOR PERSONS 65 YEARS OF AGE AND OLDER				
	WHITE	BLACK	AMERICAN INDIAN	ASIAN OR PACIFIC ISLANDER	HISPANIC
1.	Heart disease	Heart disease	Heart disease	Heart disease	Heart disease
2.	Cancer	Cancer	Cancer	Cancer	Cancer
3.	Stroke	Stroke	Diabetes	Stroke	Stroke
4.	Chronic obstructive pulmonary disease (COPD)	Diabetes	Stroke	Diabetes	Diabetes
5.	Alzheimer's disease	COPD	COPD	Pneumonia/influenza	COPD

From Gorina Y, Hoyert D, Lentzner H, Goulding M: *Trends in causes of death among older persons in the United States* (Aging Trends no. 6), 2006. Retrieved from <www.cdc.gov/nchs/data/ahcd/agingtrends/06olderpersons.pdf>.

by the American Geriatrics Society (AGS, 2012). An easy-to-use pocket card is available at http://www.americangeria trics.org/files/documents/beers/PrintableBeersPocketCard. pdf. The full document and accompanying resources may be viewed online at www.americangeriatrics.org.

One of the roles of nurses is to closely monitor medication use in the home to ensure safety (NIA, n.d.b.). An easy-to-use pill organizer may be helpful to older adults. In addition, such clients should be educated about potential adverse reactions as well as drug-drug and drug-food interactions.

ADDITIONAL HEALTH CONCERNS

Sensory Impairment

Vision and hearing impairments are among the most common age-related conditions affecting the elderly population (NIA, 2012a). Sensory disabilities increase with age and may seriously affect an older person's ability to carry out routine daily activities. The prevalence of vision impairment in individuals older than 65 years is as follows: 17% of individuals 65 to 74 years and 26% of individuals older than 75 report some form of vision impairment (Lighthouse International, 2013). And it is predicted that by 2030 the prevalence rate will double along with the country's aging population (American Foundation for the Blind, 2013). A study by physicians at Johns Hopkins University in Baltimore found the prevalence of hearing loss in patients 70 years and older to be 60% (Linnet al., 2011). These conditions impair the accomplishment of simple daily tasks and put the person at increased risk for declining social abilities, depression, falls, and an inability to communicate effectively.

The four leading eye diseases affecting older individuals are age-related cataracts, macular degeneration, diabetic retinopathy, and glaucoma.

Cataracts

Cataracts are the leading cause, as well as the most reversible cause, of visual impairment in older adults. A *cataract* is a clouding of the normally clear lens of the eye. Age is the single greatest risk factor for cataracts. By age 65 years, some degree of lens clouding has developed in half of all Americans, although it may not impair vision. Other risk factors that increase a person's risk of cataracts include diabetes, family history of cataracts, previous eye injury or inflammation, prolonged use of corticosteroids, excessive exposure to sunlight, and smoking. Older adults should have annual eye examinations, which allow early detection of cataracts and tracking of

their development. The only effective treatment for a cataract is surgical removal of the clouded lens and replacement with a clear lens implant. Interventions that may be able to reduce risks are regular eye examinations, cessation of smoking, wearing of sunglasses, maintaining a healthy weight, choosing a healthy diet, and taking care of other coexisting health problems (Mayo Clinic Staff, 2010).

Macular Degeneration

There are two types of macular degeneration: dry and wet. Dry macular degeneration is more common. It causes blurred central vision or a blind spot in the central vision. It may affect one or both eyes (Mayo Clinic Staff, 2012a). With wet macular degeneration, symptoms appear suddenly and progress rapidly, and objects appear smaller or farther away than they really are (Mayo Clinic Staff, 2012c). Any changes in central vision and the ability to see colors and fine details indicate that the individual should be seen by an eye doctor. Treatment differs for the two macular degeneration conditions. Wet macular degeneration cannot be cured, but if treated early, it may slow down its progression. Dry macular degeneration usually progresses slowly, and many people with it can live relatively normal, productive lives. Nurses can recommend the following ways to cope with changing vision: use magnifiers, use alternative options for books, use brighter lights, join a support group, and make arrangements for traveling.

Glaucoma

Glaucoma is one of the leading causes of blindness in America. The most common form of glaucoma, primary or chronic open-angle glaucoma, develops gradually without warning and progresses with few or no symptoms until the condition reaches an advanced stage. The drainage angle formed by the cornea and the iris remains open; however, the aqueous humor drains too slowly. This leads to fluid backup and a gradual buildup of pressure within the eye. Increased eye pressure continues to damage the optic nerve, and more and more peripheral vision is lost. Glaucoma cannot be cured, and its damage cannot be reversed, but treatment and regular eye examinations can prevent vision loss if the disease is found early, or can slow the disease or prevent further vision loss. Treatment consists of prescribed eyedrops or, if medications are ineffective, surgery (Mayo Clinic Staff, 2012b).

Nurses should educate clients about recommended vision screening. To determine the influence of visual impairment, the nurse should inquire about activity limitations associated with poor vision. Determining whether the client is using visual assistive devices such as glasses, contact lenses, magnifying lenses, or large-print books can be beneficial in recognizing the degree of adaptation. The nurse should know about resources that help older adults with eye care and assistive devices. Organizations that provide information include the National Eye Institute, the American Foundation for the Blind, and Lighthouse International.

Hearing Loss

Hearing loss is one of the most common conditions affecting older adults. Approximately 17% of or 36 million American adults report some degree of hearing loss; 30% of adults 65 to 74 years of age, and 47% of adults 75 years old or older have a hearing impairment (NIHseniorhealth.gov, 2012a). There are two general categories of hearing loss: presbycusis and tinnitus. Presbycusis is due to changes in the middle ear due to aging, loud noises, heredity, head injury, infection, illness, certain prescription drugs, and circulation problems such as hypertension. Tinnitus is a ringing, roaring, clicking, hissing or buzzing sound. It is a symptom not a disease, and the individual should seek medical evaluation for the cause (NIHseniorhealth.gov, 2012a).

Nurses should assess older adults for hearing impairment. The nurse should ask the individual whether he or she is having trouble hearing over the telephone, finds it hard to follow conversation when two or more people are talking, often asks people to repeat what they are saying, needs to turn up the volume of the radio or TV, or thinks that others are mumbling. If the individual is experiencing three or more of these problems, then he or she should be referred to the physician (National Institute on Deafness and Other Communication Disorders, 2012). Box 19-3 contains tips for health care providers who work with older adults who have hearing difficulties.

Dental Concerns

Age brings a host of dental problems that are often neglected because of inadequate dental care, limited mobility and transportation, poor nutrition, the myth that it is natural for older adults to become edentulous, and lack of finances and reimbursement (Medicare and some states' Medicaid programs do not provide adequate reimbursement for dental needs). With proper care it is possible to retain one's natural teeth if one adheres to good dental hygiene and has regular dental checkups. Dental problems of the elderly are: dry mouth, receding gums, tooth cavities, hypersensitivity of the teeth, and tooth discoloration (SeniorHealth365.com, 2011).

Prevention is the key to dental health because the teeth cannot be regrown and even the best dental intervention can only limit or minimize damage. Regular dental visits for cleaning and dental evaluation are essential prevention strategies.

Incontinence

Aging does not cause incontinence; however, at least one in ten people 65 years or older has this problem (National Institute on Aging [NIA], 2008). Urinary incontinence can occur for many reasons. Urinary tract infections, vaginal infection or irritation, constipation, and certain medicines can cause short-term bladder control problems. Weak bladder muscles, overactive bladder muscles, blockage from an enlarged prostate, and damage to nerves that control the bladder may cause longer-lasting incontinence. However, in most cases, urinary incontinence can be treated or controlled if not cured.

The choice of treatment depends on the type of bladder control problem. Types of urinary incontinence are stress incontinence, urge incontinence, and overflow incontinence or functional incontinence. One of the treatments that health care providers may suggest is Kegel exercises. (NIA, 2013).

An individual may also experience fecal incontinence. Loss of control of the bowels leads to leakage of stool from the large intestine. Medical evaluation to determine the cause should be recommended. Treatment varies, depending on the cause. Self-treatment is rarely successful (FamilyDoctor.org, 2011).

ELDER SAFETY AND SECURITY NEEDS

Each year, many elderly are injured in and around their homes. Older people are often targets for robbery, purse snatching, pickpocketing, car theft, and home repair scams. There are safety measures that the individual can take to avoid crime and to stay safe.

Falls

More than one in three people 65 years or older experience falls each year. The risk of falling rises with age. **Falls** are the number one cause of fractures, hospital admissions for trauma, loss of independence, and injury deaths (Centers for Disease Control and Prevention [CDC], 2010b). Many of the physiological changes that normally occur with aging, as well as a variety of chronic illnesses, can affect balance and make falls more likely. Medications such as blood pressure pills, heart medicines, diuretics, and tranquilizers may increase the risk of falling. Osteoporosis, a disease that causes a gradual loss of bone tissue or bone density, makes bones more susceptible to breaking. There is a link between osteoporosis and broken bones from falls.

A person who falls and sustains a fracture may become afraid of falling again and thus will limit his or her activities.

> **BOX 19-3** **WORKING WITH THE OLDER ADULT WHO HAS HEARING DIFFICULTIES**
>
> - Include the person with hearing loss in the conversation.
> - Find a quiet place to talk to help reduce background noise, especially in restaurants and social gatherings.
> - Stand in good lighting and use facial expressions or gestures to give clues.
> - Face the person and talk clearly.
> - Speak a little more loudly than normal, but do not shout.
> - Speak at a reasonable speed; do not hide your mouth, eat, or chew gum.
> - Repeat yourself if necessary, using different words.
> - Try to make sure only one person talks at a time.
> - Be patient. Stay positive and relaxed.
> - Ask how you can help.

From National Institute on Aging: *Age page: hearing loss,* 2009. Retrieved from <http://www.nia.nih.gov/health/publication?tid=All&field_pub_type_value=AgePage&tid_1=>.

Seniors living independently before a fall may be institutionalized for as long as a year after a fracture. Loss of footing and loss of traction are factors that can lead to a fall. Uneven surfaces such as sidewalks, curbs, and floor elevations, wet or slippery ground, and climbing up on household items not intended for climbing can result in loss of footing or loss of traction. In addition, drinking alcoholic beverages increases the risk of falling because alcohol slows reflexes and response time; causes dizziness, sleepiness, or lightheadedness; and alters balance (NIHsneiorhealth.gov, 2013).

Steps can be taken to reduce the chance of falls. Simple exercises that strengthen leg muscles and exercises that can improve balance are recommended (Box 19-4). Seniors can also improve their environment in order to reduce their risk of falling by checking floor surfaces and curb heights; identifying weather-related problems before venturing outside; wearing supportive, low-heeled shoes; making sure that rooms are well lit; and ensuring that safety equipment is installed in bathrooms and stairwells. A factor older adults should consider is having a cellular phone with them at all times to call for help directly. Telephone systems providing personal emergency response services may be available on a subscription basis, thus allowing seniors to be monitored; if such a service receives no answer to the call, help can be sent.

Traumatic Brain Injury

Traumatic brain injury (TBI) is also called acquired brain injury or simply head injury. In 2005, TBI caused nearly 8,000 deaths and 56,000 hospitalizations among those 65 years and older (CDC, 2010b). TBI results when the head is suddenly and violently hit or when an object pierces the skull and enters brain tissue (CDC, 2010b).

TBI symptoms may be mild, moderate, or severe. Symptoms of mild TBI include headache, confusion, lightheadedness, dizziness, blurred vision or tired eyes, ringing in the ears, bad taste in the mouth, fatigue or lethargy, and a change in sleep patterns or thinking. Moderate or severe TBI may cause the same symptoms as mild TBI plus a headache that gets worse or does not go away, repeated vomiting or nausea, convulsions or seizures, an inability to awaken from sleep, dilation of one or both pupils of the eyes, slurred speech, weakness or numbness in the extremities, loss of coordination, and increased confusion, restlessness, or agitation (National Institute of Neurological Disorders and Stroke, 2005). Medical attention should be sought for monitoring and treatment of symptoms. Referral for rehabilitation may be required for persons with disabilities resulting from TBI.

Driver Safety

One of the quality-of-life factors that is important to the senior is the ability to drive. Many older adults depend on driving in order to maintain independence and personal mobility. Seniors overwhelmingly prefer to drive as their means of transportation, with being a passenger their second preferred option. The number of elderly drivers will be increasing with the extension of life expectancy.

Age alone should not be the determining factor of whether or not a senior can drive safely. Driving skills vary from one elderly person to another. Age-related declines in vision, hearing, and other abilities as well as certain medical conditions and medications can affect driving skills (NIHseniorhealth.gov, 2012c). Most older drivers monitor their own driving ability and gradually limit or stop driving; others risk personal injury rather than give up their driver's licenses. The risk of being injured or killed in a motor vehicle crash increases with age (CDC, 2011c).

The nurse should be alert to signs of driving impairment in older clients and should offer practical advice so that the driver may either continue to drive safely or be encouraged to find alternative transportation (Box 19-5). The nurse can

---

BOX 19-4 IMPROVING BALANCE

Focus on the Following Areas
Perform muscle-strengthening exercises.
Obtain maximum vision correction.
When using bifocal or trifocal glasses, practice looking straight ahead and lowering the head.
Practice balance exercises daily.

Balance Exercises
While holding onto a stable item like a chair or counter, practice standing on one leg at a time for a minute. Gradually increase time, try balancing with eyes closed, and try balancing without holding onto anything.
Practice standing on toes, then rock back to balance on heels. Hold each position for count of 10.
Hold onto a stable item with both hands, then make a big circle to the left with hips. Repeat to the right. Do not move the shoulders or feet. Repeat five times.

Modified from National Institutes of Health Osteoporosis and Related Bone Diseases, National Resource Center: *Preventing falls and related fractures,* 2005. Available from http://www.niams.nih.gov/Health_Info/Bone/Osteoporosis/Fracture/prevent_falls.asp.

BOX 19-5 WARNING SIGNS THAT INDICATE A PERSON SHOULD BEGIN TO LIMIT OR STOP DRIVING

- Almost crashing, with frequent "close calls"
- Finding dents and scrapes on the car, on fences, mailboxes, garage doors, curbs, etc.
- Getting lost, especially in familiar locations
- Having trouble seeing or following traffic signals, road signs, and pavement markings
- Responding more slowly to unexpected situations, or having trouble moving their foot from the gas to the brake pedal; confusing the two pedals
- Misjudging gaps in traffic at intersections and on highway entrance and exit ramps
- Experiencing road rage or causing other drivers to honk or complain
- Easily becoming distracted or having difficulty concentrating while driving
- Having a hard time turning around to check the rear view while backing up or changing lanes
- http://www.aarp.org/home-garden/transportation/info-05-2010/Warning_Signs_Stopping.html

discuss issues with the senior driver, family, or friends such as drifting out of a lane, becoming confused when entering or exiting a highway, getting lost in familiar places, stopping inappropriately, failing to yield the right of way, and speeding or driving too slowly.

Some interventions that older adults could implement are limiting their driving to daylight hours, planning their trips to avoid rush hour, not listening to the radio, and avoiding talking with passengers while driving. The driver should also be encouraged to find other methods of transportation, such as family and friends, public transportation, taxis, and other private transportation options available in the community.

When the question of driving safely becomes personal, elderly drivers might become very defensive. Therefore it is important that elderly persons, if at all possible, be involved in the decision-making process of identifying their ability and deciding what should be done. However, if the individual is greatly impaired and, therefore, is dangerous to self or others, it may be necessary to involve the family, family physician, or department of motor vehicles in determining whether to suspend or revoke an older person's license. In addition, it may be necessary to take the keys, disable the car, or move it to a location beyond the individual's control to protect the senior and others from injury or accidents.

Residential Fire–Related Injuries

In the United States, more than 1,000 older adults 65 years and older die each year in home fires, and more than 2,000 are injured. In addition, older adults are two times more likely to die in a residential fire than the rest of the population. This risk may be attributed to reduced sensory abilities such as smell, touch, vision, and hearing, diminished mental faculties, slower reaction time, increased disabilities, and economic and social concerns that may prevent necessary home improvements that could reduce fire risk. The predominant causes of fires that result in injuries to older adults are cooking, open flames, smoking, and heating (National Fire Data Center, 2012). Nurses making home visits can assess their elderly client's home for fire risk and teach fire safety, including the importance of home smoke detectors and fire extinguishers. In many communities, the fire department installs free smoke detectors for older adults. In addition to the U.S. Fire Administration's public information campaign, A Fire Safety Campaign for People 50-Plus, organizations such as the National Fire Protection Association and the American Burn Association have active fire prevention and education programs for older adults.

Cold and Heat Stress
Cold Stress Disorders

Hypothermia is the most serious of the cold stress–related disorders and is the one elderly individuals might experience in the home because of failure of the heating systems or lack of financial resources to pay for sufficient heat. Factors that contribute to the development of hypothermia are age, health, nutrition, exhaustion, exposure and duration of exposure, wind, temperature, wetness, and medications that may decrease heat production, increase heat loss, or interfere

with thermostability. Signs of hypothermia are confusion or sleepiness, slowed, slurred speech, weak pulse, a lot of shivering, and poor control over body movements (NIA, 2010b).

Initial management is to prevent further loss of heat. Rewarming of the core temperature at a safe, slow rate is important in order to avoid lethal side effects. The reason for rewarming the core first is to prevent vasodilation that would put the individual into ventricular fibrillation (CDC, 2012a). Measures that can be taken are: (1) remove the individual from the cold area as soon as possible; (2) add more clothing, especially to the head (e.g., use a hat or scarf); (3) provide a warm sweetened drink (no coffee or tea); and (4) apply mild heat to the head, neck, chest, and groin areas using hot water bottles or warm moist towels. Medical help is imperative, and hospitalization may be needed, depending on the stage of hypothermia.

Heat Stress Disorders

The heat stress disorders are heatstroke, heat syncope, heat exhaustion, and heat cramps. As the environment becomes warmer, all methods of heat elimination become less effective, especially for older adults, who may have altered thermoregulation, diminished sweating, and decreased thirst sensation. These conditions should be taken seriously and they require immediate medical attention; heatstroke is life-threatening. Heat cramps are painful spasms of muscles of the arms, legs, or abdomen that occur during or after work. Signs and symptoms of heat exhaustion are fatigue, nausea, headache, and giddiness. The skin is clammy and moist, and the complexion may be pale or flushed. The individual may faint on standing, with a rapid, thready pulse and low blood pressure. Signs and symptoms of heatstroke include hot dry skin that is usually red, mottled, or cyanotic; confusion, loss of consciousness, or convulsions might occur (CDC, 2012c). All of these heat stress disorders may occur in the home without fans or air conditioning, or from being in the sun for prolonged periods, either in recreation or working in extremely hot temperatures and humidity. In all instances, the individual should be moved to a cooler environment and encouraged to lie down and rest. With heatstroke, immediate and rapid cooling with chilled water or by wrapping in a wet sheet, as well as being moved to a cooler area, should be done while immediate medical attention is being sought (NIA, 2010a).

Elder Abuse

Elder abuse is a serious problem throughout the United States. It is important to remember that abuse is not only a health concern but also a legal problem. States have laws defining abuse and identifying who is required to report abuse to the local Adult Protective Services. *Abuse* is generally defined as the willful infliction of pain, injury, or debilitating mental anguish; unreasonable confinement; or deprivation by a caretaker of services that are necessary to maintain mental and physical health. The categories of abuse are domestic, institutional, and from self-neglect. Domestic abuse is abuse that occurs in the home. Institutional abuse is abuse that occurs in a nursing home or other residential care facility. Self-neglect is defined as abuse that occurs when a person living alone threatens his or her own health or safety.

There are four common types of elder abuse: physical abuse, psychological/emotional abuse, financial or material exploitation, and neglect. Physical abuse involves slapping, pushing, pinching, and beating or use of physical restraint that results in broken bones, sprains, dislocations, bruises, black eyes, cuts, and rope marks, or sexual assault. Psychological or emotional abuse includes humiliation, intimidation, threats, and destruction of belongings (e.g., glasses). Financial or material exploitation refers to the improper or illegal use of the resources of an older person without consent (e.g., use of automated teller machine card). The most common type of abuse is neglect, which may be self-imposed or caused by another person. Signs of neglect include dehydration, malnutrition, untreated health problems, bedsores, unclean or inappropriate clothing, and weight loss.

More than 1 in 10 elders may experience some type of abuse but only 1 in 23 cases are reported (National Center on Elder Abuse [NCEA], 2013). This problem will steadily increase as more and more elderly are living longer and remaining in their homes. Abuse of the elderly is underreported for a number of reasons, including denial, fear of retaliation and further abuse, no other place to go, love of the abuser and not wanting him or her arrested, dependence on an abuser, shame and embarrassment that a loved one could act in an abusive manner, and lack of physical and/or cognitive ability to report the abuse. Another reason is that elder abuse may be missed by professionals working with older adults because of lack of training on detecting abuse (NCEA, 2013).

Diagnosis is very difficult because many of the signs and symptoms may truly be the result of normal physiological aging. Ways to tell the difference include conflicting stories about how physical injuries were obtained, "physician shopping," clusters of signs and symptoms, increasing depression of the elder, new poverty, poor personal care, malnutrition, unresponsiveness, hostility, anxiety, confusion, new health problems, improper medication, dehydration, and longing for death.

The abuser is frequently the spouse, adult child, sibling, friend, or caregiver. The family member profile of an abuser is an individual who is middle-aged or older, a daughter or son of the elder, someone with low self-esteem and impaired impulse control. Caregiver behavior to look for includes aggression, defensive or increasingly resentful attitude toward the elder, blaming of the victim for an injury, and treating the elder like a child; alternatively, the caregiver may show new affluence while withholding food or medication from the elder. Factors that lead to abuse are a lack of knowledge about normal aging, caregiver exhaustion, anger and frustration with the elder, financial problems, and drug and alcohol use by the caregiver. The elders who are most vulnerable are women who are widows or single, and more than 75 years of age; those dependent on a caregiver for their shelter and food or incontinent; and individuals who are frail, ill or mentally disabled.

Prevention activities include professional training of health care personnel, public education about elder abuse and its seriousness, and use of reliable assessment tools for the detection of abuse. The Elder Assessment Instrument (EAI) developed by Fulmer is one accessible assessment for reviewing signs, symptoms, and subjective complaints of elder abuse, neglect, exploitation, and abandonment; appropriate in all clinical settings, this tool may be retrieved from http://consultgerirn.org/. Nurses should report suspected abuse to the local Adult Protective Services through their state's hotline. Suggestions the community health nurse can give to the elder are to stay sociable, maintain friendships, and participate in senior citizen activities; have pension and Social Security checks deposited directly into bank accounts and obtain a durable power of attorney when no longer able to manage property and assets; consider co-guardians so more than one person knows the elder's situation and can act on the elder's behalf; ask for help if needed; keep records, property, and a will in order; and plan ahead for possible disability. Community health nurses also should advise elders to avoid leaving cash, jewelry, and other valuables lying around visible; refuse to sign a document unless someone the elder trusts reviews it first; and resist letting anyone isolate them from others. Additional resources that can be used for further information can be found on the websites of the Administration on Aging (www.aoa.gov) and the National Center on Elder Abuse (www.ncea.aoa.gov).

Crime

Older adults are less likely to be victims of **crime** than teenagers and young adults; however, the older person who becomes a victim of a crime is more likely to be seriously hurt than someone who is younger. Crime against the elderly occurs in the form of robbery, purse snatching, pocket picking, car theft, and home repair scams (NIA, 2009).

The key to crime prevention for the senior is to be careful and alert to what is going on in the environment and to the types of crimes to which elders are vulnerable. The elderly person can take measures to lessen the risk of experiencing crime. In the home, safety measures include making sure that door and window locks are strong. Bars on doors and windows need to be installed with caution because they may increase the risk of harm in the event that public officials need to access the home during a fire or to assist the elderly person who may be ill or injured from a fall. The use of a safe deposit box should be recommended to store a list and pictures of expensive belongings and other important documents, such as a copy of the individual's will. Installation of a monitored alarm system with its accompanying outdoor security sign would also help deter criminals. Caution should always be used before answering the door. The elder should note who is at the door before opening it and, if it is a stranger, have the person show identification. Nurses should remind elders that if they are uneasy about a visitor, they should not answer the door.

Measures that elderly people should observe when out in the community are to stay away from unsafe places, to keep car doors locked and windows up at all times, and to park in well-lit areas. Inside pockets of clothing should be used for valuables such as a wallet, money, and credit cards. A purse should be carried close to the body and kept closed. In addition, the elderly person should be advised not to resist a thief, but to hand over immediately what the person is requesting.

Fraud is the crime that is frequently mentioned in the media as happening to elders. Older people are vulnerable to con games, insurance scams, home repair scams, and telephone scams. Types of Internet fraud include auction fraud, nondelivery of products ordered, securities fraud, credit card fraud, identity theft, bogus business opportunities, and unnecessary professional services. One strategy to recommend to seniors to prevent fraud from happening to them is to hang up the phone on telephone salespeople. Today, the elder can get caller identification service for the telephone; if no number or individual is identified, the elder may choose not to answer the call. No personal or financial information should be given over the phone unless the elder made the phone call. When in doubt about an inquiry or opportunity, the elder should be encouraged to say no and in this way protect himself or herself. The elder should check the references of anyone seeking to do home repairs and should be sure to obtain, in writing, the details of the work to be completed as well as the cost. A job should never be paid for in advance.

Identity theft is on the increase, and elderly individuals are particularly vulnerable. To avoid this problem, Social Security and monthly pension checks should be deposited directly into a bank account. Any information that is sent to the home with credit card offers, personal information, and so forth should be shredded so that the information cannot be used illegally. The elder should check bank statements and credit card account statements carefully for any discrepancies and report them immediately to the respective business. Caution should be used in using the Internet to buy products or pay bills because of websites without security (NIA, 2009).

PSYCHOSOCIAL DISORDERS

Psychosocial disorders account for a significant number of suicides, especially among older men. Depression is often likely to lead to suicide. The rate of Alzheimer's disease increases with age. Alcohol and drug abuse are less common in older individuals but are still a concern. Depression and abuse of drugs and alcohol can coexist with one or more anxiety disorders. These conditions are discussed in the following section.

Anxiety Disorders

Anxiety is a normal human emotion that everyone experiences at one time or another. For elderly individuals, normal age-related worries experienced are financial concerns, health problems, and reduced social interactions due to loss of friends through death and relocation, but these do not mean that the individual has an anxiety disorder. Anxiety disorders are mental illnesses that cause people to feel excessively frightened, distressed, or uneasy in situations in which most other people would not. (National Alliance on Mental Illness [NAMI], 2012). Anxiety disorders are a very real and relatively common problem among older adults. Some older

adults with anxiety disorders may have had anxiety problems for a long time, whereas others may experience such problems only later in life. Studies have shown that among older adults, anxiety disorders occur anywhere from two to seven times more often than depression problems. It is possible that depression and abuse of drugs or alcohol can coexist with one or more anxiety disorders. Generalized anxiety disorder, social phobia, and agoraphobia seem to be the most common types of anxiety in the elderly (NIHseniorhealth.gov, 2012b).

Generalized anxiety disorder is characterized by excessive, exaggerated anxiety and worry about everyday events and is accompanied by physiological problems, including headaches, muscle tension, nausea, trembling, and frequent trips to the bathroom (NAMI, 2012). The worry is often unrealistic or out of proportion to the real situation because anxiety dominates the individual's thinking to such a point that it interferes with daily activities. Social phobia involves overwhelming worry and self-consciousness about everyday social activities. Worry centers on fear of being judged by others or fear of behaving in a way that might cause embarrassment. Agoraphobia is a fear of leaving the familiar setting of home that is so invasive that the individual avoids social situations or enters into life situations reluctantly. Symptoms vary depending on the type of anxiety; as noted earlier, an anxiety disorder is diagnosed only if the symptoms are excessive, are uncontrollable, create significant distress, or interfere with daily living.

Anxiety disorders cannot be prevented. Some things that can be suggested to control or lessen symptoms are good diet, adequate sleep, regular exercise, reduced consumption of caffeine, and checking over-the-counter medicines or herbal remedies for any chemicals that can increase anxiety symptoms. Effective treatment for anxiety disorders include a combination of counseling or psychotherapy and medications (NAMI, 2012). All anxiety disorders are serious medical conditions, and elderly clients should be referred to their health care providers for evaluation and treatment. The nurse can help elders realize that what they are experiencing does not need to interfere with their lives if they seek medical help.

Depression

Depression is a common problem among older adults, but it is not a normal part of aging. It may be overlooked in some older adults because sadness may not be the main symptom or they may not be willing to talk about their feelings. The risk of depression in the elderly increases with other illnesses and when ability to function becomes limited. Estimates of major depression in older people living in the community range from less than 1% to about 5% but rises to 13.5% in those who require home health care and to 11.5% in elderly hospitalized patients (NAMI 2010). Many myths exist concerning depression. Depression may last for days, weeks, months, or even years without treatment. Depression is a serious condition that lasts longer and increases the risk of death in the elderly population. Depression may lead to suicide. Elderly white men are at greatest risk. Depression is associated with increased risk of death following a heart attack, and depression may coexist with other medical illnesses and disabilities, such as diabetes, stroke, cancer, chronic lung disease, Alzheimer's disease, Parkinson's disease, and arthritis (NAMI, 2012). *Depression* refers to a lasting (2 weeks or longer) sad mood or loss of interest or pleasure in most activities. People may experience several or all of the following symptoms: changes in appetite or weight, changes in sleep patterns, restlessness, loss of energy, feelings of worthlessness or guilt, and repeated thoughts of death or suicide. Depression is tied to low serotonin levels. Serotonin is a neurotransmitter that limits self-destructive behavior. Serotonin levels decrease with age, predisposing elders to depression (National Alliance on Mental Health, 2011). If any of these symptoms exist, the client should be referred to his or her health care provider for diagnosis. The physician and the individual determine which treatment should be used. There is medication alone or medication with psychotherapy. How long depression lasts depends a great deal on identifying the condition early and seeking treatment early. Depression is often undiagnosed or underdiagnosed. Delay in treatment in the elderly can be very dangerous.

Thus, the community health nurse can play an important part in recognizing individuals who may be experiencing depression and who need to be referred for medical diagnosis and supervision. Short assessment tools such as the Geriatric Depression Scale–Short Form (Box 19-6) may be used to assess for this problem and assist the nurse in recognizing those at risk.

Substance Abuse

Data from the 2011 National Survey on Drug Use & Health (NSDUH) sponsored by the Substance Abuse and Mental Health Services Administration's (SAMHSA, 2102) revealed that in 2011, 9.7% of the population 65 years and older reported past month cigarette use. The presence of current alcohol use was 40.3% among this population. The rate of binge drinking was 8.3% and the rate of heavy drinking was 1.7% for older adults. A *binge drinker* is defined as a person who drinks five or more drinks on the same occasion on at least 1 day in the past 30 days. Marijuana was the most commonly used illicit drug, followed by pain relievers used nonmedically (SAMHSA, 2012).

Many older adults with substance abuse problems are continuing a pattern of behavior or addiction that began earlier in life. Substance abuse that begins in later life may be due to losses associated with aging. The warning signs of abuse are less obvious in older adults (NIA, 2012b). For example, many older adults are retired and drink alone at home, so they are less likely to be noticed or get into trouble. Also, many of the diseases caused by substance misuse (e.g., hypertension, stroke, dementia, or ulcers) are common disorders in later life, so health care providers and family members may not recognize substance abuse as an underlying cause.

As a result of normal physiological changes discussed earlier in this chapter, older adults generally experience increased sensitivity and decreased tolerance to alcohol and drugs. Because of loss of body mass, reduced absorption rate in the

---

BOX 19-6 GERIATRIC DEPRESSION SCALE–SHORT FORM

Choose the best answer for how you have felt over the past week:

1. Are you basically satisfied with your life? YES / **NO**
2. Have you dropped many of your activities and interests? **YES** / NO
3. Do you feel that your life is empty? **YES** / NO
4. Do you often get bored? **YES** / NO
5. Are you in good spirits most of the time? YES / **NO**
6. Are you afraid that something bad is going to happen to you? **YES** / NO
7. Do you feel happy most of the time? YES / **NO**
8. Do you often feel helpless? **YES** / NO
9. Do you prefer to stay at home, rather than going out and doing new things? **YES** / NO
10. Do you feel you have more problems with memory than most? **YES** / NO
11. Do you think it is wonderful to be alive now? YES / **NO**
12. Do you feel pretty worthless the way you are now? **YES** / NO
13. Do you feel full of energy? YES / **NO**
14. Do you feel that your situation is hopeless? **YES** / NO
15. Do you think that most people are better off than you are? **YES** / NO

Answers in **bold** indicate depression. Score 1 point for each bolded answer.
A score > 5 points is suggestive of depression.
A score ≥ 10 points is almost always indicative of depression.
A score > 5 points should warrant a follow-up comprehensive assessment.

From Yesavage JA, Sheikh JI: Geriatric Depression Scale (GDS): recent evidence and development of a shorter version, *Clin Gerontol* 5(1/2):165-173, 1986; Yesavage JA: Geriatric Depression Scale, *Psychopharmacol Bull* 24(4):709-711, 1988; and Yesavage JA, Brink TL, Rose TL, et al: Development and validation of a geriatric depression screening scale: a preliminary report, *J Psychiatr Res* 17(1):37-49, 1982-1983. Also available at <http://consultgerirn.org/uploads/File/trythis/try_this_4.pdf>.

---

gastrointestinal system, slower kidney function, and slower metabolism, drugs and alcohol remain in the body longer and at higher concentrations, thus prolonging and increasing their effects. The problem is compounded when alcohol and illicit drugs interact with prescribed or over-the-counter medications. This situation may be dangerous, because the medications may have a stronger or weaker effect on the body.

Careful screening for such problems must include a thorough review of factors that may be directly affecting substance use and abuse. Several instruments have been utilized with the elderly population, including the CAGE, the Short Michigan Alcohol Screening Test—Geriatric Version (SMAST-G), and the Alcohol Use Disorders Identification Test (AUDIT). The CAGE is an easy-to-use, four-question interview (Box 19-7). The SMAST-G (ten questions) and AUDIT (ten items) are screening instruments that provide a more detailed description of alcohol use. All three of these instruments rely on client self-report.

Alcoholics Anonymous (AA) is a community peer self-help group that may be very beneficial; however, elderly individuals may believe that they do not fit into the group or may have differing concerns from those of younger members. In addition, they may have age-related mobility or hearing

BOX 19-7   CAGE ALCOHOL SCREENING INSTRUMENT

The CAGE screening test is short and simple to administer. Two or more positive answers are correlated with alcohol dependence in 90% of cases.

This screening instrument may not pick up problems in those who are fearful of negative consequences of disclosure such as those looking for accommodation, people who are fearful of child protection agency staff, and those with mental health problems.

A short questionnaire about your alcohol use:

C: Have you ever thought you should **CUT DOWN** on your drinking?

A: Have you ever felt **ANNOYED** by others' criticism of your drinking?

G: Have you ever felt **GUILTY** about your drinking?

E: Do you have a morning **EYE OPENER**?

From National Institute on Alcohol Abuse and Alcoholism: *Assessing alcohol problems: a guide for clinicians and researchers*, ed 2 (NIH Pub. No. 03–3745), 2003. Retrieved from <http://pubs.niaaa.nih.gov/publications/arh28-2/78-79.htm>.

problems that prevent participation in peer self-help groups. It is important that nurses recognize, assess, and screen for substance abuse in older adults so that they can refer these individuals to appropriate community resources. Nurses are in a prime position to educate clients about the dangers of substance abuse.

Suicide

Suicide, the act of intentionally taking one's own life, is a serious health concern related to the elderly, who account for 18% of all suicides. Elder suicide may be underreported by 40% or more of actual cases. Omitted are "silent suicides," for example, deaths from medical noncompliance or overdoses, self-starvation or dehydration, and "accidents." Elders at highest risk for suicide are white males older than 85 years; the second highest are American Indian and Native Alaskan men (NIMH, 2010). Elderly individuals have a high success rate for suicide because they use firearms, hanging, and drowning. "Double suicides" involving spouses or partners occur frequently among the aged.

Elder suicide is associated with depression, chronic illness, physical impairment, unrelieved pain, financial stress, loss and grief, social isolation, and alcoholism. Warning signs to watch for in the elderly are loss of interest in things or activities that are usually found enjoyable; cutting back from social interactions, self-care, and grooming activities; not following medical regimens (e.g., going off diets, not taking prescriptions); experiencing or expecting a significant personal loss (e.g., spouse or friend); feeling hopeless or worthless; putting affairs in order; giving things away; making changes in will; and stockpiling medications or obtaining other lethal means of committing suicide. The most significant warning sign is any expression of intent. Risk factors that should also be considered in determining whether an elder might be at risk are previous suicide attempts, history of mental disorders, alcohol and substance abuse, family history of suicide, and local epidemics of suicide.

Prevention activities include dispelling any myths that exist relating to suicide. Many think that winter holidays are linked to suicide, but, in fact, suicide rates in the United States are lowest in the winter and highest in the spring (CDC, 2011b). Other myths that need to be discussed and banished are that those who kill themselves must be crazy, asking someone about suicide can lead to suicide, pain goes along with aging so nothing can be done, those who talk about suicide rarely actually do it, and if someone is determined to kill himself or herself no one can stop that person. Other prevention concepts are to promote awareness, develop broad-based support, reduce stigma associated with aging and being a consumer of mental health, urge use of psychiatric resources and suicide prevention services, develop community-based suicide prevention programs if none exist, reduce access to lethal means of self-harm, promote participation in education programs related to recognition of at-risk behaviors, and, lastly, promote and support research.

Alzheimer's Disease

Alzheimer's disease is a slowly progressive brain disorder that begins with mild memory loss and progresses through stages to total incapacitation and eventually death. It is the sixth leading cause of death in the U.S. Diagnosing whether an individual has Alzheimer's disease is very difficult because it mimics other conditions such as depression and other types of dementia. Usually, a tentative diagnosis is reached after all other conditions have been ruled out. The only sure way to diagnose Alzheimer's disease is by autopsy although cerebrospinal fluid analysis and magnetic resonance imaging are being investigated for their diagnostic accuracy. There is no cure, and limited treatment options are available.

In 2012, an estimated 5.4 million Americans had Alzheimer's disease; however, the exact number is unknown because of difficulty in diagnosing dementia of the Alzheimer's type (Alzheimer's Association, 2012). The numbers are expected to increase as people are living longer. Wolf-Klein and colleagues (1989) studied 312 active outpatient geriatric clients to measure the validity of the clock drawing test in screening individuals with probable Alzheimer's disease. They found that clients with Alzheimer's disease were unable to draw a normal clock and demonstrated five characteristically abnormal patterns. As a test for Alzheimer's disease, clock drawing had a sensitivity of 86.7% and a specificity of 92.7%. There was correct identification in 97.2% of healthy individuals. The researchers reported that the findings indicate that the clock drawing test, an easily administered, low-cost screening tool, can be useful to health care professionals in characterizing cognitive loss in a general geriatric clinic population.

An additional number of screening tools to assess for cognitive impairment have been developed. The Patient Protection and Affordable Care Act added to the "annual wellness visit" a requirement for primary physicians to detect cognitive impairment. The assessment tools recommended include the Mini-Cog (Box 19-8), the Memory Impairment

BOX 19-8 THE MINI-COG

Administration

1. Instruct the patient to listen carefully to and remember 3 unrelated words and then to repeat the words. The same 3 words may be repeated to the patient up to 3 tries to register all 3 words.
2. Instruct the patient to draw the face of a clock, either on a blank sheet of paper or on a sheet with the clock circle already drawn on the page. After the patient puts the numbers on the clock face, ask him or her to draw the hands of the clock to read a specific time. The time 11:10 has demonstrated increased sensitivity.
3. Ask the patient to repeat the 3 previously stated words.

Scoring (Out of total of 5 points)

Give 1 point for each recalled word after the clock drawing test (CDT) distractor. Recall is scored 0-3.

The CDT distractor is scored 2 if normal and 0 if abnormal.

(Note: The CDT is considered normal if all numbers are present in the correct sequence and position, and the hands readably display the requested time. Length of hands is not considered in the score.)

Interpretation of Results

0-2: Positive screen for dementia
3-5: Negative screen for dementia

Screen (MIS), and the General Practitioner Assessment of Cognition (GPCOG) (Jeffrey, 2012). Research is ongoing for development of a diagnostic test that could improve recognition of the disease in early stages, resulting in better management using available drugs and therapies. The U.S. Food and Drug Administration has approved five different drugs for treatment of Alzheimer's disease. Galantamine (Razadyne), rivastigmine (Exelon), and donepezil (Aricept) are used to treat mild to moderate stages of the disease. Tacrine (Cognex) is rarely prescribed today because of safety concerns. Memantine (Namenda) and donepezil are used for moderate to severe cases (Alzheimer's Association, 2012). These drugs appear to slow down some of the symptoms, but they do not stop the progression of the disease. Research continues related to diagnosis, causes and risk factors, and treatment and care issues.

The behavioral and physical changes due to Alzheimer's disease create many challenges for caregivers, family, and friends. Fifteen percent of Americans with Alzheimer's disease and other dementias live alone. For the individual living alone, inadequate self-care, social isolation, falls, unattended wandering, and injuries occur in addition to problems such as fires from leaving the stove on and having the electricity turned off because bills have not been paid. Some of the behavioral symptoms are agitation, aggression, wandering, and sleep disturbances. The Alzheimer's Association (2012)

has a list of ten "absolutes" for the care of people with the disease: never argue—instead agree, never lecture—instead reassure, never reason—instead divert, never shame—instead distract, never say "remember" —instead reminisce, never say "I told you" —instead repeat, never say "you can't" —instead do what you can, never command or demand—instead ask or model, never condescend—instead encourage and praise, and never force—instead reinforce.

Management strategies for caring for the individual with Alzheimer's disease includes: appropriate use of available treatment options, effective management of coexisting conditions, coordination of care among health care professionals and lay caregivers, participation in activities and adult day care programs, and taking part in support groups and support service such as counseling (Alzheimer's Association, 2012). Caregivers should contact the Alzheimer's Association for their many publications, experts, and local chapter programs. Medical supervision of the physical condition and medications (if clinically indicated) is essential. In addition, Alzheimer's disease centers throughout the country offer diagnosis and treatment; provide information about the disease, services, and resources; and give volunteers an opportunity to participate in drug trials and other research projects. A number of resources are available for respite for the caregiver, support groups for both client and family, and day care facilities for the client. For the patient with Alzheimer's disease who wanders, the local police should be informed of the potential problem, current pictures of the individual should be available, and safety measures such as installing locks and bells on doors should be taken.

SPIRITUALITY

As people age and face life's challenges, such as loss of loved ones, declining physical health, and a realization that life's end may be near, spirituality may become more important (Touhy and Jett, 2012). Spirituality involves "finding core meaning in life, responding to meaning, and being in relationship with God/Other" (Manning, 2013). Spirituality is a broader concept than religion, encompassing a person's values or beliefs, search for meaning, relationships with a higher power, nature, and other people. It includes religion, which is defined as a social institution that unites people in a faith in God, a higher power, and in common rituals and worshipful acts (Touhy and Jett, 2012). According to Hodge, Bonifas, and Chou (2010), the majority of older adults describe themselves as both spiritual and religious.

Research suggests that spirituality is important to many older adults and has health benefits. Manning (2013) conducted a qualitative study to explore the interplay between spirituality and resilience in six elderly women in their 80s and 90s. Results showed that the women credited their spirituality and their connection with God for helping them reach advanced age. Furthermore, the participants exhibited resilience and regarded their spirituality as a key aspect of and mechanism for dealing with adversity and negotiating hardships over their life courses. Spirituality served as a pathway to their resilience.

Addressing the spiritual needs and concerns of a client is part of providing holistic nursing care. If nurses are comfortable with their own spirituality, they will be more attentive to the spiritual needs of their clients. Visible cues, such as the wearing of a religious article or the presence of religious symbols—Bible, Koran, rosary beads, prayer or inspirational books—can provide useful insights and a means to open discussion about spiritual needs (Eliopoulos, 2014). Furthermore, use of open-ended questions to begin dialogue about spiritual concerns and use of established spiritual assessments such as the FICA Spiritual History Tool (available at www.consultgerirn.org) are helpful. The FICA, which stands for faith, importance/influence, community, and address, provides nurses with a quick and simple means to conduct a spiritual assessment.

Nursing interventions that may be helpful in addressing spiritual needs include the nurse's presence, active listening, caring touch, reminiscence, prayer, hope, conveying a nonjudgmental attitude, facilitation of religious practices, and referral to spiritual care experts (Eliopoulos, 2014).

END-OF-LIFE ISSUES

Advance Directives

Decision making at the end of life is complex. It is recommended that all adults have advance directives. Older adults often experience multiple chronic illnesses, some life-threatening; therefore it is especially imperative that this population have advance directives. An older person who is approaching death may not be able to make end-of-life decisions. For such a person, confusion as to how to provide appropriate care may develop.

The Patient Self-Determination Act is a federal law enacted in 1990 that requires health care facilities that receive Medicare and Medicaid funds to ask patients on admission whether they possess an advance directive (Miller, 2012). The most common type of advance directive is a living will. Living wills are legal documents whose purpose is to allow individuals to specify what type of medical treatment they would or would not want if they became incapacitated or had an irreversible terminal illness. Living wills can direct physicians to withhold life-sustaining procedures and can assist family members in making decisions when they are unable to consult a comatose or medically incompetent relative. An individual must be competent to initiate a living will, and he or she can revoke or change it at any time (Miller, 2012).

A durable power of attorney is another type of advance directive that authorizes someone to act on an individual's behalf with regard to property and financial matters. A durable power of attorney for health care is an advance directive that allows an individual to designate a health care proxy or surrogate to make decisions about medical care if the person is unable to make them for himself or herself. When an individual has no advance directive, is incompetent, or is unable to handle his or her affairs adequately, a guardian may be appointed by the court to direct the individual's medical treatment, housing, personal needs, finances, and property.

Because the guardian manages all the individual's affairs and assumes legal rights, a guardianship is generally considered a last resort (Miller, 2012).

ETHICAL INSIGHTS
Making End-of-Life Decisions

Al Smith is 76 years old, lives alone, and suffered a massive stroke in his home. He was found by his older brother, Joe, who had come to visit him. Joe immediately called 9-1-1, and Al was rushed to a nearby hospital. Joe informed the health care providers at the hospital that he wanted everything done for his brother.

Complications from the stroke included irregular breathing, paralysis on one side of the body, aphasia, severe confusion, and problems with vision. Because of subsequent worsening of his breathing and nonresponsiveness, Al was started on ventilation therapy.

Joe called to inform their sister Rose, who lives out of town, about the incident and condition of their brother. Rose was very upset with Joe for allowing Al to be connected to a ventilator. She claimed that Al would not have wanted this.

Questions
1. What should Al Smith have done to make his wishes known?
2. What discussion should his siblings have had to prevent disagreement?
3. What are the ethical principles involved in this case?
4. What are the legal implications?

Last, a do-not-resuscitate (DNR) order is another kind of advance directive. A DNR order is a request not to have cardiopulmonary resuscitation (CPR) if the individual's heart stops or if the person stops breathing. Individuals should place their requests on advance directive forms and inform their physicians. Afterward, a DNR order is written in the medical chart by the physician.

Advance directives not only make a person's wishes known but may also decrease the stress of decision making experienced by family members at the end of a loved one's life. State-specific advance directives can be ordered from the national organization Caring Connections or downloaded from its website (http://www.caringinfo.org/i4a/pages/index.cfm?pageid=1).

The Nurse's Role in End-of-Life Issues

The nurse is encouraged to discuss and educate clients about end-of-life issues. These issues include advance directives and prefuneral considerations when death is imminent. When a client enters a health care facility with an advance directive, nurses should ensure that it is current and reflects the client's wishes. The nurse should inform other members of the health care team and make sure that the document is visible and accessible in the client's chart. The nurse should also encourage clients to discuss their wishes regarding the decisions in these documents with their families. Clients should provide copies of advance directives such as living wills to their family members in case of emergency. Furthermore, clients should discuss their living wills with their physicians so that the documents are made part of their medical records. A copy of advance directives should also be kept in the individual's automobile.

CASE STUDY   APPLICATION OF THE NURSING PROCESS

Mrs. Darren, a 75-year-old widow, was referred to the community health nurse by her physician, who did not believe she could care for herself sufficiently. Her diagnoses were hypertension, mild congestive heart failure, arthritis, and occasional confusion after transient ischemic attacks.

During the initial home visit, the nurse observed that Mrs. Darren lived in a run-down house in an inner-city neighborhood. The roof leaked, and the house had no functioning heat unit. A rat was scrambling in the garbage. Mrs. Darren told the nurse that she did not have children and her only relative was a sister who lived with her family in another state. She was used to the neighborhood and knew her neighbors, but she was frightened of the teenagers who lingered when she took the bus to the supermarket to cash her Social Security check.

Mrs. Darren received Supplemental Security Income, Medicare, Medicaid, and food stamps. She ate mostly bread and butter and drank coffee, but she enjoyed fried chicken and oranges after going to the supermarket. Constipation was sometimes a problem, and she took a laxative every night. She said she did not always remember whether she took her medication and held out a small bottle containing an assortment of pills of different colors, shapes, and sizes.

Assessment

With Mrs. Darren as the system, or central planning focus, the nurse identified her biopsychosocial subsystem strengths and weaknesses and looked for actual or potential connections to her family and community suprasystems. Considering aging theories, the nurse believed Mrs. Darren was undergoing disengagement from her physical and social circumstances and decided that this process might be reversed if her health could be maintained and her links to the community strengthened. On a practical level, the nurse also checked with Mrs. Darren's physician regarding the prescriptions and identified the assortment of pills by taking them to the pharmacist who filled the prescriptions.

The nurse used a problem-solving approach to data gathering and identified Mrs. Darren's assets as the following:
- Being basically able to care for herself
- Receiving medical treatment
- Receiving income from various sources
- Being accustomed to the neighborhood and knowing her neighbors Her liabilities were more extensive, as follows:
- Inadequate nutrition
- Confusion with medications and improper use of laxatives
- Condition of the house, which was not supportive of health
- Threat of violence in neighborhood and possibility of attack for her Social Security money
- Physical impairment resulting from age and illness
- No children or other family living nearby
- Probable progression of confusion
- Possibility of a major stroke at home while unattended

Diagnoses

Diagnoses and related short- and long-term goals address Mrs. Darren's situation. The nurse wrote plans at the three levels of prevention for the diagnoses and included suggestions for intervention with families.

Individual
- Inadequate nutrition, which was related to difficulty or inability to procure food.
- Risk for exploitation due to possibility of robbery for Social Security money, aging, and progression of disease.

Family
- Potential for social isolation related to unanticipated loss of interaction with only relative who lives a distance away and Mrs. Darren's declining health.

Community
- Lack of knowledge regarding community resources for nutritional services and financial assistance.
- Lack of support programs for medication consistency related to unrecognized need.

Planning
Individual
Long-Term Goals
- Mrs. Darren will maintain a nutritionally adequate diet through self-care and use of community programs as evidenced by a steady weight and normal results on tests for nutritional status during physical examinations.
- Mrs. Darren will avoid inconsistency in her medication regimen related to forgetfulness and mild confusion.
- Mrs. Darren will continue to take medications as ordered, as evidenced by stabilization of disease processes and intermittent demonstration to a nurse.
- Mrs. Darren will explore sheltered housing for older adults and continue contact with a community health nurse and neighborhood friends.

Short-Term Goals
- Mrs. Darren will improve her diet to include a recommended daily allowance of nutrients, including fiber and fluids, as evidenced by diet recall, and she will report regular bowel habits without use of laxatives.
- Mrs. Darren will utilize memory aids for consistent medication regimen.
- Mrs. Darren will identify medications and know when to take them, as evidenced by demonstration to a nurse.
- Mrs. Darren will improve her home to allow healthy habitation, avoid robbery by varying her routine and using banking services, expand her social network, and maintain health care appointments.

Family
Long-Term Goal
- Mrs. Darren will maintain family contact by mail, telephone, or possible visits.

Short-Term Goal
- Family members' addresses are included in Mrs. Darren's record to facilitate emergency contact.

Community
Long-Term Goals
- Promote publicity campaign to advertise nutritional services for older adults in the community.
- Support community pharmacists in the campaign to increase public awareness of the need to take medications as prescribed.
- Identify and support programs that will assist with provision of prescribed medications for people who have difficulty obtaining prescriptions because of a lack of insurance, money, transportation, or other problems.
- Have community groups work together to maximize use of resources.

Short-Term Goal
- Identify existing programs for older adults in the community.

Intervention
Individual
When the nurse discussed the nursing diagnoses and plans with Mrs. Darren, Mrs. Darren agreed with the short-term goals, but

Continued

she was not sure that she wanted to leave her home for other housing or to meet other people through community activities. She agreed, however, to try. During the course of the next few visits, the nurse explained basic nutritional principles and helped make a shopping list and menus for 1 week. Together, they developed a plan to assist with medication scheduling.

The nurse encouraged Mrs. Darren to talk about her earlier life during the nurse's visits. She had been widowed soon after her marriage, when her husband was killed serving in the army overseas, and she had never remarried. She lived in the neighborhood where she grew up, although it had deteriorated over the years. She had worked as a secretary until her retirement and had no pension plan.

Family

Because Mrs. Darren's family did not live close by, the nurse designed a plan to increase Mrs. Darren's social contacts by introducing her to a group that met frequently and offered several activities she might enjoy. If she were unexpectedly absent, the group would check on her. A neighbor invited her to a senior center, where she became involved in a domino-playing group. Mrs. Darren allowed her name to be put on the waiting list for an apartment for older adults. With the other changes, the apartment was no longer a priority, and Mrs. Darren could make a decision when an apartment became available.

Community

Referrals initiated by the nurse resulted in a greatly improved living situation. A financial advisor from the city's Supportive Services to the Elderly program encouraged Mrs. Darren to open a bank account for the direct deposit of her checks and showed her how to use it. A home health aide from the same program came for half a day each week to assist with shopping and cleaning. The sanitation department of the health district exterminated the rats, the local Area Agency on Aging fixed the roof, and a church-sponsored group painted the house and cleaned the yard. A small heater was purchased from the Salvation Army store, and application was made to the utility company for help with bills during the winter months.

Evaluation

Individual

With the nurse as intermediary for and coordinator of community services, Mrs. Darren easily accepted help with the problems related to security and survival. When her home improvements were completed, Mrs. Darren was able to maintain herself more comfortably with the help of the weekly visit from the home health aide.

Family

In the absence of family support, the establishment of an orderly routine, the companionship at the nutrition site, and safer financial arrangements increased Mrs. Darren's feelings of belonging and self-esteem. The nurse reduced her home visits but maintained contact with Mrs. Darren during her visits to the health clinic for blood pressure checks and preventive health care to supplement her medical care.

Community

Discussion with the home health aide informed the nurse of proposed funding cuts to the city's Supportive Services to the Elderly program, which would result in reduced services. The nurse spoke to the president of the district branch of the professional nurses' association, who notified the state level of the association to monitor funding on the state level. The association also assisted the nurse in working with other local agencies for older adults

to establish a publicity campaign against proposed funding cuts through writing letters to the editors of local newspapers, speaking at public hearings on the city budget, and speaking at city council meetings. Although funds were reduced, the cuts were much less severe than they would have been without the campaign, and most services were able to continue, although with longer waiting times for admission of new clients.

Levels of Prevention

Primary Prevention

Goal: Promote good nutrition.

Individual

- Instruct about nutritional needs.
- Plan a shopping list and menus incorporating a prescribed diet for health problems.

Primary Prevention

Goal: Promote safety and prevention of injury.

Individual

- Provide immunizations as appropriate.
- Provide community services for assistance to maintain property and prevent deterioration.
- Encourage a network of friends and family members.

Family

- Provide services of community health nurse or case manager.
- Provide counseling.
- Provide respite care.

Community

- Provide community education programs for older adults.
- Be aware of potential hazards for older adult residents and provide intervention as needed.

Secondary Prevention

Goal: Assess and treat nutrition-related disorders.

Individual

- Provide referral for assessment of possible nutrition-related disorders.
- Provide hospitalization or prescribed nutritional supplements for illness resulting from inadequate nutrition.

Family

- Provide referral for nutritional assessment and counseling.

Community

- Encourage emergency food supplies.

Secondary Prevention

Goal: Diagnose and treat medication-related injuries.

Individual

- Provide referral for apparent overmedication or undermedication symptoms.
- Diagnose and treat drug or food reactions.

Family

- Reassess the client's understanding of medications.

Community

- Provide a 24-hour poison hotline.
- Provide an emergency department with 24-hour response.
- Provide medical services.

CASE STUDY APPLICATION OF THE NURSING PROCESS—cont'd

Tertiary Prevention
Goal: Maintain improved nutrition.

Individual
- Encourage use of community services.

Family
- Encourage exchange of family recipes.
- Encourage attendance at home economics classes.

Community
- Provide campaigns for nutritional awareness and healthy eating.
- Encourage the eating of healthy snacks in food machines.
- Encourage use of funding of community food services for aggregates or emergencies.
- Encourage use of services providing access to food (e.g., food banks, Meals on Wheels, and food stamps).
- Encourage use of transportation to grocery stores or nutrition services.

Tertiary Prevention
Goal: Be consistent with prescribed medications and prevent medication error.

Individual
- When medications are dispensed, provide written and oral instructions at the level of understanding and in the language of the client.
- Have the client repeat instructions to the health care provider.

Family
- Have the client repeat instructions to family members.

Community
- Provide a community education program about understanding medications.

SUMMARY

Increasing life expectancy, coupled with the aging of the baby boomer generation, will cause a dramatic and continual rise in the number of older adults. In addition to longevity, older adults desire to function independently for as long as possible. This chapter has described aging, demographic characteristics, normal aging changes, health promotion and illness prevention interventions, common health and psychosocial concerns, end-of-life issues, and various resources that may assist older adults. Community health nurses should be aware of and address these issues and concerns so that they may help elders have a better quality of life.

LEARNING ACTIVITIES

1. Interview an elderly person you know to assess his or her physical activity level and nutritional status using the nutrition checklist and food pyramid. Review the results with the person and help him or her plan a nutritious menu for 1 day. What factors hindered or enhanced your interaction with the person?
2. Find the names, addresses, and phone numbers of local resources for someone interested in, for example, exercise programs for the elderly and smoking cessation programs.
3. Devise a nursing care plan for an elder with a visual disturbance (e.g. cataracts, glaucoma, or macular degeneration).
4. You are asked to lead a 1-hour discussion (see following topic list) for a group of ten seniors at a senior citizens center. What would be your goal? What physiological aspects would you include? What psychosocial aspects would you consider?
   - Issues related to urine control
   - Fall prevention
   - Prevention of influenza and pneumonia
   - Medications and aging
   - Normal aging changes
5. Speak with police officers in a local community about elder abuse and crimes against elders. Identify community strengths and weaknesses. Discuss needs and solutions.
6. The family of your elderly client is considering taking his car keys from him. They asked you how to decide whether their loved one should stop driving. How would you respond?
7. Your 80-year-old client has become very frail and needs assistance with several activities of daily living. No family members are able or willing to take care of him full-time. The family has asked you for advice. What information would you share with them about alternative housing options?
8. Your elderly client has a terminal illness. You note that she does not have an advance directive. What issues surrounding this topic would you discuss with her?

ⓔ EVOLVE WEBSITE

http://evolve.elsevier.com/Nies
- NCLEX Review Questions
- Case Studies
- Glossary

REFERENCES

Administration on Aging: *A profile of older Americans*, Washington, DC, 2011, U.S. Department of Health & Human Services. Also available from <www.aoa.gov/aoaroot/aging_statistics/Profile/2011/docs/2011profile.pdf>.

Alzheimer's Association: *2012 Alzheimer's disease facts and figures*, Chicago, 2012, Author.

American Foundation for the Blind: *Special report on aging and vision loss*, New York, 2013, Author.

American Geriatrics Society: *AGS updated Beers criteria for potentially inappropriate medication use in older adults*, 2012. Available from <www.americangeriatrics.org/health_care_professionals/clinical_practice/clinical_guidelines_recommendations/2012>.

Budnitz D, Lovegrove M, Shehab N, Richards C: Emergency hospitalizations for adverse drug events in older Americans, *New England Journal of Medicine* 365(21):2002–2012, 2011.

Center for Healthy Aging: *Chronic disease*, 2011. Available from <http://www.ncoa.org/improve-health/center-for-healthy-aging/chronic-disease/?print.>

Centers for Disease Control and Prevention: *Traumatic brain injuries can result from senior falls*, 2010b. Available from <http://www.cdc.gov/TraumaticBrainInjury/tbi_falls_results.html>.

Centers for Disease Control and Prevention: *Fall risks for older adults*, 2011a. Available from <http://www.cdc.gov/features/fallrisks/index>.

Centers for Disease Control and Prevention: *Injury prevention & control: Holiday suicides – fact or myth?* 2011b. Available from <http://www.cdc.gov/ViolencePrevention/suicide/holiday.html>.

Centers for Disease Control and Prevention: *New data on older drivers*, 2011c. Available from <http://www.cdc.gov/Features/dsOlderDrivers/>.

Centers for Disease Control and Prevention: *Cold stress*, 2012a. Available from <http://www.cdc.gov/niosh/topics/coldstress/>.

Centers for Disease Control and Prevention: *Heat stress*, 2012c. Available from <http://www.cdc.gov/niosh/topics/heatstress/>.

Cumming E, Henry W: *Growing old*, New York, 1961, Basic Books.

De la Fuente M: Role of neuroimmunomodulation in aging, *Neuroimmunomodulation* 15:213, 2008.

Eliopoulas C: *Gerontological nursing*, ed 8., Philadelphia, 2014, Lippincott Williams & Wilkins.

FamilyDoctor.org: *Fecal incontinence*, 2011. Available from <http://familydoctor.org/familydoctor/en/diseases-conditions/fecalinontinence_printerview>.

Federal Interagency Forum on Aging-Related Statistics: *Older Americans 2012: Key indicators of well-being*, Washington, DC, 2012, Author. Also available from <www.agingstats.gov>.

Havighurst RL, Neugarten BL, Tobin SS: Disengagement and patterns of aging. In Neugarten BL, editor: *Middle age and aging*, Chicago, 1968, University of Chicago Press.

Havighurst RL, Neugarten BL, Tobin SS: Disengagement, personality, and life satisfaction in the later years. In Hansen PF, editor: *Age with a future*, Copenhagen, 1963, Munksgaard.

Hayflick L: *How and why we age*, New York, 1996, Ballantine Books.

Hodge D, Bonifas R, Chou R: Spirituality and older adults: Ethical guidelines to enhance service provision, *Advances in Social Work* 11(1):1–16, 2010.

Jeffrey S: New guidelines on screening for cognitive impairment, 2012, *Medscape Medical News*, 2012. Available from <http://www.medscape.com?viewarticle/776548>.

Lichtenstein AH, Rasmussen H, Yu WW, et al: Modified MyPyramid for older adults, *J Nutr* 138:78–82, 2008.

Lighthouse International: *Prevalence of vision impairment*, 2013. Available from <www.lighthouse.org/research/stastics-on-vision-impairment>.

Linn FR, Thorpe R, Gordon-Salant S, et al. *Hearing loss prevalence and risk factors among older adults in the United States*, Baltimore, 2011, Johns Hopkins School of Medicine. Also available from <http://www.healthyhearing.com/content/articles/Hearing-loss/Causes/47739-Hearing-loss-in-the-elderly?print=on>.

Manning LK: Navigating hardships in old age: Exploring the relationship between spirituality and resilience in later life, *Qualitative Health Research* 23(4):568–575, 2013.

Mauk K: *Gerontological nursing competencies for care*, ed 3, Boston, 2014, Jones and Bartlett.

Mayo Clinic Staff: *Cataracts*, 2010. Available from <http://www.mayoclinic.com/health/cataracts/DS0005/>.

Mayo Clinic Staff: *Dry macular degeneration*, 2012a. Available from <http://www.mayoclinic.com/health/macular-degeneration/DS00284/>.

Mayo Clinic Staff: *Glaucoma*, 2012b. Available from <http://www.mayoclinic.com/health/glaucoma/DS00283/>.

Mayo Clinic Staff: *Wet macular degeneration*, 2012c. Available from http://www.mayoclinic.com/healh/wet-macular-degeneration/DS01086/>.

Miller CA: *Nursing for wellness in older adults: theory and practice*, ed 6, Philadelphia, 2012, Lippincott Williams & Wilkins.

Miller RA: The aging immune system: primer and prospectus, *Science* 273:70, 1996.

Morley A: The somatic mutation theory of aging, *Mutat Res* 338(1–6):19–23, 1995.

Musil C, Ahmad M: Health of grandmothers: A comparison by caregiver status, *Journal of Aging and Health* 14(1):96–121, 2002.

National Alliance on Mental Illness: *Depression in older persons fact sheet*, 2011. Available from <http://www.nami.org/Template.cfm?Section=By_Illness&template=/ContentManagement/ContentDisplay.cfm&ContentID=7515>.

National Alliance on Mental Illness: *Mental illness: Anxiety disorders*, 2012. Available from <http://www.nami.org/Template.cfm?Section=By_Illness&Template=/ContentManagement/ContentDisplay.cfm&ContentID=142543>.

National Center on Elder Abuse: *Why should I care about elder abuse?* 2013. Available from <www.ncea.aoa.gov/Resources/Publications/docs/WhatsAbuse_2010.pdf>.

National Fire Data Center: *Trends in older adult fire death rates (2000-2009)*, 2012. Available from <www.usfa.fema.gov/statistics/estimates/trend_older.shtm>.

National Institute of Neurological Disorders and Stroke: NINDS Traumatic brain injury information page, 2005, Available from <www.ninds.nih.gov/disorders/tbi/tbi.htm.>

National Institute on Aging: *Age page: urinary incontinence*, 2008. Available from <www.nia.nih.gov/ HealthInformation/Publications/urinary.htm>.

National Institute on Aging: *Age page: Crime and older people*, 2009. Available from <http://www.nia.gov/print/health/publication/crime-and-older-people>.

National Institute on Aging: *Age page: Hyperthermia: Too hot for your health*, 2010a. Available from <http://www.nia.nih.gov/print/health/publication/hyperthermia-too-hot-your-health>.

National Institute on Aging: *Age page: Hypothermia: A cold weather hazard*, 2010b. Available from <http://www.nia.nih.gov/health/publication/hypothermia-cold-weather-hazard>.

National Institute on Aging: *Age page: Aging and your eyes*, 2012a. Available from <http://www.nia.nih.gov/health/publication/aging-and-your-eyes>.

National Institute on Aging: *Age page: Alcohol use in older people*, 2012b. Available from <http://www.nia.gov/health/publication/alcoholuseinolderpeople>.

National Institute on Aging: *Age page: Hearing loss*, 2012c. Available from <http://www.nia.nih.gov/health/publication/hearing-loss>.

National Institute on Aging: *Age page: Falls and fractures*, 2013a. Available from <http://www.nia.gov/print/health/publications/falls-and-fractures>.

National Institute on Aging: *Age page: Older drivers*, 2013b. Available from <http://www.nia.nih.gov/print/health/publication/older-drivers>.

National Institute on Aging: *Age page: Medicines: Use them safely*, n.db. Available from <http://www.nia.nih.gov/print/health/publication/medicines-usse-them-safely>.

National Institute on Deafness and Other Communication Disorders: *Hearing Loss and older adults*. Available from <http://www.nidcd.nih.gov/health/hearing/pages/older.aspx.>

NIHseniorhealth.gov: *Drugs in the body*, 2011. Available from <http://nihseniorhealth.gov/takingmedicines/drugsinthebody/01.html>.

NIHseniorhealth.gov: *What is hearing loss?* 2012a. Available from <http://nihseniorhealth.gov/hearingloss/hearinglossdefined/01.html>.

NIHseniorhealth.gov: *About anxiety disorders*, 2012b. Available from <http:nihseniorhealth.gov/anxietydisorders/aboutanxietydisorders/01.html>.

NIHseniorhealth.gov: *How aging affects driving*, 2012c. Available from <http://nihseniorhealth.gov/olderdrivers/howagingaffectsdriving/01.html>.

NIHseniorhealth.gov: *About falls*, 2013. Available from <http://nihseniorhealt.gov/falls/about falls/01.html>.

Nutrition Screening Initiative: *Determine your nutritional health*, Washington, DC, Author.

Orgel LE: The maintenance of the accuracy of protein synthesis and its relevance to aging, *Proc Natl Acad Sci* 49:517–521, 1963.

Ross MET, Aday L: Stress and coping in African-American grandparents who are raising their grandchildren, *Journal of Family Issues* 27(7):912–932, 2006.

Rubin M: Grandparents as caregivers: Emerging issues for the profession, *J Hum Behav Soc Environ* 23:330–344, 2013.

SeniorHealth365.com: Dental problems in the elderly, 2011. Available from <http://www.seniorhealth365.com/2011/12/14/dental-problems-in-tge-elderly/>.

Substance Abuse and Mental Health Services Administration: *Results from the 2011 National Survey on Drug Use & Health: Summary of national findings* (NSDUH Series H-44, USDHHS Publication No. SMA 12–4713). Rockville, MD, 2012, Author.

Touhy T, Jett K: *Ebersole & Hess' toward healthy aging: Human needs & nursing response*, St. Louis, 2012, Elsevier.

Tsai P: Predictors of distress and depression in elders with arthritic pain, *J Adv Nurs* 51: 158-165, 2005.

U.S. Census Bureau: *Centenarians: 2010 Census special reports (C2010SR-03)*, Washington, DC, 2012, U.S. Government Printing Office.

U.S. Department of Agriculture: *My Plate—for adults*, 2011. Available from <www.foodpyramid.com/myplate/for-adults>.

U.S. Department of Health and Human Services: *Recommended immunizations for adults*, 2013. Available from <http://www.cdc/gov/vaccines>.

U.S. Department of Health and Human Services/ Centers for Medicare and Medicaid Services (USDHHS/CMS): *Medicare and you*, Baltimore, 2013, Author. Also available from <www.medicare. gov/publications/pubs/pdf/10050.pdf>.

U.S. Department of Health and Human Services, Office of Disease Prevention & Health Promotion: *Healthy People 2020: Leading health indicators*, Washington, DC, 2012, Author. Also available from <http://www.healthypeople.gov/2020;LHI/>.

U.S. Department of Health and Human Services, Office of Disease Prevention & Health Promotion: *Healthy People 2020: Older adults,* Washington, DC, n.d., Author. Also available from <www.healthypeople.gov/2020/topicsobjectives2020/objectiveslist.aspx?topicID=31>.

Vincent G, Velkoff V: *The next four decades, the older-population in the United States: 2010-2050* (Current Population Reports, 25–1138). Washington, DC, 2010, U.S. Census Bureau.

Williams MN: The changing roles of grandparents raising grandchildren, *J Hum Behav Soc Environ* 21:948–962, 2011.

Wolf-Klein G, Silverstone FA, Levy AP, et al: Screening for Alzheimer's disease by clock drawing, *J Am Geriatr Soc* 37:730–734, 1989.

Family Health

Beverly Cook Siegrist

Family is not an important thing, it's everything.
Michael J. Fox

OBJECTIVES

Upon completion of this chapter, the reader will be able to do the following:

1. Give a definition of *family*.
2. Identify characteristics of the family that have implications for community health nursing practice.
3. Describe strategies for moving from intervention at the individual level to intervention at the family level.
4. Describe strategies for moving from intervention at the family level to intervention at the aggregate level.
5. Discuss a model of care for families.
6. Apply the steps of the nursing process to individuals within the family, the family as a whole, and the family's aggregate.

KEY TERMS

cohabitation
ecological framework
ecomap
expressive functioning
external structure
family

family health assessment
family health tree
family interviewing
general systems theory
genogram
instrumental functioning

internal structure
nuclear family
sandwich generation
social network framework
transactional model

OUTLINE

Understanding Family Nursing
The Changing Family
  Definition of Family
  Characteristics of the Changing Family
Approaches to Meeting the Health Needs of Families
  Moving from Individual to Family
  Moving from Family to Community
Approaches to Family Health
  Family Theory
  Systems Theory
  Structural-Functional Conceptual Framework
  Developmental Theory

Assessment Tools
  Genogram
  Family Health Tree
  Ecomap
Family Health Assessment
  Social and Structural Constraints
Extending Family Health Intervention to Larger Aggregates and Social Action
  Institutional Context of Family Therapists
  Models of Care for Communities of Families
Applying the Nursing Process
  Home Visit

To understand American families, many sociologists suggest that one needs to only view television and movies. Stereotypical television families have allowed American families to identify with developmental landmarks and to understand changing family demographics and structure. ABC-Disney television's hit situation comedy *Modern Family* provides a quasi-realistic depiction of a diverse extended family: Jay, a 60-ish family patriarch in a second marriage to a much younger Colombian wife, has a new son and a 14-year-old stepson; Jay's adult daughter and her husband are a traditional

nuclear family with three children; his adult son lives with his stay-at-home same-sex partner, who is the primary caregiver for their adopted Vietnamese daughter. In reality, "modern families" may be much more complex than the television families because of chronic health issues and the changing societal forces that are affecting the family in ways never before imagined by health care professionals.

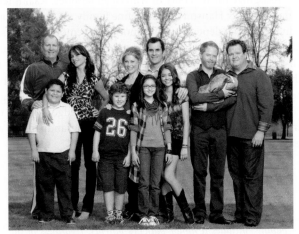

The cast of the television show *Modern Family* portray the Pritchett family, a sterotypical extended American family. (Used with permission from Disney/ABC Television Group, Burbank, California. © American Broadcasting Companies, Inc.)

The dynamic forces impacting families are not new, but when combined result in new challenges to families. For example, it is well documented that the increase in the number of aging Americans is expected to present new challenges to families and society. Forty-seven percent of the U.S. population 85 years and older is composed of women living alone, below the poverty level ($15,072), whose primary income is social security (U.S. Department of Health and Human Services [USDHHS], 2012). When combined with the declining economy, the increasing population of aging, single women has resulted in challenging living arrangements, draining economic resources, and growing numbers of families without sufficient health care coverage. The result is a **sandwich generation** or sandwich family structure, in which adults care for elderly parent(s) either in their homes or by providing financial support (Parker and Patten, 2013; Zinn, Eitzen, and Wells, 2011). Added to this financial burden is the number of adults also providing financial support to adult children. According to a report from the Pew Research Foundation, "47% of adults in their 40s and 50s have a parent aged 65 or older, are raising a young child, or financially supporting a grown child. And about one-in-seven middle-aged adults (15%) is providing financial support to both an aging parent and a child" (Parker and Patten, 2013) (Figure 20-1).

Globalization has also affected the family. In many areas manufacturing has replaced agriculture as primary employment. As in-state manufacturing jobs have decreased because of the moving of jobs offshore, the outsourcing of services, and the economy, a decreased job security has resulted in increased stress on families (Zinn et al, 2011). Loss of jobs results in financial decline, personal bankruptcies, and downward social mobility. All of these forces impact individual and family health.

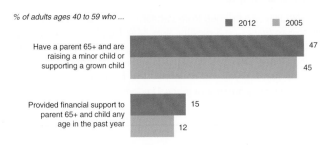

Middle-Aged Adults "Sandwiched" Between Aging Parents and Kids

% of adults ages 40 to 59 who ...

█ 2012 █ 2005

Have a parent 65+ and are raising a minor child or supporting a grown child	47
	45
Provided financial support to parent 65+ and child any age in the past year	15
	12

Note: Based on all adults ages 40 to 59: for 2012, n=844; for 2005, n=1,185.

PEW RESEARCH CENTER   Q21,27, P1,3,4

FIGURE 20-1 The sandwich generation. (From Pew Research Center: *Social and demographic trends: The sandwich generation*, 2013. Retrieved from <http://www.pewsocialtrends.org/2013/01/30/the-sandwich-generation/>).

The families described in the following Clinical Examples depict broad contemporary definitions of family and are the kinds of families carried in caseloads by undergraduate community health nursing students. Assessments made by students during home, office, and hospital visits with these families triggered interventions that linked the families to resources provided by the community and, in turn, led to questions about health needs of groups of families or larger aggregates living in the same communities.

Clinical Example

Rebecca Martin is a 72-year-old widow of 10 years who lives in a rural town in Tennessee. She resides in the home that she and her husband purchased before his death. Her primary source of income is her deceased husband's Social Security benefits, and she also receives a small income from providing child care for infants at her church. Medicare benefits are her only source of payment for health care. Her only child, a daughter from whom she has been estranged for many years, recently died. The daughter was a never-married, single mother of an 8-year-old, medically fragile child with asthma. As the only surviving relative, Rebecca has become the custodial parent for her granddaughter.

Clinical Example

Joe Hudson is a 74-year-old alcoholic who is being treated at an outpatient department in a large medical center. He lives in a hotel room in downtown Salt Lake City, Utah. He has one living relative, a 76-year-old brother. Mr. Hudson states, "I had a falling out with my brother 20 years ago. I never hear from him. I reckon he's still in Boston, if he's alive at all." Mr. Hudson frequently falls out of bed, dislodging the telephone that the desk clerk has placed precariously close to the bed, which signals the desk clerk that something is amiss. The clerk then goes to Mr. Hudson's room and puts him back in bed. Mr. Hudson's source of income is a check sent to him the first day of each month by a minister who lives in a town 75 miles away. The desk clerk cashes Mr. Hudson's check and helps him pay his bill from the hotel, which provides congregate dining facilities.

Clinical Example

Lyn Nguyen is a refugee from Vietnam who moved with her family to San Francisco 3 months ago. Mrs. Nguyen is a single parent; Mr. Chan died in an automobile accident shortly after arriving in the United States. Mrs. Nguyen has two children, an 11-year-old son and a 5-year-old daughter. The family resides in a one-room efficiency apartment in the Tenderloin district in downtown San Francisco.

Clinical Example

Jaime Gutierrez, a 72-year-old Mexican American man, lives with his 36-year-old son, Roberto; his 34-year-old daughter-in-law, Patricia; and his three grandchildren, who are 14, 13, and 12 years of age. Mr. Gutierrez was in good health until he fell from a tree while helping his son make roof repairs on the house in 1995. He suffered a concussion, right hemothorax, and fracture of vertebrae T11 and T12. Confined to bed, he is receiving home health care. He requires intermittent catheterization but feels uncomfortable when the nurse suggests that his daughter-in-law is willing to carry out this procedure for him. Therefore Roberto quit work to provide this personal care to his father. Consequently, the family of six lives on Mr. Gutierrez's retirement income, which consists of $239 from Social Security and $244 from a pension plan per month. Roberto would like to improve his job skills while at home. He has finished the fourth grade and has failed the Graduate Equivalency Degree (GED) examination twice. Patricia also would like to return to school and pursue job training. Although agreeable to Patricia's interests, Roberto is hesitant to support active steps taken by Patricia to initiate her plan.

Working with families has never been more complex or rewarding than now. Nurses understand the actual and potential impact that families have in changing the health status of individual family members, communities, and society as a whole. Additionally, families have challenging health care needs that are not usually addressed by the health care system. Instead, the health care system most frequently addresses the individual. This holds true for nursing interventions within the health care system. This chapter helps the nurse understand and address complex issues that impact family health and suggests methods to improve family health.

UNDERSTANDING FAMILY NURSING

Family nursing is not a new concept and has been taught in schools of nursing since Nightingale's "district nursing" concept (Cook, 1913) and Lillian Wald's (1904) principles on how to nurse families in the home. The National League for Nursing (NLN) has emphasized the importance of family nursing in standard curriculum guides for schools of nursing since 1917 (Beard, 1999; NLN, 1937). Early NLN publications directed nurses in "household science" and later required that 10 to 15 hours of study should be directed toward understanding the "modern family," in which the nurse must consider the family as a unit (NLN, 1937). Modern nurse theorists such as

Newman, King, Orem, and Roy, extensively discuss the family and its importance to individuals and society. Previously, nurses defined the family conceptually in the following ways: as the environment affecting individual clients; as small to large groups of interacting people; as a single unit of care with definable boundaries; or as a unit of care within a specific environment of a community or society. Current family theorists recognize the diversity of American families. Kaakimen, Gedaly-Duff, & Hanson (2009) define family as "two or more individuals who depend on one another for emotional, physical, and economical support. The members of the family are self-defined". Wright and Leahey (2012) state, "the family is who they say they are" (p. 70). Current advocacy groups find these definitions even too narrow. The Human Rights Campaign (2014) urges that health professions acknowledge all types of families, including gay, lesbian, and even grandparents as heads of family, by using this definition:

> "Family" means any person(s) who plays a significant role in an individual's life. This may include a person(s) not legally related to the individual. Members of "family" include spouses, domestic partners, and both different-sex and same-sex significant others. "Family" includes a minor patient's parents, regardless of the gender of either parent ... without limitation as encompassing legal parents, foster parents, same-sex parent, step-parents, those serving in loco parentis, and other persons operating in caretaker roles. (Human Rights Campaign, 2014, Inclusive definition of family)

These recommendations can be seen in the revised definitions related to who are family members and immediate relatives in the modification to U.S. Office of Personnel Management, Guidelines for family Medical Leave Act (75 FR 33491), by which family is to include: spouse and parents of spouse, sons and daughters and spouses, brothers and sisters and spouses, grandparents and grandchildren and spouses, domestic partners and parents of, and any individual related by blood or affinity whose close association with the employee is equivalent of a family relationship.

These later definitions are perhaps more useful to the nurse and allow the focus on the needs of the family. Family nursing care may be focused on the individual family member, within the context of the family, or the family unit. Regardless of the identified client, the nurse establishes a relationship with each family member within the unit and seeks to understand the influence of the unit on the individual and society.

The family is composed of many subsystems and, in turn, is tied to many formal and informal systems outside it. The family is embedded in social systems that have an influence on health (e.g., education, employment, and housing). Many disciplines are interested in the study of families; interdisciplinary perspectives and strategies are necessary to understand the influence of the family on health and the influence of the broader social system on the family. Traditionally, nursing and even community health nursing has relied heavily, if not solely, on theoretical frameworks for intervention with families from the disciplines of psychology or social psychology, which target individuals (Cody, 2000; Duvall, 1977; Erikson, 1963;

Maslow, 1970). This chapter addresses how community health nurses work with families within communities to bring about healthy conditions for families at the family, social, and policy levels. It focuses on the following five areas:

1. The changing family
2. Approaches to meeting the health needs of families
3. Family theory approach to meeting the health needs of families
4. Extending family health intervention to larger aggregates and social action
5. An example of the nursing process applied to a family

THE CHANGING FAMILY

Definition of Family

Many definitions of family exist, such as the traditional definition from U.S. Census Bureau (2005): "A family consists of two or more people, one of whom is the householder, related by birth, marriage, or adoption and residing in the same housing unit." The nurse's definition of *family* is influenced by personal involvement with his or her own family and clinical experiences. Definitions of *family* vary by professional discipline and type of family described. For example, psychologists may define *family* in terms of personal development and intrapersonal dynamics; the sociologist has used a classic definition of *family* in terms of a "social unit interacting with the larger society." Other professionals have classically defined *family* in terms of kinship, marriage, and choice: "a family is characterized by people together because of birth, marriage, adoption, or choice" (Allen, Fine, and Demo, 2000, p. 7). Friedman, Bowden, and Jones (2003) incorporate the idea of many nontraditional definitions: "A family is two or more persons who are joined together by bonds of sharing and emotional closeness and who identify themselves as being part of the family" (p. 10). Again, this definition supports the idea of letting the family define their composition and relationships (Wright and Leahey, 2012). The National Institute of Mental Health (2005) defines family simply as a "network of mutual commitment" (p. 2).

In the past, the dominant American definition focused on the intact nuclear family. African American families focus on a wide network of kin and community. The "nuclear" family does not exist for Italian families. To them, *family* means a strong, tightly knit three- or four-generational group that includes godparents and old friends. Some families of early- (e.g., first- or second-) generation Chinese Americans go beyond this and include in their definition of *family* multigenerational family members and ancestors (Li et al, 2009).

The community health nurse (CHN) interacts with communities made up of many types of families. When faced with great diversity in the community, the community health nurse must formulate a personal definition of *family* and must be aware of the changing definition of *family* held by other disciplines, professionals, and family groups. The CHN who interacts with Mr. Hudson, the alcoholic described in the Clinical Example who lives in a hotel, must have a broad conceptualization of the family. Both the surveillance activity by the hotel manager and the financial support from the minister could be accounted for in the definition of McDaniel and colleagues: "We define family as any group of people related either biologically, emotionally, or legally. That is, the group of people that the patient defines as significant for his or her well-being" (2005, p. 2).

Regardless of the definition of *family* accepted, what is evident is the importance of the family unit to society. The family fulfills two important purposes. The first is to meet the needs of society, and the second is to meet the needs of individual family members (Friedman et al, 2003). The family meets the needs of society through procreation and socialization of family members. "The basic unit (family) so strongly influences the development of an individual that it may determine the success or failure of that person's life" (Friedman et al, 2003, p. 4). The family is the "buffer" between individuals and society. The family meets individual needs through provision of basic needs (food, shelter, clothing, affection). The family supports spouses or partners by meeting affective, sexual, and socioeconomic needs. For children, the family is the "first teacher," instructing the children in societal rules and providing values needed for growth and development.

Characteristics of the Changing Family

The characteristics of the U.S. family continue to change. Historically the typical family, the nuclear family, has been defined as "the family of marriage, parenthood, or procreation; it is composed of a husband, wife, and their immediate children—natural, adopted or both" (Friedman et al, 2003, p. 10). The stereotypical view of this family as father, mother, and non-adult children currently represents 66% of U.S. families (Pew Research Center, 2010). A Pew Research Center Social and Demographic Trends report also describes the return of the multigenerational family household, which is probably due to the economy. Nearly 16.1% of the total U.S. population in 2012 lived in families composed of at least two adult generations or a grandparent and one other adult (Pew Research Center, 2010). In the last decade, recognition of various types of kinship families has resulted in available data that describe common types of families found in the United States. Table 20-1 presents significant family information.

The rate of cohabitation, which is defined as "a living arrangement in which an unmarried couple live together in a long-term relationship that resembles a marriage," has also increased over time (U.S. Census Bureau, 2008, 2011). The U.S. Census Bureau (2010) reported a 15% increase in the number of cohabitating families with significant changes in the family structure. The household more likely included at least an adult parent of one of the individuals and it was more likely that one half of the couple was unemployed. This was a significant change from 2007 findings, in which both individuals were employed in more than half of the couples. It is hypothesized that this change is due to the economy (Pew Research Center, 2010). The nurse should be aware of the potential need for additional family support and intervention with such families.

Single parenting has also increased over time. The birth rate among teenagers continues to raise concern. During

TABLE 20-1	A COMPARISON OF FAMILIES BY TYPE IN THE UNITED STATES, 2003, 2007, AND 2011		
FAMILY TYPE	2003	2007	2011
Married-couple households	50,130,111 (68%)	49,932,000 (69%)	48,328,000 (66%)
Father-only households	4,425,000 (6%)	5,076,000 (7%)	5,508,000 (7%)
Mother-only households	21,138,000 (31%)	22,282,000 (32%)	19,325,000 (26%)
Children in care of grandparents	3,194,000 (4%)	3,457,000 (5%)	2,871,000 (4%)
Children living with cohabiting domestic partners	4,186,000 (6%)	4,343,000 (6%)	5,512,000 (7%)
Children living with neither parent	4,126,000 (6%)	4,343,000 (6%)	3,456,000 (5%)
Children living in married-couple immigrant-family households	10,935,000	12,774,000	12,933,000
Children living in single-parent immigrant-family households	2,944,000	3,680,000	4,417,000
US born children living in single-parent immigrant families	17,967,000	18,602,000	20,301,000

Data from Annie E. Casey Foundation: *National Kids Count key indicators*, 2009. Available from <datacenter.kidscount.org>.

TABLE 20-2	PERCENTAGE (%) OF U.S. FAMILIES THAT ARE SINGLE-PARENT FAMILIES BY ETHNIC GROUP, 2007 AND 2011	
	2007	2011
Non-Hispanic white	23	25
Black or African American	65	67
American Indian	49	53
Asian and Pacific Islander	17	17
Hispanic or Latino	37	42

Data from Annie E. Casey Foundation: *Kids Count data center*, 2009. Available from <datacenter.kidscount.org>.

TABLE 20-3	TEEN BIRTH RATE (PER 1000) AGES 15 TO 17 YEARS BY ETHNIC GROUP, 2010
Non-Hispanic white	23
Black or African American	51
American Indian	39
Asian or Pacific Islander	11
Hispanic or Latino	56
Total	34

Data from Annie E. Casey Foundation: *Kids Count data center*, 2010. Available from <datacenter.kidscount.org>.

the years 1980 to 2006, the birth rate for unmarried women 15 to 17 years of age increased from 21 to 41.9 per 1000 in the United States, before dropping back to 29.4 in 2012 (Centers for Disease Control and Prevention [CDC], 2012). The Annie E. Casey Foundation (2013) reports that the incidence of teen parenting continues to rise in all ethnic groups. Single parenting is associated with greater risks because of reduced social, emotional, and financial resources, which affect the general well-being of children and families. In 2012, 34% of all U.S. children lived in single-parent homes. Single parenting is a key indicator of risk for well-being in children (Annie E. Casey Foundation, 2013).

The proportion of children younger than 18 years who are living with their grandparents has decreased slightly, by 1%, since 2007 (Annie E. Casey Foundation, 2013). In 2007, grandparent-headed families accounted for 5% of all families. The American Academy of Child & Adolescent Psychiatry (2009) suggests that parenting by grandparents may be "due to serious societal issues and problems including increasing numbers of single parent families, the high rate of divorce, teenage pregnancies, AIDS, incarcerations of parents, substance abuse by parents, death or disability of parents, parental abuse and neglect" (p. 3). The gay or lesbian family is made up of a cohabiting couple of the same sex who have a sexual relationship. The 2010 U.S. Census reports 594,000 same-sex

couple households, 84% of which include children. Table 20-2 shows statistics for single-parent families by ethnic group, and Table 20-3 shows teen birth rates by ethnic group. Both of these groups have the potential to be considered families at risk for health problems and may require additional CHN nursing interventions.

APPROACHES TO MEETING THE HEALTH NEEDS OF FAMILIES

Community health nursing has long viewed the family as an important unit of health care, with awareness that the individual can be best understood within the social context of the family. Observing and inquiring about family interaction enables the nurse in the community to assess the influence of family members on one another. However, direct intervention at the family rather than the individual client level is a new frontier for many nursing students, most of whom have experience in acute care settings before the community setting. A family model, largely a community health nursing or psychiatric–mental health intervention model, also includes the areas of birthing and parent-child interventions, adult day care, chronic illness, and home care. Nursing assessment and intervention must not stop with the immediate social context of the family; it must also consider the broader social context of the community and society. Friedman and colleagues (2003, pp. 5-6) suggest reasons why it is important for nurses to work with families:

The family is a critical resource: The importance of the family in providing care for its members has already been established. In this caregiver role, the family can also improve individual members' health through health promotion and wellness activities.

In a family unit any dysfunction (illness, injury, separation) that affects one or more family members will affect the members and unit as a whole: Also referred to as the "ripple effect," changes in one member cause changes in the entire family unit. The nurse must assess each individual and the family unit.

Case finding is another reason to work with families: As the nurse assesses an individual and family, he or she may identify a health problem that necessitates identifying risks for the entire family.

Improving nursing care: The nurse can provide better and more holistic care by understanding the family and its members.

Moving from Individual to Family

The rationale of Friedman and colleagues (2003) for the importance of moving to family nursing is still relevant. Community health and home care nurses have traditionally focused on the family as the unit of service. With health care system changes throughout the United States, many CHNs continue to focus their practices on individuals residing in the home. As a result of the current era of cost containment, constraints on the CHN and on nurses working within hospitals and in other settings will increase. For example, reimbursement, which is almost entirely calculated for services rendered to the individual, is a major constraint against moving toward planning care for the family as a unit. However, current methods of reimbursing hospitals depend on keeping patients at home, so all nurses must consider the importance of not only the entire health care team but also the patient's family unit in meeting health and rehabilitation goals. Moving from individual to family nursing becomes more important than ever. Various creative approaches to meeting the health needs of families are needed, also reflecting interventions appropriate to the needs of the population as a whole.

Family Interviewing

Approaches to the care of families are needed and must be creative, flexible, and transferable from one setting to another. Community health nurses are generalists who bring previous preparation in communication concepts and interviewing to the family arena. Wright and Leahey (2012) proposed the realm of **family interviewing** rather than family therapy as an appropriate model. In this model, the community health nurse uses general systems and communication concepts to conceptualize the health needs of families and a family assessment model to assess families' responses to "normative" events such as birth and retirement or to "paranormative" events such as chronic illness and divorce. Intervention is straightforward, as in helping parents educate prepubescent teenage family members about sex by providing appropriate educational materials, or consists of making a referral to another health professional if the level of intervention is beyond the preparation of the nurse. For the purposes of this text, the model is extended to include intervention at the level of the larger aggregate. For example, the index of suspicion based on the health needs of a particular family would prompt the community health nurse to assess the need for similar information and the resources for intervention with other families in the community, schools, churches, or other institutions. Family interviewing requires thinking "interactionally," not only in terms of the family system but also in terms of larger social systems.

Wright and Leahey (2005, 2012) identify the following critical components of the family interview: manners, therapeutic conservation and questions, family genogram (and ecomap when indicated), and commendations. Family theorists and practitioners suggest that with experience, the nurse can accomplish the family interview in 15 minutes (Bell, 2012; Martinez, D'Artoism, Rennick, 2007; Wright and Leahey, 2012).

Manners. Manners are common social behaviors that set the tone for the interview and begin the development of a therapeutic relationship. Wright and Leahey (2012) believe that erosion of these social skills prevents the family nurse from collecting essential data. Many nurses argue that too much formality establishes artificial barriers to communication; however, studies have shown that the essentials of a therapeutic relationship begin with manners. The nurse introduces himself or herself by name and title, always addresses the client (and family members) by name and title (i.e., Mr., Mrs., or Ms., unless otherwise directed by client), keeps appointments, explains the reason for the interview or visit, and brings a positive attitude. Other behaviors (manners) that invite rapport include being honest with the client and checking attitude (the nurse's) before each client encounter.

Therapeutic Conversations. The second key element in the interview is the therapeutic conversation. This type of conversation is focused and planned and engages the family. The nurse must listen and must remember that even one sentence has the potential to heal or help a family member. The nurse encourages questions, engages the family in the interview and assessment process, and commends the family when strengths are identified. Every encounter, whether brief or extended, has "healing potential." Therapeutic conversation may initiate further discussion that brings the family together on issues (Wright and Leahey, 2012).

Genogram and Ecomap. The genogram and ecomap constitute the third element and are described in detail later in this chapter. These tools provide essential information on family structure and together are an efficient way to gather information such as family composition, background, and basic health status in a way that engages the family in the interview process.

Therapeutic Questions. Therapeutic questions are key questions that the nurse uses to facilitate the interview. The questions are specific for the context or family situation but have the following basic themes (Wright and Leahey, 2012): family expectations of the interview or home visit; challenges, concerns, and problems encountered by the family at the time of the interview; and sharing of information (e.g., who will relate the family history or information).

Commending Family or Individual Strengths. The fifth element of the family interview is commending the family or individual strengths. Wright and Leahy (2012) suggest identifying at least two strength areas and, during each family interview, sharing them with the family or individual. Sharing strengths reinforces immediate and long-term positive relationships between the nurse and family. Interviews that identify and build upon family strengths tend to progress to more open and trusting relationships and often allow the family to reframe problems, thereby increasing problem solving and healing (Wright and Leahey, 2012).

Issues in Family Interviewing. Creative family interviewing requires interviewing families in many types of settings. The prediction of decreased hospitalization, supplemented by a wide variety of health care settings ranging from acute to ambulatory to community centers, calls for flexible, transferable approaches. Clinical settings for family interviewing are reviewed by Wright and Leahey (2012) and include inpatient and outpatient ambulatory care and clinical settings in maternity, pediatrics, medicine, surgery, critical care, and mental health. According to Wright and Leahey, community health nurses have many opportunities besides the traditional home visit to engage the family in a family interview. CHNs are employed in ambulatory care centers, occupational health and school sites, housing complexes, day care programs, residential treatment and substance abuse programs, and other official and nonofficial agencies. At each of these sites, CHNs meet families and can assess and intervene at the family and community levels.

Astedt-Kurki, Paavilainen, and Lehti (2001) studied methodological issues in interviewing families. They recommend the following considerations when scheduling family interviews, with the understanding that access and timing may direct who among the family members are available to the nurse: Consider that when one family member is the informant, he or she provides only that one point of view on the family member (i.e., identified patient) or family unit. In some cases this may be preferable, such as if the CHN requires information about a child from a mother. If information is needed about the family system, it is preferable to interview at least two family members because the unit of assessment is the family unit. The involvement of too many family members, in a large unit, may result in chaos if the interviewee is inexperienced. If the purpose of the assessment is to assess communication, it may be preferable to schedule an interview when all family members are present. Involving children depends on the age of the children and the purpose of the interview. Are the children of an age that the parents can be honest if needed, or will the children hide issues in front of the parents? All of these situations must be considered (Astedt-Kurki et al, 2001).

The family interview assists the nurse in identifying family health risks since the family experiences similar risk factors (i.e., physiological, behavioral, and environmental). Studies have documented the familial predisposition to the three major diseases resulting in morbidity and mortality in the United States: cardiac disease, cancer, and diabetes. Family health practices also influence lifestyle habits among family members. Recognizing the importance of a family health history related to individual and public health, the U.S. Surgeon General initiated the National family History Initiative in 2003 with a goal to educate individuals about inherited predispositions to disease (McNeill et al, 2008). This website has proved to be successful in engaging American families in learning about their family history and familial and genetic health risk for family members. The project was renamed "My family Health Portrait Tool" and has been redesigned to more user friendly for individuals (USDHHS, 2010). Another example would be a Hispanic-American family in which a family member has diabetes; the nurse could implement a family health promotion plan based on the needs of the individual within an at-risk family. The family plan for diabetes prevention is based on the nurse's understanding that the National Institutes of Health (NIH) reports that this group has the highest rate of diabetes among a nonwhite ethnic group in the United States (NIH, 2009).

Involving family members in newborn assessments can aid the community health nurse in determining the family's adjustment to the newborn and parenthood. The nurse can do this in the home, clinic, or other health care center. Family members should be involved during the first contact or visit, and, if they do not attend, a telephone call explaining the nurse's interest in them should take place (Wright and Leahey, 2012).

Children and parents in these families need a chance to express their concerns; the family interview is important and may provide the nurse with necessary information needed to care for these families.

Intervention in Cases of Chronic Illness

Perhaps as many as 90% of families are dealing with chronic illness in a family member (Martire and Schulz, 2007). The CDC (2013) reports that one of every two Americans lives with a chronic disease and that seven of every 10 U.S. deaths result from chronic illnesses. For the family with a member who has a chronic illness, it is important to the individual and family's adjustment, as well as to the patient's symptom management, that the family is prepared to be emotionally and physically supportive. The CHN can intervene to assist the family coping with related stressors. Also significant is the fact that a resource such as third-party reimbursement forces most families to learn to manage the chronic problems with limited or infrequent intervention from health professionals. The community health nurse working with families coping with chronic illness in a child, adult, or older adult is aided by the family interview. As Glaser and Strauss (1975) stated, chronic illness injects change into various areas of family life:

> *Sex and intimacy can be affected. Everyday mood and interpersonal relations can be affected. Visiting friends and engaging in other leisure time activities can be affected. Conflicts can be engendered by increased expenses stemming from unemployment and the medical treatment…. [D]ifferent illnesses may have different kinds of impact on such areas of family life, just as they probably will call for different kinds of helpful agents.* (p. 67)

Changes in family patterns, fears, emotional responses, and expectations of individual family members can be assessed in the family interview. Special needs of the primary caretaker (i.e., often the spouse, daughter, or daughter-in-law) can be assessed. The community health nurse making family visits to older adults and the terminally ill is able to assess intergenerational conflict and stress and positively influence family interaction (Wright and Leahey, 2012).

Moving from Family to Community

The health of families can affect the health of society as a whole, in both positive and negative ways. The health of a community is measured by the well-being of its people and families. Circumstances such as low-birth-weight infants, lack of health insurance, homelessness, violence, poverty, and low employment rates provide a description of families and nations. Community health nurses provide family nursing to improve individual and family health; however, the potential result may be improving the health of society. The care of entire populations is the major focus, as stated by Freeman (1963) in her classic work, *Public Health Nursing Practice:*

> The selection of those to be served ... must rest on the comparative impact on community health rather than solely on the needs of the individual or family being served.... The public health nurse cannot elect to care for a small number of people intensely while ignoring the needs of many others. She must be concerned with the population as a whole, with those in her caseload, with the need of a particular family as compared to the needs of others in the community. (p. 35)

The challenge to the community health nurse is to provide care to communities and populations and not to focus only on the levels of the individual and the family. The community health nurse, who traditionally carries a caseload of families, extends his or her practice to the community. To do so, an aggregate, community, and population focus must serve as a backdrop to the entire practice.

For example, families must be viewed as components of communities. The community health nurse must know the community. As stated in previous chapters, a thorough community assessment is necessary to practice in the community. By way of review, the nurse must remember that communities must be compared not only in terms of different health needs but also in terms of different resources to effect interventions that influence policies and redistribute resources to ensure that community and family health needs are met.

Community health nurses must then compare city data with county data and then county data, state data, and national data. In addition, they may need to compare local census tract data and areas of a city or county with other areas of the city or county.

For example, community health nursing students in San Antonio, Texas, who were planning home visits to families of pregnant adolescents attending a special high school, compared local, state, and national statistics on infant mortality rates as a part of a community assessment. They found higher rates of infant mortality in San Antonio in census tracts on the south side of the city, in which the population was predominantly Mexican American. They also found this population to be younger, to have a higher rate of functional illiteracy among adults, to be less educated, to be more likely to drop out of high school, to have higher fertility rates, to have higher birth rates among adolescents, and to be more likely to be unemployed. They found that specific health needs varied among census tracts. Common major health needs of this subpopulation were identified from the community assessment, which helped the students plan care for these families. For example, their goals were broadened from carrying out interventions at the individual level to interventions at the family and community levels. In addition to targeting good perinatal outcomes for the individual teenage parent, nursing students planned to include assessments of functional literacy at the individual and family levels and arranged for group sessions in clinic waiting rooms that offered information about and referral of individuals and family members to alternative resources to enable teenage parents to complete school, take classes in English as a second language, and use resources for family planning and employment at the community level.

In addition to the cross-comparison of communities, the community health nurse also cross-compares the needs of the families within the communities and sets priorities. The nurse in the community finds that specific health needs vary among families. The nurse must account for time spent with families and choose those families on the basis of their needs in comparison with the needs of others in the community.

 HEALTHY PEOPLE 2020

Access to Health Care

In relation to improving family health, all of the leading health indicators listed as priority in *Healthy People 2020* can serve as a guide for family nursing interventions. Access to quality health care affects every aspect of family nursing because it impacts prevention of disease and disability, quality of life, preventable death, and overall life expectancy. The objectives for measurement of this goal include the following:

- Increase the proportion of persons with health insurance.
- Increase the proportion of insured persons with coverage for clinical preventative services.
- Increase the proportion of persons with a usual primary care provider.
- Increase the proportion of persons who have a specific ongoing care.

This chapter has discussed the disparities that exist among families and populations with regard to health care access. The community nurse should use political skills, advocacy, and education to influence policy that will result in increased access to health care. The nurse can educate families about available resources and help communities develop resources to improve health care access.

Data from U.S. Department of Health and Human Services: *Healthy People 2020: Objectives.* Available from <http://www.healthypeople.gov/2020/topics objectives2020/overview.aspx?topicid=1>.

Delegation of Scarce Resources

Although the community health nurse serves the community or population as a whole, fiscal constraints hold the nurse accountable for the best delegation of scarce resources. Time spent on home visits has traditionally allowed the community health nurse to assess the environmental, social, and biological determinants of health status among the population and the resources available to them. Fiscal accountability, nevertheless, means setting priorities. In 1985, Anderson, O'Grady, and Anderson listed the factors that influence public health nursing practice, especially home visits, as "the need to justify personnel costs in a time of fiscal constraint, the increasing number of medically indigent who turn to local public health services for primary care, and the change in reimbursement mechanisms by the federal government and some states" (p. 146). These observations still hold true. In 2009, more than 46 million Americans, including 9 million children, lacked health insurance (Robert Wood Johnson Foundation, 2009). In 2010 the number of uninsured rose to 49.9 million, or 16.3% of the U.S. population; however, in 2011 there was a drop to 48.6 million (U.S. Census Bureau, 2013). This drop is attributed to the increase in the number of young adults ages 19 to 26 who could for the first time remain on their parents' primary insurance following graduation from college. The Children's Health Insurance Program (CHIP) of 1997 has greatly increased access to health care for many low-income children. When the CHIP program was initiated, there were 10 million children in the United States, and 14% were uninsured; in 2008, 7.4 million children were enrolled in state CHIP plans (Centers for Medicare and Medicaid Services, 2009). The majority of these children lived in families with working, low-income parents. On February 4, 2009, President Obama signed the Children's Health Insurance Program Reauthorization Act (CHIPRA), which renewed and expanded coverage of CHIP from 7 million children to 11 million children. The Affordable Care Act of 2010 keeps the CHIP program in place until 2019 (Medicaid.gov, n.d.).

APPROACHES TO FAMILY HEALTH

Many schools of thought regarding the approaches to meeting family health needs exist among community health, community mental health, and public health nursing professionals. Dreher (1982) wrote that the traditional basis for community health nursing intervention has a focus that has long endorsed psychological and social-psychological theories to explain variations in health and patterns of health care, such as those set forth by Erikson (1963), Maslow (1970), and Duvall (1977). Dreher (1982) stated that what is needed are "more encompassing theories which explain the relationship between society and health [and] the policies which will be most effective in assuring health and health care" (p. 508). To help bridge this gap, four frameworks for meeting family health needs are presented here: family theory, systems framework, structural-functional conceptual framework, and developmental theory.

Clinical Example

Ten-year-old Jean Wilkie was referred by her teacher to the school nurse. She was withdrawn, had no school friends, and was dropping behind in her schoolwork. The school nurse talked to Jean in her office. Jean said that she had no friends because the other girls stayed overnight with one another "all the time" and that she did not want to bring her friends home because her father "drank all the time." The school nurse decided that Jean's problems needed assessment within the context of the family and arranged to visit the family at home. The father refused to participate in the family interview, but Jean's mother, her 13-year-old brother Peter, and Jean expressed concerns that the father had changed jobs several times in the past year, was frequently absent from work, and had been in two recent car accidents while "drinking." The school nurse was able to verify the family context as the basis of Jean's "problems," continue her family assessment, and plan for intervention at the family level. In addition, she was prompted to assess the community's preventive efforts directed toward drinking and the ability to provide ongoing care for families of alcoholics.

Family Theory

Many reasons exist for why the community health nurse should work with families. Friedman (1998) listed the following six reasons:

1. Any "dysfunction" (e.g., separation, disease, or injury) that affects one or more family members probably affects other family members and the family as a whole.
2. The wellness of the family is highly dependent on the role of the family in every aspect of health care, from prevention to rehabilitation.
3. The level of wellness of the whole family can be raised through care that reduces lifestyle and environmental risks by emphasizing "health promotion, 'self-care,' health education, and family counseling" (p. 5).
4. Commonalities in risk factors and diseases shared by family members can lead to case finding within the family.
5. A clear understanding of the functioning of the individual can be gained only when the individual is assessed within the larger context of the family.
6. The family as a vital support system to the individual member needs to be incorporated into treatment plans.

Nurses have relied heavily on the social and behavioral sciences for approaches to working with families. These approaches include psychoanalytical, anthropological, systems or cybernetic, structural-functional, developmental, and interactional frameworks (for reviews, see Friedman, 2003, and Wright and Leahey, 2012). The use of a framework for assessing a family helps the nurse understand the health potential for the family. Three conceptual frameworks (systems, structural-functional, and developmental), often used by nurses in providing health care to families, are described here. These models help the nurse empower the family in the process of family health promotion.

Systems Theory

The systems approach has been used in such diverse areas as education, computer science, engineering, and communication.

General systems theory (Minuchin, 2002; von Bertalanffy, 1968, 1972, 1974) has been applied to the study of families. General systems theory is a way to explain how the family as a unit interacts with larger units outside the family and with smaller units inside the family (Friedman, 2003). The family may be affected by any disrupting force acting on a system outside the family (i.e., suprasystem) or on a system within the family (i.e., subsystem). Parke (2002) stated that there are three subsystems of the family that are most important: parent-child subsystem, marital subsystem, and sibling-sibling subsystem. Dunst and Trivette (2009) review 20 years of systems theory and its importance to early childhood interventions, adding that systems theory provides direction for understanding how health care providers can expand family capacity by changing parenting, and therefore changing child behaviors. Table 20-4 presents definitions of the major terms used in the systems approach.

The past two decades have resulted in what many sociologists identify as imposing community subsystems with actual or potential negative influence on the family system. These include communities where violence has become the norm, dangers related to community-acquired diseases both manmade and natural, disasters, biohazards, and so on. These subsystems have the potential to complicate the care planned by the CHN and require interventions from several subsystems interacting with the family system and community. It is important that the CHN understand systems theory as a tool for both assessing families and communities and identifying resources and support services for families.

Characteristics of Healthy Families

Otto (1973) and Pratt (1976) characterized healthy families as "energized families" and provided descriptions of healthy families to guide the assessment of strengths and coping. DeFrain

TABLE 20-4 MAJOR DEFINITIONS FROM SYSTEMS THEORY

TERM	DEFINITION
System	"A goal-directed unit made up of interdependent, interacting parts which endure over a period of time" (Friedman, 1992, p. 115). A family system is not concrete. It is made up of suprasystems and subsystems and must be viewed in a hierarchy of systems. The system under study at any given time is called the *focal*, or *target*, system. In this chapter, the family system is the focal system.
Suprasystem	The larger system of which the family is a part, such as the larger environment or the community (e.g., churches, schools, clubs, businesses, neighborhood organizations, and gangs).
Subsystem	Smaller unit within the family, such as the relationship between spouses, parent and child, sibling and sibling, or extended family.
Hierarchy of systems	The levels of units within the system and its environment, which, in their totality, make up the universe. Higher-level units are composed of lower-level units (e.g., the biosphere is made up of communities, which are made up of families). Families are made up of family subsystems, and, in turn, family subsystems are made up of individuals, who are made up of organs, which are made of cells, which are made of atoms.
Boundary	An imaginary definitive line that forms a circle around each system and delineates the system from its environment. Auger (1976) conceptualized the boundary of a system as a "filter" that permits the constant exchange of elements, information, or energy between the system and its environments. "The more porous the filter, the greater the degree of interaction possible between the system and its environment" (p. 24). Families with rigid boundaries may lack information necessary to and resources pertinent to maintaining family health or wellness.
Open system	A system that interacts with its surrounding environment and gives outputs and receives inputs necessary to survival. An exchange of energy occurs. All living systems are open systems. However, if a boundary is too permeable, the system may be too open to input of new ideas from the outside and may be unable to make decisions on its own (Wright and Leahey, 1994).
Closed system	A system that theoretically does not interact with the environment. This is a self-sufficient system; no energy exchange occurs. Although no system has been found that exists in a totally closed state, if a family's boundaries are impermeable (i.e., less open as a system), needed input or interaction cannot occur. An example is a refugee family from Vietnam living in San Francisco; they may remain a closed family for some time because of their differences in culture and language.
Input	Information, matter, or energy that the open system receives from its environment that is necessary for survival.
Output	Information, matter, or energy dispensed into the environment as a result of receiving and processing the input.
Flow and transformation	The system's use of input may occur in two forms. Some input may be used in its original state, and some input may have to be transformed before it is used. Both original and transformed input must be processed and flow through the system before being released as output (Friedman, 1992).
Feedback	"The process by which a system monitors the internal and environmental responses to its behavior (i.e., output) and accommodates or adjusts itself" (Friedman, 1992, p. 117). The system controls and modifies inputs and outputs by "receiving and responding to the return of its own output" (Friedman, 1992, p. 117). Internally, the system adjusts by making changes in its subsystems. Externally, the system adjusts by making boundary changes.
Equilibrium	A state of balance or steady state that results from self-regulation or adaptation. As with the concept of a system as a mobile in the wind, balance is dynamic and, with change, is always reestablishing balance.
Differentiation	The tendency for a system to actively grow and "advance to a higher order of complexity and organization" (Friedman, 1992, p. 117). Energy inputs into the system make this growth possible.
Energy	Energy is needed to meet a system's demands. Open systems require more input through porous boundaries to meet the high energy levels needed to maintain high levels of activity.

(1999) and Montalvo (2004) helped to identify healthy families. These writers suggest the following traits of a healthy family:

- Members interact with one another; they communicate and listen repeatedly in many contexts.
- Healthy families can establish priorities. Members understand that family needs are priority.
- Healthy families affirm, support, and respect each other.
- The members engage in flexible role relationships, share power, respond to change, support the growth and autonomy of others, and engage in decision making that affects them.
- The family teaches family and societal values and beliefs and shares a religious core.
- Healthy families foster responsibility and value service to others.
- Healthy families have a sense of play and humor and share leisure time.
- Healthy families have the ability to cope with stress and crisis and to grow as a result of positive coping. They know when to seek help from professionals.

Structural-Functional Conceptual Framework

With the structural-functional conceptual framework approach to the family, the family is viewed according to its structure, or the parts of the system, and according to its functions, or how the family fulfills its roles.

Structural

Wright and Leahey (2005, 2012) stated that three aspects of family structure can be examined (internal structure, external structure, and context). **Internal structure** of the family refers to the following five categories:

1. Family composition, the family members, and changes in family constellation
2. Gender
3. Rank order, or positions of family members by age and sex
4. Subsystem or labeling of the subgroups or dyads (e.g., spouse, parental, and interest) through which the family carries out its functions
5. Boundary, or who participates in the family system and how he or she participates (e.g., a single-parent mother who does not allow her 17-year-old son to have his girl-friend spend the night in their home)

External structure refers to the extended family and larger systems (Wright and Leahey, 2005). It consists of the following two categories:

1. Extended family, including family of origin and family of procreation
2. Larger systems, such as work, health, and welfare

Context refers to the background or situation relevant to an event or personality in which the family system is nested (Wright and Leahey, 2005, 2012). It comprises the following five categories:

1. Ethnicity
2. Race
3. Social class
4. Religion
5. Environment

Clinical Example

Role Relationships

When Edna Smith, a 64-year-old client with severe arthritis, received a diagnosis of diabetes, her longtime friend, Frank Gardens, a widower of several years, moved in with her and assumed a caregiver role. The community health nurse assessed the dietary habits of Mr. Gardens and Mrs. Smith and found that Mr. Gardens did the shopping and the cooking because Mrs. Smith's mobility was severely restricted by her arthritis. Mr. Gardens did the cooking; therefore he purchased canned fruits and vegetables rather than fresh or frozen. Mr. Gardens perceived cooking, which was a new role for him, as demanding. After several visits, he disclosed to the nurse that his resistance to preparing fresh or frozen fruits and vegetables came from "the time it takes to clean the darn things, cook 'em, store 'em, and clean up the fridge when they go bad on ya." He stated unequivocally that it was stressful caring for Mrs. Smith and that he wanted to do it, but it was "much easier" to just "open a can" and "heat it in a pan" than to take the time and energy that preparation of fresh or frozen foods would require. The shift in roles that is often required of couples when a chronic illness is diagnosed in one can have an influence on the health of the family. Lubkin and Larsen (2013) provide additional reading about how couples manage with chronic illness.

Functional

Wright and Leahey (2005, 2012) also dichotomized family functional assessment, or how family members behave toward one another, into two categories, instrumental functioning and expressive functioning. **Instrumental functioning** refers to routine activities of daily living (e.g., elimination, sleeping, eating, giving insulin injections) (Box 20-1). This area takes on important meaning for the family when one member of the family becomes ill or disabled, is unable to carry out daily functions, and must rely on other members of the family for assistance. For example, an older adult may need assistance getting into the bathtub, or a child may need to have medications measured and administered.

The second type of family functional assessment is **expressive functioning**, or affective or emotional aspects. This aspect has the following nine categories:

1. *Emotional communication*: Is the family able to express a range of emotions, including happiness, sadness, and anger?
2. *Verbal communication* focuses on the meaning of words. Do messages have clear meanings rather than distorted meanings? Wright and Leahey (2005, 2012) gave the example of masked criticism when a father states to his child, "Children who cry when they get needles are babies."
3. *Nonverbal communication*, which includes sounds, gestures, eye contact, touch, or inaction. An example is a husband remaining silent and staring out the window while his wife is talking to him.
4. *Circular communication* is commonly observed between dyads in families. A common example is the blaming, nagging wife and the guilty, withdrawn husband.

BOX 20-1   SUMMARY OF FAMILY FUNCTIONAL ASSESSMENT

I. Instrumental functioning (i.e., activities of daily living)
II. Expressive functioning
   A. Emotional communication
   B. Verbal communication
   C. Nonverbal communication
   D. Circular communication
   E. Problem solving
   F. Roles
   G. Influence
   H. Beliefs
   I. Alliances and coalitions

Data from Wright LM, Leahey M: *Nurses and families: a guide to family assessment and intervention*, ed 2, Philadelphia, 1994, FA Davis.

5. *Problem solving* refers to how the family solves problems. Who identifies problems? Someone inside or outside the family? What kinds of problems are solved? What patterns are used to solve and evaluate tried solutions?

6. *Roles* refers to established patterns of behavior for family members (Wright and Leahey, 2000, 2012). Roles may be developed, delegated, negotiated, and renegotiated within the family. It takes other family members to keep a person in a particular role. Formal roles, with which the larger community agrees, may come into conflict with roles set by family members and influenced by religious, cultural, and other belief systems.

7. *Influence* refers to methods used to affect the behavior of another. Instrumental influence is the use of reinforcement via objects or privileges (e.g., money or use of technology tools). Psychological influence is the influence of behavior through the use of communication or feelings. Corporeal control is the use of body contact (e.g., hugging and spanking).

8. *Beliefs* refer to assumptions, ideas, and opinions that are held by family members and the family as a whole. Beliefs shape the way families react to chronic or life-threatening illness. For example, if a family of a person with colon cancer believes in alternative treatments, then acupuncture may be a viable option.

9. Alliances and coalitions are important within the family. What dyads or triads appear to occur repeatedly in the family? Who starts arguments between dyads? Who stops arguments or fighting between dyads? Is there evidence of mother and father against child? When does this change to parent and child against the other parent? The balance and intensity of relationships between subsystems within the family are important. Questions may be asked regarding the permeability of the boundary. Does it cross generations?

Developmental Theory

Nurses are familiar with developmental states of individuals from prenatal through adult. Duvall a noted sociologist, is the forerunner of a focus on family development (Duvall and Miller, 1985). In her classic work, she identified stages that normal families traverse from marriage to death (Box 20-2).

BOX 20-2   FAMILY LIFE CYCLE

1. Leaving home
2. Beginning family through marriage or commitment as a couple relationship
3. Parenting the first child
4. Living with adolescent(s)
5. Launching family (youngest child leaves home)
6. Middle-aged family (remaining marital dyad to retirement)
7. Aging family (from retirement to death of both spouses)

Adapted from Duvall EM, Miller BC: *Marriage and family development*, ed 6, New York, 1985, Harper and Row; and Carter B, McGoldrick M: *The expanded family life cycle: individual, family, and social perspectives*, 2005, Pearson Allyn & Bacon.

To assess the family, the community health nurse must comprehend these phases and the struggles that families experience while going through them. Wright and Leahey (2005, 2012) called attention to the need to distinguish between "family development" and "family life cycle." They stated that the former is the individual, unique path that a family goes through, whereas the latter is the typical path many families go through.

The developmental categories listed in Box 20-3 outline the six stages of the middle-class North American family life cycle (Carter and McGoldrick, 1988; Wright and Leahey, 2005) and the tasks necessary for the family's resolution of each stage. Nurses may use the stages to delineate family strengths and weaknesses.

RESEARCH HIGHLIGHTS

Work Hours and Perceived Time Barriers to Healthful Eating Among Young Adults

Young adults, though identified as underinsured and having limited access to primary care, are also identified as a group knowledgeable about the benefits of healthy eating. This age-group (20-31 years) has been confirmed in numerous national surveys as not regularly engaging in healthy eating habits, especially eating fewer than the recommended daily servings of fruits and vegetables and consuming a diet high in fast foods. Earlier studies among college students identified the following barriers: cost, stress, lack of knowledge related to food preparation, peer influence, and lack of time to balance busy lives.

A population study survey involved responses from 2287 individuals who were originally among a population of 4776 high school junior and seniors participating in a program call Project EAT-III (Eating and Activity in Teens and Young Adults), a program that looked at dietary intake, weigh control, and weight control behaviors during 1998 and 1999. Ten years later, the original participants were mailed letters asking them to participate in a new questionnaire, to which 1030 men and 1257 women agreed. Information was collected on time-related beliefs and behaviors about healthful eating, their fast food intake, fruit and vegetable intake, work hours, and socio-demographics.

This group reported time-related beliefs such as being too rushed to eat breakfast, eating on the run, and no time to eat healthy. They reported eating fast food weekly. Working at least 40 hours per week was associated with with an increase in time-related poor eating habits for men but not for women. Recommendations included workplace programs—free fruit and vegetables for break, flex time, and other interventions.

Data from Escoto KH, Laska MN, Larson N, et al: Work hours and perceived time barriers to healthful eating among young adults, *Am J Health Behav* 36(3):786-789, 2012.

ASSESSMENT TOOLS

There are many tools for the community health nurse to use in assessing the family (Butler, 2008; Friedman et al, 2003; Wright and Leahey, 2005, 2012). Reviewed here are the genogram, family health tree, and ecomap. The nurse can use these tools for family assessment with families in every health care setting. They help increase the nurse's awareness of the family within the community and help guide the nurse and the family in the assessment and planning phases of care.

Genogram

The **genogram** is a tool that helps the nurse outline the family's structure. It is a way to diagram the family. Generally, three generations of family members are included in a family tree, with symbols (Figure 20-2) denoting genealogy. Children are pictured from left to right, beginning with the oldest child.

The community health nurse may use the genogram during an early family interview, starting with a blank sheet of paper and drawing a circle or a square for the person initially interviewed. The nurse tells the family that he or she will ask several background questions to gain a general picture of the family. The nurse may draw circles around family members living in separate households.

For example, as depicted in the Case Study at the end of the chapter (Figure 20-3), family order across generations can be illustrated and specific personal characteristics can be noted in the drawing. Mr. and Mrs. Garcia are non–English-speaking, a factor that will be of importance to the nurse as he or she plans nursing interventions. At times, the usefulness of the genogram is limited by how freely the family member relates significant information such as divorces and remarriages and family health concerns. Other families may be sensitive to the sharing of such information, particularly when it is shown to recur with each generation. For example, a family history of alcohol or substance abuse or depression may be a sensitive issue. For other families, the development of the genogram is an excellent opening to the discussion of family history or hereditary health problems, or highlights the need for health education and promotion.

Family Health Tree

The **family health tree** is another tool that is helpful to the community health nurse. Based on the genogram, the family health tree provides a mechanism for recording the family's medical and health histories (Butler, 2008; Friedman 2003, 1992; USDHHS, 2005, 2010). The nurse should note the following information on the family health tree:

- Causes of death of deceased family members
- Genetically linked diseases, including heart disease, cancer, diabetes, hypertension, sickle cell anemia, allergies, asthma, and mental retardation
- Environmental and occupational diseases
- Psychosocial problems, such as mental illness and obesity
- Infectious diseases
- Familial risk factors from health problems
- Risk factors associated with the family's methods of illness prevention, such as having periodic physical examinations, Papanicolaou smears, and immunizations
- Lifestyle-related risk factors (elicited by asking what family members do to "handle stress" and "keep in shape")

The family health tree can be used in planning positive familial influences on risk factors such as diet, exercise, coping with stress, and the pressure to have a physical examination. The USDHHS (2005), under the direction of U.S. Surgeon General Richard Carmona, launched the Family History Initiative. Included in this initiative is an online interactive tool, My Family Health Portrait, to help families learn about their risk for disease (www.hhs.gov/familyhistory). Included are questions to ask family members about common diseases, questions that suggest health promotion activities, and goals as established in *Healthy People 2020.* When completed, the "family tree" can be printed. This tool could be incorporated into the family assessment and utilized by the nurse to plan family interventions to improve health.

Genogram Symbols

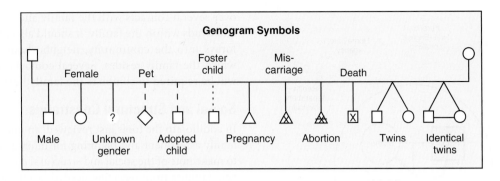

Sample Genogram: Woman with Multiple Husbands

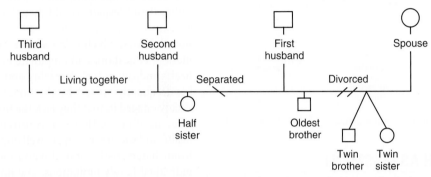

FIGURE 20-2 Commonly used genogram symbols. (Redrawn from Genopro Software: *Symbols used in genograms, 2009.* Available from <www.genopro.com>.)

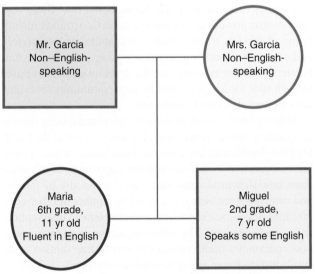

FIGURE 20-3 Sample genogram of the Garcia family (see Case Study).

Ecomap

The **ecomap** (Figure 20-4) is another classic tool that is used to depict a family's linkages to their suprasystems (Hartman, 1979; Wright and Leahey 2000, 2005, 2012). As originally stated by Hartman (1979):

The ecomap portrays an overview of the family in their situation; it depicts the important nurturant or conflict-laden connections between the family and the world. It demonstrates the flow of resources, or the lacks and deprivations. This mapping procedure highlights the nature of the interfaces and points to

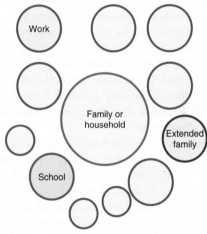

FIGURE 20-4 ecomap. (Redrawn from Hartman A: Diagrammatic assessment of family relationships, *Soc Casework* 59:496, 1978.)

conflicts to be mediated, bridges to be built, and resources to be sought and mobilized. (p. 467)

As with the genogram, the nurse can fill out the ecomap during an early family interview, noting people, institutions, and agencies significant to the family. The nurse can use symbols used in attachment diagrams (see Figure 20-2) to denote the nature of the ties that exist. For example, in Figure 20-5, the sample ecomap of the Garcia family suggests that few contacts occur between the family and the suprasystems. The community health nursing student was able to use the ecomap to discuss with the Garcia family the types of resources available in the community and the types of relationships they wanted to establish with them.

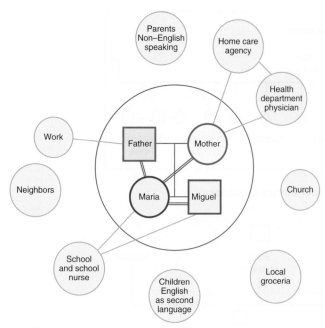

FIGURE 20-5 Sample ecomap of the Garcia family (see Case Study).

FAMILY HEALTH ASSESSMENT

Many agencies in the community have developed guidelines for assessment of the family that help practitioners identify the health status of individual members of the family and aspects of family composition, function, and process. Often included in family health assessment guidelines is information about the environment, or community context, and information about the family. A **family health assessment** form can be used as a guide to help the nurse with both collection of data and organization of the data collected from families over time. (See ⓔ **Resource Tool 20A**, Health Assessment Form on the book's Evolve site.)

The nurse can obtain information for the family health assessment through interviews with one or more family members individually, or with interviews of subsystems within the family (e.g., dyads of mother-child, parent-parent, and sibling-sibling. The nurse can also obtain information through observation of the environment in which the family lives, including housing, the neighborhood, and the larger community.

Family assessment tools are used with many health disciplines and are useful to assess a range of dimensions of the family, such as marital satisfaction, parental coping abilities, and family dysfunction.

The family health assessment addresses family characteristics, including structure and process and family environment (i.e., residence, neighborhood, and community). Not all dimensions of the family health assessment will be appropriate for every family; therefore the nurse should modify content of the assessment guideline and adapt it as necessary to fit the individual family. The guidelines are a means to record pertinent information about the family that will assist the nurse in working with the family. The nurse should gather information in the assessment spontaneously over several contacts with the family and various members and dyads within the family. It should also include multiple forays into the community, neighborhood, and home in which the family resides. Several contacts with the family will be required to complete the family health assessment.

Social and Structural Constraints

In addition to the tools just reviewed, an important aspect of family assessment and planning for intervention is the need to make note of the social and structural constraints that prevent families from receiving needed health care or achieving a state of health. These constraints explain why some families differ in mortality rates, ability to achieve "integrity" rather than "despair," or ability to "self-actualize." Social and structural constraints are usually based in social and economic causes, which affect a wide range of conditions (e.g., literacy, education, and employment) associated with major health indicators (i.e., mortality and morbidity rates). Families frequently served by the community health nurse are disadvantaged in that they lack the financial resources to purchase health care. However, constraints to obtaining needed health and social services are well documented and may come from characteristics of health and social services rather than individual family limitations. The nurse can note these constraints on the ecomap because they influence each family's ability to interact with a specific agency. For example, in addition to noting the strength of the relationship between family and agency or institution, the nurse should note those constraints that prevent use of the resource. Constraints include hours of service, transportation, availability of interpreters, and criteria for receiving services (e.g., age, sex, and income barriers). Specific examples are the different guidelines posed by each state for Medicaid and by each community for home-delivered meals to the homebound.

Helping families understand constraints and linking them to accessible resources is necessary, but intervention at the family level is not sufficient. The common basic human needs of families in a community add up, and the community health nurse must tally structural constraints faced repeatedly by families and compare them with those faced by families in other communities. The nurse can then plan and implement interventions at the aggregate level. The following section is an overview of how community health nurses can extend intervention at the family level to larger aggregates and social action.

EXTENDING FAMILY HEALTH INTERVENTION TO LARGER AGGREGATES AND SOCIAL ACTION

Institutional Context of Family Therapists

Many theories exist to help bridge the gap between the application of nursing and family theory to the family and broader social action on behalf of communities of families. Most family theorists view the family as a system that interfaces with outside suprasystems or institutions only when a problem is to be addressed, such as in the school or a courtroom. The following three approaches go beyond the family as a system to address the interaction between the family and the larger social system:

- Ecological framework
- Network therapy
- Transactional model

Ecological Framework

The **ecological framework** is a blend of systems and developmental theory that focuses on the interaction and interdependence of humans (families) as biological and social beings with the environment. Using this framework the CHN would assess the family as a system within the context of its environment. Bronfenbrenner (2005) identified four basic systems that make up our ecological environment. The *microsystem* is our immediate environment that supports our development–the family, school, church, etc. The environment interacts with "age, health, sex, genetic predispositions." The *mesosystem* recognizes the links between two or more microsystems and the individual. The *exosystem* are those settings or institutions that may not directly come in contact with an individual but still influence development in less direct ways, such as government agencies, what is happening in the world, and the media. Lastly, there is the *chronosystem,* or the future development. This takes into account the notion of time. What happens to the individual and family over time depending upon events, and so on (Smith and Harmon, 2011)?

This approach explains the results of health care specialization and fragmentation of care based on Western concepts of time and space. It focuses on providing a more complex and flexible structure. For example, Kogan and associates (2004) investigated parent–health care provider discussions of family and community health risks during well-child examinations. Additionally, they studied the gaps between the issues discussed by the practitioner and the information the parent desired. On the basis of the results of the National Survey of Early Childhood Health, health topics for discussion were identified, including family financial difficulties, the presence of a support partner, parent's emotional support, alcohol and/or drug use in the home, cigarette smoking in the home, the parent's physical health, and community violence. Cigarette smoking was discussed nearly 80% of the time, and alcohol and drug use was discussed 45% of the time; however, community violence was discussed less than 10% of the time, and financial needs 12%. The results indicate the need for better communication and education between health care providers and clients.

Social Network Framework

The **social network framework** (Christakis and Fowler, 2011) is based on earlier network therapy work involving all the connections and ties within a group. In network theory, an identified family member feels marginalized and seeks to replace the family network with others from the wider system to provide more support, hoping to enhance his or her role or functioning in the family. The concept of social network

in this instance is related to social support. "Social network refers to a weblike structure comprising one's relationships and social support focuses on the nature of the interactions taking place within social relationships" (Friedman et al, 2003, p. 462). A family's social network includes friends, community groups, church, and agencies. Social network also can be explained as the structure of relationships and social support as the function of relationships. Examples of network therapy are drawn from community mental health. In the social network framework, a *group* is defined as a collection of individuals with a common attribute. A social network is composed of connected groups. A network has structure (also called typology); contagion that flows across connections (e.g., money, violence, fashion, organs, obesity, etc.); connection, who is connected to whom (e.g., family, friends, colleagues); and homophily, or the tendency we have to be with those who are similar to ourselves. To some extent individuals and families control the density of our connectedness, our centrality to the group, and how we are viewed by others. This model has been used to explain health-related issues, such as the spread of sexually transmitted diseases, and the obesity epidemic in the United States. It has also been used to understand the issue of hyperconnectivity and technology. Christakis and Fowler (2011) state that the average Facebook user has only 110 friends, very close to the number in the "real world."

Perhaps then, using the research on social marketing, the CHN needs to become familiar with the use of social networks and other technology to ensure individuals and families have accurate health information. The Pew Research Center's Internet and American Life Project (2013) is studying Americans use of the Internet to seek health information, find medical diagnoses, and discuss medical treatments. The researchers have found that individuals with the following demographics are more likely to seek medical answers online: women, younger, white, income of $75,000 or more, and a college degree. Fifty-nine percent of Americans looked online for health information in 2012 (Parker and Patten, 2013), and the majority began with a search engine, such as Google, Bing, or Yahoo, instead of a website that a CHN might identify as a reliable source such as the National Institutes of Health or the CDC. Nearly one half of this group was seeking a diagnosis; these individuals are called "online diagnosers." Thirty-eight percent of this group believed that they could take care of the problem at home and did not seek the advice of a health professional (Parker and Patten, 2013). This presents new issues for the CHN, such as teaching families how to evaluate appropriate online sites.

Transactional Model

In the **transactional model**, the term *transaction* refers to a system that focuses on family processes. The family as an institution, along with other institutions (e.g., religious, educational, recreational, or governmental), is culturally anchored (i.e., each holds a distinct set of beliefs and values about the nature of the world and human existence). An awareness of culture (e.g., beliefs and values) as it is expressed in each system is important (i.e., as it is expressed in mainstream U.S. values versus the value patterns of the family).

VanderValk and colleagues (2007) used a transactional model to explore the relationship between parental marital distress and adolescent emotional adjustment. In a 6-year prospective study of 531 parent-adolescent dyads, they found such a relationship, especially for late adolescent and young adult girls and less so for males. The findings suggest that "girls' greater sensitivity to interpersonal problems may be reciprocal and that the parental marriage is still associated with adjustment for girls in late adolescence and early adulthood" (p. 130).

Models of Care for Communities of Families

Models exist to guide the community health nurse in providing care to communities of families in special need of services that improve access, equality between consumer and provider, and sensitivity to human need. There is generally an increase in the number and type of models that emerge as traditional public and private models of health care decline due to shrinking funding and resources. Many of the programs develop as the result of community efforts or partnerships with existing health care providers. The following are examples of such models.

The Kentucky Partnership for Farm Family Health and Safety

The Kentucky Partnership is a community coalition, originally funded by W. K. Kellogg Foundation, involving farm families, universities, and various community-based organizations. The coalition was originally established to improve the health of farm families in rural Kentucky. Farming is identified as one of the most dangerous occupations in the United States, and few resources have been developed to support the unique needs of farm families. The Partnership identified farm women as the primary "health officers" for farm families. The farm women were provided with opportunities to develop skills in leadership, conflict resolution, and teambuilding. Nurse educators and nursing students provided health education and assisted the farm women in developing a self-sustaining structure to support their efforts to improve family health. Cardiopulmonary resuscitation and first aid classes, the development of unique emergency medical subsystems, and other activities helped improve the health of the farm families. The local members reported an increase in personal knowledge, self-esteem, and personal satisfaction through the Partnership efforts. The Kentucky Partnership for Farm Family Health and Safety continues to affect the health of farm families in south-central Kentucky. The efforts are supported through the help of the South Central Kentucky Area Health Education Center at Western Kentucky University. The coalition has been replicated in three states (Texas, Louisiana, and Florida) and continues to connect universities and farm families in research efforts. Outcome assessment research was conducted to evaluate the impact of the coalition efforts on farm family health (Palermo and Ehlers, 2001; Siegrist and Jones, 2005). This organization continues as a positive force improving the health of farm families.

The Health Access Nurturing Development Services Program

The Health Access Nurturing Development Services (HANDS) program is a voluntary home visitation program targeting at-risk families that include first-time parents. Implemented through interdisciplinary teams consisting of social workers, nurses, and parent resource persons, the program serves first-time pregnant mothers and their families. HANDS was originally funded through tobacco settlement monies allocated through the state legislature to the Kentucky Cabinet for Health and Family Services. The program services are provided through district health departments and currently are available throughout the Commonwealth of Kentucky. Counseling, education, and support services are provided until the child reaches school age (4-5 years). On the basis of a systems approach, home visits are made for the purpose of screening, assessment, referrals, care coordination, case management, and policy advocacy. The program implements the "Growing Great Kids" curriculum, based on building family strengths through parenting, child safety, and connecting families with many resources. Initially the Program focused on teen and first-time mothers, but data collected have revealed that at-risk mothers include individuals with previous children but poor support and parenting skills.

Programs such as HANDS require time in order to show outcomes. Ten years after the inception of the program the Kentucky Cabinet for Health and Family Services documented the positive impact of HANDS services, which can be seen in decreases in the number of preterm births, emergency department uses, rates of child abuse and neglect, and infant mortality rates in Kentucky as well as a cost savings to the Kentucky Medicaid program (Pew Center on the States, 2012) (Table 20-5). Currently, services have been expanded in eight counties targeting mothers identified as at-risk or diagnosed with depression or other mental illness. Home visitors have been taught to use Home Cognitive Behavior Therapy to integrate into the HANDS curriculum for these families (Kentucky Cabinet for Health and Family Services, 2009; Pew Center on the States, 2012).

These alternative health programs are strategies to change the structural barriers that prevent low-income families' access to care. Professional role functions changed as nurses, rather than physicians, provided health care. Active self-care was promoted, and health and medical knowledge was shared. Assistance by family and social networks was encouraged. Both of these programs address aspects of the health needs of populations at risk, but they do not "address the social determinants of disease." Neither program addresses the health-damaging conditions that poor people face, such as poor housing, malnutrition, and environmental hazards at the workplace and in the community. Although these programs represent steps in the right direction, changes in access to medical and health services are not enough. Social changes also are necessary.

TABLE 20-5	HEALTH ACCESS NURTURING DEVELOPMENT SERVICES (HANDS) PROGRAM: OUTCOMES AND POTENTIAL RELATED MEDICAL COST SAVINGS		
OUTCOME	ESTIMATED COST PER CASE*	HANDS IMPACT	ESTIMATED ANNUAL COST SAVINGS
Preterm birth	$49,000	32% reduction	$16,900,000
Emergency department use	$420	50% reduction	$5,700,000
Child abuse	$10,400	n/a	$685,940
Child neglect	$1,900	33% reduction	$90,900
Infant mortality	N/A	70% reduction	N/A

*The original calculations used estimated costs per case drawn from the Children's Safety Network. The estimated cost per case for child abuse and child neglect are hospitalization costs only and do not consider costs associated with Child Protective Services or other expenditures.
Source: Kentucky Cabinet and Family Services and Department for Public Health: *Home visiting: a Healthy return on investment—a presentation for the Prichard committee,* 2011; table reprinted from The Pew Center on the States: *Home Visiting Issue Brief, Kentucky: joining HANDS for a comprehensive system of care,* 2012, page 8. Retrieved from <http://www.pewstates.org/uploadedFiles/PCS_Assets/2012/020_12_HOME%20Kentucky%20Brief_web.pdf> © 2012 The Pew Charitable Trusts.

APPLYING THE NURSING PROCESS

Home Visit

The case study presents the application of the nursing process to a family on a home visit. The example notes the use of the home visit to identify health needs of the family within the community and programs planned to meet those needs, which ultimately will benefit a population of families in the future.

The home visit is a crucial experience for the nursing student and family (Friedman et al, 2003). Important factors that may influence the home visit include the family's background experience with the health care system, the agency in which the nursing student is working, the family's experience with previous nursing students who have visited the family, and the student's background. For example, nursing student characteristics may vary; students bring differing levels of knowledge of medical and nursing practice, self, and the community.

The nursing student brings previous learning about families, family-related theory, the growth and development of members of different ages within a family, disease processes, and access to the health care system. Curricula within schools of nursing vary; therefore some students will also bring preparation in all specialties—medical-surgical nursing, childbearing, parent-child nursing, and psychiatric and mental health nursing—to the experience. Others may be taking basic clinical courses, such as pediatrics and psychiatric–mental health nursing, concurrently with community health. Thus the need for review of appropriate theory, health education, and standard assessment tools for individuals and families will vary.

The nursing student's knowledge of self, previous life experiences, and values also are important in planning for home visits. Nursing students must recognize their strengths and weaknesses in preparation for entering a new community and working with families. Additional preparation by all nursing students is necessary before the first home visit, depending on the content of the referral. The student should gather referral information, review assessment forms, and intervention tools (e.g., screening materials, supplies) before going to the home.

Flexibility is important in working with families because the nursing student will not know the family's priority needs until the home visit.

SUMMARY

This chapter highlights the community health nurse's work with families and identifies the major family-related health care needs that the health care system has not adequately addressed. The nature of the family is changing and challenging traditional definitions and configurations. Approaches to meeting the health needs of families must go beyond that of the traditional health care system, which addresses the individual as the unit of care. Strategies are given in this chapter for expanding notions of care from the individual to the family and from the family to the community. To guide intervention with families, nurses have traditionally relied on common theoretical frameworks from the disciplines of psychology and social psychology. These frameworks often target individuals; frameworks are needed that go beyond the individual to the family and community and that address social and policy changes needed to alter the social, economic, and environmental conditions under which families must function. This chapter provides tools for assessing the family and the family within the community and gives examples of the extension of family health intervention to larger aggregates, which involves social action to overcome constraints to accessing health services. Nonnursing and community health nursing models of care provided for communities of families are presented and critiqued. The nursing process is applied in a case study at individual, family, and community levels on a home visit. Examples of interventions by the community health nurse at individual, family, and community levels are presented.

Families remain the core of society, with diversity as the constant for families in the United States. Family nursing must be understood and practiced by community health nurses. An understanding of family theory provides a mechanism for assessing and intervening with families to improve their level of wellness and increase the health of the community as a whole.

FAMILY HEALTH ASSESSMENT: THE GARCIA FAMILY

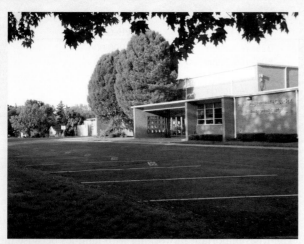

The school nurse, Jana, works with multiple city schools, including this inner-city school, which has a low-income, ethnically diverse population.

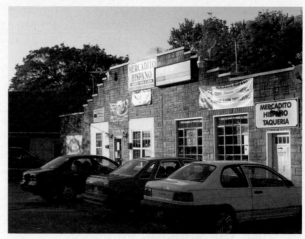

Jana assesses the community as she drives to the Garcias' home, noting the availability of resources such as the local groceria.

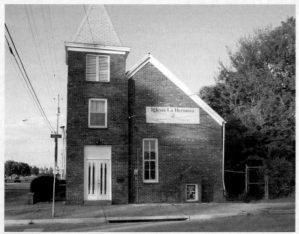

Local churches are a community resource, offering socialization and spiritual support for immigrant families such as the Garcia family.

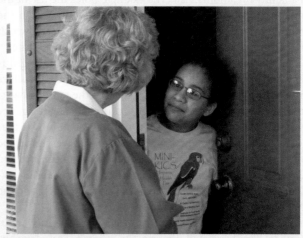

Jana arrives at the Garcias' home. Maria answers the door and invites Jana in.

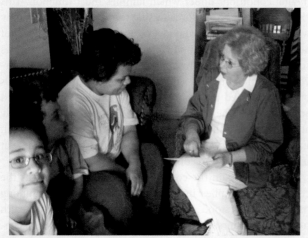

Jana completes the family assessment of the Garcia family with the help of Maria as interpreter for Mrs. Garcia. Mrs. Garcia listens intently as Jana asks questions about the family's health needs.

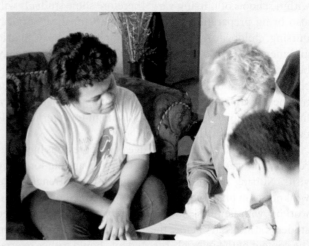

Jana reviews the plan of care and confirms the family's commitment to the plan of care they developed with her.

CASE STUDY APPLICATION OF THE NURSING PROCESS

Jana Parks is a community health nurse employed by the District Health Department. She is a school health nurse, providing services for six schools in a moderately sized community. After receiving a referral from school officials related to a student's absenteeism, Jana plans to assess the student and family. (See the Photo Novella in this chapter 398 for photos that depict this case study.)

Assessment

Jana knows that the school is located in the inner city school where 75% of the children come from families with a median family income at or below the federal poverty level. English is the second language for approximately 25% of the students, and 5% are not fluent in spoken or written English. Each year, more than 20% of the student body moves into or out of the school district.

She reviews the school records for the student, Maria Garcia, and learns that this is the first year of enrollment for the sixth grader and her second-grade brother, Miguel. Maria's family moved to the area 6 months ago from the Dominican Republic. School records note that the girl is adequately fluent in spoken English but that the parents do not speak English. The student's father works part-time at a local furniture manufacturer. There has been a noticeable decline in grades over the previous quarter, there have been no disciplinary actions, and teacher comments are positive regarding the student's classroom performance. The health record indicates that she is up-to-date with required immunizations; no chronic illnesses are noted on the school physical examination record. Jana notes that Maria's brother does not have the same school absence pattern.

Jana contacts the family and identifies her role as school health nurse. She explains the need for a meeting with the student and family to discuss concerns about Maria's school attendance. A time is scheduled when both parents and the student are available. She confirms the home address and directions.

Jana notes that the house is in need of paint and some windows have been replaced with cardboard; however, the yard is free of clutter and there are containers of blooming plants on the small porch. Maria Garcia opens the door, and Jana enters a small, dimly lit room. As the student makes introductions, Mr. Garcia stands and greets Jana with a nod and handshake while Mrs. Garcia remains recumbent on the sofa but raises her hand in greeting. Mrs. Garcia's appearance surprises Jana, as she appears much older than Mr. Garcia. Her skin is pale, her eyes are sunken, and she appears frail, with a distended abdomen and generalized muscle wasting.

Jana is aware that the exchange of social conversation is important in establishing a relationship with Hispanic clients. She mentions the beautiful picture in the room and learns that a family member painted it as a wedding gift for the Garcias. Jana learns that the family has no other relatives in the community and moved to the city through the work of a refugee assistance organization. In this interview, Jana plans to collect information related to individual, family, and/or community functioning.

Throughout the conversation, Jana has noted that both Maria and Mr. Garcia appear tense; Mrs. Garcia is quiet and rarely speaks or smiles. Maria has translated throughout the conversation, although Jana senses that the parents may have limited understanding of spoken English. To lessen anxiety, Jana begins the interview by saying, "I am here because the school and I are concerned about Maria's absences. I want to learn why Maria misses school and to see if there are ways that the school can help."

Through the interview process, Jana learns that Maria likes school and has made friends there. She observes that Miguel stays close to Maria and frequently hides his face into her shoulder when Jana speaks to him. She also notes that Mr. and Mrs. Garcia rarely look at each other, and Mr. Garcia chooses a seat on the opposite side of the room. The family rents the home, and the father has been able to supplement his part-time income by working as a day laborer

for a lawn service. The family was beginning to establish connections at a local church and with neighbors when Mrs. Garcia was diagnosed with an abdominal tumor that has required numerous operations over the past 3 months. She is still receiving home care visits for a surgical wound that has not healed. Although Medicaid has covered most physician and hospital expenses, the family has experienced out-of-pocket expenses for noncovered medications. These problems have contributed to family financial stress. Mr. Garcia has to drive his wife to medical appointments; as a result, he is in danger of losing his job. Maria also attends these appointments to serve as the interpreter, resulting in her frequent school absences.

In addition, Jana learns that Maria has assumed responsibility for the household cooking, cleaning, and laundry since her mother's illness. Mr. Garcia shops at a small neighborhood groceria. Jana determines that with food stamps the family has adequate resources to purchase food, although Maria admits that she is still learning to cook. The family eats the evening meal together, frequently rice and beans. Maria and Miguel are eligible for subsidized breakfast and lunch at school. Maria believes that it is her responsibility to help Miguel complete his homework, get to bed on time, and attend school regularly. Mr. Garcia disciplines both children. Jana asks questions regarding family health practices and learns that they see a provider at the health department only when ill or for school requirements and do not seek dental care. She observes a number of medication bottles on a table near the sofa.

Diagnosis
Individual
- Risk for excessive stress related to time-consuming activities, insufficient finances, and insufficient recreation (Mr. Garcia and Maria)
- Risk for personal injury related to improperly stored medications (Miguel)
- Ineffective health promotion related to language and cultural differences and lack of routine dental hygiene (Mr. and Mrs. Garcia, Maria, and Miguel)

Family
- Risk for poor parenting and family crisis related to change in Mrs. Garcia's ability to function, financial burden of treatments for ill family member, and disruption of family routines, mother's illness, and mother's prolonged illness

Community
- Inadequate systematic programs for linking Hispanic families to community resources

Planning
A plan of care is developed to meet the needs of the individuals, family, and community. Planning involves mutual goal setting between the nurse and family; mutual setting of objectives to meet goals; *prioritizing*, or setting short- and long-term goals with the family; contracting, or establishing the division of labor between nurse and family that will meet the objectives; and evaluation of the process and outcome.

Individual
Long-Term Goals
- Mr. Garcia will recognize appropriate roles and responsibilities for Maria. He will identify and use resources to allow her to resume suitable educational, social, and family duties.
- Mr. Garcia will identify and use community resources to assist with transportation needs and medication costs.
- Jana noted a long-term need to discuss dental care.
- Mr. and Mrs. Garcia will improve their English comprehension and speaking skills.

Continued

CASE STUDY APPLICATION OF THE NURSING PROCESS—cont'd

Short-Term Goals
- Relieve Maria of interpreting at medical appointments by identifying alternate interpretive resources.
- Store medications in a secure location.

Family
Long-Term Goal
- The family will be able to find and use appropriate services for physical and social support.

Short-Term Goal
- The family will learn to appropriately express their feelings related to the mother's illness, social isolation, role strain, and/or fear.

Community
Long-Term Goal
- The community will establish programs to support immigrant family needs for transportation, interpretation, and enculturation to the American medical system.

Short-Term Goal
- Mr. Garcia will identify existing programs available to support Hispanic immigrants.

Intervention
- Jana recognizes that many interventions must be carried out at the individual, family, and community levels.

Individual
- Education regarding safe medication storage.
- Referral to the Refugee Assistance Society or local churches for interpretive assistance.

Family
Direct nursing interventions directed at family functioning include the following levels:
- *Cognitive:* New information is provided to the family that promotes problem solving by the family. An example is referring the Garcias to the community free clinic for medical and dental care.
- *Affective:* Families are encouraged to express their feelings, which may be blocking their efforts at problem solving. An example would be Jana's planned validation of Mr. Garcia's concerns regarding finances and the threat of losing employment.
- *Behavioral:* Tasks are negotiated to be carried out either during the family interview or as homework between visits. An example is Mr. Garcia's planned call to the Refugee Assistance Society.

Community
Jana recognizes that her referral of Mr. Garcia to the Refugee Assistance Society to obtain support through existing programs is also an intervention at the community level. She engages in ongoing parafamily work to identify how the community can be mobilized to provide physical, mental, and social support to immigrant families. Does anyone at the community free clinic speak Spanish? Are interpreters available at health care facilities? Where do most immigrant families receive health care and social support? Are classes on English as a second language free of charge for Hispanic families? Are job skill training programs available for Mr. Garcia? Questions such as these bring up many areas of assessment that Jana will need to make with the Garcia family and the community in the future.

Evaluation
Individual/Family
Jana helps the Garcias obtain a small lockable box in which to store medications. Mr. Garcia establishes contact with a local church, which provides a volunteer interpreter and driver for medical visits and twice-weekly delivery of meals. Mr. Garcia takes Maria and Miguel to the free clinic, where dental sealants are applied to their molars. The social worker at the community's free clinic meets with Mr. Garcia to offer him assistance in obtaining low-cost medications. Through this conversation, Jana identifies his reluctance to ask for financial assistance. He states that he should provide for his family and that Maria should not have to assume the role of mother for Miguel. However, he does not see any other options at this time. She identifies that Mr. Garcia may be in need of ongoing support and suggests that he talk with a counselor about his concerns. Mr. Garcia refuses to see a counselor but agrees that he will talk to the pastor of his church. Maria and Miguel meet with the school counselor as needed to discuss feelings related to their mother's illness and the resulting family strain.

Community
Jana identified that many community resources are available to immigrant families; however, information about them is limited and not readily accessible. She contacts the director of the Refugee Assistance Society, and together they initiate a community coalition to address this issue.

Levels of Prevention
Society's expectations of the family are in transition. Application of the levels of prevention to families by the community nurse must take into account the changing family configuration; the financial, emotional, and physical burdens often compounded in the single-parent family; and the lack of resources, such as nonexistent or inadequate health insurance.

Primary Prevention
This chapter has established the importance of the family to individuals and society. Primary prevention with families becomes an essential element of any comprehensive family health plan. From the family perspective, health education must address actual and potential challenges to health, such as immunizations of all family members, educating about resources to support the family financially and emotionally, encouraging exercise and activity, and empowering the family to build upon strengths. An example is using the family genogram to teach the family about predisposition to diseases and helping the family develop a health prevention plan.

Secondary Prevention
The focus of secondary prevention for the family includes ensuring that the family has continued access to health care and resources for individual and family health problems. The changing economy in the United States has "closed the door" to regular health providers for some families. The challenge to the nurse is helping the family locate and access continued care and teaching the family to move through the system of government assistance, which may be new and unacceptable for the family. The nurse must be politically active in lobbying legislators for continued resources to support families.

Tertiary Prevention
Tertiary prevention for family includes assuring that the needed resources are available to support long-term care of each family member. An example of a community-based organization established and funded solely by volunteers is the Kelly Autism Program (KAP). KAP is "designed to provide services to adolescents and young adults diagnosed along the Autism Spectrum Continuum, as well as their families, while serving as a training opportunity for future professionals in a variety of disciplines. KAP has programs for middle school, high school and post-secondary participants including higher education, vocational training, and job support" (Western Kentucky University, 2014, p. 1, Vision). It includes a comprehensive screening program and one-on-one support for young adults with autism capable of living and studying on a university campus.

Developed by Mary Kovar, RN, MSN, and Barbara Minix, RN, MSN.

LEARNING ACTIVITIES

1. Define the term *family* with a group of three colleagues. Compare definitions and list similarities and differences. Develop a list of criteria for being a member of a family.

2. Complete a personal genogram. What are the high-risk factors in the family history? Current risk factors? Categorize current risk factors into physical, interpersonal, and environmental. Identify needed health education and determine who needs the education. Identify sources of appropriate screening in the community for the identified risk factors.

3. Complete a personal ecomap. Is the family an "open" or "closed" family system? What resources do families currently use for mental, physical, emotional, social, and community health? What referrals are needed?

4. Identify family types or situations (e.g., families of different cultures, gay or lesbian families, or never-married-mother families) that elicit "discomfort" in working situations. Identify ways to overcome barriers in working with these types of families.

ⓔ EVOLVE WEBSITE

http://evolve.elsevier.com/Nies
- NCLEX Review Questions
- Case Studies
- Glossary
- Resource Tool: 20A Family Health Assessment Form

REFERENCES

Allen DR, Fine MA, Demo HD: An overview of family diversity: controversies, questions, and values. In Demo DH, Allen KR, Fine MA, editors: *Handbook of family diversity*, New York, 2000, Oxford Press.

American Academy of Child & Adolescent Psychiatry: *Grandparents raising grandchildren*, 2009. Available from <www.aacap.org/cs/root/facts_for_families/grandparents_raising_grandchildren.htm>.

Annie E. Casey Foundation: *Kids Count Faststats data book online*, 2013. Available from <www.aecf.org/kidscount/databook/indicators.htm>.

Astedt-Kurki P, Paavilainen E, Lehti K: Methodological issues in interviewing families in family nursing research, *Methodological Issus in Nursing Research* 35(2):288–293, 2001.

Auger JR: Behavioral systems and nursing, *AJN* 77(11):1856–1857, 1976.

Beard M: Home nursing, *Public Health Nurs Q* 7:44–51, 1999.

Bell J: M: Making ideas "stick": The 15-minute family interview, *J Fam Nurs* 18:171, 2012.

Bronfenbrenner U: Making human beings human: bioecological perspectives on human development, Sage Publications, Thousand Oaks, CA 2005.

Butler JF: The family diagram and genogram: comparisons and contrast, *Am J Family Therapy* 36:169–180, 2008.

Carter E, McGoldrick M, editors: *The changing family life cycle: a framework for family therapy*, ed 2, New York, 1988, Gardner Press.

Centers for Disease Control and Prevention: Faststats: Teen births, 2012 <http://www.cdc.gov/nchs/fastats/teen-births.htm>

Centers for Disease Control and Prevention: *Chronic diseases and health promotion*, 2013. Available from <http://www.cdc.gov/chronicdisease/overview/index.htm>.

Centers for Medicare and Medicaid Services: *The children's health insurance program*, 2009. Available from <www.cms.hhs.gov/LowCostHealthInsFamChild/>.

Medicaid.gov: *Children's Health Insurance Program Reauthorization Act*, n.d. Available from <http://www.medicaid.gov/medicaid-chip-program-information/by-topics/childrens-health-insurance-program-chip/chipra.html>.

Christakis NA, Fowler JA: *Connected: The surprising power of our social networks and how they shape our lives*, Boston, 2011, Little, Brown & Company.

CLASP: see HoffmanCody WK: Nursing frameworks to guide practice and research with families, *Nurs Sci Q* 13(4):277–284, 2000.

Cook E: *The lif;e of Florence Nightingale*, vol 2, London, 1913, Macmillan.

DeFrain J: Strong families, *Family Matters* 53:6–13, 1999.

Dreher MC: The conflict of conservatism in public health nursing education, *Nurs Outlook* 30:504, 1982.

Dunst CJ, Trivette CM: Capacity-building family-systems intervention practices, *Journal of Family Social Work* 12(2):119–143, 2009.

Duvall EM: *Marriage and family relationships*, ed 5, Philadelphia, 1977, JB Lippincott.

Duvall EM, Miller BC: *Marriage and family development*, ed 6, New York, 1985, Harper and Row.

Erikson E: *Childhood and society*, ed 2, New York, 1963, WW Norton.

Escoto KH, Laska MN, Larson N, et al: Work hours and perceived time barriers to healthful eating among young adults, *Am J Health Behav* 36(3):786–789, 2012.

Freeman R: *Public health nursing practice*, ed 3, Philadelphia, 1963, WB Saunders.

Friedman MM: *Family nursing: theory and assessment*, ed 3, East Norwalk, CT, 1998, Appleton-Lange.

Friedman MM, Bowden VB, Jones EG: *Family nursing: research, theory and practice*, ed 3, Upper Saddle River, NJ, 2003, Prentice Hall.

Glaser B, Strauss AL: *Chronic illness and the quality of life*, St. Louis, 1975, Mosby.

Kaakinen JR, Gedaly-Duff V, Hanson SM: *Family health care nursing: theory, practice and research*, ed 4, Philadelphia, PA, 2009, FA Davis.

Hartman A: *Finding families: an ecological approach to family assessment in adoption*, Beverly Hills, CA, 1979, Sage.

Human Rights Campaign: Inclusive definition of family. http://www.hrc.org/resources/entry/lgbt-inclusive-definitions-of-family 2014.

Kentucky Cabinet for Health and Family Services: *HANDS program*, Frankfort, KY, 2009, Author. Available from <http://chfs.ky.gov/dph/ach/hands/htm>.

Kogan MD, Schuster MA, Yu SM, et al: Routine assessment of family and community health risks: parent views and what they receive, *Pediatrics* 113:1934–1943, 2004.

Li L, Lin C, Cao H, Lieber E: Intergenerational and urban-rural health habits in Chinese families, *Am J Health Behav* 33(2):172–180, 2009.

Lubkin IM, Larsen PD: *Chronic illness: Impact & intervention*, ed 8, Burlington, MA, 2013, Jones & Bartlett.

Martinez AM, D'Arois D, Rennick JE: Does the 15-minute or less family interview influence family nursing practice? *J Fam Nurs* 31(2):157–178, 2007.

Martire LM, Schulz R: Involving family in psychosocial interventions for chronic illness, *Current Directions in Psychological Science* 16(2):90–94, 2007.

Maslow A: *Motivation and personality*, ed 2, New York, 1970, Harper and Row.

McNeill JA, Cook J, Mahon M, et al: Family history: value-added information in assessing cardiac health, *AAOHN* 56(7):297–305, 2008.

Medicaid.gov: *Children's Health Insurance Program Reauthorization Act*, n.d. Available from <http://www.medicaid.gov/medicaid-chip-program-information/by-topics/childrens-health-insurance-program-chip/chipra.html>.

Minuchin P: Looking toward horizon: present and future in study of family systems. In McHale JP, Grolnick WS, editors: *Psychological study of families*, Mahwah, NJ, 2002, Lawrence Erlbaum.

Montalvo B: Useful coincidences and family strengths, *Contemp Fam Ther* 26(2):117–119, 2004.

National Institute of Mental Health: *NIMH International scientific conference on the role of families in preventing and adapting to HIV/AIDS*, 2005. Available from <www.nimh.nih.gov/scientific meetings/hivaids2005.cfm>.

National League for Nursing: *A curriculum guide for schools of nursing*, New York, 1937, Author.

National Institute of Health: *Better diabetes care for systems change: Cultural competency tips*, 2009. Available from <http://betterdiabetescare.nih. gov/ISSUESculturalcompetencytips.htm>.

Otto H: A framework for assessing family strengths. In Reinhard A, Quinn M, editors: *Family-centered community health nursing*, St. Louis, 1973, Mosby.

Palermo T, Ehlers J: *Coalitions: building partnerships to promote agricultural health and safety*, Washington, DC, 2001, National Institutes for Occupational Health and Safety. Also available from <www.cdc.gov/nasd/doc/d001701– d001774.html.>

Parke RP: Family & peer systems, *Psychol Bull* 128(4):596–601, 2002.

Parker K, Patten E: *The sandwich generation: Rising financial burden for middle-aged Americans* (Pew Research Social & Demographic Trends), 2013. Available from <http:www.pewsocialtren ds.org/2013/01/30/the-sandwich-generation/>.

Pew Center on the States: *Home Visiting Issue Brief, Kentucky: Joining HANDS for a comprehensive system of care*, 2012. Available from <http:// www.pewstates.org/uploadedFiles/PCS_Assets /2012/020_12_HOME%20Kentucky%20Brief_ web.pdf>.

Pew Research Center: *Social & demographic trends: The return of the multi-generational family household*, 2010. Available from <http://www.p ewsocialtrends.org/2010/03/18/the-return- of- the-multi-generational-family-household/>.

Pew Research Center: *Health online, 2013*. Available from <http://pewinternet.org/Reports/201 3/Health-online.aspx.>

Pratt RP: *Family structure and effective health behavior*, Boston, 1976, Houghton Mifflin.

Robert Wood Johnson Foundation: *Let's cover the uninsured*, 2009. Available from <http://covert heuninsured.org/>.

Siegrist B, Jones S: Nursing education beyond classroom walls: Service learning through collaboration with community partners. In *Exploring the scholarship of teaching*, Bowling Green, KY, 2005, Faculty Center for Excellence in Teaching, p 87. Available from <http:// www.wku.edu/teaching/booklets/sotl/sotl_ 0complete.pdf>.

Smith SR, Harmon RR: *Exploring family theories*, New York, 2011, Oxford University Press.

U.S. Census Bureau: *Population profile of the nation: dynamic version 2005*, Washington, DC, 2005, Author. Also available from <www.c ensus.gov/population/www/pop-profile/profile dynamic.html.>

U.S. Census Bureau: *Income, poverty and health insurance: coverage in the US in 2007*, 2008. Available from <www.census/prod/2008/pub/p60>.

U.S. Census Bureau: *2010 American community survey*, Washington, DC, 2011, Author. Also available from <http://www.census.gov/prod/2 011pubs/acsbr10-03.pdf>.

U.S. Census Bureau: 2013 Families and living arrangements, Available from <http://www.cen sus.gov/hhes/families/data/.>

U.S. Department of Health and Human Services: *New family history tool promotes prevention, Nations Health* 34(10):33, 2005.

U.S. Department of Health and Human Services: *My family health portrait: A tool from the US Surgeon General*, 2010. Available from <https: /familyhistory.hhs.gov/fhh-web/ home.action>.

U.S. Department of Health and Human Services, *Administration on Aging: A profile of older Americans*, 2012. Available from <http://aoa. gov/AoARoot/Aging_Statistics/Profile/index. aspx>.

VanderValk I, de Goede M, Spruijt E, et al: A longitudinal study on transactional relations between parental marital distress and adolescent emotional adjustment, *Adolescence* 42:116–136, 165, 2007.

von Bertalanffy L: *General systems theory: foundations, development, applications*, New York, 1968, George Braziller.

von Bertalanffy L: The history and status of general systems theory. In Klir G, editor: *Trends in general systems theory*, New York, 1972, Wiley.

von Bertalanffy L: General systems theory and psychiatry. In Arieti S, editor: *American handbook of psychiatry*, New York, 1974, Basic Books.

Wald L: The family as a unit of care: a historical review, *Public Health Nurs* 3:427–428, 515–519, 1904.

Western Kentucky University: Kelly Autism Program, 2014, http://www.wku.edu/ kellyautismprogram/index.php

Wright LM, Leahey M: *Nurses and families: a guide to family assessment and intervention*, Philadelphia, 1994, FA Davis.

Wright LM, Leahey M: *Nurses and families: a guide to family assessment and intervention*, ed 5, Philadelphia, 2005, FA Davis.

Wright LM, Leahey M: *Nurses and family: a guide to family assessment and intervention*, ed 6, Philadelphia, 2012, FA Davis.

Zinn MB, Eitxen DS, Wells G: *Diversity in families*, ed 9, Boston, 2011, Allyn & Bacon.

Populations Affected by Disabilities

Meredith Troutman-Jordan*

* The author would like to acknowledge the contribution of Linda L. Treloar, who wrote this chapter for the previous edition.

OBJECTIVES

Upon completion of this chapter, the reader will be able to do the following:

1. Differentiate between medical model and social construct definitions of disability.
2. Describe historical attitudes and perspectives surrounding disability that have contributed to treatment of people with disabilities.
3. Compare and contrast short- and long-term disabling conditions.
4. Discuss key federal legislation applicable to people with disabilities.
5. Identify selected health care and social issues that influence the ability of people with disabilities to live and thrive in the community.
6. Apply narrative experience to disability that integrates a holistic focus and promotes the health and well-being of people with disabilities and their families.

KEY TERMS

activities of daily living
ADA Amendments Act of 2008
Americans with Disabilities Act
children with disabilities
disability
functional activities

handicap
impairment
Individuals with Disabilities Education Act
individualized education plan
instrumental activities of daily living

intellectual disability
people with disabilities
reasonable accommodations
Social Security Disability Insurance
Supplemental Security Income

OUTLINE

Self-Assessment: Responses to Disability
Definitions and Models for Disability
    National Agenda for Prevention of Disabilities Model
    Four Models for Disability
    Differentiating Illness from Disability
A Historical Context for Disability
    Early Attitudes Toward People with Disabilities
    Attitudes Toward People with Disabilities in the Eighteenth and Nineteenth Centuries
    Disability in the Twentieth Century
    Contemporary Conceptualizations of People with Disabilities
Characteristics of Disability
    Measurement of Disability
    Prevalence of Disability
    Health Status and Causes of Disability
    Culture and Disability
    Aging and Personal Assistance

Disability and Public Policy
    Legislation Affecting People with Disabilities
    Public Assistance Programs
Costs Associated with Disability
    Economic Well-Being and Employment
Healthy People 2020 and The Health Needs of People with Disabilities
    Health Disparities in Quality and Access
    People with Intellectual Disabilities: Undervalued and Disadvantaged
The Experience of Disability
    Family and Caregiver Responses to a Child with a Disability
    "Knowledgeable Client" and the "Knowledgeable Nurse"
Strategies for the Community Health Nurse in Caring for People with Disabilities
Ethical Issues for People Affected by Disabilities
    When the Nurse Has a Disability

After having an incomplete spinal cord injury following an automobile accident, 29-year-old Jim progressed from visible physical disability and paralysis to continued disability without the use of a wheelchair. Jim explained his progression:

> *You know it's really weird. In some ways it's hard to enter into that wheelchair life, to go into that life and then come back out of it again. I entered into a whole other realm [life with paralysis] that I'd only observed. I stepped into the unknown and pulled back out of it again. Yet, one foot is still in that world. (Treloar, 1999a, p. 189)*

For Jim, disability may create a "whole other realm," or an "unknown" world. Like Jim, most people lack awareness of the divergence of perceptual worlds that disability creates and the historical and sociopolitical contexts and culture that surround disability. Attitudes toward disability influence people's responses to and care of others. Before reading further, consider the following self-assessment.

SELF-ASSESSMENT: RESPONSES TO DISABILITY

What comes to mind when you think of *someone with a disability?* List characteristics using adjectives or short phrases. What values, customs, and traditions may be promoted or blocked for individuals with disabilities?

Picture yourself as a *person with a disability.* How do others respond to you? Who or what kinds of supports are available to help? Consider your health care concerns and needs. How might health care professionals devalue or disempower you? How can nurses and other caregivers convey respect and concern for you while helping to fill in the gaps where you lack wisdom?

Imagine yourself as a *nurse with a visible disability,* or the client receiving care from a nurse with a disability. What thoughts and feelings flood your mind? Would anything change if the nurse were invisibly disabled? Consider a scenario in which you apply as a student with a disability to a college of nursing. Your disability requires additional time to achieve performance-based tasks. What might concern the nursing program staff and faculty about this situation?

Think about living in a *family affected by disability.* Consider the impact of a child with a disability on sibling and parental activities and family roles. What if you were an active, growing child in a family where mom or dad is disabled? Although it may seem easier to focus on difficulties, consider possible benefits, to include positive learning and growth in family members. What kinds of social and personal supports do you have or do you find are inadequate or lacking altogether? Finally, what is the experience of *living with disability within your community?* What social or environmental barriers related to disability exist? How can nurses and an interdisciplinary team form alliances with the client and family to reduce or eliminate these barriers? Health care professionals are taught to assess and provide interventions that promote health, and they usually believe they know what people with disabilities need. Regardless of the provider's professional experience or familiarity with disability, clients may question provider's ability to understand their experience.

Disability affects people irrespective of class, culture, race, and economic level. Depending on the term's definition, disability affects nearly one out of every five Americans. Disability increases with age, often influencing one's ability to maintain self-care, which is essential to remaining in his or her preferred living environment. A disability may be readily apparent (e.g., someone with mobility limitations in a wheelchair) or it may be less obvious, such as the individual who has autism or is deaf.

People who grow up with a disability describe their lived experience with disability somewhat differently from those who become disabled as the result of a health condition. For example, people having a sensory disability, a physical disability, or an intellectual disability from birth adapt to the world as they know it. Compare this situation with that of a 20-year-old who becomes blind, deaf, or paralyzed because of an accident. The loss may never be fully grieved. Adaptation may be delayed by the psychological impact of what is gone and its meaning. If an 80-year-old becomes blind because of diabetes-induced retinopathy, the loss of sight was chronic, progressive, and predictable. There will be loss and grief, but the blindness occurs as part of the aging process. Rather than seeing people with disabilities (PWD) as "all the same," nurses must be able to see each person with a disability as unique, having different goals, knowledge, and experiences.

DEFINITIONS AND MODELS FOR DISABILITY

Disability is the interaction between individuals with a health condition and personal and environmental factors (World Health Organization [WHO], 2012). The International Classification of Functioning, Disability and Health (ICF) (World Health Organization [WHO], 2013) defines the following key terms. Disability is an umbrella term, covering impairments, activity limitations, and participation restrictions. An impairment is a problem in body function or structure; an activity limitation is a difficulty encountered by an individual in executing a task or action; and a participation restriction is a problem one experiences in involvement in life situations (WHO, 2013). A disability, resulting from an impairment, involves a restriction or an inability to perform an activity in a normal manner or within the normal range. An anatomical, mental, or psychological loss or abnormality is an impairment. A handicap is a disadvantage resulting from an impairment or a disability that prevents fulfillment of an expected role. An impairment affects a human organ on a micro level, disability affects a person on an individual level, and a handicap involves society on a macro level of analysis (Batavia, 1993). Table 21-1 compares and contrasts these definitions related to disability.

The "old" paradigm for viewing disability, based on the Nagi model, used functional limitations to determine whether an individual was disabled (Pope and Tarlov, 1991). Although the WHO and Nagi frameworks recognize that one's ability to perform a socially expected activity reflects characteristics of the individual and the larger social and physical environment,

TABLE 21-1	TERMINOLOGY FOR IMPAIRMENT, DISABILITY, AND HANDICAP		
CHARACTERISTIC	IMPAIRMENT	DISABILITY	HANDICAP
Definition	Physical deviation from normal structure, function, physical organization, or development	May be objective and measurable	Not objective or measurable; is an experience related to the responses of others
Measurability	Objective and measurable	May be objective and measurable	Not objective or measurable; is an experience related to the responses of others
Illustrations	Spina bifida, spinal cord injury, amputation, and detached retina	Cannot walk unassisted; uses crutches and/or a manual or power wheelchair; blindness	Reflects physical and psychological characteristics of the person, culture, and specific circumstances
Level of analysis	Micro level (e.g., body organ)	Individual level (e.g., person)	Macro level (e.g., societal)

they are commonly criticized for their medical emphasis and definitional inconsistencies. Impairments do not necessarily result in disabilities, and disabilities do not necessarily produce handicaps. Disabilities may not be physically visible, either, as in the case of autism or dyslexia. Deafness (Mackenzie and Smith, 2009), phenylketonuria (Gentile, Ten Hoedt, and Bosch, 2010), and learning disability (Madaus, 2008) are examples of "hidden disabilities, which are disabilities that are unapparent to outside observers (Valeras, 2010). Whether a person is viewed as disabled varies according to the environmental barriers and the perspectives of the onlooker.

National Agenda for Prevention of Disabilities Model

The Committee on a National Agenda for the Prevention of Disabilities (NAPD) conceptualized a model for disability (Figure 21-1) that extends the ICF and Nagi frameworks. In the NAPD model, disability occurs when a person's physical or mental limitations, in interaction with physical and social barriers in the environment, prevent the person from taking equal part in the normal life of the community (Pope and Tarlov, 1991). Furthermore, disability develops through a complex, interactive process involving biological, behavioral, and environmental (i.e., social and physical) risk factors and quality of life (QOL). In this social model for disability, bodily impairments and functional limitations are not necessarily accompanied by disability. Disability may be preventable, and preventive measures can promote improved QOL and reduce costs related to dependence, lost productivity or unemployment, and medical care.

The Disabling Process

The NAPD model provides an alternative framework for viewing four related and distinct stages in the disabling process. Pathology at the cellular and tissue levels may produce impairment in structure or function at the organ level. An individual with an impairment may experience a functional limitation, which restricts his or her ability to perform an action within the normal range. The functional limitation may result in a disability when certain socially defined activities and roles cannot be performed.

Although the model appears to indicate unidirectional progression from pathology to impairment, to functional

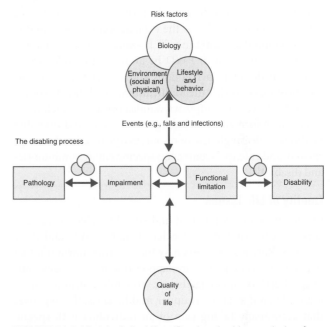

FIGURE 21-1 Model of disability. (Reprinted with permission from Pope AM, Tarlov AR, editors: *Disability in America: toward a national agenda for prevention*, Washington, DC, 1991, National Academy Press. Copyright 1991 by the National Academy of Sciences. Courtesy National Academy Press, Washington, DC.)

limitation, to disability, stepwise or linear progression may not occur. Disability prevention efforts can address any of the risk factors or stages in the disabling process. Health promotion efforts include primary prevention of disability, secondary reversal of disability and restoration of function, and tertiary prevention of complications. Disability prevention includes all actions taken to reduce the occurrence of impairment (primary) and its development into a functional limitation (secondary) and to prevent the transition of functional limitation to disability (tertiary) (Batra, 2010). Primary prevention involves prevention of the manifestation of disability (Batra, 2010). Examples of primary prevention are prenatal care and immunizations for the pregnant mother and newborn (Batra, 2010) and the use of aspirin in response to serious cardiovascular events (e.g., myocardial infarction, stroke) (Baigent et al, 2009). Secondary conditions are considered a direct consequence of having a disability, and many are presumed to be preventable (Rimmer, Chen, and Hsieh, 2011). Secondary prevention could include measures to reduce obesity that has developed as a consequence of an individual's becoming quadriplegic. A tertiary prevention example is addressing the needs of students identified as having an emotional/behavioral disability through special education services and behavior intervention plans so that they may benefit from an educational program (National Center on Education, Disability, and Juvenile Justice, 2013).

Across various cultures there are similarities and variations in conceptualizations and beliefs about causality related to disability. The Multicultural Disability Advocacy Association notes, "Cultures and religious practices are ever-changing and there are many subgroups within each culture and religion, making it impossible to give definitive answers to specific questions, such as 'What is the explanation/response to disability within that community?'" However, it is essential that the nurse working with PWD be aware of the influence of culture on disability perceptions and experiences. Students are encouraged to visit the Multicultural Disability Advocacy Association website (http://www.mdaa.org.au/), which has a wealth of information including an ethnicity and disability factbook; a clearinghouse of resources organized by language spoken; and extensive content on specific ethnic communities and disability.

Quality of Life Issues

Overcoming environmental and social barriers to needed services can frustrate and exhaust many PWD and their families. Barriers to access may include transportation to a needed service, cost of care, appointment challenges, language barriers, financial issues, and migrant/noninsured issues. Even if a family is upper middle class, the expenses that accompany taking care of an individual with special needs can quickly exceed their income. Prescriptions, therapies, and assistive devices can be very expensive, even if the family has good health insurance. Lifestyle changes have to be made, and if the family's income is over the poverty limit, there is no financial assistance. One review of the literature confirms that families of children with disabilities bear more than their "fair share" of the costs of caring for their children (Anderson, Dumont, Jacobs, and Azzaria, 2007). Having a child with a disability may make it difficult to find appropriate and affordable child care and may affect decisions about relying on public support (Reichman et al, 2008).

Literature findings portray the associations between low income and children with special needs, associations that might go both ways (Birenbaum, 2002), In other words, children with a disability are often born into low-income families; however, families who care for a children with a disability often find themselves sliding toward poverty. Furthermore, the extent of financial and other resources available, which can determine the possibility of compensatory strategies (such as home modifications), often is the key factor in determining whether effective adaptation can be achieved (Minkler and Fadem, 2002).

Moreover, denied or delayed access to needed health services can negatively affect the health and well-being of any person. The following Clinical Example illustrates an attitudinal barrier and how it influences living with disability.

Community nurses can partner with clients and families affected by disabilities to remedy barriers that negatively affect QOL for this population. Most important, nurses must look beyond health-related concerns, a significant challenge in the current managed care environment. Nurses cannot remedy health concerns without attending to interacting systems, such as knowledge and educational background, personal and family belief systems, religious/spiritual beliefs and supports, finances, social networks, physical resources, and cultural influences.

Clinical Example

Cathy sought an eye examination at an optical center in a local department store where she did much of her shopping. Although the receptionist advised her that no one could see her for several months, she noted that the woman in line behind her received an appointment for the following day. Cathy left the store feeling puzzled and angry. She called several optical offices and advised them that, unless their equipment could accommodate her motorized wheelchair, someone would need to lift her into the examining chair and hold her upright throughout the eye examination. The limitations of the optical equipment required someone to assist Cathy during the examination. After she contacted several potential providers, Cathy finally obtained an appointment.

Only one optometrist chose to see Cathy. Physically disabled himself, the optometrist had a mobility impairment, evidenced by a limp. Although his functional limitations and the extent of his disability were much less severe than Cathy's, he also experienced societal bias and discrimination related to disability. Unfortunately, when people saw Cathy's wheelchair or heard about her potential need for accommodation, their attitudes may have transformed her disability into a handicap.

Four Models for Disability

Disability is a socially constructed issue, and how it is perceived and understood often relates to perspective. Four models for viewing disability are described here:

Medical model: Disability is a defect in need of cure through medical intervention.

Rehabilitation model: A defect to be treated by a rehabilitation professional.

Moral model: Connected with sin and shame.

Disability model: Socially constructed.

The medical and rehabilitation models would attempt to correct Cathy's disability, whether indicated or desirable. The moral model would blame her for having a disability. Cathy had a college "friend" who repeatedly asked what "sin" in her life was unconfessed to God to remain unhealed. The socially constructed disability model recognizes that whether Cathy is perceived as able-bodied or disabled depends on the lenses through which she is viewed and the barriers that promote or prevent her participation in life to an equal extent with that of any other person.

Disability: A Socially Constructed Issue

Disability is a complex, multifaceted culturally rich concept that cannot be readily defined, explained, or measured (Mont, 2007). Whether the inability to perform a certain function is seen as disabling depends on socioenvironmental barriers, for example, attitudinal, architectural, sensory, cognitive, economic, and inadequate support services and other factors (Kaplan, n.d.).

Much of the complexity in defining disability stems from its socially constructed nature. Because disability is more usefully conceptualized as the inability to perform important life functions, it becomes a product of interaction between health status and the demands of one's physical and social environment. Thus, using a wheelchair is disabling in a workplace with steps and narrow doorways, but much less so in one with ramps and wide passageways. An individual with a hidden disability such as deafness may not be conscious of the disability until immersed in a social situation with others who cannot communicate via sign language. Similarly, cultural beliefs and attitudes shape the extent to which an impairment is disabling and the extent to which people with physical or mental impairments are able to function in jobs and more broadly in public life (Scotch, 1994, p. 172).

Differentiating Illness from Disability

The nurse must be able to differentiate between the person who has an illness and becomes disabled secondary to the illness and the person who has a disability but may not need treatment. A disability is not necessarily accompanied by, nor related to, an illness; neither is an illness necessarily accompanied by, or related to, a disability. Rather than assuming a need for treatment, the nurse should ask whether the client wants assistance, ask the client/family to describe the goal(s), and ask how and in what way(s) the nurse can help. Hayes and Hannold (2007) wrote:

> Although some persons with disabilities have recurrent health complications secondary to disability, the sole assignment of a disability label or diagnosis does not necessarily warrant the need for ongoing medical surveillance. Historically however, disabilities have been equated with sickness, and people with disabilities have been viewed as patients. The medicalization of disability has often relegated people with disabilities into a "sick-role" in which they are exempt from social role obligations and expectations of productivity, and instead, are viewed only as passive recipients of health care resources.

PWD often confront "medicalization" issues when others view them in the "sick role" rather than as people first. Nurses who demonstrate understanding of these issues should approach PWD and their families on an eye-to-eye level. Nurses should listen to understand, collaborating with the person/family, and make plans and goals that meet the other's needs

and that draw on strengths and improve weaknesses. Collaboration empowers and affirms the worth and knowledge of the person/family with a disability. It promotes self-determination and allows choices that foster personal values and preferences.

RESEARCH HIGHLIGHTS

Hayes and Hannold (2007) provide a historical perspective on the medicalization of disability. They claim that medicine and health care professionals (HCPs) have oppressed persons with disabilities (PWD) through a medical/knowledge power differential, reinforcement of the "sick role," and objectification of PWD. Clients who refused to follow HCP recommendations have been viewed as noncompliant, uncooperative, resistant, and/or deviant. Because PWD seek medical treatment when sickest and most in need of care, HCPs form skewed opinions about their capabilities and potential, lacking data for baseline comparison. Appropriately "aggressive" therapies may not be offered, particularly if no one can advocate for the client. These writers state that health care management, wellness, and prevention of further disability should be emphasized, as opposed to treatment that intends to cure or normalize.

Data from Hayes J, Hannold EM: The road to empowerment: a historical perspective on the medicalization of disability, *J Health Hum Services Admin* 30(3):352-377, 2007. Also available from <http://findarticles.com/p/articles/mi_m1ylz/is_3_30/ai_n25014454/>.

A HISTORICAL CONTEXT FOR DISABILITY

Current models and definitions for disability cannot be understood apart from their historical-sociopolitical context. As cultures have changed, and with them images of beauty and value, "exceptional" people have experienced a wide range of treatment. They have been loved as mascots and fascinating freaks. In other cases, people with disabilities have been isolated, ridiculed, and discriminated against or, worse, marked for extermination.

Early Attitudes Toward People with Disabilities

Since the beginning of recorded history, people with disabilities have been set apart from others and viewed as different or unusual. Carvings on the walls of Egyptian tombs contain pictures of dwarfs and blind or disabled musicians and singers. Early Greek and Roman cultures emphasized bodily and intellectual perfection. Babies who were sick, weak, or born with obvious disabilities were commonly killed or left to die (Barnes, 1996). In Biblical times, people with disabilities were often viewed as unclean and/or sinful, though Jewish culture prohibited infanticide on the basis of belief in the sanctity of life. In European history, people with disabilities sometimes served as entertainers, circus performers, and sideshow exhibitions.

Attitudes Toward People with Disabilities in the Eighteenth and Nineteenth Centuries

In the absence of a scientific model for understanding and treating disability, people saw disability as an irreparable condition caused by supernatural agency (Longmore, 1987). People with disabilities were viewed as sick and helpless, following a "medical model." They were expected to participate in whatever treatment was deemed necessary to cure or produce a reasonable level of social or vocational performance. Although contemporary perspectives for disability in Western civilization do not support these ancient views, these views persist to varying degrees, depending on culture and world location.

During the nineteenth century, the Industrial Revolution stimulated a societal need for better education. People who were unable to achieve the equivalent of a contemporary third-grade education (e.g., those with intellectual disability) were labeled as "feebleminded" (Pfeiffer, 1993). Soon, the label was applied to people with vision, hearing, speech, and mobility impairments. Schools for people who were deaf and blind were established in the early 1800s. Although these early efforts demonstrated that people with disabilities could be educated and integrated into society, institutionalization and segregation of people with disabilities were the norm.

Disability in the Twentieth Century

Special interest groups for PWD began to develop in the twentieth century. The first federal vocational rehabilitation legislation, passed in the early 1920s, focused on limitations in the amount or type of work that people with disabilities could perform (Longmore, 1987). In the early 1900s, social Darwinism and the eugenics movement conducted involuntary sterilization of many people with intellectual disabilities (Pfeiffer, 1993). A few years later, the Association for Retarded Children (Arc) began to advocate for children with intellectual disabilities. Today, the Arc (The Arc, 2013) of the United States reportedly is the "world's largest community-based organization of and for people with intellectual and developmental disabilities" (Arc, 2009).

One of the most horrendous tragedies of World War II occurred during Adolf Hitler's euthanasia or "good death" program, in which at least 5000 mentally and physically disabled children, from newborn to age 17 years, were killed by starvation or lethal overdoses. Soon the killing, through use of six gassing installations, extended to adults with mental or physical disabilities who lived in institutional settings. Following widespread public and private protest, especially by the German clergy, Hitler cancelled the adult euthanasia program in late 1941. Between January 1940 and August 1941, he had killed 70,273 adults with disabilities. This was in addition to the minimum 5000 children killed during the war years. Killing resumed in August 1942 and continued until the last days of World War II, although in a more concealed manner. An estimated 200,000 people were exterminated through Hitler's euthanasia program because they were regarded as "life unworthy of life" (Euthanasia program, 2009).

Stimulated by the deinstitutionalization movement in the 1960s and '70s, parents' groups and professionals improved institutional care and established community-based independent living centers for PWD. Although some PWD moved into a limited number of community settings, most people with ID and others with severe disabilities remained in institutional settings.

Contemporary Conceptualizations of People with Disabilities

PWD are seldom presented as having a full range of personalities and abilities. However, when the media portrays people with disabilities as fully functioning, integral members of society, the public views the portrayals as unusual or unexpected. Although some progress is evident, the PWD population is primarily portrayed as a burden to society, or from pity/pathos or heroic/"supercrip" perspectives (Martiniello, 2009).

Stigmatizing influences shape our perceptions of disability. Murphy (1990), a tenured university anthropologist who became a wheelchair user after he had a spinal tumor, reports the following in *The Body Silent* (p.106):

One cannot…shelve a disability or hide it from the world. A serious disability inundates all other claims to social standing, relegating to secondary status all the attainments of life…it is an identity, a dominant characteristic… just as the paralytic cannot clear his mind of his impairment, society will not let him forget it.

Many parents teach their children not to look at a person who is obviously disabled, reinforcing "deviance disavowal" of disability. A community health nurse describes societal stigma experienced by the families of children with disabilities as follows:

It's a huge amount. The teasing in schools. Kids are brutal to normal kids. We try to run some groups on teasing and how to cope with that. … Families talk about going to the grocery store and being sick of answering questions or having people stare at the child. I don't know that any of the families really always know how to deal with that. (Treloar, 1999b)

Experiences of school-age children may range from teasing to bullying (unwanted, aggressive behavior among school-age children, involving real or perceived power imbalance, that is repeated or has the potential to be repeated over time [stopbullying.gov, 2013]). Bullying is a very serious problem that may exist for children regardless of disability status. However, for those with disabilities, there is an increased risk; children with physical, developmental, intellectual, emotional, and sensory disabilities are more likely to be bullied than their peers (stopbullying.gov, 2013).

Whether the disability is apparent or not, and regardless of the extent of disability, bullying poses a serious threat to children with disabilities. Children with special health needs may be at greater risk of being bullied. A limited but growing amount of research validates the magnitude of the problem; children with autism spectrum are more than three times as likely to be bullied and left out by peers (Twyman et al, 2010). Along with children who have medical conditions that affect their appearance (such as cerebral palsy and spina bifida), children with epilepsy are more likely to be bullied by peers (Hamiwka et al, 2009). Children with learning disabilities are also more likely to be bullied (Twyman et al, 2010). For the child with a disability, this is an added challenge to coping with the trials imposed by a disability. Depression, anxiety, health complaints, and decreased academic achievement are among the effects of bullying (stopbullying.gov, 2013).

For individuals with disabilities, bullying may be considered "disability harassment," a behavior that is prohibited under Section 504 of the Rehabilitation Act of 1973 and Title II of the Americans with Disabilities Act of 1990. Intimidation or abusive behavior toward a child that is based on disability and creates a hostile environment by interfering with or denying the child's participation in or receipt of benefits, services, or opportunities in an institution's program constitutes disability harassment (U.S. Department of Education [USDE], 2000). If such an event occurs, there are actions parents of children with disabilities can take, including supporting the bullied child and communicating through the proper channels within the school system. Stopybullying.gov provides resources to address the problem of bullying, including strategies for bullying prevention, identification of risk factors for victimization, and resources for help. The words and actions of others reveal their regard for people with disabilities. Table 21-2 gives examples of more and less desirable language related to disability. Box 21-1 lists common misconceptions surrounding disability. Finally, Table 21-3 makes recommendations that promote effective interactions between people with and without disabilities.

CHARACTERISTICS OF DISABILITY

Whether someone has a disability depends on the criteria used. The Americans with Disabilities Act of 1990 (ADA; see later) and the Rehabilitation Act of 1973 define a disability by how it limits carrying out a major life activity. Physical disabilities, sensory disabilities (e.g., being deaf or blind), intellectual disabilities (i.e., preferred terminology for mental retardation), serious emotional disturbances, learning disabilities, significant chemical and environmental sensitivities, and health problems such as acquired immunodeficiency syndrome (AIDS) and asthma are examples of disabilities that may substantially limit at least one major life activity. Major life activities include the ability to breathe, walk, see, hear, speak, work, care for oneself, perform manual tasks, and learn. The U.S. Census Bureau (2006) defines *disability* as a long-lasting physical, mental, or emotional condition that creates a limitation or inability to function according to certain criteria.

Measurement of Disability

To monitor changes in socioeconomic conditions, the government administers four household surveys. As definitions for disability change, so must measurement criteria. For example, the Survey of Income and Program Participation (SIPP) contains an extensive set of disability questions that deal with limitations in functional activities (e.g., seeing, hearing, speaking, walking, using stairs, lifting and carrying items), activities of daily living (ADLs) (e.g., getting around inside the home, bathing, dressing, eating, or toileting), and instrumental activities of daily living (IADLs) (e.g., going outside the home, shopping, light house cleaning, preparing meals). It gathers data on whether an individual uses an adaptive mobility device (e.g., wheelchair, cane, walker) for 6 or more months; has a mental or emotional disability; or has an impairment that produces on-the-job limitations or the inability to perform housework, or that involves the disability status of children (Brault, 2008).

The American Community Survey (ACS) asks respondents whether they have a disability limitation that affects a certain function or activity, such as sensory perception, physical activities, mental or emotional state, self-care, ability to leave home, or employment options (U.S. Census Bureau, 2010). The Current Population Survey (CPS), although not specifically designed to measure disability, asks questions to determine whether people are less able or are unable to work because of a health condition or disability. Limited data relative to disability are collected from the Decennial Census of Population and Housing.

Prevalence of Disability

In 2010, approximately 56.7 million (18.7%) of the 303.9 million civilian noninstitutionalized population aged 5 years and older had a long-lasting condition or disability (U.S. Census Bureau, 2012). Of those with a disability, 38.3 million (12.6%) had a "severe" disability (Brault, 2012).

TABLE 21-2	LANGUAGE USAGE SURROUNDING DISABILITY	
LESS DESIRABLE LANGUAGE	**MORE DESIRABLE LANGUAGE**
Confined to a wheelchair; wheelchair-bound	Uses a wheelchair
Afflicted with or suffers from cerebral palsy	Has cerebral palsy
The blind, the deaf, and the disabled	People who are blind, deaf, or disabled
Mentally handicapped or mentally retarded	People with intellectual disabilities
Handicapped students and normal classmates	Students who are disabled and nondisabled or students with and without disabilities
The spinal cord injury in room 232	John, in room 232, who has a spinal cord injury

BOX 21-1	MISCONCEPTIONS SURROUNDING DISABILITY

Disability = cannot have fun
Disability = want to be pitied
Disability = cannot live in the community
Disability = menace to society
Clear voice = clear mind
You can always tell if someone has a disability by looking at the person.
All parents want to care for a child with a disability.
Wheelchair = hard of hearing
Wheelchair = intellectually disabled
Intellectually disabled = cannot learn
People with disabilities do not know when someone makes fun of them.
Most disabilities and disabling diseases are contagious.

TABLE 21-3	DOS AND DON'TS FOR INTERACTIONS WITH PEOPLE WITH DISABILITIES
DON'T	**DO**
Assume anything or offer expert advice or assistance based on what you think the person needs or can do	Ask whether the person needs help and how to assist; listen and follow his or her instructions; allow him or her to do what he or she can
Ignore or exclude the person	Treat him or her like any other person or friend; approach and include him or her
Be afraid of joking with or offending the person	Treat the individual with courtesy and respect, as with any social or professional relationship
Be afraid to ask questions	Recognize that educating others helps remove attitudinal barriers; children who ask are less likely to be afraid of people with disabilities
Focus on differences	See the person as able; accept differences and be patient; seek out similarities and shared interests
Lean on or move the person's wheelchair	Respect a wheelchair as part of the person's personal space; sit or kneel at eye level when communicating with the person
Assume that a person who is blind knows who is speaking or who is present	Inform the person who is present; say goodbye when leaving
Grab the arm of a person who is blind	Let the person take your arm so he or she does not lose balance
Become impatient and complete the speech or the action of the person	Acknowledge that the person has something important to say or do; take time to listen and understand
Repeat loudly what you want to say	Face the person; speak distinctly and slightly more slowly (this is particularly important for the person who lip-reads)
Pet a working dog; there are service dogs for people with physical, hearing, or visual disabilities	Ask for permission to pet the dog; better yet, do not interrupt the dog's work
Assume that the person can participate	Consider possible environmental obstacles (e.g., sensory, architectural, colognes or fragrances for people with chemical sensitivities)
Assume that "bad" parenting explains children's behavior	Recognize that autism and other invisible disabilities influence behavior
Assume disability and failure to be healed reflect unresolved sin and lack of faith in God	Recognize that humans as holistic beings benefit from interventions that address spiritual meaning for disability

Disability Prevalence by Race and Sex: 2005

U.S. Census Bureau SIPP data, from May through August 2010, indicate prevalence differences by race and sex (Brault, 2012). Blacks (22.2%) had a higher rate of disability than Asians (14.5%) and Hispanics (17.8%), although the higher rate was not statistically different from that of non-Hispanic whites (17.6%). Females had a higher disability rate (19.8%) than males (17.4%) in all racial groups. However, higher disability rates in females can be explained by proportionally larger groups of older women than of older men.

Selected Measures of Disability

Wheelchair users (15 years and older) constituted 1.5% (3.6 million individuals) of the population with a disability (Brault, 2012). An additional 4.8% of the population used a cane, crutches, and/or walker. In comparison, about 9.2 million people reported hearing, visual, and speech disabilities. Collectively, more than 15 million people (about 6.3%) experienced a mental disability as defined by one or more of the following: a learning disability, intellectual disability, cognitive disability (dementia), other mental/emotional condition, and/or difficulty managing money/bills. An emotional disability, experienced by nearly 8.4 million people, consisted of one or more of the following: depression and/or anxiety, interpersonal challenges, concentration difficulties, and/or difficulty coping with stress (Brault, 2012).

Prevalence of Disability in Children

According to the National Survey of Children with Special Health Care Needs (2009/10) about 15.1% of households with children had at least one child with a special health care need (disabling condition). Children with special health care needs received a broad range of comprehensive health services, including prescription medications (86%), specialty medical care (47.5%), vision care (35.3%), mental health care (27.6%), specialized therapies (21.53%), and medical equipment (11.3%) (Child and Adolescent Health Measurement Initiative, 2012). Preventive dental care was an unmet need reported by 8.9% of parents of these children.

A disability may be a communication-related difficulty, mental or emotional condition, difficulty with regular schoolwork, difficulty getting along with other children, difficulty walking or running, use of some assistive device, and/or difficulty with ADLs. Of the 62.2 million U.S. children under the age of 15, about 5.2 million (8.4%) had some kind of disability (Brault, 2012). Half of children with a disability were classified as having severe disabilities (2.6 million children). One in 88 children have an autism spectrum disorder; these disorders are about five times more common among boys than among girls (Centers for Disease Control and Prevention [CDC], 2013). Among children with special health care needs, almost 31.813% had ongoing emotional, behavioral, or developmental conditions requiring treatment; 5.8% had an intellectual disability; and 58.8% had a little or a lot of difficulty with one or more emotional or behavioral factors—feeling anxious, depression, acting out, fighting, bullying or arguing, making and keeping friends (Child and Adolescent Health Measurement Initiative, 2012). Further, 4.2% had what would be termed a severe disability (U.S. Census Bureau, 2010b).

Among children aged 6 to 14, disability is defined on a wider range of activities and impairments. Nearly 4.5 million children (12.2%) in this age group have a disability (Brault, 2012). Around 5.3% have a severe disability; 0.8% need assistance with one or more ADLs. Approximately 2.3 million children (6.2%) have difficulty doing regular schoolwork, including 1.6 million who receive special education services. Approximately 3.4 million (9.3%) have one or more selected mental, emotional, or developmental conditions.

Recommendations for the Nurse. Community nurses who listen to parental concerns about their children establish what may be the most important bond the parents will have with a health care provider. Nurses should pay attention; a well-meaning health care provider may attempt to reassure a concerned mother. However, this kind of response may create silence and delay further questions from the parent. Rather than decrease parental concern, it may increase anxiety. The nurse can serve as an intermediary, working among the family and the health care team to address parental concerns and client goals.

Whether working in a school or office setting, the nurse should regularly assess for key developmental milestones and compare current status with predicted values. The school-aged child with developmental delays or disabilities should work with a team of resource providers following an **individualized education plan** (IEP). If a child is not making progress, a parent has the right to ask for a change in the plan.

STUDENT LEARNING ACTIVITY

Parents taught their autistic son, Tim, to use sign language to communicate at home. However, public school staff rejected this communication mode. At age 8 years, Tim was mainstreamed, and, predictably, was unable to use verbal communication. Tim regressed, and his behavior deteriorated. The parents withdrew Tim from the school when school administrators refused to modify his IEP. They planned to homeschool Tim, even though he required 24-hour-a-day supervision because he lacked safety awareness. Other members include his father, who works 50 hours a week, and 6-year-old brother Roger, who helps the mother care for Tim (Treloar, 1999b).

The mother's assessment includes the following concerns:

- The family cannot locate a church that will provide supervision for Tim while they attend worship service. Initially this was not a concern until Tim became too large to be accepted in the church's nursery. This change is a significant disappointment to them.
- Tim's mother mentions that she and her husband have not had any time alone in years. She wonders whether Roger will be "normal" because he always shares her time with Tim. Although they qualify for State Developmental Disability Respite Services, the services are offered only in an institutional setting. The family believes such a setting would upset Tim.

STUDENT LEARNING ACTIVITY—cont'd

- How can the family provide 24-hour-a-day care for Tim, who is severely disabled with autism, and support the health and well-being of each family member and the family system? Consider the family's need for support:
1. Break into small groups, and select one person to play the role of the mom. The highest-priority goals should consider what key element?
2. Establish three priority nursing diagnoses based on the mother's verbalized concerns and your assessment. Family and community resources should be assessed from a holistic perspective.

RESEARCH HIGHLIGHTS

Spiritual beliefs and religious practices bring meaning and purpose, emotional and practical support, and friendships with other believers, among other benefits. Families affected by disabilities who find places of worship to be inaccessible or unfriendly lose on many levels. A person affected by a disability or another difficult situation can understand the value of believing in God, who can provide strength and wisdom to make it through another day, another night. Faith communities must explore the multiple barriers against inclusion, increase disability access, and include persons with disabilities as integral to the mission of faith communities as a national public health imperative.

Data from Cunningham JL, Mulvihill BA, Speck PM: Disability and the church: how wide is your door, *J Christ Nurs* 26(3):140-147, 2009.

Health Status and Causes of Disability

Chronic health problems are associated with aging and functional disability. Commonly, chronic respiratory conditions, hearing and vision disabilities, stroke, and fractures (both pathological, caused by osteoporosis, and accidental, from falls) increase with aging. Cognitive impairments, such as dementia, are recognized for their disabling potential. Americans in all age-groups and cultures who are sedentary and overweight or obese are more likely to experience type 2 diabetes. The nurse's involvement in health promotion and disease prevention is critical. Regardless of the cause of disability, the nurse must see beyond the disabling impairment, carefully assessing affected persons' perceptions of the disability experience. Ultimately, the personal belief system of the individual and the family and the traditions of the community influence the individual's lived experience with disability and his or her participation in health care.

Culture and Disability

Individuals from other parts of the globe may have varying perspectives and experiences of disability. For example, in Nigerian society, children with disability have been perceived as cursed by God for gross disobedience, having ancestral violations of societal norms, or being witches and wizards, among the range of common societal misperceptions, leading to poor treatment from others (Eskay, Onu, Igbo, and Ugwuanyi, 2012). Similarly, in Chinese culture, though Confucian ideology views all people as deserving respect and kindness, there has also been the recognition of social hierarchy, in which those with disabilities were regarded as having the lowest status (Campbell and Uren, 2011). Traditional Chinese culture focuses on the cause of disability because there is assumed to be a link between disability and previous wrongdoing, someone with a disability is believed to bring shame and guilt to the family (Chiang and Hadadian, 2010).

Likewise, thematic assumptions derived from qualitative research on disability in South India include the notion that increased biomedical knowledge, imparted via health education programs, will reduce the incidence of disability because people will learn to take preventive measures and will decrease suffering caused by disability (Staples, 2012). Other common beliefs are that many conditions are caused or made worse by a failure to access biomedical resources, by carelessness and that many disabled people, and especially those from rural, uneducated, and economically poor backgrounds, do not obtain suitable treatment for their bodily conditions (Staples, 2012). People in South India are regarded as personally responsible for their bodily conditions.

The overarching belief in Japan is somewhat of a contrast. On initial examination the Japanese culture might seem more accepting of PWD; contemporary Japanese society espouses a commitment to the idea that every human being is valued equally, regardless of ability (Murakami and Meyer, 2010). From the Japanese perspective, everything on the earth is considered to have a spirit, and people respect these spirits. Respecting these spirits is, in part, characterized by following nature's rules. Because being "natural" is the fundamental law of Japanese thought, the "unnatural," which includes disabilities, is rejected or avoided (Murakami and Meyer, 2010). Since individuals with both mental and physical disabilities need supplemental support to survive, and because they often have difficulty with physical productivity, they have been considered useless and are called *gokutsubushi*, translated as "good-for-nothing" or, more literally, "waste of food" (Murakami and Meyer, 2010). Moreover, Japanese educators seem confident that even so-called difficult students can be brought in line with their class. Interestingly, Japan has a lower incidence of disability, which Murakami and Meyer (2010) assert is a result of Japan's strong collectivist and paternalistic orientation and the requisite institutions' promulgation of the predominant beliefs about disability in this nation.

Aging and Personal Assistance

Disability prevalence and disability severity levels rise with aging. Thus, disability accompanies the "graying" of our elderly population, which is proportionately increasing as the "baby boomer" generation turns 65 years and older. In 2005, roughly half (49.8%) of people aged 65 years and older had a disability, and 36.6% of people 65 years and older had a severe disability (Brault, 2012). The highest incidence of disability (70.5%) occurred in people 80 years and older; of these, 55.8% had a severe disability and 30.2% needed personal assistance. As of 2005, people in nursing facilities had a disability prevalence of 97.3%

(Brault, 2008). Approximately 1.3 million of the 40.4 million people age 65 and older were living in nursing facilities in 2010 (Brault, 2012). Notably, the need for assistance with one or more ADLs or IADLs increases as severity of disability increases. In 2005, 16.56 million people needed personal care services (ADLs) and/or light housework assistance (IADLs) (Brault, 2012).

DISABILITY AND PUBLIC POLICY

Early American public policy viewed people with disabilities as "deserving poor" who required governmental protection and provision and had little capacity for self-support or independence (Rubin and Millard, 1991). Contemporary disability policy minimizes disadvantages and maximizes opportunities for people with disabilities to live productively in their communities. Public policy on disability includes civil rights protections (e.g., Title 504 of the Rehabilitation Act and the ADA), skill enhancement programs (e.g., special education, vocational rehabilitation), and income and in-kind assistance programs (e.g., Social Security Disability Insurance [SSDI], and Medicare). Box 21-2 contains foundational values and ideologies that underlie public policy related to people with disabilities.

Legislation Affecting People with Disabilities

Consistent with historical and social changes and the recognition of barriers and discrimination, key federal legislation supports the rights of people with disabilities. This section describes a few of the most significant acts.

The Individuals With Disabilities Education Act

The **Individuals with Disabilities Education Act** (IDEA) (PL 94-142) ensures a free appropriate public education to children with disabilities that is based on their needs, in the *least restrictive setting* from preschool through secondary education. Addressing special education needs requires appropriate evaluation and transition services. Parents, the student and professionals join together to develop an IEP that includes measurable special educational goals and related services for the child.

The National Association of School Nurses (NASN, 2013) asserts that the registered professional school nurse is an essential member of the team participating in the identification and evaluation of students who may be eligible for services through the implementation of Section 504 of the Rehabilitation Act and the Individuals with Disabilities Education Improvement Act (IDEIA). Under this act,

---

BOX 21-2 PUBLIC POLICY VALUES RELATED TO DISABILITY

Equal protection: All deserve equal protection under the law.
Egalitarianism: Regardless of differences in abilities, all people should receive equal treatment through equal opportunities.
Normalization: People with disabilities should be treated like non-disabled people, minimizing differences wherever possible.

the school nurse's responsibilities could include: assisting in identifying children who may need special educational or health-related services; assessing the identified child's functional and physical health status, in collaboration with the child, parent(s)/guardian(s), and health care providers; developing individualized health care plans and emergency care plans based on a nursing assessment; recommending to the team any health-related accommodations or services that may be required; assisting the team in developing an IEP or 504 Accommodation Plan that provides for the required health needs of the student and enables the student to participate in his or her educational program; assisting the parent(s)/guardians and teachers to identify and remove health-related barriers to learning; providing in-service training for teachers and staff regarding the individual health needs of the child; providing and/or supervising unlicensed assistive personnel to provide specialized health care services in the school setting; and evaluating the effectiveness of the health-related components of the IEP with the child, parent(s), and other team members, and making revisions to the plan as needed (Gibbons, Lehr, and Selekman, 2013). The school nurse who is well-informed about federal laws related to working with students with disabilities or other disorders can make significant contributions to the health and academic success of such students. It is the school nurse's responsibility to understand the laws, refer students who may be eligible for the services as outlined in the laws, and participate on school teams that determine eligibility for services covered by Section 504 and IDEIA (NASN, 2013). See the IDEA website (http://idea.ed.gov/) for additional information.

The Americans with Disabilities Act of 1990 and ADA Amendments Act of 2008

The Americans with Disabilities Act (ADA) (PL 101-336) became law in July 1990. This landmark civil rights legislation prohibits discrimination against people with disabilities in everyday activities (U.S. Department of Justice, 2009). The ADA guarantees equal opportunities for people with disabilities in relation to employment, transportation, public accommodations, public services, and telecommunications. It provides protection to people with disabilities similar to those provided to any person on the basis of race, color, sex, national origin, age, and religion. The U.S. Equal Employment Opportunity Commission (EEOC) is charged with enforcement of the employment provisions found in Title I of the ADA.

The ADA refers to a "qualified individual" with a disability as a person with a physical or mental impairment that substantially limits one or more major life activities or bodily functions, a person with a record of such an impairment, or a person who is regarded as having such an impairment. The ADA prohibits discrimination against people who have a known association or relationship with an individual with a disability. A qualified individual with a disability must meet legitimate skill, experience, education, or other requirements of an employment position. The person must be able to perform the essential job functions, such as those contained within a job description, with or without reasonable accommodation(s). Qualifying organizations must provide reasonable accommodations unless they can demonstrate that the accommodation will cause significant difficulty or expense, producing an undue hardship.

Over time, judicial decisions eroded the ADA rights of people whose disabilities were intermittent, nonvisible, or manageable with medications, prosthetics, and/or medical equipment. On January 1, 2009, the ADA Amendments Act of 2008 (PL 110-325), a bipartisan bill supported by disability advocates and employers, became effective, making it easier for a person "seeking protection under the ADA to establish that he or she has a disability within the meaning of the ADA" (U.S. Department of Justice, 2009). For additional information, see the ADA website (www.ada.gov/).

The community health nurse should develop a resource network that includes disability resource center specialists, public interest law firms, and legal advocacy groups. High-priority interventions include helping people with disabilities learn about their rights and empowering them to act on their own behalf.

Ticket to Work and Work Incentives Improvement Act

Historically, national public policy has defined disability as the inability to work. Typically, people with disabilities could qualify only for such benefits as health care, income assistance programs, and personal care attendant services if they chose not to work. To address employment and benefit issues for persons with disabilities, in December 1999, the Ticket to Work and Work Incentives Improvement Act (TWWIIA) was signed into law. The TWWIIA reduced the disincentives to work for PWD by increasing access to vocational services and provided new methods for retaining health insurance after they returned to work. Congressional efforts through the TWWIIA demonstrated evolution of attitudes and interest in the ability of PWD to work, their potential economic contributions, and their decreased reliance on public funds (Ticket to Work and Work Incentives Advisory Panel, 2007). In 2008, the Ticket to Work program experienced a significant overhaul when new regulations were produced; these regulations dramatically revised the payment structure available to employment networks, providing more money when beneficiaries make progress in their employment plans but before they reach the level of earnings that would terminate their benefits (USDE, 2008).

John, similar to many PWD, remains locked in poverty. His situation remains the "norm" despite the potential held by the TWWIIA. Complexity of rules, lack of awareness of work incentive provisions, fear of loss of health care and other support systems needed for work, and distrust associated with governmental operational issues are primary reasons the TWWIIA is poorly utilized (Ticket to Work and Work Incentives Advisory Panel, 2007). The Ticket to Work revision is intended to improve program effectiveness in order to maximize the economic self-sufficiency of beneficiaries (USDE, 2008).

TICKET TO WORK, SOCIAL SECURITY DISABILITY INSURANCE, AND SUPPLEMENTAL SECURITY INCOME ELIGIBILITY

What is a Ticket?

A Ticket to Work increases a person with a disability's available choices for obtaining employment services, vocational rehabilitation services, and other support services needed to get or keep a job. It is a free and voluntary service. A ticket may be used for its purpose, held for future use, or not used.

Where can a Ticket Be used?

The program is available in all fifty states and ten U.S. territories. Many **Social Security Disability Insurance** (SSDI) and **Supplemental Security Income** (SSI) disability beneficiaries may obtain services from a state vocational rehabilitation (VR) agency or contracted employment network.

Where can I find more information?

Contact the Social Security Administration's Ticket Program Operations Support Manager, MAXIMUS, at its toll-free numbers: 1-866-YOURTICKET (1-866-968-7842) or, for TTY/TDD, call 1-866-833-2967 between 8 AM and 10 PM Eastern time (Monday through Friday). Online information can be found at www.ssa.gov/work/aboutticket.html, www.yourtickettowork.com, or http://www.socialsecurity.gov/pubs/EN-05-10061.pdf.

Data from Social Security Administration: Ticket to Work, SSDI and SSI Eligible. In *2009 Social Security Administration Redbook*, 2009c. Available from <www.socialsecurity.gov/redbook/eng/ssdi-and-ssi-employments-supports.htm#5>.

Clinical Example

The Dilemma of Choosing Employment versus Health Care and Community Support Assistance

John uses a power wheelchair because he experiences "spastic quadriplegia" from cerebral palsy. He is college educated and chooses not to work. John weighed his options and acknowledged that, if he were to work, he would lose the state-supported social service benefits that provide his health care services and attendant caregiver services (Treloar, 1999a).

SUPPLEMENTAL SECURITY INCOME AND SOCIAL SECURITY DISABILITY INSURANCE

The Social Security Administration (2009a) defines disability as the "inability to engage in any substantial gainful activity (SGA) because of a medically determinable physical or mental impairment(s) that is expected to result in death, or that has lasted or is expected to last for a continuous period of not less than 12 months." Most people who receive disability benefits qualify on the basis of their personal inability to work because of a disability; however, exceptions include people who are blind or have low vision, benefits for widows or widowers who are disabled, and benefits for children who are disabled. The following table provides a comparison of SSI and SSDI programs.

Supplemental Security Income (SSI)	Social Security Disability Insurance (SSDI)
Funded through general tax revenues	Funded through disability trust fund monies (Social Security taxes paid by workers, employers, and self-employed workers)
To qualify for SSI, the person with disabilities (PWD) must have limited income and resources	To qualify for SSDI, the PWD must be "insured" through Federal Insurance Contributions Act (FICA) earnings of self, parents, and/or spouse
SSI disability benefits are payable to adults and children who are disabled or blind and are eligible	SSDI disability benefits are payable to workers or widow(er)s who are disabled or adults who have been disabled since childhood and are eligible
SSI recipients receive Medicaid health benefits	SSDI recipients receive Medicare health benefits
Some states may elect to pay a state supplement to some PWD in SSI programs	PWD in SSDI programs are never provided with state supplements

Information about Supplemental Security Income (SSI) and Social Security Disability Insurance (SSDI) can be accessed online (www.ssa.gov/disability/) or obtained at a Social Security office.

Data from Social Security Administration: Differentiating SSI from SSDI. In *2009 Social Security Administration Redbook*, 2009b. Available from <www.ssa.gov/redbook/eng/overview-disability.htm#4>.

Public Assistance Programs

Public assistance programs include cash assistance (e.g., SSI, Social Security), food stamps, and public/subsidized housing. For people 25 to 64 years of age, participation in public assistance programs increases with severity of disability, consistent with the highest poverty levels. In 2010, 59% of people with a severe disability received public assistance, compared with 8.8% of people with a nonsevere disability, whereas only 2.6% of people with no disability received public assistance (Brault, 2012).

COSTS ASSOCIATED WITH DISABILITY

People with disabilities continue to lag behind nondisabled Americans in most basic areas of life. There are gaps in employment, income, education, access to transportation,

attendance at religious services, and so forth. People with no disability earn the most, are more likely to be employed, and are least likely to live in poverty, whereas people with a severe disability earn the least, are less likely to be employed, and are most likely to live in poverty.

Economic Well-Being and Employment

Of people 25 to 64 years of age in 2005, 17.9% with a nonsevere disability and 28.6% with severe disabilities lived in poverty (Brault, 2012). People with no disability were most likely to be employed, and those having a severe disability were least likely to be employed. Among individuals from 21 to 64 years, only 41.1% of people with a disability and 27.5% with a severe disability were employed (Table 21-4).

TABLE 21-4 INFLUENCE OF DISABILITY ON EMPLOYMENT

LEVEL OF DISABILITY	PERCENTAGE OF PERSONS AGES 21-64 YEARS WHO ARE EMPLOYED
Any disability	41.1%
Nonsevere disability	71.2%
Severe disability	27.5%
No disability	79.1%

Data from Brault MW: *Americans with disabilities: 2010* (Current Population Reports P70–131), 2012. Available from <http://www.census.gov/prod/2012pubs/p70-131.pdf>.

Determining the actual number of PWD who are employed or unemployed at any time is challenging at best. Research outcomes vary depending on survey design, population size and characteristics, aims of the study, and interpretation of the variables. Rates of employment for PWD, compared with nondisabled counterparts, remain at significantly lower levels. Much can be done to promote employment opportunities for PWD. The Social Security Administration (SSA, 2014) offers encouragement and some incentives for employers who are willing to hire PWD. Because of the recession beginning in 2008 and persistent economic challenges; however, little improvement in employment levels has been realized, keeping many PWD in poverty, fearing loss of health care benefits and social supports.

HEALTHY PEOPLE 2020 AND THE HEALTH NEEDS OF PEOPLE WITH DISABILITIES

Persons with disabilities are one of several populations that receive poorer quality health care. This section describes health disparities and their application to *Healthy People 2020*.

Health Disparities in Quality and Access

The National Healthcare Disparities Report of 2008 (NHDR) explains that, within the scope of health care delivery, disparities are due to differences in access to care, provider biases, poor provider-patient communication, poor health literacy, and other factors (Agency on Healthcare Research and Quality, 2009). Congress mandated the NHDR to identify differences or gaps where some populations receive poor or worse care than others and to track how the gaps change over time. Because PWD experience a higher rate of chronic illness, pneumococcal vaccination of adults aged 65 years and older is a *Healthy People 2020* objective, used as a quality of care monitor. In 2010, only 22.9% of all adults 65 years and older had had a pneumococcal vaccination (Healthy People.gov, 2012) compared with 35.8% of PWD (CDC, 2011). Although PWD were immunized at a higher rate than nondisabled elders, both populations must make significant gains to approach the 90% immunization levels desired.

People with Intellectual Disabilities: Undervalued and Disadvantaged

Worldwide, unrecognized health care problems frequently are untreated in people with **intellectual disabilities** who cannot easily communicate their symptoms and demonstrate varied participation in shared decision making. Indeed, Walsh (2008) explored how people with ID compared on health measures with the general population and concluded that adults with ID were consistently undervalued and disadvantaged. Socioeconomic disadvantage accounted for a "significant proportion" of variation in health status apart from personal characteristics or other circumstance.

For example, women with ID often experience disparities in primary care services, particularly in women's health issues. Because osteoporosis develops at higher rates in women with ID, recommendations include screening at earlier and more frequent intervals, special gynecological examination techniques, and "thoughtful well-coordinated" care from primary care physicians (Wilkinson and Cerreto, 2008). Further, those with special health care needs such as ID often have less access to health services and experience great disparity in health status, health care access, and all-cause morbidity and mortality (Bodde et al, 2012). Clients with ID may exhibit behavioral problems that discourage health care providers from caring for them, or they may resist others' attempts to care for them because of their discomfort or unfamiliarity with the health care setting or equipment.

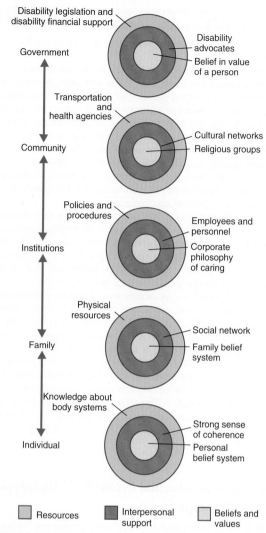

Government — Disability legislation and disability financial support

Transportation and health agencies

Community

Policies and procedures

Institutions

Physical resources

Family

Knowledge about body systems

Individual

Disability advocates
Belief in value of a person

Cultural networks
Religious groups

Employees and personnel
Corporate philosophy of caring

Social network
Family belief system

Strong sense of coherence
Personal belief system

Resources | Interpersonal support | Beliefs and values

FIGURE 21-2 Systems of support for people with disabilities.

Other problems are difficulties in obtaining a client history and in determining the nature and cause of a problem, along with inexperience and inadequate training of health care providers in specific health care problems that accompany ID (May and Kennedy, 2010). Health care for PWD must incorporate remedies that address issues surrounding their access to health care and the removal of environmental and social barriers that prevent their full participation in society. The community health nurse will use a range of support systems that promotes the health of the person with a disability and the health of his or her family. Figure 21-2 illustrates these support systems. It is only when the nurse considers a broad approach to disability that he or she can realize the objectives of *Healthy People 2020*, including caring for those who may be undervalued and disadvantaged.

THE EXPERIENCE OF DISABILITY

Persons with disabilities are commonly thought to constitute the largest minority group in the United States. In fact, most residents of the country whose lives do not end abruptly will

experience disability. Regardless of the condition associated with disability, many experiences are common to lived experience with disability. However, the personal meaning of disability differs significantly with the time frame and the event or disease process (see Table 21-5).

Those who have a temporary disability, such as a sprained ankle, have a very different experience from that of those who are permanently disabled. Although the former may experience the frustrations of mobility associated with the use of a wheelchair or crutches, they do not enter the world of people with disabilities, because they know they will soon reenter society as able-bodied. They often do not develop the skills of living with a disability, such as obtaining a disabled parking placard, and learning to perform daily activities with a disability. They view it as a temporary problem and a temporary setback.

In contrast, those who have a permanent disability from an accident or from a disease process, such as a stroke, must learn to incorporate the modifications required for living into their daily routines and identities. "Their difference from other people is inescapable and can be concealed—if at all—only at formidable cost to their energy and self-esteem" (Silvers, Wasserman, and Mahowald, 1998, p. 2). Franklin D. Roosevelt, the nation's thirty-second president, hid his disability from most Americans with the cooperation of the press. He began using a wheelchair at age 21 years after contracting polio, yet only two photographs show him profiled in a wheelchair rather than from the waist up (Health Media Lab, 2004).

People who become disabled from the progressive decline of a chronic illness may be reluctant to use assistive devices that would make life easier for them. They believe that accepting such a device would mean accepting the label of being disabled. Unfortunately, many falls could be prevented by the use of walkers or canes that were declined because the people did not want to appear disabled.

In many progressive diseases, a benchmark event forces the person to accept the label of disabled—for example, a driving accident caused by failing eyesight or mental capacity, or a leg amputation from diabetic complications, impairs mobility and the person's body becomes unreliable. The person can no longer plan daily activities and expect to accomplish them independently. Because chronic illness and disability increase with longevity, many elderly persons experience benchmark disabling changes.

When people with disabling symptoms are unable to return to work, they may lose their jobs and their benefits and exhaust personal resources. They apply for state and federal disability benefits, feeling fully qualified, but are warned to expect to be rejected. They may lose their homes; some will become homeless. Some will adapt to their experiences, choosing to live with pain, whereas others will fight their discomfort, expecting relief. Community nurses may find their best tool for helping the client through the life-altering experience is the use of self. Nurses may show they care through listening, presence, and use of holistic and spiritual resources. Finally, nurses may help clients connect with personnel at neighborhood centers that provide comprehensive social services.

TABLE 21-5	CONCEPTUALIZATION OF CHRONIC HEALTH CONDITIONS			
		LONG-TERM CONDITIONS		
	SHORT-TERM CONDITIONS	**MODEL CASE**	**RELATED CASE**	**CONTRARY CASE**
DIMENSION	**ACUTE ILLNESS**	**CHRONIC ILLNESS**	**DISABLING CONDITION**	**LIFE-THREATENING ILLNESS**
Cellular	Inflammation	Inflammation; degeneration	Destruction or atrophy	Proliferation
Time	Short	Long	Long	Short or long
Purpose of treatment (Rx)	To remove problem (i.e., cure)	To alleviate symptoms	To improve functioning	To kill cancer cells (i.e., cure)
Examples of immediate effect of treatment	Severe pain of surgery; immobility	Weight gain of prednisone therapy; dietary restrictions	Discomfort of splinting; pain of retraining muscles	Loss of hair, nausea, and weight loss
Anticipated outcome of treatment	Cure expected	Cure not expected	Cure not expected	Cure hoped for or death feared
Trajectory	Short	Exacerbations and remissions; slow progressive decline; shortened life span	Steady	Remission or cure or death
Effect on activities of daily living	Severe during Rx or none after	Regimen required	Modifications required	Severe during Rx or none during remission or cure
Mental outlook	Temporary problem	Depression or challenge	Stigma or challenge	Fear or hope
Metaphorical interpretation	A temporary setback	Chain binding; a prisoner of uncertainty because body is unreliable	Obstacle to overcome	Sword hanging over head; a sentence

Family and Caregiver Responses to a Child with a Disability

Those who have limited experience caring for children with disabilities may wonder how parents cope with the responsibility. All members of the family are affected. Parents redefine their image of and expectations for the child, and also themselves as individuals, parents, marital partners, and members of a culture and society. Sibling responses to a brother/sister who is disabled may be influenced by such factors as age of sibling, reservoir of coping strategies, strength of peer relationships, perception of parent's burden in caring for the CWD, desire of sibling to protect parents from their concerns about the CWD, and the impact of the CWD on family plans and social activities. The following comments of a mother with two children, the younger one with serious disabilities, illustrate these points (Dwight, 2001):

> *My first son, Timmy…had taught my husband, Phil, and me many things.…But I don't think I came face to face with the true meaning of motherhood until Aidan entered our lives [p. 18].…As I poured over the books and talked with these other parents, I found the factual side of Down Syndrome fairly easy to piece together.…Of course, there was nothing in those reference books that could fully explain the other side of the story— the ups and downs of raising a child with Down Syndrome in our society [pp. 34–35].…In many ways, our lives have been transformed. We have found loving support from people who used to be strangers. We look at the world differently.…We have an appreciation for a slower pace.…And we have a newfound understanding of the preciousness of all people. (p. 37)*

Ulrich and Bauer (2003) propose that the adjustment to disability experience occurs in four levels as parents gradually become aware of the impact of their child's disability.

These levels are: *the ostrich phase*, when parents do not deny a disability but also do not fully realize its impact; *special designation*, when parents begin to realize their child has a special need and seek help; *normalization*, when parents try to make the differences between their child and children without disabilities less apparent and may actually request a reduction in services; and *self-actualization*, when parents view being different not as better or worse, just different, and support their child in learning about his or her disability, along with how to be a self-advocate. These levels of adjustment reveal key opportunities for the nurse to support parents with education and referrals to community and online resources. Nurses can also encourage the parents of a child with a disability to connect with extended family, members of which make a huge difference if they provide the right kind of support (Davis and Gavidia-Payne, 2009; Morris, 2008; Reichman et al, 2008).

Family Research Outcomes

In the past, research of children with disabilities has emphasized pathology, personal deficits, and impaired family functioning (Cuskelly, 2009). Contemporary research, on the other hand, clearly establishes various benefits amid challenges in families who care for disabled children. Related research describes lived experience marked by joy amid chronic sorrow (Kearney and Griffin, 2001). Families quickly learn that neither governmental social support nor private health plans offer adequate community-based or in-home assistance for disabled family members. Parents with satisfying emotional support from families, friends, and professionals, however, tend to experience fewer potentially negative effects of unplanned or distressing events (Treloar, 2002).

Parents of a child with a disability grieve the loss of the idealized or expected child over time. Whether or not parent(s) anticipated the child's disability, the birth of any child with a disability is a shock, and denial may result. Parents are likely to be sad and may eventually embrace the child, although in some cases, the child will be rejected (more commonly by one parent). Parents will likely experience some caregiver role strain at times; caregiver role strain affects marriages and relationships with other children as well. For example, there is an 85% divorce rate among parents of autistic children (Freedman, Kalb, Zablotsky, and Stuart, 2012).

Nurses can help parents and families adjust to disability in a child by establishing a supportive relationship, educating them about the child's condition based on their readiness to learn, and referring them to a case manager for a support group as well as for pastoral/spiritual care. Empowering and enabling parent(s) for decision making on behalf of the child with a disability and establishing a partnership between the parent and health care team are also important.

"Knowledgeable Client" and the "Knowledgeable Nurse"

A person who lives with a disability commonly becomes an expert at knowing what works best for his or her body. This case differs significantly from the person with a new disabling injury or the parent of a child with a newly diagnosed disability, who needs information and time to adapt to disability. The Intersystem Model (Artinian, West, and Conger, 2011) refers to the first-described person as the "Knowledgeable Client." In this case, a client has been living with disability for an extended time and has become sensitive to the needs of his or her body. The nurse must ask the client what works best for him or her and what goals the client is pursuing. The client wants the nurse to listen to his or her concerns and may benefit from a referral to health-related resources. However, if the nurse attempts to tell the Knowledgeable Client what to do, the client may become angry and seek help elsewhere.

The clients in the second situation need the services of the "Knowledgeable Nurse" (Artinian et al, 2011). The client with a newly diagnosed condition can benefit from the nurse's information about the disability and the available community and governmental resources. If the nurse is unable to help a newly diagnosed client learn how to manage the disability and accept himself or herself as disabled, the nurse may compromise the client's adaptation and future client/nurse interactions. Table 21-6 applies this information to the Disability Paradigm (or how disability is conceptualized).

Active collaboration of the client and nurse is required to develop a plan of care that both will find acceptable. Sometimes the nurse must be flexible in his or her expectations. In the final analysis, the client will accomplish only what he or she agrees to accomplish. As one nurse observed:

⚖ ETHICAL INSIGHTS

Advances in neonatology are responsible for increasing numbers of very-low-birth-weight babies, who are at high risk for cognitive disorders and other serious health problems (Reichman et al, 2008). Consider the health care implications of caring for the infant and growing child in the home. High-quality primary and specialized, highly technological comprehensive care on a long-term basis will be required. What kinds of community resources will be needed? What anticipated challenges/obstacles to obtaining necessary services may arise? (See National Dissemination Center for Children with Disabilities [NICHCY], http://nichcy.org/).

As the child with a disability grows, early intervention services will be utilized prior to mainstreaming into public education. Consider economic issues, because families having children with disabilities across all income levels are significantly more challenged by food, housing, and health issues.

TABLE 21-6	HOW THE DISABILITY PARADIGM INFLUENCES POLICY AND ACTIONS	
DEFINING CHARACTERISTIC	**MEDICAL MODEL**	**SOCIAL CONSTRUCT**
Framework or paradigm	Disability as pathology; emphasizes functional limitations; physical limitations are primary source of problems	Disability as expected (i.e., normal); emphasizes minority-group model (i.e., discrimination and oppression) related to social attitudes and other barriers
Focus of concern	Person	Environment
Problem	Personal deficits (e.g., an impairment, lack of a vocational skill, poor adjustment, or lack of motivation)	Environmental barriers (e.g., attitudinal, architectural, sensory, economic, and inadequate social supports)
Person with a disability	Patient in need of professional help	Person is expert, knowledgeable about self, may or may not seek professional assistance
Role of the health professional	Expert and expects advice to be followed	Collaborating partner; mutually negotiated role reflects needs and desires of person and resources of professional
Perspective of discipline	Medicine, nursing, rehabilitation, medical sociology and psychology, special education, and allied health	Disability studies and disability policy
Model for decision making	Hierarchical (i.e., professional on top)	Collaboration for empowerment of person
Plan of care	Professional-centered	Person-centered
Desired outcomes	Reflect professional's goals	Reflect person's goals

Sensitivity is being able to listen, being able to hear families, being able to respond to where they're at. Not your own agenda, and that's real hard for nurses…what you think you need to do for health care and you really lose track of where the family is. …They may not do it the way we want, but they're experts in their own child's care. (Treloar, 1999b)

STRATEGIES FOR THE COMMUNITY HEALTH NURSE IN CARING FOR PEOPLE WITH DISABILITIES

Nurses who partner with people with disabilities and their families provide nursing care using a number of strategies in a variety of community sites. The individual, his or her family, and the community may be the primary client. People affected by disabilities have health care needs and resources common to people without disabilities; others are unique. Lawthers and colleagues (2003) identified five major quality of care issues for PWD: underutilization of age-appropriate preventive health care; undertreatment of comorbid health care conditions; inadequate health care provider knowledge of appropriate and effective treatments; barriers to effective communication between client, family, and providers; and risk factors for accidental injury.

The nurse's role should reflect the needs and resources of the client and his or her family. Data from interviews conducted with nurses who provide care to PWD illustrate the following guiding principles (Treloar, 1999b):

Do not assume anything. The nurse should collect data from the perspective of the person and family with a disability. A nurse case manager for families with disabled children explains:

Look at each person, client, family, each situation as a totally new and different one. …There are cultural things that you would want to respect. But, do not assume anything. …listen to what is not said. I watch people.… You go into a home and you can learn a tremendous amount by not even asking any questions.

Adopt the client's perspective. If nurses operate from their agenda or personal cultural norms rather than from those of the client, outcomes will be less productive and less satisfactory. More importantly, the nurse will fail to establish a relationship that respects the client as expert in his or her own health status. Further more, what appears to be a barrier or a limitation may not reflect the true situation or the client's perspective (priorities).

Listen and learn from the client; gather data from the perspective of the client and family. If the client has severe mental disabilities and cannot offer reliable information, ask the family or caregiver. Nurses must establish relationships that are responsive to the person's methods and the family's methods for dealing with disability. An experienced nurse explains: who explained:

That parent or caretaker is the one that is there for that child all the time. They know that child far better. I may know something medical that they do not know….That

is where you get down to sharing those kinds of things. Teach me. I am always there to learn.

Care for the client and the family, not the disability. The style and intent of client and provider communication influences the acceptability of the interaction. A "conversational" style that establishes an equal partnership with the client is preferable to an "open the textbook" approach that tells the client "here is what you need to do." The nurse should ask what the client needs help with, what the client is capable of doing, what the client would like to do, and how the nurse can help. A community health nurse describes applying these ideas in working with families of children with disabilities:

Are they able to develop a health care plan of their own for their child? This, again, may not be ours [plan]. Are they able to follow through on the important pieces of health care for their child, or at least identify that they don't have the resources to do that?… At times we make families feel that if they don't follow our plan, then they're bad parents.

Be well informed about community resources. People often respond differently to requests by someone they know and respect; therefore, it may be beneficial for the community health nurse to contact agency personnel about a client and family need. Lawthers and colleagues (2003) describe care coordination as the "lubricant" that facilitates links for all areas of quality for a person with a disability and provides the most significant opportunity for improvement in care delivery by multidisciplinary health care providers.

Become a powerful advocate. The community health nurse's advocacy for the PWD extends beyond being a resource and referral coordinator or speaking on the other's behalf. People with disabilities want to speak for themselves. They want to be in control of their lives and their health care. One person with a disability stated:

They [health care providers who act in an advocacy role] provide the information, but they leave the choice up to the person. And then even if the person chooses against what has been suggested, they still provide the same support.

The community health nurse's perspective on disability will influence the nursing role and the level of care he or she provides to people with disabilities and their families. A variety of systems, ranging from government, community, institutions, and family, to the individual (see Figure. 21-2), influences the experience of living with a disability. Regardless of whether the nurse chooses to work in a setting that specializes in health care services for people affected by disabilities, disability is a common experience that all practicing nurses will encounter.

ETHICAL ISSUES FOR PEOPLE AFFECTED BY DISABILITIES

PWD and their families are concerned about the same contemporary ethical and legal issues that concern nondisabled people. However, some of the associated issues carry particular interest for people with disabilities and their families, including questions and problems surrounding definitions of personhood, respect for human beings, and the rights of PWD.

Associated issues include choosing between abortion and continuing the pregnancy when prenatal screening suggests the presence of impairments and health problems and determining the appropriate medical care for infants, children, and adults with disabilities. In 2009, parents filed a $14 million malpractice suit when prenatal testing failed to correctly diagnose Down's syndrome. They stated that an accurate test result would have led them to end the pregnancy, and that although the child is a "dear," they fear public perception of them as "heartless" for their actions (Green, 2009). The Prenatally and Postnatally Diagnosed Awareness Act of 2008 (PL 110-374) uses federal resources to produce and distribute information about prenatally and postnatally diagnosed conditions (Dresser, 2009). Because health care professionals may convey negative attitudes about life with a disability, accurate and balanced information must be provided. People's spiritual perspectives play an important role in decision making when there is a change in health status or a life-threatening illness. People who establish hope and meaning in their lives may choose to positively reframe the difficulties associated with functional limitations that others may find intolerable. Holistic caregiving requires the nurse to assess and promote spiritual health along with physical and psychological well-being, as described in Box 21-3.

Differences in quality of life and justice perspectives intersect with concerns about the control of health care costs. For example, people with disabilities and their families may be concerned with how many and what kind of health care services they should be entitled to receive; and whether or not these expenditures should be capped, and, if so, under what criteria. Many people with lifelong disabilities establish a "disability identity" in their adaptation to their limitations and may desire (costly) life-sustaining treatment. In contrast, people who are either newly disabled or nondisabled may see future life as a disabled person as so burdensome that they may refuse extraordinary medical treatments and/or actively seek to end their lives (Hahn and Belt, 2004).

Newer genetic technologies offer hope for the prevention and cure of disease. However, people with disabilities caution that these scientific advances could be used to eliminate people with disabilities. Advocacy groups, such as Not Dead Yet, have taken a strong stance against physician-assisted suicide, fearing it will lead to the early or forced death of people with disabilities. Parents who seek cochlear implants for their deaf children often encounter opposition from deaf advocacy groups, which argue that people should accept deafness because deafness benefits the client through deaf culture and additional skills, such as sign language. People with disabilities who need assistance with ADLs and IADLs commonly find that social welfare programs have limited funding for

---

BOX 21-3   SPIRITUAL ISSUES AND DISABILITY

Assessment

Theresa is a 29-year-old, single, separated mother of two children, an 8-year-old daughter and a 5-year-old son. Her husband left her shortly after the premature birth of Joseph. He has cerebral palsy with serious intellectual and physical disabilities. In the months and early years following Joseph's birth, Theresa experienced an intense and prolonged questioning of God. She remarks:

In the beginning, I used to ask Him, "Why me?" I was upset. I had little hope, little faith, but I stuck to it. I knew it was going to get better, I just didn't know when. ... It's been tough for me as a single parent. What I've been through has made me stronger. Now I thank God for my boy. But when he was born, I thought God was punishing me. ...I didn't understand how God could give me a problem like this, when I had so many problems to begin with. (Treloar, 1999a, p. 111)

Nursing Diagnosis

Spiritual suffering related to establishing meaning for disability as manifested by repeated questioning and blaming of God

Commentary

Disability is an unexpected event, often with what feel like tragic consequences. Although disability may not be easy to adapt to, declining capabilities more commonly occur with aging and chronic illness. However, we do not expect disability to strike in the prime of our lives or with the birth of a new child.

Regardless of our religious perspectives, we are all spiritual beings who seek meaning for the events that occur in our lives. Even people with established spiritual beliefs may question their relationship with God. Community health nurses who are comfortable with their own spirituality should assess for spiritual needs and provide appropriate spiritual care for people affected by disabilities. In talking directly with the person or family about these needs, the nurse does not push his or her version of spiritual beliefs. The nurse creates a climate that invites people to incorporate religious rituals, connect with clergy, and address spiritual needs according to their preferences. However, when people's spiritual needs are unrecognized and unmet, spiritual distress may linger, causing disruption in other parts of their lives.

---

community-based living and judge it less expensive to place PWD in long-term care settings. According to Hahn and Belt (2004), the disability rights movement was started by students who refused to live in nursing homes.

Like any ethical problem, issues related to disability do not have easy solutions. However, societal attitudes toward and bias against people with disabilities may negatively influence policies and decisions related to the interests and fair treatment of PWD. Disability rights proponents recognize that the devaluation of PWD may promote their unnecessary and untimely deaths. In 2009, plans for health care reform heightened their concerns, knowing that PWD might be viewed as "life unworthy of life" or "burdens upon society" (Ne'eman, 2009). Ethical decision making cannot be separated from discussions that include the meaning associated with life and life's accompanying challenges. The case of Terri Schaivo, described in the Ethical Insights box, illustrates some of these issues.

When Is Life Worth Continuing?

The world watched while Terri Schiavo's situation unfolded amid numerous legal and legislative challenges surrounding whether her feeding tube should be discontinued, and conflict developed between her parents and her husband and guardian, Michael. Disability rights groups and right-to-life advocates kept vigil for weeks outside the nursing home where Terri resided. Terri, a 41-year-old brain-damaged woman, died on March 31, 2005, 7 years after experiencing an anoxic event that led to her condition. Although previous court decisions have clearly established a person's right to discontinuation of treatment, including the provision of food and fluids, there was no documentation or advance directive indicating Terri's wishes. Terri's parents offered to assume guardianship of their daughter, believing her to be both responsive to her environment and desiring life in her current condition. Michael fought to have her feeding tube removed, stating that in previous discussions Terri had said that, in a similar situation, she would not want to continue living. Medical discussions focused on the extent of her "vegetative state" and capacity to respond to her environment. Seven years later, amid numerous court challenges and Michael's obtaining a reported million-dollar-plus malpractice settlement designated for his wife's care, the court ordered that Terri's feeding tube and all hydration be stopped as requested by her husband. She died several days later.

What do you think? When is life meaningless? What are the relevant issues when families are in conflict about what medical treatment the person with a severe disability would want in the absence of written advanced directives? What values and ethical principles should be considered? Williams (2005), a physician, suggests that a key question to be considered is "How should we have looked at Terri? Was she a person (or nonperson) in a persistent vegetative state, perhaps with diminished rights, or was she a severely handicapped person with rights that were not considered fairly?" When medical care is futile (i.e., useless or burdensome), it *should* be stopped; however, what guides our practice when treatment, such as artificial nutrition through a feeding tube, is withdrawn because a life is seen to have no value or the care of that person is deemed excessively burdensome?

Many hoped that the Patient Self-Determination Act of 1990 would motivate people to prepare advance directives for decision making in life-threatening illness. However, many people do not consider these issues, leaving families as surrogates to decide what the individual would want. Hopefully, Terri's case, which polarized the nation on what should be done in her situation, has stimulated people to think through, discuss with loved ones, and complete advance directives that are communicated to a health care provider.

LIVING WITH A DISABILITY

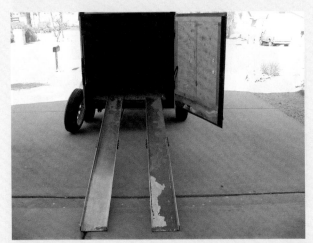

Creative wheelchair transport. People with disabilities and their families become experts at adapting to their environment. Joy's father built these folding ramps for use with her wheelchair. Unfortunately, many families lack easy access to a vehicle equipped with a wheelchair lift, or accessible public transportation. This lack affects their ability to obtain health care, to accomplish instrumental activities of daily living, and to compete with others on an equal level.

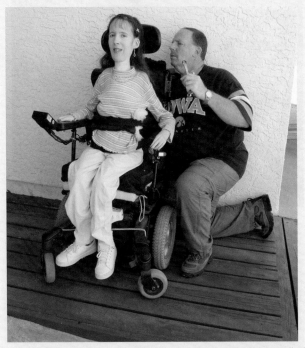

Father Bob adjusting Joy's wheelchair. Obtaining durable medical equipment that fits properly and meets a disabled person's specific needs often challenges therapist and client alike. Commonly, families with disabled members learn to modify and repair wheelchairs and other adaptive equipment—another way in which family and client become experts in the care of the person with a disability.

LIVING WITH A DISABILITY—cont'd

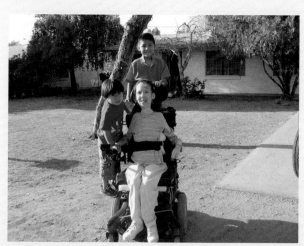

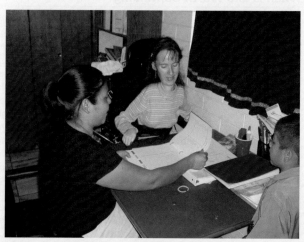

I want a ride, too! Joy rents a home that she shares with her care-giver family. The Hispanic couple's children began riding on Joy's lap in a carrier harness when they were babies. As young children, they delight in climbing onto Joy's wheelchair and helping her shop for groceries at the corner fruit and vegetable market. Joy comments, "When children see me they ask questions out of curiosity, while adults practice avoidance." Joy comments further, "Being in a wheelchair is one part of me—it doesn't define who I am. After a while, people don't see my wheelchair."

Preparing teacher lesson plans. Joy teaches underprivileged students in an inner-city grade school. As a college student, she faced bias from education faculty, who questioned the appropriateness of her dream to be a teacher. Admittedly, they lacked experience in working with a teacher or student with a disability. A few advocated for her, and she persevered and fulfilled her career goal. Despite the Americans with Disabilities Act, discrimination and misunderstanding continue to influence the lives of people with disabilities, stimulating some to fight and others to give up.

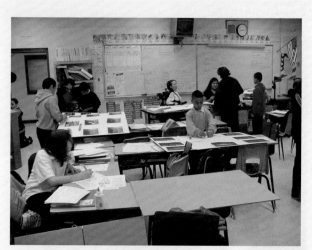

Science fair preparations.

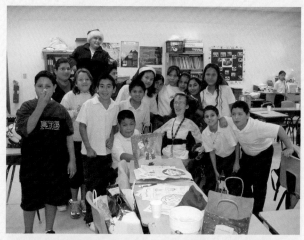

Teacher Joy and her class. Joy's students like the fact that they are at her eye level (although some tower over her). Students quickly learn to actively help their teacher and one another. Joy uses a variety of resources to teach concepts that may be challenging because of her physical limitations. They include the use of volunteers like Joy's dad (Bob) who assist students with science experiments.

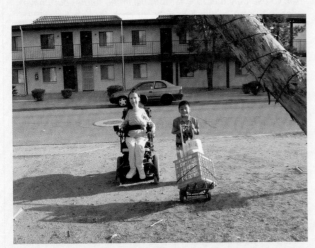

Unloading after a day of teaching. Joy uses "Dial-A-Ride" (commonly described as "Dial-A-Wait") to travel to and from her job and to run errands. Local bus service is another option but can be problematic because of bus route scheduling, broken-down lifts, and sometimes surly bus drivers.

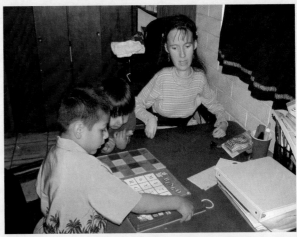

Joy lives in a multicultural world where Spanish is the dominant language spoken by people in her home and at school. Joy contributes to and benefits from being part of two families—that of her parents and her Hispanic caregiver family. Nurses with a community focus recognize and support human networks that encourage and move one another toward well-being.

When the Nurse Has a Disability

Under the ADA, nursing education programs and employers must provide reasonable accommodations for qualified students and nurses, unless doing so would impose an undue burden or hardship on the institution or employer as established by law. A qualified student or nurse must be able to meet the requirements of the clinical experience or job with reasonable accommodations, removal of barriers, and provision of appropriate aids (e.g., amplified stethoscope for someone with a hearing impairment) and services (e.g., scribe or translator). Institutions are not expected to lower their standards for an unqualified student or nurse.

Because "technical" aspects of nursing practice (e.g., bed making) tend to discriminate against nurses with physical or sensory disabilities, nursing should emphasize its "humanistic" capacities (Carroll, 2004). The art and science of nursing practice reflect a specialized knowledge base applied through interpersonal caring. Skilled nurses continuously gather and critically analyze data about their clients and families. The type of setting influences whether a nurse with a disability is qualified to perform the essential functions of the job. For example, a nurse with serious physical disabilities may be qualified to practice nursing when providing telephone triage. However, the same nurse may be unqualified to practice nursing in a medical-surgical setting or emergency department, where physical lifting and similar movements are essential functions of the job.

Although concerns about client safety and competing rights (individual vs. societal) must be considered, people with disabilities are excluded too often from nursing educational programs and practice on the basis of what a person cannot do rather than how or where access could be created to allow the person to practice nursing. Nurses must consider how personal attitudes toward people with disabilities influence not only their client care but also their responses to nursing students and colleagues with disabilities. Sowers and Smith (2004), who surveyed 88 nursing faculty members in eight programs on their perceptions, knowledge, and concerns regarding nursing students with disabilities, wrote:

Perhaps the most positive and hopeful finding of this study was that respondents recognized that they needed to learn more about disability issues and how to teach and accommodate students with disabilities....There is still a desperate need for faculty training, not only about the law, but also about the ability of people with disabilities to successfully complete nursing school and to be practicing nurses, as well as about the strategies that are effective in making this a reality for them. (p. 218)

CASE STUDY   APPLICATION OF THE NURSING PROCESS

Assessment

This narrative report on lived experience in an acute care setting provides community-based nurses with rich material for application as a case study.

Situation: Joy, shown in the photo novella in this chapter and at the end of this Case Study, is 33 years old. On June 30, 2008, Joy went to her primary care physician (PCP) who sent her for a swallowing test when she reported experiencing progressive swallowing difficulties. She shares her story:

I already knew the diagnosis. I'd had the beginning of symptoms since October of 2007. The swallowing test on July 2 confirmed the epiglottis no longer functioned and advised me to stop eating and drinking. There was no surgeon appointment for a week, so the PCP recommended I go to the emergency department (ER) the evening of July 4 and faxed the records for a feeding tube to be placed that evening.

When I reached the ER, the doctor chose to give me intravenous sedation for the percutaneous endoscopic gastrostomy (PEG) tube placement, but I stopped breathing. After that my heart stopped as well. They resuscitated me. They tried to put a tube down my mouth for the ventilator, but couldn't, so they did a tracheotomy. I went into a coma. They told Cristofer (my caregiver) to go home; that I wouldn't wake up. The doctors did not give any hope, but Cristofer came back to the house and spent the night praying for me. He called my mom the next morning. When I came out of the coma the following day, I was swollen all over with fluid. Cristofer provided me with the details of what was happening and communicated my wishes to the staff. His priority was to honor my wishes and support me completely in all ways. I was in the intensive care unit (ICU) for 1 week, and then transferred to a smaller hospital where I began the process of weaning off the ventilator.

A week later they attempted with twilight anesthesia to put the tube down my throat in order to place the PEG tube, but they were unsuccessful. A week later, they placed a feeding jejunostomy tube (J tube) with radiologic guidance and without using anesthesia. I didn't want to be put asleep, which was against their recommendations, but I didn't want the risk of my lungs or heart stopping even though I was on a ventilator. So I signed a consent with a stipulation that I was not to be under anesthesia. [Q: How bad was the pain?] Horrible, like nothing you can imagine, but better than the risk. They tried to give me pain medication or things to relax me but I refused. I choose to live without medication, with the constant support of my caregivers and their creativity in making me comfortable and content.

Now a balance had to be found for the continuous-feed formula used in the feeding tube. I am allergic to milk and milk products, so special food had to be ordered. Despite signs and reports to avoid milk in my formula, a mistake was made, causing continual abdominal pain and nausea. We looked at the formula can in the trash and discovered the cause. It contained milk products. On another occasion, a change was made in the formula, increasing the fat content from 3% to 35%, due to my lack of muscle tissue, so that my body could more effectively store and use proteins and amino acids. However, my body could not digest this level of fat, and this again resulted in abdominal pain and nausea. Hospital staff did not realize this was the cause of my reaction. I refused the new formula and asked for the old formula, suspecting this was the cause. It was. However, I could not stay on 3% fat without long-term damage to my liver and pancreas. So, my dad and I made a simple plan to mix the formulas. The dietary staff wanted the

plan to use only the 35% fat formula in the future, but I have chosen to stay on the 50%/50% of each formula for a 17% daily fat intake. My weight remains stable on that formula.

My only means of communication was by someone reading my lips or speaking with an alphabet board. Cristofer made an alphabet board on paper when I was in ICU so that I could communicate my wants and needs. Within a matter of days, he learned to read my lips, allowing us to communicate for a couple of hours at a time. This allowed me to express myself beyond just my basic physical needs. Each evening I moved from the hospital bed to a recliner chair brought from my home, which allowed me to change positions and be more comfortable for a time. This was possible because my caregiver was with me every night and moved me. With support and encouragement, God provided people in my life to give me the strength for each step in my recovery.

I weaned off the ventilator in about 6 weeks, despite medical beliefs that it was not possible due to poor lung function. I liked my pulmonologist. He was willing to look outside the box and consider how my body reacted and trust my instincts and my knowledge about my own body.

When in the hospital, even after weaning off the ventilator, I was unable to speak audibly. I was given a Passy-Muir [speaking] Valve, but was unable to tolerate it without choking in order to speak. About 6 weeks after coming home, I was able to use the valve for a few hours at a time. Gradually, I increased the time of usage.

After 2 months in the hospital, I went home using a feeding tube, 2 L oxygen, and a custom Jackson tracheostomy, which had to be cut and shaped to fit in my trachea. When I left the hospital, the recommendation was a nursing home but I did not consider that as an option. I was going home and had live-in caregivers responsible for my care. Equipment and supplies were delivered and my room was set up with all the things I would use. My caregiver family took responsibility for my 24-hour care, always having someone with me. Two months after arriving home, I stopped using oxygen and the humidified air. I have always struggled with breathing when it is humid. Despite warning [from medical personnel] that humidity is necessary for the trach, I discontinued its use because it stimulated the overproduction of secretions and required continual suctioning due to choking. Shortly after, my need for suctioning decreased to a few times a week. I made this decision, as all others, with the support of my caregivers, without doctor consent.

Although I am unable to return to teaching classes in person, I am still able to provide knowledge and experience to others through the computer and Internet. This provides distraction for me and a sense of normalcy. People in my community assist me with these activities, while others share the responsibility of my 24-hour care.

Author's note: The original chapter author, Dr. Linda Treloar (2011), assumed the role of community-based nurse in helping Joy write her plan of care.

Diagnosis

Individual

- Lifestyle adaptation required related to inability to resume role responsibilities
- Compromised verbal ability related to weakened respiratory muscles (speaking requires expiring adequate air through Passy-Muir Valve over trach)
- Receptiveness for increased comfort related to thin body habitus, immobility, and bed rest

CASE STUDY APPLICATION OF THE NURSING PROCESS—cont'd

- Risk for inadequate airway status related to collection of secretions in trach
- Risk for inadequate nutritional status: less than body requirements related to formula mixture and/or feeding tube

Caregiver Family
- Risk for caregiver burnout related to 24-hour care of Joy

Community
- Adequate community-based resource support related to history of support

Planning
Joy considers the recommendations of health care providers; alters care on the basis of knowledge of what works best for her with the support of caregivers.

Individual
Long-Term Goals
- Joy will verbalize acceptable adaptation to limitations related to immobility, trach, and feeding tube as indicated by, "I am still able to provide knowledge and experience to others."
- Joy will report ability to verbally communicate 3 hours at a time related to trach as indicated by increasing ease and time of use for Passy-Muir [speaking] Valve over trach.
- Joy will verbalize an acceptable level of comfort related to thin body habitus, immobility, and bed rest.
- Improved airway clearance related to trach as indicated by reduced collection of secretions and frequency of suctioning.
- Nutritional status, balanced related to feeding tube as indicated by maintenance of weight and absence of GI upset.

Short-Term Goals
- Joy will resume limited activities (e.g., educational) of 1-2 hours per day as tolerated within 6 weeks after hospital discharge.
- Joy will report an additional 15 minutes of verbal communication per week using the trach speaking valve until able to tolerate periods of 3 hours.

Caregiver Family
Long-Term Goal
- Effective family therapeutic regimen related to caring for Joy and family unit as indicated by harmonious, collaborative relationship with clear roles, intact boundaries, etc.

Short-Term Goals
- Caregivers and Joy make collaborative decisions based on needs of Joy and caregivers on ongoing basis.
- Caregivers and Joy verbalize mutual benefits of their relationship within 1 month.

Community
Long-Term Goal
- Joy's neighborhood community will provide caregivers and assistance as needed.

Short-Term Goal
- Caregivers, in collaboration with Joy, will educate other caregivers, as needed.

Intervention and Evaluation
Individual
- *Intervention:* Within 6 weeks following hospital discharge, Joy reduced the feeding tube rate from 55 mL/hr to 40 mL/hr due to abdominal discomfort.

- *Evaluation:* She reports feeling "less overfull," but not hungry.
- *Intervention:* Within 6 weeks following hospital discharge, Joy discontinued use of Prevacid (for reflux) after it repeatedly plugged the feeding tube.
- *Evaluation:* Joy no longer experiences acid reflux with the lower feeding tube rate.
- *Evaluation:* One year after being home, Joy's trach typically requires weekly suctioning unless there is increased humidity.
- *Intervention:* Joy comments, "On most weekends, one of my caregivers carries me from my bed to a recliner in the living room so that I can be in a different position and setting. The equipment is moved as well."
- *Evaluation:* This promotes Joy's personal well-being and provides additional comfort and normalcy. "My care is based on my needs and my schedule, rather than on a predetermined generic plan. One size does *not* fit all."

Caregiver Family
- *Intervention:* Cristofer learned suctioning and trach care in the hospital and taught other caregivers.
- *Evaluation:* Joy and caregivers adapted her care to meet her needs.

Community
- Joy budgets and directs the use of her disability benefits to provide for self (e.g., includes household rent and expenses) and pays caregivers.

Levels of Prevention

Primary
Prevention of choking and potential aspiration through 24 hr/day caregivers and oral suctioning as needed (primary level modified according to situation).

Secondary
Inspect skin and change position no less than every 2 hours to prevent skin breakdown secondary to immobility.

Tertiary
Caregivers' priority is to maintain Joy as head of household, providing information required for fully informed decisions

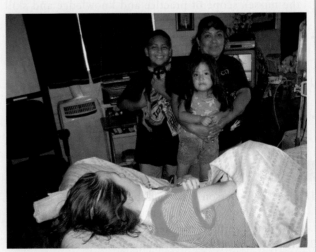

Joy and her caregiver family: Cristina and children, 10-year-old Carlos holding Paco, and 2½-year-old Alejandra.

Continued

CASE STUDY APPLICATION OF THE NURSING PROCESS—cont'd

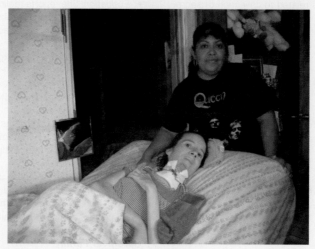

Joy and caregiver Cristina.

Photos taken by Dr. Linda Treloar.

SUMMARY

Community health nurses must recognize that there are a variety of personal and societal perspectives on disability with accompanying moral or ethical issues. They should practice holistic nursing care that incorporates mind, body, and spiritual care considerations into health care practice. To this end, nurses can do the following:

- Become familiar with a variety of ethical frameworks for decision making, and learn a strategy to analyze ethical problems related to health care for people with disabilities.
- Help the client and family access needed information from the health care team to make informed decisions that reflect their interests and priorities.
- Help educate the public on health care issues within the nurse's scope of practice and knowledge and skill level.
- Participate in the development of institutional policies and procedures for ethical and legal issues related to disability.
- Take a position on an ethical issue with political implications.
- Work to influence governmental policies and laws related to disability.

LEARNING ACTIVITIES

1. Interview a person with a disability or his or her family member about their experiences with health care providers and the health care system.
2. Shadow a nurse in a community health clinic that serves children with disabilities. Observe the roles and the interactions of the multidisciplinary team members. Follow a family through their clinic visit. If possible, meet the family at their home before the clinic visit, and observe their preparations for it. Accompany them from clinic check-in to departure. After returning to their home, ask them for their thoughts on the clinic experience.
3. Interview a community resident with a serious disability. How does the resident view himself or herself? What challenges or concerns does the resident mention? Interview a caregiver about the caregiving experience.
4. Ask an experienced nurse about his or her encounters with people with disabilities. Listen to his or her language and perceptions of disability. Compare these with the perspectives reflected in the social construct model for disability.
5. Visit with the residents and staff in a community-based living environment for people with disabilities. Assist with caregiving for the residents.
6. Visit one or two community agencies that provide services to people with disabilities. How do families gain access to services and what services are offered? How do available services and resources address the needs of a person with a disability and his or her family?
7. Spend time in the home of a family who has a child with intellectual disabilities. Note the family relationships. Interview the parents and siblings about their experiences with the child. Spend time with the child.

REFERENCES

Agency on Healthcare Research and Quality: *2008 National healthcare disparities report*, 2008. Available from <http://www.ahrq.gov>.

Anderson D, Dumont S, Jacobs P, et al: The personal costs of caring for a child with a disability: a review of the literature, *Public Health Rep* 122(1):3–16, 2007.

Arc: *The first 50 years*, 2009. Available from <www.thearc.org/NetCommunity/Page.aspx?pid=269>.

Arc: *History of the Arc*, 2013. Available from <http://www.thearc.org/page.aspx?pid=2344>.

Artinian BM, West K, Conger M, editors: *The Artinian Intersystem Model: intergration theory and practice for the professional nurse*, ed 2, NY, NY, 2011, Springer Publishing Company.

Baigent C, Blackwell L, Collins R, et al: Aspirin in the primary and secondary prevention of vascular disease: collaborative meta-analysis of individual participant data from randomised trials, *Lancet* 373(9678):1849–1860, 2009.

Barnes C: Theories of disability and the origins of the oppression of disabled people in Western society. In Barton L, editor: *Disability and society: emerging issues and insights*, New York, 1996, Longman.

Batavia AI: Relating disability policy to broader public policy: understanding the concept of "handicap,", *Policy Stud J* 21(4):735–739, 1993.

Batra S: Defining disability: development milestones and interventions for primary prevention, *Learning Community: An International Journal of Education and Social Development* 1(2):157–166, 2010.

Birenbaum A: Poverty, welfare reform, and disproportionate rates of disability among children, *Ment Retard* 40:212–218, 2002.

Bodde A, Seo D, Frey G, et al: The effect of a designed health education intervention on physical activity knowledge and participation of adults with intellectual disabilities, *Am J Health Promotion* 26(5):313–316, 2012.

Brault MW: *Americans with disabilities: 2005 (Current Population Reports P70–117)*, 2008. Available from <www.census.gov/2008pubs/p70-117.pdf>.

Brault MW: *Americans with disabilities: 2010 (Current Population Reports P70–131)*, 2012. Available from <http://www.census.gov/prod/2012pubs/p70-131.pdf>.

Campbell A, Uren A: 'The invisibles'... : Disability in China in the 11st Century, *Intl J of Special Ed* 26(1):12–24, 2011.

Carroll SM: Inclusion of people with physical disabilities in nursing education, *J Nurs Educ* 43(5):207–212, 2004.

Centers for Disease Control and Prevention: *Disability data: pneumonia vaccine-1 year at a time*, 2011. Available from <http://dhds.cdc.gov/dataviews/tabular?viewId=952&geoId=4&subsetId=&z=1>.

Centers for Disease Control and Prevention: *Autism spectrum disorders: data and statistics*, 2013. Available from <http://www.cdc.gov/ncbddd/autism/data.html>.

Chiang LH, Hadadian A: Raising children with disabilities in China: the need for early interventions, *International Journal of Special Education* 25(2):113–118, 2010.

Child and Adolescent Health Measurement Initiative: *2009/10 National Survey of Children with Special Health Care Needs*, 2012. Available from <http://www.childhealthdata.org/browse/survey/>.

Cuskelly M: Challenging the myths and redressing the missteps in family research, *Journal of Policy Practice in International Disabilities* 6(2):86–88, 2009.

Davis K, Gavidia-Payne S: The impact of child, family, and professional support characteristics on the quality of life in families of young children with disabilities, *Journal of Intellectual and Development Disability* 34(2):153–162, 2009.

Dresser R: Prenatal testing and disability: a truce in the culture wars? *Hastings Cent Rep* 39(3):7–8, 2009.

Dwight V: Aidan's gift. In Klein SD, Schive K, editors: *You will dream new dreams: inspiring personal stories by parents of children with disabilities*, New York, 2001, Kensington, pp 31–37.

Eskay M, Onu VC, Igbo JN, et al: Disability within the African culture, *US-China Review* B4:473–484, 2012.

Euthanasia program, Megargee GP, editor: *The United States Holocaust Memorial Museum Encyclopedia of Camps and Ghettos, 1933–1945* (vol. 1). 2009. Available from < www.ushmm.org/wlc/article.php?lang=en&;ModuleId=10005200.>.

Freedman BH, Kalb LG, Zablotsky B, et al: Relationship status among parents of children with autism spectrum disorders: a population-based study, *Journal of Autism Developmental Disorders* 42:539–548, 2012, http://dx.doi.org/10.1007/s10803-011-1269-y.

Gentile JK, Ten Hoedt AE, Bosch AM: Psychosocial aspects of PKU: hidden disabilities—a review, *Molecular Genetics and Metabolism* 99(Suppl):S64–S67, 2010.

Gibbons LJ, Lehr K, Selekman J: Federal laws protecting children and youth with disabilities in the schools. In Selekman J, editor: *School nursing: a comprehensive text*, ed 2, Philadelphia, PA, 2013, F.A. Davis & Company, pp 257–283.

Green A: Prenatal testing goes to court, *Oregon-Live.Com/The Oregonian* June 14, 2009. Available from <www.oregonlive.com/news/oregonian/index.ssf?/base/news/1244872511325030.xml&;coll=7&thispage=3>.

Hahn H, Belt TL: Disability identity and attitudes toward cure in a sample of disabled activists, *J Health Soc Behav* 45:453–464, 2004.

Hamiwka LD, Yu CG, Hamiwka LA, Sherman EMS, Anderson B, Wirrell E: Are children with epilepsy at greater risk for bullying than their peers? *Epilepsy & Behavior* 15:500–505, 2009.

Hayes J, Hannold EM: The road to empowerment: a historical perspective on the medicalizationof disability, *J Health Hum Serv Adm.* 30(3):352–377, 2007.

Health Media Lab: *Franklin Delano Roosevelt (1933–1945), the dying president*, 2004. Available from <www.healthmedialab.com/html/president/roosevelt.html>.

Healthy People.gov: *Healthy People 2020: immunization and infectious diseases*, 2012. Available from <http://healthypeople.gov/2020/topicsobjectives2020/objectiveslist.aspx?topicId=23>.

Kaplan D: *The definition of disability*, n.d. Available from <www.accessiblesociety.org/topics/demographics-identity/dkaplanpaper.htm>.

Kearney PM, Griffin T: Between joy and sorrow: being a parent of a child with developmentaldisability, *J Adv Nurs* 34:582–592, 2001.

Lawthers AG, Pransky GS, Peterson LE, et al: Rethinking quality in the context of persons with disability, *Int J Qual Health Care* 15(4):287–299, 2003.

Longmore PK: Uncovering the hidden history of people with disabilities, *Rev Am Hist* 15(3)355–364, 1987.

Mackenzie I, Smith A: Deafness-the neglected and hidden disability, *Annals of Tropical Medicine and Parasatology* 7:565–571, 2009.

Madaus J: Employment self-disclosure rates and rationales with university graduates with learning disabilities, *Journal of Learning Disabilities* 41(4):291–299, 2008.

Martiniello N: *Disability in the media [see chapters 6–8]*, 2009. Available from <www.trinimex.ca/disabilityinmedia/index.htm>.

May M, Kennedy C: Health and problem behavior among people with intellectual disabilities, *Behavior Analysis in Practice* 3(2):4–12, 2010.

Minkler M, Fadem P: "Successful aging": a disability perspective, *Journal of Disability Policy Studies* 12:229–235, 2002.

Mont D: Measuring health and disability, *Lancet* 369:1658–1663, 2007.

Morris B: *Synapse: Reconnecting lives: how friends and extended family can help*, 2008. Available from <http://www.autism-help.org/family-friends-support-autism.htm>.

Multicultural Disability Advocacy Association (MDAA): *Ethnic Diversity and Disability*, 2010. Available from <http://www.mdaa.org.au/resources/ethnic-diversity-and-disability>.

Murphy RF: *The body silent*, New York, 1990, Henry Holt.

Murakami Y, Meyer H: Culture, institutions, and disability policy in Japan: the translation of culture into policy, *Comparative Sociology* 9:202–221, 2010.

National Association of School Nurses: *Section 504 and individuals with disabilities education improvement act – the role of the school nurse*, 2013. Available from <http://www.nasn.org/PolicyAdvocacy/PositionPapersandReports/NASNPositionStatementsFullView/tabid/462/ArticleId/491/Section-504-and-Individuals-with-Disabilities-Education-Improvement-Act-The-Role-of-the-School-Nurse>.

National Center on Education, Disability and Juvenile Justice: *Prevention.* Available from <http://www.edjj.org/prevention/LevelsPrevention.html>.

National Dissemination Center for Children with Disabilities: *Home page.* Available from <www.nichcy.org>.

National Survey of Children with Special Health Care Needs: *Child and adolescent health measurement initiative,* 2009/10. Available from <www.childhealthdata.org/learn/NS-CSHCN>.

Ne'eman A: *Health care reform and the disability community, The Huffington Post* May 21, 2009. Available from <www.huffingtonpost.com/ari-neeman/health-care-reform-and-th_b_206492.html>.

Pfeiffer D: Overview of the disability movement: history, legislative record, and political implications, *Policy Stud J* 21(4):724–734, 1993.

Pope AM, Tarlov AR, editors: *Disability in America: toward a national agenda for prevention,* Washington, DC, 1991, National Academy Press.

Reichman NE, Corman H, Noonan K: Impact of child disability on the family, *Matern Child Health J* 12(6):679–683, 2008. Also available from <www.medscape.com/viewarticle/581577_2>.

Rimmer J, Chen MD, Hsieh K: A conceptual model for identifying, preventing, and managing secondary conditions in people with disabilities, *Physical Therapy* 91(12):1728–1739, 2011.

Rubin SE, Millard RP: Ethical principles and American public policy on disability, *J Rehabil,* January-March 1991. Available from <http://findarticles.com/p/articles/mi_m0825/is_n1_v57/ai_10684712/?tag=content;col1>.

Scotch RK: Understanding disability policy: varieties of analysis, *Policy Stud J* 22(1):170–175, 1994.

Silvers A, Wasserman D, Mahowald MB: *Disability, difference, discrimination: perspectives on justice in bioethics and public policy,* Lanham, MA, 1998, Rowman & Littlefield.

Social Security Administration: Definition of disability. In *2009 Social Security Administration Redbook,* 2009a. Available from <www.ssa.gov/redbook/eng/overview-disability.htm#5>.

Social Security Administration: *The Red Book: Guide to Work Incentives,* 2014. Available from <http://www.gsocialsecurity.gov/redbook/index.html>.

Sowers J, Smith MR: Nursing faculty members' perceptions, knowledge, and concerns about students with disabilities, *J Nurs Educ* 43(5):213–218, 2004.

Stopbullying.gov: *Bullying definition,* 2013. Available from <http://www.stopbullying.gov/what-is-bullying/definition/index.html>.

Staples J: Culture and carelessness: constituting disability in South India, *Medical Anthropology Quarterly* 26(4):557–574, 2012.

Ticket to Work and Work Incentives Advisory Panel: *Annual report to the President, Congress, and the Commissioner of SSA, Year Eight,* 2007. Available from <www.ssa.gov/work/panel/panel_documents/FORMAT%20-%20Final%20Report-;121707.pdf>.

Treloar LL: *Perceptions of spiritual beliefs, response to disability, and the church, Unpublished doctoral dissertation,* Cincinnati, Ohio, 1999a, Union Institute and University.

Treloar LL: *Unpublished interviews,* 1999b.

Treloar LL: Disability, spiritual beliefs and the church: the experiences of adults with disabilities and family members, *J Adv Nurs* 40(5):594–603, 2002.

Treloar, LL: Populations affected by disabilities. In Nies, M and McEwen M. (eds). Community/public health nursing: Promoting the health of populations. 2011, St. Louis,Elsevier.

Twyman KA, Saylor CF, Saia D, Macias MM, Taylor LA, Spratt E: Bullying and ostracism experiences in children with special health care needs, *J Developmental Behavioral Pediatrics* 31:1–8, 2010.

U.S. Census Bureau: *American community survey: population: question on disability,* 2010a. Available from <http://www.census.gov/acs/www/Downloads/QbyQfact/disability.pdf>.

U.S. Census Bureau: *Survey of income and program participation,* 2010b. Available from <http://www.census.gov/prod/2012pubs/p70-131.pdf>.

U.S. Census Bureau, Housing and Household Economic Statistics Division: *Definition of disability varies by survey,* 2006. Available from <http://www.census.gov/hhes/www/disability/disab_defn.html#CPS>.

U.S. Census Bureau, Newsroom: *Nearly 1 in 5 people have a disability in the U.S., Census Bureau reports,* 2012. Available from <http://www.census.gov/newsroom/releases/archives/miscellaneous/cb12-134.html>.

U.S. Department of Education: *Prohibited disability harassment: reminder of responsibilities under Section 504 of the Rehabilitation Act of 1973 and Title II of the Americans with Disabilities Act,* 2000. Available from <www.ed.gov/about/offices/list/ocr/docs/disabharasslt r.html>.

U.S. Department of Education: *Family educational rights and privacy; final rule,* 2008. Available from <http://www2.ed.gov/legislation/FedRegister/finrule/2008-4/120908a.html>.

U.S. Department of Justice, Civil Rights Division: *ADA home page,* 2009. Available from <www.ada.gov/>.

Ulrich ME, Bauer AM: Levels of awareness: a closer look at communication between parents and professionals, *Teaching Exceptional Children* 35(6):20–24, 2003.

Valeras AB: "We don't have a box": Understanding hidden disability identity utilizing narrative research methodology, *Disability Studies Quarterly* 30(3/4), 2010. Also available from <http://dsq-sds.org/article/view/1267/1297>.

Walsh PN: Health indicators and intellectual disability, *Curr Opin Psychiatry* 21(5):474–478, 2008. Also available from <www.medscape.com/viewarticle/581738?src=emailthis>.

Wilkinson JE, Cerreto MC: Primary care for women with intellectual disabilities, *J Am Board Fam Med* 21:215–222, 2008.

Williams H: Afterthoughts on Terri Schaivo. *Center for Bioethics and Culture Electronic Newsletter* May 5, 2005. Available from <www.thecbc.org/enewsletter/index.html>.

World Health Organization: *Disability and health,* 2012. Available from <http://www.who.int/mediacentre/factsheets/fs352/en/index.html>.

World Health Organization: *Disabilities,* 2013. Available from <http://www.who.int/topics/disabilities/en/>.

Homeless Populations

Nellie S. Droes and Diane C. Hatton

OBJECTIVES

Upon completion of this chapter, the reader will be able to do the following:

1. Discuss conceptual and legal approaches used to define *homelessness*.
2. Describe strategies used to estimate the prevalence of homelessness in the United States.
3. Identify demographic characteristics of the homeless population and its subpopulations.
4. Analyze three factors that contribute to homelessness.
5. Identify major health problems among various homeless aggregates.
6. Analyze the health status of populations who are homeless using the World Health Organization (WHO) definition of health.
7. Describe the federal health centers that provide health care services to homeless populations.
8. Plan community health nursing services based on knowledge of the social determinants of health and health status in this population.

KEY TERMS

Annual Homeless Assessment Report
Chronically homeless
continuum of care
Education for Homeless Children and Youth
European Federation of Organisations Working with the Homeless
Federally Qualified Health Centers
FQHC Look-A-Likes
military sexual trauma
point-in-time (PIT) count
U.S. Conference of Mayors

OUTLINE

Definitions, Prevalence, and Demographic Characteristics of Homelessness
    Definitions of Homelessness
    Prevalence of Homelessness
    Demographic Characteristics
Factors that Contribute to Homelessness
    Shortage of Affordable Housing
    Income Insufficiency
    Inadequacy and Scarcity of Supportive Services
    Homelessness and Causation
Health and Homeless Populations
    Federal Health Centers
Health Status of Homeless Population
    Adults
    Families with children
    Youth
    Chronically Homeless
Community/Public Health Nursing: Care of Homeless Populations
    Framework for Community/Public Health Nursing Care for Homeless Populations

The purpose of this chapter is to describe the scope of the homeless problem. The chapter presents definitions, prevalence, and it demographic characteristics of homelessness, and it describes the health status of selected aggregates of the homeless population. The chapter includes a discussion of the relationship between the factors that contribute to homelessness and the social determinants of health and of the implications of this relationship for community health nursing practice.

DEFINITIONS, PREVALENCE, AND DEMOGRAPHIC CHARACTERISTICS OF HOMELESSNESS

Definitions of Homelessness

Defining "homeless" and "homelessness" is not only complex but contested. Although a generally accepted agreement on the meaning of these terms is lacking, definitions are important in determining who should be counted, described, planned for, and assisted (Burt, Aron, and Lee, 2001; Murphy and Tobin, 2011; Shumsky, 2012). An exploration of the national and international homeless literature for the past decade reveals two approaches to defining homelessness, conceptual and legal. A brief overview of the conceptual approach used in Europe and Canada is presented next followed by discussion of the legal approach used in the United States.

Conceptual Approaches to Defining Homelessness

In 2005, the **European Federation of Organisations Working with the Homeless** (FEANTSA) launched the *European Typology of Homelessness and Housing Exclusion* (ETHOS) (European Federation of National Associations Working with the Homeless, 2011). In developing ETHOS, members of the *European Observatory on the Homeless*, the research arm of FEANTSA, used "home" as a basis for developing a definition of homelessness. From the ETHOS perspective, home was conceptualized as having three domains, *physical, social*, and *legal*. The *physical domain* meant having an adequate dwelling for which a person/family has exclusive possession; the *social domain* meant being able to maintain privacy and enjoy relations; the *legal domain* meant having exclusive possession, security of occupation, and legal title to occupation (Edgar, 2009). Building on the three domains of home, the European researchers designated four broad types of living situations to classify homeless people: *rooflessness, houselessness, insecure housing*, and *inadequate housing*. Each of these four categories is subdivided into more specific living situations to provide classifications useful for different purposes, such as determining for example, determining the extent of homelessness, developing policies, and evaluating interventions (European Federation of National Associations Working with the Homeless, 2011).

In 2012, building on ETHOS, the Canadian Homelessness Research Network provided a conceptual definition of homelessness that has four major categories: *unsheltered, emergency sheltered, provisionally accommodated, and at risk of homelessness*: Similar to the ETHOS, the Canadian definition is divided into more specific living situations, thereby providing more details to facilitate its use by different groups, such as governmental agents, service providers, and researchers. In contrast to ETHOS, the Canadian Research Network's definition includes a category that indicates an at-risk population (Canadian Homelessness Research Network, 2012).

For a more complete understanding of these two conceptual approaches to defining homelessness the reader is encouraged to visit the websites of the respective organizations. Setting the browser to search for FEANTSA and then searching within the site search for ETHOS should provide access to the complete typology. To locate the Canadian definition, one should access the Research Hub website and search for "homeless definition."

Legal Approaches to Defining Homelessness

In contrast to these previously discussed European and Canadian definitions of homelessness, which were developed by researchers, the U.S. definition has been determined by federal governmental legislative and administrative actions. These federal actions provide the statutory and regulatory basis for local homeless service providers, including program direction, funding resources, and eligibility criteria. Responsibility for implementing and managing the many federal homeless initiatives is assigned to seven different departments within the executive branch of the federal government, the Departments of: (1) Housing and Urban Development (HUD); (2) Education (ED); (3) Health and Human Resources (HHS); (4) Veterans Affairs (VA); (5) Homeland Security (DHS); (6) Justice (DOJ); and (7) Labor (DOL) (Perl et al, 2012).

Both HUD and ED administer homeless programs that hold considerable significance for community health nursing—HUD's *Homeless Assistance Grants* (U.S. Department of Housing and Urban Development [USHUD], Office of Community Planning and Development [OCPD], 2009b) and the ED's *Education for Homeless Children and Youth* (U.S Department of Education, 2001). A brief overview of these two programs and their definitions of homelessness follow.

HUD's Definitions of Homelessness. The *U.S. Code*, Title 42, Chapter 119 (U.S. House of Representatives, Office of the Law Revision Center, 2012) which is named "Homeless Assistance," contains two subchapters that provide homeless definitions. These are Subchapters I General Provisions and Subchapter VI Education and Training. The definitions in Subchapter I were broadened by the *McKinney-Vento Homeless Assistance (MVHA) Act as Amended by the Homeless Emergency Assistance and Rapid Transition to Housing (HEARTH) Act of 2009* (USHUD, OCPD, 2009b). Subsequent to the enactment of the HEARTH Act, the HUD issued regulations that summarized the statutory definitions in four descriptive categories, as follows (USHUD, OCPD, 2011):

Category 1. *Literally Homeless:* Individuals and families who lack a fixed, regular, and adequate nighttime residence and includes a subset for an individual who resided in an emergency shelter or a place not meant for human habitation and who is exiting an institution where he or she temporarily resided;

Category 2. *Imminent Risk of Homelessness:* Individuals and families who will imminently lose their primary nighttime residence;

Category 3. *Homeless Under Other Federal Statutes:* Unaccompanied youth and families with children and youth who are defined as homeless under other federal statutes who do not otherwise qualify as homeless under this definition; and

Category 4. *Fleeing/Attempting to Flee Domestic Violence (DV):* Individuals and families who are fleeing, or are attempting to flee, domestic violence, dating violence, sexual assault, stalking, or other dangerous or life-threatening conditions that relate to violence against the individual or a family member.

ED's Definition of Homeless Student. The ED administers the law known as McKinney-Vento Homeless Education Assistance Improvements Act of 2001, which is located in Subchapter VI of the *U.S. Code*. One of the intents of this law is to direct state and local educational agencies to take action to ensure that each child and each homeless youth has equal access to the same free, appropriate public education, including a public preschool education, as provided to other children and youths. The definitions, located in Part B, Section 11434a, are broader than the HUD definitions listed previously. These definitions include children and youth who are (USDE, 2001):

- Sharing the housing of other persons (frequently referred to as "doubling up")
- Abandoned in hospitals or
- Awaiting foster care placement

U.S. Department of Health and Human Services Definition of Homelessness. The U.S Department of Health and Human Services (HHS) also has definitions of who is considered homeless. The Runaway and Homeless Youth (RHY) Program is located in the Administration for Children & Families, Family and Youth Service Bureau, which are agencies within the HHS. The RHY program operates under legislation that has definitions for who is eligible for services; as defined in the statute, *runaway youth* is "a person under 18 years of age who absents himself or herself from home or place of legal residence without the permission of his or her family" and *homeless youth* is "a person under 18 years of age who is in need of services and without a place of shelter where he or she receives supervision and care" (USDHHS, Administration for Children & Families, Family and Youth Service Bureau, 2012).

In addition to these two definitions of youth, USDHHS uses a different definition in determining who is eligible for services provided through the Health Care for the Homeless (HCH) Program (see later section Health and Homeless Populations).

The next section presents information related to the number of people in the total U.S. homeless population and also in smaller subpopulations. HUD and ED are the two primary federal agencies with responsibility for reporting U.S. homeless prevalence estimates. The departments use their own, but differing definitions in their enumeration efforts.

Prevalence of Homelessness

Determining prevalence of homelessness requires not only definitions of who is counted but also how data are collected. Given the characteristics of the population and subpopulations of homeless people, obtaining accurate counts is difficult. Efforts to enumerate the homeless have evolved the over the past three decades. Earlier efforts included the U.S. Census Bureau's collections of national data on the homeless population in Census 1990 and Census 2000 (Smith and Smith, 2001) and an Urban Institute study conducted in 1996 (Burt et al, 2001). A brief sketch of more recent approaches to counting the homeless—those conducted by HUD and ED—follows.

HUD's Efforts to Count the Homeless

Two strategies used by HUD to strengthen the nation's efforts to reduce homelessness, including improvement in collecting

HEALTHY PEOPLE 2020

Objectives for Social Determinants of Health

Economic Stability
SHOH-1: Proportion of children aged 0-17 years living with at least one parent employed year round full time.
SDOH-3: Proportion of persons living in poverty.

Education
SDOH -2: Proportion of high school completers who were enrolled in college the October immediately after completing high school.

From U.S. Department of Health and Human Services: *Healthy People 2020: Social determinants of health,* 2013. Retrieved from <http://www.healthypeople.gov/2020/topicsobjectives2020/overview.aspx?topicid=39>.

prevalence data, are the **continuum of care** (CoC) concept and the Homeless Information Management System (HMIS). A brief overview of these two strategies follows.

HUD requires homeless service providers in each local community to collaborate and submit just one Continuum of Care application to HUD for funding, rather than allowing multiple providers to submit individual applications. If successful in obtaining funding, these CoC providers are then responsible for providing, to persons in the local area who are experiencing homelessness, a range of housing and related services, including emergency and preventive responses (USHUD, OCPD, 2009a).

The CoC providers are also responsible for implementing and managing the HMIS at the local level. The HMIS is a computerized database designed to facilitate collection of client-level data used to plan for service needs of homeless populations.

As a requirement of HUD funding, all groups of CoC providers conduct a **point-in-time (PIT) count** of *sheltered* homeless people on a single night in late January of *every year* and submit these data to HUD via HMIS (USHUD, 2012). In addition to the annual PIT count of sheltered homeless people, HUD requires that *every 2 years*, on odd years, the PIT count include both *sheltered and unsheltered* homeless people. Although not required, some CoC providers include unsheltered homeless people in their PIT counts on both even and odd years.

Since 2007, HUD has used the data submitted by local CoC providers via the HMIS to prepare an *Annual Homeless Assessment Report* (AHAR) that is delivered to Congress. The populations and subpopulations HUD used in the AHAR reflect the legislative and administrative definitions outlined previously. In addition to total population prevalence, the AHAR includes subpopulations—individuals, families, the chronically homeless, and veterans. Homeless children and youth enrolled in public schools are not included in HUD's HMIS. Responsibility for reporting information about this important subpopulation lies with the ED.

ED's Efforts to Count the Homeless

One of the main differences between the HUD and ED approaches to counting homeless people is based on definitions of who is considered homeless. As previously described, the ED uses a broad definition of homelessness that includes youth and families that are living with other households, or "doubled up." Consequently, the ED provides services to homeless children and youth who are not included in HUD's programmatic services. Children and youth whom the ED defines as homeless receive services through the Education for Homeless Children and Youth (ECHY) program.

To meet ECHY requirements the ED collects data on program performance from all state education agencies (SEAs) and local education agencies (LEAs). The number of homeless students enrolled in LEAs during each school year is part of the annual performance report. In addition, the ED collects information on students' night-time residence at the time they were determined eligible for EHCY services. This information is included in the Consolidated State Performance Record (CSPR), which the ED issues on an annual basis (National Center for Homeless Education, 2012).

Homeless Prevalence Estimates

These two federal departments, HUD and ED, issue summary reports of the sizes of homeless populations and subpopulations. Both departments provide annual estimates. HUD provides a PIT count as well; the results of the January 2012 count are summarized in Table 22-1.

The prevalence estimates outlined in Table 22-1 provide a "snapshot" of the homeless population taken on one night in January 2012 as reported in volume I of the 2012 AHAR. HUD also uses a different lens—the annual estimate—to produce another picture of the homeless population. In contrast to the one-night view, HUD's annual estimate is a count of the total number of people who used either shelters or

transitional housing during the course of a year. As of this writing, the most recently available annual estimates are for fiscal year 2010-2011; this information follows.

Annual National Estimate of Homeless Persons Use of Shelters and Transitional Housing 2010-2011

HUD reported the following numbers of people in the total population and in subpopulations who used shelters or transitional housing between October 1, 2010, and September 30, 2011 (USHUD, OCPD, 2012):

- 1,502,196 people in the total homeless population, a decrease of 5.4% since 2007;
- 984,469 *individuals,* a decrease of 11% since 2007;
- 537,414 *people in families,* an increase of 13.5% since 2007;
- 141,499 *veterans,* a decrease of 5.5% since 2007.

The population and subpopulations HUD included in the 2011 annual estimate of shelter use are based on the legislatively and administratively derived definitions outlined previously. The ED, using a broader definition of homeless families than HUD, provides information on the population of children and youth enrolled in public schools.

ED's Annual National Estimate of Homeless Students for 2010-2011 School Year

According to the ED (National Center for Homeless Education, 2012):

1,065,794 *homeless students* were enrolled during the 2010-2011 school year (SY), an increase of 11% over the 3-year period 2008-2009 to 2010-2011.

The *night-time residences* of homeless students at the time of establishing service eligibility were:

- 187,675 in shelters
- 767,968 doubled up
- 51,897 unsheltered
- 55,388 Hotels/Motels.

The following subpopulations of homeless students received services during SY 2010-2011:

- 55,066 *unaccompanied youths,* a 4% increase since SY 2008-9
- 12,717 *migratory children/youths,* a 55% increase since SY 2008-9
- 109,872 *children with disabilities,* a 51% increase since SY 2008-9
- 121,795 *limited-English-proficient students,* a 51% increase since 2008-2009.

The subpopulations listed here are not mutually exclusive; homeless students may be counted in one or more subpopulations.

U.S. Conference of Mayors' Hunger and Homelessness Survey 2012

In addition to the previously outlined national counts based on data generated by HUD and ED, the U.S Conference of Mayors provides an urban-local perspective on homelessness. Information on homeless populations in the cities whose mayors are members of the U.S. Conference of Mayors Taskforce on Hunger and Homelessness is reported each year.

TABLE 22-1	**PIT ESTIMATES OF HOMELESS PEOPLE JANUARY 2012**		
POPULATION	SHELTERED & UNSHELTERED SINGLE NIGHT, JANUARY 2012	CHANGE	PREVIOUS YEAR OF ESTIMATES
Households			
Individuals[1]	394,379	−6.8%	2007
Families with children	239,403	−3.7%	2007
Total	633,782	−5.7%	2007
Subpopulations[2]			
Veterans	62,619	−17.2%	2009[3]
Chronically homeless	99,894	−19.3%	2007

[1]Person who is not part of a family; single adults, unaccompanied youth, or in multiple-adult or multiple-child households.

[2]Categories are not mutually exclusive; it is possible for a chronically homeless person to be a veteran.

[3]Change for years prior to 2009 not reported for veterans.

Data from U.S. Department of Housing and Urban Development: *The 2012 point-in-time estimates of homelessness,* 2012. Retrieved from <http://abtassociates.com/CMSPages/GetFile.aspx?guid=77fdb6fa-6e6b-4524-8b5a-8e68c68caca9>.

According to the 2012 report, between September 1, 2011, and August 31, 2012, homelessness increased by an average of 7% in the 25 reporting cities; family homelessness increased by an average of 8%. The majority (16 of 24) of the cities that responded to the survey question that was related to family homeless reported an increase; 4 cities reported a decrease and 3 cities indicated no change in the number of families who were homeless. The authors of the Mayor's report recommend caution in interpreting the information because they note that the cities reporting data are not a representative sample of cities and hence the report is not a national report (U. S. Conference of Mayors, 2012).

A Caveat

This section presented a sketch of HUD's and ED's approaches to enumerating homeless populations and the latest available national prevalence estimates. Also included were pertinent prevalence rates in cities represented in the annual Mayors' report. Although structure and processes for enumerating the homeless are important and have improved, Kozol (1988, p. 10) cautioned a quarter-century ago:

> We would be wise to avoid the numbers game. Any search for the "right number" carries the assumption that we may at last arrive at an acceptable number. There is no acceptable number. Whether the number is "1 million or 4 million," there are too many homeless people in America.

Demographic Characteristics

This section reports selected demographic characteristics of the sheltered homeless population and subpopulations. The data CoC providers reported to HUD through the HIMS, from October 1, 2010, to September 30, 2011, provided the demographic characteristics of the following subpopulations: all homeless people, individuals, families with children, and veterans.

All Homeless People

Among all sheltered homeless adults, approximately 63% were men and 37% women. Men were overrepresented in comparison with general population. The sheltered homeless population is younger than the general population. Most homeless adults were between 31 and 61 years of age, and 22.1% were less than 18 years of age. Three percent were older than 62 years; 16% of the general U.S. population are older than 62 years. Minorities accounted for 60% of the total sheltered population. African Americans represented 38.1% and were overrepresented in comparison with their proportion of the general population. More sheltered homeless people had disabilities than members of the general population, 38.1% versus 15%, respectively.

Individuals

"Individual" as used by HUD refers to a person "who is not part of a family during his/her episode of homelessness. They are homeless as single adults, unaccompanied youth, or in multiple-adult or multiple-child households." Among this group, 72% were men, and 28% women; each gender

constitutes about half the general U.S. population. Most individuals (70%) were between 31 and 61 years of age, and 25% were younger than 18 years. Four percent were older than 62 years; 31% of the general U.S. population are older than 62 years. Minorities accounted for about 55% of sheltered individuals; African Americans (35.1%) were overrepresented in comparison with the racial composition of the general population. Disability rates of sheltered individuals were higher than those of the general population, 42.6% compared with 19.2% (USHUD, OCPD, 2012).

Families

A family is composed of at least one adult and one child. Women accounted for 80% of adult family members in shelters, which is a larger percentage than the 64% of women in poor families. Adults in homeless families are younger than adults in poor families; 22.3% of homeless adult family members are between 18 and 30 years of age, in contrast to 14.5% of adults in the general population's families. Minorities (71.9%) were overrepresented in sheltered homeless families in comparison to the general population (45%). African Americans made up 43.6% of the sheltered homeless population. The 20.6% of Hispanic/Latino sheltered families was lower than the rate of Hispanic/Latino families in the general population (22.7%). The homeless family disability rate, 16%, is twice that in all U.S. families (8%) (USHUD, OCPD, 2012).

Veterans

Men accounted for 90.2% of the sheltered homeless veteran population, which is less than the 92.8% in the entire U.S. veteran population (see Veterans' Health box). Among sheltered homeless veterans, 9.1% were between 18 to years old, 39.1% were 31 to 50 years old, 42.3% were between 51 and 61 years old, and 9.5% were 62 or older. This pattern differs from that of the entire veteran population, more than half which were 62 years or older. Minority sheltered veterans were overrepresented in comparison with the total veteran population. Of sheltered veterans, African Americans accounted for 35.5%, compared with 11.0% of all veterans. Although Hispanic/Latino veterans are 3% of the entire veteran population, they accounted for 6.3% of sheltered veterans. Minorities were also more likely to be in poverty and to have a disability than the general veteran population (USHUD, OCPD, 2012).

FACTORS THAT CONTRIBUTE TO HOMELESSNESS

In the larger society, three broad factors singly and interactively *contribute* to homelessness. They are: (1) shortage of affordable housing, (2) insufficient income to meet basic needs, and (3) inadequate and scarce support services.

Shortage of Affordable Housing

Housing is considered affordable if it costs a renter or owner no more than 30% of his or her income. In cooperation with

VETERANS' HEALTH
Poor and Homeless Veterans

Poor and homeless veterans present a challenge to health care providers. Coming from a military milieu, veterans do not trust easily, so their trust must be earned over time. In working with homeless veterans, health care providers must respect the humanity of each person and appreciate his or her unique story. We must ask about veteran status, because many homeless veterans complain that no one has ever asked whether they served in the military. Nurses must collaborate with community agencies and veterans groups to provide the care and services needed by veterans to prevent problems and circumstances that contribute to homelessness.

- 23% of homeless are veterans
- 47% served in Vietnam
- 33% served in a war zone
- 89% have an honorable discharge
- 45% are mentally ill
- 70% have substance abuse problems

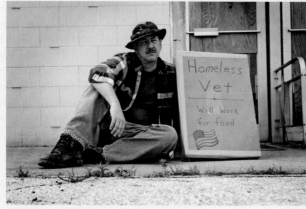

Modified from End of Life Nursing Education Consortium for Veterans Curriculum: *Cultural considerations in palliative care,* 2012. Retrieved from <http://www.aacn.nche.edu/elnec.> Created by Bridgette Crotwell Pullis, PhD, RN, CHPN.

state and local governments and nonprofit housing organizations, HUD operates programs that provide financial housing assistance to low-income families. This assistance may be provided as (1) direct payment to apartment owners, who in turn lower rents for low-income tenants; (2) access to apartments located in public housing facilities; or (3) housing choice vouchers, which may be used by low-income persons to "pay" all or part of the rent. Option 3's arrangements continue to be more commonly known as "Section 8 housing" (Center on Budget and Policy Priorities, 2013). Although these programs are intended to alleviate housing problems for low-income renters, the demand for these assisted housing programs has far exceeded the supply.

Factors contributing to the shortages include market forces that inhibit the private housing sector's production of affordable rental housing, decreases in the federal government's spending on assisted housing for low-income families, and the increasing inequality of incomes among groups within the larger population. The foreclosure crisis that began in 2007 exacerbated the obstacles that people with low incomes face

in obtaining affordable housing. As noted by HUD, the rates of worst case housing need—a renter whose income is 50 per cent of the Area Median Income and who paid more than half of his or her income for rent—increased dramatically between 2009 and 2011 (Joint Center for Housing Studies of Harvard University, 2012; National Alliance to End Homelessness, 2013; National Low Income Housing Coalition, 2013a; USHUD, Office of Policy Development and Research [OPDR], 2013).

Income Insufficiency

More than 10 years ago, Burt and colleagues (2001) documented that insufficient incomes and lack of employment prevented people from leaving homelessness. A 2012 U.S. Census Bureau Current Population Report reveals that (1) in 2011, the real median household income was $50,054 (adjusted to reflect 2011 dollars) and (2) this was the second consecutive year that it had declined (DeNavas-Walt, Proctor, and Smith, 2012). This 2011 level was 8.1% lower than in 2007, the year prior to the "great recession." Although the number of people in poverty and poverty rates in 2011 did not differ statistically from those in 2010, both the number and rates had increased during the prior 3 years. Overall, the percentage of people living below the poverty line was 15.0%. The poverty rate in 2011 among children younger than 18 years was 21.9%. Moreover, in 2011 among the poor, 44.08% had incomes below half of their poverty threshold; the U.S. Census Bureau's weighted average poverty threshold for a family of four in 2011 was $23,021 (DeNavas-Walt et al, 2012).

A consequence of the shortage of affordable housing and insufficient income is that an increasing number of low-income people end up paying much more than they can afford for rent. Since 2009, the number of renters who pay more than half of their income for rent has increased dramatically (USHUD, OPDR, 2013). In many areas of the country, the hourly wages needed to afford housing are three to five times higher than the federal minimum hourly wage, which is $7.25 (Kaiser Commission on Medicaid and the Uninsured, 2012; National Low Income Housing Coalition, 2013b).

With the lack of affordable housing in combination with insufficient income, people have to spend much of their income on rent, leaving them without adequate resources for other necessities, such as food, clothing, and health care. This situation substantially increases their risk for homelessness (Kaiser Commission on Medicaid and the Uninsured, 2012).

Inadequacy and Scarcity of Supportive Services

Some people experiencing homelessness have individual characteristics that, in interaction with the structural conditions of shortage of affordable housing and insufficient income, perpetuate their homeless condition. Supportive services for these people are deficient in quality and quantity. Some people need services to work and earn money. They are able to function in the workforce, whereas others need services to maintain their housing status. Included in this latter group are people whose serious chronic mental health and/or substance abuse problems preclude their functioning in the workforce and whose behaviors frequently interfere with their ability to obtain housing stability. People in this group need income assistance and comprehensive and accessible behavioral and physical health care.

What these two groups have in common is the need for affordable health care—that is, care that reflects health in its broadest sense as outlined by the World Health Organization, a state of complete, physical, mental and social well-being (Kilmeret et al, 2012; World Health Organization, 1948). In 2011, 25.4% of households with an annual income less than $25,000 had no health insurance (DeNavas-Walt et al, 2012).

Homelessness and Causation

This section has addressed three broad factors—shortage of affordable housing, insufficient income, and scarcity of supportive services—as societal conditions that *contribute* to homelessness rather than *cause* homelessness. Within both popular literature and scholarly literature, these factors are frequently referred to as "causes" of homelessness. As authors of this chapter, we assert that evidence is insufficient to infer causation. We have also encountered in lay and professional discussions situations in which participants claim that some people are homeless because they choose to be. Closer analysis of these claims reveals that persons as active agents do make decisions that result in homelessness. However, these decisions are made in highly contextualized conditions—frequently, in midst of addiction to alcohol and/or other substances (Nicholls, 2009; Parsell and Parsell, 2012). Whether or not these addictive conditions permit free choice entails philosophical issues that are beyond the scope of this chapter.

HEALTH AND HOMELESS POPULATIONS

As discussed in Chapter 1, the World Health Organization (WHO) has defined health from a broad perspective. This classic definition, which purports that health is "a state of complete physical, mental, and social well-being and not merely the absence of disease or infirmity" (WHO, 1948), is particularly useful when considering the health status of the homeless. For these individuals, a continual interaction exists among these three dimensions (physical, mental, and social) that has enormous consequences for health. The boundaries of these dimensions overlap; therefore, it is difficult, if not impossible, to address health among the homeless without a concomitant analysis of physical, mental, and social dimensions.

The definitions of homelessness, prevalence rates, and demographic characteristics previously outlined were based for the most part on activities of two federal agencies, HUD and ED. To provide a background for exploring health and homeless populations, this section presents a sketch of three aspects of the HHS, the federal agency with designated responsibility for provision of primary health care services to underserved populations. The three aspects of HHS's homeless services are (1) federal health centers, (2) the Health Care for the Homeless (HCH) program, and (3) the definition of the homeless individual used by the HCH program.

Federal Health Centers

Two types of federal health care centers provide services to generally underserved populations (low income), **Federally Qualified Health Centers** (FQHCs) and **FQHC Look-A-Likes** (FQHCLAs). Although both types of centers are located administratively within the HHS's Health Resources and Service Administration (HRSA), Bureau of Primary Health Care (BPHC), and both serve underserved populations, their sources of funding differ. FQHCs receive federal grants to fund services to underserved populations, whereas FQHCLAs do not. Both types of health centers may receive reimbursement under Medicare and Medicaid (USDHHS, HRSA, BPHC, n.d.).

Health Care for the Homeless

Some FQHCs receive additional federal funding to provide primary health care and substance abuse services to homeless populations through the HCH program. In addition to the homeless population, there are two other categories of special populations that federal health centers may serve—migrant seasonal farmworkers and their families and/or residents of public housing.

The definition used by health centers funded by HHS, as cited by National Health Care for the Homeless Council (2012), follows:

> A homeless individual is defined in section 330(h) (4) (A) as "an individual who lacks housing (without regard to whether the individual is a member of a family), including an individual whose primary residence during the night is a supervised public or private facility (e.g., shelters) that provides temporary living accommodations, and an individual who is a resident in transitional housing." A homeless person is an individual without permanent housing who may live on the streets; stay in a shelter, mission, single room occupancy facilities, abandoned building or vehicle; or in any other unstable or non-permanent situation. [Section 330 of the Public Health Service Act (42 U.S.C., 254b)]
>
> An individual may be considered to be homeless if that person is "doubled up," a term that refers to a situation in which individuals are unable to maintain their housing situation and are forced to stay with a series of friends and/or extended family members. In addition, previously homeless individuals who are to be released from a prison or a hospital may be considered homeless if they do not have a stable housing situation to which they can return. Recognition of the instability of an individual's living arrangements is critical to the definition of homelessness (HRSA/Bureau of Primary Health Care, Program Assistance Letter 1999-12, Health Care for the Homeless Principles of Practice; National Health Care for the Homeless Council, 2012).

The HHS definition of a homeless individual differs from the HUD and ED definitions. The differences are based on the specific legislative and administrative actions that authorize each agency's services. Both ED and HHS operate with broader definitions of homeless individuals than HUD. Using WHO's definition of health and HHS's definition of homeless individuals provides a perspective from which to view the health status of homeless populations.

HEALTH STATUS OF HOMELESS POPULATION

This section is organized according to the most prominent subpopulations within the larger homeless population: adults, women, families, youth, veterans, and persons experiencing chronic homelessness.

Adults

An exploration of the literature over the past two decades related to health of homeless population reveals that morbidity rates in the adult homeless population are higher than those occurring in comparable groups in the general population. Acute physical health problems occurring at higher rates in adults in the homeless population include respiratory infections and trauma. Chronic disorders experienced at higher rates than in the general population include hypertension, musculoskeletal disorder, gastrointestinal problems, respiratory problems (asthma, chronic bronchitis, emphysema), neurological disorders including seizures, and poor dentition. Serious mental illnesses and minor emotional problems also occur more frequently in the homeless population than in the general population. High rates of alcohol and drug use exacerbate the existing acute and chronic physical and mental health problems (Breakey et al, 1989; Burt, Aron, and Douglas, 1999; Ferenchick, 1992; Gelberg and Linn, 1989; Institute of Medicine, 1988; Wright, 1990).

Later reports of the health status of homeless populations agree with these older studies. The excessive morbidity rates are associated with mortality rates that are also higher than those in the general population (Baggett et al, 2013; Burt et al, 2001; Metraux et al, 2011; Rayburn, Pals, and Wright, 2012; Wiersma et al, 2010).

Lebrun-Harris and associates (2013) published a study that provides a national perspective on the self-reported health status of adult homeless patients in comparison with that of non-homeless federal health center patients. The researchers analyzed data collected in 2009 by the BPHC for the *Health Center Patient Survey*. Trained interviewers elicited respondents' housing status by asking patients whether they currently had a place to live, such as a house, apartment, or room. If they answered "yes" they were classified as non-homeless. Those patients who indicated they lived in an emergency or transitional shelter or hotel/motel room were categorized as homeless. In addition to housing status, interviewers elicited information regarding sociodemographic characteristics, medical conditions, access to care, and utilization of services.

On the basis of their analysis, Lebrun-Harris and associates (2013) reported that more males were homeless (57%) than were housed (37%). Unmarried patients made up 93% of the homeless group, compared with 70% in the housed group. In the group of homeless patients, 6% were employed, in contrast to 37% of the housed group. More patients in the homeless group (84%) were 100% below the federal poverty level, in contrast to 50% of the house group. Seventy-two percent of patients in the homeless group had experienced at least two homeless episodes versus 7.6% in the housed group.

A larger proportion of homeless patients reported substance use problems than their housed counterparts. Problems included higher rates of smoking, binge drinking, risk of alcohol and drug dependence, ever having injected drugs, and receiving treatment for alcohol or drug use in the past year. Larger percentages of homeless patients (52%) than of housed patients (36%) judged their health status as fair/poor. A higher proportion of patients in the homeless group (26%) than in the housed group (10%) reported that sometimes or often they did not get enough to eat—the definition of food insufficiency.

A larger proportion of individuals in the homeless group reported mental health problems in comparison with the housed individuals. The mental problems included psychological distress in past month, lifetime anxiety, and receipt of mental health treatment in the past year. A higher proportion of homeless patients than housed patients reported needing medical care and using hospital emergency departments as their usual sources of care.

Summarizing the results of the study, Lebrun-Harris and associates (2013) stated that a larger proportion of homeless patients reported worse health status and more chronic physical disease, mental health problems, and substance use problems than non-homeless patients. This conclusion substantiates results of previous research on the health status of a large segment of the homeless population—adults. Within the homeless population that the Leburn-Harris group's work addresses, there are subpopulations that, although they share similar mortality and morbidly problems, also have characteristics and circumstances that render a different health status.

Women

As noted earlier in this chapter, national data suggest that approximately 37% of sheltered individuals are women (USHUD, 2012). Women constituted nearly 30% of the 2938 homeless persons sampled in the National Survey of Homeless Assistance Providers and Clients (NSHAPC). Of these women, nearly 55% were accompanied by at least one minor child and the remaining 45% were living as unaccompanied adults; one third of the women reported experiences indicative of long-term homelessness (Zlotnick, Tam, and Bradley, 2012).

Homeless women have higher rates of pregnancy, including unintended pregnancy, than their housed counterparts, and researchers have demonstrated that the severity of homelessness increases the likelihood of preterm births and low-birth-weight infants. An accumulation of research evidence indicates that in comparison with men, homeless women report more stressful life events, foster care as children, intimate partner violence as adults, and hospitalizations for psychiatric problems (Caton, Wilkins, and Anderson, 2007).

In the 1990s, studies clearly documented the extraordinary histories of violence, from childhood through adulthood, among women experiencing homelessness (Anderson, 1996; Bassuk et al, 1997; Bassuk, Melnick, and Browne, 1998). Bassuk and colleagues (1996) reported that an estimated 92% of homeless women have experienced physical or sexual assault sometime in their lives. Advocates for the homeless continue to argue that the immediate cause of homelessness among women is typically violence and that the vast majority has experienced violence at some point in their lives. Sexual assaults are associated with worse physical and mental health outcomes, including use/abuse of alcohol and other drugs (Austin, Andersen, and Gelberg, 2008; Wenzel, Leake, and Gelberg, 2000) and, as may be expected, women living in unsheltered locations on the street have higher risk for victimization than women living in shelters. Unsheltered women also have greater odds of having multiple sexual partners and are less likely to utilize health services. Other factors that increase the risk of physical and sexual victimization include history of mental illness, substance use/abuse, and engaging in survival strategies such as selling sex and drugs (Nyamathi, Leake, and Gelberg, 2000; Wenzel et al, 2000).

Women Veterans. Men and women veterans, two groups within the homeless veteran subpopulation, have health problems similar to those of nonveteran individuals experiencing homelessness. However, women veterans who experience homelessness have problems specific to their military service experience and their roles as child caregivers. A brief sketch of these problems follows. Women veterans are three to four times more likely to be homeless than their non-veteran counterparts in virtually all age groups (Gamache, Rosenheck, and Tessler, 2003). The U.S. Government Accountability Office (2011) reported a study in which minor children accompanied 33% of homeless women veterans; almost two thirds of the women were between the ages of 40 and 59 years; and more than one third had disabilities. Additional research has demonstrated that being unemployed, disabled, or unmarried strongly predicts homelessness among women veterans (Washington et al, 2010).

Washington and colleagues (2010) found that 53% of the women veterans in their study reported a history of **military sexual trauma** (MST). Military sexual trauma is defined as "sexual assault or repeated, threatening sexual harassment that occurred while the Veteran was in the military. It includes any sexual activity where someone is involved against his or her will" (U.S. Department of Veterans Affairs, 2012). These researchers concluded that the added effect of MST explained why women veterans have a high risk for homelessness.

The U.S. Government Accountability Office (2011) also documented that 60% of the housing programs serving homeless women veterans did not accommodate children and that women reported concerns about their safety in the housing facilities with regard to incidents of sexual harassment or assault. The report recommended that services for women veterans address privacy, safety, and gender-specific concerns, including accommodations for minor children. Such services are essential for homeless women who are not veterans as well.

Families

The health status of adults and women, the two subpopulations discussed in the previous sections, is also relevant to the health status of families experiencing homelessness. The histories of chronic physical and mental health conditions, substance abuse, victimization, and low education and job training of adults are also risk factors for compromised caregiver-child relations. Because women are the single or major

caregivers in homeless families, their compromised physical, mental, and social health status is of even more concern.

Reviews of published literature about children in families experiencing homelessness show that research-based studies indicate these children have physical health problems, including asthma, iron deficiency anemia, and obesity, mental health problems, including behavior problems, and developmental delays at rates higher than those reported for children in the general population. These reviews also note that such problems interact and adversely affect homeless children's educational achievement on standardized tests covering reading, language usage, and/or mathematics. Missing days of school owing to family mobility, homeless children are more likely than other children to repeat grades. Homeless children may lack resources for clothing and school supplies and access to facilities for maintenance of personal hygiene. As a consequence, they may be at risk of nonacceptance or teasing by other students, thereby compounding the effects of their physical and mental problems (Bowman, Dukes, and Moore, 2012; McCoy-Roth, Mackintosh, and Murphey, 2012; National Center on Family Homelessness, 2011; Zlotnick, Tam, and Zerger, 2012).

Homeless children had higher rates of physical, mental health and behavior, and educational problems than children in the general population, but these rates were similar to those of poor but housed children. In other words, the difference in housing status was not a contributing factor. Other writers report that there are significant differences within the population of homeless children. There is a subpopulation of homeless children that is doing well, and another subpopulation that is experiencing multiple problems (Huntington, Buckner, and Bassuk, 2008; Obradovic et al, 2009; Park, Fertig, and Allison, 2011).

Youth

This section sketches the health problems occurring within the subpopulation of homeless youth. It includes those individuals federally defined as unaccompanied, runaway, and homeless youth.

As indicated by several substantial reports and reviews of studies, youth from all sectors of society engage in health-risking behaviors that result in serious health problems (Eaton et al, 2012). These problems include unintended pregnancy, sexually transmitted disease (STDS, including human immunodeficiency virus/acquired immunodeficiency syndrome [HIV/AIDS]), alcohol and drug abuse, depression, and suicide. For the most part, these problems are related to risk-taking behaviors. However, homeless youth experience these problems at higher rates than youth in the general population (Burt, 2007; Lawrence, Gootman, and Sim, 2009; Toro, Dworsky, and Fowler, 2007).

Homeless youth experience STDs, physical and sexual abuse, skin disorders, anemia, drug and alcohol abuse, and unintentional injuries at higher rates than their counterparts in the general population. Depression, suicidal ideation, and disorders of behavior, personality, or thought also occur at higher rates among homeless youths. Family disruption, school failures, prostitution or "survival sex," and involvement with the legal system indicate that homeless youths' social health is severely compromised (Burt, 2007; Busen and Engebretson, 2008; Edidin et al, 2012; Kennedy et al, 2012a; Lawrence et al, 2009; Nyamathi et al, 2012; Rew et al, 2008a; Rew, Rochlen, and Murphey, 2008b; Tevendale, Lightfoot, and Slocum, 2009; Toro et al, 2007; Tucker et al, 2012a).

Homeless youth who are pregnant, engage in prostitution, or identify themselves as gay, lesbian, bisexual, transgender, or questioning (LGBTQ) experience more health problems than other homeless youth. Pregnant homeless youth have more severe mental health problems and use alcohol and drugs more than nonpregnant homeless peers. Not surprisingly, they have higher rates of negative pregnancy outcomes than nonhomeless youth (Lawrence et al, 2009; Rew et al, 2008b; Tucker et al, 2012b).

Both female and male homeless youth make up a large percentage of all youth involved in prostitution. Many become involved because they need money to meet subsistence needs—the situation that is the source of the term "survival sex." They are more likely to have serious mental health problems and to be actively suicidal. Alcohol and drug use occurs at higher rates among this group than among homeless youth not engaged in prostitution. Those involved in prostitution are more likely to report histories of physical and sexual abuse (Fernandes, 2007; Lawrence et al, 2009; Molino, 2007).

Rates of attempted suicide are higher among gay homeless youth. A large majority of males involved in survival sex identify themselves as gay or bisexual. Many of these young people are on the streets because of the effects of homophobia and prejudice. Facing problems similar to those of other homeless youth, the gay-identified face an additional set of problems as a result of rejection by others because of their sexual orientation (Lawrence et al, 2009).

Homeless youth who have a history of foster care are at increased risk of psychiatric disorders. They are more likely to report psychiatric disorders than homeless youth without a history of foster placement (Thompson & Hasin, 2012).

Youth in the general population are at risk, those who are homeless are at even higher risk, and the special subpopulations of youth—including those who are LGBTQ-identified, those who are pregnant, those who are practicing survival sex, and those who have a history of foster care—are particularly vulnerable. Health for many of these groups is severely jeopardized.

Chronically Homeless

As noted previously, many homeless individuals experience both mental and substance use disorders. These are the individuals included in the HUD definition of the **chronically homeless**. More specifically, they are unaccompanied adults who are homeless for extended or numerous periods and have one or more disabling conditions. The disabling conditions that chronically homeless people experience are very often severe mental and substance use disorders (Caton et al, 2005; Caton et al, 2007; Larimer et al, 2009; Sadowski et al, 2009; Weinstein et al, 2013). This subpopulation is also at increased risk for the health problems outlined in previous sections on the health status of subpopulations of adults and women.

As of 2011, approximately 63% of the chronically homeless were unsheltered—sleeping on the street or in places not meant for human habitation. Homeless service providers, concerned about the high mortality risk among "street" homeless population, constructed the Vulnerability Index, a screening tool for identifying and prioritizing the need for housing. Those at high risk for death are individuals who have been homeless for 6 months or more with one or more of the following features (Cels and de-Jong, 2010; Kanis et al, 2012):

- More than three hospitalizations or emergency room visits in a year
- More than three emergency room visits in the previous 3 moths
- 60 years or older
- Cirrhosis of the liver
- End-stage renal disease
- History of frostbite, immersion foot, or hypothermia
- HIV/AIDS
- Co-occurring psychiatric, substance abuse, and chronic medical conditions.

COMMUNITY PUBLIC HEALTH NURSING: CARE OF HOMELESS POPULATIONS

An examination of the reports of the health status of persons experiencing homelessness reveals that physical and mental health problems predominate. Stated differently, the studies reflect a biological-psychological basis—social health is rarely addressed. Although many of the studies noted that homelessness, as a form of extreme poverty, contributed to poor health and poor health in turn was a risk for homelessness, the interventions focused on resolving the physical and mental health problem rather than ameliorating the conditions that contributed to homelessness. This section discusses concepts that suggest directions for community/public health nursing care of the homeless population that is broader in scope than the biological-psychological approach.

Framework for Community/Public Health Nursing Care for Homeless Populations

This section presents a framework for developing approaches to providing community/public health nursing care of homeless populations. The framework has four elements: models of justice, thinking upstream, social determinants of health, and the Public Health Intervention Wheel that supports upstream interventions for homeless populations.

Models of Justice

Beauchamp (1979) distinguished between the two types of justice (i.e., **market justice** and **social justice**) that influence public health policy in the United States. Market justice, which has been the dominant model, purports that people are entitled to valued ends (i.e., status, income, and happiness) according to their own individual efforts. Moreover, this model stresses individual responsibility, minimal collective action, and freedom from collective obligations other than respect for another person's fundamental rights. In contrast, under a social justice model, all people are equally entitled to key ends (i.e., access to health care and minimum standards of income). Consequently, all members of society must accept collective burdens to provide a fair distribution of these ends. Moreover, social justice is a foundational aspect of public health (Krieger and Birn, 1998) and nursing (Grace and Willis, 2012). Others have noted the limits of the market approach; citing the many problems inherent in the current health care system, they call for a social justice approach to health care (Budetti, 2008; Pauly, MacKinnon, and Varcoe, 2009).

Thinking Upstream

McKinlay's (1979) work of more than 30 years ago (see Chapter 3) suggests conceptualizing homelessness as the river and the people in the river as the homeless. Building on McKinlay's "river" metaphor, McKinlay and Marceau (2000) hold that government and private efforts to address homeless health care problems largely focus on "pulling the bodies out of the river of homelessness." Such downstream interventions, aimed at treating or alleviating health care problems such as physical disease and mental illnesses, are worthy and needed. However, these interventions when used alone are far less adequate in alleviating homeless people's social health problems. To improve the social health of the homeless, it is necessary to go upstream and focus on the primary contributors to homelessness itself (i.e., lack of affordable housing, inadequate income, and insufficient services). An upstream approach to homelessness is provided by the concept *social determinants of health*.

Social Determinants of Health

In 2008 the World Health Organization Commission on Social Determinants of Health published its final report, *Closing the Gap in a Generation: Health Equity through Action on the Social Determinants of Health*. As defined by WHO, "The social determinants of health are the circumstances in which people are born, grow up, live, work and age, and the systems put in place to deal with illness. These circumstances are in turn shaped by a wider set of forces: economics, social policies, and politics" (WHO, 2014).

Building on WHO's extensive work, the United States included in *Healthy People 2020* a new overarching goal to "create social and physical environments that promote good health for all" (Koh et al, 2011 p. 563) and a new topic area, the social determinants of health (SDH)) (USDHHS, 2013).

Five broad dimension of SDH are defined within *Healthy People 2020* as follows: (1) economic stability, (2) education, (3) social and community context, (4) health and health care, and (5) neighborhood and built environment. Each of these dimensions includes key issues that identify more specific factors (USDHHS, 2013). Two of the dimensions, economic stability and health and health care, hold significant relevance for homelessness in that the key issues are those defined as contributing to homelessness. Table 22-2 lists the key issues that *Healthy People 2020* identifies as underlying economic stability, health and health care, and the associated factors contributing to homelessness.

TABLE 22-2	**SOCIAL DETERMINANTS OF HEALTH AND FACTORS CONTRIBUTING TO HOMELESSNESS**
***HEALTHY PEOPLE 2020* SOCIAL DETERMINANT OF HEALTH DIMENSIONS AND KEY ISSUES**	**FACTOR(S) CONTRIBUTING TO HOMELESSNESS**
Economic Stability	
Poverty	Income insufficiency
Employment status	Income insufficiency
Access to employment	Income insufficiency
Housing stability (e.g., homelessness foreclosure)	Shortage of affordable housing
Health and Health Care	
Access to health services—including clinical and preventive care	Inadequacy and scarcity of supportive services
Access to primary care—including community-based health promotion and wellness programs	Inadequacy and scarcity of supportive services

Adapted from U.S. Department of Health and Human Services: *Healthy People 2020: Determinants of health*, 2012. Retrieved from <http://www.healthypeople.gov/2020/about/DOHAbout.aspx>.

SDH, as noted by the Centers for Disease Control and Prevention (CDC, 2010, p. 1), are the ". . . complex, integrated and overlapping social structures and economic systems that include the social and physical environments, and health services. . . ." These determinants are shaped by the levels of income, power, and resources at global, national, and local levels. They are also often influenced not only through personal choices but through policy choices as well. As defined, the SDH call for an upstream approach to deal with the "causes of the cause"—those factors embedded in the social fabric of communities at all levels. However, as cautioned by governmental entities and individual writers, both upstream and downstream approaches are needed (CDC, 2010; Koh et al, 2011; Martins & Burbank, 2011; UDSHHS, 2012, 2013). Interventions are needed upstream at community or systems levels and downstream at the individual or family levels.

Public Health Intervention Wheel

Developed more than 10 years ago, the Public Health Intervention Wheel provides guidance in identifying the types of interventions and the most appropriate level for providing public health nursing care to homeless populations (Minnesota Department of Health Division of Community Health Services, 2001). The 17 interventions are graphically displayed and defined in Chapter 1. One of the major strengths of the Intervention Wheel is that it directs practice at individual and family levels, a downstream approach, as well as at the community or systems level, an upstream approach.

Although nurses may use all interventions at all three levels, community/public health nurses, working downstream with individuals, families, or groups use surveillance, disease and other health event investigation, outreach, screening, case finding referral and follow-up, case management, delegated functions, health teaching, counseling, and consultation. In contrast, community/public health nurses working more upstream at the system level employ collaboration, coalition building, community organizing, advocacy, social marketing, and policy development and enforcement.

Summary

This section discussed concepts of social justice, upstream thinking, SDH, and the Intervention Wheel—four elements comprising a framework for community/public health nursing care of homeless populations. Based on principles of social justice the framework emphasizes upstream thinking in addressing the SDH factors contributing to homelessness. The interventions identified reflected macro-upstream factors and more micro-downstream condition of individuals and families experiencing homelessness.

SUMMARY

This chapter provides an overview of homelessness from a national perspective. Definitions of homeless, prevalence estimates, and demographic characteristics of subpopulations, adults, families with children, veterans, and the chronically homeless are presented. Factors contributing to homelessness, lack of affordable housing, insufficient income, and lack of supportive services are compared with the social determinants of health. Health status of homeless subpopulations, as reported in the literature, is outlined and noted to be focused mainly on physical health, reflecting a downstream focus. A framework for community/public health nursing care of the homeless population based on social justice, upstream thinking, social determinants of health, and the Public Health Intervention Wheel and supporting both upstream and downstream interventions is outlined.

LEARNING ACTIVITIES

1. Compare the information contained in the most recent U.S. Conference of Mayors Annual Report on Hunger and Homelessness with the information contained in the previous 3 years. What has changed?
2. Analyze at least three or four factors that contribute to homelessness in the United States.
3. Discuss common health problems found among homeless adults, families, women, and youth.
4. Identify two special subgroups of the homeless and describe their health problems.
5. Describe social determinants of health. What is their significance for community health nursing practice with homeless individuals and families?
6. Discuss at least two community health nursing interventions and locate the interventions on the Public Health Intervention Wheel.

EVOLVE WEBSITE

http://evolve.elsevier.com/Nies
- NCLEX Review Questions
- Case Studies
- Glossary

REFERENCES

Anderson DG: Homeless women's perceptions about their families of origin, *Western Journal of Nursing Research* 18(1):29–42, 1996.

Austin EL, Andersen R, Gelberg L: Ethnic differences in the correlates of mental distress among homeless women, *Womens Health Issues* 18(1):26–34, 2008.

Baggett TP, Hwang SW, O'Connell JJ, et al: Mortality among homeless adults in Boston: shifts in causes of death over a 15-year period, *JAMA Internal Medicine* 173(3):189–195, 2013.

Bassuk EL, Buckner JC, Weinreb LF, et al: Homelessness in female-headed families: childhood and adult risk and protective factors, *American Journal of Public Health* 87(2):241–248, 1997.

Bassuk EL, Melnick S, Browne A: Responding to the needs of low-income and homeless women who are survivors of family violence, *Journal of the American Medical Womens Association* 53(2):57–64, 1998.

Bassuk EL, Weinreb LF, Buckner JC, et al: The characteristics and needs of sheltered homeless and low-income housed mothers, *JAMA* 276(8):640–646, 1996.

Beauchamp DE: Public health as social justice. In Jaco EG, editor: *Patients, Physcians, and Illness,* ed 3, New York, 1979, Free Press.

Bowman D, Dukes C, Moore J: *Summary of the state of research on the relationship between homelessness and academic achievement among school-aged children and youth.* 2012. Available from <http://center.serve.org/nche/downloads/nche_research_pub.pdf>.

Breakey WR, Fischer PJ, Kramer M, et al: Health and mental health problems of homeless men and women in Baltimore, *JAMA* 262(10):1352–1357, 1989.

Budetti PP: Market justice and US health care, *JAMA* 299(1):92–94, 2008.

Burt MR: *Understanding homeless youth: numbers, characteristics, multisystem involvement and intervention options* (testimony submitted to Subcommittee on Income Security and Family Support, U.S. House Committee on Ways and Means), 2007. Available from <http://www.urban.org/UploadedPDF/901087_Burt_Homeless.pdf>.

Burt MR, Aron LY, Douglas T, et al: *Homelessness: programs and the people they serve: A summary report of the findings of the National Survey of Homeless Assistance Providers and Clients,* 1999. Available from <http://www.urban.org/url.cfm?ID=310291>.

Burt MR, Aron LY, Lee E: *Helping America's homeless: emergency shelter or affordable housing?,* Washington, DC, 2001, Urban Institute Press.

Busen NH, Engebretson JC: Facilitating risk reduction among homeless and street-involved youth, *Journal of the American Academy of Nurse Practitioners* 20(11):567–575, 2008.

Canadian Homelessness Research Network, The Homeless Hub: *Canadian definition of homelessness,* 2012. Available from <http://www.homelesshub.ca/Library/Canadian-Definition-of-Homelessness-54225.aspx>.

Caton CL, Dominguez B, Schanzer B, et al: Risk factors for long-term homelessness: findings from a longitudinal study of first-time homeless single adults, *American Journal of Public Health* 95(10):1753–1759, 2005.

Caton CL, Wilkins C, Anderson JA: People who experience long-term homelessness: characteristics and interventions. Presented The National Symposium on Homelessness Research, Washington, DC, March 1-2, 2007. Available from <http://aspe.hhs.gov/hsp/homelessness/symposium07/caton/report.pdf>.

Cels S, de-Jong J: *Just a tool? Implementing the vulnerability index in New Orleans,* 2010. Available from <http://www.lectoraatinnovatie.nl/wp-content/uploads/2009/03/VulnerabilityIndex.pdf>.

Center on Budget and Policy Priorities: *Policy basics: federal rental assistance*, 2013. Available from <http://www.cbpp.org/cms/index.cfm?fa=view&id=3890>.

Centers for Disease Control and Prevention: *Establishing a holistic framework to reduce inequities in HIV, viral hepatitis, STDs, and tuberculosis in the United States*, 2010. Available from <http://www.cdc.gov/socialdeterminants/docs/SDH-White-Paper-2010.pdf>.

DeNavas-Walt C, Proctor BD, Smith JC: *Income, poverty, and health insurance coverage in the United States: 2011* (Current Population Reports, P60–243). Washington, D.C., 2012, U.S. Census Bureau. Also available from <http://www.census.gov/prod/2012pubs/p60-243.pdf>.

Eaton DK, Kann L, Kinchen S, et al: Youth risk behavior surveillance—United States, 2011, *MMWR Surveillance Summaries* 61(4):1–162, 2012.

Edgar W: *European review of statistics on homelessness*, 2009. Available from <http://eohw.horus.be/files/freshstart/European%20Statistics%20Reports/2009%20European%20Review%20of%20Statistics/chapter2_EN.pdf>.

Edidin JP, Ganim Z, Hunter SJ, et al: The mental and physical health of homeless youth: a literature review, *Child Psychiatry & Human Development* 43(3):354–375, 2012.

European Federation of National Associations Working with the Homeless: *ETHOS typology on homelessness and housing exclusion*, 2011. Available from <http://www.feantsa.org/spip.php?article120>.

Ferenchick GS: The medical problems of homeless clinic patients: a comparative study, *Journal of General Internal Medicine* 7(3):294–297, 1992.

Fernandes AL: *Runaway and homeless youth: demographics, programs and emerging issues (No. RL33785)*, Washington, DC, 2007, Congressional Research Services.

Gamache G, Rosenheck R, Tessler R: Overrepresentation of women veterans among homeless women, *American Journal of Public Health* 93(7):1132–1136, 2003.

Gelberg L, Linn LS: Assessing the physical health of homeless adults, *JAMA* 262(14):1973–1979, 1989.

Grace PJ, Willis DG: Nursing responsibilities and social justice: an analysis in support of disciplinary goals, *Nursing Outlook* 60(4):198–207, 2012.

Huntington N, Buckner JC, Bassuk EL: Adaptation in homeless children: an empirical examination using cluster analysis, *American Behavioral Scientist* 51(6):737–755, 2008, Available from <http://dx.doi.org/10.1177/0002764207311985>.

Institute of Medicine: *Homelessness, health, and human needs*, Washington, DC, 1988, National Academy Press.

Joint Center for Housing Studies of Harvard University: *State of nation's housing 2012*, 2012. Available from <http://www.jchs.harvard.edu/sites/jchs.harvard.edu/files/son2012.pdf>.

Kaiser Commission on Medicaid and the Uninsured: *The uninsured and the difference health insurance makes*, 2012. Available from <http://www.kff.org/uninsured/1420.cfm>.

Kanis R, Mccannon J, Craig C, et al: An end to chronic homelessness: an introduction to the 100,000 homes campaign, *Journal of Health Care for the Poor & Underserved* 23(1):321–326, 2012.

Kennedy DP, Tucker JS, Green Jr HD, et al: Unprotected sex of homeless youth: results from a multilevel dyadic analysis of individual, social network, and relationship factors, *AIDS & Behavior* 16(7):2015–2032, 2012.

Kilmer RP, Cook JR, Crusto C, et al: Understanding the ecology and development of children and families experiencing homelessness: implications for practice, supportive services, and policy, *American Journal of Orthopsychiatry* 82(3):389–401, 2012.

Koh HK, Piotrowski JJ, Kumanyika S, et al: Healthy People: a 2020 vision for the social determinants approach, *Health Education & Behavior* 38(6):551–557, 2011.

Kozol J: *Rachel and her children: homeless families in America*, New York, 1988, Crown.

Krieger N, Birn AE: A vision of social justice as the foundation of public health: commemorating 150 years of the spirit of 1848, *American Journal of Public Health* 88(11):1603–1606, 1998.

Larimer ME, Malone DK, Garner MD, et al: Health care and public service use and costs before and after provision of housing for chronically homeless persons with severe alcohol problems, *JAMA* 301(13):1349–1357, 2009.

Lawrence RS, Gootman JA, Sim LJ: *Adolescent health services: missing opportunities*, Washington, DC, 2009, National Academies Press.

Lebrun-Harris LA, Baggett TP, Jenkins DM, et al: Health Status and Health Care Experiences among Homeless Patients in Federally Supported Health Centers: findings from the 2009 Patient Survey, *Health Services Research* 48(3):992–1017, 2013. Available from <http://dx.doi.org/10.1111/1475-6773.12009>.

Martins D, Cocozza, Burbank PM: Critical interactionism: an upstream-downstream approach to health care reform, *Advances in Nursing Science* 34(4):315–329, 2011. Available from <http://dx.doi.org/10.1097/ANS.0b013e3182356c19>.

McCoy-Roth M, Mackintosh BB, Murphey D: *When the bough breaks: the Effects of homelessness on young children*, 2012. Available from <http://www.caction.org/CAN-Research/Reports/2012/Child_Trends-2012_02_16_ECH_Homelessness.pdf>, 2012.

McKinlay JB: A case for refocusing upstream; the political economy of illness. In Jaco EG, editor: *Patients, physicians, and illness*, ed 3, New York, 1979, Free Press.

McKinlay JB, Marceau LD: To boldly go..., *American Journal of Public Health* 90(1):25–33, 2000.

Metraux S, Eng N, Bainbridge J, et al: The impact of shelter use and housing placement on mortality hazard for unaccompanied adults and adults in family households entering New York City shelters: 1990-2002, *Journal of Urban Health* 88(6):1091–1104, 2011.

Minnesota Department of Health Division of Community Health Services: *Public health interventions: Applications for public health nursing practice*, 2001. Available from <http://www.health.state.mn.us/divs/cfh/ophp/resources/docs/phinterventions_manual2001.pdf>.

Molino A: *Characteristics of help-seeking street youth and non-street youth*, 2007. Available from <http://aspe.hhs.gov/hsp/homelessness/symposium07/molino/index.htm;>.

Murphy J, Tobin K: *Homelessness comes to school*, CA, Corwin, 2011, Thousand Oaks.

National Alliance to End Homelessness: *The state of homelessness in America 2013*, 2013. Available from <http://www.endhomelessness.org/library/entry/the-state-of-homelessness-2013>.

National Center for Homeless Education: *Education for homeless children and youths program: data collection summary school year 2010-11*, 2012. Available from <http://center.serve.org/nche/downloads/data_comp_0909-1011.pdf>.

National Center on Family Homelessness: *America's youngest outcasts 2010*, 2011. Available from <http://www.homelesschildrenamerica.org/media/NCFH_AmericaOutcast2010_web.pdf>.

National Health Care for the Homeless Council: *Frequently asked questions about health care for the homeless*. Available from <http://bphc.hrsa.gov/technicalassistance/taresources/hchfaqupdated.pdf>, 2012.

National Low Income Housing Coalition: America's affordable housing shortage, and how to end it, *Housing Spotlight* 3(2):1–6, 2013a. Also available from <http://nlihc.org/sites/default/files/HS_3-1.pdf>.

National Low Income Housing Coalition: *Out of reach 2013*, 2013b. Available from <http://nlihc.org/sites/default/files/oor/2013_OOR.pdf>.

Nicholls CM: Agency, transgression and the causation of homelessness: a contextualized rational action analysis, *International Journal of Housing Policy* 9(1):69–84, 2009.

Nyamathi A, Hudson A, Greengold B, et al: Characteristics of homeless youth who use cocaine and methamphetamine, *American Journal on Addictions* 21(3):243–249, 2012.

Nyamathi A, Leake B, Gelberg L: Sheltered versus nonsheltered homeless women differences in health, behavior, victimization, and utilization of care, *Journal of General Internal Medicine* 15(8):565–572, 2000.

Obradovic J, Long JD, Cutulia A, et al: Academic achievement of homeless and highly mobile children in an urban school district: longitudinal evidence on risk, growth, and resilience, *Development and Psychopathology* 21:493–518, 2009. *21*, 493–518.

Park JM, Fertig AR, Allison PD: Physical and mental health, cognitive development, and health care use by housing status of low-income young children in 20 American cities: a prospective cohort study, *American Journal of Public Health* 101(Suppl 1):S255–S261, 2011.

Parsell C, Parsell M: Homelessness as a choice, *Housing, Theory and Society* 29(4):420–434, 2012. Available from <http://dx.doi.org/10.1080/14036096.2012.667834>.

Pauly BM, MacKinnon K, Varcoe C: Revisiting "Who gets care?": health equity as an arena for nursing action, *Advances in Nursing Science* 32(2):118–127, 2009.

Perl L, Bagalman E, Fernandes-Alcantara A, et al: *Homelessness: targeted federal programs and recent legislation* (CRS Report for Congress No. 7–5700), 2012. Available from <http://www.fas.org/sgp/crs/misc/RL30442.pdf>.

Rayburn RL, Pals H, Wright JD: Death, drugs, and disaster: mortality among New Orleans' homeless, *Care Management Journals* 13(1):8–18, 2012.

Rew L, Grady M, Whittaker TA, et al: Interaction of duration of homelessness and gender on adolescent sexual health indicators, *Journal of Nursing Scholarship* 40(2):109–115, 2008a.

Rew L, Rochlen AB, Murphey C: Health educators' perceptions of a sexual health intervention for homeless adolescents, *Patient Education & Counseling* 72(1):71–77, 2008b.

Sadowski LS, Kee RA, VanderWeele TJ, et al: Effect of a housing and case management program on emergency department visits and hospitalizations among chronically ill homeless adults: a randomized trial, *JAMA* 301(17):1771–1778, 2009.

Shumsky NL: *Homelessness: a documentary and reference guide*, Santa Barbara, CA, 2012, Greenwood.

Smith AD, Smith DI: *Emergency and transitional shelter population 2000 (Special Reports No. CENSR/01–2)*, Washington, DC, 2001, U.S. Census Bureau. Also available from <http://www.census.gov/prod/2001pubs/censr01-2.pdf>.

Tevendale HD, Lightfoot M, Slocum SL: Individual and environmental protective factors for risky sexual behavior among homeless youth: an exploration of gender differences, *AIDS & Behavior* 13(1):154–164, 2009.

Thompson RG, Hasin D: Psychiatric disorders and treatment among newly homeless young adults with histories of foster care, *Psychiatric Services* 63(9):906–912, 2012.

Toro P, Dworsky A, Fowler P. Homeless youth in the United States: recent research findings and intervention approaches. Presented by The National Symposium on Homelessness Research, Washington, DC, March 1-2, 2007. Available from <http://aspe.hhs.gov/hsp/homelessness/symposium07/Toro/report.pdf>.

Tucker JS, Hu J, Golinelli D, et al: Social network and individual correlates of sexual risk behavior among homeless young men who have sex with men, *Journal of Adolescent Health* 51(4):386–392, 2012a.

Tucker JS, Ryan GW, Golinelli D, et al: Substance use and other risk factors for unprotected sex: results from an event-based study of homeless youth, *AIDS & Behavior* 16(6):1699–1707, 2012b.

U. S. Conference of Mayors: *Hunger and homelessness survey: a status report on hunger and homelessness in America's cities*, 2012. Available from <http://usmayors.org/pressreleases/uploads/2012/1219-report-HH.pdf;>.

U.S. Department of Education: *Education for homeless children and youths*, 2001. Available from <http://www2.ed.gov/policy/elsec/leg/esea02/pg116.html#sec725>.

U.S. Department of Health and Human Services: *Healthy People 2020: determinants of health*, 2012. Available from <http://www.healthypeople.gov/2020/about/DOHAbout.aspx>.

U.S. Department of Health and Human Services: *Healthy People 2020: social determinants of health*, 2013. Available from <http://www.healthypeople.gov/2020/topicsobjectives2020/overview.aspx?topicId=39>.

U.S. Department of Health and Human Services, Administration for Children & Families, Family and Youth Service Bureau: *Runaway and homeless youth program authorizing legislation*, 2012. Available from <http://www.acf.hhs.gov/programs/fysb/resource/rhy-act>.

U.S. Department of Health and Human Services, Health Resources and Services Administration, Bureau of Primary Health Care: *Health center program terminology tip sheet*, n.d. Available from <http://bphc.hrsa.gov/technicalassistance/healthcenterterminologysheet.pdf>.

U.S. Department of Housing and Urban Development: *The point-in-time estimates of homelessness*, 2012. Available from <http://abtassociates.com/CMSPages/GetFile.aspx?guid=77fdb6fa-6e6b-4524-8b5a-8e68c68caca9>.

U.S. Department of Housing and Urban Development, Office of Community Planning and Development: *Continuum of care 101*, 2009a. Available from <https://www.onecpd.info/resources/documents/coc101.pdf>.

U.S. Department of Housing and Urban Development, Office of Community Planning and Development: *McKinney-Vento Homeless Assistance Act as amended by S.896 HEARTH Act of 2009*, 2009b. Available from <http://portal.hud.gov/hudportal/documents/huddoc?id=HAAA_HEARTH.pdf;>.

U.S. Department of Housing and Urban Development, Office of Community Planning and Development: Homeless emergency assistance and rapid transition to housing: defining "homeless", *Federal Register* 76(233), 2011. 75994–70619, Also available from <http://www.gpo.gov/fdsys/pkg/FR-2011-12-05/pdf/2011-30942.pdf>.

U.S. Department of Housing and Urban Development, Office of Community Planning and Development: *The 2011 annual homeless assessment report to Congress*, 2012. Available from <https://www.onecpd.info/resources/documents/2011AHAR_FinalReport.pdf;>.

U.S. Department of Housing and Urban Development, Office of Policy Development and Research: *Worst case housing needs 2011: report to Congress—summary*, 2013. Available from <http://www.huduser.org/portal/publications/affhsg/wc_HsgNeeds11.html>.

U.S. Department of Veterans Affairs: *Military sexual trauma*, 2012. Available from <http://www.mentalhealth.va.gov/msthome.asp>.

U.S. Government Accountability Office: *Homeless women veterans: actions needed to ensure safe and appropriate housing* (Report to Congressional Requesters No. GAO-12–182), Washington, DC, 2011, Author. Also available from <http://www.gao.gov/assets/590/587334.pdf>.

U.S. House of Representatives, Office of the Law Revision Center: *U.S. Code*, 2012. Available from <http://uscode.house.gov/download/pls/42C119.txt>.

Washington DL, Yano E, McGuire J, et al: Risk Factors for Homelessness among Women Veterans, *Journal of Health Care for the Poor and Underserved* 21(1):81–91, 2010.

Weinstein LC, LaNoue M, Collins E, et al: Health Care Integration for Formerly Homeless People with Serious Mental Illness, *Journal of Dual Diagnosis* 9(1):72–77, 2013. Available from <http://dx.doi.org/10.1080/15504263.2012.750089>.

Wenzel SL, Leake BD, Gelberg L: Health of homeless women with recent experience of rape, *Journal of General Internal Medicine* 15(4):265–268, 2000.

Wiersma P, Epperson S, Terp S, et al: Episodic Illness, Chronic Disease, and Health Care Use among Homeless Persons in Metropolitan Atlanta, Georgia, 2007, *Southern Medical Journal* 103(1):18–24, 2010.

World Health Organization: *Constitution of the World Health Organization: preamble* (Official Records of the World Health Organization, no. 2, p. 100), 1948. Available from <www.who.int/entity/governance/eb/who_constitution_en.pdf>.

World Health Organization: *Social determinants of health: key concepts*, n.d. Available from <http://www.who.int/social_determinants/thecommission/finalreport/key_concepts/en/>.

World Health Organization, Commission on Social Determinants of Health: *Closing the Gap in a generation: health equity through action on the social determinants of health, final report*, 2008. Available from <http://www.who.int/social_determinants/thecommission/finalreport/en/index.html>.

World Health Organization: Progress on the implementation of the Rio Political Declaration, 2014. Available from <http://www.who.int/social_determinants/en/>.

Wright JD: Poor people poor health: the health status of the homeless, *Journal of Social Issues* 46(4):49–64, 1990.

Zlotnick C, Tam T, Zerger S: Common needs but divergent interventions for U.S. homeless and foster care children: Results from a systematic review, *Health & Social Care in the Community* 20(5):449–476, 2012, Available from <http://dx.doi.org/10.1111/j.1365-2524.2011.01053.x>.

Rural and Migrant Health

*Patricia L. Thomas and Lori Wightman**

OBJECTIVES

Upon completion of this chapter, the reader will be able to do the following:

1. Compare and contrast characteristics of rural and urban communities.
2. Describe features of the health care system and population characteristics common to rural aggregates.
3. Discuss the impact of structural and personal barriers on the health of rural aggregates.
4. Identify factors that place farmers and migrant workers at risk for illness and accidents.
5. Discuss the importance of the informal care network to rural health and social services.
6. Describe the characteristics of rural community health nursing practice.
7. Apply an upstream perspective to health promotion and illness prevention for rural and migrant populations.

KEY TERMS

disparities
frontier
metropolitan

migrant
pesticide
rural

seasonal
urban

OUTLINE

Rural United States
    Defining Rural Populations
    Describing Rural Health and Populations
Rural
    Minority Health and *Healthy People 2020*
Rural Health Disparities: Context and Composition
    Context: Health Disparities Related to Place
    Composition: Health Disparities Related to Persons
    Perceptions of Health
Specific Rural Aggregates
    Agricultural Workers
    Migrant and Seasonal Farmworkers
Application of Relevant Theories and "Thinking Upstream" Concepts to Rural Health
    Attacking Community-Based Problems at Their Roots
    Emphasizing the "Doing" Aspects of Health
    Maximizing the Use of Informal Networks
Rural Health Care Delivery System
    Health Care Provider Shortages
    Managed Care in the Rural Environment

Community-Based Care
    Home Health and Hospice Care
    Faith Communities and Parish Nursing
    Informal Care Systems
    Rural Public Health Departments
    Rural Mental Health Care
    Emergency Services
Legislation and Programs Affecting Rural Public Health
    Programs that Augment Health Care Facilities and Services
Rural Community Health Nursing
    Characteristics of Rural Nursing
Rural Health Research
    Capacity of Rural Public Health to Manage Improvements in Health
    Information Technology in Rural Communities
    Performance Standards in Rural Public Health
    Leadership and Workforce Capacity for Rural Public Health
    Interaction and Integration of Community Health Systems, Managed Care, and Public Health
New Models of Health Care Delivery for Rural Areas

*The authors would like to acknowledge the work of Kathleen Chafey, Wade Hill, Glenna Burg, and Patti Shoe in previous editions of this chapter.

RURAL UNITED STATES

There are many different versions of rural America, in that each rural area is somewhat unique but shares certain features with other rural regions. Geographic, demographic, environmental, economic, and social factors all influence health, access to health care, and quality of health care. When aggregated, these characteristics may be contrasted with those of urban populations. In this section, we present a "snapshot" of rural population and health characteristics that contribute to challenging health disparities for many of the people living in the most rural areas of America.

Although the urban growth rate has been steadily climbing since 1890, with numbers of urban dwellers surpassing those in rural areas around 1920, the number of rural residents is the highest in the country's history (U.S. Department of Agriculture [USDA], 2007). The number and size of rural counties are highest in the South (35%), followed by the Midwest and West (23%), and the Northeast (19%) (USDA, Economic Research Service [ERS], 2013). Current census estimates are that 20% of the nation's children younger than 18 years live in rural areas (O'Hare, 2009), as do 15% of the nation's elderly and more than 50% of the nation's poor (USDA ERS, 2013).

The economic base of rural America is changing rapidly. See ⓔ **Resource Tool 23A** for a map of the United States detailing Health Insurance Coverage Status.

Rural residents have long been thought to be family farmers and ranchers, but today, rural America is a diverse and important marketplace to marketers of consumer products, and demographers and economists consider trends in farm and farm-related employment much more broadly. They characterize agriculture as a "food and fiber system" that encompasses all aspects of agriculture, from core materials sectors (farm, food processing, textiles, and other manufacturing) to wholesale and retail trade and the food service sector (USDA, National Institute of Food and Agriculture, 2009). Despite the shrinking number of family farms and full-time farmers, agriculture continues to be an important part of the rural and U.S. economy.

Poverty, a key health determinant, continues to be greater in rural America than in urban areas. Whereas the nonmetropolitan population had a poverty rate of 14.5%, the rural population had a poverty rate of 16.5% in 2010. This overall gap may not seem large, but when the degree of rurality or the poverty rate for particular subpopulations (e.g., minorities, children under 18 years of age, or the elderly) are examined, the gap increases greatly. For example, the poverty rate for non-Hispanic blacks in nonmetropolitan areas in 2012 was 41%, compared with a rate of 25% for the same group in metropolitan areas (U.S. Census Bureau, 2013). Rural poverty was highest in the South (22%) followed by the West (16%), with the Midwest and Northeast at 14% each (USDA, Rural Poverty in America, 2014). (See Box 23-1 for the 2013 U.S. Department of Health and Human Services' Poverty Guidelines).

Not only is the economic base shifting, the age composition is as well. Many rural areas are growing, especially in the

---

BOX 23-1   THE 2013 U.S. DEPARTMENT OF HEALTH AND HUMAN SERVICES POVERTY GUIDELINES

In concept, the U.S. Department of Health and Human Services (DHHS) determines the poverty guidelines by estimating the minimum income level needed by a family or individual to just meet the basic needs of food, shelter, clothing, and other essential goods and services. Official poverty guidelines adjusted for family size and composition are set by DHHS for use by all federal agencies to determine financial eligibility for certain federal programs (e.g., Medicaid). Some programs (e.g., State Children's Health Insurance Program) also use multiples of the guidelines to determine eligibility of participants. For example, participants may be eligible for programs if they are classified as being at or near poverty, *poverty* being defined as 100%, and *near poverty* as 125% or 150%, of the poverty level. Poverty guidelines are adjusted periodically by DHHS to reflect price changes, and are published in the *Federal Register*. The 2013 guidelines reflect just the size of the "family unit" rather than the family composition. The poverty level for a family unit of one, for example, was $11,490; it was $23,550 for a family unit of four, and $39,630 for a family of eight. Each household's cash income (including pretax income and cash welfare assistance, but excluding in-kind welfare assistance, such as food stamps and Medicare) is compared with the poverty line for the household.

From U.S. Department of Health and Human Services: *The 2013 HHS poverty guidelines: one version of the [U.S.] federal poverty measure,* 2013. Available from <http://aspe.hhs.gov/poverty/13poverty.cfm>.

West and South, and many rural counties, especially in the Great Plains states, are losing population because of a decline in agricultural and manufacturing jobs. Younger people are leaving rural areas for jobs in urban centers, so that those who remain behind are increasingly older and isolated and have diminished access to health care. Recent demographic changes in rural areas have also included an influx of retirees and others from urban areas, who are able to live in rural areas and conduct business through telecommunication and travel (Malecki, 2003). Newer demographic data indicate that the number of rural persons aged 60 years and older constitute 20% of the population of nonmetropolitan areas, in contrast to 15% of the population of urban areas (Rogers, 2002). Of the nation's rural elderly, the largest clusters live in the South (45%) and the Midwest (31%) (Rogers, 2002). See ⓔ **Resource Tool 23B** for a map of the older adult population in the United States.

Three trends, aging-in-place, out-migration of young adults, and immigration of older persons from metro areas (Cromartie and Nelson, 2009), present challenges to already stressed communities that must provide adequate health care, housing, transportation, and other human services (Aldwin and Gilmer, 2013; Cromartie and Nelson, 2009).

The rural population is also becoming more ethnically diverse. Generations ago, many families began farming when they came to the United States as European immigrants. In the 1990s, new immigrants began buying and operating their own small family farms, and others found employment in rural agriculture and manufacturing. Today, more than one half of rural Hispanics live outside the Southwest, and "high-growth Hispanic counties" are mostly in the South and Midwest (U.S. Census Bureau, 2011). Hispanics are now the most rapidly growing demographic group in rural and small-town America.

Policies and programs developed to close the health disparities gap must take a population health view of the special circumstances of rural life. Although 75% of U.S. counties are classified as rural, they contain only 20% of the U.S. population. Members of rural populations also are more likely to be older, to be less educated, to live in poverty, to lack health insurance, and to experience a lack of available health care providers and access to health care (Farrigan and Parker, 2012). Only 10% of U.S. physicians practice in rural counties, and the ratio of physicians in rural population size is 36 per 100,000 people, compared with nearly double that number in urban settings (American Academy of Family Practitioners [AAFP], 2014).

Rural residents more often assess their health as fair or poor and have more disability days associated with acute conditions than their urban counterparts. Rural people also tend to have more problems related to negative health behaviors (e.g., untreated mental illness, obesity, and alcohol, tobacco, and drug use) that contribute to excess deaths and chronic disease and disability rates. The literature suggests, for example, that the highest death rates for children and young adults are in the most rural counties. Residents of rural areas are nearly twice as likely to die from unintentional injuries, including motor vehicle accidents, than urban residents (National Rural Health Association [NRHA], n.d.b).

Noting a prominent and persistent pattern of risky health behaviors in rural dwellers, McClelland et al, (2010) suggests that "rural culture" may itself be a key determinant of health in rural communities and that these behaviors vary along the rural-urban continuum and within rural populations by geographical areas. These behaviors, including unintentional injury, smoking, and suicide, are discussed in more detail in the section titled "Health Disparities Related to Persons."

Defining Rural Populations

Multiple definitions of rural populations have been formulated to describe the characteristics of areas with low population density. Previous definitions have simply included either those towns with a population of less than 2500 or towns located in open country as rural. This definition has often been further differentiated into the subcategories farm and rural nonfarm. A second classification of interest used the term *rural* for populations with less than 45 persons per square mile and the term frontier for geographical areas with less than 6 persons per square mile (Rural Assistance Center, n.d.). Many counties of the Great Plains, Intermountain West, and Alaska are designated frontier.

The rural-urban continuum distinguishes counties by population and adjacency to metropolitan areas. Residences can range from small towns to large metropolitan areas. Statistical reporting has been in use since 1990 with the term *metropolitan statistical areas (MSAs)* used to differentiate nonmetropolitan and metropolitan areas. In June 2003, the Office of Management and Budget (OMB) released a new classification scheme to better reflect trends in population distribution across the nation (OMB, 2009). The MSA designation has been replaced by county-level *core based statistical areas (CBSAs)*, to simplify the multilevel designations. Within CBSAs, *metropolitan areas* are those counties that contain at least one urbanized area of 50,000 or more people. A *micropolitan area* contains a cluster of 10,000 to 50,000 persons. Counties that are neither metropolitan nor micropolitan are called "outside CBSAs," also known as noncare areas (US Census, 2013a).

Describing Rural Health and Populations

Rural populations differ in complex geographical, social, and economic ways. Although older, poorer, and less educated people are usually overrepresented in rural areas, this finding may not apply to all rural areas or to everyone in a particular rural area.

The health profiles discussed here are shared by rural areas in general and may be contrasted with overall patterns of health, health habits, and health care in urban settings. However, the reader should note that it is difficult to interpret differences between urban health and rural health. First, statistically significant differences between urban and rural health indicators may seem small when data are aggregated to "rural areas" in general. The differences tend to become larger when data are available for particular rural areas (e.g., certain counties), particular rural subgroups (e.g., minorities), or specific characteristics (e.g., percentage of uninsured children). Second, heterogeneity of race, age, economic status, regional distribution, and cultural groupings makes health data for rural populations useful only as estimates of individual health. For example, in 2011, about 15.9% of the U.S. population had income below the poverty level, an increase from 15.3% in 2010. The number of people in poverty rose from 46.2 million to 48.5 million during the same time, representing the fourth consecutive increase in the poverty rate (Bishaw, 2012). The family poverty rate in 2011 was 11.8% (representing 9.5 million), not statistically different from the 2010 estimates (U.S. Census Bureau, 2012).

Infant mortality, a major health status indicator, varies greatly by geographical area, even within rural areas, and dramatizes the importance of both contextual and compositional data. The infant mortality rate plateaued between 2005 and 2010 and then declined from 6.86 deaths per 1000 live births to 6.14 between 2005 and 2010. The largest decline was for non-Hispanic-Black women (from 13.63 to 11.46) followed by non-Hispanic whites (5.76 to 5.18) and Hispanic women (from 5.62 to 5.25). During 2000 and 2005, the non-Hispanic black infant mortality rates were 2.4 times the non-Hispanic white rates but the difference narrowed in 2010 with a non-Hispanic black rate 2.2 times that of non-Hispanic whites (Mathews and MacDorman, 2013).

The rate of infant deaths in 2009 for black Americans is 2.3 times that for whites and Hispanics per 1000 births. In both the South and West, rural counties experienced the highest rates (24% and 30% higher, respectively, than fringe areas of large metro areas) (Office of Minority Health, 2013). Overall, the infant mortality rate declined 10% between 1995 and 2004 (7.57); however, the rate has not declined much since 2000 (6.89). From 1995 until 2004, small declines were observed for all races and ethnic groups. Significant decreases were noted for infants of Central and South American (16%), Puerto Rican (12%), Asian or Pacific Islander (11%), non-Hispanic white (10%), Mexican (9%), and non-Hispanic black (7%) mothers (Centers for Disease Control and Prevention [CDC], 2011).

Mortality rates for white infants in rural areas adjacent to population centers with less than 2500 people varied from a high of 9.85 per 1000 in the South to 6.46 per 1000 in the West. Although infant mortality rates have changed since 1993, infant mortality data provide insight into the heterogeneity of rural populations and show why national or even regional data may or may not reflect the status quo for a particular county or local population.

One might also consider the health disparities that exist among rural racial and ethnic minorities. Although limited because the phenomenon has only recently been studied, research findings support the conclusion that rural racial and ethnic minorities—Native Americans, Alaska Natives, Hispanics/Latinos, and African Americans—concentrated in the South and West are more disadvantaged not only relative to rural majority members but also relative to urban racial and ethnic minorities. The disparities include employment, income, education, health insurance, mortality, morbidity, and access to health care (*Healthy People 2020* Disparities, 2010).

Because population numbers are small, national rural data, limited as they are, can only suggest the health needs of a particular area, racial or ethnic mix, or age distribution, for example. Program planners still need to determine whether certain health or health care delivery problems apply to their specific service area. Useful data sources include state, county, and census tract level data on health and demographics available from state and federal government agencies, such as those cited in the References of this chapter. In planning for health-related programs, nurses can also gather community-level data from health care providers, local records, focus groups, and older residents who know the area's history.

RURAL

Minority Health and *Healthy People 2020*

Healthy People 2020 represents the health promotion and disease prevention agenda for the nation (U.S. Department of Health and Human Services [USDHHS], Office of Disease Prevention and Health Promotion, n.d.) Additionally, *Healthy People 2020* is the United States' contribution to the World Health Organization (WHO) "Health for All" program. The framework for *Healthy People 2020*, developed through public consensus, builds upon the national health program established since the 1980s. It has the broad goals of increasing quality of life and years of life, eliminating disparities in health

among different population groups, and improving access to preventive health services (see Figure 1-1 in Chapter 1).

Healthy People 2020 is an evidence-based 10-year plan with the goal to "attain high-quality, longer lives free of preventable disease, disability, injury, and premature death." Achieving this goal will accomplish health equity, elimination of disparities, and improvement of the health of all groups through social and physical environments to promote quality of life, healthy development, and healthy behaviors across all life stages (*Healthy People 2020*, 2013, paragraph 4). The challenges are great, but public health professionals and planners in every state have a plan patterned on *Healthy People 2020* goals to direct their efforts.

RURAL HEALTH DISPARITIES: CONTEXT AND COMPOSITION

To improve understanding of the health of populations and health disparities, there is also a growing emphasis on the distinction between *context*, which is defined by the characteristics of places of residence, and *composition*, which is the collective health effects that result from a concentration of persons with certain characteristics. Most public health problems include elements of both context and composition, though they may be predominantly one or the other (Braveman, 2010).

Health issues in rural areas are contextual when they derive from characteristics of place. Characteristics of place include not only natural features of geography and environment, but also the political, social, and economic institutions that build and support communities within a given geographical areas. For example, limited economic opportunities, low wages, or agricultural accidents might be considered to have contextual effects on the health of populations. Problems in rural areas are compositional when they derive from individual characteristics of groups of people residing in rural settings. Examples of compositional sources of health disparities include such characteristics as age, education, income, ethnicity, and health behaviors.

Consideration of both context and composition enable us to take a more deliberate and refined approach to study, plan programs for, and deliver health care services to rural populations. Although the overall health of rural Americans is worse than that of urban Americans, the relationship between rurality and health is not necessarily linear. Many differences exist among rural areas in both the nature and extent of health problems. Furthermore, some rural populations share more in common with people in urban core areas than with people in other rural areas. Effective planning depends on understanding and documenting needs that take into account context, composition, and their interaction. The next section presents data for problems of both contextual and compositional sources of health disparities in rural America.

Context: Health Disparities Related to Place

Regardless of their diverse demographic and geographical attributes, rural groups share certain health patterns, difficulties, and delays in obtaining health care (see Ethical Insights box). Many of the contextual issues that contribute to rural health disparities are described in the introduction to the chapter ("Rural United States"). Many rural regions that are already sparsely populated are losing residents, a process that often triggers a downward spiral. People leave and services are lost; the local drugstore closes; the tax base will not support an ambulance service, so most seriously ill persons must be transported long distances to get health care; jobs become scarce and younger people leave the area. Retirees may be attracted to the lower costs, but they need public health and other services that must be provided by counties without the tax base to support them. Racial and ethnic minorities are migrating to rural areas to find employment

opportunities. Structural, financial, and personal barriers to accessing health care services exist in all environments, but rural residents are unique in how they experience structural barriers.

Access to Care

Rural health leaders have identified ten priorities for health care in rural America, with access to and affordability of care topping the list. Because most people in rural America are self-employed or part of small businesses, insurance tied to employment will not serve them (Bailey, 2009). Ziller, Lenardson, and Coburn (2012), using data from the 2002-2007 Medical Expenditure Panel Survey to examine uninsured rural and urban residents and the factors associated with

---

⚖ ETHICAL INSIGHTS

Racial and Ethnic Disparities in Health Care

Because public health is a societal approach to protecting and promoting health that usually acts through social rather than individuals means (Kass, 2001), many of the most pressing ethical dilemmas are considered in public domains. Perhaps no more important ethical challenge facing our public today revolves around the just distribution of health care resources.

For example, among 34.6 million rural minority adults in 2000, 32% of black, 35% of "other" race persons, and 45% of Hispanics were uninsured, compared with only 18% of whites (Glover et al, 2004). These data may help explain why minorities are more likely to be denied authorization for care (Lowe et al, 2001), to use less prenatal care (Barfield et al, 1996), and to make fewer visits to physicians (Tai-Seale, Freund, and LoSasso, 2001).

Differences in care resulting from patient or care process-level variables (e.g., patient attitudes, preferences or expectations, provider bias, stereotyping, or uncertainty) are problems of professional ethics. *Disparities in care* resulting from system-level variables, such as financing, accessibility and geographical location, are problems of justice (Institute of Medicine, 2003). Subsequently, solutions for justice issues in *disparities in care* require public discourse aimed at solving system level problems.

From an ethical perspective, the theory of justice as fairness was formulated to specify terms of social cooperation that are "fair" and ensure that people of equal basic liberties have equal opportunity (Daniels, Kennedy, and Kawachi, 1999). The Civil Rights Act of 1964 specifically bars discrimination in health care for all entities that receive federal funds, and both the American Nurses Association and American Medical Association codes of ethics endorse the principle of justice. However, despite overall agreement that justice is an important practice concept, difficulty arises in implementing changes in the health system to address *disparities in care*.

Solutions to disparities in care have been suggested by the Institute of Medicine (2003) and include the following policy, health system, and patient education and empowerment interventions.

Policy Interventions

1. Medical care financing should discourage fragmentation of health care into separate tiers of providers who adhere to different standards of care and serve separate racial and ethnic

minority segments of society. Government programs that require enrollment in managed care should be prepared to pay plans at rates comparable to those paid to plans for privately insured patients.

2. Strengthen the stability of patient-provider relationships in publicly funded health plans and create policy to create consistency, limit patient loads for providers, and provide reasonable time allowances for initial and follow-up visits.
3. Increase the proportion of underrepresented U.S. racial and ethnic minorities among health professionals.
4. Apply the same managed care protections to publicly funded health maintenance organization (HMO) enrollees that apply to private HMO enrollees.
5. Provide greater resources to the U.S. Department of Health and Human Services Office for Civil Rights to enforce civil rights laws.

Health Systems Interventions

1. Promote the consistency and equity of care through evidence-based guidelines. These guidelines should be published to allow public and professional scrutiny.
2. Construct payment systems to enhance available services to minority patients, and limit provider incentives that may promote disparities.
3. Enhance patient-provider communication and trust by providing financial incentives for practices that reduce barriers.
4. Support the use of interpretation services where community need exists.
5. Institute programs that use community health workers among medically underserved and racial and ethnic minority populations.
6. Support greater use of multidisciplinary treatment and preventive care teams to improve and streamline care for racial and ethnic minority patients.

Patient Education and Empowerment Interventions

1. Implement patient education programs to increase patients' knowledge of how to access care and participate in treatment decisions.

Data from Barfield WD, Wise PH, Rust FP, et al: Racial disparities in outcomes of military and civilian births in California, *Arch Pediatr Adolesc Med* 150(10): 1062-1067, 1996; Daniels N, Kennedy BP, Kawachi I: Why justice is good for our health: the social determinants of health inequalities. Daedalus 128:215-251, 1999; Glover S, Moore CG, Samuels ME, et al: Disparities in access to care among rural working-age adults, *J Rural Health* 20(3):193-205, 2004; Institute of Medicine: *Unequal treatment: confronting racial and ethnic disparities in healthcare*, Washington, DC, 1988, National Academy Press; Kass NE: An ethics framework for public health, *Public Health Matters* 91(11):1776-1782, 2001; Lowe RA, Chhaya S, Nasci K, et al: Effect of ethnicity on denial of authorization for emergency department care by managed care gatekeepers, *Acad Emerg Med* 8(3):259-266, 2001; Tai-Seale M, Freund D, LoSasso A: Racial disparities in service use among Medicaid beneficiaries after mandatory enrollment in managed care: a difference-in-differences approach, *Inquiry* 38(1):49-59, 2001.

access to care, found the rural uninsured more likely to have a usual source of care than their urban counterparts. Controlling for demographic and health characteristics, the access and use differences between the uninsured and insured in rural areas are smaller than those observed in urban areas, suggesting that providers in rural areas may impose fewer barriers on the uninsured who seek care.

Primary Care. Rural areas have fewer primary care physicians than urban areas, fueling concerns about inadequate access and gaps in U.S. health care equity in many rural areas. It is estimated that rural residents have 53 primary care physicians (PCPs)—internists, family/general practitioners, and pediatricians—per 100,000 people, compared with 78 PCPs per 100,000 urban residents (Ferrer, 2007; Reschovsky and Staiti, 2005). Only 10% of physicians, 22% of nurse practitioners (NPs) (13% of psychiatric NPs), and 23% of physician assistants (PAs) practice in rural areas (Hanrahan and Hartley, 2008). This pattern of practitioner distribution resembles the distribution of providers in urban areas with growing shortages in rural and underserved areas (Ricketts, 2008). In a joint statement, the NRHA and the American Academy of Family Physicians said medicine has become specialized, centralized, and urban and challenged educators to be responsive to the needs of rural underserved communities (AAFP, 2013).

Availability of providers and health care facilities in rural areas is an important determinant of the quality of the health care delivery system and the likelihood of positive health outcomes for rural residents (Bailey, 2009). A good example of the lack of specialists is the lack of mental health services available for rural dwellers of any age. The incidence of mental illness in rural areas is the same as that of urban areas, but there is far less access to mental health services in rural areas. Additionally, primary care doctors, nurses, and physician assistants, rather than mental health specialists, provide most of the mental health care in rural regions (Bailey, 2009; Hanrahan and Hartley, 2008).

General Health Services. Population decline in rural areas in the Great Plains and lower South, for example, has resulted from an out-migration of younger people, leaving a greater concentration of older people in a dwindling population. An Institute of Medicine (IOM) study reported rural medical access problems in these areas, with some hospital and pharmacy closures, greater distances to travel for physician services, and limited if any choice of providers (IOM, 2005). Lack of local access to primary care and health care facilities forces rural residents to either go without or travel long distances—often over rural roads in dangerous weather conditions—to access needed care. Access to health care may become a particularly challenging and expensive proposition for the elderly who do not drive and depend on limited public transportation. Geography, health care costs, and lack of available services also are contextual problems that keep many rural adults and children from obtaining needed primary, secondary, and tertiary preventive services.

Health Insurance. With economic decline and rising costs of health care, health insurance—or more importantly the lack of health insurance—for Americans has become a major issue for the health of the nation. An estimated 45.7 million people were without health insurance in 2010 (U.S. Census Bureau, 2011).

As with poverty and unemployment data, insurance coverage varied with race and ethnicity coverage in 2007, as did age and residence (rural or urban). For example, 10.4% of non-Hispanic whites, 19.5% of blacks, and 16.8% of Asians were uninsured for all or part of 2007; young adults were more likely to lack health insurance than older persons; and 18% of poor or near-poor children lacked coverage (U.S. Census Bureau, 2012). Lack of insurance coverage was greatest in the South (14.2%) and West regions (12%) in 2007, and in general, rural residents were more likely than urban residents to lack insurance (20% versus 17%) (IOM, 2005). Two thirds of the persons living in the most rural counties are low-income families, and 30% are children (USDA, 2004). See ℮ **Resource Tool 23C** for a map of the United States detailing estimations of populations in poverty.

Health insurance coverage influences health patterns. For example, in a study by Becker, Gates and Newsom (2004), those who had some form of health insurance reported the influence of physicians and health education programs on self-care regimens much more frequently than did those who were uninsured. In addition, obtaining health insurance can pose a financial barrier to adequate health care for rural dwellers. Research points to a strong relationship among health insurance status, chronic illnesses, and poverty (Bailey, 2009; DeNavas-Walt, Proctor, and Smith, 2012). Rural people are often employed in industries characterized by seasonal work, economic uncertainty and decline, high unemployment risk, and occupational accidents and death (e.g., agriculture, mining, forestry, and fisheries). Rural industries are often small and offer low wages, thereby contributing to the growing number of uninsured rural families. For example, self-employed farm families need to purchase private health insurance; however, in periods of hardship they often cannot afford the increasingly high premium costs (Center on Budget and Policy Priorities, 2012). Farm families also tend to be two-parent households, so they are less likely to qualify for Medicaid, even with incomes below the federal poverty level.

Health insurance has been identified as one of the 10 leading health indicators because it is generally a reliable predictor of overall health status (Bailey, 2009; Center on Budget and Policy Priorities, 2012). Public health professionals and health planners are most concerned with the impact of increasing numbers of uninsured children. In 2010, the overall percentage of children who were uninsured was 9.4%, which works out to 7 million (DeNavas-Walt et al, 2012). The uninsured rate of children has declined, in large part because of state programs, between 2009 and 2011; however, rural children are still uninsured at a slightly higher rate (7.7%) than the national average (7.5%) and their urban counterparts (7.4%) (Alker, Mancini, and Heberlein, 2012). In the absence of health insurance, poverty becomes an even more powerful predictor of poor health for all age-groups and particularly for children.

In 1997, the State Children's Health Insurance Program (CHIP) was enacted to improve health insurance coverage of children less than 19 years of age in poor and near poor families (see the "Legislation and Programs Affecting Rural Public Health" section in this chapter). In the years following passage of this program, the overall percentage of children who were uninsured fell and the number of uninsured children declined. The number of uninsured children declined to 5.5 million in 2011 from 6.4 million in 2009, and the percentage of children with insurance increased to 93% in 2011 (Alker et al, 2012). Health insurance coverage of children as well as adults varies from state to state and is influenced by employment patterns, the percentage of children in the population, state Medicaid policies, poverty levels, and racial and ethnic composition.

Composition: Health Disparities Related to Persons

To review, health problems in rural areas are compositional when they result from a concentration of persons with certain characteristics. Examples of compositional sources of health disparities include such characteristics as income, health behaviors, education, occupation, gender, and ethnicity. In the *Rural Healthy People 2010* survey, 73% of respondents listed access to health care as the top rural health priority (Bolin and Gamm, 2003). An additional 13 priorities listed by respondents as leading health problems are largely compositional but may also have a contextual dimension. For example, such problems as obesity, chronic pulmonary disease, and higher levels of infant mortality have a strong compositional component because their variation is related to the health behaviors and the educational, socioeconomic, racial, and ethnic characteristics of the rural groups. The variation may also be contextual, because the groups have fewer educational opportunities, have low-wage jobs, lack insurance, or have genetic propensities for certain health problems.

Income and Poverty

Income, education, and type of employment help determine socioeconomic status, and in the aggregate, rural dwellers have lower educational levels, higher unemployment rates, higher poverty rates, and lower income levels than urban aggregates (*Healthy People 2020*, 2013). The poverty rate is one of the most important indicators of the health and well-being of all Americans, regardless of where they live (see Ethical Insights box).

The U.S. Department of Agriculture's Economic Research Service tracks economic trends and demographic characteristics of rural dwellers to help develop policies and services. In the most recent report, the ERS contrasted the economic growth and downward trend in poverty rates during the 2000s. Figures from the U.S. Census Bureau show that 13.2% of Americans were living in poverty in 2008, the highest rate since 1997. In rural counties, however, that rate climbed to 16.3%. The gap between poverty rates in urban and rural America widened, doubling between 2003 and 2008 with an urban rate of 12.7% and the rural rate at 16.3%. The gap between the rates of urban and rural poor was 1.6 percentage points in 2003. Just 5 years later, however, the difference had grown to 3.4 percentage points (Bishop, 2009).

Poverty rates for rural people have always been higher than those for urban dwellers (Figure 23-1 and Table 23-1). As

Percent of total population in poverty, 2011

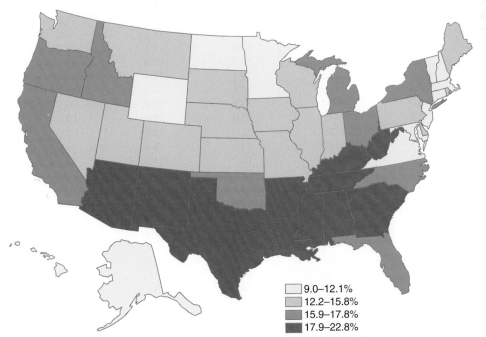

9.0–12.1%
12.2–15.8%
15.9–17.8%
17.9–22.8%

FIGURE 23-1 Percentage of total population in poverty, 2011. (From U.S. Department of Agriculture, Economic Research Service: *Profiles of America: data, 2010,* 2010. Available from <http://www.ers.usda.gov/data-products/county-level-data-sets/poverty.aspx?reportPath=/State_Fact_Sheets/PovertyReport&stat_year=2009&stat_type=0&fips_st=37#.U1MqpaLwnWc>.)

TABLE 23-1	PERCENTAGE OF POPULATION IN POVERTY BY STATE (2012)					
STATE	ALL PEOPLE IN POVERTY (2011)			CHILDREN AGES 0-17 IN POVERTY (2011)		
	PERCENTAGE	90% CONFIDENCE INTERVAL OF ESTIMATE		PERCENTAGE	90% CONFIDENCE INTERVAL OF ESTIMATE	
		LOWER BOUND	UPPER BOUND		LOWER BOUND	UPPER BOUND
Alabama	19.1	18.7	19.5	27.6	26.8	28.4
Alaska	10.8	10.3	11.3	14.7	13.6	15.8
Arizona	19.0	18.6	19.4	27.2	26.3	28.1
Arkansas	19.3	18.9	19.7	27.8	26.9	28.7
California	16.6	16.4	16.8	22.8	22.5	23.1
Colorado	13.4	13.1	13.7	17.7	17.0	18.4
Connecticut	10.8	10.5	11.1	14.6	13.8	15.4
Delaware	12.6	12.1	13.1	18.8	17.6	20.0
District of Columbia	19.1	18.2	20.0	30.9	28.1	33.7
Florida	17.0	16.8	17.2	25.1	24.6	25.6
Georgia	19.2	18.9	19.5	26.6	25.9	27.3
Hawaii	12.1	11.6	12.6	16.8	15.7	17.9
Idaho	16.5	16.0	17.0	21.3	20.2	22.4
Illinois	14.9	14.7	15.1	21.3	20.8	21.8
Indiana	15.8	15.5	16.1	22.6	21.9	23.3
Iowa	12.7	12.4	13.0	17.1	16.3	17.9
Kansas	13.8	13.4	14.2	18.8	18.0	19.6
Kentucky	19.1	18.7	19.5	27.2	26.3	28.1
Louisiana	20.5	20.1	20.9	28.8	28.1	29.5
Maine	14.2	13.7	14.7	19.3	18.3	20.3
Maryland	10.2	9.9	10.5	13.9	13.2	14.6
Massachusetts	11.6	11.3	11.9	15.3	14.7	15.9
Michigan	17.5	17.3	17.7	24.6	24.0	25.2
Minnesota	11.8	11.5	12.1	15.3	14.7	15.9
Mississippi	22.8	22.3	23.3	32.4	31.5	33.3
Missouri	15.8	15.5	16.1	22.3	21.6	23.0
Montana	15.2	14.7	15.7	20.9	19.8	22.0
National	15.9	15.8	16.0	22.5	22.3	22.7
Nebraska	12.9	12.5	13.3	17.6	16.7	18.5
Nevada	15.8	15.3	16.3	22.2	21.2	23.2
New Hampshire	9.0	8.6	9.4	12.2	11.2	13.2
New Jersey	10.4	10.2	10.6	14.6	14.0	15.2
New Mexico	20.9	20.4	21.4	29.4	28.3	30.5
New York	16.1	15.9	16.3	22.8	22.4	23.2
North Carolina	17.8	17.5	18.1	25.4	24.7	26.1
North Dakota	12.0	11.5	12.5	14.8	13.7	15.9
Ohio	16.3	16.1	16.5	23.9	23.3	24.5
Oklahoma	17.3	17.0	17.6	23.9	23.1	24.7
Oregon	17.3	16.9	17.7	23.4	22.5	24.3
Pennsylvania	13.7	13.5	13.9	19.4	18.9	19.9
Rhode Island	14.7	14.2	15.2	21.5	20.4	22.6
South Carolina	18.8	18.4	19.2	27.5	26.6	28.4
South Dakota	14.1	13.6	14.6	19.2	18.1	20.3
Tennessee	18.4	18.1	18.7	26.5	25.8	27.2
Texas	18.5	18.3	18.7	26.6	26.2	27.0
Utah	13.6	13.2	14.0	16.2	15.4	17.0
Vermont	11.9	11.4	12.4	15.8	14.6	17.0
Virginia	11.6	11.4	11.8	15.6	15.0	16.2
Washington	13.9	13.6	14.2	18.5	17.9	19.1
West Virginia	18.7	18.2	19.2	26.1	25.1	27.1
Wisconsin	13.1	12.8	13.4	18.4	17.7	19.1
Wyoming	11.3	10.7	11.9	15.5	14.3	16.7

Data from U.S. Census Bureau: *Small area income and poverty estimates.* Table modified from U.S. Department of Agriculture, Economic Research Service: *County-level data sets: Poverty,* 2013. Available from <http://www.ers.usda.gov/data-products/county-level-data-sets/poverty.aspx>.

noted earlier in this section, however, data averaged across all rural counties in the United States do not give planners and providers much information about their own counties, or even regions. The following discussion gives examples of available data that can be used to make a analysis of local and regional conditions and characteristics.

Rural Poverty: Regional Differences. Consistent with the idea that there are many rural Americas in rural America, rural poverty varies by rural region. For example, there are 353 counties with persistent poverty rates in the United States (*persistent poverty* is defined as being in poverty over the last 30 years), comprising 11% of all US counties. Of these, 301 are in non-metropolitan areas. Persistent poverty is highest in the South (22%) followed by the West (16.2%) and then the Northeast and Midwest (13%). The higher persistent poverty rate in the South is particularly important because an estimated 43% of the nonmetro population lived in this region in 2010 (USDA, ERS, 2014). Poverty is also highest in the most rural areas and in completely rural counties (i.e., not adjacent to any metropolitan counties), the poverty rate is 35% with 26% residing in persistent poverty counties (USDA, 2014).

Rural Poverty: Racial and Ethnic Minorities. When poverty rates among rural dweller are analyzed by race, ethnicity, age, and family structure, the statistics on poverty are even more dramatic than residence or region. Racial and ethnic minorities (mainly non-white Hispanics, blacks, and Native Americans) constitute 22% of the rural population, according to the 2010 Census (USDA, ERS, 2012f). This segment of the rural population has grew 30% from 1990 to 2000, largely due to the dramatic increase in non-white Hispanics (up 70.4%) (IOM, 2005). In 2012, according to the Economic Research Service (ERS), poverty rates among rural and racial minorities were two to three times higher (67%) than poverty rates for rural whites (13%) (USDA, ERS, 2012c).

Rural Poverty: Family Composition. Families with two or more adults are less likely to be poor, whether in rural or urban areas, because they are more likely to have multiple sources of income. Families with more than one adult have lower out-of-pocket child care costs and are less likely to have to limit their working hours. More than 75% of rural families are headed by a married couple, and these constitute only 7% of families living in poverty. On the other hand, people living in female-headed families have higher poverty rates (40%) than single male–headed families (21.2%) in rural areas. The Economic Research Service attributes the high rate of poverty for female-headed families to "lower labor force participation rates, shorter average work weeks, and lower earnings" (USDA, ERS, 2011).

Rural Poverty: Children. Children are particularly vulnerable to outcomes of poverty, and they are among the poorest citizens in rural America, constituting 2.8 million or 27.4% of the overall population of rural poor in 2010 (USDA, Farrigan and Parker, 2012). The heaviest concentrations of child poverty are in the South and West. Understanding how poverty is distributed in rural populations is important for planning and delivering programs that ameliorate the impact of poverty, such as food stamps, school lunch programs, school

health nursing interventions, and health insurance coverage (USDA, Farrigan and Parker, 2012).

When race and ethnicity are taken into account, the poverty profile of children worsens dramatically. Racial and ethnic minorities fare far worse than the general rural population of children from birth to 18 years of age. When family composition is also taken into account, we find that almost half of non-Hispanic black children, 34% of Native American children, and 18% of rural children who live in a female-headed household are poor (USDA, Farrigan and Parker, 201).

Health Risk, Injury, and Death

Health behaviors vary along the rural-urban continuum and within rural populations by geographical area. For example, researchers have noted that adults in nonmetropolitan areas use seat belts less often and are less likely to use preventive screening (although the latter trend is confounded by access problems). Elliot, Ginsberg and Winston (2008) compared the prevalence of unlicensed teenaged drivers and that of licensed drivers and found that the former were more likely to be black or Hispanic and to live in rural areas. Rural teens are equally likely with or more likely than both suburban and urban teens to report being victims of violent behavior, to engage in suicide behaviors, and to use drugs (Johnson et al, 2008). Rural residents in the Southern states are more likely to be obese, to smoke more heavily if they do smoke, to use smokeless tobacco, and to engage in sedentary lifestyles. In the rural West, rates of smoking, seat belt use, and obesity are lower, and those of alcohol and smokeless tobacco use are higher. For example, 19% of adolescents living in the most rural counties are smokers, compared with 11% in large metropolitan counties (National Rural Health Association, n.d.).

Other risk factors include alcohol use (higher in rural areas and highest among persons living in the most rural areas, and more commonly among men than women), obesity (higher in rural areas, most particularly rural areas of the South), and physical inactivity during leisure time, which varies by level of urbanization (National Rural Health Association, 2014).

Intentional injuries, against the self or another, are most often the result of firearms usage. In rural counties, nonfatal firearm injuries occur most often at home, whereas in urban counties such injuries occur most often in the streets. Furthermore, numerous studies have noted that firearm suicide in rural counties is an important public health concern. Nationally, suicide is the eleventh leading cause of death, but in rural America, it is the second leading cause of death. The rate of suicide in some rural areas is 800% higher than the national average. Nationally, 14 people in 100,000 died by suicide between the years 1901 and 2009, the latest year for which data is available from the CDC (CDC, Injury Center, 2013). But in Nome County, Alaska, more than 84 people for every 100,000 died by their own hands, the highest suicide rate in any U.S. county. Montana, Wyoming, Nevada, and New Mexico had suicide rates above the national average (Advancing Suicide Prevention, 2005). There was also variation by race and ethnicity. Decreased access to mental health services for treatment of depression may contribute to these higher rates. Among suicide victims, racial and ethnic disparities exist. Suicide rates among American Indian/Alaskan Native ages 15 to 34 years are 2.2 times higher than the national average for that age-group, and Hispanic female high school students in grades 9 through 12 reported more suicide attempts (14.0%) than non-Hispanic white (7.7%) or non-Hispanic black (9.9%) students (CDC, 2008). The suicide rate for non-Hispanic white men 65 years of age and over is higher than that rate for other groups. In 2004, the suicide rate for older non-Hispanic white men was about two to three times the rate for older men in other race or ethnicity groups and nearly eight times the rate for older non-Hispanic white women (CDC, 2007).

Unintentional injuries are the leading cause of death in the United States for both sexes, for all races and ethnicities, and for all age-groups from ages 1 to 44 years. Overall, unintentional injuries occur most often as the result of driving a vehicle (automobile, all-terrain vehicle, bicycle). In the latest available reports, unintentional injuries continue to be higher in rural areas of the United States. The mortality rate for unintentional injuries reported in the *Urban and Rural Health Chartbook* was 54.1 per 100,000 rural residents, which is twice the rate for large metropolitan counties (CDC, 2007). Unintentional injuries are highest among males and in rural counties with the lowest population densities (Castillo and Alexander, 2004).

According to the CDC's National Center for Health Statistics (NCHS), unintentional injury was ranked fifth in the leading causes of death in 2009. This category of death includes "transport accidents," including motor vehicle accidents, and "non-transport accidents," which include falls, firearm accidents, drowning, fire-related deaths, and accidental poisoning, Males aged 15 to 24 years are the most likely victims of unintentional injuries.

In four of the least populated states, the percentage of deaths from unintentional injuries was much higher than the national average: 7.7% in Idaho, 8.0% in Montana, 9.1% in Wyoming, and 14.3% in Alaska. Overall, deaths from unintentional injuries were approximately 80% to 85% higher for females and males in the most rural counties than for those in suburban areas of metropolitan counties in 1996 to 1998, and highest of all in the West (Castillo and Alexander, 2004). Driving at high speeds, driving long distances, driving in winter conditions, not using seat belts, and consuming alcohol have been cited as contributing to higher levels of injury deaths and disability for rural residents in the West. Lack of ready access to counseling, emergency medical services, and rehabilitation are also thought to be contributing factors to these high levels.

Vulnerable Groups

Demographic and personal characteristics, such as age, education, gender, race, ethnicity, language, and culture, round out the examples of factors that affect health and may block access to existing services. Age is an important consideration in the planning of health care services for rural communities. As noted in previous sections, many retirees are moving into rural areas, and many younger people are moving out. Because the incomes of many elderly may be lower, the tax base of counties and municipalities may be inadequate to cover the disproportionate share of the health care services used by the elderly (age 65 years and over) (Bailey, 2009).

The population of the elderly is expected to double by 2050. Elderly women tend to live at or near the poverty level and to achieve poverty status twice as often as men (Cawthorne, 2010, USDA, ERS, 2012c). Along with educational attainment, this is a critical indicator of well-being for the elderly and the young. The elderly poor tend to be isolated and to lack access to support services, health care, prescription drugs, adequate nutrition, and transportation.

The number of children in rural areas increased by 2% from 2008 to 2009 and another 0.9 percentage points from 2009 to 2010. More than 2.8 million children in nonmetro areas were in poverty in 2010 (USDA, ERS, 2012c). In addition to population growth, racial and ethnic diversity has increased. Today, the proportion of Hispanic children is the fastest-growing component of the rural population regardless of region. The population of black children has remained steady, and the majority of rural black children are still concentrated in the South. Native American children constitute only 3% of the total nonmetropolitan population, although in areas of the country (mainly West and Central) with high concentrations of Native Americans, this percentage is, of course, much higher. Evidence suggests that fetal, infant, and maternal mortality rates are slightly higher in nonmetropolitan than metropolitan areas, and that prenatal care in the later pregnancy stages is problematic. Nonmetropolitan children, like nonmetropolitan adults, are more likely to live in poverty, and proportionately fewer rural children were covered by health insurance (Kandel, 2005; USDA, ERS, 2012c).

Education and Employment

Research on the socioeconomic determinants of health has revealed a strong positive correlation between health and length of schooling (Cutler and Lleras-Muney, 2006, USDA, ERS, 2012d). Demographics of a minority group often influence and result from social and economic factors. Age and education are indicators for employment. For the aged and for ethnic and racial minorities, a pattern of lower educational attainment and unfavorable economic circumstances emerges with increasing rurality (Figure 23-2). Although the education picture is changing, many women now in their 70s and 80s grew up before public education was mandatory. Families could not afford to send them to school, or they were simply expected to learn to read and write, seek employment, and marry. Education, with its links to economic and health variables, is still a serious problem for rural America (Figure 23-3). Low education and employment levels characterize all rural minority groups except Asians. Children living in precarious economic conditions have additional challenges to doing well in school and remaining in school through high school graduation. In 2010, 70% of rural dwellers held high school diplomas or Graduate Equivalency Diplomas (GEDs),

Educational attainment for the population age 25 and older, 2000 and 2006-10

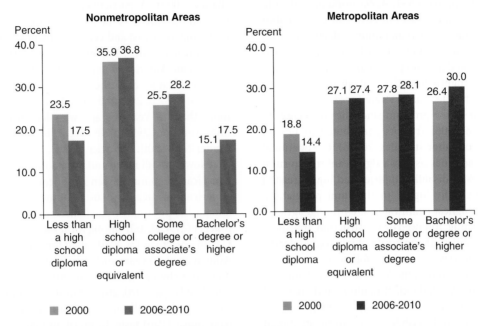

Note: Counties were classified using the 2003 metro and nonmetro definitions.
Source: USDA, Economic Research Service calculations based on data from the 2000 Census and the 2006-10 American Community Survey.

FIGURE 23-2 Educational attainment rates for rural adults. (From U.S. Department of Agriculture, Economic Research Service: *Employment & education: High school completion rates, (adults 25 and older)*, 2012. Available from <http://www.ers.usda.gov/topics/rural-economy-population/employment-education/rural-education.aspx>.)

Poverty rates, by educational attainment, 2005-09

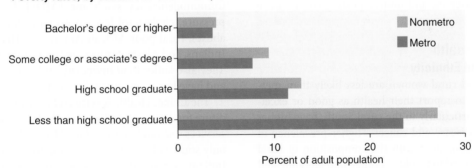

Source: Census Bureau, 2005-09 American Community Survey.

FIGURE 23-3 Rural poverty rates by educational level. (From McDonald K: *Metro and nonmetro poverty rates according to education level 2005 to 2009*, 2011. Available from <http://www.bigpictureagriculture.com/2011/11/metro-and-nonmetro-poverty-rates.html>.)

compared with 77% in 2000 (USDA, 2012a). The college completion rate of rural students was almost half (17%) that of urban students (30%). There are also large gaps in educational completion by region, race, and ethnicity, with the Western and Midwestern rural students exceeding the high school completion rates of students in the rural South (USDA, 2012a). Rural and central city students, especially minorities other than Asians, lag behind suburban children on most indicators of adequate progress in schools (IOM, 2005). Low educational attainment is a challenge in rural America. Skill

requirements for rural employment continue to rise, lack of education is correlated with persistent poverty, and poverty is a predictor of poor health.

Furthermore, counties that have a low-wage economy have difficulty providing the infrastructure needed to provide education, public health, and health care services for low-wage families. They also have difficulty attracting new employers who might contribute to the economic development of a rural area but need a more highly educated workforce.

Occupational Health Risks

In the United States, approximately 4,693 workers died from work-related illnesses and injuries in 2011 (Bureau of Labor Statistics, 2012a). Fatal occupational injuries declined 23.1% from 1992 to 2002. The overall fatal work injury rate for the U.S. in 2011 was 3.5 fatal injuries per 100,000 full-time equivalent workers, down slightly from the final rate of 3.6 reported for 2010. The published fatal injury rate for 2011 equals the lowest rate reported by the program since the conversion to hours-based rates in 2006. Tractors contributed to 12% of the deaths (Bureau of Labor statistics, 2012b). Occupational injuries, fatalities, and illnesses play a significant role in rural health, because rates of disabling injuries and injury-related mortality are dramatically higher in the rural population. Industries with the highest death rate were mining, agriculture, forestry, and fishing, followed by construction, transportation, and public utilities. The majority of job-related deaths due to workplace injuries were in the following categories: transportation-related motor vehicle accidents, machinery-related events, homicides, falls, electrocution, and chemical and thermal injuries (Castillo and Alexander, 2004).

Occupational death and disability can also be attributed to nonfatal injuries, and occupational diseases, such as cancer, asbestosis, silicosis, and anthracosis associated with both organic and inorganic exposures (CDC, NIOSH Program, 2012). Work-related injuries, deaths, and illness data must be interpreted with caution. Although surveillance of occupational injuries, illnesses, and fatalities has improved through the collaboration of the states and National Institute for Occupational Safety and Health (NIOSH), data still come from many sources, and underreporting continues to be problematic.

Perceptions of Health
Gender, Race, and Ethnicity

Both rural men and rural women are less likely than metropolitan residents to report their health as good or excellent. Rural areas, particularly in the rural South, have higher incidents of heart disease and cancer. Higher prevalence of chronic disease is consistent with the composition of rural populations, which tend to be older, poorer, and less educated (Artnak, McGraw, and Stanley, 2011). Rural men and women also smoke or use smokeless tobacco more. In the aggregate, they exercise fewer preventive behaviors, have less contact with physicians, and often have less access to care than people with similar problems in urban areas (NRHA, 2014). Rural men and youths are also more likely to die or become disabled from unintentional injuries due to risky behavior or work-related causes, and are more likely to commit suicide, than women or urban men and youths.

Although rural populations overall are at lower risk for most cancers, certain rural subpopulations are at greater risk. For example, Appalachia has a much higher rate than the national figure. Residents in low-income areas and the uninsured, particularly African Americans, tend to have more late-stage cancer diagnoses; and rural residents in general may have less access to quality health care, including both medical care and screening and prevention programs (Bailey, 2009). A particularly serious problem for minorities and the elderly is the lack of cancer screening, including screening for breast and cervical cancer for women and prostate cancer for men. Preventive care is especially important for African-American men, for whom the prostate cancer rate is higher than for any other racial or ethnic group.

From 1987 to 2005 the age-adjusted percentage of women more than 40 years of age who had had a mammogram improved from 29% to 70% according to the CDC's National Center for Health Statistics (CDC, 2009b). The percentages were lower for all racial and ethnic minorities: 55% for Asian American, 65% for African American, and 58% for Hispanic American women. Use of mammography was the lowest among the poor, most particularly in the 40- to 49-year age bracket (47.4%), and among the least educated (CDC, 2009b). Health objectives for 2010 called for at least 80% of American women aged 40 years and older to have received a mammogram and clinical breast examination in the previous 2 years (*Healthy People 2020,* 2013). Similarly, women who are poor, elderly, and less educated are less likely to receive Papanicolaou smear (Pap) tests. In racial and ethnic groups, the percentages of women who get Pap tests are lower for Hispanics, American Indians, and Alaska Natives. The lowest percentage is found in Asian women.

Coupled with poverty and lack of access to care, rural minorities are among the nation's least healthy citizens. African American and Native American children and children of migrant workers are among the poorest of rural residents. By almost any measure or index (e.g., incidence of acquired immunodeficiency syndrome [AIDS], birth weight, blood pressure, cholesterol level, cancer incidence, and substance abuse), rural poor African Americans, Hispanics, American Indians, and Alaska Natives are less healthy than rural whites. They also suffer food insecurity and hunger more frequently and have less access to quality health care.

The Indian Health Service (IHS), whose per capita expenditure for American Indian and Alaska Native (AI/AN) health services is about half that of the U.S. civilian population, is the only source of health care funding for many rural American Indians. Marked disparities persist between American Indians and whites. The death rate for American Indians is 1.5 times that for whites, and the former are more likely to suffer a chronic health condition. These higher rates of morbid conditions use significant medical resources from both primary and specialty care physicians. In addition, rural American Indians are less likely to have private health insurance coverage, less likely to use health services, and more likely to have transportation difficulties. Among perceived barriers to rural American Indians' access to important specialty services, financial constraints top the list (Baldwin et al, 2008).

The percentage of Hispanics and Latinos in the U.S. population was about equal to that of African Americans (13% vs. 16% during the year 2011) and the former will soon become the largest minority group in the United States (U.S. Census Bureau, 2010). They are already the predominant minority in the West. Hispanics have diverse cultures, histories, and socioeconomic and health status. The largest Hispanic sub-groups are of Mexican, Cuban, and Puerto Rican descent, although Mexican is the largest by far (accounting for 58% of the Hispanic population living in the United States). In non-metropolitan areas, the population of Hispanics has doubled, and almost half of all Hispanics in rural areas are living outside the traditional areas of settlement in the Southwestern states. As emphasized previously, this growing segment of the population continues to be overrepresented among the rural poor. In 2010, the U.S. Census Bureau reported that 27% of Hispanics live below the federal poverty level, compared with 13% of the white non-Hispanic population. Elderly Hispanics were also 2.5 times more likely to live below the poverty line than white non-Hispanics. Hispanics are most likely to report barriers to obtaining needed health care and are least likely to have a usual source of care; for those blacks and Hispanics reporting a usual source of care, the source is most likely to be hospital-based (U.S. Census Bureau, 2010).

SPECIFIC RURAL AGGREGATES

Agricultural Workers

Health Disparities

An example of health disparities among agricultural workers is the group of farm workers that supports fruit and vegetable production. In general, migrant and seasonal farmworkers (MSFWs) may have the poorest health of any aggregate in the United States and the least access to affordable health care. Eighty-five percent of MSFWs are Hispanic, Latino, or African American. The rest are largely white seasonal workers who follow the harvests to drive combines or haul crops from the fields to storage, market, or seaports. These populations, estimated as between 3 and 5 million people each year, are vulnerable to a host of health problems and diseases that center on occupational and environmental hazards and other health correlates (USDA, 2013c &d).

Accidents and Injuries

Working in highly variable environmental conditions (e.g., temperature extremes, a wide variety of work tasks, and unpredictable circumstances) is associated with an increased frequency of accidents and fatalities. Farm-related activities are extremely heterogeneous and vary significantly with the season, types of crops produced, and types of machinery used. Farmers are located in geographically isolated areas and often work alone. This constellation of factors puts farmers and their families at increased risk for accidental injury and delayed access to emergency or trauma care.

In 2012, the rate of fatal injuries per 100,000 full-time equivalents employed in the agricultural sector was 21.2 compared to manufacturing (2.1), retail trade (1.9), transportation (13.3), and governmental employees (2.0) (Bureau of Labor Statistics, 2012a). According to the CDC's NIOSH Program (2012), agricultural machinery is the most common cause of fatalities and nonfatal injuries of U.S. agricultural workers, including on-farm fatalities among youth (< 20 years). Tractor-related accidents, especially rollovers, are the most frequent causes of farm accidents, accounting for more than one fourth of farm fatalities. The actual causes of death and serious injury are associated with rollovers of equipment that lacks rollover protective structures (ROPSs) and seat belts (CDC, NIOSH Program, 2012). With such statistics, it is easy to see why accident prevention programs for farm children and families have focused heavily on tractor safety awareness.

Acute and Chronic Illnesses

Several types of farming activities are associated with more occurrences than expected of acute and chronic respiratory conditions. Individuals with long-term exposure to grain dusts, such as grain elevator workers and dairy workers, have diminished respiratory function and increased frequency of respiratory symptoms (National Center for Farmworker Health [NCFH], 2013). Occupational asthma and more exotic fungal or toxic gas–related conditions also occur in higher frequency in agricultural than nonagricultural populations. Community health nurses, who are familiar with local farming practices in rural areas, often make links between farm work and respiratory symptoms. In such situations, the role of the nurse is to refer patients to appropriate health care providers and to provide support and education for affected people and their families.

Exposure to pesticides, herbicides, and other chemicals is also a major concern for farmers and their families. From an occupational perspective, farming is unusual because the home and the worksite are the same. Exposure risks to children and spouses may be heightened when farmers wear contaminated clothing and boots into the home. Homes are often located in close proximity to fields and animal containment facilities, which are treated with a variety of chemicals.

Nurses in rural emergency rooms or other ambulatory care settings may be the first providers to encounter farmers and others with acute pesticide poisoning. During discussions with farmers, ranchers, or other high-risk groups (e.g., nursery workers and tree planters), community health nurses may note a pattern of headaches and nausea that occur during planting or spraying seasons. In such an instance, the nurse can serve as an important resource by obtaining a careful history of signs and symptoms, the temporal nature of symptom occurrence, and the types of pesticides and personal protection used (e.g., respirators and protective clothing). When evidence suggests pesticide-related illness, appropriate referral and follow-up are imperative to ensure the safety of the affected person and the family.

Signs and symptoms of acute pesticide poisoning are fairly clear, and most health providers in rural communities would recognize them. Common symptoms include headache, dizziness, diaphoresis, nausea, and vomiting. If left untreated, those affected may experience a progression of symptoms, including dyspnea, bronchospasm, and muscle twitching. Deaths are relatively uncommon, but they do occur.

Alterman, Steege, Petersen and Muntaner, (2008), who studied ethnic, racial, and gender variations among U.S. farmers, found a high prevalence of musculoskeletal discomfort, followed by respiratory problems, hearing loss, and hypertension. Latino and Asian American operators had lower prevalences of health problems than white non-Latino and white farmers. Hypertension and osteoarthritis were more prevalent in black farmers but hearing loss, skin problems, and heart problems were less so. Cancer was less prevalent in black than in white farmers. In American Indian or Alaska Native farmers, musculoskeletal problems, skin problems, and hypertension were most common.

Migrant and Seasonal Farmworkers

Although the discussion of agricultural issues has focused primarily on farmers and farm families, it is important to understand the role of migrant (i.e., migrate to find work) and seasonal (i.e., reside permanently in one place and work locally when farm labor is needed) farmworkers in U.S. agricultural production and the health risks to this population. Older references to farmworkers often referred to three "migrant streams," in which workers entered the country through Mexico and migrated north. The current reality is that migrant workers enter the country through a variety of access points and follow any route necessary to obtain work. Seasonal workers reside in agricultural areas permanently and take various farm jobs during harvesting times. For example, a seasonal worker may be employed in restaurant work during the winter and may spend the summer months picking apples or working in a local apple shed or cannery (USDA, ERS, 2013).

MSFWs comprise a vulnerable population in regard to health risks because they have low income and migratory status. In many rural areas, community health nurses form the central link between farmworkers and health services. Through standing or mobile clinic sites, nurses have established a leadership role in the provision of episodic and preventive services for workers and their families. Lacking access to many types of preventive services, farmworkers often visit a migrant clinic with any number of health problems, including severe dental problems, unresolved communicable diseases, and untreated injuries. In addition to the direct provision of care, nurses in many communities have served as important advocates on behalf of farmworkers and have worked to ensure health care access for those traveling through their areas.

Cultural, linguistic, economic, and mobility barriers all contribute to the nature and magnitude of health problems observed in farmworkers. Cultural and linguistic barriers are the most overt because many of the communities where farmworkers work consider them outsiders. In many settings, migrant workers live isolated from the agricultural communities they serve. Although some workers travel in extended family groups and have the support that comes with being together, other workers leave their families at home. Often the latter are male workers who work and live together. A common misconception among U.S. health care providers is that these farmworkers are from Mexico and that Spanish is their primary language. Farmworkers originate from many communities in Mexico, the Caribbean, and Central and South America, and they may speak the language of their home country, English, or several languages.

Enumeration of Migrant and Seasonal Farmworkers

To increase access to primary and preventative care for MSFW populations, information is needed on the numbers and distribution of farmworkers at the national, state, and local levels. Because MSFWs move frequently for work, census estimates generally provide a poor assessment of this population's needs for health care services. Additionally, the legislation that created the Migrant Health Program (MHP) (Section 330g of the Public Health Service Act), under the direction of the Bureau of Primary Health Care (BPHC) (2000) and the Health Resources and Services Administration (HRSA), requires that priorities be established according to where the greatest need exists. Hence the MHP has supported the ongoing and comprehensive assessment of the numbers of MSFWs and published the Migrant and Seasonal Farmworker Enumeration Profile Study (MSFWEPS) (Bureau of Health Professions, 2003). Enumeration data from the MSFWEPS are available for Michigan, Arkansas, California, Florida, Louisiana, Maryland, North Carolina, Mississippi, Oklahoma, Texas, and Washington.

Health Needs and Opportunities for Preventive Care

Similarities in exposure and work practices make some of the farmworkers' health needs similar to those of farmers and their families. Generally, these health needs reflect the increased rates of accidents and injuries, dermatological conditions, and pulmonary problems observed in the two populations. However, there are additional challenges in both the identification and the treatment of farmworkers with health problems. One of the biggest problems that nurses face in designing health programs is understanding the full magnitude of these health problems. Many farmworkers who become ill eventually return to their countries of origin to obtain treatment and to be with family. This phenomenon makes it difficult to get complete, reliable numbers about disease rates. A variety of public health indicators are likely to undercount farmworkers as a group, ranging from tumor registries to Workers' Compensation injuries (NCFH, 2013). In addition, farmworkers may be less likely to seek treatment for health problems that do not require emergency treatment or surgery.

Studies of farmworkers' health status have provided data indicating that they are less likely to receive preventive care from any health source. Preventive needs include dental care, vision screening and treatment, and gynecological and breast examinations. Many farmworkers, because they move from community to community, are often unaware of clinical and social services they could receive and that are available at reduced or no cost to low-income families.

Hearing Farmworkers' Voices

Several studies and pilot projects have used focus groups, community meetings, or other qualitative research methods to listen to farmworkers' concerns and give these concerns a voice through publication and advocacy. Several years ago, the Farmworker Justice Fund brought female farmworkers together in a national effort to give them a forum for their concerns and their impressions of health needs. The women identified priority concerns in the areas of child and family issues, health care services, workplace issues, and empowerment. The group's recommendations in the area of health care included keep clinics open during evening hours, provide transportation to clinics, increase access through mobile health units, provide social and health services in one building, increase home visits by students, encourage careers in farmworker health, enhance nutrition education to families, teach first aid, enforce farm labor health laws, and give farmworkers a copy of the record after each clinic visit (Farm Worker Health, 2006).

APPLICATION OF RELEVANT THEORIES AND "THINKING UPSTREAM" CONCEPTS TO RURAL HEALTH

Upstream and prevention-oriented approaches have several implications for nurses in rural practice. Descriptions of three strategies for upstream interventions follow: attack community-based problems at their roots, emphasize the "doing" aspects of health, and maximize the use of informal networks.

Attacking Community-Based Problems at Their Roots

Upstream approaches to community health problems direct the nurse toward an understanding of the precursors of poor health within populations of interest. Individual nurses can be effective forces in uncovering and enhancing community awareness of health-endangering situations. Environmental health issues in rural communities, such as pesticide exposure and health hazards from point-source factory emissions, are more effectively assessed and remedied on a community level than on a case-by-case basis. Nurses' involvement in helping people understand health problems in a larger context can be the genesis of change. Nurses and other community members can take social action on behalf of those affected. For example, by heightening awareness of sulfur dioxin levels from a local refinery and the relationship of those emission levels to respiratory problems in vulnerable populations, nurses can help citizens gain an understanding of the collective rather than individual burden of the refinery on their community's health.

Emphasizing the "Doing" Aspects of Health

There are consistent differences between the ways rural and nonrural residents perceive health. The primary one may be the relative importance of "work" and "being able to work" in self-reported definitions of health (Weinert and Long, 1987). Rural attitudes generally emphasize the "doing" aspects of health in functioning and performing the daily activities fundamentally important in their daily lives. The high value placed on "being able to do" can give astute nurses intervention opportunities for both families and communities. Examples of nursing intervention strategies that capitalize on this attitude include accident prevention programs for children,

exercise and nutrition programs for seniors, and participation of local industries in risk reduction programs for workers. Active involvement of the target population in all phases of program planning and implementation is key to the success of these programs.

Maximizing the Use of Informal Networks

Recognizing and using informal networks in the community is essential to the "doing" concept of prevention programs. The name used, such as empowerment model or community action model, is less important than soliciting the involvement of informal networks and local leaders in planning health interventions. As most people who have been involved in community empowerment programs will attest, accomplishing the involvement of these important entities is not easy or straightforward. Turf issues and collateral agendas can obstruct rather than facilitate change. However, failure to elicit community involvement in population-based health interventions will have unfavorable consequences. Frequently, superimposed change tends to fit poorly with the community it is intended to serve. Rural change strategies will be short-lived unless community members understand them and invest in their own well-being.

RURAL HEALTH CARE DELIVERY SYSTEM

Health Care Provider Shortages

The Bureau of Health Professions (2003) states that the size and characteristics of the future health workforce are determined by the interaction of various forces acting on the health environment, including economic factors, technology, regulatory and legislative actions, epidemiological factors, the health care education system, and demographics. Current shortages of health care professionals in rural areas are likely to become worse with the increase in demand caused by population aging and growing racial and ethnic diversity. In actual numbers, the shortage has been growing since 1990. Although approximately 25% of the U.S. population lives in nonmetropolitan counties, only 18% of registered nurses (RNs) practice there. See Primary Care.

Clearly the growing nursing shortage will affect all of America. This is both a supply shortage and a demand shortage. Declining school enrollments, retirement of current nurses, and the increased need for care of an aging population make the situation especially critical (Sigma Theta Tau International, n.d.). A survey by the American Organization of Nurse Executives (AONE) found that it takes significantly longer to fill vacancies in small hospitals, usually located in rural areas, than in larger urban facilities (Thrall, 2007). Rural nurses earn less than their urban counterparts, compounding recruitment difficulties. Nurses with baccalaureate and master's degrees, other than master's degree–prepared NPs, are compensated less for this additional education (Thrall, 2007).

A solution proposed for the shortage of health care providers is for rural communities to "grow their own." A rural community, a group of small communities, or a county could support local students attending college and recruit students currently attending professional schools. The students would make a commitment to work in the community in return for monetary support for their educations (Thrall, 2007). Tuition reimbursement and access to distance learning programs can assist practicing nurses. Continuing education and baccalaureate and master's degrees are available through e-mail, Internet-based courses, interactive video classes, and by-mail videos. Some programs are provided exclusively via the Internet. Nebraska's rural communities are enthusiastic about the University of Nebraska College of Nursing Internet courses. The program is helping them grow their own nurses. Research shows that nurses educated in rural communities are more apt to stay and work there than those who move away to attend school (Thrall, 2007).

Telemedicine

In light of provider storages and recruitment difficulties with the physician, nurse, and other health care worker shortages coupled with the difficulty in recruiting them to rural areas, alternatives to improve access must be identified. Telemedicine is an alternative that is expanding across the country. Telemedicine is viewed as a cost-effective alternative to the more traditional face-to-face way of providing medical care (Medicaid.gov, 2013).

Recent projects geared toward extending telemedicine services to rural areas include the Frontier Health Projects support of new models of health care. Distinctions are made between telehealth and telemedicine. *Telehealth* includes technologies such as telephones, facsimile machines, electronic mail systems, and remote patient monitoring devices for the collection and transmission of patient data for monitoring and interpretation. Conversely, *telemedicine* seeks to improve a patient's health by permitting two-way, real-time interactive communication between the patient and the physician or practitioner at the distant site and is centered on efficiency, effectiveness, and safety. This electronic communication means the use of interactive telecommunications equipment that includes, at a minimum, audio and video equipment. This definition is modeled on Medicare's definition of telehealth services (Medicaid.gov, 2013).

Although several states in the Midwest and West have taken advantage of telemedicine in rural areas, the patchwork approach in legislation has contributed to varying degrees of implementation and financial support for its implementation (Braum, 2013).

Managed Care in the Rural Environment

Managed care has recently changed health care delivery in the United States. In rural areas, health care delivery networks with managed care elements are being developed. Potential benefits and risks of managed care for rural areas have been identified, with recognition of the difficulty rural providers in solo or small group practices face in delivering cost-effective, complex health care needed. Possible benefits to managed care include lowering primary care costs, improving the quality of care, and stabilizing the local rural health care system. Risks are also apparent, including probable high start-up and administrative costs and the volatile effect of large, urban-based for-profit managed care companies (Allender, Rector, and Warner, 2010).

Outside of Medicaid, managed care has yet to become a major presence in much of rural America because small disperse populations, few visits per individual, and large numbers of elderly on Medicare with low-level reimbursements do not make the aggregate financially attractive to a managed care organization (MCO). In fact, despite the existence of federally qualified health centers that provide care to underserved populations through Medicare or Medicaid or on sliding fee scales, there were few rural people enrolled in sponsored health plans (Allender et al, 2010). Providers in rural markets face severe financial constraints as health maintenance organizations (HMOs) increasingly cope with smaller numbers of enrollees and continue to reduce provider reimbursement (IOM, 2005). Communities that make the most progress toward partnerships or integration are those whose local leaders and providers have strong incentives to work together and are motivated to bring about change to the health care system. Authorities in rural health and managed care report that it is too soon to know whether managed care will become a significant way of delivering health care in rural areas, like it has become in urban America (Allender et al, 2010; IOM, 2004).

COMMUNITY-BASED CARE

In the mid-1990s, the phrase *community-based care* became a popular term for the myriad of services provided outside the walls of an institution. Health care services are no longer provided exclusively in the hospital setting. Community-based care includes services that are provided where individuals live, work, or go to school. Examples of community-based services are home health and hospice care, occupational health programs, community mental health programs, ambulatory care services, school health programs, faith-based care, and elder services, such as adult day care. The concept also includes community participation in decisions about health care services, a focus on all three levels of prevention, and an understanding that the hospital is no longer the exclusive health care provider.

Home Health and Hospice Care

Home health and hospice programs vary in structure. A national study on Medicare hospice use found that only one third of rural counties have a hospice based within the county, but nearly two thirds of urban counties do (Vernig et al, 2004). Urban hospices are more likely to be freestanding, whereas rural hospices tend to be hospital-based. Larger communities may support a hospital-based home care agency with hospice service, a freestanding full-service agency, or both. In sparsely populated rural locations, home health and hospice services may be contracted from a larger regional agency, with a local nurse hired to provide services.

Vernig and associates (2004) found that the more remote the rural environment, the less likely hospice services were used. Nurse case management and development of local resources, using the county extension services as a bridge for outreach services, can improve home care for patients needing hospice care and provide support for their families. A partnership between the public health nurse and county extension service could provide support and information groups and caregiving classes for the important informal provider network. Chapter 33 discusses home health and hospice in greater detail.

Faith Communities and Parish Nursing

Rural residents are perceived as having strong traditional values. At the heart of these values is a strong sense of community, family life, and religious faith. Since the conceptualization of parish nursing in the early 1980s, registered nurses have developed and expanded the role. Parish nurses integrate nursing expertise and faith-based knowledge to provide holistic care to members of congregations. More than 7000 nurses have completed formal training programs in parish nursing. The exact number of parish nurses working as paid and unpaid staff in both urban and rural faith communities is not known, because many nurses have not been formally prepared for the role (International Parish Nurse Resource Center, n.d.). Both professional nursing and parish nursing are based on health and healing (American Nurses Association, 2005).

In a comparison of experiences of rural and urban faith-based programs, DeHaven and colleagues (2004) found that faith-based health programs can have positive effects—notably, they can significantly increase knowledge of disease, improve screening behavior and readiness to change, and reduce risks associated with disease and disease symptoms. Rural nurses are more likely to be involved in case management and coordination of services than their urban counterparts (Molanari, Jaiswal, and Hollinger-Forrest, 2011). In urban settings, contact with parishioners is primarily at the church, whereas contacts in rural settings are most often in the home, on the phone, or in other community-based settings. Collaboration between faith communities and other organizations can help extend limited rural community health resources. Such partnerships have been promoted by federal and state governments to enhance the public health efforts (Zahner and Corrado, 2004). Chapter 32 provides an in-depth discussion of parish nursing.

Informal Care Systems

Limited availability of and accessibility to formal health care resources in rural areas, combined with the self-reliance and self-help traits of rural residents, have resulted in the development of strong informal care and social support networks in rural communities. Rural residents are more apt to entrust care to established informal networks than to new formal care systems. Examining perceptions of rural health and social systems, Thorngren (2003) found that rural residents agreed that experiences inherent in rural life both contribute to and ameliorate health-related concerns attributed to higher levels of family and community involvement, problem-solving abilities, and connections to the land, that may be a factor in the formation and use of informal systems.

Informal care systems or networks include people who have assumed the role of caregiver on the basis of their individual qualities, life situations, or social roles. People who participate in these networks may provide direct help, advice, or information. Rural residents identify spouses, adult children, other family members, friends, and neighbors as informal providers of care (Coen Buckwalter et al, 2002).

Informal caregivers often find themselves in stressful circumstances (Sanford, 2004). Rural residents who are in need of assistance are usually elderly, have chronic illness, have few resources, and must travel long distances for health care. Rasheed and Rasheed (2003) suggest that by 2050, 21% of all Americans will be members of a minority group. Disparities already exist in the physical and mental health status, service availability, service access, and socioeconomic status for minorities. Americans in rural communities and in the black community rely heavily on community-based informal care systems,

Van Exel, de Graaf, and Brouwer (2008) studied caregiver attitudes toward respite care and found that those who could potentially benefit were reluctant to seek it for various reasons. This finding has enormous implications for nursing practice. Because informal health care is an important, cost-effective component of health care systems, different forms of respite care have been implemented to support caregivers. Not only do many patients have a preference for receiving care from someone familiar in their home environment; in many cases such care will help them avoid placement in a long-term care facility. Nurses have a role in discussing the potential benefits of support for both the family and the care recipient.

Rural Public Health Departments

There are more than 2,800 local health departments in the United States, yet fewer than 5% serve populations of less than 50,000 people (Weisbecker, 2010). The purpose of *Healthy People 2010* objective 23-11 was to increase the proportion of state and local public health departments that meet national performance standards for public health services. In *Healthy People 2020*, the health disparities in rural health have been highlighted and specific areas of focus for rural health have been established (*Healthy People 2020*, Disparities, 2013).

In a study of 99 local health departments in three rural states, Rosenblatt and colleagues (2002) found that public health nurses were the core providers of public health services. Many smaller local health departments do not have the economic base to employ other professional public health providers, such as physicians, epidemiologists, sanitarians, and nutritionists, at the local level. Frequently the services of such providers are instead provided at the state level or collaboratively between groups of local health departments. A local physician may serve as a part-time, unpaid health officer. The lack of additional onsite public health providers poses two problems. First, the ability to collaborate with others about potential or actual public health problems is decreased or nonexistent. Second, the ranges of services provided are less comprehensive. Often, these small facilities can offer only federally funded programs with few locally funded services.

Environmental health, maternal and child health, and communicable disease control are the three highest-priority programs of rural local health departments (Bailey, 2009).

Rural Mental Health Care

The economic crisis that affected much of the rural population in the 1980s contributed to mental health problems. Natural disasters, such as drought and flood, and economic downturns in the late 1990s have contributed to continuing chronic stress. Those affected are most apt to work in the traditional ranching, farming, mining, forestry, and fishing industries. Although mental health disorders widely affect rural and urban residents throughout the lifespan, factors such as poverty, race, age, and rural dwelling lower the prospect of accessing mental health services. Clearly, large sections of at-risk rural populations are without mental health care (Bailey, 2009).

Three key factors have been identified as contributing to mental illness in rural areas. First, there is a lack of specialized mental health providers in rural areas. The most recent figures show that 75% of rural counties with populations between 2500 and 20,000 do not have a psychiatrist and that 95% do not have a child psychiatrist. Next, because of the lack of qualified mental health care providers, rural residents often receive services from primary care providers. Many rural primary care providers are ill-equipped to provide mental health services, and there are limited nurse practitioner and physician assistant resources to support the mental health care that is needed. Both specialized mental health care and primary health care providers are confronted with barriers related to rural practice. These include a more diverse practice, fewer opportunities for ongoing education, and fewer professionals to consult than their colleagues in urban practice. Lastly, rural residents often do not seek mental health services because of perceived stigma and because they do not always recognize a need for mental health services (Bailey, 2009).

Emergency Services

Access to emergency medical services (EMS) has been identified as one of the most significant health care issues for rural residents (Bailey, 2009; Bryant, 2009). Emergency medical services include pre-hospital care, hospital- or health center–based emergency care, and trauma systems.

Rural residents depend on EMS because of their high risk for unintentional injury. Low population density has been shown to be a strong predictor of higher injury-related morbidity and mortality rates in rural areas (Peek-Asa, Zwerling, and Staliones, 2004). In medically underserved areas, EMS systems play an increasingly important role in decreasing the morbidity and mortality of individuals needing emergency care. Getting patients from the place of injury to the trauma center within the "golden hour" is frequently not possible in rural areas because of barriers imposed by distance, terrain, climatic conditions, and communication methods. Some rural facilities are more than 1 hour away by air from the nearest trauma center or tertiary care hospital (Hsia and Shen, 2011). For those rural residents, the death rate remains twice that of urban residents.

Challenges faced by rural EMS systems include a shortage of volunteers, a lower level of training than among urban providers, training curricula that often do not reflect rural hazards (e.g., farm equipment trauma), lack of guidance from physicians, and lack of physician training about and orientation to the EMS system (Bryant, 2009). Low population density, large, isolated, or inaccessible areas, severe weather, poor roads, and lower density of telephones or other communication methods also contribute to difficult public access for emergency care. These problems make the challenges of developing EMS in rural areas substantial (Branas et al, 2005).

Emergency Preparedness in Rural Communities

Emergency preparedness refers to actions that should be performed prior to an emergency, such as planning and coordination meetings, procedure writing, team training, emergency drills and exercises, and positioning of emergency equipment. *Emergency response* refers to actions taken to deal with an actual, ongoing event (Rural Assistance Center, n.d.). Rural areas are not exempt from disasters. Challenges of emergency preparation and management are different for rural communities from those for urban ones. Bryant (2009) categorized these challenges into four major themes: resource limitation, separation and remoteness, low population density, and communication.

Resources needed in a disaster include human capital, financial capital, and social capital. Owing to the increase in urbanization, the decline in rural overall population, and the rise in rural population age, the human and financial resources available to prepare and respond to disasters are limited. Social capital becomes the focus to meet the challenges of rural communities. Building relationships among emergency agencies, community organizations, and local businesses is essential to secure human and financial resources. Rural areas also depend on networks of volunteers (e.g., first responders).

The remoteness of rural areas results in longer response times. Population density may impact funding of rural communities emergency preparedness. State and federal programs often consider population size and density in many funding decisions, so densely populated areas receive the most attention for mitigation and recovery activities (Bryant, 2009). Finally, communication education about emergency preparation is more expensive in rural areas. This higher cost leads to reduced outreach prior to disasters and throughout the event. Warning systems are often absent or neglected in remote areas, placing the burden on the individual to access emergency information.

LEGISLATION AND PROGRAMS AFFECTING RURAL PUBLIC HEALTH

Programs that Augment Health Care Facilities and Services

Several programs are particularly important for meeting the public health needs of rural people. One is the Community Health Centers (CHC) program administered by the United

States Public Health Service (USPHS). The CHC program benefits underserved areas and populations by providing primary health care and, in some cases, supplemental secondary and tertiary health care, such as hospital care, long-term home health care, and rehabilitation. Rural health clinics (RHCs) are designed to improve access to primary care. As an incentive to rural communities to apply for RHCs, Medicare and Medicaid are reimbursed at a higher rate than usual at such centers.

The Migrant Health Clinic (MHC) program and the Migrant Health Program (MHP) also come under the Division of Community and Migrant Health and HRSA. The MHC program provides comprehensive nursing and medical care and support services to MSFWs and their families. The centers provide culturally sensitive care to a racially and culturally diverse farm labor force from many countries in Latin America and the Caribbean. Bilingual, bicultural health personnel, including lay outreach workers, use culturally appropriate protocols to provide primary care, preventive health care, transportation, dental care, pharmaceuticals, and environmental health services. The MHCs must provide the same services as the CHC and may also offer supplemental services, such as environmental health services, infectious disease and parasite control, and accident prevention programs.

Medicare's Rural Hospital Flexibility (RHF) grant program replaces earlier demonstration programs. According to information provided by the Office of Rural Health Policy (ORHP), the RHF program "allows small hospitals the flexibility to reconfigure operations and be licensed as Critical Access Hospitals (CAHs)" (HRSA, Medicare Rural Hospital Flexibility Grant, n.d.). The program also provides cost-based reimbursement for inpatient Medicare and outpatient services. Grants are also awarded for planning, implementing, and establishing networks of care and improving emergency medical services.

Primary care cooperative agreements facilitate the development of primary care services and attract primary care providers to rural health professional shortage areas (HPSA). Special legislation for HPSAs has also created programs to provide acute care facilities and services. The Rural Transition Grants Program, administered by HCFA, helps small rural communities with nonprofit hospitals adjust to changes in clinical practice patterns and in-hospital use, shifts from hospital- to community-based care, and changes in emergency care delivery patterns.

RURAL COMMUNITY HEALTH NURSING

Perhaps a more accurate title than *rural community health nursing* would be "community health nursing along the rural continuum." Nonmetropolitan areas would be at one end of the continuum, with metropolitan areas at the other end.

Practice in a rural area may require working as the only nurse at a health department in a remote Western Great Plains frontier county with a population of 6000, at a full-service health department in a town of 50,000 people, or at a large health department in a rural area next to an urban

population. A practice in a rural area adjacent to a large metropolitan area often appears to have more in common with the urban end of the continuum in terms of agency size, distances, and resources. For the purposes of this discussion, the practice setting is at the more "rural" end of the continuum.

The following definition illustrates the broad-based, generalist focus of the modern rural community health nurse. It includes the important geographical and cultural environment in which community health practice is implemented and helps define appropriate nursing interventions.

Rural nursing is the practice of professional nursing within the physical and sociocultural context of sparsely populated communities. It involves the continual interaction of the rural environment, the nurse, and his or her practice. Rural nursing is the diagnosis and treatment of a diversified population of people of all ages and a variety of human responses to actual (or potential) occupational hazards or to actual or potential health problems existent in maternity, pediatric, medical/surgical and emergency nursing in a given rural area (Bigbee, 1993; Lee and Winters, 2004; Rosenthal, 2005; Williams et al, 2012).

Characteristics of Rural Nursing

The uniqueness of rural nursing practice has been in question. Some believe that nursing care for rural clients is the same as for other individuals, and that health problems and patient care needs are similar regardless of the setting. Others argue that rural practice should be designated as a specialty or subspecialty area because of factors such as isolation, scarce resources, and the need for a wide range of practice skills that must be adapted to social and economic structures. Whether generalist or specialist, nurses being prepared for rural practice must be equipped with other community health assessment skills (Kulbok et al, 2012).

Molanari, Jaisiwal, and Hollinger-Forrest (2011) identified several positive aspects of rural nursing in the ability to provide holistic care, to know everyone well, and to develop close relationships with the community and coworkers where they enjoyed rural lifestyle as reasons to practice rural nursing. Autonomy, professional status, and being valued by the agency and community have been reported components of positive job satisfaction. Of those components identified as negative, agencies and professional organizations are most actively addressing professional isolation. The use of distance education technologies is one way to address the isolation many rural nurses experience. University degree programs and continuing education courses are readily available online or through full-motion interactive television. Using these technologies, rural nurses are able to update their skills and network with other nurses without having to leave their home communities.

Scharff (1998) considered the distinctive nature of the rural nurse's practice. She found that the rural nurse is a generalist, and remarked that "generalist" is not synonymous with "boring." Interviews with rural nurses show that they feel an "intensity of purpose" that makes rural nursing distinctive. Nurses living and practicing in the same place have a strong sense of integration and continuity between practice and community:

The newcomer practices nursing in a rural setting, unlike the more experienced nurse, who practices rural nursing. Somewhere between these extremes lies the transitional period of events and conditions through which each nurse passes at her or his own pace. It is within this time zone that nurses experience rural reality and move toward becoming professionals who understand that having gone rural, they are not less than they were, but rather, they are more than they expected to be. Some may be conscious of the transition, and others may not, but in the end, a few will say, "I am a rural nurse." (Scharff, 1998, p. 38)

Rural community health nursing is rewarding and challenging. Services can include maternal and child health, elder health, school health, mental health, and occupational health. The nurse practicing with the autonomy common in rural practice brings knowledge and competence in other clinical specialties. The work requires a discriminating, solid practitioner who can perform general nursing at a skill level beyond that of the outdated "mile wide and inch deep" general nursing. The rural nurse must be an "expert generalist."

RURAL HEALTH RESEARCH

Contemporary developments in the health care delivery system and advances in science suggest the need for an active agenda in rural health research. Berkowitz, Ivory, and Morris (2002) comment that rural health policy and research agendas must at the very least address the following issues:

1. The capacity of rural public health to manage improvements in health.
2. Information technology capacity in rural communities.
3. Development and monitoring of performance standards in rural public health.
4. Development of leadership and public health workforce capacity within rural public health.
5. Interaction and integration of community health systems, managed care, and public health in rural America.

Capacity of Rural Public Health to Manage Improvements in Health

Healthy People 2020 (HealthyPeople.gov, 2013) outlines health-related objectives for Americans and forms the rationale for efforts to intervene in disease trends to improve health where disparities have been identified. Determining the status of health indicators, such as rates of morbidity, mortality from common diseases or injury, and, perhaps most important, access to health care services, allows for priorities to be determined for which improvements in health are needed. Importantly, *Healthy People 2020* objectives and intervention strategies have been analyzed for rural-urban disparities that may exist along geographic, demographic, and cultural dimensions to provide a more specific picture of potential research priorities concerning improvements in health. The *Healthy People* box presents data from a survey of 44 national and state rural health experts that identify percentages of respondents who indicated giving priority status for various health issues.

♥ HEALTHY PEOPLE 2020
Rural Health Priorities

Rural Priorities (Identified By 25% Or More)	Percentage (%) of Respondents (N = 44)
Access to health care (includes one of the following):	73
Access to emergency medical services	32
Access to health workforce	29
Access to health services (general)	29
Access to health insurance	26
Access to primary care	24
Mental health	49
Oral health	41
Educational and community-based programs	29
Diabetes	26
Injury and violence prevention	26
Nutrition and overweight	21
Public health infrastructure	21
Tobacco	21
Maternal, infant, and child health	18
Occupational safety and health	18
Cancer	15
Environmental health	15
Heart disease and stroke	15

Data from Gamm LD, Hutchison L, Dabney RJ, Dorsey AM, editors: *Rural Healthy People 2010: A Companion Document to* Healthy People 2010, Volumes 1-3. College Station, TX, 2003, The Texas A&M University System Health Science Center, School of Rural Public Health, Southwest Rural Health Research Center.

Research questions directed toward improving health may be suggested for any of the *Healthy People 2020* objectives but may have the greatest potential to address salient rural trends if they relate to issues of access to care, mental health, oral health, educational and community-based programs, diabetes, or injury and violence prevention. Additionally, investigators may want to consider how these established rural priorities may be consistent or different within specific populations of concern. Because availability of surveillance data are often limited as researchers concern themselves with increasingly smaller populations (e.g., from state to county), efforts to gather additional primary data may be needed to set research priorities for improvements to health.

Information Technology in Rural Communities

As the distribution of technology expands across rural populations, more research is needed to examine the impacts of readily accessible information on both rural citizens and the health care delivery system. Rural patients are able to access specialty services such as radiological or dermatological examinations through telemedicine, and rural people are increasingly taking advantage of the World Wide Web to access information to make health decisions. The federal government has tied health care reimbursement to compliance with requirements of hospitals and physician practices to implement an electronic health record (EHR). Federal efforts directed toward disaster and terrorism preparedness have strengthened rural technological infrastructure so that communication pathways remain open during times of need. Just as patients access health care services from isolation, rural citizens are accessing health education through distance programs both for continuing education for entry-level and advanced degree programs in various health sciences. The need to address new research questions has grown alongside rapid expansion of information technology (IT), and questions abound relating to the application and evaluation of technology for improving systems of care and care outcomes (see the Research Highlights box).

Telehealth (or telemonitoring) is the use of telecommunications and IT to provide access to health assessments, diagnosis, intervention, consultation, supervision, and information across distance. Telehealth includes technologies such as interactive video (e.g., teleconsultation, teleradiology), patient monitoring (e.g., home monitoring, electronic ICU), and medication order review (Frontier Community Health Integration Project, Telehealth, 2014).

RESEARCH HIGHLIGHTS

Defining Rural Areas: Old and New Classifications

Old System (Before Census 2000)

Metropolitan (metro) areas:
- Cities of 50,000 or more residents *or*
- Urbanized areas of 50,000 or more residents and total area population of 100,000 or more

Nonmetropolitan (nonmetro) areas:
- All counties not classified as metropolitan

New Core-Based System (Starting with Census 2000)

Metropolitan (metro) areas:
- Central counties with 50,000 or more residents, regardless of total area population; includes outlying counties with 25% or more of the employed population commuting daily

Micropolitan (micro) areas:
- Central counties with one or more urban clusters of 10,000-50,000 persons; includes outlying counties with 25% or more of the employed population commuting daily

Noncore areas:
- All counties not meeting the new "metro" or "micro" classification are classified as "outside core-based statistical areas."

Data from Slifkin RT, Randolph R, Ricketts TC: The changing metropolitan designation process and rural America, *J Rural Health* 20(1):1-6, 2004.

Questions related to IT for public health in rural areas include:
- What is the role of telehealth in public health?
- What impact is distance learning having on the skills of rural public health professionals?
- What are the costs and infrastructure implications of ensuring access to IT in rural areas?
- How can IT be used to fill the gaps in epidemiology and surveillance capacity in rural health departments?

Performance Standards in Rural Public Health

The National Public Health Performance Standards Program (NPHPSP) was a collaborative effort, organized through the CDC, whose mission is to improve the quality of public health practice and the performance of local public health systems by providing and evaluating standards of performance.

The NPHPSP utilized the Ten Essential Public Health Services to establish three assessment instruments that can be used by local and state public health systems for evaluation and improvement. Standards describe an optimal level of performance by public health systems, which include all public, private, and voluntary entities that contribute to activities directed toward public health in an assessment area. The assessment can be used to improve collaborations among key public health partners, educate participants about public health, strengthen the network of public health partners, identify strengths and weaknesses, and provide benchmarks for public health practice improvements (CDC, 2012a).

In 2012, the Public Health Act and Prevention and Public Health Fund (PPHF), were created as part of the Patient Protection and Affordable Care Act (Public Law 111-148). With this law and allocation of resources, the National Public Health Improvement Initiative—part of the CDC's larger effort to increase the performance management capacity of public health departments to ensure that public health goals are effectively and efficiently met—was born. The focal point of this work will be to strengthen the public health infrastructure so as to improve health outcomes. Research questions that need to be addressed in rural areas may focus on the extent to which state and local performance assessments outlined by NPHPSP have been carried out as well as on the ability of rural public health systems to respond to needed changes to comprehensively address essential services. Additionally, rural areas may benefit from research examining resource constraints and the need to expand partnerships to address essential services that may be difficult to provide in isolated populations.

Leadership and Workforce Capacity for Rural Public Health

In 2003, the IOM published results of a project intended to improve our understanding of what is needed to prepare the public health workforce for the twenty-first century (Gebbie, Rosenstock, and Hernandez, 2003). Workforce capacity challenges cited by the IOM report include globalization, which increases travel and allows for distribution of emerging and reemerging diseases (e.g., human immunodeficiency virus [HIV] and acquired immunodeficiency syndrome, tuberculosis, hepatitis B, malaria, cholera, diphtheria, and Ebola virus); advances in scientific and medical technologies that challenge the public health workforce in areas of ethics, data security, and communication; and demographic transformations that require new skills and services as our population ages and becomes more diverse.

The CDC's Public Health Improvement Initiative (CDC, 2012b) aims to accelerate public health accreditation readiness activities, to provide additional support for performance management and improvement practices, and to develop, identify, and disseminate innovative and evidence-based policies and practices. This program supports the *Healthy People 2020* focus area of addressing public health infrastructure. Cross-jurisdictional (state, local, tribal, territorial, regional, community, and border) collaboration is encouraged to increase the impact of limited resources, to improve efficiency, and to leverage other related health reform efforts and projects. This initiative suggests that an initial strategy should be to monitor workforce composition and conduct research to validate methodology for public health worker enumeration.

Interaction and Integration of Community Health Systems, Managed Care, and Public Health

The evolution of managed care into rural environments has limited the safety-net role of some local health departments to provide primary care by preventing fee-for-service reimbursement and contracting care to networks of providers or organizations. This statement is especially true for Medicaid managed care, which serves the same population of people that traditionally receive primary care services through local public health departments. As Hurley, Crawford, and Praeger (2002) note, Medicaid's importance for rural areas is likely to grow as broader health care developments, such as declining inpatient use of rural hospitals and reductions in Medicare reimbursement, provoke more interest in using the Medicaid system to support threatened rural infrastructure.

Consequently, the administration of the Medicaid program will increasingly seek the cost savings promised by managed care, and the role of rural public health departments may increasingly narrow into areas that are currently without any type of reimbursement. For this reason, Berkowitz, Ivory, and Morris (2002) argue that finding ways to integrate public health into rural primary care at the community level will become more and more important. Many questions will have to be answered by additional research. What are the factors associated with successful integration of public health and managed care in rural environments? What capacity do rural health departments have for contracting arraignments with managed care organizations? What are the effects of local public health and managed care contracts on direct provision of services?

NEW MODELS OF HEALTH CARE DELIVERY FOR RURAL AREAS

In recent years, several innovative pilot projects have been implemented to address care delivery in rural areas. The Frontier Community Health Integration Project (F-CHIP), authorized by the Public Health Service Act and guided by the Medicare Improvements to Patients and Provider Act of 2008 (MIPPA), is testing new models of care delivery to frontier areas in critical access hospitals and through the use of telemedicine. Four frontier states have been identified: Alaska, Montana, North Dakota, and Wyoming. A *frontier area* is defined as a county with 6 or fewer people in a square mile and a daily hospital census of 5 or less (Frontier Community Health Integration Project, 2014.). The telehealth application can include home monitoring and electronic intensive care unit services; other applications include remote medication review by a pharmacist and consultation by a specialist at a distance. Payment for these services vary by third party payer, and distinct challenges in credentialing providers and leveraging technology exist.

SUMMARY

This chapter provides an overview of rural and migrant health. People who live in rural areas make up about 25% of the U.S. population. The reader must not assume that all rural people are similar; diversity exists in age, ethnicity, income, education, and geography.

Not all rural residents are disadvantaged. The data show that in some ways such populations are penalized as a whole, no matter how diverse the rural population. Health care access and income levels are areas where disadvantages generally exist. Provider shortages, an ineffective health care system, hospital-based and community-based care, and little in the way of health promotion and disease prevention services represent a marginal health care network. One half of the poor in the United States live in rural areas. The combination of poor health care access and low income level results in higher morbidity and mortality rates in rural populations. The high-risk nature of such occupations as farmworkers, miners, and loggers also contributes to disability and death rates. This chapter describes the structural, financial, and personal barriers to poor health care access.

Nurses who work with rural people must assess each aggregate's characteristics. A ranching community in Wyoming will have different needs from those of a migrant community in Arizona. Demographic information, aggregate morbidity and mortality data, emerging rural nursing theory, knowledge of barriers, and rural health care research are all necessary to plan appropriate upstream community health nursing interventions. Integrating these concepts gives nurses the tools to improve the health of rural people.

LEARNING ACTIVITIES

1. University libraries commonly subscribe to newspapers published within the state. Visit the library and select three to four small town or rural county newspapers. Read them for information about health care activities and concerns related to the health of the individuals, families, and community.
   - Report findings to the class about rural health concerns and activities.
   - Identify one priority problem that could be researched in the community and has relevance to rural community health nursing practice.
2. Select a rural community health nurse (i.e., public health or home care), and conduct an interview in person or by telephone if distance prohibits a face-to-face meeting.
   - Identify what the nurse sees as the pros and cons of rural nursing.
   - If negative aspects of rural nursing are identified, discuss how the nurse deals with them.
   - Ask the nurse to discuss the three highest-priority efforts related to his or her rural practice.

3. Choose one of the major causes of morbidity and mortality in migrant populations.
   - On the basis of risk factor and natural history, specify interventions for primary, secondary, and tertiary prevention of this problem.
   - Identify which of these interventions are examples of upstream thinking.
4. Locate a telephone book, a community resource directory, or a resource website from a rural community.
   - List and evaluate the resources that are available for prevention, assessment, intervention, and follow-up care for the major cause of mortality and morbidity identified in Learning Activity 3.
   - Would it be necessary to go outside the rural town or county for any of the needed resources? Which ones? Where might they be located?

ⓔ EVOLVE WEBSITE

http://evolve.elsevier.com/Nies
- NCLEX Review Questions
- Case Studies
- Glossary
- **Resource Tool 23A:** Health Insurance Coverage Status in the United States-2010
- **Resource Tool 23B:** Population of Older Adults Living in the United States-2010
- **Resource Tool 23C:** Estimated Percentage of Population Living in Poverty in the United States-2011

REFERENCES

Advancing Suicide Prevention: *Dying by their own hand in rural America: suicide is the second leading cause of death in states with primarily rural populations*, 2005. Available from <http://www.advancingsp.org/Press_Release_8_11_05.pdf.>.

Advancing Suicide Prevention: *Suicide in rural areas: lost in rural America—the challenges, the progress, and the hope*, 2005. Available from <http://advancingsp.org/ASP_July_August_2005.pdf>.

Aldwin C, Gilmer D: *Health, Illness, and Optimal Aging: biological and Psychosocial Perspectives*, ed 2, New York, 2013, Springer Publishing.

American Academy of Family Practitioners: *Rural practice, keeping physicians in (position paper)*, 2002. Available from <http://www.aafp.org/online/en/home/policy/policies/r/ruralpracticekeep.html>.

Alker J, Mancini T, Heberlein M: *Uninsured children 2009-2011: charting the nation's progress*, 2012. Available from <http://ccf.georgetown.edu/wp-content/uploads/2012/10/Uninsured-Children-2009-2011.pdf>.

Allender JA, Rector C, Warner KD: *Community Health Nursing: promoting and Protecting the Public's Health 7th edition*, Lippincott, 2010, Wolters Kluwer, Williams & Wilkins: Philadelphia.

Alterman T, Steege A, Petersen M, et al: Ethnic, racial, and gender variations in health among farm operators in the United States, *Annals of Epidemiology* 18(3):179–186, 2008.

American Academy of family practitioners: Rural Practice, keeping physicians (position paper), 2014. Available from <http://www.aafp.org/about/policies/all/rural-practice-paper.html>.

American Nurses Association: Scope and standards of parish nursing practice, Washington, DC, 2005.

Artnak K, McGraw R, Stanley V: Health care accessibility for chronic illness management and end-of-life care: a view from rural America, *Journal of Law, Medicine & Ethics* 39(2):140–155, 2011.

Bailey J: *The Top 10 rural issues for health care reform: a series examining health care in rural America*, 2009. Available from <http://files.cfra.org/pdf/Ten-Rural-Issues-for-Health-Care-Reform.pdf>.

Baldwin LM, Hollow WB, Casey S, et al: Access to specialty health care for rural American Indians in two states, *Rural Health* 24(3):269–278, 2008.

Becker G, Gates RJ, Newsom E: Self-Care Among Chronically Ill African Americans: culture, Health Disparities, and Health Insurance Status, *American Journal of Public Health* 94(12):2066–2073, 2004.

Berkowitz B, Ivory J, Morris T: Rural public health: policy and research opportunities, *J Rural Health* 18(Suppl):186–196, 2002.

Bigbee J: The uniqueness of rural nursing, *Nurs Clin North Am* 28:131–144, 1993.

Bishaw A: Poverty 2010 and 2011, American Community Service Briefs, 2012. Available from <http://www.census.gov/prod/2012pubs/acsbr11-01.pdf>.

Bishop B: *Poverty rate jumps in rural America*, 2009. Available from <http://www.dailyyonder.com/poverty-rate-jumps-rural-america/2009/11/23/2466>.

Bolin J, Gamm LG: Access to quality health services in rural areas: insurance. In *Rural Healthy People 2010: a Companion Document to Healthy People 2010*, Vol 1, College Station, TX, 2003, The Texas A&M University System Health Science Center, School of Rural Public Health, Southwest Rural Health Research Center.

Branas CC, MacKenzie E, Williams JC, et al: Access to Trauma Centers in the United States, *JAMA* 293(21):2626–2633, 2005.

Branas CC, Nance MD, Elliott MR, Richmond TS, and Schwab WS, Urban–Rural Shifts in Intentional Firearm Death: different Causes, Same Results, American Journal of Public Health, Vol 94, No. 10 1750-1755.

Braum S: *Where do states stand on private coverage of telemedicine?*, 2013. Available from <http://medcitynews.com/2013/05/where-do-states-stand-on-private-coverage-of-telemedicine-check-out-this-map/>.

Braveman P: Social conditions, health equity, and human rights, *Health and Human Rights: An International Journal* 12(2):31–48, 2010.

Bryant D: *Challenges of rural emergency management*, Homeland1 News, 2009. Available from <http://www.homeland1.com/print.asp?act=print&vid=480917>.

Bureau of Health Professions: *Changing demographics: implications for physicians, nurses, and other health workers*, 2003. Available from <ftp://ftp.hrsa.gov/bhpr/nationalcenter/changedemo.pdf>.

Bureau of Labor Statistics (2012a). Number of Fatal Work Injuries 1992-2011. Available from <http://www.bls.gov/iif/oshwc/cfoi/cfch0010.pdf>.

Bureau of Labor Statistics (2012b). National Census of Fatal Occupational Injuries in 2012 (Preliminary Results). Available from <http://www.bls.gov/news.release/pdf/cfoi.pdf>.

Bureau of Primary Healthcare: *Migrant and seasonal farmworker enumeration profiles study*, 2000. Available from <http://bphc.hrsa.gov/migrant/Enumeration/EnumerationStudy.htm>.

Castillo G, Alexander J: Injury and violence prevention in rural areas. In Gamm L, Hutchison L, editors: *Rural Healthy People 2010: a companion document to Healthy People 2010*, College Station, TX, 2004, The Texas A&M University System Health Science Center, School of Rural Public Health, Southwest Rural Health Research Center. Also available from <www.srph.tamhsc.edu/centers/rhp2010/>.

Cawthorne, A. (2010). The Not-So-Golden Years Confronting Elderly Poverty and Improving Seniors' Economic Security. Available from <http://www.americanprogress.org/wp-content/uploads/issues/2010/09/pdf/not_so_golden_years.pdf>.

Centers for Disease Control and Prevention: *Health, United States, 2007, with chartbook of trends in the health of Americans*, 2007. Available from <http://www.cdc.gov/nchs/data/hus/hus07.pdf>.

Centers for Disease Control and Prevention: *Health, United States, 2008, with chartbook on trends in the health of Americans*, 2008. Available from <http://www.cdc.gov/nchs/data/hus/hus08.pdf>.

Centers for Disease Control and Prevention: *Health, United States, 2011, with a special feature on socioeconomic status and health*, 2011. Available from <http://www.cdc.gov/nchs/data/hus/hus11.pdf#091>.

Centers for Disease Control and Prevention: *Behind international rankings of infant mortality: how the United States compares with Europe* (NCHS Brief no. 23), 2009a. Available from <http://www.cdc.gov/nchs/data/databriefs/db23.htm>.

Centers for Disease Control and Prevention: *Mammography use*, 2009b. Retrieved from <http://www.cdc.gov/nchs/data/health_policy/mammography.pdf>.

Centers for Disease Control and Prevention: *National Public Health Performance Standards Program*, 2012a. Available from <http://www.cdc.gov/nphpsp/index.html>.

Centers for Disease Control and Prevention: *PPHF National Public Health Improvement Initiative*, 2012b. Available from <http://www.cfda.gov/?s=program&mode=form&tab=step1&id=64d3ba3bc07bea2d79d07bf7650ba066>.

Centers for Disease Control and Prevention, Injury Center: Violence Prevention, *National suicide statistics at a glance: trends in suicide rates among persons ages 10 years and older, by sex, United States, 1991–2009*, 2013. Available from <http://www.cdc.gov/violenceprevention/suicide/statistics/trends01.html>.

Centers for Disease Control and Prevention, National Center for Health Statistics: *HHS issues report on community health in rural, urban areas* (HHS News), 2001. Available from <http://www.cdc.gov/nchs/pressroom/01news/hus01.html>.

Centers for Disease Control and Prevention, NIOSH Program Portfolio: *Occupational health disparities: occupational safety and health risks*, 2012. Available from <http://www.cdc.gov/niosh/programs/ohd/risks.html>.

Coen Buckwalter K, Lindsey Davis L, Wakefield BJ, et al: Telehealth for elders and their caregivers in rural communities, *Fam Community Health* 25(3):31–40, 2002.

Cutler, D., Lleras-Muney, A. (2006). NBER Working Paper Series, Education and Health Evaluating health theories and evidence. Available from <http://www.nber.org/papers/w12352.pdf?new_window=1>.

Daniels N, Kennedy BP, Kawachi I: Why justice is good for our health: the social determinants of health inequalities, *Daedalus* 128:215–251, 1999.

Cromartie J, Nelson P: *Baby boom migration and its impact on rural America* (USDA Economic Research Report no. ERR-79), 2009. Available from <://<www.ers.usda.gov/publications/err-economic-research-report/err79/report-summary.aspx>.

DeHaven M, Hunter I, Wilder L, et al: Health Programs in Faith-Based Organizations: are They Effective? *American Journal of Public Health* 94(6):1030–1036, 2004.

DeNavas-Walt C, Proctor B, Smith J: *Income, poverty and health insurance coverage in the United States in 2011*, 2012. Available from <http://www.census.gov/prod/2012pubs/p60-243.pdf>.

Elliott MR, Ginsburg KR, Winston FK: Unlicensed Teenaged Drivers: who Are They, and How Do They Behave When They Are Behind the Wheel? *PEDIATRICS* 122(5):994–1000, 2008.

Farm Worker Fund: *Innovative outreach practices report*, 2006. Available from <http://www.farmworkerhealth.org/docs/IOPR2006.pdf>.

Farrigan T, Parker T: *The concenteration of poverty is a growing rural problem*, 2012. Available from <http://www.ers.usda.gov/amber-waves/2012-december/concentration-of-poverty.aspx>.

Ferrer RL: Pursuing equity: contact with primary care and specialist clinicians by demographics, insurance, and health status, *Ann Fam Med* 5(6):492–502, 2007.

Frontier community health integration project, White Paper #2 Case study on Frontier Telehealth, 2014. Available from <http://www.raconline.org/new-approaches/pdf/case-study-on-frontier-telehealth.pdf>.

Gamm LD, Hutchison L: Rural Healthy People 2010: evolving interactive practice, *Am J Public Health* 94(10):1711–1712, 2004. Also available from <http://www.pubmedcentral.nih.gov/articlerender.fcgi?artid=1448522>.

Gebbie K. Rosenstock L, Hernandez L. National Research Council. Who Will Keep the Public Healthy? Educating Public Health Professionals for the 21st Century. Washington, DC: The National Academies Press,

Gosschalk A, Carozza S: Cancer in rural areas. In Gamm LD, Hutchison L, Dabney RJ, et al, editors: *Rural Healthy People 2010: a companion document to Healthy People 2010*, Vols 1–3, College Station, Tex, 2003, The Texas A&M University System Health Science Center, School of Rural Public Health, Southwest Rural Health Research Center.

Hanrahan N, Hartley D: Employment of advanced-practice psychiatric nurses to stem rural mental health workforce shortages, *Psychiatr Serv* 59(1):109–111, 2008.

HealthyPeople.gov: *Home*, 2013. Available from <http://www.healthypeople.gov/2020/default.aspx>.

HealthyPeople 2020, Disparities, 2010. Available from <http://www.healthypeople.gov/2020/about/DisparitiesAbout.aspx>.

Hoyer DL, Kung HC, Smith BL: *Deaths: preliminary data for 2003 (National Vital Statistics Report vol. 53 no. 15)*, Hyattsville, MD, 2005, National Center for Health Statistics.

HRSA, Medicare Rural Hospital Flexibility Grant Program, n.d. Available from <http://www.hrsa.gov/ruralhealth/about/hospitalstate/medicareflexibility_.html>.

Hsia R, Shen Y: Possible Geographical Barriers to Trauma Center Access for Vulnerable Patients in the United States: an Analysis of Urban and Rural Communities, *Archives of Surgery* 146(1):46–52, 2011. Available from <http://dx.doi.org/10.1001/archsurg.2010.299>.

Hurley RE, Crawford H, Praeger S: Medicaid and rural health care, *J Rural Health* 18(Suppl):164–175, 2002.

Hutchison L, Blakely C: Substance abuse: trends in rural areas. In Rural People 2010: Available from <http://sph.tamhsc.edu/centers/rhp2010/11Volume2substanceabuse.pdf>.

Institute of Medicine: *Quality through collaboration: the future of Rural Health Care*, Washington, DC, 2005, National Academy Press.

International Parish Nurse Resource Center: *Information for clergy*, n.d. Available from <http://ipnrc.parishnurses.org/forcl.phtml>.

Johnson AO, Mink MD, Harun N, et al: Violence and Drug Use in Rural Teens: National Prevalence Estimates From the 2003 Youth Risk Behavior Survey, *Journal of School Health* 10(78):554–561, 2008.

Jones C, William K, Parker T: Population Dynamics are Changing the Profile of Rural Areas, *Amber Waves* 5(2):30–35, 2007.

Jones CA, Parker TS, Ahearn M, et al: *Health status and health care access of farm and rural populations* (ERS Report Summary), 2009. Available from <http://www.ers.usda.gov/media/155449/eib57_reportsummary_1_.pdf>.

Kaiser Family Foundation: *State health facts*, 2014. Available from <http://www.statehealthfacts.org/>.

Kandel W: Rural Hispanics at a glance (Economic Information Bulletin No. EIB-8 2005), 2003. Available from <http://www.ers.usda.gov/publications/eib8/>.

Kulbok P, Thatcher E, Park E, et al: Evolving public health nursing roles: focus on community participatory health promotion and prevention, *Online Journal of Issues in Nursing* 17(2), 2012. Available from <http://www.nursingworld.org/MainMenuCategories/ANAMarketplace/ANAPeriodicals/OJIN/TableofContents/Vol-17-2012/No2-May-2012/Evolving-Public-Health-Nursing-Roles.html>.

Lee H, Winters C: Testing rural nursing theory: perceptions and needs of service providers, *Online Journal of Rural Nursing and Health Care* 4(1):51–63, 2004. Available from <http://www.rno.org/journal/issues/Vol-4,/issue-1/Lee_article.htm>.

Malecki E: Digital development in rural areas: potentials and pitfalls, *Journal of Rural Studies* 9(2):201–214, 2003.

Mathews T, MacDorman M: Infant mortality statistics from the period linked birth/infant death data set. Natational Vital Statistic Report, 2013;62(8) 2010.

McClelland S, Steel S, Marsh L, et al: (2010). Dimensions in Health : A Sample of Rural and Global Health Issues, Available from http://hdl.handle.net/1928/11329

Medicaid.gov: *Telemedicine*, 2013. Available from <http://www.medicaid.gov/Medicaid-CHIP-Program-Information/By-Topics/Delivery-Systems/Telemedicine.html>.

Molanari D, Jaiswal A, Hollinger-Forrest T: Rural Nurses: lifestyle Preferences and Education Perceptions, *Online Journal of Rural Nursing and Health Care* 11(2):16–26, 2011. Available from <http://rnojournal.binghamton.edu/index.php/RNO/article/view/27>.

National Center for Farmworker Health: *Farmworker occupational health and safety fact sheet*, 2013. Available from <http://www.ncfh.org/docs/fs-Occ%20Health.pdf>.

National Rural Health Association: *Mental health in rural America: what's different about rural healthcare,* n.da. Available from <http://www.ruralhealthweb.org/go/left/about-rural-health/what-s-different-about-rural-health-care>.

National Rural Health Association: *what's different about rural health care?* 2014. Available from < http://www.ruralhealthweb.org/go/left/about-rural-health/what-s-different-about-rural-health-care>.

U.S. Department of Health and Human Services, Office of Disease Prevention and Health Promotion. Available from <http://www.healthypeople.gov/>

Office of Management and Budget: *Metropolitan and micropolitan statistical areas main,* 2009. Available from <http://www.census.gov/population/www/metroareas/metroarea.html>.

Office of Minority Health: *Infant mortality and African Americans,* 2013. Available from <http://minorityhealth.hhs.gov/templates/content.aspx?ID=3021>.

O'Hare W: *Poverty is a persistent reality for many rural children in U.S,* 2009. Available from <http://www.prb.org/Articles/2009/ruralchildpoverty.aspx>.

Peek-Asa C, Zwerling C, Stallones L: Acute traumatic injuries in rural populations, *Am J Public Health* 94(10):1689–1693, 2004.

Rasheed MN, Rasheed JM: Rural African American older adults and the black helping tradition, *Journal of Gerontological Social Work* 41:137–150, 2003.

Reschovsky JD, Staiti A: Access and quality of medical care in urban and rural areas: does rural America lag behind? *Health Affairs* 24(4):1128–1139, 2005.

Ricketts TC: Education of Physician Assistants, Nurse Midwives, and Nurse Practitioners for Rural Practice, *The Journal of Rural Health* (6)4,537–543, 2008.

Rogers CC: The older population in 21st century rural America, *Rural America* 17(3), 2002. Available from <http://www.ers.usda.gov/publications/ruralamerica/ra173/ra173b.pdf>.

Rosenblatt RA, Casey S, Richardson M: Rural-urban differences in the public health workforce: local health departments in 3 Western states, *Am J Public Health* 92(7):1102–1105, 2002.

Rosenthal K: What rural nursing stories are you living? *Online Journal of Rural Nursing and Health Care* 5(1), 2005. Available from <http://www.rno.org/journal/issues/Vol-5/issue-1/Rosenthal_article.htm>.

Rural Assistance Center: What is rural? n.d. Available from <http://www.raconline.org/topics/what-is-rural/>.

Sanford JT, Townsend-Rocchiccioli J: The perceived health of rural caregivers, *Geriatr Nurs* 75(3):145–148, 2004.

Scharff KE: The distinctive nature and scope of rural nursing practice: philosophical bases. In Lee HJ, editor: *Conceptual basis for rural nursing,* New York, 1998, Springer.

Sigma Theta Tau International: *Facts on the nursing shortage,* n.d. Available from <http://www.nursingsociety.org/MEDIA/Pages/shortage.aspx>.

Slifkin RT, Randolph R, Ricketts TC: The changing metropolitan designation process and rural America, *J Rural Health* 20(1):1–6, 2004.

Thorngren J: Rural mental health: a qualitative inquiry, *Journal of Rural Community Psychology* E6(2):1–6, 2003. Available from <http://muwww-new.marshall.edu/jrcp//JRCP_E6_2_Thorngren.htm>.

Thrall T: Rural recruitment, *Hosp Health Netw* 81(12):45–48, 2007.

U.S. Census Bureau: Overview of Race and Hispanic Origin: 2010; Census Briefs. Available from <http://www.census.gov/prod/cen2010/briefs/c2010br-02.pdf>.

U.S. Census Bureau: *Income, poverty, and health insurance coverage in the United States: 2011,* 2011. Available from <http://www.census.gov/hhes/www/poverty/data/incpovhlth/2011/index.html>.

U.S. Census Bureau: *Income, poverty and health insurance coverage in the United States: 2011; correction to Table A,* 2012. Available from <http://www.census.gov/newsroom/releases/archives/income_wealth/cb12-172.html>.

U.S. Census Bureau: *Small area income and poverty estimates,* 2013. Available from <http://www.census.gov/did/www/saipe/>.

U.S. Census Bureau, Metropolitan and Micropolitan: *Metropolitan and Micropolitan Statistical Areas Main,* 2013a. Available from < http://www.census.gov/population/metro/>.

U.S. Department of Agriculture, Economic Research Service: *Measuring what is rural,* 2007. Available from <http://www.ers.usda.gov/Briefing/rurality/Whatisrural>.

U.S. Department of Agriculture, Economic Research Service: *Rural income, poverty, and welfare: poverty geography,* 2011. Available from <http://webarchives.cdlib.org/sw1rf5mh0k/http://www.ers.usda.gov/Briefing/IncomePovertyWelfare/PovertyGeography.htm>.

U.S. Department of Agriculture, Economic Research Service: *Employment & education: rural education,* 2012a. Available from <http://www.ers.usda.gov/topics/rural-economy-population/employment-education/rural-education.aspx>.

U.S. Department of Agriculture, Economic Research Service: *Rural economy & population.* Available from <http://www.ers.usda.gov/Emphases/Rural/>.

U.S. Department of Agriculture, Economic Research Service: *Rural income, poverty, and welfare: poverty demographics,* 2012c. Available from <http://webarchives.cdlib.org/sw1rf5mh0k/http://www.ers.usda.gov/Briefing/IncomePovertyWelfare/PovertyDemographics.htm>.

U.S. Department of Agriculture, Economic Research Service: *Rural labor and education: farm labor,* 2012d. Available from <http://www.ers.usda.gov/topics/rural-economy-population/employment-education/rural-education.aspx>.

U.S. Department of Agriculture, Economic Research Service: *The concentration of poverty is a growing rural problem,* 2012f. Available from <http://www.ers.usda.gov/amber-waves/2012-december/concentration-of-poverty.aspx>.

U.S. Department of Agriculture, Economic Research Service: *Farm labor: background,* 2013. Available from <http://www.ers.usda.gov/topics/farm-economy/farm-labor/background.aspx>.

U.S. Department of Agriculture, Economic Research Service: Immigration and the Rural Workforce, 2013c. Available from <http://www.ers.usda.gov/topics/in-the-news/immigration-and-the-rural-workforce.aspx#.U12qyKLwnWc>.

U.S. Department of Agriculture, Economic Research Service: Farm Workers Background, 2013d. Available from <http://www.ers.usda.gov/topics/farm-economy/farm-labor/background.aspx>.

U.S. Department of Agriculture, Economic Research Service: *Rural poverty & well-being: Geography of Poverty.* Available from <http://www.ers.usda.gov/topics/rural-economy-population/rural-poverty-well-being/geography-of-poverty.aspx>.

U.S. Department of Agriculture, National Institute of Food and Agriculture: *Agricultural systems overview,* 2009. Available from <http://www.csrees.usda.gov/nea/ag_systems/ag_systems_all.html>.

U.S. Department of Health and Human Services, Health Resources and Services Administration: *Emergency medical services in frontier areas: volunteer community organizations,* 2006. Available from <ftp://ftp.hrsa.gov/ruralhealth/FrontierEMS.pdf>.

van Exel J, de Graaf G, Brouwer W: Give me a break!: informal caregiver attitudes towards respite care, *Health Policy* 88(1):73–87, 2008.

Vernig B, Moscovice I, Durham S, et al: Do Rural Elders Have Limited Access to Medicare Hospice Services, *Journal of the American Geriatrics Society,* 52(5), 731–735, 2004.

Weinert C, Long KA: Understanding the health care needs of rural families, *Fam Relat* 36:450–455, 1987.

Weisbecker A: Local health departments hit hard by budget woes, *Food Safety News,* May 6, 2010. Available from <http://www.foodsafetynews.com/2010/05/local-health-departments-hit-hard-by-budget-woes/>.

Williams M, Andrews J, Zanni K, et al: Rural nursing: searching for the state of the science, *Online Journal of Rural Nursing and Health Care* 2(12):102–117, 2012.

Zahner SJ, Corrado SM: Local health department partnerships with faith-based organizations, *J Public Health Manag Pract* 10(3):258–265, 2004.

Ziller E, Lenardson J, Coburn A: Health care access and use among the rural uninsured, *Journal of Health Care for the Poor and Underserved* 23(3):1327–1345, 2012.

Populations Affected by Mental Illness

*Kim Jardine-Dickerson**

OBJECTIVES

Upon completion of this chapter, the reader will be able to do the following:

1. Explain the concepts of community mental health, and discuss the importance of community mental health promotion in special populations.
2. Discuss the historical context for contemporary community mental health care.
3. Describe biological, social, and political factors associated with mental illness.
4. Illustrate the impact of natural and human-made disasters on the mental health of communities.

5. Describe some of the most common types of mental illnesses encountered in community settings.
6. Discuss the problem of suicide and recognize suicide warning signs.
7. Describe different types of evidence-based treatment for mental disorders, including use of psychotropic medication management, community case management, and crisis intervention.
8. Describe the role of mental health nurses in the community.

KEY TERMS

2008 Mental Health Parity and
   Addiction Equity Act
Affordable Care Act
agoraphobia
anorexia nervosa
anosignosia
Assertive Community Treatment
attention deficit disorder
attention deficit/hyperactivity
   disorder
bipolar disorder

bulimia nervosa
case management
Community Mental Health
   Centers Act
co-occurring
comorbidity
Crisis Intervention Team
deinstitutionalization
depression
generalized anxiety disorder
major depression
mental health

mental health consumer
mental illness
obsessive-compulsive disorder
panic disorder
phobia
post-traumatic stress disorder
psychotropic/psychotherapeutic
   medications
schizophrenia
severe emotional disorder
severe mental illness
stigma

OUTLINE

Overview and History of Community Mental Health: 1960
  to the Present Day
   Deinstitutionalization Cause and Effects
   Present-Day Community Mental Health Reform
   Medicalization of Mental Illness
   Brain Neuroimaging, Genetics, and Hope for New
    Treatments
HEALTHY PEOPLE 2020: Mental Health and Mental
  Disorders
Factors Influencing Mental Health
   Biological Factors

Social Factors
Gender, Racial, and Sexual Orientation Disparities
Natural and Human-made Disasters and Mental Illness
Political Factors
Mental Disorders Encountered in Community Settings
  Overview of Selected Mental Disorders
  Depression
Identification and Management of Mental Disorders
  Identification of Mental Disorders
Community-Based Mental Health Care
Role of the Community Mental Health Nurse

*The author would like to acknowledge the contributions of Jane Mahoney and Nancy Diacon, who wrote this chapter for the previous edition.

Mental health refers to the absence of mental disorders and to the ability to function socially and occupationally. Mental illness consists of diagnosable mental disorders that affect alterations in thinking, mood, or behavior associated with distress and impaired functioning. Other effects of mental illnesses including disruptions of daily function and lifestyle, such as incapacitating personal, social, and occupational impairment as well as premature death. Mental health can be affected by numerous factors, such as biological and genetic vulnerabilities, acute or chronic physical dysfunction, environmental conditions, and stressors. Twenty-first century community mental health necessitates comprehensive mental health services, inpatient, outpatient, home-based, school, and community-based programs for individuals, families, and populations at need. Threats such as vulnerability, poverty, homelessness, cost and limited accessibility to community mental health care can be pervasive. Whether populations in need live in rural or urban settings, people need mental health services. Community mental health care can exist throughout all levels of prevention and can be designed to supplement and decrease the need for more costly inpatient mental health care delivered in hospitals. A community's mental health is a reflection of community as a whole. Community mental health professionals work with populations at risk such as homeless veterans, families, children and the elderly.

It is estimated that up to 25% of all U.S. adults have a mental illness and that nearly 50% of U.S. adults will experience at least one mental illness during their lifetimes (Reeves et al, 2011). Mental illness is a significant public health problem affecting not only the person with mental illness but their family, friends, schoolmates, work mates, and others. Mental illness is associated with lower use of health care, reduced adherence to treatment therapies for chronic diseases, and higher risks of adverse health outcomes. The costs of mental health care can be estimated much the way that other health care costs are determined. There are significant studies that look at co-occurring mental illness and chronic diseases such as cardiovascular disease, diabetes, obesity, asthma, epilepsy, and cancer. There is increased co-occurring use of tobacco products and abuse of alcohol in mental illness populations. Rates for intentional and unintentional injuries are two to six times higher among people with a mental illness than in the general population. The knowledge that many mental illnesses can be managed successfully offers hope, and increasing access to and use of mental health treatment services could substantially reduce the associated morbidity. There are evidence-based practice (EBP) models consisting of community-based programs of intervention, education, and collaboration. Continual monitoring of mental illness is critical in providing appropriate organizations the data they require to assess the need for mental and behavioral health services and to inform the provision of those services.

The Affordable Care Act (ACA) builds on the 2008 Mental Health Parity and Addiction Equity Act to extend federal parity protections to 62 million Americans (HealthCare.gov, 2013). This parity law aims to ensure that when coverage for mental health and substance use conditions is provided, it is generally comparable to coverage for medical and surgical care. The ACA builds on the parity law by requiring coverage of mental health and substance use disorder benefits for millions of Americans who currently lack these benefits.

More than ever, community mental health nurses and interdisciplinary community teams face multiple challenges such as complex patient comorbidity, lack of resources, competent mental health professional workforce and law enforcement, physical facility inadequacies, and the stigma of mental illness. The purpose of this chapter is to describe critical issues that affect the mental health of individuals, families, groups, and special populations and to explore the potential influences and advocacy issues that nurses can be involved with. The chapter depicts issues that affect individuals, families, groups, and populations and explores promising EBP programs and educational models utilized in community mental health.

Severe mental illness (SMI) is a diagnosis applied to any adult who currently or at any time during the past year has had a diagnosable mental, behavioral, or emotional disorder with moderate, severe, or extreme functional behavior in specific lifestyle areas. These mental health disorders of persons 18 years of age or older present emotional or behavioral functioning that is so impaired as to interfere substantially with their capacity to remain in the community without supportive treatment or services of a long-term or indefinite duration. SMI mental disability is severe and persistent, resulting in a long-term limitation of functional capacities for primary activities of daily living, such as interpersonal relationships, homemaking, self-care, employment, and recreation. There are hopeful models of care that integrate team approaches with patients with SMI and families (LeVine, 2012).

OVERVIEW AND HISTORY OF COMMUNITY MENTAL HEALTH: 1960 TO THE PRESENT DAY

The National Institute of Mental Health (NIMH) initially developed a Community Mental Health Center (CMHC) program in the 1960s. CMHCs were designed to provide comprehensive services for people with mental illness, locate these services closer to home, and provide an umbrella of integrated services for catchment areas of 125,000 to 250,000 people. These centers were intended to provide prevention, early treatment, and continuity of care in communities, promoting social integration of people with mental health needs. In 1963 President John F. Kennedy signed the Community Mental Health Centers Act (CMHCA) which resulted in deinstitutionalization and the closing of mental institutions. As a result, patients were released into communities too often without supporting community services. Further cuts in housing and other services throughout the 1980s resulted in a new population of homeless individuals in the United States.

The 1999 Surgeon General's Report on Mental Health defined mental health as a state of successful performance of mental function that results in productive activities, fulfilling relationships with others, and an ability to adapt to change and cope with adversity.

Table 24-1 provides a snapshot of the development of community mental health from the 1960s to present day.

TABLE 24-1	Community Mental Health Movement from the 1960 to the Present Day	
1960	Blue Ribbon Panel report *Action for Mental Health*	Recommendations for intensive care of acutely ill mental patients and community mental health clinics
1963	Community Mental Health Clinics Legislation	Community mental health centers in some urban communities
1960s	Deinstitutionalization	Discharged mentally ill from state hospitals, patients returned to communities with inadequate resources (i.e., finances, housing, health care, supportive employment)
1981	Mental Health Block Grant, as part of the Omnibus Reconciliation Act	States develop comprehensive mental health plans for persons with serious mental illness
1986	State Mental Health Planning Act	
1999	U.S. Surgeon General's Report on Mental Health	Acknowledging mental illness as a disease
2008	Mental Health Parity and Addiction Equity Act of 2008	Insurance coverage for mental health and substance use conditions
2010	Affordable Care Act	Builds on the Mental Health Parity and Addiction Equity Act of 2008 to extend federal parity protections to 62 million Americans

Deinstitutionalization Cause and Effects

Deinstitutionalization is the release of institutionalized people, especially mental health patients, from an institution for placement and care in the community. From 1955 to 1980, the number of mentally ill patients in state facilities fell from 559,000 to 154,000 as patients were moved back into their communities. Even though national deinstitutionalization was initiated in 1965 through the community mental health centers program, there had been significant movement of dislocated patients from state institutions for some 10 years prior. This national movement was also concerned with civil rights issues and the conditions of the state institutions. These questions and concerns led courts throughout the country to limit involuntary institutionalization and to set minimum standards for care in institutions. At this time there were not sufficient community resources, such as adequate housing, supported employment, community mental health professional workforce, and other community mental health care services, available throughout the country to meet the needs of patients coming back to communities. There was a beginning evolution in the structure, practice, experiences, and purposes of community mental health care in the United States. The Community Mental Health Centers Act of 1964 provided federal support for mental health services. The Act supported measures to implement facilities to care for those who were mentally retarded and to construct community mental health centers.

Following passage of the Act, individuals with serious mental illness were returned to families and communities who were ill prepared to care for them, and funding did not follow the change in policy. Too many individuals with mental illness found themselves homeless, in shelters, or in prisons or jails. There was a critical need for more effective mental health treatment, improvements in the social welfare system, and provision of community support for this population, and shortly thereafter, the federal government recommended linking community mental health services with informal community support services to improve treatment options.

Present-Day Community Mental Health Reform

Mental health reform works toward monitoring federal legislation, administration activity, and public education initiatives. Such reform policies make community mental health a national priority and establish early access, recovery, and quality in mental health services as quality standards in our nation's mental health care delivery systems. For example, the epidemic of gun violence and school safety is being addressed on a federal level with Project AWARE from the U.S. Department of Health and Human Services' (USDHHS's) agency from Behavioral Health Workforce (HHS Project AWARE). For military veterans and their families, the U.S. Department of Veterans Affairs (VA) is attempting to bring attention to education and community resources through the National Center for PTSD (Post-Traumatic Stress Disorder). The National Alliance on Mental Illness (NAMI) is the nation's largest grassroots mental health organization, dedicated to educate and advocate for access to services, treatment, support services, and research. President Barack Obama has initiated BRAIN (Brain Research through Advancing Innovative Neurotechnologies), new research effort to revolutionize our understanding of the human mind.

Medicalization of Mental Illness

The American Psychiatric Association (APA) work *Diagnostic and Statistical Manual of Mental Disorders, Fourth Edition, Text Revision* (DSM V, 2013; APA, 2013) has supported the medicalization of mental illness and has helped put mental disorders on parity with other diseases. With mental health parity, schizophrenia and depression may be treated as forcefully with treatment as diabetes. There is hope that federal laws barring health insurers from imposing lower coverage limits on mental health services than they do on other medical treatments will change. Medicalization of mental health looks at holism, health, and understanding of illness on a functioning level and is seen as treatment toward the absence of disease (Smith, 2012; Vilhelmsson and Svensson, 2011).

Brain Neuroimaging, Genetics, and Hope for New Treatments

Brain imaging scans, also called neuroimaging scans, are being used more and more to help detect and diagnose a number of medical disorders and illnesses. Currently, the main use of brain scans for mental disorders is in research studies to learn more about the disorders.

Researchers use neuroimaging to study healthy brain development and the effects of mental illnesses or the effects of mental health treatments on the brain. Brain scans alone, however, cannot be used to diagnose a mental disorder, such as autism, anxiety, depression, schizophrenia, or bipolar disorder (NIMH, 2010).

HEALTHY PEOPLE 2020: MENTAL HEALTH AND MENTAL DISORDERS

Healthy People 2020 is a collaboration among federal, state, and territorial governments and private, public, and nonprofit organizations to set national disease prevention and health promotion objectives (USDHHS, 2013). The *Healthy People 2020* box lists several objectives that cover issues related to mental health. Major mental health objectives target decreasing suicides and reducing the numbers of person with major depressive episodes. There are objectives for treatment expansion, and providing adequate community resources for adults, children, and families struggling with mental illnesses.

 HEALTHY PEOPLE 2020

Objectives Related to Mental Illness and Health

Mental Health Status Improvement
MHMD–1: Suicide
MHMD–2: Adolescent suicide attempts
MNMD–3: Eating disorders
MHMD–4: Major depressive episodes

Treatment Expansion
MHMD–5: Mental health treatment provided in primary care facilities
MHMD–6: Treatment for children with mental health problems
MHMD–7: Juvenile justice facility screening
MHMD–8: Employment of persons with serious mental illness
MHMD–9: Treatment of adults with mental health disorders
MHMD–10: Treatment for co-occurring substance abuse and mental disorders
MHMD–11: Depression screening by primary care providers
MHMD–12: Receipt of mental health services among homeless adults

From HealthyPeople.gov: *Healthy People 2020: Topics & objectives: Mental health and mental disorders, 2013.* Retrived from <http://www.healthypeople.gov/2020/topicsobjectives2020/objectiveslist.aspx?topicId=28.>

FACTORS INFLUENCING MENTAL HEALTH

Although treatment of mental disorders has dramatically improved, the cause of most mental illnesses is not well understood. Research has identified a number of biological and sociological factors that contribute to mental health and mental illness. Some of these factors are discussed here.

Biological Factors

For centuries, mental illnesses were viewed as conditions that needed to be contained in institutions. Neuroscience research has provided a better understanding of the biology of mental illnesses; however, many questions remain unanswered. Biological factors associated with mental illness include genetic factors, neurotransmission, and abnormalities of brain structure and functioning.

Genetic Factors

Genetic expressions, combined with neurochemical and metabolic changes and environmental insults, may result in the display of mental disorder characteristics. Genetic testing and counseling offers promise for understanding the complexities associated with gene variation, brain structure, and the physiological response to information processing (Baune and Thome, 2011). There is evidence of predisposition to mental illnesses in families, suggesting that people who have a family member with a mental illness are more likely to experience one themselves. Experts believe that many mental illnesses are linked to abnormalities in many genes, not just one. People may inherit a susceptibility to a mental illness and do not necessarily go on to have a mental illness. Mental illnesses more likely occur from the interaction of multiple genetic factors and some other factors, such as stress, abuse, and traumatic events. These factors can influence, trigger, or exacerbate an illness in a person who has an inherited susceptibility to it.

Abnormalities of Brain Structure and Functioning

Evidence indicates that structural brain abnormalities can be related to some mental illnesses, such as schizophrenia, depression, and Alzheimer's disease. As the science of neuroimaging evolves, a more refined view of the role of brain structure and functioning is unfolding. For example, neuroimaging studies are beginning to explain the role of different central nervous system structures in regulating the hypothalamic-pituitary-adrenal axis that controls responses to stress (Pruessner et al, 2010). Scientists are also recognizing how other systems of the body can impact brain functioning. For example, in one study, researchers found a greater than 60% activation of the amygdala in sleep-deprived subjects than in controls (Pruessner et al, 2010).

Although a number of theories on the etiology of mental disorders have been developed, information is insufficient to establish a definitive biological cause for mental illness. Scholars have concluded that mental disorders are multifactorial, complex phenomena. The important point for community health nurses to understand is that mental illnesses have a very strong biological basis, much like other chronic conditions such as diabetes and heart disease, but that other factors are highly influential.

Social Factors

Some community occurrences and phenomena, such as school shootings, public bombings, bullying, domestic violence, and other tragic events, have identified critical gaps in the need for public education, advocacy, and treatment of mental illness (Bazelon Center, 2013). Throughout history, the symptoms of mental illness have been perceived as permanent, dangerous, frightening, and shameful. People with a diagnosis of mental illness have been described as lazy, idle, weak, immoral, irrational, and too often criminal. On the basis of these characterizations and assumptions, many people with a diagnosis of mental illness have experienced widespread social rejection that may lead to isolation and more social stigma (Kondrat and Early 2011).

Another social concern is the tendency of communities to make use of prisons rather than psychiatric hospitals as a solution to the "mental health problem." Approximately 10 million people spend time in correctional facilities at some point each year. They are more likely than people in the general population to have mental health problems and addictions. Many of these individuals lack access to treatment for these problems outside of jails and prisons.

About half of all people in jails and prisons have mental health problems, and about 65% meet medical criteria for alcohol or other drug abuse and addiction. Prisons are woefully unprepared to provide adequate care to the mentally ill. To help address this problem, in 2008, Senate Bill S.2304, the Mentally Ill Offender Treatment and Crime Reduction Reauthorization and Improvement Act, was signed into law. This bill provided grants aimed at improving the mental health treatment provided to criminal offenders with a mental illness. Other related initiatives have focused on establishing specialty courts or problem-solving courts. There may be mental health courts in communities to address the needs of the community and those who are charged with a criminal offense and also experience a mental illness (Mental Health America, 2013).

Gender, Racial, and Sexual Orientation Disparities

Racial and ethnic minorities are the fastest-growing communities in the United States. The NIMH's Office for Research on Disparities and Global Mental Health (ORDGMH) is active in reducing mental health disparities. ORDGMH collects local and global mental health disparities data, including movements of populations, global economic relationships, and communication technologies. Culturally diverse groups often bear a disproportionately high burden of disability due to mental disorders. For example, in schizophrenia and mood disorders, there is a high probability of misdiagnosis because of differences in how African Americans express symptoms of emotional distress (APA, 2012).

Because of the lack of access in their communities, Hispanic Americans use mental health services far less than other ethnic and racial groups. This population also constitutes the largest group of uninsured in the United States. American Indian and Alaska Natives experience the higher rates of mental disorders compared to the overall population. These groups experience far greater psychological distress are at greater risk for mental disorders such as depression, substance abuse, anxiety, and PTSD. In some American Indian groups, the rates of alcoholism and illicit drug use disorder are much higher than the U.S. average. Significantly greater

percentages of lifetime major depression have been reported among women (11.7%) than men (5.6%). Lifetime percentages of depression reveal ethnic differences: 6.52% among whites, 4.57% among blacks, and 5.17% among Hispanics (APA, 2012).

Although a majority of gay, bisexual, and other men who have sex with men (MSM) have good mental health, there are MSM populations at greater risk for mental health problems. Homosexuality is not a mental disorder. Homophobia, stigma, and discrimination, however, have negative effects on the health of MSM, lesbians, and other sexual minorities. The negative effects of social stigma and discrimination can be found in adolescent and adult MSM. The lesbian, gay, bisexual, and transgendered (LGBT) community are at increased risk for a number of mental health problems. MSM are at increased risk of: major depression, bipolar disorder, and anxiety disorders (Reeves et al, 2011). Lesbian and bisexual women report higher rates of depression and anxiety than other women do. Bisexual women are even more likely than lesbians to have had a mood or anxiety disorder; depression and anxiety in lesbian and bisexual women may be due to stigma, discrimination, rejection, abuse and violence, or being uninsured (Reeves et al, 2011).

Natural and Human-made Disasters and Mental Illness

Natural and human-made disasters, such as hurricanes, floods, violence, terrorism, war, and the global economic crisis, are profound stress-inducing events that can lead to mental illness. Researchers reported high levels of PTSD among survivors of Hurricane Katrina which devastated New Orleans in 2005. Community mental health nurses must be prepared not only to respond to the mental health needs of a community during a disaster but also to maintain vigilance in caring for survivors many years thereafter.

PTSD is highly prevalent among combat veterans returning from war. PTSD is associated with extreme anxiety that can result in suicide. Male veterans in communities are twice as likely to die by suicide as their civilian counterparts (NIMH, 2013) (see Veterans' Health box on suicide). During 2012, there were 60 suicides among active-duty members of the Navy, 59 in the Air Force, and 48 in the Marine Corps. Throughout the U.S. military, suicides increased by nearly 16% from 2011 to 2012 (U.S. Department of Defense, 2012). The Army's suicide rate rose dramatically, as the service reported more than 320 suicides in 2012. The rise in the number of reported suicides prompted the service to take a closer look at its suicide prevention program. Early intervention is key to prevention and treatment. The *2012 National Strategy for Suicide Prevention: Goals and Objectives for Action* was released by the U.S. Surgeon General and of the National Action Alliance for Suicide Prevention (USDHHS, 2012) (Box 24-1). This plan is being utilized by the VA (see Veterans' Health box on raising awareness of PTSD).

BOX 24-1   2012 NATIONAL STRATEGY FOR SUICIDE PREVENTION

- Create supportive environments that promote healthy and empowered individuals, families, and communities
- Enhance clinical and community preventive services
- Promote the availability of timely treatment and support services
- Improve suicide prevention surveillance collection, research, and evaluation

From U.S. Department of Health and Human Services, Office of the Surgeon General and National Action Alliance for Suicide Prevention: *2012 National Strategy for Suicide Prevention: Goals and Objectives for Action*. Washington, DC, 2012, Author.

VETERANS' HEALTH

Suicide Among Veterans

A 2010 report by the U.S. Department of Veterans Affairs (VA) states that an estimated 18 veterans die by suicide every day and that there are 950 suicide attempts by veterans every month. Repeated deployments in Iraq and Afghanistan with resulting post-traumatic stress disorder (PTSD) among veterans who served in these theaters are the main reasons for the sharp increases in suicides among veterans aged 19 to 25. The suicide rate is lower for those who are receiving services through the VA. Veterans are less likely to complete treatment if they are male, under age 25, living in a rural area, or receive a diagnosis of PTSD from a primary care provider rather than a mental health program.

Nurses must be aware of the signs of depression and possible suicide and must be knowledgeable about their clients' military status. Always ask whether your client is a veteran and refer him or her to VA resources in the community.

Remember "ACE":

Ask the veteran, "Do you think about hurting yourself?"

Care about the veteran by listening to his or her story in a non-judgmental way.

Escort the veteran. Encourage the veteran to get help and provide information on resources available in the community. Escort the veteran to the nearest emergency room or VA facility if he or she is expressing suicidal thoughts or plans.

There are many resources available for veterans in distress. The VA's Veteran's Crisis Line is available 24 hours a day, 7 days a week. Veterans and their families can also access mental health assistance through an online chat at http://www.veteranscrisisline.net/ or by sending a text to 838255 to access assistance 24/7. All of these resources are confidential and connect the veteran or the veteran's family to resources at the VA.

Modified from a presentation created by Bridgette Crotwell Pullis, PhD, RN, CHPN. Data from The U.S. Department of Veterans Affairs: *Mental health*, n.d. Available from <http://www.mentalhealth.va.gov/suicide_prevention/index.asp>.

The global economic crisis that began in late 2008 has had enormous mental health consequences. The sense of hopelessness and powerlessness that accompanied the financial losses associated with dwindling retirement accounts for some, and layoffs for others, has contributed to much emotional distress throughout the world. The World Health Organization (2009), warning that the economic crisis will have a detrimental effect on the mental health of citizens of all nations, called for enhanced monitoring for indications of mental health decline.

VETERANS' HEALTH

Raising Awareness of Post-Traumatic Stress Disorder (PTSD)

The National Center for PTSD sponsored by the U.S. Department of Veterans Affairs is the national clearing house and resource center for PTSD. Veterans and professionals who work with veterans are encouraged to "Take the Step" to raise awareness of PTSD:

Step 1: Learn about PTSD

Symptoms of PTSD:

- Sadness or depression
- Guilt that you did not do more to prevent the trauma
- Shame over your actions during the trauma
- Anger
- Drug or alcohol abuse
- Avoiding people or certain situations

Step 2: Challenge Your Beliefs

Think about the benefits of treatment for PTSD. Realize that treatment is not just for people with severe problems but that treatment can allow everyone suffering from PTSD to get back into control of their lives.

Veterans often worry that getting help will make them look weak or hurt job opportunities and may not seek help until their families or their careers suffer as a result of PTSD symptoms. Getting treatment for PTSD during deployment or immediately after returning home from deployment is optimum.

Step 3: Explore Options

There are many options for treatment and support for PTSD. Veterans may access services through the VA specific to their needs, such as women's mental health services, as well as resources for their families. There are self-help tools available online and through mobile "apps."

Step 4- Reach Out and Make a Difference

- Raise awareness of PTSD
- Support veterans through Joining Forces, About Face, or other community programs
- Learn about PTSD
- Encourage veterans and their families to get treatment and support for PTSD

Modified from a presentation created by Bridgette Crotwell Pullis, PhD, RN, CHPN. Learn all of the facts about PTSD at <http://www.ptsd.va.gov/index.asp>, and learn how veterans with PTSD changed their lives for the better at <http://www.ptsd.va.gov/apps/AboutFace/>.

Political Factors

Political factors can dramatically influence how mental disorders are managed. One significant factor in the politics of mental illness is parity in health care coverage—that is, the equal access to health care for physical and mental illnesses. Historically, health insurance companies have provided less access to treatment for a mental disorder than for a physical disorder. Since 2008, when the Paul Wellstone and Pete Domenici Mental Health Parity and Addiction Equity Act was enacted, there are laws requiring health insurance to cover treatment for mental illness on the same terms and conditions as physical illness. Although this legislation was a victory for mental health, there has been inconsistency in how the the legislation has moved forward.

Health care disparities have become a key issue in public health policy discussions. As previously discussed, members of ethnic minority groups have less access to mental health services than do their white counterparts. Minorities are more likely to delay seeking mental health care and are more likely to receive poor care when they are treated (Stacciarini et al, 2011).

MENTAL DISORDERS ENCOUNTERED IN COMMUNITY SETTINGS

The influence of untreated mental illness on communities and their social structure has been vastly understated. The NIMH estimates that 44.7 million adults aged 18 or older, or 19.8% of all U.S. adults, have experienced any diagnosable mental illness in the past year. Mental illness is one of the leading causes of disability in the United States and mental illness accounts for more than 10% of the disease burden worldwide, ranking it second, following all forms of cardiac disease (USDHHS/SAMHSA, 2012). In the United States, the estimated cost of mental illness exceeds $100 billion for diagnosing and treating mental disorders, and $193 billion in lost productivity (NIMH, 2010).

Because most mental illnesses are identified and managed in community settings, it is essential that community health nurses be familiar with frequently occurring mental disorders. There is a need for screening, referring, and follow-up for people with mental health problems in order to meet these mental health needs (Happell and Cleary, 2012).

Overview of Selected Mental Disorders

The *DSM* V (American Psychiatric Association [APA], 2013), classifies mental illnesses and outlines diagnostic criteria for more than 300 disorders. Children with mental disorders are often referred to as children with severe emotional disorder (SED). SED disturbance suggests broad ranges of behaviors that might result in classification of a student with SED as eligible for special education. A child with SED may demonstrate emotional disturbance with hallucinations, may have a very short attention span, may hurt others physically, may destroy property, or may have severe presentations of depression, anger, or fear. Among students with SED, externalizing behaviors such as acting out are significantly more prevalent than internalizing behaviors such as withdrawal or depression.

Clinical Example

Michael Nye, a photographer, spent hundreds of hours photographing and taping illness narratives of individuals living with serious mental illness. Viewing his photographs and listening to the accounts of those living with these conditions are valuable experiences for nurses who care for this population (http://michaelnye.org/fineline/index.html). Fleming and colleagues (2009) analyzed the photographs and narratives from the exhibit and concluded that suffering, stigma, and loss of identity were the central experiences depicted by this project.

Schizophrenia

Schizophrenia is the most severe and most profound of all mental illnesses; globally, it affects about 1% of the population (Brain and Behavior Research Foundation, 2013). The effect of this condition on the community is enormous in terms of social and economic burden. To the individual and families affected by schizophrenia, the impact is incalculable. The affected person may present with positive symptoms, including hallucinations, delusions, disorganized thinking and speech, and bizarre behavior, or negative symptoms, such as flat affect, poor attention, lack of motivation, apathy, lack of pleasure, and lack of energy. Onset typically occurs during late adolescence and early adulthood in males and somewhat later in females. There is an increased risk for alcohol use, depression, suicide, and diabetes among persons with schizophrenia. These factors compound the problems associated with living with a psychotic disorder.

Among people diagnosed with schizophrenia, an estimated 20% to 40% attempt suicide; between 5% and 13% actually succeed. Patients with schizophrenia may have anosognosia (Treatment Advocacy Center, 2012), an impaired awareness of illness, so they may not recognize that they are ill (Amador, 2007, 2008). This impaired awareness of illness affects approximately 50% of individuals with schizophrenia. Anosognosia contributes to noncompliance with medications and treatment.

Treatment for schizophrenia must be intensive and generally involves hospitalization (initially), antipsychotic medications, and psychotherapy/counseling. Long-term follow-up by mental health professionals is necessary to monitor medication compliance and to watch for side effects and complications, which may be severe and life threatening, and to evaluate the patient's ability to integrate into the community.

Depression

Depression is the most frequently diagnosed and one of the most disabling mental illnesses in the United States. Depressive disorders affect approximately 18.8 million American adults, or about 9.5% of the U.S. population age 18 and older, in a given year. The disorders include major depressive disorder, dysthymic disorder, and bipolar disorders. Depression often co-occurs with serious physical disorders, such as heart attack, stroke, diabetes, and cancer. About 25% of women and 12% of men have at least one episode of depression during their lifetimes. Although effective treatments exist, most people (almost two thirds) with depressive illness do not seek help (NIMH, 2013). Having a family or personal history of depression, suicide attempt, or sexual abuse, or having current substance abuse or a chronic medical condition increases the risk for depression (APA, 2013). Health education for patients with depression should include risk factor identification as well as when and how to obtain treatment. Symptoms of depression are listed in Box 24-2.

BOX 24-2   SYMPTOMS OF DEPRESSION

- Persistent sad, anxious, or "empty" feelings
- Feelings of hopelessness or pessimism
- Feelings of guilt, worthlessness, or helplessness
- Irritability, restlessness
- Loss of interest in activities or hobbies once pleasurable, including sex
- Fatigue and decreased energy
- Difficulty concentrating, remembering details, and making decisions
- Insomnia, early-morning wakefulness, or excessive sleeping
- Overeating or appetite loss
- Thoughts of suicide, suicide attempts
- Aches or pains, headaches, cramps, or digestive problems that do not ease even with treatment

From National Institute of Mental Health: *Depression* (NIH Publication No. 11-3561), Rockville, MD, 2000, Revised 2011, Author.

RESEARCH HIGHLIGHTS

Measuring Mental Illness–Related Stigma Imposed by Health Care Providers

Knowing that mental illness-related stigma can lead to low rates of seeking help, lack of access to care, under-treatment and social marginalization, Kassam and associates (2012) developed and tested the *Opening Minds Scale for Health Care Providers* (OMS-HC). 787 health care providers/trainees across Canada. The OMS–HC provides hope in demonstrating that it that can be utilized in evaluation of programs with goals to reduce mental illness–related stigma imposed by health care providers.

Data from Kassam A, Papish A, Modgill G, Patten S: The development and psychometric properties of a new scale to measure mental illness related stigma by health care providers: The Opening Minds Scale for Health Care Providers (OMS-HC). *BMC Psychiatr* 12:62, 3-12, 2012.

Depression In Children and Adolescents. The incidence of depression in children is 0.9% in preschool-age children, 1.9% in school-age children, and 4.7% in adolescents (Healthy Place, 2013). According to the Centers for Disease Control and Prevention (2013) almost 4% of children 3-17 have ever been diagnosed with depression and as many as 12% of adolescents may have depression. A family history of depression is a major risk factor for childhood depression. Other associated factors that may increase the risk of depression in children and adolescents are a history of verbal, physical, or sexual abuse; frequent separation from, or loss of, a loved one; poverty; mental retardation; attention deficit/hyperactivity disorder; hyperactivity; and chronic illness.

Treatment for depression includes pharmacological therapy, psychotherapy, behavior therapy, electroconvulsive therapy, or a combination of these (APA, 2013; NIMH, 2012). In general, the most effective, first-line treatment is a combination of antidepressant medication and psychotherapy.

Bipolar Disorder

Bipolar disorder refers to a group of mood disorders that manifest as changes in mood from depression to mania. The depressed phase manifests as symptoms seen in major depressive disorder. The manic phase is characterized by a persistent abnormally elevated or irritable mood, impaired judgment, flight of ideas, pressured speech, grandiosity, distractibility, excessive involvement in goal-directed activities, spending few hours sleeping, and impulsivity. These symptoms may co-occur with psychotic features such as hallucinations and delusions. Persons with bipolar disorder are at increased risk for alcohol and substance abuse as well as suicide. The presence of bipolar disorder results in poor occupational and social functioning.

Management of bipolar disorder must be ongoing and must involve close monitoring. Treatment generally involves use of mood-stabilizing medication, often in combination with antipsychotic and antidepressant therapy (APA, 2012). When working with persons with bipolar disorder, nurses need to monitor symptoms and response to psychopharmacological treatment.

Anxiety Disorder

Anxiety disorders are a group of conditions characterized by feelings of anxiety. Anxiety disorders affect up to 16% of the general population at any time. Anxiety disorders may be attributed to the genetic makeup and life experiences of the individual. Some of the more commonly encountered anxiety disorders are generalized anxiety disorder, panic disorder (sometimes accompanied by agoraphobia), phobias, obsessive-compulsive disorder, and PTSD (APA, 2013). They are discussed briefly here.

Generalized Anxiety Disorder. Generalized anxiety disorder (GAD) is characterized by chronic, unrealistic, and exaggerated worry and tension about one or more life circumstances lasting 6 months or longer (APA, 2013). Approximately half of cases of GAD begin in childhood or adolescence, and the disorder is more common in women than in men. Symptoms of GAD include trembling, twitching, muscle tension, headaches, irritability, sweating or hot flashes, dyspnea, and nausea. Periods of increasing symptoms are usually associated with life stressors or impending difficulties. GAD is probably the most underdiagnosed mental disorder.

Panic Disorder. Approximately 6 million American adults have panic disorder (NIMH, n.d.). Panic disorder can occur at any age, but it most often begins in young adulthood (average age, 17-30 years). A panic attack consists of a period of intense fear that develops abruptly and unexpectedly. The initial attack may occur suddenly and unexpectedly while the client is performing everyday tasks. Typically, he or she experiences tachycardia; dyspnea; dizziness; chest pain; nausea; numbness or tingling of the hands and feet; trembling or shaking; sweating; choking; or a feeling that he or she is going to die, go crazy, or do something uncontrolled. It can be extremely frightening. A diagnosis of panic disorder is made when attacks occur with some degree of frequency or regularity.

As the disorder evolves, the anxiety attacks become increasingly frequent and severe, and anticipatory anxiety (fear of having a panic attack) develops. During this phase, events and circumstances associated with the attack may be selectively avoided, leading to phobic behaviors. Thus, the client's life may become progressively constricted.

As the avoidance behavior intensifies, the client begins to withdraw further to avoid being in places or situations from which escape may be difficult or embarrassing or in which help may be unavailable in the event of a panic attack (e.g., church, elevators, movie theaters). The fear of being in these situations or places can lead to agoraphobia (literally, fear of the marketplace or open places). Individuals with agoraphobia frequently progress to the point that they cannot leave their homes without experiencing anxiety.

Rates for co-occurring major depression range from 10% to 65% in persons with panic disorder (APA, 2013). Cognitive behavioral treatment and short-course benzodiazepines therapy are used to treat panic disorder.

Phobias. A phobia is an irrational fear of something (an object or situation), and as many as 8% of Americans are affected by phobias at any given time. Adults with phobias realize that their fears are irrational, but facing the feared object or situation might bring on severe anxiety or a panic attack. Although phobias may begin in childhood, they usually first appear in adolescence or adulthood.

Social phobia, or social anxiety disorder, is a persistent and intense fear of, and compelling desire to avoid, something that would expose the individual to a situation that might be humiliating and embarrassing (APA, 2013). It has a familial tendency and may be accompanied by depression or alcoholism. The most common social phobia is a fear of public speaking. Other examples include being unable to urinate in a public bathroom and not being able to answer questions in social situations. Most people with social phobias can be treated with cognitive-behavioral therapy and medication.

Simple phobias involve a persistent fear of, and compelling desire to avoid, certain objects or situations. Common objects of phobias are spiders, snakes, dogs, cats, and situations such as flying, heights, and closed-in spaces. The person often recognizes that the fear is unreasonable but avoids the situation or endures it with intense anxiety. Systematic desensitization and normal exposure are the most effective treatments for simple phobias.

Obsessive-Compulsive Disorder. Obsessive-compulsive disorder (OCD) is characterized by anxious thoughts and rituals that the individual has difficulty controlling. The person with OCD feels compelled to engage in some ritual to avoid a persistent frightening thought, idea, image, or event. *Obsessions* are recurrent thoughts, emotions, or impulses that cannot be dismissed. *Compulsions* are the rituals or behaviors that are repeatedly performed to prevent, neutralize, or dispel the dreaded obsession. When the individual tries to resist the compulsion, anxiety increases. Common compulsions include hand washing, counting, checking, and touching (APA, 2013). Most individuals recognize that what they are doing is senseless but are unable to control the compulsion. About 2% of Americans are afflicted with OCD, which often appears in the teenage years or early adulthood. Depression and other anxiety disorders often accompany OCD. Behavioral therapy and medication aimed at reducing accompanying symptoms have been found to be helpful.

Post Traumatic Stress Disorder. Post-traumatic stress disorder is a debilitating condition that follows a terrifying event. It affects about 3.5% of U.S. adults. Individuals with PTSD have recurring, persistent, frightening thoughts and memories of their ordeal. The event may involve "shell shock" or "battle fatigue" common to war veterans, a violent attack, serious accident, or natural disaster, or having witnessed a mass destruction or injury, such as an airplane crash. Sometimes the individual is unable to recall an important aspect of the traumatic event. The highest incidence of PTSD occurs among combat-experienced military personnel.

People with PTSD repeatedly relive the trauma in the form of nightmares or disturbing recollections or flashbacks during the day, resulting in sleep disturbances, depression, feelings of detachment or emotional numbness, or being easily startled. They may avoid places or situations that bring back memories (e.g., a woman raped in an elevator may refuse to ride in elevators), and anniversaries of the event are often very difficult. PTSD occurs at all ages and may be accompanied by depression, substance abuse, and/or anxiety. It usually begins within 3 months of the trauma, and the course of the disorder varies. Some individuals recover within 6 months; the condition becomes chronic in others. Infrequently, the illness does not manifest until years after the traumatic event. Treatment includes antidepressants and antianxiety medications and psychotherapy. Support from family and friends can be very beneficial.

Eating Disorders

Eating disorders—anorexia nervosa and bulimia nervosa—are increasingly prevalent in the United States, affecting about 3 million U.S. residents. Anorexia affects about 0.5% to 3.7% of females in their lifetimes (NIMH, 2010), and as many as 4% to 15% of female high school and college women have some symptoms of bulimia.

Eating disorders primarily affect females; males account for 5% to 10% of cases, although the disorders in males may be underreported. Most clients with a diagnosis of eating disorders are white; however, the reason may be socioeconomic factors rather than race. Anorexia and bulimia are often triggered by developmental milestones (e.g., puberty, first sexual contact) or another crisis (e.g., death of a loved one, ridicule over weight, starting college).

Bulimia nervosa refers to binge eating: discreetly consuming an abnormally large amount of food and then using maladaptive compensatory methods to prevent weight gain (APA, 2013). For example, a person with bulimia might eat an entire pie, half a cake, or a half gallon of ice cream at one sitting. Snacking throughout the day is not considered bingeing. To lose or maintain weight, the person with bulimia practices purging, which usually involves self-induced vomiting, caused by gagging, using an emetic, or simply mentally willing the action. Laxatives, diuretics, fasting, and excessive exercise may also be employed to control weight.

Bulimia nervosa typically begins in adolescence or during the early 20s, usually in conjunction with a diet. High school and college students, as well as members of certain professions that emphasize weight and/or appearance (e.g., dancers, flight attendants, cheerleaders, athletes, actors, models), are at risk. The condition may lead to electrolyte imbalance, resulting in fatigue, seizures, muscle cramps, arrhythmias, and decreased bone density. Vomiting can damage the esophagus, stomach, teeth, and gums.

The person with anorexia nervosa becomes obsessed with a fear of fat and with losing weight. Anorexia nervosa often develops as a fairly gradual decrease in caloric intake. However, the decrease continues until the person is consuming almost nothing. Anorexia usually begins in early adolescence (12 to 14 years is the most common age-group) and may be limited to a single episode of dramatic weight loss within a few months, followed by recovery, or may last for many years.

Risk factors for eating disorders are perfectionism, low self-esteem, stress, poor coping skills, sexual/physical abuse, poor self-image, dependency on others' opinions and deference to others' wishes, and being emotionally reserved. In response to the severely decreased caloric intake, the body tries to compensate by slowing down body processes. Menstruation ceases; blood pressure, pulse, and respiration rates slow; and thyroid activity diminishes. Electrolyte imbalance can become very severe. Other symptoms are mild anemia, joint swelling, and reduced muscle mass. Anorexia nervosa can be life threatening and has a mortality rate of 5% to 21%.

Treatment for eating disorders involves long-term nutrition counseling, psychotherapy, and behavior modification. Hospitalization may be required for clients with serious complications. Self-help groups and support groups can be very beneficial for both the client and the family.

Nurses need to be aware of the resources available from the American Academy of Child and Adolescent Psychiatry (AACAP), which has a section for families and youth. Such knowledge is important, as community health nurses assess the social influences that contribute to the condition.

Attention Deficit/Hyperactivity Disorder

Two of the most common conditions encountered by nurses who work with children in community settings are attention-deficit/hyperactivity disorder (ADHD) and attention deficit disorder (ADD). About 11% of school-age children in the United States—and 19% of high school–age boys—have been diagnosed ADHD, according to CDC data. Behaviors that might indicate ADHD/ADD usually appear before age 7 years and are often accompanied by related problems, such as learning disability, anxiety, and depression. The three major characteristics of ADHD/ADD are inattention, hyperactivity, and impulsivity.

The cause of ADHD/ADD is not known, but it is important to note that the disorder is not caused by minor head injuries, birth complications, food allergies, too much sugar, poor home life, poor schools, or too much television watching. Maternal substance use and abuse (e.g., alcohol, cigarettes, cocaine) may affect the brain of the developing baby and produce symptoms of ADHD/ADD later in life. This possibility, however, accounts for only a small percentage of those affected. Attention disorders run in families.

Although parents may notice symptoms and signs, it is often teachers who recognize the behaviors consistent with attention deficit disorders and suggest referral for assessment and treatment (NIMH, 2013. Experts caution that diagnosis of attention disorders should be made following a comprehensive physical, psychological, social, and behavioral evaluation and should not be based solely on anecdotal reports from parents or teachers. The evaluation should rule out other possible reasons for the behavior (e.g., emotional problems, poor vision or hearing, physical problems) and should include input from teachers, parents, and others who know the child well. Intelligence and achievement testing may also be performed to rule out or identify a learning disability.

Symptoms of ADHD/ADD are typically managed through a combination of behavior therapy, emotional counseling, and practical support. Use of medication is now becoming increasingly commonplace in the management of ADHD/ADD. It is very important, however, that children with attention disorders and their families understand that medication does not cure the disorder; it just temporarily controls symptoms.

Stimulants have been shown to be successful in treating attention disorders. The most commonly used medications are methylphenidate (Ritalin) and amphetamines. Appetite suppression and poor sleep are common side effects.

Suicide

There are approximately 1 million deaths by suicide per year throughout the world. The Centers for Disease Control and Prevention (2012) reported there were more than 38,000 deaths by suicide in the United States in 2010. Suicide is the third leading cause of death among those aged 15 to 24 years. The highest rate of suicide occurs in males older than 65 years; white males older than 85 years are particularly vulnerable.

Historically, risk and protective factors have been used to identify those at highest risk for suicide. The American Association of Suicidology (AAS) (2013) has recommended recognition of warning signs as more relevant than risk and protective factors in preventing death by suicide. The AAS has organized the warning signs according to the easily remembered mnemonic, IS PATH WARM (Table 24-2). Warning signs that indicate acute risk for suicidality may be observed in individuals who are threatening to hurt or kill themselves, attempting to identify access to lethal weapons or other means that could result in death, or communicating about dying when these thoughts or actions are out of the ordinary for them.

Risk factors include previous suicide attempts, mental illness, substance abuse, and barriers to accessing mental health treatment. Protective factors may decrease the risk of suicide include appropriate mental health care, easy access to treatment, community support, and continuing support from medical and mental health care providers. Box 24-3 lists protective factors and risk factors that all community health nurses should recognize, and Box 24-4 provides warning signs of suicide.

TABLE 24-2 Suicide Warning Signs: "IS PATH WARM"

Ideation	Does the person state that he or she is having thoughts of suicide?
Substance abuse	Is the person demonstrating increased use of alcohol or drugs?
Purposelessness	Does the person state that he or she feels as if there is no purpose in his or her life?
Anxiety	Is the person demonstrating anxiety-related behaviors such as: talking about being overly worried about things, ruminating, difficulty concentrating, or exhibiting increased psychomotor agitation?
Trapped	Does the person state that he or she feels trapped, that there is no way out of the current situation except to die?
Hopelessness	Does the person state that he or she feels hopeless? Is the person able to describe something to look forward to?
Withdrawal	Is the person withdrawing from others such as family and friends? Is the person isolating?
Anger	Is the person demonstrating uncontrolled anger? Is the person acting with rage or seeking revenge?
Recklessness	Is the person engaged in risk-taking behaviors? Is the person acting as if he or she "doesn't care" or isn't thinking about the consequences of the risk-taking behavior?
Mood changes	Is the person experiencing dramatic mood changes?

From American Association of Suicidology: *Know the warning signs*, 2009. Retrieved from <www.suicidology.org>. Contact information: American Association of Suicidology 5221 Wisconsin Ave. NW 2nd Floor Washington, DC 20015-2032 Phone (202) 237-2280 Fax (202) 237-2282 www.suicidology.org info@suicidology.org

BOX 24-3 SUICIDE: PROTECTIVE FACTORS AND RISK FACTORS

Protective Factors
- Effective clinical care for mental, physical, and substance abuse disorders
- Easy access to a variety of clinical interventions and support for help seeking
- Family and community support (connectedness)
- Support from ongoing medical and mental health care relationships
- Skills in problem solving, conflict resolution, and nonviolent ways of handling disputes
- Cultural and religious beliefs that discourage suicide and support instincts for self-preservation

Risk Factors
- Family history of suicide
- Family history of child maltreatment
- Previous suicide attempt(s)
- History of mental disorders, particularly clinical depression
- History of alcohol and substance abuse
- Feelings of hopelessness
- Impulsive or aggressive tendencies
- Cultural and religious beliefs (e.g., belief that suicide is noble resolution of a personal dilemma)
- Local epidemics of suicide
- Isolation, a feeling of being cut off from other people
- Barriers to accessing mental health treatment
- Loss (relational, social, work, or financial)
- Physical illness
- Easy access to lethal methods
- Unwillingness to seek help because of the stigma attached to mental health and substance abuse disorders or to suicidal thoughts

Adapted from Substance Abuse and Mental Health Services Administration, National Suicide Prevention Lifeline: *Risk factors for suicide,* n.d. Available from <http://www.suicidepreventionlifeline.org/learn/riskfactors.aspx>.

Thus, it is important that all community health nurses become familiar with assessing for suicide warning signs and accessing appropriate resources. Nurses should refer the person exhibiting suicide warning signs to a mental health clinic or provider as soon as possible. This may involve taking emergency action by calling the local emergency services number in the community and staying with the person until help arrives. Table 24-3 provides a list of suicide information resources.

IDENTIFICATION AND MANAGEMENT OF MENTAL DISORDERS

Early identification, appropriate treatment, and rehabilitation can significantly reduce the duration and level of disability associated with mental disorders and decrease the possibility of relapse. Interventions to promote mental health and decrease mental disorders include focusing on decreasing stressors and/or increasing the capacity of the individual to cope with stress. Other interventions include the use of pharmacological agents and psychosocial interventions such as strengthening interpersonal, psychological, and physical resources through counseling, support groups, and psychoeducation.

BOX 24-4 WARNING SIGNS OF SUICIDE

Seek help as soon as possible by contacting a mental health professional or by calling the National Suicide Prevention Lifeline at 1-800-273-TALK if you or someone you know exhibits any of the following signs:
- Threatening to hurt or kill oneself or talking about wanting to hurt or kill oneself
- Looking for ways to kill oneself by seeking access to firearms, available pills, or other means
- Talking or writing about death, dying, or suicide when these actions are out of the ordinary for the person
- Feeling hopeless
- Feeling rage or uncontrolled anger or seeking revenge
- Acting reckless or engaging in risky activities—seemingly without thinking
- Feeling trapped—like there's no way out
- Increasing alcohol or drug use
- Withdrawing from friends, family, and society
- Feeling anxious, agitated, or unable to sleep or sleeping all the time
- Experiencing dramatic mood changes
- Seeing no reason for living or having no sense of purpose in life

From Suicidepreventionlifeline.org: *When it seems like there is no hope, there is help* (Brochure CMHS-SVP-0141), 2006. Available from <http://www.cbp.gov/linkhandler/cgov/careers/benefits_employees/frc/suicide_prevention/suicide_prevention_materials/prevention_brochure.ctt/prevention_brochure.pdf>.

TABLE 24-3	Suicide Prevention and Referral Resources
National Suicide Prevention Lifeline	1-800-273-TALK (8255) www.suicidepreventionlifeline.org/
American Association of Suicidology	www.suicidology.org/home
Suicide Prevention Resource Center	www.sprc.org/
Suicide Awareness Voices of Education	www.save.org/
Suicide Prevention: A Resource Manual for the Army	http://www.armyg1.army.mil/dcs /docs/Suicide%20Prevention %20Manual.pdf
Veterans Crisis Line	1-800- 273- 8255 Text to 838255 www.veteranscrisisline.net/ ChatTermsOfService.aspx? account=Veterans%20Chat
American Foundation for Suicide Prevention	www.afsp.org/
Local emergency resource	Dial 911

The accessibility of mental health service is pivotal in promoting and maintaining the health. Decreased funding for services, managed care limitations on mental health coverage, and the inequality of coverage by the insurance industry have caused downsizing or forced closure in the traditional places of treatment, such as community mental health centers and community hospitals. Consequently, the accessibility to community mental health services has become an issue of significant concern. In addition, the symptoms of mental illness often interfere with an individual's ability to access services. Alterations in thoughts and perceptions, anxiety, and decreased energy are common symptoms of mental illness, all of which interfere with negotiating the complex systems that currently surround the provision of mental health services. This section describes actions that may be taken by community health nurses to identify mental illness and outlines potential treatment options.

Identification of Mental Disorders

Whether the nurse is working in a physician's office, a community clinic, a school, or home health and hospice, occupational health, or other setting, recognition of signs and symptoms that might indicate a mental disorder is an important component of practice. More than ever, public health nurses work in collaboration with crisis housing agencies and school district managers for homeless families. In these situations, the nurse should continue to assess for other signs and symptoms that might indicate a mental disorder and should be prepared to intervene if they appear.

Often, the assessment process includes direct questioning or observation. At other times, a standardized assessment tool or questionnaire might be employed. Figures 24-1 and 24-2 contain examples of instruments that are available to elicit information about symptoms of anxiety or depression. Whenever using these or other screening tools, the nurse

should be prepared in advance to intervene on the basis of assessment data. Often, this intervention incorporates referral to other health professionals for further assessment, testing, counseling, treatment, and follow-up by all health professionals involved.

Evidence-Based Practice Management of Mental Disorders

The website of the Substance Abuse and Mental Health Services Agency's (SAMHSA) National Registry of Evidence Based Programs and Practices (NREPP) lists EBP programs and interventions that demonstrate positive outcomes in community mental health. The goals of treatment for mental illness are to reduce symptoms, improve occupational and social functioning, develop and strengthen coping skills, and promote behaviors to improve the individual's life. Crisis housing programs, supportive employments programs, Assertive Community Treatment (ACT) team models, Crisis Intervention Team (CIT) models, psychotropic medication management programs, community case management programs, mobile crisis units, Cognitive Behavioral Intervention for Trauma in Schools programs, and many more are listed. Basic approaches to the treatment of mental disorders are detailed; see the website <http://www.nrep p.samhsa.gov/SearchResultsNew.aspx?s=b&q=smi.>

Psychotropic or Psychotherapeutic Medications

Psychotropic/psychotherapeutic medications treat symptoms of mental illness. The appropriateness of psychopharmacological agents and their prescribed regimen depends on the diagnosis, side effects, and client response. Some of the psychotropic medications prescribed are classified as antipsychotics, antidepressants, mood stabilizers, anticonvulsants, antianxiety agents, and hypnotics. Information about medication profiles and treatment regimens often changes as new information becomes available, so nurses should be aware of up-to-date medication information from Internet resources such as www.nlm.nih.gov/medlineplus/druginfor mation.html or www.rxlist.com.

Psychotherapy

Psychotherapy refers to a process of discovery that helps alleviate troubling emotional symptoms and assists individuals in returning to a healthy life (APA, 2013). In nursing, psychotherapy is an intervention used predominantly by psychiatric/mental health advanced practice nurses. Psychotherapy involves the use of a professional, therapeutic relationship and the application of psychotherapy theories and best practices to change a client's attitudes, feelings, beliefs, defenses, personality, and behaviors. Therapy approaches vary among schools of psychotherapy and with the nature of the client's problem. Psychotherapy is often used in conjunction with medication to treat many mental disorders. Various types of psychotherapy include the following (NIMH, 2014):

Individual therapy focuses on the client's current life and relationships within the family, social, and work environments.

Family therapy involves problem-solving sessions with members of a family.

During the Past Week	Rarely or None of the Time (Less than 1 Day)	Some or a Little of the Time (1-2 Days)	Occasionally or a Moderate Amount of the Time (3-4 Days)	Most or All of the Time (5-7 Days)
1. I was bothered by things that don't usually bother me.	0	1	2	3
2. I did not feel like eating; my appetite was poor.	0	1	2	3
3. I felt that I could not shake off the blues even with the help of my family or friends.	0	1	2	3
4. I felt that I was just as good as other people.	3	2	1	0
5. I had trouble keeping my mind on what I was doing.	0	1	2	3
6. I felt depressed.	0	1	2	3
7. I felt everything I did was an effort.	0	1	2	3
8. I felt hopeful about the future.	3	2	1	0
9. I thought my life had been a failure.	0	1	2	3
10. I felt fearful.	0	1	2	3
11. My sleep was restless.	0	1	2	3
12. I was happy.	3	2	1	0
13. I talked less than usual.	0	1	2	3
14. I felt lonely.	0	1	2	3
15. People were unfriendly.	0	1	2	3
16. I enjoyed life.	3	2	1	0
17. I had crying spells.	0	1	2	3
18. I felt sad.	0	1	2	3
19. I felt that people disliked me.	0	1	2	3
20. I could not get "going."	0	1	2	3

FIGURE 24-1 Center for Epidemiologic Studies depression scale. Interpretation: A total score of 22 or higher is indicative of depression when the scale is used in primary care. (From Radloff LS: The CES-D scale: a self-report depression scale for research in the general population, *Appl Psychol Meas* 1:385-401, 1977. Copyright 1977, West Publishing Company/Applied Psychological Measurement, Inc.)

Couple therapy is used to develop the relationship and minimize problems through understanding how individual conflicts are expressed in the couple's interactions.

Group therapy involves a small group of people with similar problems who, with the guidance of a therapist, discuss individual issues and help one another with problems.

Play therapy is a technique used for establishing communication and resolving problems with young children.

Cognitive-behavioral therapy may be used in individual, family, couples, or group therapy. The goal is to identify and correct distorted thought patterns that can lead to troublesome feelings and behaviors.

Behavioral therapy uses learning principles to change thought patterns and behaviors systematically; it is used to encourage the individual to learn specific skills to obtain rewards and satisfaction.

Rank	Life Event	Mean Value	Rank	Life Event	Mean Value
1	Death of spouse	100	23	Son or daughter leaving home	29
2	Divorce	73	24	Trouble with in-laws	29
3	Marital separation	65	25	Outstanding personal achievement	28
4	Jail term	63			
5	Death of close family member	63	26	Wife begins or stops work	26
6	Personal injury or illness	53	27	Begin or end school	26
7	Marriage	50	28	Change in living conditions	25
8	Fired at work	47	29	Change in personal habits	24
9	Marital reconciliation	45	30	Trouble with boss	23
10	Retirement	45	31	Change in work hours or conditions	20
11	Change in health of family member	44			
12	Pregnancy	40	32	Change in residence	20
13	Sex difficulties	39	33	Change in schools	20
14	Gain of new family member	39	34	Change in recreation	19
15	Business readjustment	39	35	Change in church activities	19
16	Change in financial state	38	36	Change in social activities	18
17	Death of close friend	37	37	Mortgage or loan less than $10,000	17
18	Change to different line of work	36			
19	Change in number of arguments with spouse	35	38	Change in sleeping habits	16
			39	Change in number of family get-togethers	15
20	Mortgage over $10,000	31			
21	Foreclosure on mortgage or loan	30	40	Change in eating habits	15
22	Change in responsibilities at work	29	41	Vacation	13
			42	Christmas	12
			43	Minor violations of the law	11

Life Crisis Categories and LCU Scores*

No life crisis	0-149
Mild life crisis	150-199
Moderate life crisis	200-299
Major life crisis	300 or more

*The LCU score includes those life event items experienced during a 1-year period.

FIGURE 24-2 Social readjustment rating scale. *LCU,* Life change unit(s). (From Holmes TH, Rahe RH: The social readjustment rating scale, *J Psychosom Res* 11:213-217, 1967, Elsevier Science Inc.)

Psychotherapy may be short-term or long-term, depending on the nature of the problem and the availability of resources.

COMMUNITY-BASED MENTAL HEALTH CARE

Over the past several decades, there have been a number of initiatives directed toward improving and promoting community-based care of those with mental illness. One of those initiatives is the President's New Freedom Commission on Mental Health (NFCMH). The New Freedom Initiative was first envisioned as a promise to tear down the barriers to equality that face millions of Americans with disabilities, including those with mental illness. The goal of the commission was to advise the president on strategies aimed at improving the mental health system so that persons with serious and persistent mental illnesses can enjoy full access to community life. The commission determined that in a transformed mental health system, the following would be true (NFCMH, 2003, p. 8):

1. Americans understand that mental health is essential to overall health.
2. Mental health care is consumer and family driven.

3. Disparities in mental health services are eliminated.
4. Early mental health screening, assessment, and referral to services are common practice.
5. Excellent mental health care is delivered, and research is accelerated.
6. Technology is used to access mental health care and information.

The commission acknowledged that mental illness comprises the only type of illness that defies a comprehensive delivery approach. The commission called for a shift in the fragmented system to an integrated comprehensive approach to mental health care delivery. Table 24-4 provides an overview of the recommendations of the commission. One of the areas addressed by the commission pertained to the need for school-based mental health (SBMH) programs. In an overview of key elements related to SBMH, Paternite and Johnston (2006) identified the need for (1) partnerships between and among schools, families, and communities; (2) a pledge to support a full continuum of mental health services that include education, health promotion, assessment, and early intervention; and (3) services for all children and adolescents.

TABLE 24-4	Goals and Recommendations of the New Freedom Commission on Mental Health
GOAL	**RECOMMENDATIONS**
1. Americans understand that mental health is essential to overall health.	Advance and implement a national campaign to reduce the stigma of seeking care and a national strategy for suicide prevention. Address mental health with the same urgency as physical health.
2. Mental health care is consumer and family driven.	Develop an individualized plan of care for every adult with a serious mental illness and child with a serious emotional disturbance. Involve consumers and families fully in orienting the mental health system toward recovery. Align relevant federal programs to improve access and accountability for mental health services. Create a comprehensive state mental health plan. Protect and enhance the rights of people with mental illnesses.
3. Disparities in mental health services are eliminated.	Improve access to quality care that is culturally competent. Improve access to quality care in rural and geographically remote areas.
4. Early mental health screening, assessment, and referral to services are common practice.	Promote the mental health of young children. Improve and expand school mental health programs. Screen for co-occurring mental and substance use disorders and link with integrated treatment strategies. Screen for mental disorders in primary health care across the lifespan, and connect to treatment and support.
5. Excellent mental health care is delivered and research is accelerated.	Accelerate research to promote recovery and resilience and ultimately to cure and prevent mental illnesses. Advance evidence-based practices using dissemination and demonstration projects and create a public-private partnership to guide their implementation. Improve and expand the workforce providing evidence-based mental health services and supports. Develop the knowledge base in four understudied areas: mental health disparities, long-term effects of medications, trauma, and acute care.
6. Technology is used to access mental health care and information.	Use health technology and telehealth to improve access and coordination of mental health care, especially for Americans in remote areas or in underserved populations. Develop and implement integrated electronic health record and personal health information systems.

From New Freedom Commission on Mental Health: *Achieving the promise: transforming mental health care in America, Final report* (USDHHS Pub No SMA 03-3832), Rockville, MD, 2003, Author. Also available from <http://govinfo.library.unt.edu/mentalhealthcommission/reports/FinalReport/downloads/FinalReport.pdf.>.

ETHICAL INSIGHTS

Valuing Human Beings

A study by Eriksen and colleagues (2012) demonstrates how users of mental health services describe and make sense of their meetings with other people. Acknowledging and valuing one other is an essential human characteristic that promotes individual dignity and vulnerability in relationships. The group utilized the Interpretative Phenomenological Analysis (IPA) to explore peoples' relationship to the world and how they make sense of their life experiences. Participants represented people living with mental health problems who depended on others for support and help in their everyday lives. Participants often would report the process "to be recognized" as a phenomenon in their life. To be recognized as a human being and be recognized as a human being struggling with a chronic mental health problems was helpful in their struggle in *self-preservation*. Mental health professionals may be challenged to recognize the struggle of the person with a serious mental illness (SMI). Mental health professionals can be helpful and instrumental in health promotion with SMI populations.

Data from Eriksen KA, Sundfor B, Karlsson B, et al: Recognition as a valued human being: Perspectives of mental health service users, *Nursing Ethics* 19(3) 357–368, 2012.

In an earlier initiative, the Center for Mental Health Services (CMHS) was formed in the early 1990s to improve prevention and mental health treatment services for all Americans. The CMHS helps states improve and increase the quality and range of treatment, rehabilitation, and support services for people with mental health problems, their families, and their communities (SAMHSA, 2014).

One of the programs promoted by the CMHS is the Community Support System. The Community Support System uses case management strategies to comprehensively provide care for those with serious mental illness. Components of the Community Support System include client identification and outreach, mental health treatment, crisis response service, health and dental care, housing, income support and entitlement, peer support, family and community support, rehabilitation services, and protection and advocacy. The case management approach serves to link the service system to the client and to coordinate their service received (Kondrat and Early, 2011). Other initiatives and programs sponsored by the CMHS are listed in Table 24-5.

The **Assertive Community Treatment (ACT)** model is another example of a community-based initiative to help meet the needs of those with mental illness. ACT, which has been in existence since the late 1960s, has become the exemplar of community mental health treatment models. The ACT program moves the traditional 24-hour treatment model of acute care settings into the community and serves people with mental illness in a highly individualized fashion (National Alliance on Mental Illness [NAMI], 2013). The ACT model provides supportive therapy, mobile crisis intervention, psychiatric medications, hospitalization, education, and skill teaching for consumers and their families. Currently, seven states and the District of Columbia have statewide ACT programs, and many more have at least one

TABLE 24-5	Center for Mental Health Services: Examples of Programs and Initiatives
PROGRAM/INITIATIVE	PURPOSE AND ACTIVITIES
Prevention of substance abuse and mental illness	Creating communities where individuals, families, schools, faith-based organizations, and workplaces take action to promote emotional health and reduce the likelihood of mental illness, substance abuse including tobacco, and suicide.
Trauma and justice	Reducing the pervasive, harmful, and costly health impact of violence and trauma by integrating trauma-informed approaches throughout health, behavioral health, and related systems and addressing the behavioral health needs of people involved in or at risk of involvement in the criminal and juvenile justice systems.
Military families	Supporting America's service men and women—active duty, National Guard, Reserve, and veteran—together with their families and communities by leading efforts to ensure that needed behavioral health services are accessible and that outcomes are positive.
Recovery support	Partnering with people in recovery from mental and substance use disorders and family members to guide the behavioral health system and promote individual-, program-, and system-level approaches that foster health and resilience; increase permanent housing, employment, education, and other necessary supports; and reduce discriminatory barriers.
Health reform	Increasing access to appropriate high quality prevention, treatment, and recovery services; reducing disparities that currently exist between the availability of services for mental and substance use disorders compared with the availability of services for other medical conditions; and supporting integrated, coordinated care, especially for people with behavioral health and other co-occurring health conditions.
Health information technology	Ensuring that the behavioral health system, including states, community providers, and peer and prevention specialists, fully participates with the general health care delivery system in the adoption of health information technology (HIT) and interoperable electronic health records.
Data, outcomes, and quality	Realizing an integrated data strategy and a national framework for quality improvement in behavioral health care that will inform policy, measure program impact, and lead to improved quality of services and outcomes for individuals, families, and communities.
Public awareness and support	Increasing the understanding of mental and substance use disorders and the many pathways to recovery to achieve the full potential of prevention, help people recognize mental and substance use disorders and seek assistance with the same urgency as any other health condition, and make recovery the expectation.

From Substance Abuse and Mental Health Services Administration, *Leading change: A plan for SAMHSA's roles and actions 2011-2014* (HHS Publication No. [SMA] 11-4629), Rockville, MD, 2011, Substance Abuse and Mental Health Services Administration. Also available from <http://store.samhsa.gov/shin/content//SMA11-4629/01-FullDocument.pdf>.

BOX 24-5 KEY FEATURES OF THE ASSERTIVE COMMUNITY TREATMENT (ACT) PROGRAM

- Psychopharmacological treatment
- Individual supportive therapy
- Mobile crisis intervention
- Hospitalization
- Substance abuse treatment
- Behaviorally oriented skill teaching
- Supported employment
- Support for resuming education
- Collaboration with families and assistance to clients with children
- Direct support to help clients obtain legal and advocacy services

---

BOX 24-6 CORE ELEMENTS OF CRISIS INTERVENTION TEAMS (CITS)

Ongoing Elements
1. Partnerships: law enforcement, advocacy, mental health
2. Community ownership: planning, implementation & networking
3. Policies and procedures

Operational Elements
4. CIT: officer, dispatcher, coordinator
5. Curriculum: CIT training
6. Mental health receiving facility: emergency services

Sustaining Elements
7. Evaluation and research
8. In-service training
9. Recognition and honors
10. Outreach: developing CIT in other communities

From the University of Memphis, School of Urban Affairs and Public Policy, Department of Criminology and Criminal Justice, CIT Center CIT International, Randolph Dupont, PhD, Major Sam Cochran MS, and Sarah Pillsbury, MA: Crisis Intervention Team Core Elements, 2006, Retrieved from http://www.citinternational.org/images/stories/CIT/SectionImplementation/CoreElements.pdf.

---

pilot project (NAMI, 2013). Box 24-5 gives additional details about ACT programs.

The Crisis Intervention Team (CIT) program originates from the Memphis Model, an educational and advocacy training program. The Memphis Police Department joined with the Memphis Chapter of the NAMI, mental health providers, the University of Memphis, and the University of Tennessee in organizing, training, and implementing a specialized unit. CIT programs partner with mental health consumers and family members, mental health professionals, and advocacy organizations. Law enforcement personnel are trained in developing a more intelligent, understandable, and safe

approach to mental crisis events. (See Box 24-6 for the core elements of the Crisis Intervention Team).

Specialty courts—also called treatment courts, accountability courts, and problem-solving courts—deal with a number of problem areas within the criminal justice system. These specialty courts can deal with adult, juvenile, users, and family drug problems, mental health disorders, military veterans, and people found to be driving under the influence (DUI) of

TABLE 24-6 Organizations that Promote Education and Advocate for Mental Health

RESOURCE	SERVICES	CONTACT INFORMATION
Substance Abuse and Mental Health Services Administration (SAMHSA)	Programs, policies, information and data, contracts and grants Vision: Behavioral health is essential for health, prevention works, treatment is effective, people can recover from mental illness diagnosis and substance abuse	http://www.samhsa.gov/
National Alliance on Mental Illness (NAMI)	Consumer education regarding various mental health disorders, medication and treatment, research, public policy issues; links to find support at state and local level including support groups and online discussion groups; tips for becoming politically involved in mental health public policy issues	http://www.nami.org/
Mental Health America (MHA)	Inform, advocate and enable access to quality behavioral health services for all Americans	http://www.mentalhealthamerica.net/
National Institute of Mental Health (NIMH)	Education on mental health topics and research Vision: Understanding and treatment of mental illnesses through basic and clinical research, paving the way for prevention, recovery, and cure	http://www.nimh.nih.gov/index.shtml
Depression and Bipolar Support Alliance	Education on depression and bipolar disorder; online discussion and support groups; assistance in finding treatment resources	http://www.dbsalliance.org
National Education Alliance for Borderline Personality Disorder	Education about borderline personality disorder and treatment	www.borderlinepersonalitydisorder.com/
Obsessive-Compulsive Foundation	Education about obsessive compulsive and anxiety disorders and treatment	www.ocfoundation.org/
Postpartum Support International	Education and resource information for individuals experiencing symptoms of prenatal or postpartum mood or anxiety disorders	http://postpartum.net/
U.S. Department of Veteran Affairs National Center for PTSD	Public and professional sections for education, training materials as well as information and tools to help you with assessment and treatment	http://www.ptsd.va.gov/
Brain and Behavior Research Foundation, formerly called National Association for Research on Schizophrenia And Depression (NARSAD)	Alleviating the suffering caused by mental illness by awarding grants that will lead to advances and breakthroughs in scientific research	http://bbrfoundation.org/
National Council for Community Behavioral Healthcare	Behavioral health care, holistic approach to meet needs of the individuals and families	www.thenationalcouncil.org/cs/home

alcohol or drugs. These programs incorporate assessment and screening to examine problematic behavior due to mental health problems and substance abuse. Specialty courts provide education regarding mental and substance use disorders and medication monitoring and drug testing.

ROLE OF THE COMMUNITY MENTAL HEALTH NURSE

More than ever, there are opportunities for the community mental health nurse to make a difference. For the psychiatric–mental health nurse there are EBP models of care providing promising outcome in communities. Applications of the nursing process are and always can be facilitated to help special populations affected by mental illness in the community. There certainly are challenges to the effective provision of mental health services in the community, such as accessibility, disparity, and cost. When nurses are providing care to individuals, families, groups, and communities, there is a hope for change, progress, and improved health promotion for everyone. In spite of multiple challenges, the role of a community mental health nurse can be extremely rewarding (Sheerin, 2011). Perhaps the most critical impact made by nurses in community settings is

through the establishment of interpersonal relationships with the community as professional, knowledgeable, responsible care providers (Happell et al, 2011, 2012).

Community mental health nursing roles are multidimensional (e.g., participant in mental health courts, veterans courts, other specialty or problem-solving courts; educator, researcher, collaborator, consultant, case managers, content expert, administrator, activist, politician, advocate, initiator, evaluator, grant writer, practitioner, and coordinator). Mental health nurses serve on ACT, Crisis Intervention, community case management, mobile crisis, and crisis housing coordination teams. Community mental health nurses as educators and activists dispel myths, provide accurate information about mental illness, and influence policy and legislation advocating for those with mental illness.

As practitioner and coordinator, the nurse works directly with individuals, groups, and families. Besides intervening to assist consumers in controlling or alleviating the symptoms of mental illness, the practitioner and coordinator also helps the consumer "navigate" the segmented web of agencies and other service providers. A list of organizations that advocate for mental health is shown in Table 24-6. Community mental health nurses not only take action to solve an immediate problem but also plan and intervene to ensure safety, continuity, and quality of care for consumers. Therefore, the practitioner and coordinator roles require skills in anticipating and evaluating the actions of other providers and communicating with consumers, families, rehabilitation services, and government or social agencies.

Within this aspect of community mental health nursing, individual-, family-, and community-level crises are anticipated and prevented or, failing these, contained. For example, as practitioners and coordinators, nurses might organize people taking psychotropic medications to share experiences about interacting with a psychiatrist, managing side effects of medications, and enhancing their coping strategies. Such a proactive stance may help prevent problems that lead clients to discontinue medications and the consequences of such actions. In the practitioner and coordinator roles, community mental health nurses work toward matching consumers and families with culturally appropriate and sensitive providers to achieve the "best fit."

CASE STUDY   APPLICATION OF THE NURSING PROCESS

Joseph Green, a divorced 52-year-old veteran of Operation Iraqi Freedom, was discharged from the hospital with a referral to cardiac rehabilitation. Joseph has a ventricular pacemaker that was inserted 2 years ago. Last week he was brought into the emergency department for failure of the pacemaker. He was experiencing syncope and hypotension. His pacemaker was corrected and he was discharged back into the community, where he is currently living at a men's shelter.

Joseph has a history of a congestive heart failure (CHF), depression, alcoholism, chronic obstructive pulmonary disease (COPD), traumatic brain injury (TBI), and posttraumatic stress disorder (PTSD). He has prescriptions for citalopram, carvedilol, and an Advair inhaler. He admits to being noncompliant at times with taking his prescriptions. He has access to health care services from the nearest VA medical center, which is 350 miles away. He takes a Disabled American Veterans (DAV) van to the medical center once or twice a month where he fills his prescriptions and sees mental health counselors. There is cardiac rehabilitation at the center, but Joseph does not want to go as often as the VA doctors have recommended. Joseph has no income and cooks meals at the men's shelter for his room and board. Because he cannot drink alcohol at the shelter, he has been abstinent for 9 months. He smokes a pack of cigarettes daily when he has cigarettes.

Joseph has difficulty sleeping most nights and awakens from nightmares. He was diagnosed with major depression and PTSD 5 years ago and reports having suicidal thoughts occasionally. He has been estranged from his grown children for several years. He has a sister living in the same city and his relationship with her strained. The Assertive Community Treatment (ACT) team makes visits to the shelter to assist other men, and Joseph has inquired how to become a consumer of ACT services. There is a local veterans' support group at the Veterans of Foreign Wars (VFW) building that Joseph and others from the shelter go to several nights a week.

Assessment
On his first trip to the VA medical center after his recent discharge, the outpatient clinic nurse notes that Joseph was noncompliant with his mediations only 2 days the previous week. He reports that he is not depressed, and he denies having suicidal thoughts. He has had no syncope or chest palpations.

Diagnosis
Individual
- History of mental illness (depression, PTSD, and alcoholism)
- Difficulty following treatment regimen
- Less than adequate social skills
- Poor self-worth
- History of suicidal ideation

Family and Social Relationships
- Inability to communicate with family members effectively
- Jeopardy of reoccurring homelessness

Planning
Planning for Joseph is primarily through collaboration in the community where he resides at the men's shelter. His relationships with others at the shelter and the VFW are important. The staff at the men's shelter are familiar with the VA's homeless program information: 1-877-4AID-VET (1-877-424-3838) and http://www.va.gov/HOMELESS/for_homeless_veterans.asp.

The men's shelter also supports Joseph by helping him get to the DAV van when he has appointment at the VA medical center. The shelter offers chaplain services and also utilizes the community Crisis Intervention Team (CIT) law enforcement officers at times to help talk with residents when they are experiencing stress or need de-escalation of their behavior. A CIT officer who is a veteran stops in once in awhile to see the men as a proactive visit.

Individual
Long-Term Goal
- Joseph will progress with community supportive services and relationships with people

Short-Term Goals
- Joseph will remain medication compliant
- Joseph will remain abstinent from alcohol

Family and Social Relationships
Long-Term Goals
- Safe housing
- Compliance with medications
- Sobriety
- Case management with ACT Team and VA

Short-Term Goals
- Working with shelter staff and ACT Team
- Sobriety
- Compliance with medications

Intervention
The staff at the men's shelter meet with Joseph regularly to evaluate compliance with medications. The staff also will know when his appointments are at the VA in order to plan transportation on the DAV van. The relationships that Joseph has with other veterans is helpful in a support milieu.

Individual
- Joseph has agreed to work with the staff at the shelter in a team effort to keep him in safe housing. He has agreed to work with the ACT Team, VA case management, and his Alcoholics Anonymous (AA) community.

CASE STUDY   APPLICATION OF THE NURSING PROCESS—cont'd

Family and Social Relationships
- Joseph will continue to work with VA case management, the ACT Team, and the staff at the shelter.
- He will call his sister weekly.

Evaluation
Joseph verbalized understanding of the importance of safe housing, the ACT Team intervention, and social relationships with VA peers and AA peers. He also agreed to call his AA or VA contact when needed if he is beginning to feel agitated or wanting to isolate himself. The ACT Team will consistently contact Joseph and be available on weekends. Joseph has agreed to give permission for the ACT Team to report his status to the VA case managers.

Levels of Prevention
Primary
- Maintaining housing at shelter
- Assisting Joseph with compliance with medications

Secondary
- Encouraging maintenance of social relationships (shelter staff, other veterans, AA peers) and relationship with sister

Tertiary
- Monitoring of medical health status and psychological health status
- Group therapy at AA meetings and the VA medical center

SUMMARY

Like all other aspects of nursing, community mental health nursing is developing, applying and utilizing EBP models of community treatment, such as ACT, community case management, or Crisis Intervention teams. The twenty-first century community mental health multidisciplinary team approaches can promote improvement in the identification of and care for those with mental illness. Improved information and EBP may result in greater understanding of the factors that contribute to mental disorders and lead to more effective treatment.

As discussed in this chapter, the vast majority of individuals with diagnosable mental disorders are found in the community, and many, if not most, never seek professional help. The framework for community mental health nursing presented in this chapter should prove useful in improving the lives of individuals, families, and groups of people with mental illness. Further, it is hoped that all nurses will become advocates for the mentally ill and will support social and political change to improve the mental health of all.

LEARNING ACTIVITIES

1. Reflect on your personal experience interacting with individuals with mental illness. What thoughts or feelings did these experiences produce? What are several issues that nurses can advocate for in caring for this special population?
2. Locate the National Alliance for Mental Illness (NAMI) and Suicide Prevention Action Network (SPAN) chapters in your community. What services do these agencies offer? How might those services be helpful in the community mental health nursing role?
3. List five topics or issues for which the community mental health nurse can facilitate individual, family, or group education about in the community.

ⓔ EVOLVE WEBSITE
http://evolve.elsevier.com/Nies
- NCLEX Review Questions
- Case Studies
- Glossary

REFERENCES

Amador X: *I am not sick, I don't need help! Peconic*, NY, 2007, Vida Press.

Amador X: *I'm right, you're wrong, now what?: Break the impasse and get what you need. Peconic*, NY, 2008, Vida Press.

American Psychiatric Association: *Helping children and youth who have experienced traumatic events*, 2012. Available from <http://www.psychiatry.org/mental-health/people/children>.

American Psychological Association: *Understanding psychotherapy and how it works*, 2013. Available from <http://www.apa.org/>.

American Psychiatric Association: *Diagnostic and statistical manual of mental disorders*, 5th ed., Arlington, VA, 2013, American Psychiatric Publishing. 2013.

Baune BT, Thome J: Translational research approach to biological and modifiable risk factors of psychosis and affective disorders, *The World Journal of Biological Psychiatry* 12(S1):28–34, 2011.

Bazelon Center for Mental Health Law, 2013: Available from <http://www.bazelon.org/>

Brain and behavior research foundation: *Schizophrenia*. Available from http://bbrfoundation.org/schizophrenia, 2013.

Centers for Disease Control and Prevention (CDC): Mental Health Surveillance Among Children – United States, 2005-2011, *MMWR* 62(2):1–35, 2013. Available from http://www.cdc.gov/mmwr/preview/mmwrhtml/su6202a1.htm?s_cid=su6202a1_w.

Centers for Disease Control and Prevention (CDC): *Suicide: Facts at a Glance*, . Available from http://www.cdc.gov/ViolencePrevention/pdf/Suicide_DataSheet-a.pdf, 2012.

Department of Health and Human Services (USDHHS): *Healthy People 2020*, 2013. Available from http://www.healthypeople.gov/2020/default.aspx, .

Eriksen KA, Sundfor B, Karlsson B, et al.: Recognition as a valued human being: Perspectives of mental health service users, *Nursing Ethics* 19(3):357–368, 2012.

Fleming JA, Mahoney JS, Carlson E, et al.: An ethnographic approach to interpreting a mental illness Photovoice exhibit, *Arch Psychiatr Nurs* 23(1):16–24, 2009.

Happell B, Cleary M: Promoting health and preventing illness: Promoting mental health in community nursing practice, *Contemporary Nurse* 41(1):88–89, 2012.

Happell B, Palmer C, Tennent R: The mental health nurse incentive program: desirable knowledge, skills and attitudes from the perspective of nurses, *Journal of Clinical Nursing* 20:901–910, 2011, http://dx.doi.org/10.1111/j.1365-2702.2010.03510.x.

Happel B, Hoey W, Gaskin CJ: Community mental health nurses, caseloads, and practices: a literature review, *International Journal of Mental Health Nursing* 21(2):131–137, 2012.

Healthy Place: *Depression in children: Causes and treatment of childhood depression*, 2013. Available from http://www.healthyplace.com/depression/children/depression-in-children-causes-treatment-of-child-depression/.

Healthcare.gov: *The healthcare law and you*, . Available from <http://www.healthcare.gov/law/index.html>, 2013.

HealthyPeople.gov: *Healthy People 2020: Topics & objectives: Mental health and mental disorders*, . Available from <http://www.healthypeople.gov/2020/topicsobjectives2020/objectiveslist.aspx?topicId=28>, 2013.

Kassam A, Papish A, Modgill G, et al.: The development and psychometric properties of a new scale to measure mental illness related stigma by health care providers: The opening minds scale for Health Care Providers (OMS-HC), *BMC Psychiatry* 12(62):3–12, 2012.

Kondrat DC, Early TJ: Battling in the trenches: Case managers' ability to combat the effects of mental illness stigma on consumers' perceived quality of life, *Community Mental Health Journal* 47:390–398, 2011, http://dx.doi.org/10.1007/s10597-010-9330-4.

LeVine ES: Facilitating recovery for people with serious mental illness employing a psychobiosocial model of care, *Professional Psychology: Research and Practice* 43(1):58–64, 2012.

National Alliance on Mental Illness: *Assertive community treatment (ACT)*, 2013. Available from<http://www.nami.org/Template.cfm?Section=ACT-TA_Center&Template=/TaggedPage/TaggedPageDisplay.cfm&TPLID=4&ContentID=28611>

National Institute of Mental Health: *Neuroimaging and mental illness: A window into the brain: Frequently asked questions about brain scans*, 2010. Available from <http://www.nimh.nih.gov/health/publications/neuroimaging-and-mental-illness-a-window-into-the-brain/neuroimaging-faq.pdf>.

National Institute of Mental Health: *Psychotherapy*, 2014. Available from http://www.nimh.nih.gov/health/topics/psychotherapies/index.shtml.

National Institute of Mental Health: *Alliance for research progress: February 8, 2013 meeting*, 2013. Available from <http://www.nimh.nih.gov/outreach/alliance/alliance-report-february-2013/alliance-for-research-progress-february-8-2013-meeting.shtml>.

National Institute of Mental Health: *Panic disorder among adults*, n.d. Available from <http://www.nimh.nih.gov/statistics/1PANIC_ADULT.shtml>

Paternite CE, Johnston TC: Rationale and strategies for central involvement of educators in effective school-based mental health programs, *Journal of Youth and Adolescence* Vol. 34, 2006. No. 1, February 2005, pp. 41–49 (C2005) DOI: 10.1007/s10964-005-1335-x 2006.

Pruessner JC, Dedovic K, Pruessner M, et al.: Stress regulation in the central nervous system: evidence from structural and functional neuroimaging studies in human populations, *Psychoneuroendocrinology* 35(1):179–191, 2010.

Reeves WC, Strine TW, Pratt LA, et al.: Mental illness surveillance among adults in the United States, *MWR Surveill Summ* 60(Suppl 3):1–29, 2011.

Sheerin F: The nurse's role as specialist practitioner and social activist, *Learning Disability Practice* 14(10):31–37, 2011.

Smith DE: The medicalization of therapeutic communities in the era of health care reform, *Journal of Psychoactive Drugs* 44(2):93–95, 2012.

Stacciarini JM, Shattell MM, Coady M, et al.: Review: Community-based participatory research approach to address mental health in minority populations, *Community Mental Health Journal* 47:489–497, 2011, http://dx.doi.org/10.1007/s10597-010-9319-z.

Substance Abuse and Mental Health Services Administration (SAMSHA): *Center for Mental Health Services*, 2014. Available from http://beta.samhsa.gov/about-us/who-we-are/offices-centers/cmhs.

Treatment Advocacy Center: *The anatomical basis of anosignosia: lack of awareness of illness*, 2012. Available from <http://www.treatmentadvocacycenter.org/storage/documents/Anosognosia–Anatomical_Basis_-_August_2012.pdf>.

U.S. Department of Defense: *Suicide prevention and awareness*, 2012. Available from http://www.defense.gov/home/features/2012/0812_suicide-prevention/.

U.S. Department of Health and Human Services, Office of the Surgeon General and National Action Alliance for Suicide Prevention: *2012 National Strategy for Suicide Prevention: Goals and Objectives for Action*, Washington, DC, 2012, Author.

USDHHS/SAMHSA: *Behavioral health, United States*, 2012. http://www.samhsa.gov/data/2012BehavioralHealthUS/Index.aspx.

Vilhelmsson A, Svensson T: Mental ill health, public health, and medicalization, *Public Health Ethics* 4(3):207–217, 2011.

World Health Organization: *The financial crisis and global health*, 2009. www.who.int/topics/financial_crisis/financialcrisis_report_200902.pdf.

OBJECTIVES

Upon completion of this chapter, the reader will be able to do the following:

1. Review principles related to the occurrence and transmission of infection and infectious diseases.
2. Describe the three focus areas in *Healthy People 2020* objectives that apply to infectious diseases.
3. Describe the chain of transmission of infectious diseases.
4. Apply the chain of transmission to describing approaches to control infectious disease.
5. Review types of immunity, including herd immunity.

6. Review principles of immunization, and specify the immunization recommended for all age-groups in the United States.
7. Describe the legal responsibility for control of communicable diseases in the United States.
8. Describe the chain of transmission and control for priority infectious disease.
9. Identify nursing activities for control of infectious diseases at primary, secondary, and tertiary levels of prevention.

KEY TERMS

acquired immunity
active immunity
agent
antigenicity
carriers
case
cold chain
communicable disease
communicable period
control
direct transmission
elimination
endemic
environment
epidemic
eradication
fomites
herd immunity

host
immunity
immunization
incidence
incubation period
indirect transmission
infection
infectious disease
infectivity
isolation
latency
multicausation
natural immunity
notifiable infectious diseases
outbreak
pandemic
passive immunity
pathogenicity

portal of entry
portal of exit
primary vaccine failure
quarantine
reservoir
resistance
secondary vaccine failure
subclinical infection
susceptible
toxigenicity
universal precautions
vaccination
Vaccine Adverse Event Reporting
    System
vectors
virulence

OUTLINE

Communicable Disease and *Healthy People 2020*
Principles of Infection and Infectious Disease Occurrence
   Multicausation
   Spectrum of Infection
   Stages of Infection
   Spectrum of Disease Occurrence

Chain of Transmission
   Infectious Agents
   Reservoirs
   Portals of Exit and Entry
   Modes of Transmission
   Host Susceptibility

OUTLINE—cont'd

Breaking the Chain of Transmission
Controlling the Agent
Eradicating the Nonhuman Reservoir
Controlling the Human Reservoir
Controlling the Portals of Exit and Entry
Improving Host Resistance and Immunity
Public Health Control of Infectious Diseases
Terminology: Control, Elimination, and Eradication
Defining and Reporting Communicable Diseases
Vaccines and Infectious Disease Prevention
Vaccines: Word of Caution
Types of Immunizations
Vaccine Storage, Transport, and Handling
Vaccine Administration
Vaccine Spacing

Vaccine Hypersensitivity and Contraindications
Vaccine Documentation
Vaccine Safety and Reporting Adverse Events and
Vaccine-Related Injuries
Vaccine Needs for Special Groups
Healthy People 2020 **Focus on Immunization and
Infectious Diseases**
Healthy People 2020 **Focus on Sexually Transmitted
Diseases**
Healthy People 2020 **Focus on HIV/AIDS**
Prevention of Communicable Diseases
Primary Prevention
Secondary Prevention
Tertiary Prevention

Throughout history, epidemics have been responsible for the destruction of entire groups of people. Despite amazing advances in public health and health care, control of communicable diseases continues to be a major concern of health care providers. The emergence of new pathogens, the reemergence of old pathogens, and the appearance of drug-resistant pathogens are creating formidable challenges worldwide.

Despite global eradication campaigns, malaria and other vector-borne diseases and life-threatening gastrointestinal infections continue to cause significant morbidity and mortality in the developing world. Although the incidence rate of tuberculosis (TB) has been declining, in 2012 there were an estimated 8.6 million new cases of TB worldwide, with 1.3 million people dying from the disease (World Health Organization [WHO], 2013). Measles, when coupled with vitamin A deficiency, is a leading cause of blindness in many developing countries in the Eastern Hemisphere. To add to the world's growing infectious disease burden, human immunodeficiency virus (HIV) and acquired immunodeficiency syndrome (AIDS) continue to spread unchecked throughout the world, as evidenced by the estimate that 34.0 million adults and children were living with HIV/AIDS globally at the end of 2011. Although new HIV infections have been declining slowly since 2001, there are approximately 2.5 million new infections worldwide each year (UNAIDS, 2012).

Great strides have been made in the United States with respect to vaccine-preventable diseases, yet segments of the population remain unimmunized or under-immunized. Both measles and pertussis can be prevented with a vaccine, and indigenous measles has been virtually eliminated in the United States, with only 43 cases reported in 2007. This number increased to 222 cases reported to the Centers for Disease Control (CDC) in 2011, 90% of which were imported from other countries (CDC, 2012a). Pertussis incidence increased from 10,454 cases of pertussis reported in 2007 in the U.S. (Hall-Baker et al, 2009) to 48,277 cases in 2012 (CDC, 2013). Cases of hepatitis A, B, and C have

been significantly reduced since the 1990s, through administration of vaccines for hepatitis A and B and testing of the blood supply for hepatitis C. Yet these diseases persist. Treatable sexually transmitted diseases (STDs), such as gonorrhea, *Chlamydia*, and syphilis, are still occurring at significant rates. Gonorrhea plateaued or declined until 2009 but has increased steadily since then. Reported infections with *Chlamydia* reached an all-time high in 2011 (CDC, 2012c). Syphilis had increased during the 2000s but began to decrease slightly in 2010 (CDC, 2012c). In the United States, there have been significant accomplishments in preventing food-borne and waterborne infections through environmental sanitation, but the incidence of vector-borne infections, such as Lyme disease, Rocky Mountain spotted fever, St. Louis encephalitis, and West Nile encephalitis, appear to be increasing. Furthermore, although the advent of effective antiretroviral treatment for AIDS in the mid-1990s briefly slowed the incidence of AIDS diagnosis, about 30,000 new AIDS cases were reported yearly between 2008 and 2011 in the United States. Approximately 50,000 new HIV infections were diagnosed annually in the United States during the same period (CDC, 2013).

Probably one of the most profound failures in infectious disease control in the United States and elsewhere is that the successes are not equally distributed in the general population. Infectious diseases continue to be differentially distributed by income and ethnic groups, and the poor and minorities continue to experience the greater burden.

Although there has been marked improvement, infectious and communicable diseases persist. Scientific discoveries about the infectious etiology of stomach ulcers, coronary artery disease, and cervical cancer, for example, suggest that infectious agents may be responsible for more morbidity and mortality than previously recognized. New concerns include the rapid proliferation of drug-resistant organisms (Box 25-1) and the threat that deadly pathogens may be weaponized by terrorists (Box 25-2). Other threats are emerging infectious diseases, those diseases for which the incidence in humans

BOX 25-1   DRUG-RESISTANT PATHOGENS/DISEASES

Bacteria

- *Acinetobacter* spp.: Nosocomial bacteremia, septicemia
- *Bacillus anthracis*: Anthrax
- *Bordetella pertussis*: Pertussis
- *Campylobacter* (fluoroquinolone-resistant): Enteritis
- *Enterococcus* spp. (multidrug-resistant, including vancomycin-resistant [VRE])
- *Enterobacter* spp.
- Group B streptococcus
- *Klebsiella* spp., *Klebsiella pneumoniae*
- *Mycobacterium tuberculosis* (multidrug-resistant [MDR-TB]): Tuberculosis
- *Neisseria gonorrhoeae* (fluoroquinolone-resistant): Gonorrhea
- *Neisseria meningitides*: Meningitis
- *Pseudomonas aeruginosa*
- *Salmonella* spp.: Typhoid fever and salmonellosis
- *Shigella*: Shigellosis
- *Staphylococcus aureus* (methicillin-resistant [MRSA], vancomycin-resistant [VRSA])
- *Staphylococcus epidermidis* (vancomycin-resistant [VRSE], methicillin-resistant [MRSE])
- *Streptococcus pneumoniae* (multidrug-resistant): Pneumonia, meningitis, and otitis media
- *Treponema pallidum* (azithromycin-resistant): Syphilis
- Other gram-negative bacteria developing drug resistance: *Citrobacter freundii, Escherichia coli, Morganella morganii, Providencia* spp., and *Serratia* spp.

Viruses

- Human immunodeficiency virus (HIV): HIV infection and acquired immunodeficiency syndrome (AIDS)
- Influenza: some forms are resistant to one or more of the four antiviral drugs approved by U.S. Food and Drug Administration (amantadine, rimantadine, zanamivir, and oseltamivir)

Fungi

- *Candida*: Candidiasis

Parasites

- *Pediculus humanus capitis*: Head lice
- *Plasmodium falciparum* and *Plasmodium vivax*: Malaria

Data from Centers for Disease Control and Prevention: *Diseases/pathogens associated with antimicrobial resistance*, 2013. Available from <www.cdc.gov/drugresistance/DiseasesConnectedAR.html.>; and Heymann DL, editor: *Control of communicable diseases manual*, ed 18, Washington, DC, 2008, American Public Health Association.

BOX 25-2   CENTERS FOR DISEASE CONTROL AND PREVENTION LIST OF POTENTIAL BIOTERRORISM AGENTS AND DISEASES BY PRIORITY CATEGORY

Category A

Highest priority; easily transmitted with high mortality and social disruption:

- Anthrax (*Bacillus anthracis*)
- Botulism (botulinum toxin)
- Plague (*Yersinia pestis*)
- Smallpox (variola virus)
- Tularemia (*Francisella tularensis*)
- Viral hemorrhagic fevers (Ebola, Lassa, and Marburg viruses)

Category B

Moderately easy to disseminate; high morbidity with low mortality:

- Brucellosis (*Brucella* spp.)
- Epsilon toxin of *Clostridium perfringens*
- Food safety threats:
  - Salmonellosis (*Salmonella* spp.)
  - Escherichia coli 0157:H7
  - Shigellosis (*Shigella* spp.)
- Glanders (*Burkholderia mallei*)
- Melioidosis (*Burkholderia mallei*)
- Psittacosis (*Chlamydia psittaci*)
- Q fever (*Coxiella burnetii*)
- Ricin toxin
- Staphylococcal enterotoxin B
- Typhus fever (*Rickettsia prowazekii*)
- Viral encephalitis (alphaviruses)
- Water safety threats:
  - Cholera (*Vibrio cholerae*)
  - *Cryptosporidium parvum*

Category C

Emerging pathogens that could be engineered for mass dissemination because of availability and ease of production and dissemination

Modified from Centers for Disease Control and Prevention: *Bioterrorism agents/diseases*, 2013. Available from <http://www.bt.cdc.gov/agent/agentlist-category.asp>.

has increased within the past two decades or threatens to increase in the near future. (For more information, see the CDC website on emerging infectious diseases, at www.cdc.gov/ncidod/diseases/eid/disease_sites.htm.)

This chapter is written to provide nurses with the knowledge necessary to help control infectious diseases. The terms *communicable disease* and *infectious disease* are synonymous and will be used interchangeably (Heymann, 2008).

COMMUNICABLE DISEASE AND *HEALTHY PEOPLE 2020*

The U.S. Department of Health and Human Services (USDHHS) program *Healthy People 2020* contains several

hundred objectives to improve health; these are organized into 38 topic areas. Three of the topic areas (Immunization and Infectious Diseases, Sexually Transmitted Diseases, and HIV) are specific to infectious diseases (HealthyPeople.gov, n.d.a). These objectives have been used to evaluate national prevention and control efforts and can guide local prevention and control efforts. The *Healthy People 2020* box lists examples of objectives for immunizations and infectious diseases, objectives related to sexually transmitted diseases, and a few of the objectives covering HIV/AIDS. These lists suggest strategies for prevention and control of infectious diseases. Additional information, including baseline and target data for all objectives, can be found on the *Healthy People 2020* website: www.healthypeople.gov/2020/topicsobjectives2020.

HEALTHY PEOPLE 2020

Communicable Disease

Topic Area—Immunization and Infectious Diseases

IID-1: Reduce, eliminate or maintain elimination of cases of vaccine preventable diseases

IID-2: Reduce early-onset group B streptococcal disease

IID-3: Reduce meningococcal disease

IID-4: Reduce invasive pneumococcal infections

IID-5: Reduce the number of courses of antibiotics for ear infections in young children

IID-6: Reduce the number of courses of antibiotics prescribed for the sole diagnosis of the common cold

IID-7 to IID-11: Achieve and maintain effective vaccination coverage levels for universally recommended vaccines among children and adolescents

IID-12: Increase the percentage of children and adults who are vaccinated annually against seasonal influenza

IID-13: Increase the percentage of adults who are vaccinated against pneumococcal disease

IID-14: Increase the percentage of adults who are vaccinated against zoster (shingles)

IID-15: Increase hepatitis B vaccine coverage among high-risk populations (hemodialysis patients, men who have sex with men, health care personnel and injection drug users)

IID-23 to IID-28: Reduce hepatitis A, hepatitis B and hepatitis C

IID-29 to IID-32: Reduce tuberculosis; increase treatment completion rate

Topic Area—Sexually Transmitted Diseases

STD–1: Reduce the proportion of adolescents and young adults with *Chlamydia trachomatis* infections

STD-5: Reduce the proportion of females aged 15 to 44 years who have ever required treatment for pelvic inflammatory disease (PID)

STD-6: Reduce gonorrhea rates

STD-7: Reduce sustained domestic transmission of primary and secondary syphilis

STD-8: Reduce congenital syphilis

STD-9: Reduce the proportion of females with human papillomavirus (HPV) infection

STD-10: Reduce the proportion of adults with genital herpes infection due to herpes simplex type 2

Topic Area—Human Immunodeficiency Virus (HIV)

HIV-1 to HIV-3: Reduce new HIV infection, transmission and diagnosis among adolescents and adults

HIV-4 to HIV-7: Reduce new cases of acquired immunodeficiency syndrome (AIDS) among all adolescents and adults

HIV-8: Reduce perinatally acquired HIV and AIDS

HIV-9: Increase the proportion of new HIV infections diagnosed before progression to AIDS

HIV-10: Increase the proportion of HIV-infected adolescents and adults who receive HIV care and treatment consistent with current standards

HIV-11: Increase the proportion of persons surviving more than 3 years after a diagnosis with AIDS

HIV-12: Reduce deaths from HIV infection

HIV-13: Increase the proportion of persons living with HIV who know their serostatus

HIV-14: Increase the proportion of adolescents and adults who have been tested for HIV in the past 12 months

HIV-15: Increase the proportion of adults with tuberculosis who have been tested for HIV

HIV-16: Increase the proportion of substance abuse treatment facilities that offer HIV /AIDS education, counseling, and support

HIV-17: Increase the proportion of sexually active persons who use condoms

HIV-18: Reduce the proportion of men who have sex with men who reported unprotected anal sex in the past 12 months

From HealthyPeople.gov: *Healthy People 2020: Topics & objectives,* n.d. Retrieved from <http://www.healthypeople.gov/2020/topicsobjectives2020/objectiveslist.aspx?topicId=23>.

PRINCIPLES OF INFECTION AND INFECTIOUS DISEASE OCCURRENCE

Nurses in all settings must be aware of potential threats related to communicable diseases and be prepared to intervene (see Ethical Insights box). To help prepare nurses for this responsibility, biological and epidemiological principles inherent in infection and infectious disease occurrence are reviewed and major terms defined in this section.

 ETHICAL INSIGHTS

Nurse's Responsibility Regarding Communicable Diseases

Rapid proliferation of drug-resistant organisms, bioterrorism, and emerging infectious diseases are all concerns that have great implications for nursing practice. Every nurse should be knowledgeable about recognizing, reporting, preventing, and controlling infectious diseases. Infectious disease control can no longer be limited to the jurisdiction of the public health department or the hospital infection control nurse; it is every nurse's responsibility.

Multicausation

During the early years of medical and nursing history, science promulgated cause-and-effect theories of disease that relied on specifying one cause for each disease. Today, it is understood that disease etiology is complex and multicausal. Infectious diseases are the result of interaction among the human **host**, an infectious **agent**, and the **environment** that surrounds the human host where transmission can occur. This interaction is pictured in the epidemiological triangle of agent, host, and environment described in Chapter 5 (Epidemiology). The principle of **multicausation** emphasizes that an infectious agent alone is not sufficient to cause disease; the agent must be transmitted within a conducive environment to a susceptible host.

Spectrum of Infection

Not all contact with an infectious agent leads to infection, and not all infection leads to an infectious disease. The processes, however, begin in the same way. An infectious agent may contaminate the skin or mucous membranes of a host, but not invade the host. Or it may invade,

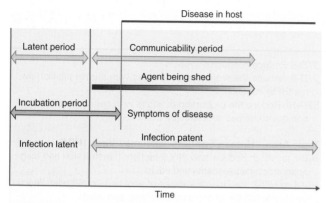

FIGURE 25-1 Stages of infection. (From Grimes DE: *Infectious diseases*, St Louis, 1991, Mosby.)

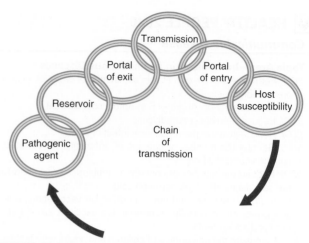

FIGURE 25-2 Chain of transmission. (From Grimes DE: *Infectious diseases*, St Louis, 1991, Mosby.)

multiply, and produce a subclinical infection (unapparent or asymptomatic) without producing overt symptomatic disease. Or the host may respond with overt symptomatic infectious disease. Infection, then, is the entry and multiplication of an infectious agent in a host. Infectious disease and communicable disease refer to the pathophysiological responses of the host to the infectious agent manifesting as an illness. When the disease is diagnosed in a person, the occurrence would be considered a case. Once infectious agents replicate in a host, they can be transmitted from the host irrespective of the presence of disease symptoms. Some persons become carriers and continue to shed the infectious agent without any symptoms of the disease.

Stages of Infection

An infectious agent that has invaded a host and found conditions hospitable will replicate until it can be shed from the host. This period of replication before shedding is called the latent period or latency. The communicable period, or communicability, follows latency and begins with shedding of the agent. The incubation period is the time from invasion to the time when disease symptoms first appear. Frequently the communicable period begins before symptoms are present. Understanding the distinctions among these terms is important in controlling transmission. These stages of infection are depicted in Figure 25-1.

Spectrum of Disease Occurrence

The principles covered to this point apply to individuals and their acquisition of infections and infectious diseases. Control of infectious diseases in a population requires identifying and monitoring the occurrence of new cases (incidence) in a population. Some infectious diseases are endemic and occur at a consistent, expected level in a geographic area. Such is the case with some STDs and with TB. An outbreak is an unexpected occurrence of an infectious disease in a limited geographic area during a limited period. Outbreaks of pertussis and salmonellosis, for example, are not uncommon. An epidemic is an unexpected increase in occurrence of an infectious disease

in a geographic area over an extended period. Epidemics are defined relative to the infectious agent and the history of the disease in the area. One case of smallpox anywhere would constitute an epidemic, whereas 1000 new cases of gonorrhea would not be considered an epidemic in an area where gonorrhea is common. A pandemic is a steady occurrence of a disease, or an epidemic, that covers a large geographic area or is evident worldwide. In July 2009, for example, the WHO designated the occurrence of H1N1 influenza as a pandemic.

CHAIN OF TRANSMISSION

Transmission is frequently conceptualized as a chain with six links, all connected, as in Figure 25-2. Each of the links (infectious agent, reservoir, portal of exit, mode of transmission, portal of entry, and host susceptibility) represents a different component that contributes to transmission. The chain of transmission and its elements are summarized in Table 25-1.

Infectious Agents

Because the process of transmission is different for every infectious agent, one might envision a different configuration of the chain and its links for each infectious agent and infectious disease that exists. Infectious agents act differently, depending on their intrinsic properties and interactions with their human host. For example, an agent's size, shape, chemical composition, growth requirements, and viability (ability to survive for extended periods) have an impact on transmission and the type of parasitic relationship it establishes with its host. These characteristics determine the classifications of different agents (e.g., prions, viruses, bacteria, fungi, and protozoa), and knowing the classification is helpful in understanding how specific agents are transmitted and produce disease. Also important are how the agent interacts with its host and its mode of action in the body. For example, it may kill cells, like *Mycobacterium tuberculosis*, or interfere with circulation, like the

TABLE 25-1	CHAIN OF TRANSMISSION	
LINK OF THE CHAIN	**DEFINITION**	**FACTOR(S)**
Infectious agent	An organism (virus, rickettsia, bacteria, fungus, protozoan, helminth, or prion) capable of producing infection or infectious disease	Properties of the agent: morphology, chemical composition, growth requirements, and viability; interaction with the host: mode of action, infectivity, pathogenicity, virulence, toxigenicity, antigenicity, and ability to adapt to the host
Reservoir(s)	The environment in which a pathogen lives and multiplies	Humans, animals, arthropods (bugs), plants, soil, or any other organic substance
Portal(s) of exit	Means by which an infectious agent is transported from the host	Respiratory secretions, vaginal secretions, semen, saliva, lesion exudates, blood, and feces
Mode(s) of transmission	Method whereby the infectious agent is transmitted from one host (or reservoir) to another host	*Direct:* Person to person *Indirect:* Implies a vehicle of transmission (biological or mechanical vector, common vehicles or fomites, airborne droplets)
Portal(s) of entry	Means by which an infectious agent enters a new host	Respiratory passages, mucous membranes, skin, percutaneous new host space, mouth, and through the placenta
Host susceptibility	The presence or absence of resistance to an infectious agent	Biological and personal characteristics (e.g., gender, age, genetics), general health status, personal behaviors, anatomical and physiological lines of defense, immunity

spirochete that causes syphilis. Or maybe it produces a toxin (**toxigenicity**) as does *Clostridium botulinum*, or stimulates an immune response in the host (**antigenicity**), as does rubella virus. Other considerations for understanding the action of agents are their power to invade and infect large numbers of people (**infectivity**), their ability to produce disease in those infected with the agent (**pathogenicity**), and their ability to produce serious disease in their hosts (**virulence**). If we apply the preceding concepts to the chickenpox virus, we see that it has high infectivity, high pathogenicity, and very low virulence. On the other hand, *M. tuberculosis* has low infectivity, low pathogenicity, but high virulence if untreated. Smallpox virus is high on all three concepts. Last, one must consider how adaptable an agent is to its human host and whether the agent changes, or mutates, over time, as HIV does.

Reservoirs

The environment in which a pathogen lives and multiplies is the **reservoir**. Reservoirs can be humans, animals, arthropods, plants, soil, water, or any other organic substance. Some agents have more than one reservoir. Knowing the reservoirs for infectious agents is important, because in some cases, transmission can be controlled by eliminating the reservoir, such as eliminating the standing water where mosquitoes breed.

Portals of Exit and Entry

Agents leave the human host through a **portal of exit** and invade through a **portal of entry**. Portals of exit include respiratory secretions, vaginal secretions, semen, saliva, lesion exudates, blood, and feces. Portals of entry are associated with the portal of exit and include the respiratory passages, mucous membranes, skin and blood vessels, oral cavity, and the placenta.

Modes of Transmission

Direct transmission is the immediate transfer of an infectious agent from an infected host or reservoir to an appropriate portal of entry in the human host through physical contact, such as a touch, bite, kiss, or sexual contact. Direct projections of mucous secretions by droplet spray to the conjunctiva, or mucous membranes of the eye, nose, or mouth during coughing, sneezing, or laughing are also considered direct transmission. Direct person-to-person contact is responsible for the transmission of many communicable diseases (e.g., sexually transmitted disease [STDs,] influenza).

Indirect transmission is the spread of infection through a vehicle of transmission outside the host. These may be contaminated fomites or vectors. **Fomites** can be any inanimate objects, materials, or substances that act as transport agents for a microbe (e.g., water, a telephone, or a contaminated tissue). The infectious agent may or may not reproduce on or in the fomite. Substances such as food, water, and blood products can provide indirect transmission through ingestion and intravenous transfusions. Botulism is an example of an indirectly transmitted food-borne enterotoxin disease.

Vectors can be animals or arthropods, and they can transmit through biological and mechanical routes. The mechanical route involves no multiplication or growth of the parasite or microbe within the animal or vector. Such is the case when a housefly carries gastrointestinal agents from raw sewage to uncovered food. Biological transmission occurs when the parasite grows or multiplies inside the animal, vector, or arthropod. Examples of diseases spread by this method of transmission include arthropod-borne diseases such as malaria, hemorrhagic fevers, and viral encephalitis. Transmission from a vector to the human host usually occurs through a bite or sting. Such is the case with the mosquito vector that transmits St. Louis encephalitis and West Nile virus.

Fecal-oral transmission can be direct or indirect. It can occur indirectly through the ingestion of water that has been fecally polluted or through consumption of contaminated food. Direct transmission occurs through engagement in oral sexual activity. Poliovirus and hepatitis A are spread through fecal-oral routes.

Airborne transmission occurs mainly through dissemination of microbial aerosols and droplet nuclei (small residues that result from evaporation of droplets of fluid from an infected host). The timeframe in which an airborne particle can remain suspended greatly influences the virility and infectivity of the organism. The size of the particle can also determine how long it remains airborne and how successful it will be at penetrating the human lung. Aerosols are extremely small solid or liquid particles that may include fungal spores, viruses, and bacteria. Droplet nuclei, such as the spray from sneezing or coughing, may make direct contact with an open wound or with a mucous membrane, or they may be inhaled into the lung. TB is spread through inhalation of contaminated droplets.

Host Susceptibility

Not all humans are equally **susceptible** to or at risk for contracting an infection or development of an infectious disease. Biological and personal characteristics play an important role. Just as the young are at greater risk for diphtheria, older adults are at greater risk for bacterial pneumonia. General health status is important, as evidenced by the increased risk for gastrointestinal parasites in children living in poverty. Personal behaviors certainly influence susceptibility, as does the presence of healthy lines of defense. The immune system and immunization status play important roles in the increased number of infections in unimmunized and immunocompromised persons.

BREAKING THE CHAIN OF TRANSMISSION

Picture a situation in which one of the links in the chain of transmission is broken (see Figure 25-2). Breaking just one link of the chain at its most vulnerable point is, in fact, what is done to control transmission of an infectious agent. Of course, where the chain is broken depends on all of the factors that have just been discussed—characteristics of the agent, its reservoir, portals of exit and entry, how the agent is transmitted, and susceptibility of the host.

Controlling the Agent

Controlling the agent is an area in which technology and medical science have been extremely effective. Inactivating an agent is the principle behind disinfection, sterilization, and radiation of fomites that may harbor pathogens. Antiinfective drugs, such as antibiotics, antivirals, antiretrovirals, and antimalarials, play important roles in controlling

infectious diseases. Not only do they permit recovery of the infected person but they also play a major role in preventing transmission of the pathogens to another. The first step in preventing transmission of tuberculosis and syphilis is to treat the infected person with antibiotics. Early treatment of an HIV infection with antiretrovirals suppresses the virus and thus has the potential to reduce transmission of the virus (CDC, 2013a; International Association of Physicians in AIDS Care IAPAC, 2012).

Eradicating the Nonhuman Reservoir

Common nonhuman reservoirs for pathogens in the environment include water, food, milk, animals, insects, and sewage. Treating or eliminating them is an effective method of preventing replication of pathogens and thus preventing transmission.

Controlling the Human Reservoir

Treating infected persons, whether they are symptomatic or not, is effective in preventing transmission of pathogens directly to others. **Quarantine** is an enforced isolation or restriction of movement of those who have been exposed to an infectious agent during the incubation period; this is another method of controlling the reservoir. Quarantine was used effectively during the outbreak of severe acute respiratory syndrome (SARS) in 2003, when some hospitals required that their staff exposed to patients with SARS remain at the hospital until proven to be symptom-free at the end of the incubation period.

Controlling the Portals of Exit and Entry

The transmission chain may be broken at the portal of exit by properly disposing of secretions, excretions, and exudates from infected persons. Additionally, **isolation** of sick persons from others and requiring that persons with tuberculosis wear a mask in public can be effective.

The portal of entry of pathogens also can be controlled by using barrier precautions (masks, gloves, condoms); avoiding unnecessary invasive procedures, such as indwelling catheters; and protecting oneself from vectors, such as mosquitoes. In response to the risk of exposure to bloodborne pathogens (e.g., HIV, hepatitis B, and hepatitis C) in the late 1980s, the CDC developed a set of guidelines, called **universal precautions**, to prevent transmission of diseases found in blood and other body fluids. These guidelines were developed because infected people may be asymptomatic and have no knowledge of their conditions; therefore health care workers must assume that every patient is infectious and must protect themselves.

Improving Host Resistance and Immunity

Many factors, such as age, general health status, nutrition, and health behaviors, contribute to a host's **resistance**, or ability to ward off infections. Immunity, however, is an incredible defense against infection. There are several kinds of **immunity**, each providing resistance in different ways to different pathogens. **Natural immunity** is an innate resistance to

TABLE 25-2	TYPES OF ACQUIRED IMMUNITY		
TYPE OF IMMUNITY	**HOW ACQUIRED**	**EXAMPLE**	**DURATION OF RESISTANCE**
Natural			
Active	Natural contact and infection with the antigen	Acquiring measles	May be temporary or permanent
Passive	Natural contact with antibody transplacentally	Infant born with temporary antibodies to measles	Temporary or through colostrum and breast milk
Artificial			
Active	Inoculation of antigen	Tetanus vaccine to stimulate production of antibodies to tetanus	May be temporary or permanent
Passive	Inoculation of antibody or antitoxin	Injection of tetanus antitoxin to an unimmunized person	Temporary

Modified from Grimes DE: Infectious diseases. In Thompson JM et al, editors: *Mosby's clinical nursing*, St Louis, 1991, Mosby.

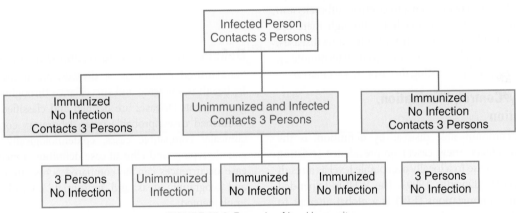

Herd Immunity: 66% immunized (10/13 or 77%) protected

FIGURE 25-3 Example of herd immunity.

a specific antigen or toxin. **Acquired immunity** is derived from actual exposure to the specific infectious agent, toxin, or appropriate vaccine. There are two types of acquired immunity: active and passive. **Active immunity** occurs when the body produces its own antibodies against an antigen, from either infection with the pathogen or introduction of the pathogen in a vaccine. **Passive immunity** is the temporary resistance that has been donated to the host either through transfusions of plasma proteins, immunoglobulins, or antitoxins or transplacentally (from mother to fetus). Passive immunity lasts only as long as these substances remain in the bloodstream. Types of acquired immunity with examples are summarized in Table 25-2.

When administered according to established guidelines and protocols, vaccines provide acquired immunity in most cases. However, there are exceptions. **Primary vaccine failure** is the failure of a vaccine to stimulate any immune response. It can be caused by improper storage that may render the vaccine ineffective, improper administration route, or exposure of a light-sensitive vaccine to light. Additionally, seroconversion never occurs in some immunized persons, either because of failure of their own immune system or for some other unknown reason. **Secondary vaccine failure** is the waning of immunity following an initial immune response. It often occurs in patients with immunosuppression and in

those who have undergone organ transplantation, in whom the immune memory is essentially destroyed.

Herd immunity is a state in which those not immune to an infectious agent are protected if a certain proportion (generally considered to be 80%) of the population has been vaccinated or is otherwise immune (Figure. 25-3). This effect applies only if those who are immune are distributed evenly in the population. This is especially true for the transmission of diseases, such as diphtheria, that are found only in the human host and that have no invertebrate host or other mode of transmission. Without the presence of a susceptible population to infect, the organism will be unable to live because the vast majority of the population is immune.

PUBLIC HEALTH CONTROL OF INFECTIOUS DISEASES

Most human diseases (e.g., cancer or diabetes) can be classified as personal health problems. Individuals with personal health problems can be treated by the health care system one person at a time. By contrast, infectious diseases are categorized as public or community health problems. Because of their potential to spread and cause community-wide or worldwide emergencies, infectious diseases require organized, public efforts for their prevention and control.

Such organized public efforts are under the jurisdiction of official public health agencies at local, state, national, and international levels. Each government unit obtains its powers through a complex array of laws. It is important to remember that in areas of health within a state, state laws usually prevail over federal law. The reason for this hierarchy is that the U.S. Constitution did not address health and the Tenth Amendment reserved power to the states over all issues not addressed in the Constitution (Schneider, 2006). Historically, states have accepted this responsibility. For example, all states have laws addressing infectious disease control, such as what diseases must be reported and who has authority to implement quarantines. Every state has a board of health and a department of health to implement state laws.

The CDC is the national public health entity responsible for infectious disease control across the states. The CDC has responsibility for monitoring infectious diseases and for supporting local and state governments to control outbreaks and epidemics if such assistance is needed. Although there are many aspects of public health control of infectious diseases, only three are presented here—common control terminology, reporting diseases, and preventing diseases by vaccination.

Terminology: Control, Elimination, and Eradication

Control of a communicable disease, by definition, is the reduction of incidence (new cases) or prevalence (existing cases) of a given disease to a locally acceptable level as a result of deliberate efforts (Dowdle, 1999). The WHO's Expanded Programme on Immunizations (EPI) is a global attempt to control morbidity and mortality for many vaccine-preventable diseases, with each country adapting these guidelines as necessary. An example of control of pertussis would be to achieve 80% immunization coverage of children against pertussis.

Elimination of a communicable disease occurs when it is controlled within a specified geographic area such as a single country, an island, or a continent, and the prevalence and incidence of the disease is reduced to near zero. Elimination is the result of deliberate efforts, but continued intervention measures are required (Dowdle, 1999). Such would be the case if no new cases of polio were reported in the United States during the year following an aggressive immunization campaign.

The International Task Force for Disease Eradication (ITFDE) defines eradication as reducing the worldwide incidence of a disease to zero as a function of deliberate efforts, without a need for further control measures (Dowdle, 1999). Eradication is possible under certain conditions. Criteria for assessing eradicability are listed in Box 25-3.

Smallpox was eradicated in 1977, and the virus now exists only in storage in laboratories. Many factors contributed to the successful eradication of the disease, including the mode of transmission of the disease, the isolated geographic distribution of the infection, the ease of administration of the freeze-dried vaccine, the establishment of an effective surveillance system, the increase in national and international political will, and tremendous community participation.

BOX 25-3   CRITERIA FOR ASSESSMENT OF DISEASE ERADICABILITY

Criteria for assessment of the possibility of disease eradication include the following:

- Human host only; no host in nature
- Easy diagnosis; obvious clinical manifestations
- Limited duration and intensity of infection
- Natural lifelong immunity after infection
- Highly seasonal transmission
- Availability of vaccine, curative treatment, or both
- Substantial global morbidity and mortality rates
- Cost-effectiveness of campaign and eradication
- Integration of eradication with additional public health variables
- Eradication is preferred over use of control measures only

From Centers for Disease Control and Prevention: Recommendations of the international task force for disease eradication, *MMWR Morb Mortal Wkly Rep* 42:1-38, 1993; and Dowdle WR: The principles of disease elimination and eradication, *MMWR Morb Mortal Wkly Rep* 48(Suppl 1):23-7, 1999.

Defining and Reporting Communicable Diseases

Standardized definitions of diseases are necessary for public health monitoring and surveillance throughout all levels of government. Diseases are defined and classified according to confirmed cases, probable cases, laboratory-confirmed cases, clinically compatible cases, epidemiologically linked cases, genetic typing, and clinical case definition. Once defined, disease occurrences can be compared across time, populations, and geographic areas, and appropriate control efforts can be implemented.

The CDC is responsible for monitoring communicable disease in the United States. Along with the Council of State and Territorial Epidemiologists, the CDC has designated notifiable infectious diseases, meaning that health care providers who encounter cases of these diseases must report them to, or notify, the local or regional health department. These notifiable diseases are listed in Box 25-4.

Because state health departments have the responsibility for monitoring and controlling communicable diseases within their respective states, they determine which diseases will be reported within their jurisdictions. Although not all nationally notifiable diseases are reportable in every state or territory, some states have notifiable disease lists that are longer than the CDC's list. All health professionals are advised to check the websites of their state health departments for specifics about reporting laws in their states. The processes for reporting also vary by state, and this information usually is available on the state health department's website. Generally, providers are encouraged to report cases of infectious diseases to their local or regional health departments, who then report to the state and to the CDC.

The CDC publishes a weekly list of notifiable diseases reported by region, state, and nation in *Morbidity and Mortality Weekly Report* (MMWR). MMWR can be found in medical libraries, local health departments, infection control departments in hospitals and medical centers, and on the Internet at http://www.cdc.gov.

BOX 25-4	INFECTIOUS DISEASES DESIGNATED AS NOTIFIABLE AT THE NATIONAL LEVEL, 2011

- Anthrax
- Arboviral neuroinvasive and nonneuroinvasive diseases: California serogroup virus disease, Eastern equine encephalitis, Powassan virus disease, St. Louis encephalitis, West Nile virus disease, and Western equine encephalitis
- Babesiosis
- Botulism (food-borne, infant, and other)
- Brucellosis
- Chancroid
- *Chlamydia trachomatis*, genital infections
- Cholera
- Coccidioidomycosis
- Cryptosporidiosis
- Cyclosporiasis
- Dengue virus infections (Dengue Fever, Dengue Hemorrhagic Fever, Dengue Shock Syndrome)
- Diphtheria
- Ehrlichiosis/anaplasmosis
- Giardiasis
- Gonorrhea
- *Haemophilus influenzae*, invasive disease
- Hansen's disease (leprosy)
- Hantavirus pulmonary syndrome
- Hemolytic uremic syndrome, post-diarrheal
- Hepatitis, acute (hepatitis A, hepatitis B, perinatal, hepatitis C)
- Hepatitis, chronic (hepatitis B and hepatitis C)
- Human immunodeficiency virus (HIV) infection
- Influenza-associated pediatric mortality
- Legionellosis
- Listeriosis
- Lyme disease
- Malaria
- Measles
- Meningococcal disease
- Mumps
- Novel influenza A virus infections

- Pertussis
- Plague
- Poliomyelitis, paralytic
- Poliovirus infection, nonparalytic
- Psittacosis
- Q fever (acute and chronic)
- Rabies (animal and human)
- Rubella
- Rubella, congenital syndrome
- Salmonellosis
- Severe acute respiratory syndrome–associated coronavirus (SARS-CoV) disease
- Shiga toxin–producing *Escherichia coli* (STEC)
- Shigellosis
- Smallpox
- Spotted fever rickettsiosis (formerly Rocky Mountain Spotted Fever)
- Streptococcal toxic-shock syndrome
- *Streptococcus pneumoniae*, invasive
- Syphilis (all stages)
- Syphilis, congenital
- Tetanus
- Toxic shock syndrome (other than streptococcal)
- Trichinellosis (trichinosis)
- Tuberculosis
- Tularemia
- Typhoid fever
- Vancomycin-intermediate *Staphylococcus aureus* (VISA)
- Vancomycin-resistant *Staphylococcus aureus* (VRSA)
- Varicella (morbidity and death)
- Vibriosis
- Viral hemorrhagic fevers (Crimean-Congo hemorrhagic fever virus, Ebola virus, Lassa virus, Lujo virus, Marburg virus, New World Arenaviruses [Guanarito, Machupo, Junin, and Sabia viruses])
- Yellow fever

From Centers for Disease Control and Prevention: Infectious diseases designated as notifiable at the national level during 2011, *MMWR Morb Mortal Wkly Rep* 60(53), 1-118, 2013. Retrieved from <http://www.cdc.gov/mmwr/PDF/wk/mm6053.pdf

VACCINES AND INFECTIOUS DISEASE PREVENTION

This section contains comprehensive information on vaccines and vaccine-preventable diseases. Diseases for which there are vaccines are listed in Box 25-5. Recommended vaccination schedules for selected groups are available on the CDC website, which is listed in Box 25-6 along with other resources.

Vaccines: Word of Caution

As with other areas of health care, information and recommendations on immunizations and vaccine usage change regularly. Therefore health care providers should seek the most current information on the CDC website. Recommendations, policies, and procedures concerning international immunization practices are determined by the WHO. In the United States, national governance is provided by the American Academy of Pediatrics Committee on Infectious Diseases and the U.S. Public Health Service Advisory Committee on Immunization Practices (ACIP). Occasionally these agencies differ in their recommendations.

Precautions must be taken when giving any immunization. The most recent recommendations—which immunizations to give; to whom they should be given; how they should be given; and how they are to be transported, stored, and administered—can be obtained from the CDC.

The CDC produces Vaccine Information Statements (VISs) that explain the benefits and risks of a vaccine to vaccine recipients, their parents, or their legal representatives. Federal law requires that VISs be handed out before each dose whenever certain vaccinations are given. VISs can be downloaded from the Internet at http://www.cdc.gov/vaccines/hcp/vis/index.html.

Types of Immunizations

Immunization is a broad term used to describe a process by which active or passive immunity to an infectious disease is induced or amplified. Immunizing agents can include vaccines, immune globulins, or antitoxins. **Vaccination** is a narrower term referring to the administration of a vaccine or toxoid to confer active immunity by stimulating the body to produce its own antibodies.

BOX 25-5 VACCINE-PREVENTABLE DISEASES

- Anthrax
- Cervical cancer
- Diphtheria
- *Haemophilus influenzae* type b (Hib)
- Hepatitis A
- Hepatitis B
- Human papillomavirus (HPV)
- H1N1 Flu (Swine flu)
- Influenza (seasonal flu)
- Japanese encephalitis (JE)
- Lyme disease
- Measles
- Meningococcal disease
- Monkeypox
- Mumps
- Pertussis
- Pneumococcal disease
- Poliomyelitis
- Rabies
- Rotavirus
- Rubella
- Shingles (herpes zoster)
- Smallpox
- Tetanus
- Tuberculosis
- Typhoid Fever
- Varicella (chickenpox)
- Yellow fever

From Centers for Disease Control and Prevention: *Vaccines & preventable diseases*, 2012. Retrieved from <http://www.cdc.gov/vaccines/vpd-vac/>.

BOX 25-6 RESOURCES FOR RECOMMENDED VACCINE SCHEDULES FOR SELECTED POPULATION GROUPS

Children/adolescents	http://www.cdc.gov/vaccines/schedules/hcp/child-adolescent.html
Adults	http://www.cdc.gov/vaccines/schedules/hcp/adult.html
Travelers	http://www.cdc.gov/travel/destinations/list
Pregnant women	www.cdc.gov/vaccines/pubs/preg-guide.htm
Health care workers	www.cdc.gov/vaccines/spec-grps/hcw.htm
Specific health conditions	www.cdc.gov/vaccines/spec-grps/conditions.htm
Other special groups	www.cdc.gov/vaccines/spec-grps/default.htm

Vaccines can be prepared in several ways. They may be suspensions in a variety of solutions; protected with preservatives, stabilizers, or antibiotics; or mixed with adjuvants, which are used to increase immunogenicity. Vaccines can be live and attenuated (with the virulence reduced), or they may be killed or inactivated (with the virulence removed), leaving only the antigenic property necessary to stimulate the human immune system to produce antibodies. Types of inactivated vaccines include toxoids and polysaccharide vaccines. Inactivated conjugate vaccines, containing chemically linked polysaccharides and proteins, and genetically engineered "recombinant" vaccines are also now being administered. Inactivated vaccines can be fractions or subunits or whole "killed" bacteria or viruses. Immune globulins and antitoxins are solutions that contain antibodies from human or animal blood and are introduced into a patient to provide passive protection without initiating the immune system to produce an immunogenic response. Table 25-3 presents information on types of available vaccines.

Vaccine Storage, Transport, and Handling

Vaccines should be safely stored, transported, and handled at all times to ensure their efficacy. A cold chain is a system used to ensure that vaccines are kept at a designated temperature from the time they are manufactured until they are used for vaccination. Failing to maintain the cold chain and exposing the vaccines to higher or lower temperatures than recommended may result in loss of potency and vaccine failure. Several methods are available for ensuring that the appropriate temperature has been maintained throughout vaccine transport and storage. These include liquid crystal thermometers, dial thermometers, recording thermometers, digital thermometers, ice pack indicators, shipping indicators that change color if the temperature exceeds or falls below the recommended level, freeze-watch indicators, and cold chain monitors. Vaccine storage and handling information can be obtained at www.cdc.gov/vaccines/recs/storage/default.htm.

Vaccine Administration

The efficacy of a vaccine can be adversely affected if it is not administered appropriately. Information on the correct dosage can be found on the package insert. If more than one vaccine is being administered simultaneously, different anatomical sites should be used. Additionally, it is important to follow the same safety procedures one would use to administer any intramuscular or subcutaneous injection (i.e., use sterile technique, use the correct size needle, avoid injecting in a blood vessel, and dispose of the needle and syringe properly).

Vaccine Spacing

Wherever possible, all children should be age-appropriately immunized and their immunization status kept up-to-date according to current recommendations. The same applies to adolescents, adults, persons with chronic illness, pregnant women, health care workers, and international travelers.

The number of injections for any one immunobiological substance should be administered according to recommendations of the Advisory Committee on Immunization Practices. An interruption in the schedule does not require that the entire series begin again. However, if vaccines are administered at less than the recommended intervals, they should not be counted as part of the primary series of immunization. Completion of the primary vaccine series and receiving periodic booster doses as recommended are necessary to ensure protective levels of immunity. Additional information is available at www.CDC.gov/vaccines.

Vaccine Hypersensitivity and Contraindications

Although adverse reactions are not common following immunization, they can occur in some individuals. These reactions can be to vaccine components such as eggs, egg proteins, antibiotics, preservatives, and adjuvants. Patient allergies should be considered before administration of specific vaccines. For additional precautions and contraindications, refer to the vaccine package insert and the latest instructions from the CDC, at www.cdc.gov/vaccines/recs/vac-admin/contraindications-vacc.htm.

TABLE 25-3 AVAILABLE VACCINES BY TYPE

TYPE	DESCRIPTION
Live Attenuated	
Viral	Measles, mumps, rubella, oral polio, vaccinia, yellow fever, and varicella
Bacterial	*BCG* (bacille Calmette-Guérin)
Recombinant	Oral typhoid
Inactivated	
Viral	Influenza, polio, rabies, and hepatitis A
Bacterial	Typhoid, cholera, and plague
Subunit (fractional)	Influenza, acellular pertussis, typhoid VI, and Lyme disease
Toxoid	Diphtheria and tetanus
Recombinant	Hepatitis B
Conjugate polysaccharide	*Haemophilus influenzae* type b, and pneumococcal 7-valent
Pure polysaccharide	Pneumococcal 23-valent, meningococcal, and *Haemophilus influenzae* type b

From Centers for Disease Control and Prevention: *Epidemiology and prevention of vaccine-preventable diseases (pink book)*, ed 6, Atlanta, 2000, Public Health Foundation.

Mild illness with or without low-grade fever is not a contraindication to vaccination. However, vaccination should be postponed in cases of moderate or severe febrile illness to avoid any confusion between a vaccine side effect and an unknown underlying cause.

Pregnancy is not a contraindication to immunization using inactivated vaccines, antitoxins, or immune globulins. However, pregnant women should avoid live vaccines, including those for measles-mumps-rubella (MMR), varicella, and yellow fever, unless the risk of infection is very high (see the link to guidelines for vaccinating pregnant women in Box 25-6).

Immunocompromised patients should not receive live vaccines; however, MMR can be administered to asymptomatic HIV-infected people, and varicella can be given to people with humoral immunodeficiency and some HIV-asymptomatic people as determined by their physician. Killed or inactivated vaccines can be given, but they may not produce an optimal antibody response (see the link to guidelines for vaccinating specific groups of people in Box 25-6).

Vaccine Documentation

Legal documentation of vaccinations is important for both the individual and the provider for future administration and follow-up of hypersensitivity reactions. Both individual and provider immunization records should be maintained. The health care provider is responsible for maintaining accurate records, including patient name, dates immunized, vaccine type, vaccine manufacturer, vaccine lot number, date of the Vaccine Information Statement (VIS), and the name, title, and address of the person administering the vaccine. VISs can be downloaded from http://www.cdc.gov/vaccines/hcp/vis/index.html.

Vaccine Safety and Reporting Adverse Events and Vaccine-Related Injuries

No drug is perfectly safe or effective, and vaccines are no exception. They are biological rather than chemical, and when introduced into the human biological system, they can and do produce a variety of responses, both positive and negative. Furthermore, vaccines are administered to healthy people; they are given to prevent illness and not treat it; and they are given to far greater numbers of people than other pharmaceuticals.

Public concern regarding the health risks associated with vaccines has increased as the risk of contracting the diseases has declined. For example, wild virus polio has been eliminated in the United States, yet between 1979 and 1997 cases of poliomyelitis were reported in the U.S. in association with use of the oral, live virus vaccine. The health risk of the oral vaccine exceeded that of the risk of the disease. This led to a change in vaccine policy from the use of the live oral vaccine to the inactivated polio vaccine (IPV) (CDC, 1999). Likewise, whole cell pertussis vaccine has been changed to an acellular pertussis vaccine because of the adverse side effects, most notably convulsions, associated with the whole cell vaccine.

To enable monitoring of actual and potential vaccine-related problems, health care providers must report specific postvaccination "adverse events" to the Vaccine Adverse Event Reporting System (VAERS). Information and reporting forms are available at www.cdc.gov/vaccinesafety/Activities/vaers.html.

The National Vaccine Injury Compensation Program reviews all VAERS reports and provides assistance for individuals and families who experience a vaccine-related injury, including disability and death.

VACCINE NEEDS FOR SPECIAL GROUPS

Recommendations on immunizations and schedules for vaccination are routinely updated and published by the CDC on its website. Practitioners are encouraged to check regularly for updates. Travelers can obtain the most current recommendations from the CDC through its telephone hotline, 1-800-CDC-info (1-800-232-4636), or at its website, http://wwwnc.cdc.gov/travel.

HEALTHY PEOPLE 2020 FOCUS ON IMMUNIZATION AND INFECTIOUS DISEASES

Healthy People 2020 objectives, discussed earlier in this chapter, detailed three topic areas for infectious diseases. Immunization and Infectious Diseases (IID), as listed in the *Healthy People 2020* table, highlights vaccine-preventable and other priority infectious diseases (Healthypeople.gov, n.d. c), excluding STDs and HIV. This section provides tables summarizing the chain of transmission and control of such conditions. Table 25-4 covers childhood vaccine-preventable diseases, excluding hepatitis, which is summarized in Table 25-5. Table 25-6 summarizes tuberculosis.

Text continued on p. 506.

TABLE 25-4   CHAIN OF TRANSMISSION AND CONTROL: CHILDHOOD VACCINE-PREVENTABLE DISEASES

	CHICKENPOX	DIPHTHERIA	PERTUSSIS	TETANUS	POLIO
Occurrence	Worldwide and universal in all populations, primarily in children	Rare where immunization rates are high; affects unimmunized children under 15 yr and adults whose immunity has waned	Worldwide and common in children; declined with immunization; some outbreaks in recent years in U.S. adults whose immunity has waned	Worldwide; occurs sporadically and affects all ages; more common in agricultural areas and among parenteral drug users; rare in areas with high immunization rates	Worldwide before immunization; is now rare in countries with adequate immunization rates
Etiological agent(s)	Human (alpha) herpesvirus 3 (varicella zoster virus)	Corynebacterium diphtheriae, of gravis, mitis, or intermedius biotypes	Bordetella pertussis	Clostridium tetani (an anaerobic pathogen)	Poliovirus, types 1, 2, and 3; all are paralytogenic
Reservoir	Humans	Humans	Humans	Intestines of humans and animals	Humans, particularly children with subclinical infections
Transmission	Direct and indirect contact with droplets from respiratory passage or vesicle fluid; extremely contagious	Direct or indirect contact with exudates from mucous membrane lesions of infected person or carrier; raw milk has served as a vehicle	Direct contact with droplets from respiratory passages	Tetanus spores enter body through a wound (usually puncture wound) contaminated with soil and feces; necrotic tissue favors the growth of the anaerobic bacillus	Direct and indirect contact with respiratory discharges and feces; fecal-oral route more common than respiratory transmission
Incubation period	14-16 days; range 2-3 wk; prolonged in immunocompromised persons	2-5 days; occasionally longer	9-10 days; range 6-20 days	10 days; range 3-21 days; rarely, several months	7-14 days; range 3-35 days
Communicability period	1-2 days before onset of rash to 5 days after lesions have crusted	Until bacilli have disappeared from discharges and lesions (usually 2 wk); effective antibiotic therapy interferes with shedding; a carrier may transmit for 6 mo	Highly communicable during early catarrhal and coughing stages; gradually decreasing until week 3; communicability is negligible after 5 days with effective antibiotic therapy	Not transmitted directly	Highly communicable during first days after onset of symptoms; virus is in throat secretions within 36 hr and in feces 72 hr after infection; remains 1 wk in throat and 6 wk in feces
Susceptibility and resistance	General population not previously infected or vaccinated are at risk; can be severe or fatal in adults and immunocompromised persons	General unimmunized population are at risk; infants born of immune mothers have passive immunity for 6 mo; recovery from disease or asymptomatic infection usually confers lifetime immunity; immunization confers prolonged, but not lifetime, immunity	General unimmunized population are at risk; unimmunized children under 5 yr are most susceptible; no passive immunity from mother; disease confers prolonged, but not lifetime, immunity	General unimmunized population are at risk; active immunity from tetanus toxoid persists for 10 yr; tetanus immune globulin confers temporary immunity; infants born to immune mothers are protected at birth; active disease does not confer lifetime immunity	General unimmunized population is at risk; active immunization confers lifetime immunity; disease or subclinical infection confers type-specific lifetime immunity

Prevention and control	Two-dose vaccination of children: 1st dose between 12 and 15 mo. of age; 2nd dose between 4 and 6 yr (see Box 25-6)	After initial immunization with diphtheria-pertussis-tetanus vaccine (DPT), immunization with diphtheria toxoid boosters every 10 yr (see Box 25-6)	Childhood immunization with DPT (see Box 25-6) Immunization with whole cell vaccine prophylaxis with a 7-day course of erythromycin should be given to all exposed persons, including health care workers, regardless of vaccination status	Active immunization with tetanus toxoid boosters every 10 yr, and as prophylaxis following penetrating injuries for those whose last booster was more than 10 yr ago	Active immunization with inactivated polio virus (IPV) in childhood as recommended (see Box 25-6)
Disease manifestations	Sudden mild fever, and malaise, rash, or both; rash is progressive changing from maculopapular to vesicular, and then forming a crust or scab; lesions tend to be more numerous on covered parts of the body; can be on all mucous membranes and are highly pruritic; complications are more common in persons over 15 yr old, infants under 1 yr old, and immunocompromised persons; virus can persist in a dormant state in sensory nerve endings and can reactivate, causing herpes zoster, or shingles	Acute onset; usually affecting the upper respiratory tract. Lesions are caused by the release of a cytotoxin and manifest as a patch or patches of inflammation surrounding a grayish membrane; complications may result in severe swelling of the neck, thrombocytopenia, neuritis, and myocarditis	Pertussis (whooping cough) begins with an upper respiratory cough and proceeds to a paroxysmal stage of coughing, often ending in vomiting; paroxysmal stage may last 1-2 mo or longer; complications include seizures, pneumonia, encephalopathy, and death	Tetanus (lockjaw) is an acute neurological illness caused by an anaerobic bacterium that produces an exotoxin in the portal of entry in the human host; tetanus causes gradually worsening neurological symptoms, including painful muscle contractions and spasms frequently resulting in death	Symptoms may range from inapparent illness to severe paralysis or death
Diagnosis	By symptoms	Bacteriological culture of nasal and throat secretions and from lesions	Bacteriological culture of nasal or throat secretions	History of injury plus clinical symptoms; bacterium is rarely found in wound cultures	Isolation of the virus from fecal or oropharyngeal specimens
Treatment	Antiviral drugs within 1 wk of exposure may modify severity; varicella-zoster immune globulin administered within 96 hr of exposure can modify or prevent the disease	Single dose of equine antitoxin followed by a full course of antibiotic therapy	Treatment with antibiotics reduces the period of infectivity and may lessen the severity of the disease if given before the paroxysmal stage	Tetanus antitoxin or tetanus immune globulin (TIG), preferably human; supportive care	Supportive care
Report to local health authority?	Yes	Yes	Yes	Yes	Yes

Continued

TABLE 25-4 CHAIN OF TRANSMISSION AND CONTROL: CHILDHOOD VACCINE-PREVENTABLE DISEASES—cont'd

	MEASLES (RUBEOLA)	MUMPS	RUBELLA	*Haemophilus influenzae* TYPE B MENINGITIS	PNEUMOCOCCAL DISEASE	INFLUENZA
Occurrence	Worldwide; endemic and epidemic occurrences where immunization rates are low; still a major killer of children worldwide	Worldwide; incidence decreasing where immunization rates are high; one third of infected persons have subclinical infections	Worldwide and endemic where immunization rates are low; epidemics occur every 5-9 yr; primarily a disease of children	Worldwide; most common in children 2 mo to 5 yr of age; rare with widespread immunization	Worldwide; most common in children 2 mo to 3 yr of age, the elderly, and immunocompromised adults	Worldwide; in pandemics, epidemics, localized outbreaks, and sporadic cases
Etiological agent(s)	Measles virus, a paramyxovirus	Mumps virus, a paramyxovirus	Rubella virus	*H. influenzae* serotype B (Hib)	*Streptococcus pneumoniae*	Three types of influenza virus (A, B, and C), each with many subtypes
Reservoir	Humans	Humans	Humans	Humans	Humans (often found in respiratory passages of healthy persons)	Humans; some mammals and birds suspected as sources of new subtypes
Transmission	Direct or indirect contact with nasal or throat secretions of infected person; highly communicable	Direct contact with saliva (airborne or droplets) from infected person	Direct or indirect contact with nasopharyngeal secretions of infected person; transplacental transmission leads to congenital rubella syndrome (CRS)	Direct or indirect contact with droplets of nasopharyngeal secretions of infected person	Direct or indirect contact with droplets of nasopharyngeal secretions of infected person	Airborne spread
Incubation period	10 days until fever; 14 days until rash; range 7-18 days	16-18 days; range 14-25 days	14-17 days; range 14-21 days	Unknown; probably 2-4 days	Unknown: probably 1-4 days	1-3 days
Communicability period	1 day before the prodromal period to 4 days after appearance of the rash	2 days before to 4 days after onset of parotitis; but the range can be 7 days before to 15 days after onset; can be transmitted by persons with subclinical infections	7 days before to 4 days after onset of rash; highly communicable; infants with CRS may shed virus for months after birth	Variable as long as organisms are in nasopharynx; noncommunicable within 24-48 hr after onset of effective antibiotic therapy	As long as organism is found in nasopharynx; may be prolonged in immunocompromised persons	3-5 days from clinical onset in adults; up to 7 days in children
Susceptibility and resistance	General population who has not had disease or immunization is at risk; lifetime immunity after illness; infants of mothers who have had the disease are protected for 6-9 mo; infants of immunized mothers have variable level of passive antibody; length of immunity following immunization is unknown	Lifetime immunity develops after subclinical or clinical illness	General unimmunized or previously uninfected population is at risk; lifetime immunity after illness; infants born to immune mothers are protected for 6-9 mo; long-term immunity following immunization	General unimmunized or previously uninfected population is at risk; immunity acquired transplacentally, from infection, and by immunization	General population is probably at risk; immunity is acquired transplacentally, from prior infection, or from immunization	General population is at risk; infection and immunization produces immunity to only one subtype of the virus

	Measles	Mumps	Rubella	Hib	Pneumococcal	Influenza
Prevention and control	Active immunization with live, attenuated measles vaccine (see Box 25-6)	Active immunization with live, attenuated mumps virus vaccine (see Box 25-6)	Active immunization with live, attenuated rubella virus vaccine in childhood (see Box 25-6); immunity in adolescent girls should be ensured	Active immunization with Hib conjugate vaccine (see Box 25-6)	Pneumococcal conjugate vaccine (PCV) for infants and children; pneumococcal polysaccharide vaccine (PPV) for high-risk groups (see Box 25-6)	Active immunization yearly prior to influenza season
Disease manifestations	Acute-onset fever of 101° F or higher, cough, coryza, conjunctivitis, Koplik's spots on the buccal mucosa, and a red rash lasting longer than 3 days that begins on the face and becomes generalized; measles can progress into severe complications, including pneumonia, encephalitis, and death	Acute-onset fever and painful swelling of the salivary and parotid glands; may be asymptomatic; complications range from meningoencephalitis to permanent hearing impairment and orchitis in postpubescent males, but rarely sterility	Maculopapular rash and postauricular, occipital, and posterior cervical lymphadenopathy; children are usually relatively asymptomatic, but adults may experience fever, headache, and malaise; rare complications include encephalitis and thrombocytopenia; congenital defects in fetuses of pregnant women who are infected	Hib can affect multiple organ systems, resulting in meningitis, epiglottitis, otitis media, pneumonia, arthritis, and cellulitis, with symptoms associated with those conditions; complications are serious and include septic arthritis, life-threatening airway obstruction, fulminating infection, and death	Acute-onset symptoms of meningitis or pneumonia	Acute-onset dry cough, fever, headache, myalgia, sore throat, and other generalized symptoms; symptom severity depends on the subtype of the virus; complications include pneumonia, otitis media, meningitis, Reye's syndrome, and death
Diagnosis	Tissue culture of nasopharyngeal secretions and serological testing	Isolation of virus from oral and throat spray, urine, and cerebrospinal fluid	Serological testing	Identification of organisms in blood or cerebrospinal fluid	Isolation of the organism from the blood or other sterile body site	Isolation of virus from nasal or pharyngeal secretions, serological testing, antigen detection, gene amplification, and rapid diagnostic test
Treatment	Supportive care	Supportive care	Supportive care	10-14 days of antibiotics	Antibiotics	Antiviral drugs started within 48 hr of onset of symptoms
Report to local health authority?	Yes	Yes	Yes	Yes	Epidemics only	Epidemics only

Modified from Grimes DE, Grimes KA, Zack CM: Infectious diseases. In Thompson JM et al, editors: *Mosby's clinical nursing,* ed 5, St. Louis, 2002, Mosby; with data from Heymann DL, editor: *Control of communicable diseases manual,* ed 19, Washington, DC, 2008, American Public Health Association; and from Centers for Disease Control and Prevention: Advisory Committee on Immunization Practices (ACIP) recommended immunization schedules for persons aged 0 through 18 years and adults aged 19 years and older—United States, 2013. *MMWR Morb Mortal Wkly Rep* 62(Suppl 1):1, 2013.

TABLE 25-5 CHAIN OF TRANSMISSION AND CONTROL: HEPATITIS

	HEPATITIS A	HEPATITIS B	HEPATITIS C	HEPATITIS D	HEPATITIS E
Occurrence	Worldwide; sporadic and epidemic with cyclic recurrence; outbreaks in institutions where sanitation is poor	Worldwide; endemic; highest in young adults, homosexually active men, persons engaging in unprotected sex, injection drug users, health care and public safety workers	Worldwide; directly related to prevalence of injection drug use in the population, HCV in the donated blood supply, and lack of use of parenteral precautions in health care	Worldwide; occurs epidemically and endemically in population at risk for HBV infection; declining in areas where chronic carriers of HBsAG	Epidemic and sporadic cases, particularly in developing countries; highest in young adults; rare in children or the elderly
Etiological agent(s)	Hepatitis A virus (HAV)	Hepatitis B virus (HBV); made up of a core antigen, HB-cAG, and a surface antigen, HBsAG; HBV has at least 8 different genotypes	Hepatitis C virus (HCV), which has 6 genotypes and 100 subtypes	Hepatitis delta virus (HDV), which consists of a coat of HBsAG and an internal antigen, the delta antigen	Hepatitis E virus (HEV)
Reservoir(s)	Humans and captive primates	Humans and possibly captive primates	Humans; virus has been transmitted experimentally to chimpanzees	Humans; virus can be transmitted experimentally to chimpanzees and to woodchucks	Humans and nonhuman primates, pigs, chickens, and cattle
Transmission	Person-to-person by fecal-oral route; contaminated food, water, shellfish, etc.	Direct and indirect contact with blood and serum-derived fluids; sexual contact; perinatal	Parenteral; sexual and perinatal transmission are less likely to occur	Similar to that of HBV; must co-infect with HBV	Person-to-person by fecal-oral route; contaminated food or water
Incubation period	28-30 days; range 15-50 days	60-90 days; range 45-180 days	6-9 wk; range 2 wk to 6 mo	2-8 wk	26-42 days; range 15-64 days
Communicability period	Latter half of incubation period to 1 wk after onset of jaundice	During incubation period and throughout clinical course of disease; carrier state may persist for years	Virus persists indefinitely	Throughout acute and chronic disease	Unknown; virus has been detected in stools 14 days after onset of symptoms and 4 wk after ingestion of contaminated food or water
Susceptibility and resistance	General population is at risk; usually affects children and young adults; probable lifetime immunity following infection	General population is at risk; disease is mild in children; lifetime immunity follows infection if antibody to HBV develops and test for HBV is negative	General population is at risk; degree of immunity following infection is not known	All persons susceptible to HBV or who have an HBV infection and are co-infected with HDV	Unknown
Prevention and control	Eliminate common sources of infection with sanitation; improve hygienic practices and hand washing; cook shellfish; immunize high-risk groups or persons in high-risk situations with HAV vaccine; for post-exposure: administer vaccine and immune globulin (IG) within 2 wk; use universal precautions	Routinely immunize infants, children, and high-risk groups (see Box 25-6); at birth give HBIG and Hep B vaccine to infants born to HBsAg-positive mothers, followed by additional vaccine doses at 1 and 6 months of age; immunize persons exposed to HBV; test all donated blood for HBV antigen; practice safe sex; use universal precautions	Apply HBV control measures except immunization; no vaccine exists at this time, and IG does not prevent HCV infection	Apply HBV prevention and control measures; however, HBIG, IG, and hepatitis B vaccine do not prevent HDV infection in those already infected with HBV	No vaccine; IG not effective; sanitation appears to be the only effective measure of prevention

Disease manifestations	Acute-onset fever, anorexia, malaise, dark urine, and jaundice, usually lasting 2 mo; has a very low fatality rate and, although rare, can last up to 6 mo	Insidious onset that ranges from asymptomatic illness to generalized nonspecific symptoms, such as anorexia, nausea, and vomiting followed by jaundice and occasionally resulting in fulminant fatal hepatitis	Like HBV, has an insidious onset; symptoms vary from completely asymptomatic (80%) to the rare fulminating, fatal disease; mild symptoms are same as those for HBV; chronic hepatitis develops in 75%-85% of those who are acutely ill	Abrupt onset with range of symptoms similar to those of HBV; always associated with HBV infection, either co-infection or as a supra-infection in persons with chronic hepatitis B	Clinical course similar to that of HAV; no chronic form
Diagnosis	Serum antibodies (anti-HAV) detectable 5-10 days post-exposure	Presence in sera of HBsAG, anti-HBsAG (antibodies), HBcAG and anti-HBcAG, HBeAG and anti-HBeAG	Presence of serum antibodies to HCV (anti-HCV)	Presence of serum antibodies to HDV (anti-HDV)	Exclusion of other causes of hepatitis, particularly HAV; presence of serum antibodies, anti-HEV; presence of HEV RNA in feces and serum
Treatment	Supportive care	Supportive care	Treatment with ribavirin and slow-release interferons (pegylated interferons)	Supportive care	Supportive care
Report case to local health authority?	Yes	Yes	Yes	Yes	Yes

Modified from Grimes DE, Grimes KA, Zack CM: Infectious diseases. In Thompson JM et al, editors: *Mosby's clinical nursing*, ed 5, St. Louis, 2002, Mosby; with data from Heymann DL, editor: *Control of communicable diseases manual*, ed 19, Washington, DC, 2008, American Public Health Association; and from Centers for Disease Control and Prevention: Advisory Committee on Immunization Practices (ACIP) recommended immunization schedules for persons aged 0 through 18 years and adults aged 19 years and older—United States, 2013. *MMWR Morb Mortal Wkly Rep* 62(Suppl 1):1, 2013.

TABLE 25-6   CHAIN OF TRANSMISSION AND CONTROL: TUBERCULOSIS

TUBERCULOSIS	
Occurrence	Worldwide; tuberculosis (TB) cases have declined in the U.S. since 1993; drug-resistant cases continue to be reported; most newly reported cases in the U.S. occur in foreign born, immunosuppressed, homeless, and disadvantaged persons or are a reactivation of a latent infection in older age-groups and those with chronic diseases; in areas of world with high incidence of new transmission cases occur in working-age adults, children, and disadvantaged populations
Etiological agent	*Mycobacterium tuberculosis*; less often *Mycobacterium bovis* or *Mycobacterium africanum*
Reservoir	Humans; diseased cattle for *M. bovis*
Transmission	Inhalation of airborne droplets from the sputum of persons with active disease; children rarely transmit TB because they do not cough forcefully; infrequently by ingestion or skin penetration

	INFECTION	ACTIVE DISEASE (CASE)
Incubation period	2-10 wk	Anytime during one's lifetime
Communicability period	Not communicable unless there are viable bacilli in the sputum	As long as bacilli are in sputum; may be communicable for years in inadequately treated persons
Susceptibility and resistance	Anyone, such as health care workers, family members, or the institutionalized, working or living in close contact with a person who has active disease can become infected	Vulnerable persons such as children and persons who are older than 65 years, have chronic diseases or compromised immune systems, are malnourished, etc.
Prevention and control	Perform skin testing in high-risk groups (e.g., health care workers), and treat those with new infections to prevent progression to active disease; routine skin testing, particularly of children, is no longer recommended in U.S.; bacille Calmette-Guérin (BCG) vaccine is still used in some parts of the world	Promptly identify, diagnose, and treat those with active disease; ensure compliance with treatment; initiate respiratory isolation until sputum is clear of bacilli; have patient wear a mask; examine close contacts of TB cases and treat, if infected
Disease manifestations	Initial infection goes unnoticed; 5%-10% of infected persons eventually have active disease, 50% of those within the first 2 yr	Onset of active disease can occur immediately following an initial infection or after a variable latency period for untreated persons; disease onset is usually insidious, with fever, night sweats, and weight loss; cough with pulmonary disease; extrapulmonary symptoms correspond with the location of disseminated bacilli and lesions
Diagnosis	TB skin test reaction within 2-10 wk of infection; immunosuppressed persons may have a negative skin test reaction owing to anergy. Skin test results: 5-mm induration = positive for the immunosuppressed and close contacts with active cases; 10 mm induration = positive for infections <2 yr and persons with high-risk conditions; 15 mm induration = positive for all low-risk persons	10%-20% of those with active disease have a negative skin test reaction; demonstration of acid-fast bacilli in stained smears of sputum or other body fluids; isolation of organism from cultured specimen; radiological evidence of TB in lungs or elsewhere
Treatment	Treat with isoniazid (INH) for 6-12 mo, or with other drug combinations for persons with human immunodeficiency virus	Treat with combination of antimicrobial drugs to which the strain of *Mycobacterium* is susceptible, such as isoniazid (INH), rifampin (RIF), pyrazinamide (PZA), and ethambutol (EMB), for 6-12 mo or until sputum cultures are negative; monitor adherence to therapy carefully because nonadherence is increasing drug resistance
Report to local health authority?	No	Yes

Data from Heymann DL, editor: *Control of communicable diseases manual*, ed 19, Washington, DC, 2008, American Public Health Association; and Centers for Disease Control and Prevention: Trends in tuberculosis—United States, 2012, *MMWR Morb Mortal Wkly Rep* 62(11):201-205, 2012.

HEALTHY PEOPLE 2020 FOCUS ON SEXUALLY TRANSMITTED DISEASES

STDs include the more than 25 infectious organisms that are transmitted primarily through sexual activity. STDs, even those for which treatment exists, continue to be a major public health problem. The rates of STDs in the United States are among the highest in the industrialized world, approaching those in some developing countries. Indeed, an estimated 20 million cases of STDs occur each year in the United States, almost half of them in persons aged 15 to 24 years (CDC, 2013b).

Men and women of all ages, racial and ethnic backgrounds, and income levels contract STDs. However, the following populations are disproportionately affected: adolescents, young adults, women, minorities, and the poor (CDC, 2012c). Teenage girls in particular may be more susceptible to STDs because they have fewer protective antibodies to STDs and their cervixes are biologically immature. Women are at higher risk for contracting STDs than men because they have anatomical differences that enhance transmission of disease and make diagnosis difficult. In addition, women are less likely to experience symptoms.

Furthermore, complications from undiagnosed STDs occur more frequently and are more severe in women. For example, pelvic inflammatory disease (PID), largely resulting from an undetected STD, is diagnosed in more than 1 million women annually. Scarring from PID may lead to infertility, ectopic pregnancy, or chronic pelvic pain. An infected woman who transmits an STD to her fetus during pregnancy or childbirth may experience spontaneous abortion, premature delivery, stillbirth, neonatal death, and her infant may have low birth weight, chronic respiratory problems, blindness, or mental retardation.

Concern over the persistence and increases in STDs led those formulating the *Healthy People 2020* objectives to create a Topic Area specific to STDs (Healthypeople.gov, n.d d). For easy reference, the chain of transmission and control of STDs addressed in the *Healthy People 2020* objectives is presented in Table 25-7. The CDC regularly updates STD treatment guidelines, which are available on the CDC website.

HEALTHY PEOPLE 2020 FOCUS ON HIV/AIDS

No other infection or infectious disease in recent history has inflicted as much destruction and pain on individuals, families, and communities, and created as many challenges for health care professionals as HIV/AIDS. Indeed, HIV stands out as the one condition that touches nurses everywhere. HIV affects persons of every age, ethnicity, socioeconomic status, gender, and occupation. Eventually, HIV/AIDS has an impact on every organ and function of

---

RESEARCH HIGHLIGHTS

Human Papillomavirus Immunization

Humans are subject to infection from more than 100 human papillomaviruses (HPVs). HPV infects skin and mucous membrane cells and is transmitted by direct contact. Pathogenic HPV has been recovered from fingertips, nails, breast tissue, sinonasal areas, nipples, and hair follicles. Pathogenic HPV has been found in 6.5% of the oral cavities of a random sample of Americans and can readily be transmitted from infected mothers to their children during childbirth and by touch after birth The vast majority of HPV viruses are not pathogenic, but a small number are known to be oncogenic. Two—HPV 16 and HPV 18—are known to be causative agents for cancers of the cervix, vulva, vagina, anus, penis, and oropharynx; they may also contribute to prostate and breast cancer. In addition, HPV 6 and HPV 11 are known to cause genital warts.

Vaccines that protect against HPVs 6, 11, 16, and 18 have been approved for use in the U.S. Currently, the Centers for Disease Control (CDC) recommend that both boys and girls between 9 and 11 years of age be immunized against HPV. For those who did not receive the vaccine at these ages, it can be administered up to age 26. Although widespread HPV vaccine use in other countries has proved to be extremely effective, less than a third of young adolescents in the U.S. have received the recommended three doses, and less than 10% of women older than 17 years have been immunized. Fewer males have been immunized. Uptake of the vaccine in the U.S. has been poor for several reasons, including cost; parental concerns that children will become sexually active; concerns about the safety of the vaccine; lack of understanding of the nature of transmission of HPV; and failure of health professionals to promote and adhere to the recommendations.

Many of the cost concerns will disappear with implementation of the Affordable Care Act of 2008, which requires that health insurers pay for the vaccine for young women. As for other concerns, research has shown that girls who were vaccinated did not have higher rates of pregnancy or sexually transmitted disease than did those who were not vaccinated. Unfortunately, many health professionals are not aware of the widespread nature of HPV, or of the vaccine and its safety. Some health professionals have viewed the transmission of HPV as occurring only during sex and have not allayed parental concerns about potential increases in sexual behavior or the safety of the vaccine. Education is critical, because research shows that young women are three times more likely to undergo immunization if it is strongly recommended by their health care providers. Furthermore, even partial immunization, both at the individual level and within a community, has been very effective in reducing overall prevalence of HPV through the effects of herd immunity.

Implications for Nurses

1. Nurses need to educate patients and others that HPV is not only sexually transmitted but can be transmitted by other means.
2. Nurses can be central to reduction of a number of cancers by encouraging widespread use of the HPV vaccine for both males and females as recommended by the CDC.

Further Reading

Centers for Disease Control and Prevention: *Vaccine safety: Human papillomavirus (HPV) vaccine*, n.d. Available from <http://www.cdc.gov/vaccinesafety/Vaccines/HPV/index.html>.

Centers for Disease Control and Prevention: National and state vaccination coverage among adolescents aged 13 through 17 years—United States, 2010, *MMWR Morb Mortal Wkly Rep* 60:1117, 2011.

Caskey R, Lindau ST, Alexander GC: Knowledge and early adoption of the HPV vaccine among girls and young women: results of a national survey, *J Adolesc Health* 45:453, 2009.

Read TRH, Hocking JS, Chen MY, et al: The near disappearance of genital warts in young women 4 years after commencing a national human papillomavirus (HPV) vaccination programme, *Sex Transm Infect* 87:544, 2011.

Grimes RM, Benjamins LJ, Williams KL: Counseling about the HPV vaccine: Desexualize, educate, and advocate, *J Pediatr Adolesc Gynecol* 26(4):243, 2013.

Bednarczyk RA, Davis R, Ault K, et al: Sexual activity-related outcomes after human papillomavirus vaccination of 11- to 12-year-olds, *Pediatrics* 130:798, 2012.

Rosenthal SL, Weiss TW, Zimet GD, et al: Predictors of HPV vaccine uptake among women aged 19-26: Importance of a physician's recommendation. *Vaccine* 29:890, 2011.

TABLE 25-7	CHAIN OF TRANSMISSION AND CONTROL: SEXUALLY TRANSMITTED DISEASES (STDS)				
	GONORRHEA	*Chlamydia trachomatis*	**SYPHILIS**	**GENITAL HERPES**	**WARTS, HUMAN PAPILLOMAVIRUS (HPV) INFECTION**
Occurrence	Worldwide; highest in males and females 15-30 yr old	Worldwide; most prevalent STD; continues to increase	Worldwide and increasing; highest in males and females 20-30 yr old	Worldwide and increasing; highest in males and females 15-30 yr old	Worldwide; most common STD (see Research Highlights box)
Etiological agent	*Neisseria gonorrhoeae*, the gonococcus	*Chlamydia trachomatis*	*Treponema pallidum*	Herpes simplex virus (HSV) types 1 and 2	HPV, which has 100 types
Reservoir	Humans	Humans	Humans	Humans	Humans
Transmission	Contact with exudates from mucous membranes of infected persons; usually by direct sexual contact, although the pathogens can be transmitted during childbirth	Contact with exudates from mucous membranes of infected persons; usually by direct sexual contact, although the pathogens can be transmitted during childbirth	Direct sexual contact with infectious exudates from lesions; transplacental; blood transfusion early in infection of donor	Direct contact with secretions from mucous membranes and lesions; transplacental	Direct contact with infected skin and mucous membranes; autoinoculation; during childbirth
Incubation period	2-7 days	7-10 days	3 wk; range 10 days to 3 mo	2-12 days	2-3 mo; range 1-20 mo
Communicability period	Months if untreated	Unknown	When moist lesions are present during the primary and secondary stages, generally 1 yr	During and up to 7 wk after primary lesions; transient shedding of virus occurs in absence of lesions for years	Unknown, probably as long as lesions persist
Susceptibility and resistance	General population is at risk; antibodies are not protective against reinfection	General population is at risk; no acquired immunity	General population is at risk; however, only 30% of exposures lead to infection; some immunity develops over time	General population is at risk; immune response does not prevent recurrence	General population is at risk; immunosuppressed persons are more susceptible
Prevention and control	Safer sexual practices; detect and treat cases and contacts; test pregnant women for infection and treat			Safer sexual practices; cesarean delivery if lesions are present during late pregnancy	Routinely immunize females and males aged 11-12 yr against HPV, with "catch-up" vaccination for females 13-26 yr; HPV vaccination may be recommended for some males aged 9-26 yr; safer sexual practices
Disease manifestations	*Males:* urethritis with purulent discharge from anterior urethra *Females:* mucopurulent cervicitis, often asymptomatic; 20% progress to endometritis, salpingitis, and pelvic peritonitis Both genders may have pharyngeal or anorectal infections, depending on their sexual practices; individuals are frequently co-infected with *N. gonorrhoeae* and *C. trachomatis*	*Males:* urethritis with purulent discharge from anterior urethra *Females:* mucopurulent cervicitis, often asymptomatic; 20% progress to endometritis, salpingitis, and pelvic peritonitis Both genders may have pharyngeal or anorectal infections, depending on their sexual practices; individuals are frequently co-infected with *N. gonorrhoeae* and *C. trachomatis*	*Primary:* moist lesion appearing within 3 wk at area of contact *Secondary:* symmetrical maculopapular rash in 4-6 wk *Latency:* indefinite time, no symptoms *Tertiary:* late lesions of bone, viscera, central nervous system (CNS), and cardiovascular system	Local, primary, vesicular lesions, period of latency and recurring, localized lesions; lesions start at area of contact but may spread to surrounding tissues or be disseminated in body, even to the CNS; other disease symptoms depend on extent of dissemination	Skin and mucous membrane lesions that are circumscribed, hyperkeratotic, and of varying sizes and shapes; certain types of HPV warts (16,18,31,33, and 45) have been found to be associated with cancer of the cervix, vulva, anus, penis, vagina, and oropharynx

TABLE 25-7	CHAIN OF TRANSMISSION AND CONTROL: SEXUALLY TRANSMITTED DISEASES (STDS)—cont'd				
	GONORRHEA	*Chlamydia trachomatis*	**SYPHILIS**	**GENITAL HERPES**	**WARTS, HUMAN PAPILLOMAVIRUS (HPV) INFECTION**
Diagnosis	Gram staining of discharges, bacteriological cultures, or tests that detect gonococcal nucleic acid	Failure to detect *N. gonorrhoeae* in discharges from symptomatic persons; mononuclear antibody tests of discharges	Serological testing of blood and cerebrospinal fluid, if indicated	Detection of cell changes in tissue scrapings or biopsy specimens; isolation of virus from lesions or other affected tissue; serological tests	Visualization of the lesion; excision and histological examination of the lesion
Treatment	Treat with antibiotics, preferably with single dose, intramuscular antibiotics, such as ceftriaxone; treatment depends on extent of infection; follow-up testing is recommended	Treat with antibiotics such as single-dose azithromycin or 7 days of doxycycline; advisable to treat for gonorrhea and chlamydia concurrently	Treat with antibiotics; treatment differs with stage of the disease	Treatment with antivirals; treatment varies depending on area of lesions and whether they are disseminated	Removal of the warts by freezing with liquid nitrogen or other chemical; treatment of cancers
Report to local health authority?	Yes	Yes	Yes, including congenital syphilis	No	No

Modified from Grimes DE, Grimes KA, Zack CM: Infectious diseases. In Thompson JM et al, editors: *Mosby's clinical nursing,* ed 5, St. Louis, 2008, Mosby; with data from Heymann DL, editor: *Control of communicable diseases manual,* ed 19, Washington, DC, 2008, American Public Health Association; from Centers for Disease Control and Prevention: *HPV vaccine,* 2009. Available from <www.cdc.gov/vaccines/vpd-vac/hpv/default.htm#vacc>; and from Centers for Disease Control and Prevention: *Sexually transmitted diseases (STD): Human papillomavirus (HPV),* n.d. Available from <http://www.cdc.gov/std/hpv/>.

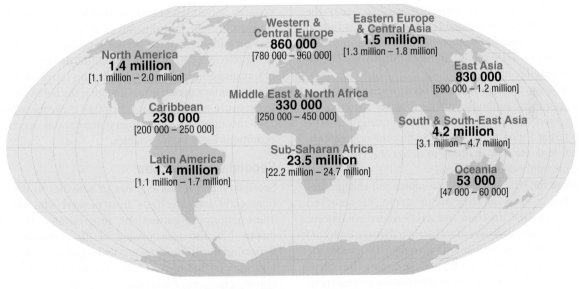

Total: 34.2 million [31.8 million –35.9 million]

FIGURE 25-4 Human immunodeficiency virus/acquired immunodeficiency syndrome (HIV/AIDS) worldwide, 2011. (From World Health Organization/UNAIDS: *July 2012 core epidemiology slides,* 2012. Retrieved from <http://www.unaids.org/en/media/unaids/contentassets/documents/epidemiology/2012/201207_epi_core_en.pdf>.)

the human body. Every nurse, regardless of area of practice, will eventually care for someone with HIV infection. Currently, there is no cure or vaccine, and minimal hope of stemming the continuing spread throughout the world (Figure. 25-4). It is not surprising, then, that *Healthy People 2020* objectives have an entire Topic Area specific to HIV/AIDS (Healthypeople.gov, n.d b).

HIV, a retrovirus, is the organism that causes the syndrome known as AIDS. Following initial infection, the disease is typically asymptomatic for months to years. Usually the infected person does not know that he or she is infected and continues to transmit the virus to others. The timeline for the usual course of HIV infection without adequate and persistent treatment with antiretroviral agents can be seen in

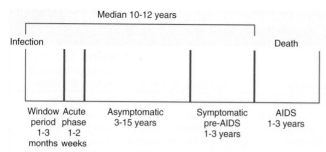

FIGURE 25-5 Usual course of human immunodeficiency virus (HIV) infection for persons not treated with antiretroviral medications. (Modified from Grimes DE, Grimes RM: *AIDS and HIV infection*, St Louis, 1994, Mosby.)

Figure 25-5. HIV usually manifests gradually as conditions that result from inadequate immune system function, as the virus slowly attacks the body's immune system. Over time, the body loses its ability to fight illnesses, and opportunistic infections occur and become recurrent. A standardized case definition for AIDS was specified by CDC in 1993. An updated case definition for AIDS as well as revised classifications for HIV infection can be found at http://www.cdc.gov/hiv/statistics/recommendations/. The critical elements for both HIV and AIDS are summarized for easy reference in Table 25-8.

HIV infection is usually determined by the HIV antibody test, and the most commonly used form is the enzyme-linked immunosorbent assay (ELISA) for antibodies in the blood. There may be false-positive findings, so Western blot analysis is frequently used to verify the results. Since 2004 a more rapid test for antibodies in oral fluid, as well as blood, has been available. Further information on testing for HIV can be found at http://www.cdc.gov/hiv/testing/index.html.

False-negative findings still may occur, especially before the body produces antibodies after exposure; therefore an exposed person who tests negative should undergo the HIV antibody test at 1 month and 3 months after the original test. Additional tests are now available to detect the virus in the blood before antibodies are present.

Treatment for HIV and AIDS is complex and changes frequently. The U.S. Food and Drug Administration has approved many drugs for HIV infection and AIDS-related conditions. At present there are six classes of antiretroviral drugs, each corresponding to different mechanisms whereby HIV invades the cells of the immune system. It is beyond the scope of this chapter to review them all here. Current information on treatment is always available from the CDC. One source is the HIV/AIDS Treatment Information Service, at www.aidsinfo.nih.gov.

Exposure of health care personnel to HIV, although rare, remains a concern for the CDC and health care workers. The CDC continues to update recommendations for postexposure prophylaxis (PEP) for occupational exposures. Although the principles of immediate treatment following exposure have not changed, the drugs and drug combinations have changed. These guidelines are among the many that can be downloaded from the CDC's website. Additional resources include a postexposure hotline for clinicians, the PEPline at 1-888-448-4911, which is available 24 hours a day, 7 days a week.

Before the development of effective antiretroviral therapies in the late 1990s, reported cases of AIDS provided a good indicator of the progression of the epidemic. With effective treatment, persons with HIV infection have taken longer to progress to having AIDS, and the incidence of AIDS has declined. This change has given the false impression that the epidemic was coming under control. Reporting cases of HIV infection has been incomplete and has varied by state. In 2011, all states reported HIV infection as well as AIDS cases by name (CDC, 2013a).

Eradication of HIV/AIDS depends on development of a vaccine and the infrastructure necessary to vaccinate populations at risk worldwide. Neither possibility is foreseen in the near future. Given that reality, control of HIV/AIDS currently depends on preventing transmission of the virus. One current approach is to successfully treat those who are infected to lower their viral load, thus lowering their risk of transmitting the virus. Problems with adherence to the therapy are interfering with the "treatment as prevention" approach.

PREVENTION OF COMMUNICABLE DISEASES

All practicing nurses have a role in primary, secondary, and tertiary prevention of communicable diseases. Examples of appropriate interventions are reviewed here and in Table 25-9.

Primary Prevention

Primary prevention of communicable diseases involves measures to prevent transmission of an infectious agent and to prevent pathology in the person exposed to an infection. All of the activities described in the section on breaking the chain of transmission are primary prevention activities. Immunization is primary prevention. Changing the behaviors that lead to exposure to a pathogen is primary prevention. See Tables 25-4 through 25-8 for primary preventions specific to the conditions listed in those tables.

Secondary Prevention

Secondary prevention consists of activities to detect infections early and effectively treat persons who are infected. These actions prevent not only progression of the infectious disease but also transmission of the pathogen to others. Reporting infectious diseases, investigating contacts, notifying partners, finding new cases, and isolating infected people also are examples of secondary prevention.

Tertiary Prevention

Tertiary prevention includes activities involved in caring for persons with an infectious disease to ensure that they are cured or that their quality of life is maintained. Perhaps the most important part of the treatment process is to ensure that people take their antimicrobial agents completely and effectively. In a time of increased resistance to pathogens, helping patients adhere to a drug regimen is critical. Additionally, caregivers should be taught to protect themselves and their environment by using appropriate precautions when caring for an infected family member.

TABLE 25-8	CHAIN OF TRANSMISSION AND CONTROL: HUMAN IMMUNODEFICIENCY VIRUS/ACQUIRED IMMUNODEFICIENCY SYNDROME (HIV/AIDS)

HIV/AIDS

Occurrence	Worldwide; in 2011 about 34.2 million persons estimated to be living with HIV, 69% residing in sub-Saharan Africa, 12% in South and Southeast Asia, 4% in Latin America, and 4% in North America; 2.5 million new infections in 2011; 1.7 million deaths
Etiological agent	HIV is a retrovirus with two serologically and geographically distinct types (HIV-1 and HIV-2); HIV-1 makes up 90%-95% of the world's cases; it may be more pathogenic, lead to more rapid disease progression, and have higher mother-to-infant transmission than HIV-2 does; multiple subtypes (sometimes called clades) have been identified for both HIV-1 and HIV-2
Reservoir	Humans; HIV may have evolved from a chimpanzee virus
Transmission	Direct person-to-person through unprotected sexual contact or from mother to fetus or mother to infant (during birth or by breastfeeding) Indirect through contact of abraded skin or mucous membranes with infected blood or body fluids, injection of contaminated blood or fluids, use of contaminated needles, or transplantation of organs from infected person

	HIV INFECTION	AIDS
Incubation period	1-3 mo before antibodies are detectable	<1 yr to 15 yr; may be longer with effective anti-retroviral therapy
Communicability period	Presumed to be <10 days after infection and lasting throughout life; may be highest in early infection when viral load is highest, and again later when clinical status worsens	
Susceptibility and resistance	General population is at risk; increased risk for infection with untreated ulcerative STDs and in uncircumcised males; evidence that some persons are less susceptible because of chemokine-receptor polymorphisms; very small percentage of infected persons do not progress to AIDS, for an unknown reason	
Prevention and control	Practice universal precautions and safer sex; treat pregnant women with antiretrovirals to prevent transmission to fetus; teach infected women to avoid breastfeeding; treat drug users and provide needle exchange programs for injection drug users; treat STDs to decrease chance of acquisition of HIV through sores on mucous membranes; maintain a safe blood supply; encourage autologous blood transfusions, when possible Early treatment of HIV-infected persons suppresses the virus enough to decrease risk of transmission to others	Adherence to effective antiretroviral therapy delays progression to AIDS; prophylactic treatment for opportunistic infections delays onset of conditions associated with AIDS diagnosis
Disease manifestations	Acute, self-limiting illness lasting for 1-2 wk with symptoms that mimic other conditions (fever, rash, pharyngitis, myalgia, lymphadenopathy, and malaise); although immune deficiency may progress, the person may be without further symptoms for years	Progressive immune deficiency and increasing susceptibility to life-threatening infections and cancers in untreated populations
Diagnosis	*Early after infection:* the p24 and polymerase chain reaction blood tests identify the presence of viral nucleic acids *Within 1-3 months after infection:* serologic tests (enzyme-linked immunosorbent assay, western blot) identify antibodies to HIV in the blood; a more rapid test is now available to detect antibodies in saliva.	A standardized case definition for AIDS was specified by the Centers for Disease Control and Prevention (CDC) in 1993 An updated case definition for AIDS and revised classifications for HIV infection can be found in the CDC document cited in "Resources" below
Treatment	Treatment with antiretroviral drugs to suppress the virus, not eradicate it; Currently six classes of drugs are available: nucleoside reverse transcriptase inhibitors, nonnucleoside reverse transcriptase inhibitors, protease inhibitors, integrase inhibitors, fusion inhibitors, and CCR5 antagonists; each attacks a different target in the reproduction process of the virus; current treatment strategies use at least 3 drugs from at least 2 classes; Requires almost perfect adherence to regimen because development of drug-resistant HIV is common Current guidelines recommend early treatment to suppress the virus to prevent transmission and treatment as pre-exposure prophylaxis (PrEP) for high-risk persons	
Report to local health authority?	Yes in all states	Yes in all states

RESOURCES FOR INFORMATION ON HIV/AIDS

Case Definition:
CDC definition (http://www.cdc.gov/hiv/pdf/statistics_HIV_Case_Def_Consult_Summary.pdf) **OR** *2012 UNAIDS Report on the Global AIDS Epidemic* (http://www.unaids.org)
Testing: www.cdc.gov/hiv/testing
Treatment: www.cdc.gov/hiv/topics/treatment **OR** www.aidsinfo.nih.gov
Treatment as prevention and pre-exposure prophylaxis: www.iapac.org

Data from Heymann DL, editor: *Control of communicable diseases manual*, ed 19, Washington, DC, 2008.

TABLE 25-9 EXAMPLES OF PRIMARY, SECONDARY, AND TERTIARY PREVENTION ACTIVITIES FOR CONTROL OF INFECTIOUS DISEASES AT THE INDIVIDUAL AND POPULATION LEVELS

INFECTIOUS DISEASE	INDIVIDUAL	POPULATION
Primary Prevention		
Sexually transmitted disease	Teach safe sex practices. Provide education and access to human papillomavirus (HPV) vaccine.	Place condom machines in accessible areas in places where young adults congregate.
Diseases caused by blood-borne pathogens	Teach barrier precautions to all health care workers. Teach injecting drug users about dangers of sharing needles.	Provide an adequate supply of gloves and sharps containers in patient care areas. Initiate city-wide needle exchange programs and methadone programs.
Vaccine-preventable diseases	Ensure that all children who come to the clinic have age-appropriate immunizations.	Work with community groups to cosponsor immunization clinics in areas where immunization rates are low. Work to counteract parental fears of vaccines. Educate on the value and safety of HPV vaccine.
Hepatitis A, gastrointestinal infections	Teach safe food-handling practices in the home.	Require, as part of the licensing of restaurants, that food handlers take a course in safe food handling.
Hepatitis A and B	Provide immune globulin after exposure to hepatitis A or B.	Mandate immunization of health care workers for hepatitis A and B.
Secondary Prevention		
STDs	Screen and treat for all STDs.	STD partner notification program
Tuberculosis	Screen close contacts of persons with TB. Treat persons with a recent skin test "conversion" (from negative to positive).	Initiate a program of yearly testing of health care workers for TB. Provide treatment to all with recent skin text conversions free of charge at their workplace.
Human immunodeficiency virus/acquired immunodeficiency syndrome (HIV/AIDS)	Provide testing and treatment for HIV in local clinics. Monitor patient adherence to antiretroviral therapy	Educate public about the concept of treatment as both prevention and pre-exposure prophylaxis
Meningitis	Provide immunization and chemoprophylaxis to persons exposed to meningitis.	Provide immunization and chemoprophylaxis to all students in a school following an exposure.
Tertiary Prevention		
Tuberculosis	Provide therapy for persons with active TB. Teach patients to take all doses of prescribed antibiotics, and monitor adherence.	Initiate a directly observed therapy (DOT) program in the community shelters and jails. Initiate community education campaigns about the problem of drug resistance associated with incomplete antibiotic use.

CASE STUDY

ASSESSMENT

Adrienne Zack is the Employee Health Nurse for a large city hospital. On a recent workday, she saw Beverly Yancy, a staff nurse in the newborn nursery of the hospital, who presented to the employee health clinic with a productive cough, wheezing, low-grade fever, chills, and fatigue lasting more than 1 month. Beverly stated that she had been treating her symptoms with over-the-counter antihistamines, cough suppressants, and antipyretics. When weighed in the clinic, Beverly was surprised that she had lost 10 lb since she was weighed last. She told Adrienne that she has no history of asthma or lung disease.

Beverly's employee health record revealed that she had had a positive tuberculin skin test (TBST) reaction of 15-mm induration when she was screened 11 years earlier for employment at the hospital. A chest radiograph at that time showed no evidence of tuberculosis (TB). Because Beverly was without TB symptoms at the time of employment and declined to take isoniazid (INH) for treatment of the latent tuberculosis infection (LTBT), she believed that the positive TBST reaction was the result of having received bacille Calmette-Guérin (BCG) vaccination at birth in the Philippines.

Furthermore, she has had no symptoms during her annual symptom screen by the Employee Health Clinic.

A chest x-ray showed suspicious areas indicating that Beverly most likely had active, infectious pulmonary TB. The diagnosis was confirmed when a sputum smear examination was positive for acid-fast bacilli (AFB). On the basis of the timing of Beverly's symptoms, Adrienne determined that Beverly's disease probably has been communicable for 3 months.

Diagnosis
Individual
- Active TB
- Potential for spread of TB to close contacts

Family
- Potential for undiagnosed TB

Community
- At risk for exposure to TB

CASE STUDY ASSESSMENT—cont'd

Planning

Mycobacterium tuberculosis (MTB) is transmitted by airborne droplets of sputum from persons with active disease who cough or otherwise discharge respiratory droplets into the air. Health care workers are at risk for TB infection because of frequent exposure to patients with active TB disease. Beverly could not have been infected by the newborns in the nursery where she worked. Most likely she was exposed to TB before her screening 11 years previously. The skin test reaction of 15-mm induration suggested a latent TB infection rather than a BCG vaccination at birth. Latent TB infection can become active tuberculosis disease at any time. In this case, latency lasted more than 11 years.

Health care workers, like anyone with active TB, can transmit the infection to close contacts such as coworkers, high-risk patients, and personal contacts. Newborns and children younger than 2 years are at high risk for acquiring TB infection and for progressing to TB disease. Such contacts must be found, screened, and treated as soon as possible. The incubation period for a detectable infection is 2 to 10 weeks following exposure. Recent contacts whose skin test results are negative now should be retested in 2 to 3 months.

Goals

Individual

Short-Term Goals

- Beverly will begin her course of medications immediately.
- Beverly will take short-term disability and will not return to work until her sputum culture results are negative and she is cleared by the employee health clinic.

Long-Term Goals

- Beverly will complete her course of medications as directed.
- Beverly will provide sputum cultures and undergo chest x-ray examination at 3, 6, and 9 months and will be free of evidence of active TB.

Family

Short-Term Goals

- All of Beverly's family members will be tested for TB within 3 days.
- Any family member testing positive will be started on a course of medication as recommended by the health department and his or her health care provider.

Long-Term Goal

- All family members will be retested in 6 months.

Community (Hospital)

Short-Term Goals

- Beverly's coworkers will be tested for TB within 3 days.
- The parents of all of Beverly's patients from the past 3 months will be contacted to encourage that they be tested and have their babies tested.
- Any contact or patient testing positive will be started on a course of medications as recommended by the local health department and his or her health care provider.

Long-Term Goal

- All contacts will be retested in 6 months.

Intervention

Tuberculosis must be reported to local public health authorities, who are responsible for control of TB in the community. Control relies on identifying and adequately treating all active TB cases and those with latent infections. The public health department will investigate Beverly's contacts inside and outside the hospital during the previous 3 months. This process will identify and treat persons, including the discharged newborns, to whom Beverly might have transmitted MTB. Adrienne and the other health clinic employees may be asked to assist with screening hospital workers exposed to Beverly and providing education about treatment.

Tuberculin skin test reactions are determined to be positive under the following conditions:

1. Induration of 5 mm in persons with HIV infection, those in close personal contact with someone with active TB, or persons who have fibrotic chest radiographs.
2. Induration of 10 mm in other high-risk persons, such as injecting drug users and persons with chronic disease or other causes of immune suppression and those from countries or communities where TB prevalence is high.
3. Induration of 15 mm for anyone who does not meet the preceding criteria.

All persons with a positive skin test reaction should be tested for active disease. Those for whom AFB are identified in a stained smear of sputum, mycobacteria are isolated from a cultured specimen, or there is radiological evidence of TB must be treated for active disease with a combination of drugs according to protocols established by the Centers for Disease Control and Prevention (CDC).

Multidrug-resistant TB (MDRTB) is an ever-increasing problem. Of active TB cases, 1% to 2% are now resistant to all available drugs. Patients must be helped to meticulously adhere to the prescribed regimen. Studies have demonstrated that health care workers are as poor as the general public at adhering to long-term drug therapy.

Persons with a recent "conversion" to a positive TBST result should undergo treatment for latent TB according to CDC protocols. Such treatment reduces lifetime risk that a latent infection will progress to active disease. Persons taking isoniazid should be taught the symptoms of side effects to the drug, including hepatotoxicity, peripheral neuropathy, and central nervous system (CNS) changes.

Teaching should include the following information:

- The importance of isolating oneself from contact with others and wearing a mask in public until sputum is clear of bacilli—around 4 to 8 weeks with effective treatment.
- Proper discharge of sputum and materials contaminated with sputum.
- Drug therapy must be continued uninterrupted for designated period even after sputum tests are negative for bacilli.
- Drug toxicity and side effects must be reported to the physician immediately. These include, but are not limited to the following:
  - *Isoniazid (INH):* Hepatotoxicity, peripheral neuropathy, CNS changes
  - *Ethambutol:* Reduced visual acuity with inability to see the color green
  - *Streptomycin:* Rash, fever, malaise, vertigo, deafness, gastrointestinal disturbance, CNS changes
  - *Pyrazinamide:* Hypersensitivity, hepatotoxicity, gastrointestinal disturbances, renal failure
  - *Rifampin:* Red-orange urine, hepatotoxicity, CNS symptoms
  - *Ethionamide:* Gastrointestinal disturbance and symptoms of hepatotoxicity
  - *Cycloserine:* CNS effects
- Sputum must be reexamined monthly until it tests negative for bacilli, then every 3 months for the duration of therapy.

Evaluation

Beverly and anyone else with active TB can return to work when the results of AFB testing of three sputum smear specimens collected 8 to 24 hours apart, at least one of which is an early morning specimen, are negative. Adrienne will refer to the CDC's latest guidelines for preventing transmission of tuberculosis in health care settings, available at www.cdc.gov/tb/topic/infectioncontrol/default.htm, and will update the hospital's infection control plan in accordance with the guidelines.

CASE STUDY ASSESSMENT—cont'd

Levels of Prevention

Primary

- Educate health care workers and others about TB infection and disease.
- Educate staff on airborne precautions and the proper use of respiratory protection.
- Design and implement signage throughout the hospital to remind staff and patients about respiratory hygiene, cough etiquette, and hand hygiene.

Secondary

- Establish regular screening of health care workers for positive skin test conversions.
- Establish mechanisms for detection, referral, and treatment of staff with latent TB infections and with active TB.
- Implement procedures for rapid detection and treatment of patients with active TB.
- Coordinate efforts with the local health department.

Tertiary

- Monitor medication compliance and follow-up testing.

Adapted from Centers for Disease Control and Prevention: Guidelines for preventing the transmission of *Mycobacterium tuberculosis* in health-care settings, *MMWR Morb Mortal Wkly Rep* 54(RR17):1-141, 2005. For more information on treatment of tuberculosis, go to: www.cdc.gov/tb/topic/treatment/default.htm.

SUMMARY

This chapter presents the challenges of infectious diseases that face community health nurses everywhere. It reviews principles that are the foundation for the occurrence, transmission, and control of infectious diseases and applies those principles to infectious diseases that are emphasized in the *Healthy People 2020* objectives. Most important, because nurses will be affected by infectious diseases wherever they practice, resources from which any nurse can obtain up-to-date information on any infectious disease at any time are included.

LEARNING ACTIVITIES

1. Subscribe to the e-mail Listserv to receive *Morbidity and Mortality Weekly Report* (www.cdc.gov/mmwr).
2. Attend an immunization clinic at your local health department to observe a nurse screening children for immunizations.
3. Obtain and evaluate health education materials regarding childhood immunizations from your local health department.

4. Log on to the website of an advocacy group against immunizations to understand the messages that they are communicating to the public.
5. Log on to your state health department website to learn about the process of reporting notifiable diseases in your state. Who is responsible for the reporting process? To whom do they report, what information is reported, and how often are diseases reported?
6. Log on to the CDC website to obtain the most recent guidelines for treating persons with HIV/AIDS, STDs, or tuberculosis.
7. Purchase a 1-year subscription to a public health nursing journal.

ⓔ EVOLVE WEBSITE

http://evolve.elsevier.com/Nies

- NCLEX Review Questions
- Case Studies
- Glossary

REFERENCES

Centers for Disease Control and Prevention: Recommendations of the advisory committee on immunization practices: revised recommendations for routine poliomyelitis vaccination, *MMWR Morb Mortal Wkly Rep* 48(27):590, 1999.

Centers for Disease Control and Prevention: Measles—United States, 2011, *MMWR Morb Mortal Wkly Rep* 61(15):253–257, 2012a.

Centers for Disease Control and Prevention: *2012 final pertussis surveillance report*, 2013. Available from <www.cdc.gov/pertussis//reporting.html>.

Centers for Disease Control and Prevention: *2011 sexually transmitted diseases surveillance*, 2012c. Available from <www.cdc.gov/std/stats11/default.htm>.

Centers for Disease Control and Prevention: Diagnoses of HIV infection in the United States and dependent areas, 2011, *HIV Surveillance Report* vol. 23, 2013a. Available from <http://www.cdc.gov/hiv/topics/surveillance/resources/reports>.

Centers for Disease Control and Prevention: *Incidence, prevalence, and cost of sexually transmitted infections in the United States*, 2013b. Available from www.cdc.gov/std/stats/STI-Estimates-Fact-Sheet-Feb-2013.pdf.

Dowdle WR: The principles of disease elimination and eradication, *MMWR Morb Mortal Wkly Rep* 48(Suppl 1):23–27, 1999.

Hall-Baker PA, Nieves Jr E, Jajosky RA, et al.: Summary of notifiable diseases: United states, 2007, *MMWR Morb Mortal Wkly Rep* 56(53):1–100, 2009.

HealthyPeople.gov: *Healthy People 2020: Topics & objectives*, n.da. Available from <www.healthypeople.gov/2020/topicsobjectives2020/> .

HealthyPeople.gov: *Healthy People 2020: Topics & objectives: HIV*, n.db. Available from <http://www.healthypeople.gov/2020/topicsobjectives2020/overview.aspx?topicid=22>.

HealthyPeople.gov: *Healthy People 2020: Topics & objectives: Immunization and infectious diseases*, n.dc. Available from <http://www.healthypeople.gov/2020/topicsobjectives2020/overview.aspx?topicid=23> .

HealthyPeople.gov: *Healthy People 2020: Topics & objectives: Sexually transmitted diseases*, n.dd. Available from <http://www.healthypeople.gov/2020/topicsobjectives2020/overview.aspx?topicid=37> .

Heymann DL, editor: *Control of communicable diseases manual*, ed 19, Washington, DC, 2008, American Public Health Association.

International Association of Physicians in AIDS Care (IAPAC): *Controlling the HIV epidemic with antiretrovirals: Consensus statement*, 2012. Available from www.IAPAC.org.

Schneider M-J: *Introduction to public health*, ed 2, Boston, 2006, Jones and Bartlett.

UNAIDS: *Report on the global AIDS epidemic*, 2012. Available from <http://www.unaids.org/en/media/unaids/contentassets/documents/epidemiology/2012/gr2012/20121120_UNAIDS_Global_Report_2012_en.pdf>.

World Health Organization: *Global tuberculosis report 2013*, 2013. Available from <http://www.who.int/tb/publications/global_report>.

Substance Abuse

Kim Jardine-Dickerson *

KEY TERMS

abstinence
addiction
Alcoholics Anonymous
case management
co-occurring disorders
delirium tremens
detoxification
dual diagnosis

harm reduction
initiation
intensive outpatient treatment
intervention
mutual help groups
National Institute on Drug Abuse
professional enablers
social consequences

Substance Abuse and Mental Health Services
substance abuse
substance abuse treatment
War on Drugs

OUTLINE

Etiology of Substance Abuse
Historical Overview of Alcohol and Illicit Drug Use
Prevalence, Incidence, and Trends
    Alcohol
    Illicit Drug Use
    Gender Differences
    Demographics
    Trends in Substance Use
Adolescent Substance Abuse
Conceptualizations of Substance Abuse
    Definitions
Sociocultural and Political Aspects of Substance Abuse
Course of Substance-Related Problems
Legal and Ethical Concerns Related to Substance Abuse
Modes of Intervention
    Prevention
    Treatment

    Pharmacotherapies
    Mutual Help Groups
    Harm Reduction
Social Network Involvement
    Family and Friends
    Effects on the Family
    Professional Enablers
Vulnerable Aggregates
    Preadolescents and Adolescents
    Elderly
    Women
    Ethnocultural Considerations
    Other Aggregates
Nursing Perspective on Substance Abuse
    Nursing Interventions in the Community
    Nursing Care Standards Related to the Patients with Substance Abuse Problems

* The author would like to acknowledge the contribution of Marilyn R. Mouradjian, who wrote this chapter for the previous edition.

Perhaps no other health-related condition has as many far-reaching consequences in contemporary Western society as substance abuse. These consequences include a wide range of social, psychological, physical, economic, and political problems. Drug abuse and addiction have negative consequences for individuals, families, and communities. Estimates of the total overall costs of substance abuse in the United States, including productivity and health- and crime-related costs, exceed $600 billion annually. This figure includes approximately $193 billion for illicit drugs, $193 billion for tobacco, and $235 billion for alcohol. These numbers in dollars do not describe the extent of public health and safety implications (National Drug Intelligence Center U.S. Department of Justice, 2011). Some of these critical implications are family disintegration, loss of employment, failure in school, domestic violence, and child abuse. Each year in the US, substance-abuse costs an estimated $1000 per person for health care, law enforcement, accidents, treatment, and lost productivity. More deaths, illnesses, and disabilities are attributed to substance abuse than to any other preventable health condition in the United States (Substance Abuse and Mental Health Services Administration [SAMHSA], 2012). In 2010, 10,228 people were killed in alcohol-impaired driving crashes, accounting for nearly one third (31%) of all traffic-related deaths in the United States. Each year, approximately 5000 youth (younger than 21 years) die as a result of underage drinking from accidents (U.S. Department of Transportation, 2012). The burdens that alcohol, tobacco, and other drug problems pose are compounded when the individual abuser is one of the estimated 54 million Americans who have one or more physical or mental disabilities. For these individuals, the process of recovery is made more difficult by barriers that do not exist for others.

The social consequences of substance abuse include its role in crime, need for money to buy substances, and specific theft of drugs. Many offenders commit crimes while under the influence of drugs, alcohol, or both. Between 35% and 50% of inmates in correctional facilities reported that they had been under the influence of drugs when their crime was committed. Furthermore, almost 75% of inmates report prior drug use (Bureau of Justice Statistics [BJS], 2014).

According to the U.S. Department of Justice (DOJ) National Drug Intelligence Center (2011), 37% of almost 2 million convicted offenders then in jail reported that they were drinking at the time of their arrest. Ninety-five percent of all violent crime on college campuses involves the use of alcohol by the assailant, victim or both, and 90% of acquaintance rape and sexual assault on college campuses involves the use of alcohol by the assailant, victim, or both (Robers, Kemp, & Truman, 2013).

All aggregates in society are potentially affected by substance abuse problems. Infants exposed in utero to alcohol, amphetamines, or opiates are at risk for withdrawal syndromes and later developmental problems. Indirect social effects of substance abuse include relationship conflicts, divorce, spousal and child abuse, and child neglect.

In the past, alcoholism and drug addiction were considered problems of the urban poor; society and most health professionals virtually ignored them. Substance abuse problems now pervade all levels of U.S. society, and awareness has increased. Community health nurses must be knowledgeable about substance abuse because it is a problem that frequently intertwines with other medical and social conditions.

This chapter focuses on helping community health nurses recognize substance abuse in their clients and in the larger community. It reviews historical trends, the causes of substance abuse, the most common symptoms of these disorders, and treatment options. The chapter also suggests nursing interventions appropriate for assisting those with substance-related problems in a community context.

ETIOLOGY OF SUBSTANCE ABUSE

Substance abuse has an impact on virtually every aspect of individual and communal life, and many institutions and academic fields have addressed it. Several theories attempt to explain the cause and scope of the problem and offer solutions. Some theories address individual, physiological, spiritual, and psychological factors. Others deal with social influences involving family, ethnicity, race, access to drugs, environmental stressors, economics, political status, culture, and sex roles. Most theories suggest that a combination of factors is the underlying impetus for substance abuse.

Although previous research studies have suggested a link between genetics and alcoholism, there is growing evidence that genetic variations may contribute to the nature of alcoholism within families. Individual and environmental factors also contribute to an increased risk for alcohol abuse. On the individual level, a person's inherited sensitivity to alcohol is a predictor for the development of alcohol abuse. Two broad personality dimensions are also associated with an increased risk for alcohol abuse. Impulsivity and ease of disinhibition add to risks for substance abuse. Proneness to anxiety and depression are also risks, and these comorbidities are not well understood. Alcohol expectancies (i.e., beliefs about anticipated consequences of drinking) are also a predictor of alcohol abuse. If one expects a certain effect, such as relief, one is more likely to feel it after use of a drug. The satisfied expectancies may set up neural pathways that are interpreted as pleasurable.

Medical models of alcoholism and other substance abuse conditions may not provide an understanding of commonalities among addictive behaviors (e.g., excessive drinking, gambling, eating, drug use, and sexual behavior). Cross-addiction, or multidrug use, is more prevalent now than in the past, and more studies point to the presence of both automatic and nonautomatic factors in physiological and psychological dependence. Specific biological medical models are giving way to multicausal models.

In the biopsychosocial model, risk factors interact with protective factors to develop a predisposition toward drug or alcohol use. This predisposition is then influenced by exposure to the substance, availability, and the experiential interpretation of the drug experience (e.g., pleasant or unpleasant). Continued availability of the substances and a social support system that enables or supports their use is also necessary. These factors combine to determine whether addiction develops and is maintained.

HISTORICAL OVERVIEW OF ALCOHOL AND ILLICIT DRUG USE

During the twentieth century, fluctuations in the use of alcohol and illicit drugs were influenced by shifts in public tolerance and political and economic trends. In general, alcohol use gained more social acceptance than other drug use. Alcohol consumption in the United States was higher during World Wars I and II and decreased during Prohibition and the Great Depression. Alcohol use was highest during the 1980s, when states lowered the drinking age to 18 years. Lawmakers became alarmed at the increased rate of drinking and the greater number of alcohol-related deaths among 18- to 25-year-olds after lowering the drinking age and thereby reversed the decision. During the late 1980s, alcohol use declined after the minimum drinking age was reinstated to 21 years. The decline in alcohol consumption through the 1990s and into the twenty-first century is attributed to less tolerant national attitudes toward drinking, increased societal and legal pressures and actions against drinking and driving, and increased health concerns among Americans. The identification of, and response to, driving under the influence of alcohol or another drugs is an example of a shift in thinking from addiction as the primary concern to other problems linked with, for example, alcohol use. These problems are thus termed *substance-related problems* and have become a significant community concern.

Public attitudes and governmental policies also have influenced the history of illicit drug use. Although nineteenth-century physicians prescribed morphine for a large variety of ailments, the discovery of the addictive properties of cocaine and opiates led to increased governmental regulation at the beginning of the twentieth century. The Harrison Narcotic Act of 1914, and subsequent laws, lessened the medical profession's control over the use of addictive drugs; the legislation specified that the physician could prescribe these drugs only in the course of general practice and not to maintain an addiction. This limitation on the physician's power to prescribe and dispense addictive drugs, and restrictions on the importation of narcotics, limited the supply of these drugs until the 1950s and 1960s. At that time, an increase in illegal drug trafficking caused heroin use to proliferate, particularly in inner cities.

By the 1970s, drugs were increasingly available. During this period, a counterculture population, composed largely of young people, focused their efforts on enhancing social justice, ending the Vietnam War, and lessening "repressive" sexual mores; many conceptualized drug use as a way to liberate the mind. Marijuana use occurred in communal, social settings; alcohol use was less favored because it was associated with the "establishment" the young people were critiquing. Consequently, the use of hallucinogens, cannabis, and heroin

spread beyond urban drug subcultures to the general population. Alarmed by the social and personal problems inherent in this change, the public grew less tolerant of drug use, and prevention and treatment programs were given more attention and resources. After peaking in 1979, illicit drug use decreased among most segments of the population throughout the 1980s, reaching a low in the early 1990s. The Anti-Drug Abuse Acts of 1986 and 1988 increased funding for treatment and rehabilitation; the 1988 act created the Office of National Drug Control Policy. The director, referred to as the "drug czar," is responsible for coordinating national drug control policy.

To combat concerns about the physical, social, and psychological impacts of drug abuse and dependence, federal drug policy has emphasized law enforcement and interdiction—the War on Drugs—to reduce the supply. Trends have shown renewed interest in prevention and treatment efforts to decrease the amount of illicit drug use in society and to lessen its impact (SAMHSA, 2012). In 2012 the Office of National Drug Control Policy (ONDCP), working on a public health approach to drug control, committed more than $10 billion to drug education programs and support for expanding access to drug treatment for addicts (ONDCP, 2013).

There are numerous federal resources that nurses and other health care professionals need to be familiar with. For instance, there is the National Institute on Drug Abuse (NIDA) (http://www.drugabuse.gov/). NIDA's mission is to lead the United States in research on drug abuse and addiction. NIDA's strategic goals address substance abuse as a complex disease and underlying causes. The institute works with research programs in basic, clinical, and translational science, including genetics, functional neuroimaging, social neuroscience, medication and behavioral therapies, prevention, and health services. There are four major goal areas—prevention, treatment, decreasing the spread of human immunodeficiency virus (HIV)/acquired immunodeficiency syndrome (AIDS)—and other priority areas. Research on pain and other compulsive disorders is in developmental stage. NIDA gathers data on health disparities related to drug addiction and its many effects. The institute has many education programs encompassing criminal justice, medical, and educational systems. NIDA continues to promote research addressing nicotine addiction, HIV/AIDS, and emerging trends as well as training and dissemination of science-based information on drug abuse.

The Substance Abuse and Mental Health Services Administration (SAMHSA), at http://www.samhsa.gov/index.aspx, builds and sustains programs, policies, information and data, contracts, and grants with the intent of helping the nation act on the knowledge that promotes behavioral health treatment through all levels of prevention. SAMHSA promotes programs that work with military families as well as justice systems (SAMHSA, 2011b).

PREVALENCE, INCIDENCE, AND TRENDS

The growing recognition of the widespread effects of substance abuse has initiated extensive collection of data by multiple agencies. This section describes selected statistics and current trends. The U.S. National Survey on Drug Use and Health is an annual survey conducted by SAMHSA that estimates the prevalence of illicit drug and alcohol use in the United States. Findings from a 2011 report include the following (SAMHSA, 2011a):

Alcohol

Slightly more than half (51.8%) of Americans aged 12 or older reported being current drinkers of alcohol in the 2011 survey, making for 133.4 million current drinkers in 2011. Nearly one quarter (22.6%) of persons aged 12 or older participated in binge drinking (about 58.3 million people). Heavy drinking was reported by 6.2% of the population aged 12 or older, or 15.9 million people. Among young adults aged 18 to 25 in 2011, the rate of binge drinking was 39.8%. The rate of current alcohol use among youths aged 12 to 17 was 13.3% in 2011. Youth binge and heavy drinking rates in 2011 were 7.4% and 1.5%, respectively. An estimated 11.1% of persons aged 12 or older had driven under the influence of alcohol at least once in the past year. There were an estimated 9.7 million underage (aged 12 to 20) drinkers in 2011, including 6.1 million binge drinkers and 1.7 million heavy drinkers (drinking more than 3 times weekly). Past month, binge, and heavy drinking rates among underage persons declined between 2002 and 2011 (http://www.monitoringthefuture.org//pubs/monographs/mtf-vol1_2012.pdf). Fifty-seven percent of current underage drinkers reported that their last use of alcohol occurred in someone else's home, and 28.2% that it had occurred in their own home. About a third (30.3%) had paid for the alcohol the last time they drank, including 7.7% who purchased the alcohol themselves and 22.4% who gave money to someone else to purchase it. Among those who had not paid for the alcohol they last drank, 38.2% got it from an unrelated person aged 21 or older, 19.1% from another person younger than 21 years old, and 21.4% from a parent, guardian, or other adult family member.

Illicit Drug Use

An estimated 22.5 million Americans aged 12 or older (8.7%) were current (past month) illicit drug users, meaning they had used an illicit drug during the month prior to the survey interview (SAMHSA, 2011a). Illicit drugs included marijuana/hashish, cocaine (including crack), heroin, hallucinogens, inhalants, and prescription-type psychotherapeutics (pain relievers, tranquilizers, stimulants, and sedatives) used nonmedically. The rate of current illicit drug use among persons aged 12 or older in 2011 was similar to the rate in 2010 (8.9%). Further findings are as follows:

- Marijuana was the most commonly used illicit drug. In 2011, there were 18.1 million past month users. Between 2007 and 2011, the rate of use increased from 5.8% to 7.0%, and the number of users rose from 14.5 million to 18.1 million.
- The number of persons who were past-year heroin users in 2011 (620,000) was higher than the number in 2007 (373,000).
- Hallucinogens had been used in the past month by 972,000 persons (0.4%) aged 12 or older in 2011. These estimates were lower than the estimates in 2010 (1.2 million or 0.5%).

- In 2011, 6.1 million persons (2.4%) aged 12 or older had used prescription-type psychotherapeutic drugs nonmedically in the month before the survey. These estimates were lower than the estimates in 2010 (7.0 million or 2.7%).
- The number of past-month methamphetamine users decreased between 2006 and 2011, from 731,000 (0.3%) to 439,000 (0.2%).
- Among youths aged 12 to 17, the current illicit drug use rates were similar in 2010 (10.1%) and 2011 (10.1%), but higher than the rate in 2008 (9.3%). Between 2002 and 2008, the rate had declined from 11.6% to 9.3%.
- The rate of current marijuana use among youths aged 12 to 17 decreased from 8.2% in 2002 to 6.7% in 2006, remained unchanged at 6.7% in 2007 and 2008, then increased to 7.4% in 2009. Rates in 2010 (7.4%) and 2011 (7.9%) were similar to the rate in 2009.
- The rate of current use of illicit drugs among young adults aged 18 to 25 increased from 19.7% in 2008 to 21.4% in 2011, driven largely by an increase in marijuana use (from 16.6% in 2008 to 19.0% in 2011).
- Among young adults aged 18 to 25, the rate of current nonmedical use of prescription-type drugs in 2011 was 5.0%, which was lower than the rate in the years from 2003 to 2010. There was also a decrease from 2005 to 2011 in the use of cocaine among young adults, from 2.6% to 1.4%.
- Among those aged 50 to 59, the rate of past-month illicit drug use increased from 2.7% in 2002 to 6.3% in 2011. This trend partially reflects the "aging into" this age-group of the baby boom cohort (i.e., persons born between 1946 and 1964), whose lifetime rate of illicit drug use has been higher than those of older cohorts.
- Among unemployed adults aged 18 or older in 2011, 17.2% were current illicit drug users, which was higher than the 8.0% of those employed full time and 11.6% of those employed part time. However, most illicit drug users were employed. Of the 19.9 million current illicit drug users aged 18 or older in 2011, 13.1 million (65.7%) were employed either full or part time.
- In 2011, 9.4 million persons aged 12 or older reported having driven under the influence of illicit drugs during the past year. This corresponds to 3.7% of the population aged 12 or older, which was lower than the rates in 2010 (4.2%) and 2002 (4.7%). In 2011, the rate was highest among young adults aged 18 to 25 (11.6%).
- Among persons aged 12 or older in 2010-2011 who used pain relievers nonmedically in the past 12 months, 54.2% had gotten the drug they most recently used from a friend or relative for free. Another 18.1% reported they had gotten the drug from one doctor. Only 3.9% had gotten pain relievers from a drug dealer or other stranger, and 0.3% had bought them on the Internet. Among those who reported getting the pain relievers from a friend or relative for free, 81.6% reported in a follow-up question that the friend or relative had obtained the drugs from just one doctor.

Nonmedical Use of Prescription-Type Psychotherapeutics

Nonmedical use and abuse of prescription drugs constitute a serious public health problem in this country. An estimated 52 million people (20% of those aged 12 and older) have used prescription drugs for nonmedical reasons at least once in their lifetimes. The NIDA Monitoring the Future (MTF) survey found that about 1 in 12 high school seniors reported past-year nonmedical use of the prescription pain reliever hydrocodone (Vicodin) in 2010, and 1 in 20 reported abusing oxycodone (OxyContin)—making these medications among the drugs most commonly abused by adolescents (NIDA, 2012). There are three classes of the most commonly abused prescription drugs: opioids, central nervous system depressants, and stimulants.

There has been a significant increase in the lifetime nonmedical use of pain relievers (20.8% of individuals aged 12 years and older), specifically Percocet, Percodan, Vicodin, Lortab, Darvocet, Darvon or Tylenol with codeine, propoxyphene or codeine products, oxycodone, and hydrocodone (NIDA, 2011).

Hallucinogen, Inhalant, and Heroin Use

Hallucinogen drugs cause hallucinations by disrupting the interactions of nerve cells and the neurotransmitter serotonin. There are profound distortions of perceptions of reality. People may see things, hears sounds, and feel sensations that seem real but do not exist. Some hallucinations may also produce emotional changes in behavior. There may be changes in mood, hunger sensations, body temperature, sexual behavior, and muscle coordination.

LSD (D-lysergic acid diethylamide), which was discovered in 1938 and is manufactured from lysergic acid, has unpredictable psychological effects, "trips" that may last 12 hours. Some doses of LSD may cause delusions and hallucinations. LSD may be sold in tablets, capsules, or, occasionally, liquid form; thus, it is usually taken orally. LSD is often added to absorbent paper, which is then divided into decorated pieces, each equivalent to one dose. Behavior of someone using LSD may manifest as psychosis. There may be other symptoms, such as increases in body temperature, heart rate, and blood pressure; sleeplessness; and loss of appetite (NIDA, 2011).

Peyote is a small, spineless cactus in which the principal active ingredient is mescaline. The peyote cactus has been used by natives in northern Mexico and the southwestern United States as a part of religious ceremonies. Tops (buttons) of the peyote cactus are cut from the roots and dried, then are chewed or soaked in water to produce an intoxicating liquid. Extracts are bitter and may be prepared into a tea by boiling the cacti for several hours. A hallucinogenic dose of mescaline is about 0.3 to 0.5 grams, and its effects last about 12 hours (NIDA, 2011).

Psilocybin(4-phosphoryloxy-N,N-dimethyltryptamine) is obtained from certain types of mushrooms that are indigenous to tropical and subtropical regions of South America, Mexico, and the United States. Mushrooms containing psilocybin are available fresh or dried and are typically taken orally. They may be brewed as a tea or added to other foods to mask their bitter flavor. Hallucinatory effects may appear within 20 minutes of ingestion and may last up to 6 hours.

PCP (phencyclidine) was developed in the 1950s as an intravenous anesthetic but was never approved for human use because of problems during clinical studies, including intensely negative psychological effects. PCP is a white crystalline powder that is readily soluble in water or alcohol. PCP can also be mixed easily with dyes and is often sold on the illicit drug market in a variety of tablet, capsule, and colored powder forms that are normally snorted, smoked, or orally ingested. PCP has a distinctive bitter chemical taste. When smoked, it is often applied to a leafy material such as mint, parsley, oregano, or marijuana. Depending on concentration and route of ingestion, its effects can last approximately 4 to 6 hours.

Uses of PCP, LSD, psilocybin, and MDMA (**methylenedioxymethamphetamine**), also known as Ecstasy, increase significantly after age 17 years (NIDA, 2010a).

Approximately 2% of individuals aged 12 to 25 years abuse inhalants. The inhalants of choice are amyl nitrite, or "poppers"; followed by glue; shoe polish, or toluene; correction fluid, degreaser, or cleaning fluid; gasoline or lighter fluid; and spray paints and other aerosols. Inhalants can be found in many products readily available in the home or workplace. Spray paints, markers, glues, and cleaning fluids contain volatile substances that have psychoactive properties when inhaled. They can be used especially, but not exclusively, by young children and adolescents. Most often these substances produce a rapid high that resembles alcohol intoxication, resulting in a loss of sensation and even unconsciousness. Serious and irreversible effects include hearing loss, limb spasms, central nervous system or brain damage, and bone marrow damage. Inhaling high concentrations of these substances may result in death from heart failure or suffocation.

In 2011, 4.2 million Americans aged 12 or older (or 1.6%) said they had used heroin at least once in their lives. It is estimated that about 23% of individuals who use heroin become dependent on it. An opioid drug, heroin is synthesized from morphine. Heroin usually is a white or brown powder or as a black sticky substance, known as black tar heroin. Injection of drugs like heroin brings about the highest risk of contracting HIV and hepatitis C. These diseases are transmitted through contact with blood or other bodily fluids, which can occur with sharing of needles or other injection drug use equipment. Hepatitis C is the most common blood-borne infection in the Unites States. HIV can also be contracted during unprotected sex, which drug use makes more likely. There is close association between drug abuse and the increased of infectious diseases.

Gender Differences

Overall, more males than females abuse prescription drugs in all age-groups except those 12 to 17 years old. Females in this age group exceed males in the nonmedical use of all psychotherapeutics, including pain relievers, tranquilizers, and stimulants. Among *nonmedical users* of prescription drugs, females 12 to 17 years old are also more likely to meet abuse or dependence criteria for psychotherapeutics. Female illicit drug use for ages 12 years and older is increasing, but there is little change in male illicit drug utilization (SAMHSA, 2010).

Demographics

Demographic correlates show some regional, racial, and gender differences and changes over the past few years. For example, people living in the West have the highest percentage of past month drug use, at 12.9%, compared with 9.7% for those in the Midwest, 9% for those in the Northeast, and 9% for those in the South. Additionally, rates of current illicit drug use vary significantly among major racial/ethnic groups. Rates were highest among American Indians or Alaska Natives (19.5%), followed by African Americans (16.9%), whites (14.4%), and Hispanics (12.3%). Asians had the lowest rate, at 7.4% (SAMHSA, 2010). Visit the SAMHSA Office of Applied Studies website, at www.oas.samhsa.gov/nhsda.htm for more information about substance abuse trends and statistics.

Trends in Substance Use

Research has revealed that problems associated with substance abuse may or may not relate to classically or clinically defined dependence or addiction. Many people are turning to recovery before they have developed physiological dependence. Thus many in the field have begun to differentiate between use and misuse (*misuse* being interchangeable with *abuse*), and these terms now appear in the literature. This section describes significant trends in substances that are being abused and discusses substance abuse among special populations.

Healthy People 2020 and Substance Abuse

The U.S. Department of Health and Human Services USD-HHS) set goals and objectives related to substance abuse in *Healthy People 2020* (HealthyPeople.gov, 2013). *Healthy People 2020*'s overarching goals for all Americans are attaining high-quality, longer lives with more prevention opportunities in preventable disease, disability, injury, and premature death. Positive directions in achieving health equity, eliminating disparities, and improving the health of all groups are much more possible today. With ideas to create social and physical environments that promote good health for all, more communities are working together in health promotion education and programs. *Healthy People 2020*'s mission encompasses promoting quality of life, healthy development, and healthy behaviors across all life stages. The use of harmful substances is indirectly and directly related to all of the leading health indicators (i.e., tobacco use, alcohol and other drug abuse, physical activity, overweight and obesity, mental health, injury and violence, environmental quality, responsible sexual behavior, immunization, and access to health care). The *Healthy People 2020* box presents selected objectives and targets from *Healthy People 2020* related to substance abuse.

♥ HEALTHY PEOPLE 2020

Selected Proposed Objectives for Substance Abuse

Policy and Prevention
- Reduction of proportion of adolescents who report they rode during the previous 30 days, with a driver who had been drinking alcohol
- Increase the proportion of adolescents never using substances
- Increase the proportion of adolescents who disapprove of substance abuse
- Increase the proportion of adolescents who perceive great risk associated with substance abuse
- Increase the number of drug and other specialty courts
- Increase the number of states with mandatory ignition interlock laws for first time and repeat driving offenders

Screening and Treatment
- Increase number of admissions to substance abuse treatment for injection drug use
- Increase the proportion of persons who need alcohol and/or illicit drug treatment and received specialty treatment for abuse or dependence in the past year
- Increase the proportions of persons referred for follow-up care of alcohol problems, drug problems after diagnosis, or treatment of one of those conditions in a hospital emergency department
- Increase the number of Level I and Level II Trauma Centers and primary care settings that implement evidence-based alcohol screening and brief intervention (SBI)

Epidemiology and Surveillance
- Reduce cirrhosis death
- Reduce drug-induced deaths
- Reduce past month use of illicit substance abuse
- Reduce the proportion of persons engaging in binge drinking of alcoholic beverages
- Reduce proportion of adults who drank excessively in the past 30 days
- Reduce average annual alcohol consumption
- Decrease the rate of alcohol-impaired driving fatalities
- Reduce steroid use among adolescents
- Reduce the past-year nonmedical use of prescription drugs
- Reduce the number of deaths attributed to alcohol
- Reduce the proportions of adolescents who use inhalants

From HealthyPeople.gov: *Healthy People 2020: 2013 objectives*, 2013. Retrieved from <http://www.healthypeople.gov/2020/topicsobjectives2020/overview.aspx?topicid=28>.

Methamphetamine

Methamphetamine (MA) has evolved as the most widely produced controlled substance in the United States. It is appearing in mass quantities, in part because of the ease with which the fertilizer anhydrous ammonia can be converted into MA, which has attracted more individuals to this clandestine business. Illegal street forms of the drug, often called crank, crystal, or meth, are available as a powder that can be injected, inhaled, or taken orally. In addition, a smokable form, known as ice or glass, is widely available. Currently, the preferred route of administration is injection, possibly because of the undesirable physical difficulties related to smoking MA (NIDA, 2010b).

The pleasurable effects of MA are due to the release of high levels of dopamine in the brain, leading to increased energy, a sense of euphoria, and greater productivity. Short-term effects are increased heart rate, insomnia, excessive talking, excitation, and aggressive behavior. Prolonged use results in tolerance and physiological dependence. MA has multiple negative effects for users, their families, and communities. It appears to damage the brain in ways that are different from, and more severe than, damage from using other drugs. Negative consequences range from anxiety, convulsions, and paranoia to brain damage. The DOJ reports the use of MA is associated with an increased incidence of violence in such forms as domestic abuse, homicide, and suicide, whether the user is a victim or a perpetrator.

MA is used predominantly by white young persons, with an overrepresentation of females. Thirty-six percent indicate that they were first introduced to the drug when they were younger than 16 years (SAMHSA, 2010). Rates of admission for treatment of methamphetamine vary by region. The highest is in Utah; however, most areas of the country are reporting an exponential rise of the manufacture and use of MA.

The impact of MA abuse on communities, families, and social networks is considerable. Reported use is highest among 20- to 29-year-olds. This group often has young children, putting these children at risk for abuse and neglect. The incidence of prenatal use is also rising, increasing the risk for children to be born with developmental problems, aggression, and attention disorders. Furthermore, exposure to combustible secondhand fumes puts children at risk for not only complications related to primary ingestion but also fatalities and injuries related to the highly combustible nature of the chemicals used in manufacture of the drug.

Steroids

Anabolic steroids are synthetic variants of the male sex hormone testosterone. The proper term for these compounds is anabolic-androgenic steroids. They can build muscle and are said to be androgenic, referring to increased male sexual characteristics. These steroids are taken orally, injected into the muscles, or applied topically. Doses taken may be 10 to 100 times higher than the doses prescribed to treat medical conditions. Steroids taken continuously can decrease the body's responsiveness to the drugs, increasing tolerance as well as causing the body to stop producing its own testosterone. Evidence suggests that steroid use among adolescents is decreasing (NIDA, 2010b). In 2011, in its annual survey used to assess drug use among our nation's teens, Monitoring the Future found that 0.9% of eighth graders, 0.9% of tenth graders, and 1.5% of twelfth graders had used anabolic steroids during the previous year. Steroid use is more common in athletes and other individuals willing to risk potential and irreversible health consequences to build muscle. There are other more potentially fatal risks, including blood clots, liver damage, premature cardiovascular changes, and increased cholesterol (NIDA, 2010b). Evidence also points at behavioral changes leading to an increased potential for suicide and aggressive and risky behaviors among steroid users.

Collaborative treatment programs that monitor both psychological and physical issues, including options of the drug use route as injection, are necessary to combat steroid abuse.

ADOLESCENT SUBSTANCE ABUSE

Youth are a particularly susceptible aggregate for substance abuse. Individuals between 18 and 25 years of age have the highest prevalence of illicit drug use during their lifetimes (65% of the population). The 2012 MTF Survey reported the rate of current marijuana use among youths aged 12 to 17 increased to 7.3% in 2009 and 7.4% in 2010 (Johnston et al, 2012).

One positive development is that teen use of cigarettes and smokeless tobacco has declined. The rate of current alcohol use among youths aged 12 to 17 was 13.6% in 2010, which was lower than the 2009 rate (14.7%). Youth binge and heavy drinking rates in 2010 (7.8% and 1.7%, respectively) were also lower than rates in 2009 (8.8% and 2.1%, respectively) (Johnston et al, 2012). It is noteworthy, however, that this significant decline in adolescent smoking and use of smokeless tobacco has decelerated sharply and seems to be on the verge of halting among tenth graders (NIDA, 2010b). Cigarettes are still highly available to the young, and concerned groups continue to monitor advertising that targets new potential smokers, such as youth and women.

With nearly half of teens trying marijuana before they graduate, there is definitely skepticism about the drug's danger. There is research that marijuana use during adolescence has the potential to set young people up for a cascade of life-altering events, impeding their success and hindering them from fulfilling their potential. Teens too often do not believe this to be true. The Monitoring the Future (MTF) survey of drug use has for years demonstrated a steady drop in the number of middle- and high-school students who think occasional or even regular marijuana users risk harming themselves physically or in other ways. With this declining perception, comes the risk of increasing use. One in 15 high-school seniors now use marijuana daily. In fact, although use of most drugs and alcohol continue to decline or hold steady, marijuana is almost the only licit or illicit drug showing significant 5-year increases (NIDA, 2012a).

The 2010 National Survey on Drug Use and Health (NSDUH) measured perceived risk as the percentage of youth reporting that there is great risk in the substance use behavior (SAMHSA, 2011a). The percentage aged 12 to 17 years who perceived great risk in smoking marijuana once or twice a week decreased from 54.7% in 2007 to 47.5% in 2010. Studies demonstrated that from 2002 to 2008, almost half of 12- to 17-year-old respondents reported in 2010 that it would be fairly easy or very easy to obtain marijuana. Most of the movement in teen substance use has been in a downward direction, but generally the declines have been marginal (NIDA, 2010c).

In order to effectively plan for the present and future needs of the community, the community health nurse needs the most current overall perspective. Information on the prevalence, incidence, and trends in the amount and types of substance abuse at the general, state, and local levels is readily available on the Internet. As harmful, illicit substances come in and out of vogue, particularly among young people, the community health nurse must develop a good understanding of drug culture, terminology, and differing signs and symptoms.

CONCEPTUALIZATIONS OF SUBSTANCE ABUSE

Conceptualizations of substance abuse and dependence have changed over the years, often for political and social reasons rather than for scientific reasons. Some conceptualizations focus on the phenomenon of addiction, which is manifested by compulsive use patterns and the onset of withdrawal symptoms when substance use is abruptly stopped. Other views focus on the problems resulting from the substance use itself, regardless of whether an addictive pattern is present. Problematic consequences of substance use include intoxication, psychological dependence, relational conflicts, employment or economic difficulties, legal difficulties, and health problems. For example, addiction need not be present for individuals to experience legal consequences of illicit drug use, such as driving while intoxicated or alcohol- or drug-related domestic violence.

Drawing fine distinctions among ideas of dependence, addiction, and abuse concerning substance use may seem irrelevant if there is evidence that the substance use has become problematic. However, broadly labeling all habitual or compulsive behavior patterns as addiction or dependence may obscure the fact that interventions could precede the development of addiction, for example, in cases in which use has become misuse and a problem is evident. It is also becoming increasingly evident that specific interventions may be needed for each separate addictive problem (e.g., overeating and gambling). Moreover, in each specific group, there is wide individual diversity.

Definitions

The term *substance abuse* came into common usage in the 1970s. Earlier conceptualizations generally focused on either alcoholism or drug addiction as singular addictive disorders. Most substance abuse theories identify core commonalties that occur in regard to use of a variety of substances or in relation to compulsive behavior syndromes. There is also an emphasis on relapse prevention that may include moderate use goals and abstinence.

There remains debate about how substance use and substance abuse should be defined and what substances should be included under each definition. Traditional conceptualizations of substance abuse focus solely on alcohol and illicit street drugs. Other conceptualizations include prescription medications such as tranquilizers and analgesics. In eating disorders such as bulimia and compulsive overeating, food is viewed as the abused substance. Table 26-1 shows a classification scheme for commonly abused substances.

In addition to varying in their abuse potential, substances vary in their degree of potential harm to those who use them and to others in the immediate environment. Tobacco is an example of a substance that is unsafe to the smoker and to those who inhale secondhand smoke. Those who abuse alcohol may also harm others by driving under its influence, and its lowering of inhibitions may foster violent activities in some users (e.g., child or partner abuse).

Integrating the various opinions regarding the diagnosis of substance abuse, the American Psychiatric Association (APA) has classified substance use disorders as either "dependence" or "abuse" (APA, 2013). The APA focused on the following psychoactive substances that affect the nervous system: alcohol, amphetamines, caffeine, cannabis, cocaine, hallucinogens, inhalants, nicotine, opioids, phencyclidine, sedatives, and hypnotics or anxiolytics. Substance use disorders can also be categorized as being in partial or full remission. A diagnosis of substance abuse indicates a maladaptive pattern of substance use that is manifested as recurrent and significant adverse consequences related to repeated use of a substance. These adverse consequences include failure to fulfill major role obligations, repeated use in physically hazardous situations, multiple legal problems, and recurrent social and interpersonal problems.

The criteria for the diagnosis of dependence include a cluster of cognitive, behavioral, and physiological symptoms that indicate continued use of the substance despite significant substance-related problems. A pattern of repeated, self-administered use results in tolerance, withdrawal, and compulsive drug-taking behaviors, which are frequently accompanied by a craving or strong desire for the substance. This craving then motivates the user to be preoccupied with supply, money to purchase drugs, and getting through time between periods of use, all of which take up mental energy, effort that is diverted from work or school and from connectedness to significant others. This process is how the use becomes problematic and how others around the user become confused and eventually often feel rejected, hurt, ignored, angry, or even responsible for the user's behavior.

SOCIOCULTURAL AND POLITICAL ASPECTS OF SUBSTANCE ABUSE

Within community settings, substance-related problems are not always easy to identify. For example, the consequences of the sale and use of crack cocaine in an inner-city, African American neighborhood may be apparent through media attention. The traffic of these drugs into the middle classes, on the other hand, is less easily recognized. The increasing tendencies of elderly persons to rely on alcohol and other, even illicit, drugs may be shocking to some nurses. It can be understood contextually, however, and may be the result of multiple factors, such as isolation, fears, uncontrolled chronic pain, anxiety, and sleep disturbances. Nurses must incorporate sociocultural and political dimensions into caring for clients in the community. Nurses must also possess knowledge that is useful in countering media stereotypes and allows them to

TABLE 26-1 CLASSIFICATION OF COMMONLY USED AND ABUSED SUBSTANCES

SUBSTANCE	DESIRED EFFECT(S)	POSSIBLE WITHDRAWAL SYMPTOMS
Central Nervous System Depressants		
Alcohol	Euphoria, disinhibition, and sedation	Anxiety, irritability, seizures, delusions, hallucinations, and paranoia
Barbiturates	Euphoria and sedation	Restlessness, tremors, and anxiety
Sedative-hypnotics (e.g., benzodiazepines [Rohypnol])	Sedation and amnesia	Insomnia, anxiety restlessness and tremors
Tranquilizers (e.g., GHB [gamma-hydroxy-butyrate], the "date rape" drug)	depress consciousness	Confusion, psychosis, agitation
Central Nervous System Stimulants		
Amphetamines (e.g., methamphetamine)	Euphoria, hyperactivity, omnipotence, insomnia, and anorexia	Depression, apathy, lethargy, and sleepiness
Cocaine	Increased sense of energy and alertness	Depression and anxiety
Nicotine	Calmness concentration	Restlessness and agitation
Caffeine	Concentration, energy	Restlessness and agitation
Narcotics-Opioids	Euphoria and sedation	Restlessness, pain and agitation
Codeine	Euphoria and sedation	Anxiety, irritability, agitation, runny nose, watery eyes, chills, sweating, nausea and vomiting, diarrhea, tremors, and yawning
Meperidine and acetaminophen (e.g., Demerol)	Euphoria and sedation	Restlessness, pain and agitation
Hydromorphone (e.g., Dilaudid)	Euphoria and sedation	Restlessness, pain and agitation
Fentanyl	Euphoria and sedation	Restlessness, pain and agitation
Heroin	Euphoria and sedation	Restlessness, pain and agitation
Methadone	Euphoria and sedation	Restlessness, pain and agitation
Morphine	Euphoria and sedation	Restlessness, pain and agitation
Opium	Euphoria and sedation	Restlessness, pain and agitation
Oxycodone (e.g., Percodan)	Euphoria and sedation	Restlessness, pain and agitation
Hallucinogens		
Mescaline	Hallucinations, illusions, and heightened awareness	Depression
LSD	Hallucinations, illusions, and heightened awareness	Depression
PCP (phencyclidine) (e.g., ketamine)	PCP: violent dissociative and anesthetic effect	
STP (2,5-dimethoxy-4-methylamphet-amine) and MDMA (methylenedioxy-methamphetamine (i.e., Ecstasy)	Hallucinations, illusions, and heightened awareness	Depression
Psilocybin (e.g., mushrooms)	Hallucinations, illusions, and heightened awareness	Depression
Cannabis		
Marijuana	Hallucinations, illusions, and heightened awareness	Depression
Hashish and THC (tetrahydrocannabinol)	Hallucinations, illusions, and heightened awareness	Depression
Inhalants		
Gasoline	Euphoria	Restlessness, anxiety, and irritability
Toluene acetate	Euphoria	Restlessness, anxiety, and irritability
Cleaning fluids	Euphoria	Restlessness, anxiety, and irritability
Airplane cement	Euphoria	Restlessness, anxiety, and irritability
Amyl nitrate	Euphoria	Restlessness, anxiety, and irritability

Modified from Faltz B, Rinaldi J: *AIDS and substance abuse: a training manual for health care professionals*, San Francisco, 1987, Regents of the University of California.

model a more holistic, multifaceted approach to prevention and management of substance abuse.

Although there are subcultural and regional variations, drinking norms of the dominant culture in the United States are relatively permissive. Traditional ethnic ceremonial and symbolic substance use patterns vary significantly. As acculturation occurs, however, cultural definitions of "appropriate" use of alcohol and drugs have been dulled, leaving a void regarding social expectations. Subcultural groups such as gay, lesbian, bisexual, and transgender persons have often had a social center that was a bar, and alcohol use was historically a way of demonstrating and celebrating differentiation from a more repressive majority. These cultural conditions create ambiguity in clearly determining when a substance abuse problem exists. Furthermore, each subculture may define *abuse* differently. It can be theorized that stigmatized minorities might be under more stress, and perhaps more likely to use substances, but this cannot be assumed in any individual case.

Substances are also given economic value and are bought and sold as commodities in a variety of social arenas, both legal and illegal. The ways in which drugs, including nicotine, medications, and alcohol, are produced and distributed among the various segments of the population are determined largely by economic, cultural, and political conditions.

These dynamics of drug distribution can bring many other consequences as various subgroups attain and maintain status. A group without cultural values, or with competing cultural values, suffers from chaos and disorganization. Competing value systems lead to cultural disintegration and a sense of powerlessness and hopelessness. The group becomes susceptible to forces that further threaten its ability to survive. When they are unable to organize or determine a collective direction because of conflicting values, the group and its members are separated and disempowered. The history of cocaine abuse and dependence among people of color is an example of how these conditions are interrelated. Indeed, cocaine use was epidemic in the 1980s and early 1990s, with crack cocaine most prevalent in poor communities, but its use has declined markedly in recent years (SAMHSA, 2011a).

COURSE OF SUBSTANCE-RELATED PROBLEMS

There is no predictable course of addictive illness and no "addictive personality type." When habitual use is well established, behaviors may be clinically visible and similar; this observation has led to assumption of a singular, addiction-prone personality. However, not everyone who initiates drug or alcohol use progresses to dependence or displays associated behaviors. Because the path from initiation to dependency is multidimensional, the context of client and community experiences is key to understanding and responding to problems encountered. Nurses need to take a comprehensive health and substance use history and place it in a context of cultural, historical, family, and social factors. Neither addiction nor dependency is a unitary phenomenon with a single isolated cause; rather, it is the result of interactions among a host of variables.

The assessment process should include consideration of the triad: the person, the substance, and the context or environment (Kornreich et al, 2012). The person assessment involves demographic information, medical history, comorbidities, and known perceptions and meanings the individual displays. The drug assessment consists of the qualities of the substance itself, physiopharmacological effects, pattern of use, availability,

and toxicity. Context assessment should cover family, social, employment, legal, cultural, and economic contingencies.

The progression from initiation to continuation, transition to abuse, and, finally, addiction and dependency varies. Individuals often describe a progression that began with initiation through social interactions. For some, the substance and setting are reinforcing and prime the individual for a pattern of use. For others, the experience is unpleasant enough to prevent further use. It cannot be assumed, however, that an unpleasant initiation will always be preventive. In the case of stimulants, such as MA, the drug produces such strong feelings of euphoria, alertness, control, and increased energy that future use is enticing, especially when the drug is easily accessible.

The continuation stage of substance abuse is a subsequent period in which substance use persists but does not appear to be detrimental to the individual. In stimulant abuse, continued use often occurs in a binge pattern. Individuals are able to exercise some control over use, but use becomes more frequent. Neither the individual nor the social network views use during this stage as problematic.

A critical point is the transition stage from substance use to substance abuse. It may be evident to both the user and his or her social network that the use of the substance is having adverse effects. During this stage, users begin to use more often and in more varied settings. Rationalizations that deny the seriousness and consequences of the substance use are commonly constructed during this stage.

The research on correlates and antecedents of substance abuse points to a variety of personal and social motivations. For many young people, motivators are the attraction of a rebellious subculture, peer pressure, and nationwide fads. Considerable research exists on the self-medication aspects of individuals with comorbid mental illnesses. Once the addiction is established, unpleasant physical and emotional withdrawal symptoms are strong motivators to continue use. Abstinence in the stimulant abuser can result in symptoms such as depression, lethargy, and anhedonia (i.e., inability to feel pleasure). The depression experienced by the user when not using stimulants is contrasted with the recalled euphoria produced by the use of the drug. These factors, coupled with associated cues, help initiate the cycle of binge use, with increased craving and continued self-administration to relieve symptoms. Brain imaging techniques have demonstrated that abuse of drugs such as cocaine and amphetamine produce immediate and long-lasting physical changes that are likely to contribute to the maintenance of dependency. Nurses can learn more about this research from the NIDA's web page on addiction science, at http://www.drugabuse.gov/related-topics/addiction-science.

The development of addiction or dependency is marked by changes in both behavior and cognition. There is a growing focus on the substance and a narrowing of interests, social activities, and relationships. The process of becoming dependent or addicted requires the individual to deny or ignore evidence or information that may challenge the behavior or the rationalization of the behavior. There is a preoccupation with the substance and its procurement during this stage, even in the face of negative consequences. Table 26-2 outlines the stages in the process of stimulant addiction.

LEGAL AND ETHICAL CONCERNS RELATED TO SUBSTANCE ABUSE

For the past 30 years, the United States has pursued a drug policy based on prohibition and the active application of criminal sanctions against the use and sale of illicit drugs. During this time, the number of criminal penalties for drug offenses has climbed to 1.5 million offenses. This increase in drug-related imprisonment is a result of harsher enforcement policies and longer mandatory sentences for possession of smaller quantities of drugs. Although some individuals are in prison for violent crimes (Mattson et.al, 2012) or major drug trafficking, many drug offenders are arrested for small-scale drug deals made to support their personal use (DOJ, 2011).

Alcohol use and abuse are different issues because the possession and sale of alcoholic beverages is illegal only if the individual involved is a minor. Concerns arise when individuals are intoxicated during work, while driving, or in situations that may affect the welfare of others. Legal penalties have increased for driving under the influence of alcohol because groups such as Mothers Against Drunk Driving (MADD) have influenced legislation.

One area that has also received the attention of the legal system is the use by pregnant women of substances known to increase risks to their fetuses in terms of future long-term developmental and behavioral problems. Pregnant addicts have been imprisoned and forced into treatment, and their children have been removed from their custody after birth. Many treatment providers and patient advocates view this approach as punitive and counterproductive to assisting these women and their children. There is concern that such sanctions may prevent addicted women from seeking treatment, for fear of legal consequences.

Military veterans are an aggregate also deserving quality **substance abuse treatment** (Bray et al, 2010; Tollison et al, 2012). The U.S. Department of Veterans Affairs (VA) can address the following areas in substance abuse: screenings for alcohol or tobacco use, outpatient counseling, intensive outpatient treatment, marriage and family counseling, self-help groups, and drug substitution therapies.

TABLE 26-2	TYPICAL COURSE OF ADDICTIVE ILLNESS: STAGES IN CONTINUUM FROM INITIATION TO DEPENDENCY
STAGE	**CHARACTERISTICS**
Initiation	First use of the substance
	Exposure frequently occurs through family or friends
Continuation	Continued, more frequent use of substance
	Usually social use only, with no detrimental effects
Transition	Beginning of change in total consumption, frequency, and occasions of use
	More than just social use, with beginning of loss of control
Abuse	Adverse effects and consequences of substance use
	Rationalizations for continued use and denial of adverse effects present in user and significant others
	Unsuccessful attempts at control of use
Dependency and addiction	Physical or psychological dependency, or both, on the substance; marked by behavioral and cognitive changes
	Preoccupation with the substance and its procurement, despite negative consequences
	Narrowing of interests, social activities, and relationships to only those related to the substance use

Use of a drug, alcohol, or tobacco by a pregnant woman, thereby exposing her developing fetus to the substance, can have potentially deleterious and even long-term effects on the exposed child. Smoking during pregnancy can increase risks of stillbirth, infant mortality, sudden infant death syndrome, preterm birth, respiratory problems, slowed fetal growth, and low birth weight. Alcohol use during pregnancy can lead to the development of fetal alcohol spectrum disorders, characterized by low birth weight and enduring cognitive and behavioral problems. Prenatal use of opioids and other drugs may cause a withdrawal syndrome in newborns called neonatal abstinence syndrome (NAS). These infants are at greater risk of seizures, respiratory problems, feeding difficulties, low birth weight, and even death. There are evidence-based treatments for pregnant women (and their babies), including medications. Methadone maintenance combined with prenatal care and a comprehensive drug treatment program can improve many of the detrimental outcomes associated with untreated maternal heroin abuse. However, newborns exposed to methadone during pregnancy still require treatment for withdrawal symptoms. A medication option for opioid dependence, buprenorphine, has been shown to produce fewer NAS symptoms in babies than methadone, resulting in shorter infant hospital stays. In general, it is important to closely monitor women who are trying to quit drug use during pregnancy and to provide treatment as needed.

Data from National Institute on Drug Abuse: *Principles of drug addiction treatment: A research-based guide,* 3rd ed, 2012b. NIH Publication No. 12–4180.

MODES OF INTERVENTION

Correlating with the numerous theories about substance abuse is the wide variety of **intervention** strategies incorporating all levels of prevention. National, state, and local legislative measures have attempted to limit access to potentially addictive pharmaceuticals and illicit street drugs. The growing social demand for smoke-free environments in public buildings, restaurants, airplanes, and similar areas exemplifies how perceptions of tobacco and its risks have changed over the past 50 years. Alcohol taxes, zoning schemes for liquor outlets, a legal drinking age, and legal sanctions on driving while intoxicated are other examples of community efforts to prevent or contain substance abuse.

Media campaigns provide public service communications about the risks of substance abuse and the availability of treatment for these problems. However, these efforts must have culturally relevant and realistic goals. Some have proved to be quite successful. The Partnership for a Drug-Free America conducted an anti-inhalant media campaign. Several goals of *Healthy People 2020* are reduction of the proportion of adolescents who report they rode, during the previous 30 days, with a driver who had been drinking alcohol; and increases in the proportions of adolescents who have never used substances, who disapprove of substance abuse, and who perceive great risk associated with substance abuse. Educational programs administered through schools and penal institutions have been developed, but evaluation and evidence of success or failure of the interventions have been sporadic. National organizations such as the Partnership for a Drug-Free America and the National Alliance on Mental Illness (NAMI) have national, state, and local chapters and affiliates that support community education, research, and support.

Prevention

The principles of prevention are paramount in community nursing practice. Primary prevention in the community includes working with other providers to perform a needs assessment. This process identifies high-risk situations and potential problems that threaten the integrity of the community and its inhabitants—in particular, what factors in the community are encouraging initiation of substance abuse, how effective school- and community-based programs are, and what political issues in the community may be influencing resource allocation.

On the federal level, primary prevention efforts have been overshadowed by the ongoing "War on Drugs." A significant amount of fiscal resources has been allocated to law enforcement, interdiction, crop eradication, and harsh, punitive laws to prosecute drug users and manufacturers. Debate continues at both the state and federal levels regarding the cost-benefit ratio of drug legalization or decriminalization. Supporters argue that legalization and decriminalization would lead to a reduction in crime and would move the drug problem out of the realm in which it is regarded as the moral failure of individuals toward more humane treatment approaches.

There is no question that substance abuse is a costly medical, social, and legal problem. Until society can effectively deal with the serious effects of two lethal but legal drugs, alcohol and nicotine, there will be an argument for adding further sanctions that is difficult to accept and justify. Other preventive efforts at government and private levels include community-based programs, training of health professionals, faith-based initiatives, volunteer consumer groups, organized sports programs, and employer programs.

The secondary prevention role of the community health nurse involves screening and finding resources and solutions specific to the particular community. It is important for the community health nurse to be aware of the evidence base for certain programs and to modify or discard those programs that have not proved successful over time.

Screening tools such as the CAGE test are brief and simple and allow health providers to talk about substance abuse by incorporating relevant questions into the interview and history of any client. A positive response to any of the CAGE questions does not constitute a diagnosis of alcohol or drug dependence, but it should raise suspicion and mandate further investigation. Prevention efforts should be specific to aggregates rather than directed at the general public. The Clinical Institute Withdrawal Assessment (CIWA) is a continual assessment protocol commonly utilized in the medical setting that helps patients transition through alcohol withdrawal with less risk of delirium tremens (DTs) and other medical problems (Riddle et al, 2010). The CIWA focuses on common withdrawal symptoms, such as nausea and vomiting, anxiety, paroxysmal sweats, tactile disturbances, tremors, agitation, orientation, auditory disturbances, and headaches.

Prevention efforts focusing on minority groups such as African Americans have been only marginally successful (NIDA, 2010c). A possible reason is that such treatment programs fail to incorporate culturally sensitive and appropriate interventions and strategies. The demand for a culturally specific approach is evidence that previous approaches, and the assumptions that underlie them, are insufficient for understanding and explaining the etiology of substance abuse among members of minority groups. Successful prevention efforts are usually not focused solely on alcohol and drug abuse but are community controlled and work toward improving individuals' general competencies, communication skills, and self-esteem.

Treatment

Substance abuse problems are socially defined and frequently attributed to sufferers who do not recognize their substance use as a problem. Furthermore, the substance abuse treatment system has increasingly taken on social welfare and criminal justice tasks. In this sense, substance abuse differs from many other health-related problems. Most states have laws pertaining to involuntary treatment of substance abusers. Employers and families are often enlisted to assist or coerce the identified client into accepting treatment. This aspect of substance abuse as a health concern raises some crucial questions for health care providers in terms of the encroachment of therapeutic interventions on individual rights to privacy, informed consent, and self-determination.

On the individual level, those providing substance abuse treatment should take into consideration the cultural and educational background and resources of the person, the attitudes of significant others, the degree of invasiveness of the effects of the substance use, and the existence of alternatives. Interventions have been developed to assist some individuals in achieving moderation. Additionally, some research has shown that a small percentage of individuals who recognize a harmful pattern of substance use are able to stop using the substance or to achieve a controlled, nonpathological pattern of use. There are those who, because they experience an important life change, such as graduating from college or getting married, appear to change from excessive alcohol use to social alcohol use.

Nevertheless, people exhibit serious problems related to their use of substances and are usually not able to stop or control their use without outside intervention. Research on identified problem drinkers' ability to return to social alcohol use is still inconclusive. Consequently, most scientists and health care providers advocate **abstinence** as a cornerstone of recovery.

Abstinence is difficult to maintain on a long-term basis. Therefore, an important area of continuing research is relapse prevention (i.e., a behavioral approach that aims to prepare the client for the relapse situation in the hope of preventing it or minimizing its impact on recovery). Relapse prevention models can be applied to alcohol, drug, and behavioral addictive problems (e.g., overeating and compulsive gambling) and can have either controlled use or abstinence as their goal. In relapse prevention, relapses are reframed as learning opportunities, and the client makes plans for coping with negative mood states, meeting the challenge of craving, and stopping a relapse quickly if it should occur.

Inpatient and outpatient are the two main types of treatment programs for substance abuse. Each of these programs may or may not include a detoxification component. Treatment programs also differ in the following ways: they may be voluntary or compulsory and pharmacologically based or drug free. In general, although treatment is intricately tied to the concept of recovery, disciplinary philosophy guides specific treatment approaches. There are a variety of treatment approaches and models, which are sometimes contradictory. The treatment models vary by such factors as the composition of staff and the philosophical approach (i.e., social vs. psychological vs. medical models) to substance abuse problems.

Inpatient treatment isolates individuals from the external world and provides an opportunity to focus only on substance abuse issues. Outpatient treatment is appropriate for those who do not require such structure and protection, those with strong supportive social networks and high levels of motivation, and those who need to continue working while in recovery.

The severity of the individual's alcohol or drug problems and pertinent cultural factors determine the necessity and type of treatment. Therefore the assessment process is of primary importance and begins with an accurate social and medical history. The history taking begins with more general questions about lifestyle, employment, relationships, and self-perception. This general line of questioning permits the development of a therapeutic relationship with the client.

A therapeutic relationship based on trust is essential to collecting information about sensitive issues such as drug and alcohol use. The assessment should then proceed to determining risky behavior patterns and stressors. The interviewer assesses dietary practices; prior health problems; allergies; hospitalizations, including psychiatric disorders; and family history of similar problems, including drug- and alcohol-related problems. This general line of questioning can be followed by more specific questions about harmful behaviors, such as smoking, drinking, and illicit drug use. This ordering of questions progresses from the more socially sanctioned behaviors to more "socially disapproved" behaviors and from the general to the more specific. Positive responses to questions about drug and alcohol use should be probed in a nonjudgmental, direct way and treated as "routine" in health care encounters.

A physical examination is another valuable tool in evaluating the client for potential or actual alcohol and drug problems. Although at-risk clients may not have physical signs of alcohol and drug problems and may even deny obvious consequences of such, certain physical findings warrant further investigation. Complaints such as vague, nonspecific abdominal pain, insomnia, depression, chronic fatigue, back pain, chronic anxiety, refractory hypertension, and night sweats require more intensive investigation. Consistent and heavy users of methamphetamine commonly experience extensive and rampant tooth decay, known as "Meth Mouth," owing to the acidic nature of the drug. Although laboratory tests may not yield clues to drug or alcohol use, certain laboratory findings (e.g., abnormal liver function), in the absence of other etiological agents, may raise the index of suspicion.

Intervention strategies frequently begin with information about the effects of alcohol and drugs and a discussion of the solutions to substance abuse–related problems. This initial educational approach can defuse frequently encountered barriers to intervention, such as shame, guilt, fear, and the client's erroneous perceptions regarding risks. Presenting information and solutions in a nonjudgmental and clear manner may help minimize defensiveness. Reframing interventions within the context of health maintenance or health promotion and education minimizes the sense of stigma.

Ambivalent clients may respond to education and decide to abstain from substances or seek treatment. Other clients, however, even when confronted with legal, financial, physical, and psychological consequences of substance abuse, may resist treatment offers. Therefore the clinician must continue to work with clients and involve important members of their social network to remove internal and environmental barriers and move clients toward readiness for change and treatment. Potential discrimination in group settings and logistical problems, such as lack of child care, may be barriers to treatment.

Much of the effort for substance abuse treatment has been invested in detoxification, residential, and outpatient treatment programs. Secondary problems related to drug and alcohol abuse are intoxication, overdose, and withdrawal. Overdose may be accidental or intentional and requires acute interventions to stabilize the client. As a client advocate, the community health nurse can be an important ally in ensuring that adequate follow-up is conducted for those admitted to emergency departments for overdose. **Detoxification** is best described as a short-term treatment intervention designed to manage acute withdrawal from the substance. It involves medical management to reduce the adverse side effects of the substance and help stabilize the client. It may be performed on an inpatient or outpatient basis, depending on the substance and severity of dependence.

Addressing acute withdrawal symptoms is of utmost importance in detoxification. The cocaine abuser may experience extreme depression with suicidal ideation. Withdrawal from central nervous system depressants, including alcohol, produces the most life-threatening medical consequences, including anxiety, tremors, delirium, convulsions, and possible death, unless medically managed. Symptoms of withdrawal from narcotics, although less life threatening, are temporarily disabling and painful; they include chills, sweating, cramps, and nausea. Such feelings may cause the individual who is withdrawing from treatment to begin the cycle of abuse again. Detoxification is one of the most crucial periods in the recovery process. Clinicians should be aware of the level of services offered in any detoxification program in order to make appropriate referrals.

Outpatient and inpatient treatment programs vary, but they usually include group and individual therapy and counseling, motivational interviewing, family counseling, education, and socialization into 12-step mutual self-help groups. Many programs are integrating psychotherapy, such as cognitive-behavioral therapy, with pharmacotherapy. The medications used are discussed more fully in the next section. Other strategies are hypnosis, occupational therapy, confrontation, assertiveness training, blood alcohol–level discrimination training, and other behavior modification approaches. Relapses are common; therefore the most effective treatment programs incorporate some form of relapse prevention as a part of the healing process.

Therapy that involves the family has proved to be most effective in aiding recovery. Family and social contacts can be helped to initiate change in the abuser, to aid in recovery, and to assist in maintenance of treatment gains. A well-known family involvement motivational technique is the Johnson Institute Intervention, which involves a confrontation of the abuser with guidance from therapists. A less coercive version is called A Relational Sequence for Engagement (ARISE), whereby significant others are educated and coached over time. Another effective strategy is Community Reinforcement and Family Training (CRAFT). With this approach, a concerned significant other is trained in techniques such as positive reinforcement, identification of dangerous situations, and stress reduction. The television network Home Box Office (HBO) made a video called "Getting an Addict into Treatment: The CRAFT Approach"; it can be seen at http://www.hbo.com/addiction/thefilm/supplemental/628_addict_into_treatment.html. NIDA (2012b) published a research-based guide to drug addiction treatment. Important points from this publication are listed in Box 26-1.

Treatment programs have been unprepared for the influx of users of MA and the unique problems associated with its use. Prolonged MA use may lead to serious acute psychotic disorders with intensive physical and psychological withdrawal, characterized by protracted anhedonia and dysphoria and accompanied by severe craving. Currently, there are no medications to reverse overdoses of and no reliable drugs to treat the paranoia and psychosis associated with MA. Complications of treatment include high dropout rates, severe

BOX 26-1   GUIDELINES FOR DRUG ABUSE TREATMENT

- Drug addiction is a brain disease that affects behavior.
- Recovery from drug addiction requires effective treatment, followed by management of the problem over time.
- Treatment must last long enough to produce stable behavioral changes.
- Assessment is the first step in treatment.
- Tailoring services to fit the needs of the individual is an important part of effective drug abuse treatment for criminal justice populations.
- Drug use during treatment should be carefully monitored.
- Treatment should target factors that are associated with criminal behavior.
- Criminal justice supervision should incorporate treatment planning for drug abusing offenders, and treatment providers should be aware of correctional supervision requirements.
- Continuity of care is essential for drug abusers reentering the community.
- A balance of rewards and sanctions encourages pro-social behavior and treatment participation.
- Offenders with co-occurring drug abuse and mental health problems often require an integrated treatment approach.
- Medications are an important part of treatment for many drug abusing offenders.
- Treatment planning for drug abusing offenders who are living in or reentering the community should include strategies to prevent and treat serious, chronic medical conditions, such as human immunodeficiency virus/acquired immunodeficiency syndrome (HIV/AIDS), hepatitis B and C, and tuberculosis.

From National Institute on Drug Abuse: *Principles of drug abuse treatment for criminal justice populations: a research-based guide*, 2012. Retrieved from <http://www.drugabuse.gov/sites/default/files/podat_cj_2012.pdf>.

behavioral and psychotic states, and severe craving. Various treatments for MA abuse and addiction are being tried, with mixed results. The effect of MA on brain functioning suggests a need for longer treatment plans. The most promising is a long-term comprehensive case study approach, using home visits and assisting with transportation and emergency fund provision. Cognitive-behavioral therapy and contingency management are other promising approaches for treatment of MA abuse and dependence (NIDA, 2010c). Treatments currently being studied include aversion therapy, medication therapy, and matrix treatment plans.

Studies show that clients respond favorably to treatment for MA use, but because of the multiple dimensions, it is a very challenging problem. Women with MA problems who have young children require a higher level of care. Specifics may include an environment of security and safety with social and emotional support (Wright et al, 2012). Because many abusers lack a supportive environment, the potential for relapse is high. Also, because of MA addicts' typical inability to recognize the problematic nature of their use, combined drug court and outpatient treatment strategies are being developed.

Having a substance abuse problem does not mean that all problems are attributable to the addiction. Many substance-abusing clients also have other psychiatric problems (e.g., schizophrenia, depression, bipolar affective disorder,

BOX 26-2 CRITERIA FOR MEASURING EFFECTIVENESS OF SUBSTANCE ABUSE TREATMENT PROGRAMS

- Number of days abstinent
- Number of days without negative consequences of substance use
- Employability or work attendance
- Self-image improvement
- Spouse's assessment of client's functionality
- Regular attendance at 12-step group meetings
- Compliance with follow-up appointments
- Absence of overt psychiatric symptoms such as depression and anxiety
- Self-reports of progress
- Evidence of personal satisfaction and growth

dissociative disorder, posttraumatic stress disorder). Likewise, many of these clients have chronic medical problems (Chesher et al, 2011; Sabri, 2012). In cases with compounding problems, specialized attention involving a case management approach is warranted.

Research demonstrates that treatment for substance abuse can be more effective than no treatment, but evaluation of treatment alternatives requires establishment of appropriate criteria to measure effectiveness (Staton-Tindall et al, 2011). Examples of criteria that have been used are shown in Box 26-2. It is clear that treatment programs vary and that certain programs will be more culturally appropriate and therefore more effective than others for particular aggregates of individuals.

Pharmacotherapies

In the search for successful treatment of those susceptible to drug and alcohol problems, several pharmacotherapeutic adjuncts to formalized treatment have been developed. Medications include drugs used to assist in the initiation and maintenance of abstinence, drugs used as substitutes for illegal drug use, and drugs used to treat comorbidities. This section discusses pharmacotherapies that providers currently use. Good clinical judgment and patient motivation should guide the use of any pharmacotherapy, and therapy should be combined with psychosocial support.

Pharmacotherapeutics are used in detoxification, stabilization, and maintenance; as antagonists; and as treatment for coexisting disorders. Clinically, it is considered better to prevent withdrawal symptoms with medication than to wait for symptoms to appear. Methadone is the treatment of choice in withdrawal from heroin and other opiates. As a detoxification agent, methadone is dispensed over an 8-day period in a tapering dose. Dosage depends on the severity of opiate withdrawal symptoms present. A widely used example of the use of medication for long-term stabilization is methadone maintenance. The client is prescribed daily administration of a long-acting opioid (methadone) as a substitute for the illicit use of opiates (typically heroin). A large body of research confirms its effectiveness in treatment retention and in reduction

of risks such as human immunodeficiency virus (HIV) (http://www.drugabuse.gov/publications/drugfacts/heroin).

However, there are continuing varying philosophical opinions about abstinence versus sanctioned use in the debate over the use of methadone. Methadone maintenance is more controversial because the individual remains dependent on the drug. It is dispensed under medical supervision as part of a treatment program. Maintenance may minimize or abate illegal activity, eliminate the infection hazards of injection drug use, reduce the social disruption typically seen with opiate use, and facilitate increased levels of functioning. A myth about maintenance programs is that methadone produces a euphoric "high" and is therefore merely a legal substitute for heroin.

Naltrexone is a long-acting narcotic antagonist traditionally used as an adjunct in the treatment of opiate dependence. It blocks the effects of opiates via competitive binding, but it does not block the effects of other substances, such as benzodiazepines, cocaine, and alcohol (Center for Substance Abuse Treatment, 2005). Studies indicate that naltrexone is also effective in reducing craving, rates of relapse to alcohol, and severity of alcohol-related problems.

Buprenorphine is an opioid agonist-antagonist that has been used in the treatment of opiate-dependent clients and those with concurrent cocaine dependence. Buprenorphine does not produce severe withdrawal on abrupt cessation of its use, giving it an advantage over methadone. Its antagonist component helps reduce the possibility of lethal overdose. Clinical studies support the use of buprenorphine in reducing the frequency of heroin and cocaine self-administration.

Use of disulfiram (Antabuse) to promote cessation of alcohol abuse is rare today because of serious safety issues. A select group (i.e., those who are relapse prone, those who have supportive networks, and those who have histories of abstinence) may benefit from its short-term use. Requests for disulfiram should not be granted in the absence of treatment and supportive relationships. Disulfiram, when combined with alcohol, produces the classic disulfiram ethanol reaction (DER) (i.e., flushing, tachycardia, nausea, headache, chest tightness, and chest pain). The DER is thought to be the result of a disturbance in alcohol metabolism. The response, which typically begins within minutes after alcohol consumption, is dose dependent and highly variable. Significant risks of the DER are cardiovascular symptoms of tachycardia, hypotension, dysrhythmia, and shock. Preexisting cardiac disease is an absolute contraindication to disulfiram. Emergency treatment of the DER is symptomatic.

Benzodiazepines are considered effective tools for alcohol withdrawal because they decrease the likelihood of seizures and delirium (SAMHSA, 2010). Acamprosate (calcium acetyl homotaurinate; Campral) has been used successfully in Europe over the past decade and was approved for use in the United States in 2010. The main efficacy is in reducing frequency of drinking and maintenance of abstinence. Acamprosate reduces glutaminatergic transmission and neuronal hyperexcitability during withdrawal from alcohol. This drug has a low incidence of side effects but should be used under the care of a physician and prescribed cautiously in patients with liver or kidney problems.

Mutual Help Groups

Mutual help groups are associations that are voluntarily formed, are not professionally dominated, and operate through face-to-face supportive interaction focusing on a mutual goal. Many mutual help groups exist, and they are usually organized by recovering substance abusers or those recovering from compulsive behavior patterns. The first mutual help group was Alcoholics Anonymous (AA), founded in 1935. Initially, a small group of male alcoholics found a way to stay sober "one day at a time" through meeting regularly with others like themselves. The early AA members developed 12 steps to guide the recovery process, which are summarized in Box 26-3.

As a nonprofessional ongoing source of assistance, AA is viewed as an invaluable resource to the community. However, not all of those with alcohol problems find AA comfortable, culturally relevant, and socially supportive. Because of the realities of social discrimination and regional variation in customs, AA should not be considered a universal form of assistance for alcohol problems. Predominantly in large cities, women and members of racial, ethnic, religious, or sexual preference minority groups with alcohol problems have formed their own AA groups and other mutual help organizations for support in recovery.

Other 12-step programs have developed through the adaptation of AA's approach to similar addictive problems. Narcotics Anonymous, Gamblers Anonymous, Debtors Anonymous, Cocaine Anonymous, Overeaters Anonymous, and Sex and Love Addicts Anonymous are examples. Because they became organized more recently than AA, these groups may not be as well known or as widely available, and they may not exhibit as much diversity among their membership as AA. Children, partners, and close associates of substance abusers have also founded self-help groups, such as Al-Anon, Codependents Anonymous, and Adult Children of Alcoholics. Although these groups initially had a predominance of female members, the trend is moving toward participation by equal numbers of men and women.

AA meetings are not standardized. Customs shaping the actual format and sequence of the meeting vary according to region, group size, ethnic and sex composition, and other cultural variations of the members. In general, 12-step meetings follow one of the following formats:

- Uninterrupted talks by one or more speakers about "what it was like, what happened, and what it is like now."
- Each person at the meeting being given the opportunity to speak briefly during discussion.
- A combination of the first two options.
- Meetings either closed or open to the general public.

At least two mutual help groups have developed in response to their founders' negative experiences in AA or their failure to succeed in AA. Women for Sobriety was organized in 1976 to replace or augment AA for women; it addresses women's needs to overcome depression, guilt, and low self-esteem. Secular Sobriety Groups were organized to meet the needs of individuals who are unable to accept the concept of, or to depend on, a "higher power" in their recovery from alcohol problems.

Other mutual help groups that do not follow the 12 steps are available for a variety of addictive problems. AA does not require dues or fees, but some groups, such as Weight Watchers, require monetary commitment. Other groups, such as Recovery Incorporated, have more professional involvement. Any of these groups could be a resource for selected people with substance abuse problems.

To be effective, interventions for substance abuse must take place at multiple levels and must involve a number of individuals, activities, policies, and substances. Table 26-3 summarizes some of the many interventions available for substance abuse at various levels.

TABLE 26-3	MODES OF INTERVENTION FOR SUBSTANCE ABUSE
LEVEL	**INTERVENTION**
Individual and family levels	Education
	Treatment: detoxification, inpatient, outpatient, and residential
	Mutual help groups (e.g., Alcoholics Anonymous, Narcotics Anonymous, Cocaine Anonymous, Al-Anon)
Community level	Law enforcement measures to limit access to and distribution of addictive substances (e.g., street drugs)
	Alcohol taxes and zoning schemes for liquor outlets
	Legal drinking age and legal sanctions on driving while intoxicated
	Educational programs at schools and penal institutions
	Television and radio public service communications concerning the risks of substance abuse and the availability of treatment
State and federal levels	Formation of national associations such as the National Council on Alcoholism and Drug Dependence
	Establishment of federal research entities such as the National Institute on Drug Abuse and the National Institute on Alcohol Abuse and Alcoholism to centralize research, education, and treatment efforts
	Specialty courts/problem-solving courts (drug courts, veteran courts)

BOX 26-3	BASIC TENETS OF 12-STEP PROGRAMS

- Admission of defeat and surrender to a higher power
- Inventory of past shortcomings and strengths
- Spiritual practices (e.g., prayer and meditation)
- Willingness to change
- Making amends
- Extension of this process into daily life

Harm Reduction

New approaches reflecting a changing view of drug and alcohol addiction have been proposed for substance use problems that are not amenable to traditional approaches. Some of these have been grouped under the general term **harm reduction**. Harm reduction consists of individual and collective approaches to the treatment of substance use that are not primarily aimed at complete abstinence from all substances. Instead, incremental change is sought, which involves elimination of the more harmful effects of substance use through behavior and policy modifications. Harm reduction is a process rather than a static approach or an end in itself. It is used in various ways, depending on the context and the needs of individual clients (Lucas, 2012).

Harm reduction strategies remain controversial, although some see them as evidence of a paradigm shift with the potential to significantly improve treatment results. They are often the only options that will preserve a therapeutic relationship when people continue to use or drink problematically. An early example of harm reduction is the substitution of methadone for heroin. Although they are still using an opiate, individuals taking methadone can be functional without getting high and without the need to engage in criminal activity for drugs. Harm reduction psychotherapy aims to support the process of self-transformation through empathetic resonance, raising awareness of harm, setting goals, and understanding the multiple meanings of the substance. Harm reduction has been used in response to alcohol, illicit drugs, and tobacco use. In the case of alcohol, harm reduction might involve decreasing the number of drinks, decreasing the number of days in which drinking occurs, or avoiding drinking when driving.

On a community level, harm reduction may include attempts to legislate for decreased access to alcohol or raising the legal age for drinking. More controversial public health projects aimed at harm reduction are legalization of some illicit drugs and needle exchange programs. Needle exchange programs have had some success, and although they may not lead the intravenous drug user to abstinence, they do, in fact, serve to break the link in the deadly chain of exposure to and transmission of AIDS.

Viewed from a community health perspective, harm reduction involves planned social and policy changes. The goal of these changes is to decrease health risks consequent to alcohol and other drug use among specific aggregates (Wright et al, 2012). Although harm reduction strategies are not usually sanctioned by lay support systems (e.g., 12-step groups), they can have an important impact. Community health nurses using harm reduction strategies can help reduce drug- and alcohol-related social problems by advocating for programs that "bridge the gap" for those who cannot immediately reach the goal of abstinence.

In 2010, the rate of alcohol-impaired driving fatalities per 100,000 population was 3.3, representing a significant 20-year decrease. For every 100,000 people in the United States in 2010, slightly more than 3 people were killed in a drunk driving fatal crash, a rate that has been cut almost in half over the past two decades. Alcohol-impaired driving fatalities accounted for 31% of the total vehicle traffic fatalities in 2010. The rate of drunk driving fatalities per 100,000 population has decreased 48% nationally, and 63% among those younger than 21 years. These improved statistics are positive indicators of the gains being made to fight drunk driving. According to the National Highway Traffic Safety Administration, 33,808 people died in traffic crashes in 2010 in the United States, or on average of 1 death every 51 minutes. Among the people killed in these drunk driving crashes, 65% were drivers, 28% were motor vehicle occupants, and 7% were non-occupants.

SOCIAL NETWORK INVOLVEMENT

Family and Friends

The social network of the substance abuser either can be highly influential in helping the individual alter behavior or can aid and abet the substance abuser in self-destruction. There is evidence for both positive and negative effects of social support in either mitigating or supporting the behaviors of substance abusers (Winters et al, 2008). Evidence suggests that particularly among adolescents and young adults, substance use and abuse often occur in the context of social interactions. Adolescents may use alcohol and other substances as social lubricants during an often-troubled developmental period. Family treatment is considered essential because of the potential for enabling behavior. In addition, the family has suffered the effects of substance abuse emotionally, socially, economically, physically, and spiritually. The family's wounds must be acknowledged and treated in order for the substance abuser to return to an environment supportive of recovery.

A user's social network may play a role in allowing the substance abuse to continue. Spouses may call to work to report that their partner is "sick" or may remain silent after discovering evidence of abuse. Complex community and family interactions that serve to promote certain behaviors are commonly known as *codependency* and *enabling*. The boundaries between the nonaddicted family members and addict waver, with the result that the excessive substance-abusing behavior is covered up or excused. Social network members may compensate for the fact that the student is absent from school, the car payment is late, or an important appointment is canceled or forgotten. These distress signals are common but often go unrecognized because periods of use are often interspersed with periods of abstinence. This behavior reinforces the individual's, and often the significant other's, perceived sense of control over the substance use. There are mutual help groups for addressing codependency that are founded on the principles of AA and provide opportunities to discuss the issues germane to the alcoholic or addicted family system or network. Families participating in treatment should also be encouraged to participate in these mutual help groups.

Codependency cannot be concretely defined the same way in each culture. Cultural groups vary in the degree to which individuals are expected to anticipate the needs of others and care for them. The danger in applying a rigid definition of codependency in all cases is that it might unfairly and inappropriately label it as a disease in some cultures that value interdependency over individualism.

Through development of a therapeutic relationship and comprehensive assessment, the community nurse should identify the important members of the social network for each client and the ways in which these individuals provide support for the client. The nurse must also recognize that the concept of family refers not only to nuclear families but also to alternative family systems. Whatever the constellation of family, significant others should be included in the treatment and intervention. Substance abuse, addiction, and recovery do not occur in a vacuum, and many relapses are precipitated by interpersonal conflicts.

Effects on the Family

Substance abuse has been called a family disease because it affects the entire family system and holds potential adverse psychological and physical consequences for the family members in addition to the abuser. Family theorists view families, whether the traditional nuclear form or an alternative, as social systems that try to stay in balance (Winters et al, 2008). Professionals may see families as either functional or dysfunctional, depending on how well they fulfill the social tasks expected of them by society. Substance-abusing families are frequently observed to be dysfunctional in clinical terms. However, cultural and political factors should also be considered, because families may have developed these patterns for historical reasons rather than as the effects of substance abuse.

A functional family system is open and flexible and allows its members to be themselves. In the nuclear family model, the parents model intimacy for the children, differences are negotiated, boundaries are defined and maintained, and communication is consistent and clear. In functional family systems, whether the traditional nuclear family or other non-traditional forms, there is trust, individuality, and accountability among family members. All family members are able to have their needs met in a reasonable way.

On the other hand, dysfunctional families are closed systems with fixed, rigid roles. In the case of substance abuse, a major purpose of the system is to deny the substance abuse of the affected family member and keep it a "shameful" family secret. Generally, ego boundaries between the family members are weakened or nonexistent, with enmeshment of the members and an intolerance of individual differences. Rules are rigid and communication is unbalanced; the dynamics are either always conflicting or always superficially pleasant. Children may become involved in a "role reversal" in which they act as caretakers of their parents.

When one or more family members are substance abusers, family functions revolve around the substance abuser and accommodate or compensate the abuser's behavior (Winters et al, 2008). The individual needs of other family members are often unmet. Denial is central to a "dysfunctional" family system. The spouse of the substance abuser may gradually take over latter's role, functions, and control of the family. The children are cast into various roles in their struggle for survival in this environment and to maintain the family.

Adult children from dysfunctional families often carry these roles and coping mechanisms into adult life, with many becoming substance abusers or partners of substance abusers. The children of alcoholics are four to nine times more likely to experience alcohol use disorders than children of nonalcoholics. Frequently, they have difficulties with intimacy and parenting. Many have lifelong emotional problems, such as depression and anxiety, and physical illnesses often associated with these conditions (e.g., ulcers, colitis, migraine headaches, and eating disorders). However, some offspring exhibit thriving and resilient behavior. Using a strength-based approach, the community health nurse can work with resiliency factors (Martel et al, 2009).

In addition to psychological burdens that substance abuse places on families, there are the financial burdens related to medical costs, loss of income from job difficulties or unemployment, and the financial losses attributable to divorce. Furthermore, spousal violence and child abuse and neglect are strongly associated with substance abuse.

Professional Enablers

Health care professionals can also contribute to the initiation and continuation of substance abuse and dependency in various ways, becoming **professional enablers**. One obvious way is the physician's role in prescribing psychoactive medications. The medical model advocates the treatment of symptoms with medication. The relief of pain, anxiety, and insomnia is not an exception. The addictive potential of narcotic analgesics and antianxiety agents is often ignored if quick symptom relief is the main goal. Long-term goals for the treatment of medical problems and nonmedication management of pain and anxiety are more thoughtful approaches. However, under-medication or refusal to use "addictive" medicines can lead susceptible clients to self-medicate with illegal drugs or alcohol.

Physicians and nurses are often the first to see the physical effects of substance abuse and are in an excellent position to intervene. By focusing on the health consequences of substance abuse, they can form trusting relationships, provide information, and refer patients to the appropriate treatment. Too often, this opportunity is missed because the health care professional is reluctant to bring up this taboo subject. This reluctance may be based on professionals' inability to examine their own drinking or drug-taking behaviors, or those of significant others, or on concerns about negative responses from clients.

In the past, many psychiatrists and psychotherapists have focused on the reasons the client uses substances rather than on the dependency itself. The assumption was that insight would lead to a change in behavior. This approach has usually not proved to be effective, especially if the psychiatrist is concurrently prescribing other potentially addictive antianxiety medications or hypnotics. Complete abstinence from all mood-altering medication is a model for preventing the cross-addiction common in substance abusers (i.e., substituting one substance for another, such as a benzodiazepine for alcohol). Exceptions to this approach are patients with serious medical conditions requiring pain medication and those who also have a second psychiatric disorder that requires medication (i.e., schizophrenia, depression, bipolar affective disorder). The recovering substance abuser often needs support when he or she must take medication for these psychiatric conditions because others may criticize the use of any medication and place the patient in a difficult situation.

Caregivers have become more aware of signs of client substance abuse. Some providers are willing to begin therapy with a nonabstinent client under the stipulation that, if therapeutic gains are not made, the client will be referred for treatment or the caregiver will withdraw services. Clients who lack social support may succeed using this strategy, which allows the formation of a trusting relationship before taking the leap to abstinence. Clinical wisdom and research continue to point toward more tailored, individualized approaches to substance abuse.

VULNERABLE AGGREGATES

When viewed from a community perspective, substance abuse problems clearly affect some populations more severely than others. Some groups are more susceptible to experiencing substance abuse problems, may tend to deteriorate more quickly in the process, or may have fewer sources of support for recovery. These groups, termed *vulnerable aggregates*, require special attention in terms of prevention, intervention, and rehabilitation strategies.

Current resources for prevention, treatment, and mutual support may not be flexible enough to meet the needs of various vulnerable aggregates who are at risk of experiencing substance abuse problems and are often excluded or alienated from services by policies, provider attitudes, economic constraints, and social isolation. This section describes the issues of substance abuse with several vulnerable aggregates, including adolescents, the elderly, women, and racial and ethnic minorities.

Hispanic youth may have positive recovery outcome with family intervention programs such as "the Familia Adelante Program" (Cervantes and Goldbach, 2012). This program looks at and works with HIV prevention, risk, and family intervention.

Preadolescents and Adolescents

Why do young people use drugs? It is clear that drug and alcohol use among adolescents is a pervasive problem with many devastating consequences. The trend data in some aspects are undoubtedly worse for adolescents than for adults. The teenage years may be a turbulent time for some because of the necessary developmental tasks of discovering their own unique identity, learning how to form intimate relationships, and developing autonomy. Currently, this maturing is accomplished in a confusing era in which the cultural status of adolescents is undefined. Today's teenagers are an increasingly independent subculture with more money available than any time before, yet they have not attained full adult status.

The teenage years may be a time of experimentation, searching, confusion, rebellion, poor self-image, alienation, and insecurity. There is no such thing as the typical adolescent substance abuser, and there are multiple theories of causation for the abuse. Researchers have concluded that adolescent drug use is a symptom and not the cause of maladjustment. Those with significant difficulty are usually using substances as coping mechanisms.

Studies have identified various predictors of adolescent substance abuse. For example, use of legal substances (e.g., tobacco, alcohol) almost always precedes use of illegal drugs. Poor school performance, a social setting in which drug use is common, and drug use among peers are the strongest predictors of subsequent drug involvement, followed by strength of family bonds (NIDA, 2010c). The younger the initiation, the greater the probability of prolonged and accelerated substance use. Other contributing factors are the feeling of powerlessness and selling drugs as a viable economic solution to poverty. Subculture theory describes the status and power that charismatic leaders have to influence members of peer groups. In drug-using peer groups, such leaders have influence over inexperienced drug users and acculturate them into the drug scene. Thus it is crucial that communities work to maintain strong family and social bonds.

The community health nurse can play an important part in advocating for these vulnerable children and educating teachers on the vital importance of maintaining a validating, nonjudgmental attitude toward these students.

It is especially important that families are supported in the community. Substance abuse is less likely in families who give clear messages and have open communication and more likely in families in which parents are alcoholic, condemning, overly demanding, or overly protective. Committed family involvement helps retain the adolescent in treatment. However, it must be remembered that many well-functioning families have children who succumb to substance abuse. There is positive outcome with wraparound recovery programs (Walker and Sanders, 2011). Wraparound programs take a team approach, with children, parents, counselors, and other invested team members involved in the adolescent's successful recovery through abstinence, education, and life skills. Families whose teenagers are substances abusers also may experience significant community rejection and judgmental attitudes.

The preadolescent years are a particularly vulnerable time for initiation into and subsequent problematic substance use. The number of teens between seventh and twelfth grades being offered drugs is increasing (NIDA, 2010c). When drug use escalates in adolescents, it can have devastating long-lasting consequences. There is a strong relationship between adolescent behavior problems, such as aggressiveness, delinquency, and criminal activity, and heavy alcohol use between the ages of 12 and 17 years.

Escalating use of substances enhances the risk of school and social failure, criminal activities, violent behavior, sexual risk taking, sexual violence, depression, suicide, and unintended injuries. Primary prevention for adolescents is typically focused on education aimed toward complete abstinence, which some say is unrealistic. Education plays an important role. A striking feature is the strong inverse relationship between perceived risk and drug use. Historically for all drugs, with no change in drug availability, when students perceive a drug as harmful, fewer students actually use it. However, marijuana use has increased in use as demonstrated by the 2011 MFT study (SAMHSA, 2011a).

Responsible media efforts can bring about change but only with accompanying parental and community efforts. Early detection of predisposing factors, such as underlying psychiatric illness, is important. Other strategies are providing structured clubs and organizations and facilitating school success, career skills, family communication skills, and conflict resolution. Secondary prevention is targeted at inpatient and outpatient treatment and harm reduction.

However, almost as important as intervention and treatment is recognizing when treatment is unnecessary. Not all drug use requires therapy, nor is it even desirable. Not all young drug users are antisocial or mentally unstable, nor should they be labeled as such. Most will develop a responsible philosophy concerning substance use if given support and opportunity.

Anabolic steroids do not cause the same high as other drugs. Use of this type of steroid can lead to addiction. Steroid use may persist despite physical problems and negative effects on social relationships that it causes. Steroid abusers typically spend large amounts of time and money obtaining the drug. Individuals who abuse steroids often experience withdrawal symptoms when they stop using them, including mood swings, fatigue, restlessness, loss of appetite, insomnia, reduced sex drive, and steroid cravings. One of the most dangerous withdrawal symptoms is depression. Persistent depressive symptoms can sometimes lead to suicide attempts. Research has found that some steroid abusers turn to other drugs, such as opioids, to counteract the negative effects of steroids (NIDA, 2012b).

Elderly

Elderly men and women are considered vulnerable to substance abuse problems because of diminished physiological tolerance, increased use of medically prescribed drugs, and cultural and social isolation. Conservative estimates indicate that 6% to 11% of elderly patients admitted to hospitals exhibit symptoms of alcoholism, as do 20% of the elderly in psychiatric hospitals, and 14% of elderly patients in emergency departments (SAMHSA, 2010).

Misuse of prescription drugs may be the most common form of drug abuse among the elderly. According to NIDA (2010c), elderly persons use prescription medications approximately three times as frequently as the general population. In addition, data from the Veterans Affairs Hospital System suggest that elderly patients may be prescribed inappropriately high doses of benzodiazepines.

Women

Since the 1970s, much attention has been turned to substance abuse problems in women. Evidence is mounting that alcohol use and abuse affect women much differently from how they affect men. Women absorb and metabolize alcohol differently, partly because of body composition differences and the production of less gastric alcohol dehydrogenase in women (Center for Substance Abuse Treatment, 2009). Specific aggregates of women may be more severely affected by substance abuse problems, including those from minority groups, those with low or no income, and those of the working classes. The increased risk stems from economic, social, and cultural factors.

Lesbians are another aggregate of women in whom substance abuse may be associated with marginalization and should be understood within the diversity of lesbians individually and culturally. This issue is especially heightened in periods when homosexuality is demonized through media, churches, and legislation linking homosexuality with pathology and when lesbians and gays are denied the right to marry (e.g., civil unions, partner benefits).

Women who were abused as children are more susceptible to substance abuse problems in adolescence and adulthood than are nonabused women. They also face many more distressing consequences in substance abuse treatment and recovery. Disclosure of abuse in group treatment contexts or 12-step meetings is risky. In some cases, women are told to compartmentalize the abuse issues and speak only of addiction. In other cases, women are told that if they do not disclose in a group they will fail in their recovery program (Center for Substance Abuse Treatment, 2009). However, many current-day treatment programs designed for women now routinely address interpersonal violence in individual and group settings, leaving disclosure up to the client.

Drug-dependent women report frequent physical and medical problems, many related to their reproductive systems (Center for Substance Abuse Treatment, 2009). Women tend to experience symptoms of alcoholic hepatitis and cirrhosis sooner than men because they metabolize alcohol at a different rate. They also have higher blood alcohol levels relative to body weight and higher mortality rates from heavy drinking (Center for Substance Abuse Treatment, 2009).

Excessive alcohol use, especially binge drinking, during pregnancy continues to have long-term developmental consequences in the newborn (Center for Substance Abuse Treatment, 2009). Cocaine use during pregnancy is associated with increased risk of spontaneous abortion, premature delivery, and abruptio placentae. Infants who have been addicted to cocaine in utero are hyperirritable, subject to seizures, and possibly at increased risk for sudden infant death syndrome. Long-term learning disabilities, behavioral problems, mental retardation, and physical handicaps are other potential consequences associated with children of cocaine-using mothers (Messinger, 2004).

Getting the pregnant woman into treatment and managing her withdrawal are frequently problematic. The woman's fear of punitive legal actions complicates the process. Additionally, the addiction itself often interferes with obtaining adequate prenatal care. If addiction is linked with risky sexual behavior or sexual assault, there is an increased risk of contracting HIV and hepatitis viruses, which can infect the infant; testing should be recommended.

Ethnocultural Considerations

Community health nurses need to be culturally competent and aware of certain ethnocultural vulnerabilities and differing perspectives when considering treatments for individuals with substance abuse. Data on African Americans, Hispanics, and Native Americans suggest an increased risk for substance abuse in these groups (Echo-Hawk, 2011; Lane and Simmons, 2011; Larios et al, 2011). However, the usual ethnic/racial categories in research do not take into account the distinctions within each category. Consequently, there are limited data, especially about middle-class minorities. Creating another stereotype might undermine prevention and treatment strategies. However, it is true that, under the strain of poverty, underemployment, decreased job opportunities, macro-level and micro-level aggression, and ongoing racism, some members of these aggregates find the relief in using substances, which numb the "social pain" caused by their environments. Racial and ethnic minorities are overrepresented among the economically disenfranchised. Limited financial resources may limit alternatives to public treatment settings, which are often understaffed, underfunded, and filled to capacity and have long waiting lists. The privatization of treatment has further decreased access to treatment.

Theories of stress, social causation, and oppressed status support the belief that discrimination and racism are factors in the generation of mental illness and alcohol and drug problems in members of racial and ethnic minorities. Socioeconomic, political, and historical realities have encouraged some minorities to enter into the illegal drug trade as a means of economic survival. In working with ethnic and racial minorities, health care professionals must recognize the sociopolitical and socioeconomic factors that form the context of substance use, abuse, and dependency. These same factors will have an impact on seeking help, treatment, and outcome. Traditional substance abuse treatment modalities, designed primarily for white working men, sometimes overlook ethnic and racial minority experiences (Wells et al, 2011). Recovery for minority groups might be contextually and experientially different from that for whites, just as the environment that contributed to the initial abuse was different.

During periods of slavery, alcohol was used as a reward, and it was seen as a way to cope. The value themes for this aggregate are a oneness with nature and spirituality, the importance of extended family, a present orientation, and a spiral concept of time. Barriers to treating African Americans with substance abuse or addiction problems are listed in Box 26-4.

Myths about certain ethnicities must be critically examined. Native Americans, for example, fight the stereotype of the drunken, once-noble warrior. However, alcohol as the predominant drug of choice does pose a threat to this population, particularly among youth and young adults. Native American adolescents use drugs and alcohol earlier and with more devastating consequences than other groups (NIDA,

---

BOX 26-4 **BARRIERS TO TREATING SUBSTANCE ABUSE AND ADDICTION PROBLEMS IN AFRICAN AMERICANS**

- Weekend drinking as a reward
- Ongoing sociocultural violence
- Use of substances to escape the emotional pain caused by racism
- Poverty, underemployment, and unemployment
- Prevalence of both drugs and liquor stores within the community
- Cultural and community disintegration, which has altered traditional values and behaviors
- Allure and economic rewards of selling drugs
- Inadequate social support system for recovery
- Internalized racism harming the self-concept, along with anger and frustration
- Greater likelihood of being arrested than treated (three to six times more than whites)
- Limited role models
- Inability to "change people and places" as advocated by 12-step programs

---

2010b). Evidence for a biological predisposition is conflicting, and many stop drinking when they reach adulthood and their sense of family and social responsibility increases. Interventions for this group must involve long-term outreach that gains respect from the community.

Studies have identified that social support has a positive effect on treatment and outcome. Without this support, the individual completing treatment may return to the original social environment, undermining any gains made within the treatment setting. Environmental cues and conditioned reinforcement for continued drug and alcohol use may be extremely powerful. The individual may return to an environment of nonsupport, characterized by continued use by important members of the individual's social network. The individual needs a well-coordinated aftercare program that addresses these issues.

The treatment of ethnic and racial minority aggregates poses special challenges related to the individuals seeking treatment. Treatment providers must recognize that these vulnerable aggregates will encounter a host of barriers that will make treatment and long-term recovery extremely difficult. For example, providers should understand the effect of rituals, holidays, music, and customs and how they can hinder progress. Providers who work from the public health perspective of "thinking upstream" will examine larger, macro-level issues that increase the susceptibility of at-risk populations to alcohol and drug problems. Box 26-5 presents helpful information on working with people from diverse cultures.

Other Aggregates

Substance abuse is the most common psychopathological problem in the general population. Within this category is a smaller aggregate of people with one or more psychiatric diagnoses in addition to substance abuse; this situation is referred to as **dual diagnosis**. Nearly one third of adults with a mental disorder also experience a co-occurring substance abuse disorder (USDHHS, 2012). This may be less readily identified by health care providers, who may fail to recognize that the two problems may coexist. Treatment of the individual with a dual diagnosis is complicated when the individual must take prescribed psychotropic medications. As previously mentioned, it may be perceived as prescription drug abuse or as the substitution of one addiction for another. Special attention and flexibility are needed to meet the needs of the dual-diagnosis aggregate, and such strategies are still in the developmental phase.

In assessing the risks for substance abuse and the extent of its impact on the community, nurses must be aware that are there frequently several bases for the vulnerability in an individual or group. The adolescent, the low-income Hispanic male, the lesbian African American mother receiving public assistance, and the Native American family living on reservation land are all facing multiple sources of vulnerability that contribute to an increased potential for substance abuse.

Special attention must be paid to the impact of sexually transmitted diseases (STDs) (e.g., HIV, herpes, genital warts, and syphilis) and their relationship to substance abuse. Substance abusers are at increased risk of STDs, including HIV, in the following ways:

- Substances may cloud judgment, leading to high-risk sexual practices involving the exchange of body fluids (e.g., sex without the use of appropriate barriers such as condoms).
- Intravenous drug use may involve the sharing of hypodermic needles.
- Chronic substance use (e.g., of alcohol, heroin, amphetamines, nicotine, and cocaine) impairs the immune system and facilitates infection by HIV or by other pathogens that increase the chances of HIV infection.
- Substance abuse may hasten physical and mental deterioration from the condition of seropositivity to an AIDS diagnosis and, eventually, the terminal phase of the disease.
- Chronic substance abusers generally have few supportive relationships available to them in the process of coping with the hardships that accompany severe and chronic illnesses.

- People facing a stigmatizing, terminal, debilitating illness, in themselves or in a significant other, are more prone to experience substance abuse problems in an attempt to cope with distress.

⚖ ETHICAL INSIGHTS

Ethical Issues Related to Substance Abuse

Ethical issues regarding substance use and abuse relate to behaviors of the user/abuser that present a risk to the self, coworkers, or the public. A nurse who diverts medication from a patient, thereby depriving the patient of pain relief, is acting both unethically and illegally. Other ethical areas of concern include property theft or damage and the general welfare of others. Kunyk and Austin (2012) considered that when nurses have addiction problems, there is always the possibility of compromised safety to patients. Nurses who are living in addiction have more options than ever with assessment and treatment that may not necessarily end their professional careers. Currently 37 states offer some form of substance abuse treatment program to direct nurses to treatment, monitor their reentry into work, and continue their licensure according to the National Council of State Boards of Nursing.

Finally, substance abuse among health care professionals cannot be ignored. Physicians, nurses, dentists, and pharmacists are vulnerable to substance abuse; alcohol or narcotic use is most common (Cousins et al, 2012). Health care professionals are assumed to be "immune" to dependency because they are knowledgeable about medications. However, their increased access to drugs, belief in pharmaceutical solutions, and work-related stress increase their risk for substance abuse. Typically, they gain access to drugs through their work settings by diverting medications for their own use or by abusing drugs obtained by prescription. State regulatory boards discover the abuse by these health care professionals after drug theft or when the effects of the substance abuse impairs professional functioning.

Community health nurses should be especially vigilant about this possibility because colleagues are working in isolation and episodes of incompetence may not be easily observed. Most states have rehabilitation programs for health care professionals that consist of treatment and monitoring. They are allowed to retain their professional licenses during treatment. Despite their usually favorable recovery rate, it is difficult to get this population into treatment because they exhibit denial and shame related to their substance abuse. However, the threatened loss of their professional license to practice may be a good motivator to break through denial of the problem and encourage them to seek treatment.

NURSING PERSPECTIVE ON SUBSTANCE ABUSE

Nurses have encountered substance abuse in clients whose health problems are clearly related to alcohol abuse, such as cirrhosis of the liver, heart disease, neurologic syndromes, and nutritional deficits. Unfortunately, alcohol problems were often not addressed in these health encounters in the past because of the stigma of alcoholism and a lack of effective treatments. The nursing literature did not clearly address substance abuse as a nursing problem until the late 1960s and did not address it as a significant problem until the 1970s. Before the 1970s, substance abuse was usually viewed as a moral problem or, if it involved illicit drugs, as a legal problem.

Since the 1970s, nursing has become more involved in the spectrum of compulsive behavior problems, including substance abuse. A specialized organization, the International Nurses Society on Addictions (IntNSA; at http://www.intnsa.org/home/index.asp), has been established with the philosophy that alcohol abuse and other drug abuse, eating disorders, sexual and relational addiction, and compulsive gambling, working, and spending are closely related behavior patterns. There is a tendency in society to deal with substance abusers in stigmatizing, devaluing, coercive, and punitive ways. Negative attitudes are ubiquitous in our culture. As part of the larger culture, nurses may reflect these attitudes and have difficulty providing care to these individuals. The moral view of substance abuse implies that individuals choose to become sick, injured, or addicted.

Strong negative feelings that conflict with nursing's humanistic stance may also stem from personal experiences. Being the emotionally or physically abused spouse or child of a substance abuser can have lasting effects on a nurse's attitude toward substance-abusing clients. The nurse who uses alcohol or drugs to relieve stress or to self-medicate a dysphoric state may over-identify with the client and deny the severity of the client's substance abuse.

Frequently, substance abusers are difficult clients in health care settings. When intoxicated, they may be raucous, uncooperative, and antisocial. When not intoxicated, they may exhibit none of these negative behaviors, or they may be manipulative and demanding, using flattery or intimidation to hide drug-seeking behavior. Nurses may initially be warm and understanding, but once aware of manipulative attempts, they may have difficulty maintaining an accepting, nonjudgmental attitude. Realizing that recovery from substance abuse often comes very slowly can help nurses feel less pressured to get patients into treatment and more able simply to raise consciousness by presenting the facts about addictive illness and leaving the decision making to the client.

Nursing Interventions in the Community

The problem of substance abuse is so widespread that it affects every community and its inhabitants to varying degrees. Hence, the community health nurse is often involved with substance abusers or their significant others. Substance abuse nursing interventions with clients and their caregivers are necessary to ensure the success of other health interventions. Ignoring substance abuse problems frequently leads to lack of progress and clients' inability to perform needed health practices. This situation is especially frustrating for the community health nurse and other professionals who have collaborated on a comprehensive plan to allow an individual with a serious health problem to remain at home and avoid placement in an institution.

There are many ways in which community health nurses can assist individuals, families, and groups experiencing substance abuse problems. Community health nurses may be the first to identify or suspect an alcohol or drug problem in the clients and families with whom they are working. Nurses in all care contexts should routinely assess substance use patterns when performing client histories. The client history is a critical assessment and screening tool that can identify those at risk. Using current knowledge and theories about substance abuse etiology and risk factors should help identify those individuals predisposed to alcohol and drug use.

The community health nurse can be alert to environmental cues in the home that indicate substance abuse, such as empty liquor and pill bottles. An indication of prescription medication abuse is the patient's involvement with several physicians from whom narcotic analgesics and tranquilizers are obtained. This type of assessment can help with case finding and treatment referral, although the individual may have denied the existence of a substance abuse problem initially.

Denial of substance abuse or dependence may range from completely blocked awareness of the problem to partial disavowal of the detrimental effects of the substance use and abuse. One of the primary tasks for intervention and treatment with the substance-dependent individual is to increase the individual's awareness of the problem. Family and significant others can assist with this process by being more honest and direct with the individual about the detrimental effects of the substance abuse. Before this occurs, the significant others must overcome their own denial of the problem and its associated shame and guilt. Referrals to community education programs on substance abuse and dependence and mutual help groups such as Al-Anon and Narcotics Anonymous are helpful interventions for families and significant others.

The community health nurse may also involve the social network in getting the client into treatment. Although individuals who are forced to enter treatment may not be willing to admit the severity of the abuse, they can still benefit from exposure to the treatment program and eventually begin recovery. Experiencing serious health consequences related to dependency may constitute "hitting bottom" for the individual. This experience may also break through denial or collusion on the part of the family.

The trust that develops in a caring nursing relationship can support disclosure of substance abuse problems and decrease denial in the client or family members. A realistic and positive attitude toward the person with substance abuse can provide families with hope. Community health nurses must have knowledge of available community resources. One of the primary roles of the community health nurse in helping substance abusers is to facilitate contact with helping agencies such as local treatment programs or mutual help groups. Collaboration with the client's physician is helpful, should medical detoxification be necessary. Community health nurses should assume a validating, nonjudgmental position toward the whole family and should avoid being confrontational so as not to fan the fires of resistance. It is imperative that nurses ascribe a noble intention to their substance-abusing clients and families and avoid negativity and preaching.

Other traditional community health nursing roles and interventions also are appropriate to use with substance abusers. Examples follow:

- Health teaching regarding addictive illness and addictive effects of different substances
- Advocating that evidence-based practice treatment works in special populations through problem-solving courts (drug courts), specialized adolescent treatment, and other community case management programs
- Providing direct care for abuse-related and dependence-related co-occurring medical problems
- Educating clients and families about problems related to substance abuse
- Collaborating with other disciplines to ensure continuity of care
- Coordinating health care services for the client to prevent prescription drug abuse and avoid fragmentation of care
- Providing consultation to nonmedical professionals and lay personnel
- Facilitating care through appropriate referrals and follow-up
- Knowing how to refer to community resources working with substance abuse, mental health, and other issues

Nursing Care Standards Related to the Patients with Substance Abuse Problems

Utilization of the nursing process is critical to quality care of patients with substance abuse problems. Nurses must know how to develop therapeutic alliances with the patient and family to develop trust and rapport. There is no single treatment appropriate for all individuals, and in the development of health teaching for clients, evidence-based models meet the needs for many specific populations may be chosen. Evidence demonstrates that effective treatment must address the multiple holistic needs of the individual. Ongoing assessment is critical for continual assessment in treatment planning and services. Knowledge, skills, and attitudes of the behavioral health workforce must be adequate. More success is noted when patients remain in treatment for adequate periods and when individual and group counseling and other behavioral therapies are utilized. Medications are an important element of treatment for many patients, especially when combined with counseling and other behavioral therapies. Nurses must have the knowledge of treatment in co-occurring mental health disorders and substance use disorders. Addiction recovery usually is a long-term process and frequently requires multiple episodes of treatment.

CASE STUDY   APPLICATION OF THE NURSING PROCESS

Kate Gray, 29 years old, was having abdominal pain, nausea, and vomiting. She was admitted to the hospital thorough the emergency department. After 3 days she was discharged and referred to a community clinic and public health department. Kate has been diagnosed with hepatitis C and alcoholism. She weighs 115 pounds. She is taking a multivitamin, cimetidine for symptoms of gastroesophageal reflux disease (GERD), gabapentin for chronic pain, and Atarax for pruritus. She had abdominal pain and a low-grade fever on discharge from the hospital. Her appetite is poor and she often is nauseated. She becomes fatigued easily. She agrees to comply with discharge planning from the hospital. She is unemployed and recently started Medicaid benefits.

Kate's drug use history is as follows: Marijuana use starting at age 16, alcohol use starting at age 20, methamphetamine use at age 26; she has been injecting the drug for 2 years. She was arrested 4 months ago for drug use and mandated to participate in a community felony drug court. She has been abstinent from marijuana and methamphetamine since her arrest. However, 2 weeks ago she violated probation by drinking and received 3 days in jail for probation violation. She has two daughters ages 6 and 8. Her children live with their father in the same city.

Assessment
Individual
The drug court team nurse practitioner sees Kate 2 days after discharge. Kate is still struggling with fatigue and poor appetite. She is afebrile. The nurse practitioner will follow her through drug court. When participating in drug court, Kate will attend Intensive Outpatient Treatment (IOT) and Narcotic Anonymous (NA) meetings. She has an NA sponsor.

Family
Kate will meet with her daughters weekly for family therapy through drug court. She meets with her husband, daughters, and pastor weekly for family counseling. Kate's husband attends NA meetings. He has been clean and sober for 1 year. He also is on felony probation and has recently graduated from drug court. He works as a mechanic. Their daughters have safe and adequate housing with their father.

Community
Drug court firmly assists with keeping individuals in treatment long enough for it to work while supervising them closely. Participants are held accountable by the drug court judge for meeting their obligations to the court, society, themselves, and their families. Participants are regularly and randomly tested for drug use. Kate is required to appear in court frequently so that the judge may review her progress and reward her for doing well or sanction her when she does not live up to drug court obligations.

Diagnosis
Individual
- Altered gastrointestinal and hepatic status secondary to hepatitis C and alcoholism pain
- Poor nutritional status
- Inadequate coping related to substance abuse history
- Need for patient education regarding hepatitis C, alcoholism, and addiction

Family
- Inadequate knowledge about addictive disease and effects of alcoholism, methamphetamine abuse, and polysubstance abuse
- Inadequate knowledge of treatment approaches available for alcohol abuse and the recovery process
- Family dysfunction secondary to poor communication and denial of addiction in client

CASE STUDY   APPLICATION OF THE NURSING PROCESS—cont'd

Community

- Need for understanding of the prevalence of alcohol abuse problems in the elderly population and adverse health effects of alcohol consumption in the elderly
- Inadequate knowledge in community agencies that assist alcohol abusers (e.g., local Alcoholics Anonymous [AA] and counselors) regarding the need to make home visits and provide services

Planning

Planning for Kate and her family's care involves collaboration among her family, her case management team through drug court, probation services, her pastor, and other community treatment resources. Case management health promotion teaching, counseling, support, and advocacy are the main approaches used to directly assist the client and her family. Indirect approaches involve networking with community agencies, collaboration, communications.

Individual

Short-Term Goals

- Kate will follow her post-hospitalization IOT attendance, drug court, and case management.
- Kate will be compliant with her medications.

Long-Term Goals

- Kate will continue to be clean and sober.
- Kate's health status will improve and/or stay at optimal health status as indicated by stabilization of weight, and optimal pain control.
- Kate will complete drug court.

Family

Short-Term Goals

- Kate's family will continue family therapy.
- Communication will improve between Kate, her husband, and children.

Long-Term Goals

- Family recovery in abstinence and sobriety

Community

Long-Term Goals

- NA meetings and sponsorship
- Successful completion of and release from probation
- Optimal health status

Intervention

Individual

- Nurse practitioner appointments weekly initially to monitor the client's medication issues or problems as related to maintaining abstinence, gastrointestinal and hepatic functioning, medication compliance, nutritional status
- Health promotion and patient/family education regarding addiction, hepatitis C, and alcoholism
- Patient teaching about the client's medications, their effects and side effects, and the necessity of following recommended dosing schedules

Family

- Continued support for Kate and her family through early recovery
- Health promotion and education to the family on the course and treatment of addiction, and other medical problems associated with Kate's medical diagnosis
- Nonjudgmental support and advocacy

Community

- List of local and national referral resources for clients with substance abuse problems made available to drug court team and physicians, with a particular focus on resources providing services for drug court participants
- Educating community stakeholders about drug courts, NA and other 12-step programs, and community case management
- Collaboration with community organizations that provide outreach for other individuals and families living with addiction

Evaluation

Individual

Kate was very compliant with drug court, IOT, NA meetings, and following medical treatment.

Family

Kate's family joined her in drug court graduation. Kate continues outpatient drug once weekly, NA meetings, and family therapy.

Community

Drug court case management will follow through with compliance in IOP attendance, NA meeting compliance, family therapy compliance, and other treatment obligations.

Levels of Prevention

Primary

- Health teaching to individuals and groups on the risk factors, early symptoms, and adverse health and social consequences of substance abuse; the addictive disease process; and available treatment services
- Need to gear educational approaches to the more vulnerable aggregates

Secondary

- Screening and earlier treatment approaches aimed at minimizing health and social consequences of substance abuse
- Involvement of physicians, nurses, and other health care professionals in various community health care settings in this process

Tertiary

- More direct approaches, such as case management, IOT, family therapy, and NA meeting with sponsorship. Goals are to halt the physiologically damaging effects of hepatitis C and alcoholism in Kate's abstinence and sobriety.
- Frequent use of medications to treat the symptoms of substance abuse–related disorders or as part of aversion therapy (e.g., disulfiram)
- Services provided by medical practitioners, treatment services, and mutual help organizations generally advocate abstinence from the substance and improving the individual's health status

This case study illustrates the complexity of substance abuse and co-occurring disorders. There is hope in treatment through problem-solving courts. Substance abuse affects patients and their families. Now more than ever, substance abuse may be treated through case management involving multidisciplinary team members. In sobriety, the social situation, living situation, or social acquaintances must change to maintain long-term recovery. However, with patience, persistence, and a caring, nonjudgmental attitude, the nurse can often be effective in helping clients with substance abuse problems attain recovery and improve their health status.

SUMMARY

This chapter provides an overview of the complex, multifaceted phenomenon of substance abuse and its manifestations in the community. The focus is on social, economic, political, and health-related aspects of substance abuse. In addition, the concept of substance abuse is related to the more general concept of addictive behaviors, not just those related to drug or alcohol abuse.

From the review of the various etiological theories, it is clear that there is no one causative factor in the development of substance abuse. Consequently, one treatment approach does not apply to all substance abusers. Multiple factors as well as issues specific to vulnerable aggregates, such as women, adolescents, the elderly, and people of color, must be considered in the development of intervention plans and strategies and in the evaluation of outcomes. Resources for prevention and intervention at the individual, family, and community levels are outlined here and should be familiar to nurses practicing in the community.

LEARNING ACTIVITIES

1. Attend a local AA, Narcotics Anonymous, or Cocaine Anonymous meeting, and share impressions with classmates.
2. Local resources in your community that help veterans with substance abuse.
3. Visit a local treatment center that provides detoxification, inpatient, or outpatient treatment, and determine the center's treatment philosophy and the types of services it provides to patients and their families.
4. Visit a treatment program for women, and determine how the particular needs of this population are assessed and addressed.
5. Learn about problem solving courts in your community.
6. Contact mental health services or substance abuse treatment services at the county or city level, and obtain a list of local treatment and education resources.

⊝ EVOLVE WEBSITE

http://evolve.elsevier.com/Nies

- NCLEX Review Questions
- Case Studies
- Glossary

REFERENCES

American Psychiatric Association: *Diagnostic and statistical manual of mental disorders*, ed 5, 2013.

Bray RM, Pembetton MR, Lane ME, et al.: Substance use and mental health trends among U.S. military active duty personnel: Keyfindings from the 2008 DoD health behavior survey, *Military Medicine* 175(6):390–399, 2010.

Bureau of Justice Statistics: *Drugs and crime facts* 2014. Available from: HYPERLINK "http://www.bjs.gov/content/dcf/duc.cfm" \l "prior" <http://www.bjs.gov/content/dcf/duc.cfm #prior>.

Center for Substance Abuse Treatment: *Medication-assisted treatment for opioid addiction in opioid treatment programs* (Treatment Improvement Protocol [TIP] Series 43, DHHS Publication No. [SMA] 05–4048). Rockville, MD, 2005, Substance Abuse and Mental Health Services Administration.

Center for Substance Abuse Treatment: *Substance Abuse Treatment: Addressing the Specific Needs of Women*, Treatment Improvement Protocol (TIP) Series 51. HHS Publication No. (SMA) 09-4426. Rockville, MD, 2009, Substance Abuse and Mental Health Services Administration.

Cervantes RC, Goldbach JT: Adapting Evidence-Based Prevention Approaches for Latino Adolescents: the Familia Adelante Program- Revised, *Psychosocial Intervention* 21(3):281–290, 2012.

Chesher NJ, Bousman CA, Gale M, et al.: Chronic illness histories of adults entering treatment for co-occurring substance abuse and other mental health disorders, *American Journal on Addictions* 21:1–4, 2011, http://dx.doi.org/10.1111/j.1521-0391.2011.00916.x.

Cousins SJ, Antonini VP, Rawson RA: Utilizing, measurement, and funding of recovery supports and services, *Journal of Psychoactive Drugs* 44(4):325–333, 2012, http://dx.doi.org/10.1080/02791072.2012.718924.

Echo-Hawk H: Indigenous communities and evidence building, *Journal of Psychoactive Drugs* 43(4):269–275, 2011, http://dx.doi.org/10.1080/02791072.2011.628920.

HealthyPeople.gov: *Healthy People 2020: 2013 objectives*, 2013. Retrieved from <http://www.healthypeople.gov/2020/topicsobjectives2020/overview.aspx?topicid=28>.

Johnston LD, O'Malley PM, Bachman JG, et al.: *Monitoring the Future national results on drug use: 2012 Overview, Key Findings on Adolescent Drug Use*, Ann Arbor, 2013, Institute for Social Research, The University of Michigan.

Kornreich C, Delle-Vigne D, Campanella S, et al.: Conditional reasoning difficulties in polysubstance-dependent patients, *Psychology of Addiction Medicine* 26(3):665–671, 2012, http://dx.doi.org/10.1037/a0025841.

Kunyk D, Austin W: Nursing under the influence: a relational ethics perspective, *Nursing Ethics* 9(3):380–389, 2012.

Lane DC, Simmons J: American Indian youth substance abuse: Community-driven interventions, *Mount Sinai Journal of Medicine* 78:362–372, 2011, http://dx.doi.org/10.1002/msj.20262.

Larios SE, Wright S, Jernstrom A, et al.: Evidence-Based Practices, Attitudes, and Beliefs in Substance Abuse Treatment Programs Serving American Indians and Alaska Natives: A Qualitative Study, *Journal of Psychoactive Drugs* 43(4):355–359, 2011, http://dx.doi.org/10.1080/02791072.2011.629159.

Lucas L: Harm reduction and recovery-oriented care, *Recovery to Practice Weekly Highlights* 3(15):2012, 2012. Available from <http://www.dsgonline.com/rtp/wh/2012/2012.04.19/WH.2012.04.19.html>.

Martel MM, Pierce L, Nigg JT, et al.: Temperament pathways to childhood disruptive behavior and adolescent substance abuse: Testing a cascade model, *Journal of Abnormal Child Psychology*, 2009 (2009) 37:363 –373 DOI 0.1007/s10802-008-9269-x.

Mattson RE, O'Ferrell TJ, Lofgreen AM, et al.: The role of substance use in a conceptual model of inmate partner violence in men undergoing treatment for alcoholism, *Psychology of Addictive Behaviors* 26(2):255–262, 2012.

Messinger DS: The maternal lifestyle study: cognitive, motor and behavioral outcomes of cocaine-exposed and opiate-exposed infants through three year of age, *Pediatrics* 113(6):1677–1685, 2004.

National Institute on Drug Abuse: *Drugs, brains, and behavior: The science of addiction*, 2010a. NIH Publication No.10–5605 NIH

National Institute on Drug Abuse: *NIH health disparities strategic plan fiscal years 2009-2013*, 2010b. No. 10–5605

National Institute on Drug Abuse: *Strategic plan national institute on drug abuse*, 2010c. NIH Publication Number 10–6119

National Institute on Drug Abuse: *Research report series: Prescription drugs: Abuse and addiction*, 2011. NIH Publication No. 11–4881

National Institute on Drug Abuse: *Monitoring the future study: Trends in prevalence of various drugs*, 2012a. Available from <http://www.drugabuse.gov/related-topics/trends-statistics/monitoring-future/trends-in-prevalence-various-drugs>.

National Institute on Drug Abuse: *Principles of drug addiction treatment: A research-based guide*, 3rd ed, 2012b. NIH Publication No. 12–4180

Office of National Drug Control Policy (ONDCP): 2013. Available from <http://www.whitehouse.gov/ondcp>.

Riddle E, Bush J, Tittle M, et al.: Alcohol withdrawal: development of a standing order set, *Critical Care Nurse* 30:37–38, 2010.

Robers S, Kemp J, Truman J. (2013). Indicators of School Crime and Safety: 2012 (NCES 2013-036/NCJ 241446). National Center for Education Statistics, U.S. Department of Education, and Bureau of Justice Statistics, Office of Justice Programs, U.S. Department of Justice. Washington, DC.

Sabri B: Severity of victimization and co-occurring mental health disorders among using adolescents, *Child Youth Care Forum* 41:37–55, 2012, http://dx.doi.org/10.1007/s10566-011-9151-9.

Substance Abuse and Mental Health Services Administration: *MedTEAM: The evidence* (HHS Pub. No. SMA-10–4548). Rockville, MD, 2010, Author.

Substance Abuse and Mental Health Services Administration: *Results from the 2010 National Survey on Drug Use and Health: Mental health findings*(NSDUH Series H-42, HHS Publication No. [SMA] 11–4667) Rockville, MD, 2011a, Author. Available from <http://www.samhsa.gov/data/nsduh/2k11results/nsduhresults2011.pdf>.

Substance Abuse and Mental Health Services Administration: *SAMSHA's strategic initiatives*, 2011b. Available from <http://store.samhsa.gov/shin/content//SMA11-4666/SMA11-4666.pdf>.

Substance Abuse and Mental Health Services Administration: *The DAWN report: Highlights of the 2010 Drug Abuse Warning Network (DAWN) findings on drug-related emergency department visits*, Rockville, MD, 2012, Author.

Staton-Tindall M, McNees E, Leukefeld C, et al.: Treatment utilization among metropolitan and nonmetropolitan participants of corrections-based substance abuse programs reentering the community, *Journal of Social Service Research* 37:379–389, 2011, http://dx.doi.org/10.1080/01488376.2011.582019.

Tollison SJ, Henderson RC, Baer JS, et al.: Next steps in addressing the prevention, screening, and treatment of substance use disorder in active duty and veteran operation enduring freedom and Operation Iraqi Freedom populations, *Military Medicine* 177(8):39–46, 2012.

U.S. Department of Justice, National Drug Intelligence Center: *The economic impact of illicit drug use on American society*, Washington, DC, 2011, Author. Also available from h<ttp://www.justice.gov/archive/ndic/pubs44/44731/44731p>.

U.S. Department of Transportation, National Highway Traffic Safety Administration: *Traffic safety facts, 2010 data: alcohol-impaired driving*, . Available from <http://www-nrd.nhtsa.dot.gov/Pubs/811606.pdf>, 2012.

Walker JS, Sanders B: The community supports for wraparound inventory: An assessment of the implementation context for wraparound, *Journal of Child and Family Studies* 20:747–757, 2011, http://dx.doi.org/10.1007/s10826-010-9432-1.

Wells JE, Haro JM, Karam E, et al.: Cross national comparisons of sex differences in opportunities to use alcohol or drugs, and the transitions to use, *Substance use and misuse* 46:1169–1178, 2011, http://dx.doi.org/10.3109/10826084.2011.553659.

Winters KC, Stinchfield RD, Lee S, Latimer WW. (2008). Interplay of psychosocial factors and the long-term course of adolescents with a substance use disorder. Official Publication Of The Association For Medical Education And Research In Substance Abuse [Subst Abus], ISSN: 0889-7077, 2008; Vol. 29(2), pp. 107–119; Publisher: Routledge; PMID: 19042330;

Wright TE, Schuetter R, Fombonne E, et al.: Implementation and evaluation of a harm reduction model for clinical care of substance using pregnant women, *Harm Reduction Journal* 19(9), 2012. 5, 2012.

OBJECTIVES

Upon completion of this chapter, the reader will be able to do the following:
1. Describe the concepts of interpersonal and community violence.
2. Identify factors that influence violence.
3. Identify populations at risk for violence and the role of public health in dealing with the epidemic of violence.
4. Describe the role of the nurse in primary, secondary, and tertiary prevention of violence.

KEY TERMS

abusive head trauma
bullying
child maltreatment
date rape drugs
dating violence
elder abuse
emotional abuse

hate crimes
human trafficking
intentional injuries
interpersonal violence
intimate partner violence
neglect
physical abuse

prison violence
sexual abuse
stalking
terrorism
violence
workplace violence
youth-related violence

OUTLINE

Overview of Violence
History of Violence
Interpersonal Violence
  Homicide and Suicide
  Intimate Partner Violence
  Child Maltreatment
  Elder Abuse
Community Violence
  Workplace Violence
  Youth-Related Violence
  Gangs
  Prison Violence
  Human Trafficking

Hate Crimes
Terrorism
Factors Influencing Violence
  Firearms
  Media
  Mental Illness
Violence from a Public Health Perspective
  Healthy People 2020 and Violence
Prevention of Violence
  Primary Prevention
  Secondary Prevention
  Tertiary Prevention

Violence is a national public health problem that affects all ages from the young to the elderly. Violent deaths, however, only tell part of the problem. Although many survive, they and their families and friends often have permanent emotional and physical scars. Violence occurs around the world on a daily basis, as evidenced by the nightly newscast and stories on the Internet. For example:

April 1999: In Columbine High School, Littleton, Colorado, 13 killed by two teenagers who then committed suicide.

September 11, 2001: 2974 people from 90 different countries killed when 19 terrorists hijacked four planes and intentionally crashed two of them into the World Trade Center's twin towers, the third into the Pentagon, and the fourth in an empty field in Pennsylvania.

October 2006: 5 Amish schoolgirls killed and 6 others wounded in Nickel Mine, Pennsylvania, by a truck driver who then committed suicide.

April 2007: 32 killed, 15 wounded at Virginia Tech University in Blacksburg, Virginia, by a student who then committed suicide—the deadliest school shooting in U.S. history.

November 2009: 13 killed, 42 injured at a military base in Fort Hood, Texas, by a U.S. Army psychiatrist.

January 2011: 6 killed, including a 9-year-old girl, and 12 injured, including Congresswoman Gabrielle Giffords, at a political meeting in Tucson, Arizona.

July 2012: 12 killed, 58 injured during a midnight showing of the movie *Batman: The Dark Knight* in Aurora, Colorado.

August 2012: 6 killed at a Sikh Temple in Oak Creek, Wisconsin.

November 2012: 2 children stabbed and killed by a nanny in New York.

December 2012: 20 students and 7 adults killed, 2 wounded, at Sandy Hook Elementary School in Newtown, Connecticut—the second deadliest school shooting in U.S. history.

April 2013: 3 killed and an estimated 264 injured when 2 men set two pressure-cooker bombs at the finish line of the Boston Marathon.

September 2013:12 killed and 3 injured in a Navy Yard complex in Washington, DC, by a man who was then shot by police.

Although the preceding list shows well-publicized acts of extreme violence, violence occurs every day in communities across the country. The woman who is beaten and killed by her husband, the cousins who are kidnapped and murdered by a neighbor, the infant who is shaken to death by his mother, the young woman who is gang raped, the children who are sexually abused (such as those by former Penn State Assistant Football Coach Jerry Sandusky), and the coworkers who are killed by a disgruntled former employee are all examples of the violence that occurs every day.

The purpose of this chapter is to explore the influence of violence from a public health perspective as it relates to individuals and communities. It includes discussions of the effects of violence in terms of homicides and suicides; the direct influence of violence on individuals and communities; public health interventions to reduce violence; the roles and responsibilities of the community health nurse in dealing with those experiencing violence; and measures to increase awareness of violence in the workplace. An in-depth look at the causes, effects, interventions, and measures to increase awareness of violence is presented.

OVERVIEW OF VIOLENCE

The World Health Organization (WHO) defines **violence** as "the intentional use of physical force or power, threatened or actual against oneself, another person, or against a group or community, which either results in or has a high likelihood of resulting in injury, death, psychological harm, maldevelopment, or deprivation" (WHO, 2013). In public health, injuries from violence are referred to as **intentional injuries**. Violence threatens the health and well-being of people of all ages across the globe. Worldwide, 1.6 million people lose their lives annually as a result of violence, and it is one of the leading causes of death among people aged 15 to 44 years (Centers for Disease Control and Prevention [CDC], 2011). In 2009, in the United States, more than 16,000 people were victims of

homicide and more than 37,000 people committed suicide. Many more people survive acts of violence and are left with emotional and/or physical scars (CDC, 2012b).

The reasons for the high rate of violence in society are complex. Universally recognized factors that contribute to violence include the following:

1. Poverty, unemployment, economic dependency
2. Substance abuse
3. Dysfunctional family and/or social environment and lack of emotional support
4. Mental illness
5. Media influence
6. Access to firearms
7. Political and/or religious ideology
8. Intolerance and ignorance

HISTORY OF VIOLENCE

Violence is a global problem. From prehistoric times humans have dealt violently with other humans. In the Bible, Cain killed his brother Abel out of jealousy and anger. Throughout history, sporting events often resulted in death for the audience's pleasure, such as the gladiator events in Rome. Infanticide, or the killing of unwanted newborn children, has been practiced throughout history. For example, if a female, a twin, sickly, or deformed child was left to die of exposure. Children, especially firstborn children, were often sacrificed for religious reasons. Infanticide was not condemned until early in the fifth century; however, this did not protect children in many societies. Children were considered to be the property of the father, who could do whatever he wanted with them (Campbell and Humphreys, 1993).

Throughout the ages, corporal punishment has been used as a means of controlling children. Biblical reference to corporal punishment has often been used as justification for some types of child abuse. To some parents, "spare the rod and spoil the child" (Proverbs 13:24) implies an imperative to abusively discipline an errant child. The idea of "beating some sense into him" was considered necessary to ensure that a lesson was learned. In 1874, the first legal protection against child abuse in the United States was created when the Society for the Prevention of Cruelty to Animals intervened to protect an 8-year-old girl. As a result of the notoriety associated with this case, the New York Society for the Prevention of Cruelty to Children was organized later that year (Campbell and Humphreys, 1993).

Even nursery rhymes that adults read to small children seem to condone violence against them. Consider the following Mother Goose nursery rhyme:

> *There was an old woman who lived in a shoe,*
> *She had so many children she didn't know what to do,*
> *She gave them some broth without any bread,*
> *And whipped them all soundly and sent them to bed.*
> *(Mother Goose Nursery Rhymes, 2000, pp. 195-196)*

Wife beating was legal in the United States until 1824. Wives were seen as their husbands' chattel and could be beaten for such offenses as "nagging too much." In fact, the common phrase "rule of thumb" was derived from English law that allowed a man to beat his wife with a cane no wider than his thumb. Biblical interpretation of "wives be subject to your husband" (Ephesians 5:22) still provides some men with a faulty rationalization for wife beating. Some cultures and religions still allow, and even support, abuse of wives.

The silence that long surrounded domestic violence is derived from a historical perspective of women as their husbands' property. The problem of assault against women was not explored in America until the Civil Rights Movement of the 1960s. In fact, marital rape was not considered an offense in the United States until 1980. In the last three decades, additional cultural issues have surfaced regarding domestic abuse that includes female circumcision and genital mutilation, abuse between gay partners, and the realization that men are also victims of domestic violence.

Elder abuse is also a continuing problem. The problem is of greater magnitude now because people are living longer, resulting in increased numbers of dependent and vulnerable adults. Elder abuse frequently goes undetected because of a lack of awareness on the part of health care professionals and society. The exact prevalence of elder abuse is unknown because reporting is still not mandatory in all states.

INTERPERSONAL VIOLENCE

Homicide and Suicide

In the United States, homicide claimed the lives of 12,765 individuals in 2012. Sixty-nine percent of the deaths were firearm-related. Young people, particularly black and Hispanic males, are at higher risk than the general population. Further more, in 2012, blacks were more likely to commit homicide than whites and were more likely to be victims of homicide than whites. Of those murdered for whom race was established: 50.6% were black, 46% were white, and 3.4% were of other races; 78% were male and 22% were female. More than 50% of the victims were killed by someone they knew (Federal Bureau of Investigations [FBI], 2012).

Homicide is the third leading cause of death among all races and both sexes in the age-groups 1 to 4 years and 20 to 29 years; is the fourth leading cause of death in the 5 to 14 year age-group; and ranks fifth in the 30 to 34 year age-group. Black females are more likely to be victims than white females, but among all females, homicide ranks in the top ten causes of death in those aged 1 to 44 years (CDC, 2012a). Notably, 37% of female murder victims are killed by an intimate partner (FBI, 2013).

Homicide is the leading cause of death for black males aged 15 to 34 years, and the second leading cause for black males aged 1 to 4 and 10 to 14 years; homicide is the third leading cause of death in white males aged 15 to 29 years (CDC, 2012a).

Often ignored or overlooked, suicide is listed as the tenth leading cause of death for all Americans in all age-groups in 2010. More people die of suicide than of homicide in the United States; suicide took the lives of 38,364 people in 2010, an average of 105 people per day. This form of death affects virtually all ages. For people aged 15 to 24 years, suicide is the third leading cause of death, and for people aged 25 to 34 years, it is the second leading cause. It ranks fourth among persons aged 35 to 54 and eighth in those aged 55 to 64. Males commit suicide four times more often than females. In Native Americans and Alaska Natives, suicide is the second leading cause of death in those aged 15 to 34 years. Of suicides in men in 2010, 56% were committed with a firearm (CDC, National Center for Injury Prevention and Control [NCIPC] 2012b).

In women, the leading method of suicide was poisoning, followed by the use of firearms (CDC NCIPC, 2012b). Women with a history of sexual assault are more likely to attempt or commit suicide than other women. Studies show that women who attempt suicide are more likely to have been physically abused by intimate partners and are more likely to have posttraumatic stress disorder (PTSD).

Risk factors for suicide include:
1. Psychiatric disorders such as major depression, bipolar disorder, and/or schizophrenia
2. Substance abuse
3. Posttraumatic stress disorder
4. Bulimia or anorexia nervosa
5. Past history of attempted suicide
6. Genetic disposition to suicide
7. Age, (e.g., elderly and Caucasian males have high rates)

Refer to Chapter 24: Populations Affected by Mental Illness, for further discussion on suicide.

Intimate Partner Violence

Intimate partner violence (IPV), formerly known as *domestic violence,* is a pattern of coercive behaviors perpetrated by someone who is or was in an intimate relationship with the victim, such as a spouse, ex-spouse, boyfriend or girlfriend, ex-boyfriend or ex-girlfriend, or date. These behaviors may include battering resulting in physical injury, psychological abuse, and sexual assault that contributes to progressive social isolation and intimidation of the victim. Abuse is typically repetitive and often escalates in frequency and severity.

RESEARCH HIGHLIGHTS

Physical Dating Violence from Middle to High School

A study led by a professor at the University of Georgia examined the association of physical dating violence with relationship quality and acceptability of aggression. The study showed "that the kids who were involved in dating violence are consistently involved in dating violence and this violence starts early." The study began while the sample of students were in 6th grade and followed them through the 12th grade. Close to a third of study participants report abusive relationships, and this cycle increases over time. "Bad dating experiences particularly those related to physical violence, are associated with a plethora of negative experiences such as anxiety, depressed moods, suicidal thoughts, alcohol and drug abuse, lower educational achievement and poor relationships with parents," the researchers observed.

Data from Orpinas P, Hsieh HL, Song X, et al: Trajectories of physical dating violence from middle to high school; association with relationship quality and acceptability of aggression, *J Youth Adolesc* 42(4):551-565, 2012.

More than 12 million incidents of IPV occur each year. In 2007, 2340 people died as a result of IPV, 70% of whom were female (CDC NCIPC, 2012d). Violence may also be directed by women against women in lesbian relationships, by men against men in homosexual relationships, and by women against men.

IPV crosses all ethnic, racial, socioeconomic, and educational lines. About 30% of women and 1% of men report experiencing physical forms of IPV at some point in their lives. The following are risk factors for victims of IPV (CDC NCIPC, 2012d):

- Low self-esteem
- Poverty
- Risky sexual behavior
- Eating disorders and/or depression
- Substance abuse
- Trust and relationship issues

Victims of IPV frequently suffer in silence and accept abuse as a transgenerational pattern of normal behavior. When children witness abuse between parents, they learn that violence is a means of control.

Each year in the United States, more than 207,000 people are victims of sexual assault. In 66% of reported rapes, the women knew the perpetrators (Rape, Abuse, & Incest National Network, 2009). Women may report that they were subjected to forced intercourse when they were ill or had recently given birth. They also report forced anal intercourse and other violent sexual acts. Box 27-1 includes considerations for working with victims of intimate partner violence.

Pregnancy does not protect women from the danger of abuse. Indeed, pregnancy may increase stress within the family and provoke the first instances of battering. It is estimated that one in six pregnant women have been abused by a partner (March of Dimes, 2008).

Societal awareness of IPV during pregnancy is a relatively recent phenomenon; the mention of abuse during pregnancy began to appear in the literature in the 1980s. The image of a woman being battered during pregnancy shatters the idealized image of pregnancy as a time of nurturing and protection. All pregnant women should be routinely screened for abuse. Common signs of IPV in pregnancy are delay in seeking prenatal care, unexplained bruising or damage to breasts or abdomen, use of harmful substances (cigarettes, alcohol, drugs), recurring psychosomatic illnesses, and lack of participation in prenatal education. Violence during pregnancy can result in hemorrhage, spontaneous abortion, stillbirths, preterm deliveries, and fetal fractures.

Dating violence, which has become a national concern, refers to abusive, controlling, or aggressive behavior in an intimate relationship that can take the form of emotional, verbal, physical, or sexual abuse. It happens in straight and gay relationships. Research indicates that 9% of high school students have been victims of physical dating violence and that it occurs more frequently among black students than Hispanics or whites (CDC, 2006). Furthermore, almost 22% of women and 15% of men report some form of partner violence between ages 11 and 17 years (CDC NCIPC, 2012e).

BOX 27-1 CONSIDERATIONS FOR WORKING WITH VICTIMS OF VIOLENCE

1. Working with victims of intimate partner violence (IPV):
   - Establish rapport and trust.
   - Deal with issues of confidentiality honestly.
   - Provide current information regarding shelters and sources of support.
   - Recognize and accept that clients may "choose" to stay in an abusive relationship.
2. Working with victims of child abuse:
   - Protect the well-being of the child; this is the primary obligation of health care providers.
   - Report child abuse; it is a legal and ethical obligation in all states.
   - Establish rapport and trust; this may take time.
   - Remain objective when dealing with suspected family members.
3. Working with victims of elder abuse:
   - Establish rapport and trust; this may take time.
   - Report elder abuse; it is an ethical obligation for health care providers and a legal obligation in most states.
   - Remember that competent adults have the right to make decisions about their own care, even if it means staying in an abusive situation.
   - Support efforts to create respite programs and support groups for caregivers.
4. Advocating for the rights of vulnerable populations, which is the responsibility of all health care professionals:
   - Support research on effective interventions for violence prevention and reduction.
   - Lobby for a decrease in media violence.
   - Support community efforts to increase resources for victims of violence.
   - Lobby for effective regulation of firearms and cyberstalking.

Dating violence can involve the use of **date rape drugs**, such as gamma-hydroxybutyrate (GHB), flunitrazepam (Rohypnol), and ketamine, to reduce inhibitions and promote anesthesia or amnesia in the victim. GHB is odorless and colorless and can easily be made at home. Instructions are available in libraries and on the Internet, possibly explaining the drug's rapid rise in popularity. Although illegal in the United States, it has become available in many nightclubs, where it is sold in clear liquid form. GHB has been touted as an aphrodisiac and an anesthetic. It is actually a depressant that slows down the respiratory system and has been responsible for numerous overdoses and multiple deaths. When mixed with alcohol, it can be deadly.

Flunitrazepam, which is classified as a benzodiazepine, has been compared to methaqualone (Quaalude), the "love drug" of the 1960s and 1970s. Like GHB, flunitrazepam is not legal in the United States, but many reports have been received of its use at fraternity parties, college gatherings, and in bars. Two other drugs in the benzodiazepine family, alprazolam (Xanax) and clonazepam (Klonipin), are also used as date rape drugs. The ability to provide a quick, cheap high with long-lasting effects may explain their popularity. When they are combined with alcohol, serious side effects, including death, have been reported.

Ketamine (ketamine hydrochloride) is an anesthetic used primarily in veterinary practice. It causes a lost sense of time and problems with memory. Another drug that is becoming more common as a date rape drug is carisoprodol (Soma), a prescription muscle relaxant and central nervous system depressant.

Studies have also linked alcohol, "a hallmark of college campus social life," with dating violence. Substance abuse is often implicated in sexual assaults on college campuses. Alcohol contributes to sexual assault because it impairs the ability to think clearly, lowers inhibitions, and impairs the ability to evaluate an unsafe situation.

Stalking is a pattern of repeated and unwanted attention, contact, harassment, or any type of conduct directed at a person that instills fear. Types of stalking include messaging through the Internet or cell phone (cyberstalking), damaging the victim's property, following the victim, obtaining personal information about the victim, and making direct or indirect threats to the victim's family or friends. In one 12-month period, approximately 3.4 million people reported being stalked (U.S. Department of Justice, Office on Violence Against Women [USDOJ OFAV], 2009). Owing to the severity of the problem, in 2004, the National Center for Victims of crime proclaimed January as National Stalking Awareness Month (National Center for Victims of Crime, 2014).

Bullying is defined "as a repeated oppression, psychological or physical, of a less powerful person by a more powerful person or group of persons" (van der Zande, n.d.). Types of bullying include cyberbullying, physical threats or violence, verbal bullying, and workplace bullying. Bullying can occur in any setting, real world or online, and at any age. See Box 27-2.

IPV is about control, not anger. The objective of abuse is to exert power and control over the victim. Victims may have been exposed to violence as children. In these cases, the learned response is often one of helplessness that implies passivity and acceptance of abuse. Box 27-3 presents commonly held myths associated with IPV.

The Domestic Abuse Intervention Project (2011) in Duluth, Minnesota, has developed a wheel of violence that depicts the types of power and control that are used by perpetrators. Figure 27-1 depicts the Power And Control Wheel, "a helpful tool in understanding the overall pattern of abusive and violent behaviors that are used by a batterer to establish and maintain control over his partner. Very often, one or more violent incidents are accompanied by an array of these other types of abuse." This organization has also developed other wheels that focus on domestic abuse programs that include equality, abuse of children, and nurturing children. Their newest model focuses on using children after spousal separation to maintain power and control.

Victims of abuse often experience chronic fatigue and tension, disturbed sleeping and eating patterns, and vague gastrointestinal and genitourinary complaints. Misdiagnosis often occurs because of the obscurity of the symptoms and/or the failure to adequately assess the patient. Victims tend to stay in an abusive relationship on the basis of cultural,

---

BOX 27-2 BULLYING

Bullying includes repeated harmful acts and a real or perceived imbalance of power. Often underreported, bullying creates a climate of fear. Bullying can be physical, verbal, or psychological/relationalbullying or cyberbullying.

* Physical bullying involves assault, intimidation, and/or destruction of property
* Verbal bullying includes threats and name-calling
* Psychological/relational bullying can include all of the above and is distinguished by the power imbalance between the victim and the bully
* Cyberbullying consists of targeting the victim online

Modified from U.S. Department of Justice, *Office of Justice Programs: OJP Factsheet, 2011*. Available from <http://www.ojp.usdoj.gov/newsroom/factsheets/ojpfs_bullying.html>.

BOX 27-3 COMMON MYTHS ASSOCIATED WITH INTIMATE PARTNER VIOLENCE

* It occurs only in poor, uneducated, minority households.
* It is a private family matter (vs. a societal problem).
* It only occurs in heterosexual relationships.
* Victims deserve the abuse.
* Victims can change the abusers' behavior.
* Abusers will stop the abuse on their own without professional intervention.

---

religious, and economic factors. According to a study by Campbell and Humphreys (1993), the people more likely to leave abusive relationship s are those who have resources and power (e.g., a job, credit cards, and status outside the family), no children, and no personal history of abuse (of themselves or their mothers). The most dangerous time for victims is when they leave or attempt to leave the relationship. The victim is much more likely to be killed at this time than at any other time in the relationship.

Child Maltreatment

Most **child maltreatment** occurs within the family. Children are abused more often by parents than by other relatives or caregivers. Maltreatment is more commonly seen in families living in poverty, in families in disorganization, or with parents who are younger and are substance abusers. Risk factors for child maltreatment include but are not limited to special needs children (children with disabilities, mental retardation, or chronic illness), children less than 4 years of age, family history of violence, substance abuse, poverty, and social isolation (CDC NCIPC, 2012c). The four types of child maltreatment are:

* Neglect
* Physical abuse
* Emotional abuse
* Sexual abuse

In some families all children are equal targets, whereas in other families a particular child may be selected as the designated recipient of abuse. The child may be singled out by a particular physical characteristic that evokes negative

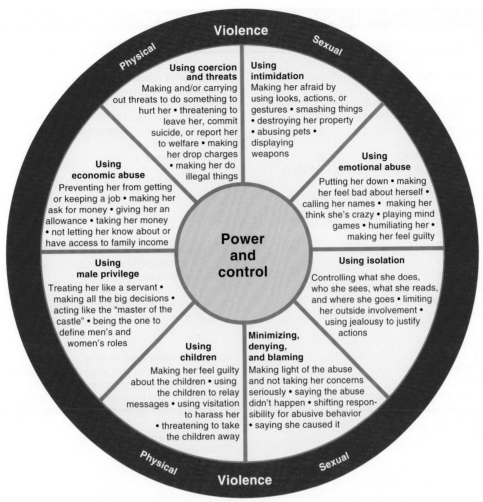

FIGURE 27-1 Power and Control Wheel. (Developed by the Domestic Abuse Intervention Project, 206 West Fourth Street, Duluth, MN 55806. Used with permission.)

emotions in the abusive parent. Although statistical reporting of child abuse is mandatory throughout the country, reported numbers are probably an underestimation. Children are not likely to report the abuse because they fear reprisal.

According to the (CDC NCIPC, 2012a), in 2010, there were more than 695,000 confirmed cases of child maltreatment in the United States. Girls were more likely to be victims than boys, and infant's less than 1 year old accounted for 21.7% of nonfatal maltreatment cases, followed by 12.9% of children who were 1 year old. More than 1500 children died in the United States of abuse and neglect in 2010. Of child maltreatment cases in 2008, 80% of deaths occurred in children younger than 4 years, whereas 10% of deaths occurred in children between the ages of 4 and 7 (CDC NCIPC, 2010a).

Neglect is the failure of the responsible person to provide basic needs such as shelter, food, clothing, education, and access to medical care. Seventy-one percent of all child maltreatment cases are classified as neglect (CDC NCIPC, 2010a). Failure to provide a nurturing environment for a child to thrive, learn, and develop and to provide for the health needs of a child can also be construed as neglect. Examples of emotional neglect include failure to cuddle and/or physically

stimulate a newborn, failure to give positive feedback, failure to pay attention to the overall emotional needs of a child, and failure to show affection.

Physical abuse is an intentional injury inflicted on a child by another person and accounts for 16% of child maltreatment cases (CDC NCIPC, 2010a). Parents who abuse often have unreasonable expectations of their children and may misinterpret children's behavior as threats to their parental self-esteem and need to control. Physical abuse includes beating, burning, biting, and bruising. The type of physical injury varies only with the adult's imagination. Patterned injuries may give some clue as to how the child was injured. A child who touches a light cord or light plug might be beaten with it, producing a looped or linear pattern. A child who plays with matches or the stove might have his or her hand placed in the flame. A crying child or a child who talks back might have hot pepper sauce poured into his or her mouth or might be suffocated with a pillow.

Abusive head trauma/inflicted traumatic head injury, also known as shaken baby syndrome, is a leading cause of death from abuse in the United States. Most victims are between 3 and 8 months of age. In this form of abuse, violent shaking of the infant causes trauma at the junction of the brainstem

TABLE 27-1	PHYSICAL AND BEHAVIORAL INDICATORS OF CHILD ABUSE AND NEGLECT
PHYSICAL INDICATORS	**BEHAVIORAL INDICATORS**
Physical Abuse	
Unexplained bruises and welts in various stages of healing that may form patterns	Wary of adult contact
Unexplained burns by cigars or cigarettes or immersion burns (e.g., socklike, glovelike, or on buttocks or genitalia)	Apprehensive when other children cry
Burns in the shapes of objects	Constantly on alert
Rope burns	Exhibiting extremes of behavior; aggressive or passive and withdrawn, or overly friendly to strangers
Unexplained lacerations or abrasions	Frightened of parents
Unexplained fractures in various stages of healing; multiple or spiral fractures	Afraid to go home
Unexplained injuries to mouth, lips, gums, eyes, or external genitalia	
Physical and Emotional Neglect	
Hunger	Begging or stealing food
Poor hygiene	Alone at inappropriate times or for prolonged periods
Poor or inappropriate dress	Delinquent behavior
Lack of supervision for prolonged periods	Stealing
Lack of medical or dental care	Arriving early to and departing late from school
Constant fatigue, listlessness, or falling asleep in class	Lack of affection
Sexual Abuse	
Difficulty in walking or sitting	Exhibiting negative self-esteem
Torn, stained, or bloody underwear	Exhibiting inability to trust and function in intimate relationships
Genital pain or itching	Exhibiting cognitive and motor dysfunctions
Bruises in or bleeding from the external genitalia, vaginal, or anal area	Exhibiting deficits in personal and social skills
Sexually transmitted disease	Exhibiting bizarre, sophisticated, or unusual sexual behavior or knowledge
Drug and alcohol abuse	Delinquent or a runaway behavior
Developmental delays	Exhibiting suicide ideation
	Reporting sexual assault
Emotional Abuse	
Failure to thrive	Exhibiting behavior extremes from passivity to aggression
Lag in physical development	Exhibiting habit and conduct disorders (e.g., antisocial behavior and destructiveness)
Speech disorders	Exhibiting neurotic traits
Developmental delays	Attempting suicide

and spinal cord that can result in death. Serious and permanent brain damage may occur, with results such as cerebral palsy, severe retardation, blindness, hearing loss, and developmental delays. In 65% to 90% of abusive head trauma cases, the father or the mother's boyfriend is the perpetrator (KidsHealth, 2011).

Emotional abuse accounts for approximately 7% of all child abuse cases and is the behavior that may damage a child's self-worth or emotional well-being (CDC NCIPC, 2010a). The child may demonstrate a substantial impairment in behavior, such as being overly compliant or passive, being very aggressive, or being inappropriately adult or infantile. Emotionally abused children frequently do not progress at a normal rate of physical, intellectual, or emotional development. They also have an increased risk of suicide. Emotional abuse usually occurs in the home, unwitnessed by others. Emotional abuse might include name calling—such as "you're stupid," "you're a slut," "you're bad," or "you're evil"—shaming, withholding love, rejection, or threatening behavior. Impairment in behavior may also occur in children who are

not abused; therefore, identification of emotional abuse is difficult.

Sexual abuse involves engaging a child in sexual acts. *Incest* is defined as sexual relations between persons considered too closely related to marry. Approximately 9% of child abuse cases are sexual abuse (CDC NCIPC, 2010a). The incidence of sexual exploitation of children by Internet pedophiles has increased in recent years. Most research has focused on girls as victims of sexual abuse, but boys are also targets. The victim may refrain from reporting abuse because he is ashamed or because cultural values expect males to be assertive and capable of self-defense.

Low self-esteem, psychiatric disorders, chronic health problems, depression, suicidal ideation, substance abuse, eating disorders, obesity, sexual maladjustment, delayed developmental processes, and high-risk sexual behaviors may result from child maltreatment (CDC NCIPC, 2011). The child may delay reporting the abuse for months or years, because it may take that long for him or her to feel safe. Table 27-1 describes physical and behavioral indicators of child abuse and neglect.

All states mandate that health care providers and teachers report suspected child abuse. Reporting child abuse may be one of the hardest things a nurse will ever have to do, but may be one of the most rewarding when an abused child is removed from a harmful situation.

Elder Abuse

Elder abuse lags far behind child abuse and IPV as a social and health care issue because society fails to recognize the cruelty many older adults experience. Failure to recognize abuse is likely attributable to the perception of elders as an "invisible" segment of the population. The exact number of abused elders is unknown because of underreporting and no uniform reporting system. Estimates indicate that 2% to 10% of the older adult population suffer some form of abuse. Reasons for underreporting include shame on the part of the victim, social and physical isolation from resources, and the failure of health care providers to routinely assess for abuse and neglect during points of contact. The most likely victims are those in poor physical or mental health, those dependent on others for physical or financial support, and those confused, depressed, or who are socially isolated (National Center on Elder Abuse [NCEA], 2005).

According to the NCEA (2011), types of abuse and neglect of older adults are as follows:

- Physical abuse (purposeful infliction of physical pain or injury or unnecessary physical or drug-induced restraints)
- Psychological-emotional abuse (verbal assault, threats, provoking fear, or isolation)
- Sexual abuse (unwanted sexual contact or taking pornographic pictures)
- Neglect (withholding of personal care, food, or medications, intimidation, humiliation, abandonment)
- Financial exploitation (theft or misuse of money or property)
- Health care fraud and abuse (charging for services not delivered, or Medicaid fraud)

Elder abuse tends to escalate in incidence and severity. When an older adult cannot care for himself or herself because of the physical or mental infirmities of age, what happens to that person may depend on whether relatives can provide care, or whether the person has financial resources to obtain care in his or her own home, a retirement home, or a residential care facility. Caregivers are often adult children or other relatives. The generation of individuals currently in their 40s, 50s, and 60s is often called the "sandwich generation" because they are caring for their children at the same time they are providing care for their aging parents. As parents age, the role reversal is often painful and demanding for both the elder and the caregiver.

Care of an aging parent requires sacrifice and commitment. As parents age, they may become more physically and cognitively impaired, increasing the likelihood of abuse. Elders who were themselves abusers are more likely to be abused by their caregivers. Older adults may undergo changes in personality that make it difficult for their adult children to care for them. They may need to be lifted, which may be difficult for someone with limited strength. They may need assistance walking, toileting, or eating that requires time the caregiver may not have. There is also an intimacy in caring for a parent that the caregiver may not be comfortable with.

All of these factors cause stress, which can be associated with abuse—especially in families in which violence is a response to stress. The needs of the older adult may exceed the family's ability to meet them.

In many ways, helpless older adults are in the same vulnerable position as children, because they are dependent on others for care. The population of the United States is aging, and by 2020, the number of adults older than 85 years is expected to account for 19% of the population (USDHHS Administration on Aging, 2012). Recognition of physical and behavioral indicators helps the professional become aware of possible abusive situations. None is conclusive in itself; however, each alerts the professional to the need for careful and complete assessment. Even though nurses are required to report instances of elder abuse, they may be reluctant to do so because assessment is not always conclusive. However, if there is a question of possible abuse, it must be reported to the appropriate authorities for further investigation. The State of New York took the lead in passing legislation with its "Granny's Law," which stiffened the penalties for assaults on elders. Table 27-2 lists the indicators of possible abuse of older adults.

COMMUNITY VIOLENCE

The United States is one of the most violent countries in the industrialized world. Every day we hear about some community, region, or state that has been affected by violent crime. Community violence may not affect everyone directly, but it affects all indirectly. In contrast to interpersonal violence, which affects only one or two individuals, community violence usually occurs suddenly and without warning and can potentially destroy entire segments of the population. Community violence includes workplace violence, youth violence, gang-related violence, hate crimes, and terrorism.

Workplace Violence

Workplace violence is a serious safety and health issue. Violence in the workplace includes physical assaults such as rape and homicide, muggings, verbal and written threats and bullying. In 2011, there were 458 workplace homicides out of a total of 4609 fatal work injuries in the United States (U.S. Bureau of Labor Statistics, 2012). Workplace violence tends to be more common in some service-oriented work environments, including health care. Such violence is widely believed to be underreported, perhaps in part because of belief that it is an expected part of certain jobs. In the health care field, frequent areas for the occurrence of violence include emergency departments, psychiatric units, geriatric units, and waiting rooms. Nurses and nursing assistants who work directly with patients are often at risk. Nurses who work in public health

TABLE 27-2 INDICATORS OF POSSIBLE ELDER ABUSE OR NEGLECT

Abuse

PHYSICAL INDICATORS	EMOTIONAL/BEHAVIORAL INDICATORS
Bruises, black eyes, welts, lacerations, and rope marks	Being emotionally upset or agitated
Bone and skull fractures	Being extremely withdrawn and noncommunicative or nonresponsive
Open wounds, cuts, punctures, untreated injuries in various stages of healing	Unusual behavior usually attributed to dementia (e.g., sucking, biting, rocking)
Sprains, dislocations, and internal injuries/bleeding	Sudden change in behavior
Signs of being subjected to punishment and signs of being restrained	Elder's report of being verbally or emotionally mistreated
Laboratory findings of medication overdose or underutilization of prescribed drugs	
Report of being hit, slapped, kicked, or mistreated	
The caregiver's refusal to allow visitors to see an elder alone	
Unexplained sexually transmitted disease	
Elders sudden change in behavior	
Elder's report of sexual assault	

Neglect

PHYSICAL INDICATORS	FINANCIAL INDICATORS (MATERIAL EXPLOITATION)
Dehydration, malnutrition, untreated bedsores, and poor personal hygiene	Sudden changes in bank account or banking practice (e.g., unexplained withdrawal of large sums of money, inclusion of additional names on an elder's bank signature card)
Unattended or untreated health problems	Unauthorized withdrawal of the elder's funds using the elder's automatic teller machine card
Hazardous or unsafe living conditions/arrangements (e.g., improper wiring, no heat, or no running water)	Abrupt changes in a will or other financial documents (e.g., power of attorney)
Unsanitary and unclean living conditions (e.g., dirt, fleas, lice, soiled bedding, fecal/urine smell, inadequate clothing)	Unexplained disappearance of funds or valuables
Elder's report of being mistreated or neglected	Bills unpaid despite the availability of adequate financial resources
Abandonment (desertion of an elder at a hospital, nursing facility, or other similar or public places or institutions)	Elder's signature being forged for financial transactions or for the titles of his/her possessions
	Sudden appearance of previously uninvolved relatives interested in the elder's affairs and possessions
	Unexplained sudden transfer of assets to a family member or someone outside the family
	The provision of services that are not necessary
	Report of financial exploitation

Modified from Administration on Aging/National Center on Elder Abuse: *Signs and symptoms of elder abuse*, 2011. Available from <www.ncea.aoa.gov/Main_Site/FAQ/Basics/Types_Of_Abuse.aspx>.

roles are not immune to violence because their work may bring them in direct contact with individuals prone to violent behavior. Identification of risk factors may offer some protection to the worker whether in the hospital or home or public health setting. Examples of risk factors include:

- Increasing numbers of acute and chronically mentally ill patients
- Working alone
- Availability of drugs at the worksite
- Low staffing levels
- Poorly lit parking areas and corridors
- Long waits for service
- Inadequate security
- Increasing numbers of substance abusers
- Access to firearms

Violence also negatively impacts the workplace, resulting in low morale, increased job stress and turnover, reduced trust of management and/or coworkers, and hostile work environments.

Youth-Related Violence

Violence is taking a toll on American youth. In 2010, juveniles (less than 18 years of age) accounted for 13.7% of all violent criminal arrests. Racial disparities are evident in youth-related violence, because blacks are more likely to be victims than either whites or Hispanics. Most of the increased homicide rates among American youth are attributable to death caused by firearms (CDC NCIPC, 2012f). Table 27-3 lists risk factors for youth-related violence.

Youth-related violence is more concentrated in minority communities and inner cities, putting a disproportionate burden on these communities. Violence is a complicated and multilayered problem. Adolescents and children increasingly use violence to settle disputes. Children are often not taught peaceful ways of resolving differences and learn by what they observe at home, on television, and in movies. Consequently, schools have become a common site for violence. See Chapter 29 for more information on violence in schools.

TABLE 27-3	RISK FACTORS FOR YOUTH-RELATED VIOLENCE
Individual Risk Factors	Involvement with drugs, alcohol or tobacco
	Antisocial beliefs and attitudes
	Low IQ
	History of violent victimization
	History of early aggressive behavior
	Attention deficits, hyperactivity or learning disorders
	Poor behavioral control
	Deficits in social, cognitive or information-processing abilities
	Exposure to violence and conflict in the family
	High emotional distress
	History of treatment of emotional problems
Community Risk Factors	Diminished economic opportunities
	High concentration of poor residents
	High level of family disruption
	Low levels of community participation
	Socially disorganized neighborhoods
	High level of transiency
Family Risk Factors	Poor family functioning
	Low emotional attachment to parents or caregivers
	Low parental education and income
	Parental substance abuse or criminality
	Poor monitoring and supervision of children
	Harsh, lax, or inconsistent disciplinary practices
	Authoritarian child-rearing attitudes
Peer/Social Risk Factors	Association with delinquent peers
	Involvement in gangs
	Social rejection by peers
	Lack of involvement in conventional activities
	Poor academic performance
	Low commitment to school and school failure

Data from Centers for Disease Control and Prevention, National Center for Injury Prevention and Control, Division of Violence Prevention: *Youth violence: Risk and protective factors,* 2013. Available from <www.cdc.gov/ViolencePrevention/youthviolence/riskprotectivefactors.html>.

Gangs

Gangs are increasingly responsible for crimes and violence throughout the United States. In 2009, the National Gang Threat Assessment reported that 94.3% of gang-related homicides involved the use of firearms. In 2011, there were an estimated 1.4 million youth gang members in the United States and the American Commonwealth (USDOJ, Bureau of Alcohol, Firearms, and Explosives [ATF], 2012).

Reasons that young people give for joining gangs include the belief that gangs will protect them, peer pressure, the need for respect, and a sense of belonging. Gangs exist in all 50 states, and it is estimated that gangs are responsible for approximately 48% of all crime, up to 90% in some areas. These crimes include illegal alien smuggling, armed robbery, assault, auto theft, drug and weapon trafficking, identity theft, and murder (USDOJ, Bureau of Alcohol, Firearms, and Explosives [ATF], 2012).

Prison Violence

The United States has one of the world's highest incarceration rate, 2.9% of adults (1 in 34 adults) being under some form of correctional supervision. Inmates are both victims and perpetrators of violence. With more than 1.5 million prisoners in federal and state prisons or local jails, **prison violence** includes allegations of physical abuse as well as reports of rape by both corrections officers and inmates (USDOJ, Bureau of Justice Statistics, 2012). The public and the judicial system have expressed little sympathy for this population for a variety of reasons, including indifference, disbelief, and denial. Little research exists to reflect the long-term effects on these victims or on society when they are released. See Chapter 31 for more information on forensic and correctional nursing.

Human Trafficking

Human trafficking is a global problem and public health issue. It may involve prostitution, sexual exploitation, forced labor, slavery, and removal of organs. Threats, coercion, abduction, fraud, and abuse of power are all methods used by human traffickers. An estimated 2.4 million people across the globe are victims of human trafficking at any given time, and 80% of them are being used as sexual slaves (HumanTrafficking.org, 2012). The United Nations Office on Drugs and Crime (2013) is actively helping states and countries legislate against and prevent trafficking.

Hate Crimes

Hate crimes are crimes in which the offender is motivated by factors such as an individual's race, sexual orientation, religious beliefs, ethnic background, or national origin. Hate crimes may include murder, sexual or physical assault, harassment, attacks on homes or on places of worship, or vandalism. Because hate crimes attack an individual's identity, the emotional effects are compounded. In 2009, 6604 hate crimes were reported in the United States even though it is estimated that only 44% of hate crimes are reported. The most commonly reported hate crimes are motivated by race, followed by religion and sexual orientation (USDOJ, Office of Justice Programs, 2011).

Terrorism

Terrorism has been present throughout history. The U.S. Department of Defense (2014) defines **terrorism** as "the unlawful use of violence or threat of violence to instill fear and coerce governments or societies. Terrorism is often motivated by religious, political, or other ideological beliefs and committed in the pursuit of goals that are usually political." All terrorist acts include at least three key elements—violence, fear, and intimidation. Nurses need to be prepared for terrorism in whatever form it takes, from an explosion at a local refinery to an act that affects an entire region or country, such as biological, chemical, or nuclear incidents. Mental and physical health issues remain a nursing concern for the victims, responders, and the community long after the act has occurred. See Chapter 28 for a more detailed discussion of terrorism.

FACTORS INFLUENCING VIOLENCE

Controversy surrounds the factors that influence violence in today's society. Three of them are easy access to firearms, the impact of media, and mental illness. Firearms are readily available, and even children are carrying guns to school.

The influence of media is pervasive in our society, especially among adolescents and young adults.

Firearms

Approximately 270 million privately owned firearms exist in the United States, and more than 1 million new handguns are sold in the United States annually. The United States ranks number one in privately owned guns among 179 countries, and statistics indicate that firearms are the weapon of choice in homicides in the United States. Of the nearly 13,000 murders in this country in 2010, 67.5% were committed with firearms (FBI, 2013).

Concern about firearms arises when it has been shown that guns kept in the home for self-protection are more likely to kill a family member or a friend than an attacker. Furthermore, the presence of a gun in the home triples the risk of homicide in the home and increases the risks of suicide three to five times and of accidental deaths by four (Edelman, 2013). The cost of gun violence is staggering. Direct cost of violence related to firearms in the United States is in millions of dollars annually. Indirect costs, including loss of productivity, mental health treatment, rehabilitation, and legal and judicial costs, adds even more. Heated discussions regarding firearms occur daily between opponents and proponents of gun control. Even the underlying meaning of the second amendment of the Constitution, "the right to bear arms," is argued.

Media

Media violence is prevalent and is accessible to all age-groups. It includes exposure to, and participation in, violent video games, music and music videos that depict rape or violence, and virtual violence that allows subscribers to harm or kill victims. Television and movies often depict people being tortured or killed in such graphic detail that may make it hard for children and adults to distinguish between reality and fantasy. Media violence has become more pronounced and graphic in nature. The public health community believes that repeated exposure to media violence leads to emotional desensitization to real-life violence.

Mental Illness

Mental illness is considered by many to be a major factor in violence. Studies, however, are inconclusive in their findings that all violence is committed by mentally unstable persons. Prosecutors and defense attorneys argue the case of whether someone is evil or mentally unstable when these cases go to court.

Following the violence in Newtown, Connecticut, there has been an increased push for legislation to fund public health strategies that identify and treat mental illness across the country. This is especially important since the budget crisis in the United States has forced many states to eliminate or reduce the availability of mental health services. See Chapter 24 for a more in-depth discussion of mental illness.

VIOLENCE FROM A PUBLIC HEALTH PERSPECTIVE

Dealing with violence has traditionally been the U.S. criminal justice system's responsibility. However, because violence is also a public health epidemic, efforts are being made to prevent and manage it using public health strategies and community approaches such as church groups, community groups, and local, state, and federal governments. Violence, as discussed previously, has a tremendous influence on morbidity and mortality rates and health care resources. The public health system is challenged to go beyond its traditional programs to include prevention and management of violence. As is true with most public health problems, many interrelated factors must be addressed.

Healthy People 2020 and Violence

Violence was one of the areas addressed by *Healthy People 2000* and again in *Healthy People 2010* and *Healthy People 2020*. Several objectives regarding violence and abuse prevention have been established. The *Healthy People 2020* table lists a few of these (HealthyPeople.gov, 2012). These objectives are intended to target causes of violence and abuse, improve national data collection and analysis, provide input for legislative funding, facilitate research efforts, and concentrate public health efforts on models that demonstrate effectiveness.

 HEALTHY PEOPLE 2020

Objectives Related to Injury and Violence Prevention

> *IVP–29:* Reduce homicides.
> *IVP–30:* Reduce firearm-related deaths.
> *IVP–31:* Reduce nonfatal firearm-related injuries.
> *IVP–32:* Reduce nonfatal physical assault injuries.
> *IVP–33:* Reduce physical assaults.
> *IVP–34:* Reduce physical fighting among adolescents.
> *IVP–35:* Reduce bullying among adolescents.
> *IVP–36:* Reduce weapon carrying by adolescents on school property.
> *IVP–37:* Reduce child maltreatment deaths.
> *IVP–38:* Reduce nonfatal child maltreatment.
> *IVP–41:* Reduce nonfatal intentional self-harm injuries.
> *IVP–42:* Reduce children's exposure to violence.
> *IVP–43:* Increase the number of states and the District of Columbia that link data on violent deaths from death certificates, law enforcement, and coroner and medical examiner reports to inform prevention efforts at the state and local levels.

From HealthyPeople.gov: *Healthy People 2020: Topics & objectives: Injury and violence prevention,* 2012. Available from <http://www.healthypeople.gov/2020/topicsobjectives2020/objectiveslist.aspx?topicId=24>.

Many of the *Healthy People 2020* objectives are difficult to achieve because of complex barriers. These barriers include lack of comparable data sources and standardized definitions as well as inadequate resources to establish consistent tracking systems and fund prevention programs.

PREVENTION OF VIOLENCE

The nurse who cares for people experiencing violence must be a skilled clinician who is knowledgeable about both the problem and available community resources. Box 27-4

BOX 27-4 SAFETY ISSUES FOR THE COMMUNITY HEALTH NURSE

Plan Ahead

- Know the area you are visiting.
- Schedule the visit ahead of time, and get the correct address, directions, and information about who will be in the home.
- Tell the office where you will be, and check in regularly.
- Carry a cell phone, possibly a pager, and a small amount of money.
- Dress for function and mobility, and wear a name tag. Avoid any provocative clothing.
- Ensure that the vehicle you drive is in good repair, has a full gas tank, and has emergency equipment. Always carry two sets of car keys.

Approaching the Home

- Notice the environment, animals, fences, activity, possible indicators of crime, and places you could go for assistance if necessary.
- Walk with confidence, and maintain a professional attitude.
- Listen for signs of fighting before knocking. If you hear sounds of fighting, leave!
- Do not enter a home if you suspect an unsafe situation.

In the Home

- Be aware of who is in the home and what is going on. If angry people are in the home, use your professional and social skills. Do not expect the client to protect you.
- Note the exits, and sit between the client and an exit of the home. Be prepared to leave quickly if the situation changes suddenly.
- If someone in the home is violent, leave and call 911.

Handling a Tight Situation

- Do not show fear; control your breathing.
- Speak calmly and in a soothing manner. Be assertive but not aggressive.
- Repeat the reason for your visit, and find a reason to leave.

Leaving the Home

- Take all of your belongings, and keep your car keys in your hand.
- Watch for cars following you when you leave. Do not stop. If you feel that you are in danger, go to the nearest police station or well-lighted business and ask for help.
- Trust your instincts. Never forget your own safety.

Modified from Oregon Public Health Association, Public Health Nursing Section, Seattle–King County Department of Public Health, and Washington State Public Health Association: *Public health nursing domestic violence protocol* [booklet], Seattle, WA, and Salem, OR, 1993, Authors.

presents tips regarding safety issues for a community health nurse. A considerable body of knowledge has been developed about trends in violence. Table 27-4 provides the components of a comprehensive program to reduce violence in individuals and the community.

Primary Prevention

The goal of primary prevention is to stop violence, abuse, or neglect before it occurs. Education plays a major part in primary prevention and may include life-skills training such as parenting and family wellness, anger management, and/or conflict resolution. Professionals should increase their awareness of violence and identification of cases. The nurse can work in or with the community to educate citizens about the problem of violence, potential causes of violence, and available community services.

Primary prevention must begin at a community level, helping to change attitudes about abuse and violence. Primary prevention focuses on stopping the transgenerational aspect of abuse, starting with young children and continuing throughout the life span. Mentoring and peer programs can be designed to promote healthy relationships and decrease conflict. For example, parenting is one of the most difficult jobs that individuals will undertake, yet there is a widespread myth that parenting "comes naturally." Classes for parents should focus on physical care of the infant, including ways to soothe and manage a "fussy" baby, the effect of fatigue on new parents, the need for support, and the fears and questions of new parents. Nurses in the hospital have little time to help new parents learn basic newborn care before discharge. Some hospitals and public health agencies provide follow-up to parents to ensure that they can adequately care for their newborn. This support is especially given to all persons deemed to be high risk for infant abuse, including teenage mothers, mothers without support, or women with a history of spousal abuse.

Secondary Prevention

The goal of secondary prevention is to assess, diagnose, and treat victims and perpetrators of violence. Consideration of the safety of the potential victim is critical.

Secondary prevention begins with assessment. For example, consistent assessment of women during health care visits will increase case finding and provide opportunities for early intervention that is particularly crucial during pregnancy. Women should be interviewed in private when asked about abuse. Questions should be asked in a matter-of-fact way and the health care provider should not show shock or dismay at the response. The Nursing Research Consortium on Violence and Abuse has developed a simple three-question abuse assessment screening. See ⓔ **Resource Tool 27A** for the Abuse Assessment Screen. These three questions should be asked of all women at each visit, and careful and detailed documentation should be done.

Victims, once identified, must be offered resources to increase their safety. However, all victims may not be ready or able to leave the situation, and available options must be explored. Victims should have knowledge of legal options and how to access them. The nurse must be ready to intervene when the abuse involves a child or someone who is cognitively impaired. Some states have developed protocols for nurses who deal with victims of violence. Review of these protocols can help the nurse become familiar with the questions to ask and suggestions that should be made to help the victim develop a safety plan. See ⓔ **Resource Tool 27B** for a sample of a safety plan.

Another example of secondary prevention involves screening for abuse in the elderly that should occur at every health care visit. Elder abuse remains underreported across the United States; therefore routine screening can facilitate early intervention. Nurses can help raise professional and community consciousness of elder abuse by participating in political activities to create or strengthen mandatory reporting laws and funding of support groups.

TABLE 27-4	EXAMPLES OF PREVENTION STRATEGIES TO REDUCE VIOLENCE FOR INDIVIDUALS AND COMMUNITIES	
INDIVIDUALS		**COMMUNITY**
Primary Prevention—Goal: Promotion of Optimal Parenting and Family Wellness		
Life-skill training in schools, churches, and communities		Community education concerning violence
Education of children, adolescents and adults on methods of conflict resolution		Reduction of media violence
Parenting classes in hospitals, schools, and other community agencies		Development of community support services such as crisis lines, respite care for families with dependent members, shelters for battered women and their children, and development and vigorous enforcement of anti-stalking measures, including cyberstalking
Mental health services for all age-groups		
Training for professionals in early detection of violence		Handgun safety education
Secondary Prevention—Goal: Diagnosis of and Service for Families in Stress		
Nursing assessment for evidence of violence in all health care settings		Education of all health professionals in assessment of violence and possible protocols for dealing with victims
A safety plan for victims		List of hospital emergency departments and trauma centers with 24-hour response Reporting of different types of abuse
Knowledge of legal options		
Shelter referral for victims		Coordination with medical authorities, Coordination with voluntary and social service agencies for provision of services
Social services for individuals or families		
Referral to self-help groups in the community		Death review teams to review deaths from injury, especially in infants and children
Referral to appropriate community agencies		Public authority involvement by police, district attorneys, and courts
		Epidemiological tracking and evaluation of violence
Tertiary Prevention—Goal: Reeducation and Rehabilitation of Violent Families		
Empowerment strategies for battered women		Foster homes, shelters, and care for dependents
Professional counseling services for individuals		Public authority involvement
Parenting reeducation (i.e., formal training in child-rearing)		Follow-up care for known cases of abuse, neglect, or violence
Counseling services for individuals and families		
Self-help groups		

The nurse should work with family members or caregivers who provide care for the elderly to promote healthier relationships. Helping the caregiver deal with stress by finding respite care, a home health aide, or counseling may help. Documentation is crucial in meeting medical-legal requirements. The nurse should record observations accurately and refrain from opinions and interpretations, because this documentation may be used in court proceedings.

The problem of violence cannot be managed by nurses alone, but rather in combination with other professionals, including physicians, child and adult protective services providers, social workers, clergy, and police. This interdisciplinary approach leads to optimal outcomes. Public health surveillance is important in obtaining accurate numbers of intentional injuries for individuals. Death review teams can analyze records to determine whether an injury was intentional or unintentional.

Tertiary Prevention

Tertiary prevention is aimed at rehabilitation of individuals, families, groups, or communities and includes both victims and perpetrators of violence. Rehabilitation may take months or even years, depending on the situation. For example, the September 11, 2001, attack on the United States disrupted thousands of lives and changed the country's sense of security. This attack affected everyone in the country, not just those in the immediate vicinity. After all these years, the effects continue. The nurse must be able to work in conjunction with a variety of mental health professionals and social service agencies to provide coordinated care. The nurse may have also been a victim and may be experiencing many of the same problems as those he or she is trying to help with. Self-care and recognition of the nurse's own limitations or needs are critical.

SUMMARY

Violence is a major public health issue in the United States and affects individuals across the life cycle. Morbidity and mortality statistics indicate that violence is epidemic in many communities. Whether it occurs at home, in the neighborhood, or at school, violence affects countless numbers of individuals. The influence of media, easy access to and proliferation of firearms, and mental illness in the United States are considered contributing factors to violence. The cycle of violence will persist if not broken. The abuser is also a victim, and the ultimate victim is society, which must care and pay for the results of violent acts.

Violence is a public health epidemic, and national objectives for reducing it have been identified. The core public health functions of needs assessment and surveillance, policy development, and assurance are useful methods of combating this epidemic. The literature describes interventions that focus on the three levels of prevention. The need for continued research in violence should be a funding priority at the local, state, and national levels. The reality of violence has been validated. Everyone is affected.

CASE STUDY   APPLICATION OF THE NURSING PROCESS

Karen, 36 years old, comes to the neighborhood clinic where you are the nurse. She is obviously distraught and is holding her head down when she enters the exam room. As you are getting her vital signs, she lifts her head and you notice multiple bruises on her face, around her left eye, and on her left cheek and the right side of her neck. She sees you looking at her and she begins to cry. You ask her what happened and she tells you that her boyfriend hit her two nights ago. As you question her further, you find out that she is divorced, has custody of her two children, a boy age 8 and a daughter age 3, and is unemployed. Her ex-husband lives three states away, about an 8-hour drive. She has been with the current boyfriend about 6 months and they have been living together about 3 months. He hit her repeatedly the night before last after he came home upset about a problem at work. The attack ended as abruptly as it started. He apologized repeatedly, hugged her, and left the house. Her children were in bed and did not witness the abuse. She took the children to a friend's house and then went to an after-hours clinic for treatment. While she was at the after-hours clinic, the police were notified, and she pressed charges against her boyfriend. He was arrested later that night and she subsequently filed a restraining order against him.

After further discussion, she tells you that this is not the first time he has hit her; that it has happened twice before, always after something has upset him. She then states that she knows he loves her and that he would not deliberately hurt her—that she must have done something to make him angry. She feels that he does really love her and she regrets having him arrested and filing the restraining order. She felt as if she had no choice once the clinic personnel and the police urged her to do something. He is now in the county jail and she is considering going to the police station and dropping the charges. She does admit, however, that she is afraid about how angry he is going to be once he gets out.

You tell her about the cycle of domestic violence and how it repeats itself. You give her information about local shelters and explain that abusers usually do not stop their cycle of violence on their own, but only after counseling and support. You also tell her that she may be in danger of serious harm and even death if she stays with him. You recommend that she leave where she is living, take her children with her, and talk with an attorney before doing anything about the legal situation.

One month later, Karen again appears in your clinic. She tells you that she did leave home and take her two children to her ex-husband's house. She also states that the boyfriend is still in county jail, that she did not drop the restraining order, and that she has moved in with her boyfriend's mother. She visits him every Sunday afternoon and talks to him once a week on the phone. His mother refuses to speak with him.

Assessment

The following are the summary assessment points:
- The boyfriend has a history of intimate partner violence (IPV)—duration unknown.
- Karen is a stay-at-home mom, with two children under the age of 9 years, who currently live with their father in another state.
- Karen does not have close family in the area.
- Karen does not believe that she is in danger.
- Karen believes she lacks employable skills.
- The boyfriend's abuse is aggravated by problems at work.

Diagnoses
- Potential for severe injury or death related to abuse
- High risk for emotional trauma from dysfunctional family dynamics
- High risk for loss of children

Planning
Short-Term Goals
- Boyfriend will be referred for anger management classes once released.
- Strategies will be identified to help Karen regain her children.
- A safe setting will be identified for Karen and the children.

Long-Term Goals
- Karen will be free of IPV.
- Karen will enter individual counseling.
- Boyfriend will enter counseling.

Intervention
Individual
Karen was assessed for injuries, and none was found to be life threatening. She was given a referral for counseling at the local counseling center where a community health nurse works. She was also given locations and numbers for local shelters. She did leave the charges against her boyfriend standing and decided not to drop the restraining order.

Karen agreed to enter counseling and continues to live with her boyfriend's mother until other arrangements can be made. She decided to leave her children at her ex-husband's house until she feels more secure about her situation. Karen has spoken with the community health nurse at the local counseling center. The nurse's goals are centered on Karen's ongoing physical and emotional well-being.

During these visits the nurse was able to engage Karen in conversation regarding her future and that of her children. Karen indicated that this most recent episode of violence had frightened her and caused her to question the wisdom of her decision to stay with her boyfriend. Her boyfriend was found guilty of domestic abuse and was released after 2 months with a probation period of 2 years and mandatory anger management classes. She and her ex-husband are discussing child care arrangements and the possibility of her moving closer to him where she should be able to find work.

Community
The community health nurse arranged to speak at the monthly breakfast meeting of community pastors where she presented an informational program on IPV. Within 3 weeks she received speaking invitations from four of the nine churches represented at the meeting. The first of the programs will take place in the next month. In two of the churches, "mother's day out" (a partial day of babysitting) services are available to church members, and after an appeal from the community health nurse, one of the churches has expressed a willingness to open its program to non–church members.

Evaluation
Individual and Community
You and the community health nurses jointly focused on safety as a priority of care for Karen. The visit to the after-hours clinic and the medical personnel's call to the police started the chain of events. Karen's injuries created an opportunity for the community health nurse to maintain contact and provide psychosocial support. During visits the nurse was able to speak openly with Karen and offer options to enhance her coping skills. One of the local pastors has encouraged Karen to focus on both her children and her own future.

Karen came back into the clinic where you are working and seems healthier. She states that she is going to move to the same area where her ex-husband is living and will be reconciled with her children. Karen also says that her ex-husband agreed to help her

CASE STUDY   APPLICATION OF THE NURSING PROCESS—cont'd

find employment in the area. Her boyfriend continues to fulfill the requirements of his probation, and he acknowledges that this will be an ongoing recovery process.

Levels of Prevention
Primary
Goal: Promote safety and prevent violence.
- Encourage contact with friends in the neighborhood and at church.
- Provide services of the community health nurse.
- Provide community education programs about anger management.
- Provide community education programs about IPV.

Secondary
Goal: Assess for signs of IPV.
- Facilitate health care for treatment of injuries.
- Provide both physical and psychosocial support.
- Provide referral for anger management.
- Provide individual and family counseling.
- Provide a 24-hour abuse hotline number.

Tertiary
Goal: Promote development of healthy family dynamics.
- Encourage continued use of community resources.
- Encourage community involvement with other young families.
- Provide community education programs on the cycle of violence.

LEARNING ACTIVITIES

1. Investigate professional responsibilities relative to reporting abuse, neglect, or violence in your state. Share findings with classmates.
2. Using the telephone directory or computer search engine, find three public or private agencies in the community that provide help for victims of violence. Make a list of the telephone numbers and post copies of it in public areas.
3. Call a child abuse center in the community and ask what services they provide.
4. Call a battered women's shelter and determine the procedure for securing shelter placement for a battered victim and her children.
5. Visit a respite center for the elderly and observe the clients and the activities that are provided. Observe behaviors that would contribute to stress in the caregiver.
6. Find out what support groups exist in the community for older adult caregivers.
7. Read your local newspaper for 1 month and clip articles that deal with violence and gun control. Determine how many individuals were killed or injured during that period. How many of the deaths and injuries were gun related?
8. Look up the laws that relate to reporting of child and elder abuse in your area.

⊜ EVOLVE WEBSITE
http://evolve.elsevier.com/Nies
- NCLEX Review Questions
- Case Studies
- Glossary
- Resource Tool 27A: Abuse Assessment Screen
- Resource Tool – 27B: Planning for Safety

REFERENCES

Campbell J, Humphreys J: *Nursing care of survivors of family violence,* St. Louis, 1993, Mosby.

Centers for Disease Control and Prevention: Physical dating violence among high school students—United States, 2003, *MMWR Morb Mortal Wkly Rep* 55:532–535, 2006. Also Available from <www.cdc.gov/mmwr/preview/mmwr.html/mm5519a3.htm>.

Centers for Disease Control and Prevention: *Injury prevention & control: CDC helps prevent global violence,* 2011. Available from <www.cdc.gov/violenceprevention/globalviolence/index.html>.

Centers for Disease Control and Prevention: *Table LCWK1: Deaths, percent of total deaths, and death rates for the 15 leading causes of death in 5-year age groups, by race and sex: United States, 2010,* 2012a. Available from <www.cdc.gov/nchs/data/dvs/LCWK1_2010.pdf>.

Centers for Disease Control and Prevention: *Violence prevention,* 2012b. Available from <www.cdc.gov/violenceprevention/index.html>.

Centers for Disease Control and Prevention, National Center for Injury Prevention and Control: *Child maltreatment: Facts at a glance,* 2010. Available from <www.cdc.gov/ViolencePrevention/pdf/CM_DataSheet-a.pdf>.

Centers for Disease Control and Prevention, National Center for Injury Prevention and Control: *Child maltreatment: Consequences,* 2011. Available from <www.cdc.gov/ViolencePrevention/childmaltreatment/consequences.html>.

Centers for Disease Control and Prevention, National Center for Injury Prevention and Control: *Child maltreatment: Facts at a glance,* 2012a. Available from <www.cdc.gov/ViolencePrevention/pdf/CM_DataSheet2012-a.pdf>.

Centers for Disease Control and Prevention, National Center for Injury Prevention and Control: *Suicide: Facts at a glance,* 2012b. Available from <www.cdc.gov/violenceprevention/pdf/Suicide_DataSheet_a.pdf>.

Centers for Disease Control and Prevention, National Center for Injury Prevention and Control: *Understanding child maltreatment: Fact sheet,* 2012c. Available from <www.cdc.gov/ViolencePrevention/pdf/CM_Factsheet2012-a.pdf>.

Centers for Disease Control and Prevention, National Center for Injury Prevention and Control: *Understanding intimate partner violence: Fact sheet,* 2012d. Available from <www.cdc.gov/violenceprevention/pdf/IPV_factsheet-a.pdf>.

Centers for Disease Control and Prevention, National Center for Injury Prevention and Control: *Understanding teen dating violence: Fact sheet,* 2012e. Available from <www.cdc.gov/violenceprevention.gov/TheViolencePrevention/pdf/TeenDatingViolence2012.a.pdf>.

Centers for Disease Control and Prevention, National Center for Injury Prevention and Control: *Youth violence: Facts at a glance,* 2012f. Available from <www.cdc.gov/ViolencePrevention/pdf/yr-datasheet-a.pdf>.

Domestic Abuse Intervention Program: *Wheel gallery,* 2011. Available from <http://www.theduluthmodel.org/index.htm>.

Edelman MW: The massive human and moral costs of gun violence, *Huffington Post,* January 11, 2013. Available from <www.huffingtonpost.com/marian-wright-edelman/the-massive-human-and-morale_b_2459693.html>.

Federal Bureau of Investigation: *Crime in the United States 2010: Expanded homicide data,* 2010. Available from <http://www.fbi.gov/about-us/cjis/ucr/crime-in-the-u.s./2012/crime-in-the-u.s.2012>.

HealthyPeople.gov: *Healthy People 2020: Topics & objectives,* October 30, 2012. Available from <www.healthypeople.gov/2020/topicsobj';s2020/objectiveslist.aspx?topicId=24>.

HumanTrafficking.org: *News and updates: U.N.: 2.4 million victims,* April 4, 2012. Available from <http://humantrafficking.org/updates/893>.

KidsHealth: *Abusive head trauma (shaken baby syndrome),* 2011. Available from <http://kidshealth.org/parent/medical/brain/shaken.html>.

March of Dimes: *Staying safe: Abuse during pregnancy,* 2008. Available from <www.marchofdimes.com/pregnancy/stayingsafe_abuse.html>.

Mother Goose nursery rhymes, Bath, England, 2000, Robert Frederick Publishing.

National Center on Elder Abuse: *Elder abuse prevalence and incidence: Fact sheet,* 2005. Available from <www.ncea.aoa.gov/main_site/pdf/publication/FinalStatistics050331.pdf>.

National Center on Elder Abuse: *Major types of elder abuse,* 2011. Available from <www.ncea.aoa.gov/ncearoot/Main_Site/FAQ/Basics/Types_Of_Abuse.aspx>.

National Center for Victims of Crime: *National Stalking Awareness Month,* 2014. Available from http://www.victimsofcrime.org/our-programs/stalking-resource-center/resources/national-stalking-awareness-month.

Rape, Abuse, & Incest National Network: *Statistics,* 2009. Available from <www.rainn.org/statistics>.

United Nations, Office on Drugs and Crime: *Human trafficking,* 2013. Available from <http://www.unodc.org/unodc/en/human-trafficking/what-is-human-trafficking.html>.

U.S. Bureau of Labor Statistics: *Injuries, illnesses and fatalities,* 2012. Available from <www.bls.gov/iif/>.

U.S. Department of Defense: Dictionary of Military and Associated Terms. Joint Publication 1-02: February 15, 2014. Available from www.dtic.mil/doctrine/dod_dictionary

U.S. Department of Justice, Bureau of Alcohol, Firearms and Explosives: *Fact sheet: Combating gang violence,* 2012. Available from www.atf.gov/publications/factsheets/factsheet-combating-gang-violence.html.

U.S. Department of Justice, Bureau of Justice Statistics: *Prisoners in 2011,* 2012. Available from <http://bjs.ojp.usdoj.gov/index.cfm?ty=pbdetail&iid=4559>.

U.S. Department of Justice, Office of Justice Programs: *Fact sheet: Hate crimes,* 2011. Available from <www.ojp.gov/newsroom/factssheets/ojpfs_hatecrimes.html>.

U.S. Department of Justice, Office on Violence Against Women: *About stalking,* 2009. Available from <www.ojp.usdoj.gov/bjs/abstract/svus.htm>.

van der Zande I: *Bullying—common questions and answers from Kidpower,* n.d. Available from <www.kidpower.org/library/article/bullying-questions-answers/?gclid=COuX-NLkqbUCFY6PPAodhTMAvw>.

World Health Organization: *Health topics: Violence,* 2013. Available from <http://www.who.int/topics/violence/en/>.

Natural and Man-Made Disasters

Edith B. Summerlin

OBJECTIVES

Upon completion of this chapter, the reader will be able to do the following:

1. Identify the types of disasters.
2. Discuss the characteristics of disasters.
3. Describe the stages of a disaster.
4. Discuss the stages of disaster management.

5. Describe the roles of federal, state, local, and volunteer agencies involved in disaster management.
6. Identify potential bioterrorist chemical and biological agents.
7. Discuss the impact of disasters on a community.
8. Describe the role and responsibilities of nurses in relation to disasters.

KEY TERMS

American Red Cross
direct victim
disaster
disaster triage
displaced persons
Federal Emergency Management
   Agency (FEMA)
first responders
frequency

imminence
indirect victim
mass casualty
mitigation
multiple casualty
natech (natural-technological) disaster
National Incident Management System
National Response Framework
Office of Emergency Management

predictability
preventability
refugees
resource map
risk map
shelter in place
terrorism
U.S. Department of Homeland Security
weapon of mass destruction

OUTLINE

Disaster Definitions
Types of Disasters
Characteristics of Disasters
   Frequency
   Predictability
   Preventability/Mitigation
   Imminence
   Scope and Number of Casualties
   Intensity

Disaster Management
   Local, State, and Federal Governmental Responsibilities
   Public Health System
   American Red Cross
Disaster Management Stages
   Prevention Stage
   Preparedness and Planning Stage
   Response Stage
   Recovery Stage

Communities throughout the world experience an emergency or disaster incident of one kind or another almost daily. The media may only mention these events or may report on them in great detail, depending on the number of dead or injured, the amount of devastation or damage to the area involved, and how much the event has disrupted normal activities within the community.

The health of a community can be affected significantly by disasters. Hurricanes Sandy, Katrina, and Rita are examples of how communities and their hospitals, clinics, nursing homes, and other health care facilities are directly affected by a disaster. During Katrina and Rita, both of which occurred in 2005, access to health care was impeded by physical barriers, such as road closures due to flooding, inadequate numbers of first responders, and limited transportation for search and rescue. Patients were evacuated from one hospital to another, sometimes more than once. Medical and nursing personnel, medicines, and needed supplies were unavailable, scarce, or depleted because of the increased demand. Temporary shelters and health care services were established in schools, churches, and a variety of other facilities throughout the area. The wind damage and extensive flooding from Hurricane Katrina resulted in panic for food, water, and rescue in the Gulf Coast regions between New Orleans, Louisiana, and Biloxi, Mississippi. First responders and rescue teams were overwhelmed in their attempts to reach the victims. The same would have been experienced during Hurricane Sandy.

The evacuation of Houston, Texas, and the surrounding coastal area because of Hurricane Rita created severe traffic jams, many lasting 18 to 20 hours, so travelers needed water, food, and gasoline before they reached shelter. As a result, many people suffered from dehydration and urinary tract infections. In addition, Hurricane Rita occurred during a period of record heat, and many travelers became victims of heat exhaustion caused by the high temperature and humidity. The lessons learned from these events resulted in changes in disaster plans that made a significant difference in how the next major hurricane—Ike in September 2008—was managed.

Hurricanes, tornadoes, floods, wildfires, and industrial accidents occur yearly in some parts of the United States. Further, in recent years, terrorist attacks have become more common. The bombings of the World Trade Center in New York City in 1991 and the bombing of the Alfred P. Murrah Federal Building in 1995 occurred two decades ago, but the combined terrorist attacks on the twin towers of the World Trade Center in New York City, the Pentagon in Washington, DC, the plane hijacking and crash in Pennsylvania in 2001, and the Boston Marathon bombings in 2013 indicate that the potential is ever present. Additionally, terrorist attacks occur all over the world on an almost daily basis, and concerns about potential terrorist attacks have increased the focus on what needs to be done in terms of prevention/mitigation, preparedness, response, and recovery—not only in the event of terrorist attacks but also in the event of disasters of all kinds (Federal Bureau of Investigation [FBI], 2013).

Because of the recognition of the need to be prepared, programs have been created to address the national, state, and local management of disasters. President George W. Bush established the U.S. Department of Homeland Security (DHS) in March 2003 and put into place the **National Incident Management System** (NIMS) the following year. The NIMS provides a systematic, proactive way for all levels of governmental and nongovernmental agencies to work seamlessly to prevent, protect against, respond to, recover from, and prevent the effects of disasters (Federal Emergency Management Agency [FEMA], 2012c). Local Citizen Corps Councils have been established throughout the country to give volunteers an opportunity to support local fire, law enforcement, emergency medical services, and community public health efforts and to contribute to the four stages of emergency management: prevention, preparedness, response, and recovery (FEMA, 2013e).

Efforts to prepare for disasters have also been significantly enhanced at the state level. In 2003, for example, the Texas Legislature passed a bill requiring nurses to attend a continuing education program related to bioterrorism. Further, the Ready Texas Nurses Emergency Response System (Ready Texas Nurses) was created to allow mobilization of volunteer nurses to support communities in times of crisis or disaster. Similar actions are occurring throughout the country.

Nurses have both a personal and a professional role in relation to disasters. Nurses' personal role is to develop a disaster plan for work, home, and family. Disaster kits for survival in each of these settings should be prepared. Professionally nurses are uniquely positioned to provide valuable information for the development of plans for disaster prevention, preparedness, response, and recovery for the facilities in which they are employed as well as the communities in which they live. Nurses, as team members, can cooperate with health and social representatives, government bodies, community groups, and volunteer agencies in disaster planning and preparedness programs (e.g., drills). Using their knowledge of nursing, public health, and cultural-familial structures, as well as their clinical skills and abilities, nurses can actively assist with or participate in all aspects and stages of an emergency or disaster, regardless of the setting in which the event may occur. Disaster nursing requires the application of basic nursing knowledge and skills in difficult environments with scare resources and changing conditions.

DISASTER DEFINITIONS

A **disaster** is any event that causes a level of destruction, death, or injury that affects the abilities of the community to respond to the incident using available resources. Emergencies differ from disasters, in that agencies, communities, families, or individuals can manage emergencies using their own resources. But a disaster event, depending on the characteristics of the disaster, may be beyond the ability of the community to respond and recover from the incident using its own resources. Disasters frequently require assistance from outside the immediate community, both for management of resulting issues and for recovery.

Some disasters (e.g., a house fire) may affect only a few persons, whereas others (e.g., a hurricane) can impact thousands. A **mass casualty** event is one in which 100 or more individuals are involved; a **multiple casualty** event is one in which more than 2 but fewer than 100 individuals are involved. A casualty can be classified as a direct victim, an indirect victim, a displaced person, or a refugee. A **direct victim** is an individual who is immediately affected by the event; the **indirect victim** may be a family member or friend of the victim or a first responder. Displaced persons and refugees are special categories of direct victims. **Displaced persons** are those who have to evacuate their homes, schools, or businesses as a result of a disaster; **refugees** are a group of people who have fled their homes or even their country as a result of famine, drought, natural disaster, war, or civil unrest.

BOX 28-1 TYPES OF DISASTERS

Natural Disasters	Man-Made Disasters
Avalanches	Terrorism
Blizzards	Civil unrest (riots)
Communicable disease epidemics	Explosions, bombings
	Fires
Droughts, wildfires	Structural collapse (bridges)
Earthquakes, tsunamis	Floods, mudslides
Hailstorms	Toxic or hazardous spills
Heat waves	Mass transit accidents
Hurricanes	Pollution
Tornadoes, cyclones	Wars
Volcanic eruptions	

TYPES OF DISASTERS

Disasters are identified as natural, man-made, or a combination of both. A natech (natural-technological) disaster is a natural disaster that creates or results in a widespread technological problem. An example of a NA-TECH disaster is an earthquake that causes structural collapse of roadways or bridges, which, in turn, leads to downed electrical wires and subsequent fires. Another example is a chemical spill resulting from a flood. Types of natural disasters and man-made disasters are listed in Box 28-1.

The American Public Health Association identified types of disasters and their consequences (Landesman, 2012). Types of disasters are blizzards, cold waves, heavy snowfalls, cyclones, tornadoes, drought, earthquakes, floods, heat waves, thunderstorms, volcanic eruptions, wildfires, man-made and technological events, explosions or blasts, and epidemics. It was noted in the report that injury or death from the disaster in question may be direct or indirect. For example, injuries from hurricanes occur because people fail to evacuate or take shelter, do not take precautions in securing their property despite adequate warning, and do not follow guidelines on food and water safety or injury prevention during recovery. Drowning, electrocution, lacerations or punctures from flying debris, and blunt trauma from falling trees or other objects are some of the morbidity concerns. Heart attacks and stress-related disorders also occur. Injuries also may occur from activities in the recovery phase, for example, from use of chain saws or other power equipment or from animal, snake, or insect bites.

Americans are familiar with most of the disasters listed in Box 28-1, but terrorism was largely unknown or unheeded prior to the bombing of the Alfred P. Murrah Federal Building in Oklahoma City in 1995. The U.S. Code of Federal Regulations defines terrorism as "the unlawful use of force and violence against persons or property to intimidate or coerce a government, the civilian population, or any segment thereof, in furtherance of political or social objectives" (FBI, 2013). The FBI is charged with the responsibility for investigating terrorism-related matters in the United States and internationally. According to the Central Intelligence Agency (2013b), terrorism "is premeditated, politically motivated violence perpetrated against noncombatant targets by sub-national groups or clandestine agents." *International terrorism* involves the territory or the citizens of more than one country (p. 1).

The FBI reported the breakdown of terrorist events in the United States from 1980-1999 as: bombings 321; 22 other; assassinations 21; arson 19; shootings 19; 15 sabotage/malicious destruction; 13 robbery; 10 hostile takeovers; assaults; 5 weapons of mass destruction; kidnapping/hijacking; 2 rocket attacks; a total of 457 incidents or planned acts (FBI, 2013). Specific incidents of terrorism include the September 11, 2001 terrorist attacks; bombing of the Alfred P. Murrah Federal Building, 1995; the nerve gas (sarin) attack in the Tokyo subway in March 1995, which killed 12 and injured more than 6000 people; the bombing of the commuter train in Spain in March 2004, which killed 191 people; the suicide bombings in the London transport system in July 2005, which killed 52 commuters and four terrorists; and the shooting and bombing attacks in the financial district of Mumbai, India, in November 2008, which killed more than 170.

Concerns now are increasingly focused on weapons of mass destruction. Weapon of mass destruction refer to any weapon that is designed or intended to cause death or serious bodily injury through release, dissemination, or impact of toxic or poisonous chemicals, or their precursors; any weapon involving a disease organism; or any weapon that is designed to release radiation or radioactivity at a level dangerous to human life. Biological organisms considered to be potential weapons of mass destruction are shown in Box 28-2, and chemicals that are potential weapons of mass destruction are listed in Table 28-1. Chemical warfare agents are classified as nerve agents, vesicants, pulmonary agents, and cyanides (formerly "blood agents"). These tables also include information about the lethality, treatment, and impact related to each.

CHARACTERISTICS OF DISASTERS

Several characteristics have been used to describe disasters (Box 28-3). These characteristics are interdependent and therefore important to consider in plans for managing any disaster event. Each is discussed briefly.

Frequency

Frequency refers to how often a disaster occurs. Some disasters occur relatively often in certain parts of the world. Terrorist activities are occurring on an almost daily basis in Iraq and elsewhere in the world. Other examples are hurricanes, which occur with variable frequency between the months of June and November in the northern hemisphere, and earthquakes, which occur periodically throughout the world. In the United States, earthquakes are generally considered to be a West Coast problem, but 45 states and territories are at moderate to high risk for an earthquake, and earthquakes have occurred in every region of the country (DHS, 2013). Other disasters, such as volcanic eruptions, are far less frequent and are geographically limited to certain regions.

BOX 28-2 BIOTERRORISM AGENTS/ DISEASES

Category A

High-priority agents include organisms that pose a risk to national security because they:

- Can be easily disseminated or transmitted from person to person;
- Result in high mortality rates and have the potential for major public health impact;
- Might cause public panic and social disruption; and
- Require special action for public health preparedness.

Agents/diseases:

- Anthrax (*Bacillus anthracis*)
- Botulism (*Clostridium botulinum* toxin)
- Plague (*Yersinia pestis*)
- Smallpox (Variola major)
- Tularemia (*Francisella tularensis*)
- Viral hemorrhagic fevers (filoviruses [e.g., Ebola, Marburg]) and arenaviruses [e.g., Lassam Nacgyoi])

Category B

Second-highest-priority agents include those that:

- Are moderately easy to disseminate;
- Result in moderate morbidity rates and low mortality rates; and
- Require specific enhancements of CDC's diagnostic capacity and enhanced disease surveillance.

Agents/diseases:

- Brucellosis (*Brucella* species)
- Epsilon toxin of *Clostridium perfringens*
- Food safety threats (e.g, *Salmonella* species, *Escherichia coli* 0157:H7, *Shigella*)

Category C

Third-highest-priority agents include emerging pathogens that could be engineered for mass dissemination in the future because of:

- Availability;
- Ease of production and dissemination; and
- Potential for high morbidity and mortality rates and major health impact.

Agents:

- Emerging infectious diseases such as Nipah virus and hantavirus

Data from National Center for Environment Health (NCEI), <http://www.cdc.gov/nceh/>; Agency for Toxic Substances and Disease Registry (ATSDR), <http://www.atsdr.cdc.gov/>; and National Center for Injury and Violence Prevention and Control (NCIPC), <http://www.cdc.gov/injury/>.

Predictability

Predictability relates to the ability to determine when and whether a disaster event will occur. Some disasters, such as floods, may be predicted in the spring through monitoring of the snowmelt. Weather forecasters can predict when conditions are right for the development of tornadoes; these generally occur between April and June, but they may occur at any time of the year or as secondary results of hurricanes. Weather forecasters can predict hurricanes with increasing accuracy. Other disasters (e.g., fires and industrial explosions) may not be predictable at all.

Preventability/Mitigation

Mitigation refers to actions taken to reduce loss of life and property by lessening the impact of disasters. It means taking action now—before the next disaster—to reduce human and financial consequences. (FEMA, 2013f). Some disasters (e.g., hurricanes, tornadoes, and earthquakes) are not preventable, whereas others can be easily controlled if not prevented entirely. For example, flooding can be controlled or prevented through construction of dams or levees or deepening bayous.

Primary prevention is aimed at preventing the occurrence of a disaster or limiting consequences when the event itself cannot be prevented (mitigation). Primary prevention occurs in the nondisaster and predisaster stages. The *nondisaster stage* is the period before a disaster occurs, and the *predisaster stage* is time when a disaster is pending. Preventive actions during the nondisaster stage include assessing communities to determine potential disaster hazards; developing disaster plans at local, state, and federal levels; conducting drills to test the plan; training volunteers and health care providers; and providing educational programs of all kinds.

Risk maps and resource maps are developed to aid in planning. A risk map is a geographic map of an area that is analyzed for the impact of a potential disaster on the population and buildings in the area that would be involved (e.g., an area in a flood plain, an area covered if a nuclear explosion would occur, an area involved in an explosion of an industrial site) (Figure 28-1). A resource map is a geographic map that outlines the resources that would be available in or near the area affected by a potential disaster (e.g., potential shelter sites, potential medical sources, and location of equipment that might be needed) (Figure 28-2).

The disaster plan is initiated predisaster, or when a disaster is imminent. Primary prevention actions during this stage include notification of the appropriate officials, warning of the population, and advising what response to take (e.g., voluntary or mandatory evacuation).

Secondary prevention strategies are implemented once the disaster occurs. They are actions aimed at preventing further injury or destruction. Safety is considered before search and rescue.

Tertiary prevention focuses on recovery of the community, that is, restoring the community to its previous level of functioning and its residents to their maximum functioning. Tertiary prevention is aimed at preventing a recurrence or minimizing the effects of future disasters through debriefing meetings to identify problems with the plan and make revisions.

Nurses should be involved in all stages of prevention and related activities. In order to respond effectively, personally, and professionally during different types of disasters, nurses need to know: (1) what kind of disasters threaten their communities, (2) what injuries to expect from different disaster scenarios, (3) evacuation routes, (4) locations of shelters, and (5) warning systems. They must be able to educate others about disasters and how to prepare for and respond to them. Finally, nurses need to keep up to date on the latest recommendations and advances in lifesaving measures (e.g., basic first aid, cardiopulmonary resuscitation [CPR], and use of automated external defibrillators).

TABLE 28-1 CHEMICAL AGENTS OF MASS DESTRUCTION

CHEMICAL AGENT	LETHALITY	TREATMENT	IMPACT
Sarin (nerve agent)	High	Move to fresh air; wash skin; drugs have limited effectiveness	Likely nerve agent; chemicals needed to produce are banned by International Chemical Weapons Convention
VX (nerve agent)	Very high	Move to fresh air; wash skin; drugs have limited effectiveness	Not likely weapon; difficult to manufacture
Tabun (nerve agent)	High	Move to fresh air; wash skin; drugs have limited effectiveness	Easy-to-manufacture nerve agent; likely agent to be used
Chlorine (pulmonary agent)	Low	Move to fresh air; wash skin; no antidote	Readily available; likely agent because of availability; breaks down with water
Hydrogen cyanide (blood agent)	Low to moderate	Move to fresh air; wash skin; some drugs mitigate effects	Industrial product; some chemicals used to produce it are banned; likely agent because of availability

Modified from Cieslak TJ, Eitzen EM: Bioterrorism: agents of concern, *J Public Health Manag Pract* 6(4):19-29, 2000.

BOX 28-3 CHARACTERISTICS OF DISASTERS

Frequency
Predictability
Preventability
Imminence
Scope and number of casualties
Intensity

Imminence

Imminence is the speed of onset of an impending disaster and relates to the extent of forewarning possible and the anticipated duration of the incident. Weather forecasters can tell when a hurricane may be developing days ahead of its expected arrival and can give the time of arrival, general direction it will take, and an approximate location for its landing and forward movement. Hurricanes, however, are subject to other weather variables and can change direction and intensity several times before making landfall. A *warning* for a hurricane means it will reach landfall in 24 hours or less, whereas a *watch* means it will reach landfall in 24 to 36 hours. A warning for tornadoes means to take shelter immediately, and a watch means to stay alert for possible tornadoes.

Some disastrous incidents (e.g., wildfires, explosions, and terrorist attacks) have no warning time. Bioterrorist attacks are generally silent, and the first awareness may be days or even weeks after exposure. For example, individuals exposed to a pathologic agent (e.g., anthrax, smallpox) may arrive at health care facilities at various times and to various providers, making diagnosis and early treatment difficult. Nurses and medical personnel need to know the signs and symptoms of biological, chemical, radiation, and nuclear exposure in order to identify the nature of the threat, report the problem to the Centers for Disease Control and Prevention (CDC) and then treat and control the spread of both biological and chemical agents (see Box 28-2 and Table 28-1).

Scope and Number of Casualties

The *scope* of a disaster indicates the range of its effect. The scope is described in terms of both the geographic area involved and the number of individuals affected, injured, or killed. From a health care perspective, the location, type, and timing of a disaster event are predictors of the types of injuries and illnesses that might occur. For example, the October 1989 earthquake in San Francisco occurred while people were on their way to work. Overall, more than 60 people died from a multitude of causes, including a motorcycle officer who was killed after the collapse of a freeway, 16 people who were killed by building collapses, 5 who died as a result of falls, and 9 who died of heart attacks.

In contrast, the earthquake and tsunami in December 2004 killed more than 174,000 people in South Asia, Southeast Asia, and East Africa; most died of drowning (CDC, 2013b). Another example of the horribly destructive power of earthquakes is the Pakistani quake of October 2005. It caused landslides that killed more than 73,000 people, many of the whom were children whose schools were buried by the mudslides.

Hurricanes generally affect a large geographic area. Nevertheless, they may cause few if any deaths if sufficient preventive measures are taken. The scope of Hurricane Katrina in September 2005 covered all of New Orleans, most of south Louisiana, and parts of Florida, Alabama, and Mississippi. Hurricane Rita, only a few days later, struck New Orleans again as well as south Louisiana and much of eastern Texas. Remarkably, despite the widespread destruction caused by these storms, the number of dead from Katrina was more than 1300, and the number of dead from Hurricane Rita was 58, including 23 elders who were killed in a bus accident while evacuating.

Intensity

Intensity is the characteristic describing the level of destruction and devastation of the disaster event. Factors contributing to the amount of damage from a disaster event such as a hurricane are the distance from the zone of maximum winds, how exposed the location is, building standards, vegetation type, and resultant flooding. Parts of New Orleans were under water from the primary effects (storm surge and rain) and secondary effects (levee failure) of Hurricane Katrina. Some buildings and homes were completely destroyed, and others were left in terrible condition by flooding and wind damage.

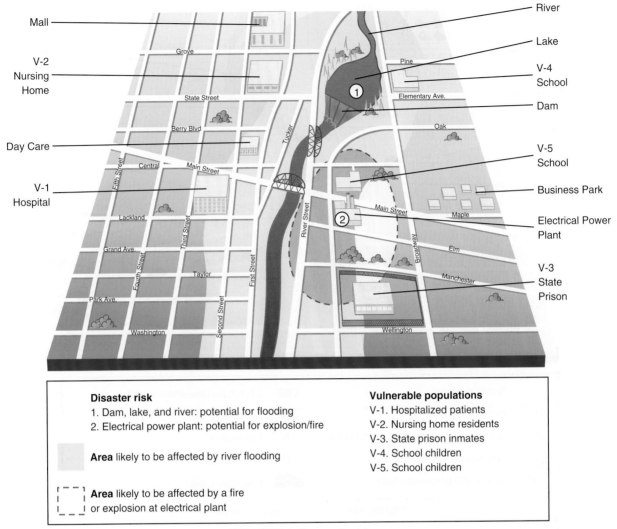

FIGURE 28-1 Community risk map.

Various hurricane and tornado scales have been developed on the basis of wind intensity and predicted level of destruction. The Fujita Tornado Intensity Scale, developed in 1971, categorized each tornado by its intensity and the area involved. In 1992, Fujita updated the scale to include an estimate of F-scale damage. The new scale, the Enhanced Fujita Scale (EF Scale), implemented in the United States on February 1, 2007, is still a set of wind estimates (not measurements) based on types of structural damage. The estimates vary with height of apparent damage above the ground and exposure (National Oceanic and Atmospheric Administration, 2012.

Hurricanes have been categorized since 1975 with use of the Saffir-Simpson Hurricane Scale, which includes sustained wind intensity, storm surge ranges, and flooding references. On an experimental basis for the 2009 tropical cyclone season, the storm surge ranges and flooding references were removed for each of the five categories (Box 28-4) because storm surge information is inaccurate. For example, Hurricane Ike in 2008 was a category 2 hurricane but had a storm surge at Galveston, Texas, equivalent to a category 4–5 storm surge, and Hurricane Katrina in 2007 was a category 3 hurricane with a storm surge equivalent to a category 5. The revised scale is called the Saffir-Simpson Hurricane Wind Scale. The new scale does not include storm surge, rainfall-induced floods, and tornadoes. The National Weather Service is currently debating whether or not to make the change (National Oceanic and Atmospheric Administration, 2012).

DISASTER MANAGEMENT

When one is aware of the types and characteristics of disasters, the question then becomes: What can be done to prevent/mitigate, prepare for, respond to, and recover from disasters? Disaster management requires an interdisciplinary, collaborative team effort and involves a network of agencies and individuals to develop a disaster plan that covers the multiple elements necessary for an effective plan. Communities can respond more quickly, more effectively, and with less confusion if the efforts needed in the event of a disaster have been anticipated, and plans for meeting them identified. The result of planning is that more lives are saved and less property is damaged. Planning ensures that resources are available and that roles and responsibilities of all personnel and agencies, both official and unofficial, are delineated.

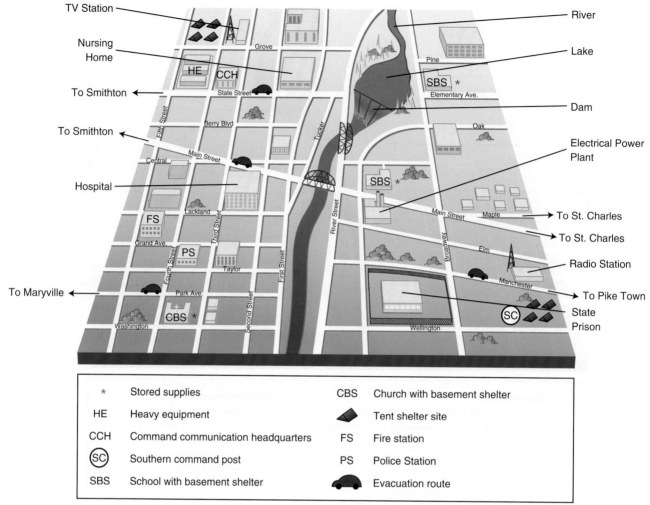

FIGURE 28-2 Community resource map.

*	Stored supplies	CBS	Church with basement shelter
HE	Heavy equipment		Tent shelter site
CCH	Command communication headquarters	FS	Fire station
SC	Southern command post	PS	Police Station
SBS	School with basement shelter		Evacuation route

BOX 28-4 THE SAFFIR-SIMPSON HURRICANE WIND SCALE

Category 1 (74-95 mph): Very dangerous winds will produce some damage.
Category 2 (96-110 mph): Extremely dangerous winds will cause extensive damage.
Category 3 (111-129 mph): Devastating damage will occur.
Category 4 (130-156 mph): Catastrophic damage will occur.
Category 5 (157 mph or higher): Catastrophic damage will occur.

Data from National Oceanic and Atmospheric Administration National Weather Service, National Hurricane Center: *Saffir-Simpson hurricane wind scale*, 2012. Retrieved from <http://www.nhc.noaa.gov/aboutsshws.php>.

Nurses need to know their personal, professional, and community responsibilities. They should realize that conflicts may arise between their personal and professional responsibilities if they have not been considered and planned for in advance (see the Ethical Insights box). Also, nurses may be direct or indirect victims and may even be displaced persons as a result of a disaster event. Recognizing this possibility, nurses need to plan, prepare, practice, and teach their family and significant others how to respond.

⚖ ETHICAL INSIGHTS

Deciding Whether to Care for Family or Care for Patients

During a disaster, a nurse might face an ethical dilemma because of competing responsibilities to self, family, employer, and patients. For example, a nurse who is a single parent with young children and has a limited support system may be forced to decide between her responsibility to care for her children and a mandate to report to work to care for patients. Choosing may result in loss of employment or danger to the children. Potential conflicts such as this should be considered and discussed, and decisions made in conjunction with the employer before a disaster event.

Local, State, and Federal Governmental Responsibilities

Local Government

The local government is responsible for the safety and welfare of its citizens. Emergencies and disaster incidents are handled at the lowest possible organizational and jurisdictional level. Police, fire, public health, public works, and

BOX 28-5   GUIDELINES FOR EARLY DETECTION OF BIOCHEMICAL TERRORIST INCIDENTS

- A rapidly increasing disease incidence (within hours or days) in a normally healthy population.
- An unusual increase in the number of people seeking care, especially with fever, respiratory, or gastrointestinal complaints.
- An endemic disease rapidly emerging at an uncharacteristic time or in an unusual pattern.
- Clusters of patients arriving from a single locale.
- Large numbers of rapidly fatal cases—patients who die within 72 hours after admission to the hospital.
- Any patient presenting with a disease that is relatively uncommon and has bioterrorism potential (e.g., pulmonary anthrax, smallpox, or plague).

From Chettle C: Recognizing bioterrorism: nurses on the frontline, *NurseWeek* 6:29-30, Nov 12, 2001.

medical emergency services are the **first responders**, responsible for incident management at the local level. Local officials and agencies are responsible for preparing their citizens for all kinds of emergencies and disasters and for testing disaster plans with mock drills. They manage events during an incident by carrying out evacuation, search, and rescue and maintaining public health and public works responsibilities. Local communities should have contingency operation plans for multiple disaster situations and for various aspects of the plan. For example, landline telephone service and cell phone service may not work because of being restricted for emergency use only or damage to the infrastructure, so other forms of communication need to be available.

In an incident other than a biological, chemical, radiation, or nuclear event, in most cases, it is the 911 communication center or the fire or police department that gets the initial message. The emergency communication center then communicates the incident to the other first responders and the director of the **Office of Emergency Management**, who determines what others may be needed (e.g., ambulances, other officials, and voluntary group representatives). Local hospitals are notified of the incident and the predicted nature of impending casualties. The hospitals may begin to receive victims via private automobiles who have not been triaged at the site of the incident. According to the CDC, a hospital can assess the expected number of victims that it may receive by counting the number that arrive within the first hour and doubling it.

For a biological or chemical terrorist incident, the process is very different. First responders generally are not involved. Rather, nurses and doctors in health care facilities may be the first to suspect that a biological or chemical agent has been released into the community. Box 28-5 lists the guidelines for detecting biochemical incidents. If any of these instances occurs in a health care provider setting, the suspicion should be immediately reported to the infection control department, the administration of the facility, or both. Each setting should post near the telephone the numbers to be called if a biochemical incident (whether internal or external) is suspected.

These numbers should include those of the CDC Bioterrorism Emergency Response, the CDC Hospital Infections program, and the U.S. Army Medical Research Institute of Infectious Diseases (Chettle, 2001).

The Office of Emergency Management involves representatives from all official and unofficial agencies in developing the community disaster plan, developing scenarios to test the plan through drills, and assessing the scope, intensity, and number of casualties (once an incident has occurred) in order to initiate the proper response. For those events that are not within the abilities of the local community or in the event of a terrorist-type incident, higher-level agencies and resources must be requested and will become involved.

State Government

When a disaster overwhelms the local community's resources, the state's Department or Office of Emergency Management is called for assistance. Prior to an event, state officials provide technical support for prevention, preparedness, response, and recovery. State officials visit local officials to assist and assess local emergency management plans, promote and conduct workshops and training courses, help with training exercises, and advise and support local government officials, and are on scene at disaster events to facilitate coordination of state resources and to disseminate information. In some cases, the National Guard may be called in to aid the community. When the scope of the event is so great that local and state resources are not adequate to meet the needs, the state calls on the federal government; at that point, the President may declare the incident a "national disaster." Once the President declares a national disaster, federal aid is made available. The National Response Plan, the 2004 core operational plan for domestic incident management, was replaced in 2008 by the National Response Framework for an all-hazards response. It describes best practices for managing incidents "that range from the serious but purely local, to large-scale terrorist attacks or catastrophic natural disasters" (DHS, 2013 p. 1).

Federal Government

U.S. Department of Homeland Security. As previously mentioned, the U.S. Department of Homeland Security was established in March 2003 to realign the existing federal departments, agencies, groups, and organizations into a single department focused on protecting the American people and their homeland.

The mission of DHS is to: (1) lead the unified national effort to secure America, (2) prevent and deter terrorist attacks, and (3) protect against and respond to threats and hazards to the nation (DHS, 2012). The organizational structure of the DHS has several divisions: the Office of the Secretary, Border and Transportation Security, Emergency Preparedness and Response Directorate, Information Analysis and Infrastructure Protection, Science and Technology, Office of Management, U.S. Citizenship and Immigration Services, U.S. Coast Guard, and the U.S. Secret Service. Within each of these divisions are multiple offices and centers (DHS, 2012).

BOX 28-6   FEDERAL EMERGENCY MANAGEMENT AGENCY RECOMMENDATIONS FOR BASIC DISASTER SUPPLIES KIT

- Three-day supply of non-perishable food
- Three-day supply of water – one gallon of water per person, per day
- Portable, battery-powered radio or television and extra batteries
- Flashlight and extra batteries
- First aid kit and manual
- Sanitation and hygiene items (moist towelettes and toilet paper)
- Matches and waterproof container
- Whistle
- Extra clothing
- Kitchen accessories and cooking utensils, including a can opener
- Photocopies of credit and identification cards
- Cash and coins
- Special needs item, such as prescription medications, eye glasses, contact lens solution, and hearing aid batteries
- Items for infants, such as formula, diapers, bottles, and pacifiers
- Other items to meet your unique family needs
- If you live in a cold climate, you must think about warmth. Be sure to include one complete change of clothing and shoes per person, including:
  - Jacket or coat
  - Long pants
  - Long sleeve shirt
  - Sturdy shoes
  - Hat, mittens, and scarf
  - Sleeping bag or warm blanket (per person)

Modified from Federal Emergency Management Agency: *Basic disaster supplies kit,* n.d. Available from <http://www.ready.gov/basic-disaster-supplies-kit>.

The DHS established its Homeland Security Advisory System to build a comprehensive and effective communication structure for disseminating threat information to public safety officials and the public at large. The previous color-coded threat level system has been replaced with the National Terrorism Advisory System. "The system provides timely, detailed information to the public, government agencies, first responders, airports and other transportation hubs, and the private sector" (DHS, 2013). The threat alert indicates whether there is an elevated threat (no specific information about timing or location) or imminent threat (impending or very soon). DHS (2011) has published a public guide with recommended steps that individuals, communities, businesses, and governments can take to help prevent, mitigate, or respond to the threat.

FEMA (2013d) has published an in-depth guide for citizen preparedness, *Are You Ready?* The focus of the contents is on how to prepare, practice, and maintain emergency plans that indicate what must be done before, during, and after a disaster. The guide explains how to prepare disaster supplies sufficient in quantity for individuals and families to survive (Box 28-6). Additionally, *Are you Ready?* lists specific natural hazards, technological hazards, and terrorism incidents with detailed information on what to do in each incident

(Box 28-7). Nurses could use this guide in developing educational programs and disaster plans related to natural and man-made disasters to which individuals, families, or communities may be exposed

In 2011 DHS announced its first national preparedness goal. The goal sets the "vision for nationwide preparedness and identifies the core capabilities and target necessary to achieve preparedness across five mission areas" in Presidential Policy Directive (PPD) 8: prevention, protection, mitigation response and recovery (DHS, 2011). Thirty-one core capabilities needed to achieve the goal have been identified where they most logically fit.

The Federal Emergency Management Agency. The Federal Emergency Management Agency became part of DHS in 2003. FEMA's mission is to support citizens and first responders to ensure that as a nation, everyone works together to build, sustain, and improve the capacity to prepare for, protect against, respond to, recover from, and mitigate all hazards, In 2006, a law was passed that significantly reorganized FEMA, giving it substantial new authority to remedy gaps that became apparent in the response to Hurricane Katrina in 2005 (FEMA, 2012a).

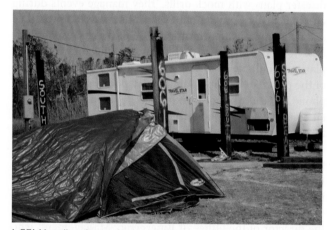

A FEMA trailer sits on the home site of Regina Fowler, who lost her home in Waveland, Mississippi, during Hurricane Katrina. (Photo by Patsy Lynch/FEMA.)

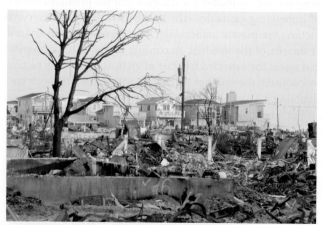

The close-knit community of Breezy Point, New York, lost more than 100 homes to fire during Hurricane Sandy. FEMA is providing ongoing support and resources to the Queens, New York, community. (Photo by Andre R. Aragon/FEMA)

BOX 28-7   WHAT TO DO IN DIFFERENT TYPES OF EMERGENCIES

Biological Attack
- Move away quickly.
- Wash with soap and water.
- Contact authorities.
- Listen to the media for official instructions.
- Seek medical attention if you become sick.

Nuclear Blast
- Do not look at the flash or fireball—it can blind you.
- Take cover behind anything that might offer protection.
- Lie flat on the ground and cover your head. If the explosion is some distance away, it could take 30 seconds or more for the blast to hit.
- Take shelter as soon as you can, even if you are many miles from ground zero—where the attack occurred; radioactive fallout can be carried by the winds for hundreds of miles. Remember the three protective factors: Distance, shielding, and time.

Chemical Attack
- If you are instructed to remain in your home or office building, you should:
  - Close doors and windows and turn off all ventilation, including furnaces, air conditioners, vents, and fans.
  - Seek shelter in an internal room and take your disaster supplies kit.
  - Seal the room with duct tape and plastic sheeting.
  - Listen to your radio for instructions from authorities.
- If you are caught in or near a contaminated area, you should:
  - Move away immediately in a direction upwind of the source.
  - Find shelter as quickly as possible.

Radiation Dispersion Device Event
Outdoors
- Seek shelter indoors immediately in the nearest building.
- If appropriate shelter is not available, move as rapidly as is safe upwind and away from the location of the explosive blast. Then, seek appropriate shelter as soon as possible.
- Listen for official instructions and follow directions.

Indoors
- If you have time, turn off ventilation and heating systems, and close windows, vents, fireplace dampers, exhaust fans, and clothes dryer vents. Retrieve your disaster supplies kit and a battery-powered radio, and take them to your shelter room.
- Seek shelter immediately, preferably underground or in an interior room of a building, placing as much distance and dense shielding as possible between you and the outdoors where the radioactive material may be.
- Seal windows and external doors that do not fit snugly with duct tape to reduce infiltration of radioactive particles. Plastic sheeting will not provide shielding from radioactivity nor from blast effects of a nearby explosion.
- Listen for official instructions, and follow directions.

Explosions
- If there is an explosion, you should:
  - Get under a sturdy table or desk if things are falling around you.
  - When they stop falling, leave quickly, watching for obviously weakened floors and stairways.
  - As you exit from the building, be especially watchful of falling debris.
  - Leave the building as quickly as possible. Do not stop to retrieve personal possessions or make phone calls.
- Do not use elevator. Once you are out:
  - Do not stand in front of windows, glass doors, or other potentially hazardous areas.
  - Move away from sidewalks or streets to be used by emergency officials or other still exiting the building.
- If you are trapped in debris:
  - If possible, use a flashlight to signal your location to rescuers.
  - Avoid unnecessary movement so you don't kick up dust.
  - Cover your nose and mouth with anything you have on hand. (Dense-weave cotton material can act as a good filter. Try to breathe through the material).
  - Tap on a pipe or wall so rescuers can hear where you are.
  - If possible, use a whistle to signal rescuers.
  - Shout only as a last resort. Shouting can cause a person to inhale dangerous amounts of dust.

Modified from Federal Emergency Management Agency: *Are you ready? an in-depth guide to citizen preparedness*, 2004. Available from <http://www.fema.gov/pdf/areyouready/areyouready_full.pdf>.

Centers for Disease Control and Prevention. After the rescue of survivors has been accomplished, the Department of Health and Human Services' CDC conducts surveillance to ensure that clean drinking water, food, shelter, and medical care are available for those affected. Whether CDC's involvement is necessary depends on the type of disaster. For example, floods pose risks of contaminated water (e.g., cholera) and food supplies (e.g., *Escherichia coli*); loss of shelter leaves people vulnerable to heat or cold and other environmental hazards (e.g., insects); and earthquakes create traumatic injuries (e.g., broken bones, head injuries) that will need to be addressed.

Public Health System

The public health system's mission is the promotion of health, prevention of disease, and protection from threats to health. *Public health system* is a broad term used to describe all of the governmental and nongovernmental organizations and agencies that contribute to the improvement of the health of populations. Public health agencies are the primary agencies for the health and medical responses to disaster incidents and therefore are a part of the initial response activities.

Public health officials provide advice and assistance to other public officials on environmental and health matters. Preparedness includes surveillance and reporting of suspicious illnesses (e.g., signs and symptoms of biological agents, food-borne diseases, and communicable diseases) in the community by physicians and nurses in local health care facilities or private offices and clinics. Public health officials then have the responsibility of detecting outbreaks, determining the cause of illness, identifying the risk factors for the population, implementing interventions to control the outbreak, and informing the public of the health risks and preventive

TABLE 28-2	SHELTER-IN-PLACE INSTRUCTIONS
LOCATION	**INSTRUCTIONS**
Home	Bring children and pets indoors immediately; close and lock all outside doors and windows; close the window shades, blinds, or curtains; turn off fans, heating, ventilation, or air conditioning system, and close the fireplace or woodstove damper; get the disaster supplies and make sure the radio is working; take everyone, including pets, into an interior room with no or few windows and shut the door; if instructed to seal the room, use duct tape and plastic sheeting (e.g., heavy-duty plastic garbage bags) to seal all cracks around the door into the room; keep the phone handy in case it is needed to report a life-threatening condition; keep listening to the radio or television until told all is safe or told to evacuate (do not evacuate unless instructed to do so).
Day care centers and schools	Close the school; activate the school's emergency plan and follow reverse evacuation procedures to bring students, faculty, visitors, and staff indoors; have all children, staff, and visitors take shelter in preselected rooms that have phone access, stored disaster supply kits, and, preferably, access to a bathroom; shut the doors and lock all windows and doors; if it is not possible for a person to monitor the telephone and the school has voice mail or an automated attendant, change the recording to indicate that the school is closed and that students and staff are remaining in the building until authorities say it is safe to leave; turn off heating, ventilating, and air conditioning systems; if children have cell phones, allow them to use them to call a parent or guardian to let them know that they have been asked to remain in school until further notice and that they are safe; one teacher or staff member in each room should write down the names of everyone in the room and call the designated contact to report who is in that room; everyone should stay in the room until school officials announce that all is safe or say everyone must evacuate.
Work	Close the office or business, making any customers, clients, or visitors in the building aware that they need to stay until the emergency is over; close and lock all windows, exterior doors, and any other openings to the outside; a knowledgeable person should use the building's mechanical systems to turn off all heating, ventilating, and air conditioning systems (systems that automatically provide for exchange of inside air with outside air, in particular, need to be turned off, sealed, or disabled); turn on call-forwarding or alternative telephone answering systems or services; if there is danger of explosion, close any window shades, blinds, or curtains; go to a predetermined sheltering room(s), and when everyone is in, shut and lock the doors; monitor radios or TVs for updates until you are told all is safe or you are told to evacuate.
Vehicle	If close to home, workplace, or a public building, go there immediately and go inside. If unable to get indoors quickly and safely, stop the vehicle in the safest place possible (e.g., stop under a bridge or in a shady spot to avoid being overheated); turn off the engine and close windows and vents; if possible, seal the heating, ventilating, and air conditioning vents with duct tape or anything else you may have available; listen to the radio periodically for updated advice and instructions; stay in place until you are told it is safe to get back on the road, and follow the directions of law enforcement officials.

Modified from American Red Cross: *Shelter-in-place during a chemical or radiation emergency,* 2006. Available from <www.redcross.org/preparedness/cdc_english/Sheltering.asp#howdo>.

measures that need to be taken. These activities relate both directly and indirectly to the ten essential public health services described in Chapter 1.

American Red Cross

The American Red Cross (ARC, or Red Cross) is not a governmental agency. It is, however, chartered by Congress to provide disaster relief. The ARC works in partnership with FEMA, DHS, the CDC, and other local, state, and federal agencies to provide and manage needed services.

The ARC is primarily a volunteer organization with chapters in all 50 states, Puerto Rico, the Virgin Islands, and the Pacific Rim; its national headquarters is in Washington, DC. Disaster Services is only one of the programs that the this agency provides. Others are International Services; Biomedical Services; Armed Forces Emergency Services; and Health, Safety, and Community Services.

The Red Cross places great emphasis on preparedness and participates with communities in developing and testing their disaster plans, maintaining and training personnel for disaster response, and responding during an actual emergency

or disaster. The ARC publishes many pamphlets and educational materials to help individuals, families, neighborhoods, schools, and businesses prepare for potential disasters. The key actions the agency recommends are: (1) identify potential disaster events, (2) create a disaster plan for sheltering in place or for evacuation, (3) assemble a disaster supplies kit, and (4) practice and maintain the plan. The disaster plan should include an emergency communications plan, a predetermined meeting place for family members or significant others, and plans for care of pets in the event that evacuation is required.

If local authorities issue a shelter-in-place communication, instructions that address what actions to take if at home, at work, at school, or in a vehicle should be followed (Table 28-2). For example, during a disaster such as hazardous gas emission from an industrial plant, anyone at home, at a business, or in a public building may be instructed to go inside and follow home or work shelter-in-place recommendations (i.e., close doors, turn off fans and air-conditioning, bring children and pets inside, and stay inside until "all clear" has been called).

RESEARCH HIGHLIGHTS

School Nurses and Emergency Preparedness

A survey of 193 school nurses was conducted to assess their knowledge of bioterrorism and educational needs for emergency preparedness (Evers and Puzniak, 2005). The researchers reported that although 80% of the respondents stated that their school had an emergency plan and an evacuation plan, only about half (48.5%) had a shelter-in-place plan. Furthermore, although most (62%) stated that their school was "somewhat prepared" for a disaster, only 6.2% rated their school as "very prepared." Knowledge of specific information on bioterrorism was only fair. For example, it was noted that only 55% of survey respondents could distinguish between signs and symptoms of anthrax and influenza. Finally, slightly more than half of respondents believed that a biological or chemical attack was "somewhat likely," and nearly 40% believed that a nuclear attack was "somewhat likely." The researchers concluded that school nurses need more training and preparation to be able to respond appropriately to an emergency or disaster situation.

Data from Evers S, Puzniak L: Bioterrorism knowledge and emergency preparedness among school nurses, *J School Health* 75(6):232-237, 2005.

TABLE 28-3	AMERICAN RED CROSS DISASTER SERVICES FROM JULY 1, 2010, TO JUNE 30, 2011
TYPE OF ASSISTANCE	**NUMBER**
Shelters opened	Approximately 490
Workers deployed	20,000
Health and mental health contacts	Nearly 95,000
Clean up, comfort, and relief supplies	2 million
Meals and snacks served	4 million

Data from American Red Cross: *Disaster services program review: Fiscal year 2011*, 2012. Available from <http://www.redcross.org/images/MEDIA_CustomProductCatalog/m8540111_Disaster-Relief-Program-Review-2011.pdf>.

The Red Cross disaster response efforts focus on meeting the immediate disaster-related needs of affected people and providing support services to the emergency rescue and recovery workers (ARC, 2012). The disaster response functions are to provide health services, mental health services, family services, and mass care, and to inquire about family well-being. Mass care involves feeding, sheltering, providing basic first aid, bulk distribution, and a Disaster Welfare Information system (ARC, 2012). Table 28-3 shows the breadth of services that the ARC provided for hurricane disaster relief in 2011.

DISASTER MANAGEMENT STAGES

Prevention Stage

The first stage in disaster management occurs before a disaster is imminent and is also known as the *nondisaster stage*. Potential disaster risks should be identified and risk maps created (see Figure 28-1). The population demographics and vulnerabilities, as well as the community's capabilities, should be analyzed. Primary prevention measures include educating the public

regarding what actions to take to prepare for disasters at the individual, family, and community levels. Furthermore, on the basis of the assessment of potential risks, the community must develop a plan for meeting the potential disasters identified.

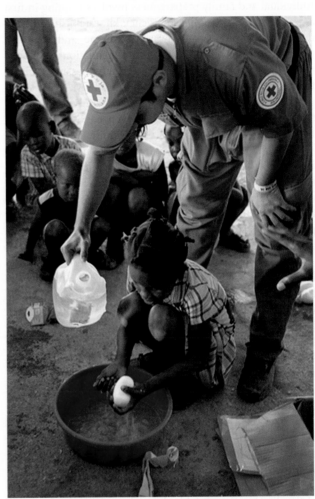

Red Cross volunteers share health and hygiene messages with young earthquake survivors. (Photo by Bonnie Gillespie/American Red Cross.)

With regard to bioterrorist attacks, *prevention* means that health care providers need to be knowledgeable about the biological and chemical agents that might be used. In addition, health care providers must be able to recognize the signs and symptoms of the various biological and chemical agents that have been recognized as potential threats and must know what to do in the event of exposure for themselves and others. As mentioned, unlike other disasters, biochemical terrorist threats may be identified only when events raise suspicions of health care providers rather than by first responders at a particular site.

Early identification of ill or exposed persons, rapid implementation of preventive therapy, special infection control considerations, and collaboration or communication with the public are essential in controlling the spread of cases. Hospitals need to identify rooms that can be converted into isolation units to meet the demand. Nurses must be instructed in decontamination and reminded of isolation techniques that might be needed, depending on the biological agent. Volunteers and professionals must remain current in first aid, cardiopulmonary resuscitation, and advanced lifesaving procedures.

Preparedness and Planning Stage

Individual and family preparedness involves training in first aid, assembling a disaster emergency kit, establishing a predetermined meeting place away from home, and making a family communication plan. Recommendations for what needs to be included in each of these activities are available from many sources (e.g., ARC, DHS, and FEMA). These are guidelines, and each individual and each family must modify the preparations to meet their personal needs. Nurses need to have plans and survival kits for work, family, and evacuation.

Although there will be some variation according to the individual community's needs, all community disaster plans should address the following elements: authority, communication, control, logistical coordination of personnel, supplies and equipment, evacuation, rescue, and care of the dead. The plan should indicate who has the power to declare that there is a disaster and who has the power to initiate the disaster plan.

Authority should be designated by the title of the person; it should not specify a person by name. There should also be backup positions identified in the event the first individual is not available. Every individual should be equally informed about the role and responsibilities that go with this authority. A clear chain of authority for carrying out the plan is critical for successful implementation of the plan. Authority may change, depending on whether the disaster is natural or man-made, and change of authority should be addressed in the plan.

Communication is recognized as a very significant problem during disasters. Misinformation and misinterpretation can occur when communication is ineffective. Reliance on telephone systems or cell phones should not be the sole planned means of communicating because these may not work or the systems might be overwhelmed. The communication section of the disaster plan should address how the authority figure will be notified of the disaster, how the emergency management team members will be notified, how the community residents will be warned about the incident, and what actions to take. This section needs to address how communication between relief workers and authorities will be maintained. Also, it should include information on the role of the media in keeping people informed and in letting people know what assistance and supplies are needed.

The analysis of the population that was completed during the nondisaster stage should identify groups that need special attention as to how they will be notified. These people should be noted in advance and plans developed to meet the varied needs of these vulnerable groups. Such groups include those who speak different languages, are homeless or poor, are without television or other means of communication, and are in institutions such as prisons, nursing homes, day care settings, or schools. Effective communication during a disaster must be credible, current, and authoritative and must give some indication of future events.

The *logistical* section should specify where supplies and equipment are located or where additional supplies and equipment can be obtained, where they will be stored or found, and how they will be transported to the disaster site (see Figure 28-2). Essential *human resources* (e.g., emergency and disaster specialists, officials of governmental and voluntary agencies, engineers, weather specialists, and community leaders) should be identified and where they will be located together determined. The plan should include information about transportation for *evacuation and rescue* (particularly taking into account vulnerable groups), documentation and record keeping, and plans for evaluation of the success or failure of the plan.

A disaster plan is a dynamic entity. Planning is a continuous process, and the plan changes with circumstances and when gaps are identified during drills or from actual disaster incidents. The plan should set realistic expectations of effects and needs, should be brief and concise, and should establish priorities and timelines for actions. It should also follow the disaster planning principles listed in Box 28-8.

For a plan to be effective, it must be tested with different disaster scenario drills. The more times realistic scenarios are created to test the plan in actual practice sessions, and not just with tabletop or paper drills, the more problems with the plan will be identified, and solutions for those problems found. Without practice drills, a plan may have many unrecognized faults, and as a result, many more individuals may be harmed and communities damaged when an actual disaster occurs.

BOX 28-8   DISASTER PLANNING PRINCIPLES

1. Measures usually taken are not sufficient for major disasters.
2. Plans should be adjusted to people's needs.
3. Planning does not stop with development of a written plan.
4. Lack of information causes inappropriate responses by community members.
5. People should be able to respond with or without direction.
6. Plans should coordinate efforts of the entire community, so large segments of the citizenry should be involved in the planning.
7. Plans should be linked to surrounding areas.
8. Plans should be general enough to cover all potential disaster events.
9. As much as possible, plans should be based on everyday work methods and procedures.
10. Plans should specify a person's responsibility for implementing segments by position or title rather than by name.
11. Plans should develop a record-keeping system before a disaster occurs, regarding:
    * Supplies and equipment
    * Records of all present at any given time (to account for everyone and to identify the missing)
    * Identification of victims and deceased, conditions and treatment documented, and to which facility victims are sent
12. Backup plans need to be in place for the following:
    * Disruption of telephone and cell phone lines
    * Disruption of computer data (should be downloaded weekly and stored off-site)
    * Protecting essential public health functions (e.g., vital records and communicable disease data)

Response Stage

The response stage begins immediately after the disaster incident occurs. The community preparedness plans that have been developed are initiated. If a disaster occurs, people should remain calm and exert patience, follow the advice of local emergency officials, and listen to the radio or television for news and instructions. If people nearby are injured, one should give first aid, seek help, and check the area for dangerous hazards. Those at home should shut off any damaged utilities, confine or secure pets, call family contact(s), and check on neighbors, especially the elderly or disabled.

The plan may call for people to shelter in place or to evacuate, or for search and rescue to begin. If the only response needed is to shelter in place, people need to know what to do if they are at home, at work, at school, or in their vehicles.

Shelter in Place

The ARC has provided explicit instructions for individuals and families to be followed when told by authorities to "shelter in place" in the event of a disaster. Table 28-2 shows these guidelines.

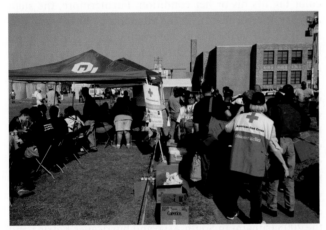

Busloads of Galveston, Texas, residents returned from temporary shelter in San Antonio after the hurricane in September 2008. (Photo by Mike Moore/FEMA.)

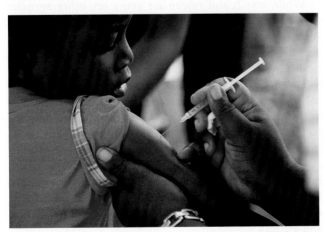

Between February 8 and March 9, 2010, 125,000 earthquake survivors in Port-au-Prince, Haiti, were vaccinated against measles, diphtheria, pertussis, and tetanus. (Photo by Bonnie Gillespie/American Red Cross.)

Evacuation

Each community should have established evacuation routes for the residents to use if evacuation from the area is necessary. In some instances, mandatory evacuation may be implemented. However, there are always some individuals who will not leave their homes for any number of reasons (e.g., fear of vandalism, denial of the potential extent of the disaster, pride in home and belongings). Education of residents as to the potential damage, deaths, and injuries that will be incurred from the potential disasters that may affect their community needs to be accomplished during the preparedness stage, and not when evacuation is ordered. In some extreme cases, it may be necessary for hospitals and other facilities, such as nursing homes, to evacuate patients. This procedure requires significant advance planning, because health practitioners must determine how to move seriously ill, and even critically ill, people and coordinate transportation and placement for their disposition to safe facilities.

Search and Rescue

Before search and rescue begin, safety must be considered. In some instances, if a criminal action is suspected as part of the disaster, law officials will be among the first to respond in order to secure the area and possibly gather evidence. While the area is being checked and then cleared of potential threats, a staging area can be set up at or near the site of the incident to direct on-site activities. Search for and rescue of victims can begin once clearance is given, a disaster triage area is established, and an emergency treatment area is set up to provide first aid until transportation for victims to hospitals or health care facilities for treatment can be coordinated (Figure 28-3).

Staging Area

The staging area is the on-site incident command station. Disaster responders should report to this area to "check in" so that everyone is accounted for and can be given an assignment. This arrangement allows for the most effective use of the skills and abilities of those responding. No one should go to the disaster site unless directed to do so by the staging area commander. The staging area is also where the authority rests for decisions as to the need for additional resources to manage the disaster incident. Such resources include construction equipment to move building materials, rescue dogs to locate

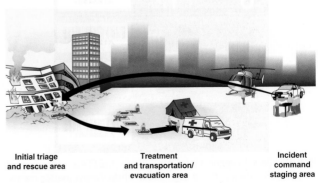

Initial triage and rescue area   Treatment and transportation/evacuation area   Incident command staging area

FIGURE 28-3 Areas of operation of disaster response.

humans who are buried in the debris, and more fire, police, or medical personnel.

Disaster Triage

Triage is identifying and separating individuals quickly according to injury severity and treatment needed. Disaster triage focuses on sorting the greatest number of people as fast as possible. Triage performed at the site and again at the treatment area is very different from triage that is routinely conducted in the emergency department. The focus of disaster triage is to do as little as possible, for the greatest number, in the shortest time. One triage system that is used by first responders is START. START stands for "simple triage and rapid treatment." This system describes what to do when first arriving at a multiple casualty or mass casualty incident. Disaster triage of an injured person should occur in less than 1 minute. This system also describes how to use people with minor injuries to help. As a decision is made regarding the status of an individual, the person is labeled with a colored triage tag (Figure 28-4).

Green on the triage tag is for the walking wounded or those with minor injuries (e.g., cuts and abrasions) who can wait several hours before they receive treatment; yellow is for those with systemic but not yet life-threatening

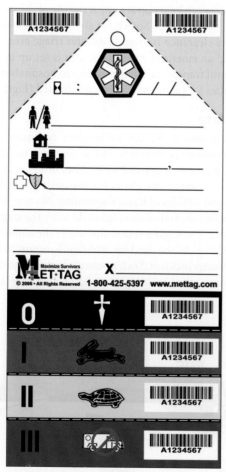

FIGURE 28-4 Disaster triage tag. (From METTAG: *The original medical emergency triage tag*, 2006. <http://www.mettag.com>. Reprinted with permission.)

complications who can wait 45 to 60 minutes (e.g., simple fractures); red is considered top priority or immediate and is for those who have life-threatening conditions but who can be stabilized and have a high probability of survival (e.g., amputations); black is for the deceased or for those whose injuries are is so extensive that nothing can be done to save them (e.g., multiple severe injuries).

A new classification of victim, those who are contaminated, will require a *hazmat* (for "hazardous materials") tag. To assess an individual within the 1-minute guideline, the START system uses three characteristics. First, *respiration* is checked; if the rate is more than 30 per minute, the individual is tagged red or immediate. If the rate is fewer than 30 per minute, the assessor moves to the second step, *perfusion*. The assessor pinches the nail bed and observes the reaction. Color should return to normal within 2 seconds; if it takes longer, the person is tagged red or immediate. The third step is checking mental status. If the person is able to answer a question, he or she is tagged yellow; the person not able to answer a question is tagged red or immediate. By doing these steps, the individual responsible for triage can very quickly assess an individual and decide which color tag fits his or her condition. Furthermore, the steps are easy to remember with the mnemonic "30—2—can do," in which "30" is the number of respirations, "2" is the number of seconds needed to check for perfusion, and "can do" relates to checking mental status.

Following triage, victims are moved to the treatment area where their condition is checked again. First aid may be provided there until transportation is available. Ambulances, helicopters, busses, or all three may be used to transport the victims to various hospitals or health care facilities. Some victims, such as those in the surrounding area that may have been affected by the incident, may even go by private vehicle to a hospital or medical facility. This process may go on for days as it did in the September 11, 2001, incidents, the 2005 tsunami in South Asia, and hurricanes Katrina and Rita. Search and rescue eventually will be called off, and the recovery stage will begin.

While search and rescue are going on, other agencies (e.g., public health agencies) are surveilling for threats such as contaminated water, vectors, and air quality. They also disseminate data on what has been found and relate health information to officials, the media, and the public as appropriate. Designated agencies gather epidemiological information as to the occurrence and distribution of health-related events associated with the disaster, describe factors contributing to health-related effects, and assess the needs of populations and facilities. They then allocate resources and work to prevent further adverse health problems that might result from the disaster. For example, following Hurricane Katrina, public health officials administered tetanus and hepatitis A immunizations to rescuers and victims.

Although triage of individuals exposed to chemical warfare agents is basically the same as for any multiple or mass casualty incident, it poses special challenges. For these events, the triage area is set up in the "hot zone" to assist in determining priorities for resuscitation, decontamination, pharmacological therapy, and site evacuation. Only specially trained emergency personnel who are familiar with chemical agents and the use of personal protection equipment should triage victims of a chemical agent. The same triage categories can be assigned to these victims.

Psychological triage presents the challenge of determining who most needs help and deciding what interventions will help. Mental health disorders related to disasters include anxiety disorders, exacerbation of existing substance abuse problems, somatic complaints, depression, and later, posttraumatic stress disorder (PTSD). Risks for PTSD include living through dangerous events or traumas, having a history of mental illness, getting hurt, seeing people hurt or killed, feeling horror, helplessness, or extreme fear, having little or no social support after the event, and dealing with extra stress after the event, such as loss of a loved one, pain and injury, or loss of a job or home. Research has identified four keys to gauging the mental health impact of such events, any two of which may result in severe, lasting, and pervasive psychological effects. The key factors are: (1) extreme and widespread property damage; (2) serious and ongoing financial problems; (3) high prevalence of trauma in the form of injuries, threat to life, and loss of life and; (4) when human intent caused the disaster. In addition, panic during the disaster, horror, separation from family, and relocation or displacement are factors that may play a part in psychological impairment. Nurses need to evaluate an individual's risk to self or others. Nurses need to know what symptoms to look for as well as what resources are available for people who need help (Patterson, 2005).

Community Responses to a Disaster

Heroic Phase. The classic four phases of a community's reaction to a disaster are the heroic phase, honeymoon phase, disillusionment phase, and reconstruction phase. During the heroic phase, nearly everyone feels the need to rush to help people survive the disaster. Medical personnel may work hours without sleep, under very dangerous and life-threatening conditions, in order to take care of their patients. Medical personnel may help out in areas with which they are not familiar and have no experience. Disaster Medical Assistance Teams, consisting of professional and paraprofessional medical personnel, provide emergency relief during a disaster and may travel long distances to help out in one. This was illustrated by the thousands of people who volunteered to help in the immediate aftermaths of September 11 and hurricanes Katrina and Rita.

Honeymoon Phase. Individuals who have survived the disaster gather together with others who have simultaneously experienced the same event; this is known as the honeymoon phase. People begin to tell their stories and review over and over again what has occurred. Bonds are formed among victims and health care workers. Gratitude is expressed for being alive.

Disillusionment Phase. When time has elapsed and a delay in receiving help or failure to receive the promised aid has not occurred, feelings of despair arise. Medical personnel and other first responders may begin to experience depression due to exhaustion from many long days of long hours. Depression may set in as a result of knowledge about what has happened to the community, friends, and family. People realize the way things were before the disaster is not the way things are now and may never be again. They recognize that many things are different and much needs to be done to adjust to the current situation.

NATURAL AND MAN-MADE DISASTERS

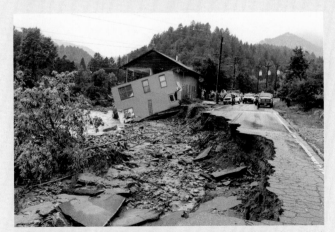

The devastation of the tsunami that occurred in Indonesia in December 2004. (Copyright Associated Press.)

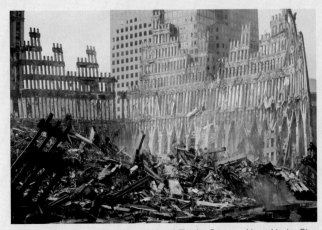

The remaining section of the World Trade Center, New York, City, is surrounded by a mountain of rubble following the September 11, 2001, terrorist attacks. (Photo by Bri Rodriguez/FEMA News Photo.)

Continued

NATURAL AND MAN-MADE DISASTERS—cont'd

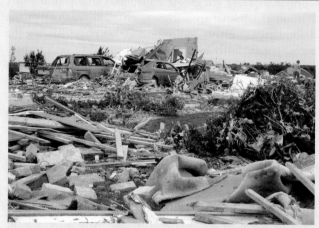

Only an interior wall remains after an F-4 tornado ripped through Manhattan, Kansas, in June 2008. (Photo by Anita Westervelt/FEMA.)

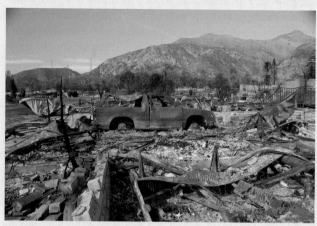

Many homes and vehicles were destroyed in a wildfire in Sylmar, California, in November 2008. (Photo by Michael Mancino/FEMA.)

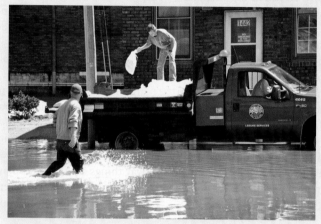

Waterloo and other towns in Iowa experienced record flooding in June 2008. (Photo by Patsy Lynch/FEMA.)

DISASTER RELIEF: HURRICANE KATRINA, SEPTEMBER 2005

When Hurricane Katrina hit the Gulf Coast in late August 2005, thousands of evacuees from New Orleans and south Louisiana were sent to Houston. Two huge shelters were set up in the city to accommodate those displaced, and the needs, as was documented in the media, were massive.

Faculty, staff, and students from the University of Texas Health Science Center at Houston (UT-Houston), personnel from the city and county health departments, and local emergency medical services personnel were joined by thousands of volunteers to care for these disaster victims. Indeed, doctors, nurses, and other health care providers came from across Texas and the Gulf Coast area and from as far away as California, Arizona, Illinois, and New York to help.

To care for the health needs of the evacuees, a clinic was established in the George R. Brown Convention Center. According to one of the officials at UT-Houston, "We got the call at 9 AM Friday [to create the clinic], and by 5 PM it was all set up." The clinic was modeled after army field hospitals, with a command center, triage areas, and various clinics. There were sections for trauma and acute care, adult medical care, women's/gynecological care, and pediatric care, as well as an area for people with mental health concerns. A full-service pharmacy was also set up.

During the next 17 days, more than 10,000 patient visits were logged, and there were more than 6000 volunteers. These photos depict how care was organized and show the efforts of the many volunteers.

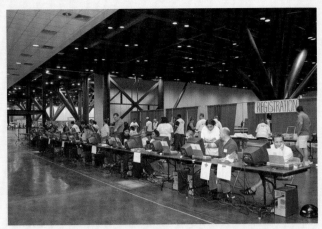

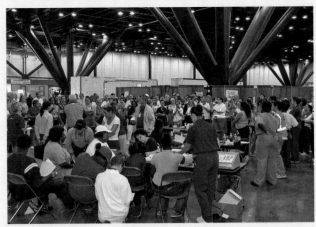

Setting up the registration area to check in clinic clients. Setting up one of the client care areas (note the portable water supply).

Registration and triage area as clients are being seen.

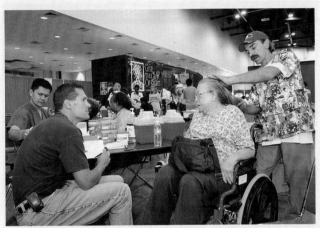

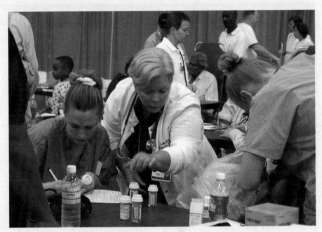

Triage area.

Nurses organizing client medications.

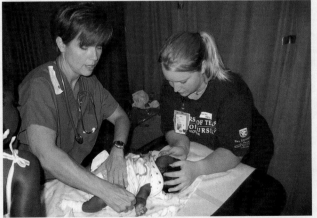

Examining an infant. (Photo courtesy of the University of Texas Health Science Center, Houston, Texas.)

Reconstruction Phase

Once the community has restored some of the buildings, businesses, homes, and services, and some sense of normality is returning, feelings of despair subside. Counseling support for victims and helpers may need to be initiated to help people recover more fully. During this phase, people begin to look to the future.

Common Reactions to a Disaster

The reactions by individuals to a disaster vary. Table 28-4 lists some of the more commonly encountered emotional, cognitive, physical, and interpersonal reactions to a disaster that anyone may experience.

Posttraumatic Stress Disorder. The reactions mentioned usually resolve in 1 to 3 months after the disaster event but, in some cases, may lead to PTSD. PTSD is a psychiatric disorder that can occur following an individual experiences or witnesses a life-threatening event, such as a disaster. Men and women, adults and children, and all socioeconomic groups can experience PTSD. People who have the disorder often relive the experience through nightmares and flashbacks. The social and psychological symptoms mentioned in Table 28-4 can be severe enough, and last long enough, to significantly impair a person's daily life. If PTSD occurs in conjunction with related disorders (e.g., depression, substance abuse, and other problems of physical and mental health), the situation becomes more complicated. Individuals experiencing PTSD require medical attention (National Institute of Mental Health, 2013).

CASE STUDY APPLICATION OF THE COMMUNITY ASSESSMENT PROCESS

Assessment

Deer Park, Texas, is a city 20 miles east of Houston, Texas. The population is approximately 32,000 people. The majority of the people are white (80.8%) and Hispanic (15.2%). The median age of the population is 34.7 years, and the median income $61,334. Eighty-nine percent of the population older than 25 years has a high school diploma or higher education degree. The unemployment rate is 5.6%. The city consists of residential homes, apartment complexes, and retail and service businesses. There are nine schools and several churches of all denominations. Many AM and FM radio stations and TV broadcast stations are available to the Deer Park area.

The Federal Communications Commission (FCC) has developed the Emergency Alert System to warn of any emergency (nuclear attack, hurricane, tornado, flood, or chemical release). The FCC has designated KTRH 740 AM as the station for the Houston area. The city has a volunteer fire department (5 full-time employees) and a city police department (55 full-time employees). The city government consists of a mayor, city council, and city manager. The city has two emergency committees: the Community Awareness and Emergency Response Committee and the Local Emergency Planning Committee.

There are no hospitals in Deer Park. The closest hospitals are 6 to 7 miles away and take 20 minutes to reach. The closest level 1 trauma center is 15 miles away, and the nearest adult care burn center is 20 miles away; the pediatric burn center is in Galveston, Texas, which is about 45 miles away.

The city is also the home of the Shell Deer Park Chemical Plant and the Shell Deer Park Refining Company. The company processes 3% of the nation's oil supply into gasoline. The Shell plants are located on 1500 acres in the Houston Ship Channel. Shell employs approximately 1100 people and 2200 contract workers. The chemical plant and the refining company have their own fire stations, an internal railroad, docks and transportation networks, small medical facilities (one physician and four nurses, 7 days a week, 24 hours a day), first responder teams, two ambulances, and a vehicle that can handle 30 casualties.

Diagnosis
Individual

Because of Deer Park's location on the Gulf Coast and the presence of the Shell Deer Park Refining Company and Shell Deer Park Chemical Plant, the residents are at risk for injury or death due to hurricane disasters and potential industrial accidents from either accidental or terrorist causes.

Family

The families of Deer Park are at risk for losing their homes, separation from family members, and having to evacuate from their homes either temporarily or permanently owing to hurricane damages or industrial accidents.

Community

The community of Deer Park is at risk for destruction of buildings and city public works due to hurricane disasters and potential explosions from either accidental or terrorist causes.

Planning
Disaster Management

Deer Park is in the storm surge zone, requiring its residents to evacuate when a category 1 hurricane is predicted to land in, or within a 100-mile radius of, the Deer Park area. The media sources available to the Deer Park area or the city officials are to give instructions about supplies and equipment to have ready and when to leave. Only one evacuation route is available to the community.

A survey was conducted during the nondisaster stage to identify vulnerable groups that would need help in evacuating.

Individual

Vulnerable individuals who would need to have special consideration for evacuation are the very young (4000 individuals between birth and 10 years), the elderly (2110 individuals aged 65 years and over), and families below the poverty level (1200). It was determined that more than 7000 individuals might need some form of transportation in order to evacuate.

Long-Term Goal
- Residents will have a disaster kit prepared according to ARC and FEMA guidelines.
- Short-Term Goals
- Residents will follow officials' instructions for sheltering in place or evacuation.
- Vulnerable individuals will know what to do in the event of an evacuation order or shelter-in-place announcement.

Family
Long-Term Goal
- Family members will continually update their family disaster plans according to family dynamics.

CASE STUDY APPLICATION OF THE COMMUNITY ASSESSMENT PROCESS—cont'd

Short-Term Goals
- Families will have a disaster plan in place for communicating.
- Families will have a disaster kit in place to accommodate each family member for a period of at least 3 days.

Community
Long-Term Goals
- Additional evacuation routes will be identified for area residents.
- Central meeting locations will be identified for those needing transportation assistance for evacuation.

Short-Term Goal
- School buses will be used for evacuation of vulnerable individuals and families who need transportation.
- Other sources must be identified that could be called upon to provide transportation.
- School bus drivers should be able to include their family members on the buses with others being evacuated, so the drivers will not have to worry about their families.
- If all individuals follow instructions, there should be no injuries to, or deaths of, Deer Park residents from a hurricane or related storm surge. Homes may be damaged or destroyed, but no lives should be lost. With the help of local, state, and possibly federal agencies, the community should recover.

Long-Term Goal
- City officials will continually update the community disaster plan as gaps are identified and keep the residents informed as the plan changes.

Onsite Management
The following figure summarizes the disaster plan in place for the Deer Park Shell plants for handling any industrial accident that occurs on their property.

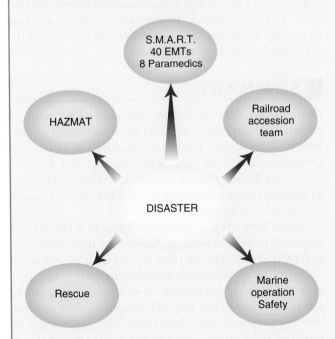

Shell has annual drills with the Harris County's Emergency Management and Channel Industries Mutual Aid organization to evaluate emergency response. This group is Shell's direct link to support in the event of a disaster. Many buildings on Shell property can serve as shelters, and no visitor or employee is allowed on the property without having a "safe shelter map" in his or her possession. If an explosion occurs that is confined to the property, and only minor casualties result, the resources available should be sufficient to manage the disaster.

Shell has developed a buffer zone between the plants and the city of Deer Park. However, if fumes were to escape as a result of the explosion, a shelter-in-place warning would be issued for Deer Park residents through a specific six sounding message system. Chemical products that are used and that might potentially escape are benzene, toluene, solvent xylene, isoprene butadiene, sulfur, phenol, hydrogen sulfide, and asbestos. Citizens would be advised about actions to take according to the chemical released. Most plants have also installed dedicated, fiberoptic telephone lines so that the city and industry can stay in touch even when normal phone circuits are overloaded or out of service.

Community and Local Response Preparedness
Deer Park's police and fire dispatchers have been trained on how to handle calls from industries about a chemical release and how to quickly activate the city's emergency warning systems. The local emergency planning committee has adopted a three-level community awareness and emergency response system to categorize the severity of each chemical release. Level 1 is information only, level 2 is standby alert, and level 3 is full emergency condition, with sheltering in place required. The final level is "all clear." Deer Park has a website featuring Wally Wise Guy, who gives instructions to the citizens about what to do if a shelter-in-place emergency is issued.

The local emergency planning committee hired a consulting group to study the impact of toxic substances on the community to ensure that shelter-in-place procedures are adequate for protecting the residents. The consulting group recommended that each home in the region have a shelter-in-place kit containing 2- to 3-inch–wide masking tape, plastic film or sheets, towels or sheets for sealing under doors, battery-powered radio and extra batteries, flashlight and extra batteries, and bottled water stored inside a designated shelter-in-place room.

The Deer Park Communications Subcommittee works with others to develop detailed procedures on how to notify and warn the public of a chemical release. The city and local industry have invested in six state-of-the-art systems to provide reliable and redundant warning to homes, schools, businesses, and visitors. Siren-type alarms have been mounted on utility poles throughout the city. This system is used only for chemical emergencies, not for tornadoes, hurricanes, or other types of emergencies. In addition, the city has contracted with First Call Interactive Network, an automated telephone notification network that can ring the telephones of homes and businesses in the immediate danger area to give prerecorded instructions about what to do.

Evaluation
Individuals and Families
- Before a hurricane, all residents will have been evacuated.
- All vulnerable individuals and families will have been evacuated to shelters.
- All residents will know and respond to shelter-in-place warnings as indicated by the siren-type alarm system in place.

Community
- City officials will evaluate and continually update the community disaster plan as gaps are identified.
- Community residents will remain informed and prepared.

The City of Deer Park and the Deer Park Shell plants have detailed plans for prevention, preparedness, and response in the event of an industrial accident. In that event, evaluation of the plan will take place to identify gaps and make appropriate changes. A plan needs to be in place for hurricane preparedness of the plants to avoid industrial accidents, and the plan evaluated for effectiveness. Drills are conducted to test their industrial accident plans; they provide training of personnel; they have identified sites for shelters both on Shell property and in the city; and they have elaborate notification and warning systems in place.

Areas that need to be enhanced include readily available city health resources (lack of a nearby trauma hospital or burn center to care for the type of injuries that would occur). Plans for preparing the plants for hurricanes and evacuation need to be developed and made available to the workers.

Prevention

Primary

- Perform periodic education of area residents regarding warning systems in place and appropriate response to take should they be implemented.
- Perform periodic review of plans in response to changing demographics.

Secondary

- Check credentials of first responders for currency.
- Screen first responders for training needs and preparedness to take action during disasters.

Tertiary

- Institute building codes that will reduce amount of damage to infrastructures.

TABLE 28-4	COMMON RESPONSES TO A TRAUMATIC EVENT
Cognitive	• Poor concentration • Confusion • Disorientation • Indecisiveness • Shortened attention span • Memory loss • Unwanted memories • Difficulty making decisions
Emotional	• Shock • Numbness • Feeling overwhelmed • Depression • Feeling lost • Fear of harm to self and/or loved ones • Feeling nothing • Feeling abandoned • Uncertainty of feelings • Volatile emotions
Physical	• Nausea • Lightheadedness • Dizziness • Gastrointestinal problems • Rapid heart rate • Tremors • Headaches • Grinding of teeth • Fatigue • Poor sleep • Pain • Hyperarousal • Jumpiness
Behavioral	• Suspicion • Irritability • Arguments with friends and loved ones • Withdrawal • Excessive silence • Inappropriate humor • Increased/decreased eating • Change in sexual desire or functioning • Increased smoking • Increased substance use or abuse

From Centers for Disease Control and Prevention: *Coping with a traumatic event: information for health professionals*, 2005. Available from <http://www.bt.cdc.gov/masscasualties/copingpub.asp>.

Recovery Stage

The recovery stage begins when the danger from the disaster has passed and all local, state, and federal agencies are present in the area to help victims rebuild their lives and the community restore public services. Cleanup of the damage and repair of homes and businesses begin. Evaluation and revision of the disaster plans based on lessons learned from the experience are made. Understanding the financial impact on the community and agencies involved is essential in developing future public health policy.

Research is needed on all aspects of prevention, preparedness, response, and recovery stages of disasters. Research is also needed on the education and training needs of first responders, health care providers, and community populations. Nurse researchers, in partnership with researchers from other disciplines, can play a significant role in conducting research on disaster management.

SUMMARY

Communities, now more than ever, need to be aware of potential disasters that may affect their residents. Comprehensive disaster plans need to be developed at all levels of government and by all communities, families, and individuals. Having disaster plans in place increases the likelihood of an effective response, resulting in saved lives and minimized destruction to the community.

Nurses have a role in and contribution to make at every stage of disaster management. Nurses need to have personal and professional plans in place for any disaster. All medical personnel must keep their credentials current and must learn the signs and symptoms of exposure to weapons of mass destruction so that they will recognize people who may have been exposed. They should learn what injuries may be sustained from various disasters and know which types of disasters are most likely to affect their communities, so that disaster triage and treatment can save lives. Finally, they must take drills in their respective health care facilities seriously. The more prepared the population and health care providers are for all kinds of disasters, the fewer lives will be lost.

LEARNING ACTIVITIES

1. Assess the community where you live for potential disasters that could result in mass casualties. What disasters are predictable? Are there measures that can be taken to prevent or minimize injuries, death, or destruction?

2. Find out who is responsible for disaster management in your community. What plans are in place for warning people and for communicating which actions to take in the event of a disaster? Are the people aware of these plans?

3. What social and cultural factors need to be considered in disaster planning in your community? Are there vulnerable populations with special needs (e.g., homeless, imprisoned, mobility impaired)? If evacuation of the community is mandated, have plans for evacuation of these groups been made?

4. Create an emergency plan for yourself, your family, or both. What factors would you consider in deciding whether to stay or leave your home? If evacuation were mandated, what important documents and mementos would you need to take with you?

5. Interview the person or persons in the ARC responsible for disaster services in your area. What is the role of their disaster nurses? What are the requirements to become a disaster nurse for the ARC?

6. Speak with police and fire department personnel about their responsibilities during a disaster. Do their roles during a disaster differ from their roles on a day-to-day basis? Do they have special teams and plans for biological, chemical, nuclear, or radiological incidents?

7. What emergency supplies does your health care facility have available in the event of a disaster? What provisions have been made available for vulnerable patients when there is no electricity? How would patients be evacuated from the facility to safe shelters?

ⓔ EVOLVE WEBSITE

http://evolve.elsevier.com/Nies
- NCLEX Review Questions
- Case Studies
- Glossary

REFERENCES

American Red Cross: *Disaster service program review, Fiscal year 2011*, 2012. Available from <www.redcross.org/what-we-do/disaster-relief/2011-disaster-relief-program>.

Centers for Disease Control and Prevention: *Emergency preparedness and response*, 2013b. Available from <http://emergency.cdc.gov/disasters/>.

Central Intelligence Agency: *Terrorism FAQs*, 2013b. Available from <www.cia.gov/about-cia/faq/index/html>.

Chettle C: Recognizing bioterrorism: nurses on the frontline, *Nurse Week* 6:29–30, 2001.

Federal Bureau of Investigation: *Terrorism in the United States 1999: Counterterrorism threat assessment and warning unit counterterrorism division*, 2013. Available from <www.fbi.gov/stats-services/publications/terror_99.pdf>.

Federal Emergency Management Agency: *About the agency*, 2012a. Available from <www.fema.gov/about/>.

Federal Emergency Management Agency: *National incident management system*, 2012c. Available from <http://www.fema.gov/about-national-incident-management-system>.

Federal Emergency Management Agency: *Are you ready?*, 2013d. Available from <http://www.fema.gov/pdf/areyouready/areyouready_full.pdf>.

Federal Emergency Management Agency: *National preparedness system*, 2013e. Available from <www.fema.gov/preparedness-1/national-prepredness-system>.

Federal Emergency Management Agency: *What is mitigation?*, 2013f. Available from <www.fema.gov/what-mitigation>.

James DC, Langan JC: *Nurses as heroes*, n.d. Available from <www.Advanceweb.com>.

Landesman LY: *Public health management of disasters: The practice guide 3rd ed.* Washington DC: American Public Health Association, 2012

National Institute of Mental Health: *Post-traumatic stress disorder (PTSD)*, 2013. Available from <www.nimh.nih.gov>.

National Oceanic and Atmospheric Administration, National Weather Service, National Hurricane Center: *Saffir-Simpson hurricane wind scale*, 2012. Available from <www.nhc.noaa.gov/aboutsshws.php>.

Patterson K: *Psychological triage: In Katrina's wake, sorting out who will need mental health care the most won't be easy*, 2005. Available from <www.nursingspectrum.com/Katrina/PsychTriage.cfm>.

U.S. Department of Homeland Security: *National response framework*, 2013. Available from <www.fema.gov/NRF>.

U.S. Department of Homeland Security: *DHS announces first national preparedness goal*, 2011. Available from <www.dhs.gov/news/2011/10/07/dhs-announces-first-national-preparedness-goal>.

U.S. Department of Homeland Security: *Homeland security*, 2012. Available from <www.dhs.gov/history>.

U.S. Department of Homeland Security: *National Terrorism Advisory System*, 2013. Available from <www.dhs.gov/alerts>.

Cathi A. Pourciau and Elaine C. Vallette

OBJECTIVES

Upon completion of this chapter, the reader will be able to do the following:

1. Discuss how *Healthy People 2020* can be used to shape the care given in a school health setting.
2. Identify and discuss the eight components of a comprehensive school health program.
3. Recognize the major stressors that can negatively affect an adolescent's mental and physical health.
4. Identify common health concerns of school-age children and associated health interventions.
5. Explore the various roles of the nurse in the school setting.
6. Be familiar with the standards according to which school nurses practice.
7. Cite several resources available to the school nurse.

KEY TERMS

early and periodic screening, diagnostic, and treatment
emergency care plan
Family Educational Rights and Privacy Act
Health Insurance Portability and Accountability Act of 1996
individualized healthcare plan
Individuals With Disabilities Education Act of 1990
Public Law 99-142
school health
school nurse
school-based health centers
Youth Risk Behavior Surveillance System

OUTLINE

History of School Health
School Health Services
  Health Education
  Physical Education
  Health Services
  Nutrition
  Counseling, Psychological, and Social Services
Healthy School Environment
Health Promotion for School Staff
Family and Community Involvement
School Nursing Practice
School-Based Health Centers
Future Issues Affecting the School Nurse

The healthy development of children and adolescents is influenced by many societal institutions. After the family, the school is the primary institution responsible for the development of young people in the United States. (Centers for Disease Control and Prevention, 2011c).

Academic success and healthy youth are closely intertwined. It is impossible to achieve success in school without maximizing the health of the students. School-age children and adolescents face increasingly difficult challenges related to health. Many of today's health challenges are different from those of the past and include behaviors and risks linked to the leading causes of death such as heart disease, injuries, and cancer. Examples of behaviors that often begin during youth and increase the risk for serious health problems are the use of tobacco, alcohol, and drugs; poor nutritional habits; inadequate physical activity; irresponsible sexual behavior; violence; suicide; and reckless driving (Box 29-1).

In the United States, approximately 52 million children attend school every day. Their presence creates a unique opportunity for school nurses to have a positive impact on

BOX 29-1   YOUTH AT RISK

- Every day nearly 4000 young people start smoking.
- Daily participation in high school physical education classes dropped from 42% in 1991 to 32% in 2011.
- Seventy-five percent of young people do not eat the recommended number of servings of fruits and vegetables.
- Marijuana use among young people increased from 15% in 1991 to 23% in 2011.*

*Data from Centers for Disease Control and Prevention: *YRBSS: Trends in the prevalence of marijuana, cocaine, and other illegal drug use, national YRBS:1991-2011,* 2012. Available from <www.cdc.gov/yrbss>.

TABLE 29-1 RACIAL AND ETHNIC BREAKDOWN OF UNINSURED CHILDREN IN THE UNITED STATES IN THE YEAR 2010

RACE	NUMBER	PERCENTAGE
White	3.2 million	38.5
Hispanic	3.1 million	37.1
Black	1.3 million	16.2
Asian and Pacific Islander	375,000	4.5
American Indian	110,000	1.3
Other (multiracial)	134,000	1.6

Data from Children's Defense Fund: *Who are the uninsured children, 2010: Profile of America's uninsured children,* 2011. Available from <http://www.childrensdefense.org/child-research-data-publications/data/data-unisured-children-by-state-2010.pdf>.

the nation's youth. The primary providers of health services in schools are school nurses, and there are approximately 73,000 registered nurses working in schools in the United States (U.S. Department of Health and Human Services [USDHHS], Health Services and Resources Administration, 2010). Although the National Association of School Nurses (NASN) recommends one school nurse for every 750 students in the general population, one for every 225 students in mainstreamed special education populations, and one for every 125 severely chronically ill or developmentally disabled students, caseloads vary widely, depending on mandated functions, socioeconomic status of the community, and service delivery model (NASN, 2010).

On a daily basis, school nurses see students with a variety of complaints. Increasing numbers of children are being seen in the school setting because they lack a source of regular medical care. According to the Children's Defense Fund (2012b), nearly 8 million U.S. children, or one in ten, do not have health insurance. This is a decrease from the nearly 12 million in previous years. Table 29-1 illustrates the racial and ethnic breakdown of uninsured children in the United States in the year 2010. Poor academic performance is strongly correlated with the uninsured status of youth, and conversely, acquisition of health insurance leads to an increase in school performance. Through education, counseling, advocacy, and direct care across all levels of prevention, the nurse can improve the immediate and long-term health of this population.

More than 22% of the nation's children are living in poverty and are less likely to have access to primary and preventive care (Children's Defense Fund, 2012a). *Poverty* is defined as annual income below $23,021 for a family of four. The poverty rate in children increased by 35% between 2000 and 2011. Decreased or inferior medical care has been linked to serious health problems resulting in an increase in absenteeism that may be correlated with failure in school. The school nurse can effectively manage many complaints and illnesses, allowing these children to return to or remain in class.

There is a need for mental and physical health services for students of all ages to improve both their academic performance and their sense of well-being. This chapter provides an overview of school health and the role of the nurse in the provision of health services and health education. It also offers an in-depth look at the components of a successful school health program and the major health problems of today's youth.

HISTORY OF SCHOOL HEALTH

Before 1840, education of children in the United States did not exist or was uncoordinated and sparse. In 1840, Rhode Island passed legislation that made education mandatory, and other states soon followed. In 1850, a teacher and school committee member, Lemuel Shattuck, spearheaded the legendary report that has become a public health classic. This report, known as the Shattuck Report, has had a profound impact on school health because it proposed that health education was a vital component in the prevention of disease.

Public health officials and others soon realized that schools played an important part in the prevention of communicable disease. When smallpox broke out in New York City in the 1860s, health officials were faced with trying to implement a widespread prevention program. They chose to target the schools and began vaccinating children. This experience led to the 1870 requirement that all children be vaccinated against smallpox before entering school (Allensworth et al, 1997).

At that time, schools were poorly ventilated and lacked fresh air, effectively spreading diseases among the children. Late in the nineteenth century, a practice of inspecting schools began to identify children who were ill and exclude them until it was deemed they were no longer infectious. Soon thereafter, compulsory vision examinations became a requirement to identify children who might have difficulty in school. In 1902, New York City hired the first nurses to help inspect children, educate families, and ensure follow-up treatment. Within a few years the renowned nurse Lillian Wald was able to show that the presence of school nurses could reduce absenteeism by 50%. By 1911, slightly more than 100 cities were using school nurses; in 1913, New York City employed 176 school nurses (Allensworth et al, 1997).

As they became more comfortable in their positions, early school nurses began to take on more active roles in the assessment of children, treatment of minor conditions, and referral for more serious problems. In addition to identification, treatment, and exclusion for communicable diseases and screening for problems that might affect learning, other issues quickly became part of school nurse practice. In the early part of the twentieth century the temperance movement led schools to teach about the effects of alcohol and tobacco. Also early in the twentieth century, "gymnastics" was introduced in schools in an effort to promote physical activity.

World War I was a pivotal point for school health services, and the call for a national effort to improve the health of schoolchildren emerged. In 1918 the National Education Association joined forces with the American Medical Association (AMA) to form the Joint Committee on Health Problems and publish the report *Minimum Health Requirements for Rural Schools.* This group also called for the coordination of health education programs, medical supervision, and physical education that some authorities contend is still lacking. By 1921 nearly every state had laws that required physical and health education in schools. Additionally, fire drills became part of safety education programs introduced during and after World War I (Allensworth et al, 1997).

Even though emphasis was placed on health services in schools, barriers still existed. Many schools and cities were unwilling to take on the task of providing primary health care for all children. The idea that schools should simply identify and refer problems to physicians was a common practice that the AMA backed. By the 1920s, medical services and preventive health services were clearly separated in the public health arena and in the schools. Not surprisingly, school health became known as school health education. The federal government did not get involved with school health until the passage of the National School Lunch Program in 1946. The School Breakfast Program was implemented 30 years later (Allensworth et al, 1997).

There was no impetus to change the direction of school health programs until the 1960s and 1970s. During these decades there was increasing publicity about children living in poverty and the move to mainstream children with disabilities. These two issues, along with an increase in the number of children of immigrants, contributed to changes in school health programs.

During the 1960s the first nurse practitioner training programs opened and made the inclusion of primary care services in schools possible. In 1976 the first National School Conference, supported by the Robert Wood Johnson Foundation, was held in Galveston, Texas. Following this conference a variety of school health service models began to emerge with new partnerships and ideas created to provide the most comprehensive health care services for school-age children. In addition, the Education for the Handicapped Act in 1975 mandated that all children, regardless of disabilities, have access to educational services.

The 1980s and 1990s saw several measures aimed at improving the health of schoolchildren. The Drug-Free Schools and Community Act was implemented in 1986 to fight substance abuse through education and was expanded in 1994 to include violence prevention measures. The Centers for Disease Control and Prevention (CDC), Division of Adolescent and School Health, began funding state education agencies to develop and implement programs aimed at

alcohol and tobacco use, physical education, and the reduction of sexually transmitted diseases (STDs) and human immunodeficiency virus (HIV) infection among the nation's youth. Also, the federal government encouraged states to use part of their maternal and child block grant monies to fund school-based health centers.

The No Child Left Behind Act of 2001 (NCLB) was signed into law by President Bush in 2002. As part of the NCLB, the Safe and Drug Free Schools and Communities Act (SDFSC) became effective that same year. SDFSC supports programs that focus on prevention of school violence and illegal use of alcohol, tobacco and drugs. This legislation promotes the involvement of parents and communities in efforts and resources to create a safe and drug-free environment in order to enhance student academic achievement.

The Patient Protection and Affordable Care Act (ACA) was signed into law March 23, 2010 by President Obama. Under this act, an initial 95 million dollars was awarded to 278 school-based health centers (SBHCs), as part of a capital program to create new sites and expand existing services in 2011. In 2012, an additional 14.5 million dollars was awarded to 45 school-based health centers for expansion of services in medically underserved areas. The new funds were expected to allow these centers to increase the number of children served by 50% (USDHHS, 2011). See later discussion of this topic.

School health services vary widely among states and school districts. There continues to be a lack of coordination among providers, with no single agency responsible for tracking services. Recognizing that there are differences among schools in the United States and that important health information must be delivered to children and adolescents, the USDHHS addressed many related issues in *Healthy People 2020* program. Objectives targeting children and adolescents are written for diverse areas, including physical activity, sex education and HIV prevention, nutrition, smoking prevention, and school absences related to asthma. The *Healthy People 2020* box lists a few of these objectives related to school health.

SCHOOL HEALTH SERVICES

The School Health Policies and Programs Study (SHPPS) describes school health services as a "coordinated system that ensures a continuum of care from school to home to community health care provider and back" (Allensworth et al, 1997, p. 153). School health services goals and objectives vary from state to state, community to community, and school to school. These differences reflect wide variations in student needs, community resources, funding sources, and school leadership preferences. Many organizations, such as the American School Health Association and NASN, are involved in the care and welfare of school-age children and have compiled and adopted definitions, standards, and statistics related to school health.

According to the National Assembly on School-Based Health Care (2010), 45 states have at least one school-based health center. Most school-based health centers are staffed

♥ HEALTHY PEOPLE 2020

Selected Objectives for School Health

AH-5.6: Decrease school absenteeism among adolescents due to illness or injury.

AH-8: Increase the proportion of adolescents whose parents consider them to be safe at school.

DH-14: Increase the proportion of children and youth with disabilities who spend at least 80% of their time in regular education programs.

EMC-1: (Developmental) Increase the proportion of children who are ready for school in all five domains of healthy development: physical development, social and emotional development, and approaches to learning, language, and cognitive development.

EMC-4: Increase the proportion of elementary, middle, and senior high schools that require school health education.

ECBP-5: Increase the proportion of the nation's elementary, middle, and senior high schools that have a full-time registered school nurse–to-student ratio of at least 1:750.

EH-16: Increase the proportion of the nation's elementary, middle, and high schools that have official school policies and engage in practices that promote a healthy and safe physical school environment.

FP-12: Increase the proportion of adolescents who received formal instruction on reproductive health topics before they were 18 years old.

IID-10: Maintain vaccination coverage levels for children in kindergarten.

IVP-27: Increase the proportion of public and private schools that require students to wear appropriate protective gear when engaged in school-sponsored physical activities.

MHMD–6: Increase the proportion of children with mental health problems who receive treatment.

NWS-10: Reduce the proportion of children and adolescents who are considered obese.

NWS-2: Increase the proportion of schools that offer nutritious foods and beverages outside of school meals.

OH-1: Reduce the proportion of children and adolescents who have dental caries in their primary or permanent teeth.

PA-4: Increase the proportion of the nation's public and private schools that require daily physical education for all students.

RD-5.1: Reduce the proportion of children aged 5 to 17 years with asthma who miss school days.

SA-18: Reduce steroid use among adolescents.

TU-3: Reduce the initiation of tobacco use among children, adolescents, and young adults.

V-2: Reduce blindness and visual impairment in children and adolescents age 17 and under.

From HealthyPeople.gov: *Healthy People 2020: Topics & objectives,* 2012. Available from <www.healthypeople.gov/2020/TopicsObjectives2020/default.aspx>.

with a nurse, a nurse practitioner, or physician assistant. The following services are frequently provided in these centers: vision, hearing, and scoliosis screening; first aid; and medication administration. Nearly all schools maintain health records on students and, at a minimum, monitor immunization status. Most authorities agree that comprehensive school health programs should have the following eight components (Figure 29-1): health education; physical education; health services; nutrition services; counseling, psychological and social services; healthy school environment; health promotion for staff; and family and community involvement.

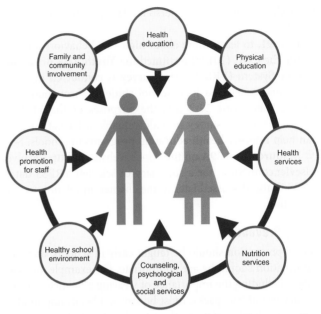

FIGURE 29-1 The eight components of school health programs.

Health Education

An objective of *Healthy People 2020* sets a goal that middle, junior, and senior high schools provide health education courses in priority areas. The CDC (2012f) identified the following six high-risk behaviors as needing to be targeted in health education courses:

1. Alcohol and drug use
2. Injury and violence (including suicide)
3. Tobacco use
4. Poor nutrition
5. Lack of physical activity
6. Sexual behavior that results in STDs or unwanted pregnancies

These problems and behaviors are preventable and often coexist. They also lead to both social and educational problems that contribute to our nation's high dropout and unemployment rates and crime statistics.

The National Health Education Standards were established to promote positive health behaviors for students in all grades (CDC, 2011a). These standards give students, families, and communities a framework for development of health education programs in schools. The standards specify that the students will: (1) comprehend concepts related to health promotion and disease prevention to enhance health; (2) analyze the influence of family, peers, culture, media, technology, and other factors on health behaviors; (3) demonstrate the ability to access valid information, products, and services to enhance health; (4) demonstrate the ability to use interpersonal communication skills to enhance health and avoid or reduce health risks; (5) demonstrate the ability to use decision-making skills to enhance health; (6) demonstrate the ability to use goal-setting skills to enhance health; (7) demonstrate the ability to practice health-enhancing behaviors and avoid or reduce health risks; and (8) demonstrate the ability to advocate for personal, family, and community health.

In 1991, to learn more about high-risk behaviors among youth, the CDC (2012e) instituted the Youth Risk Behavior Survey System (YRBSS). This survey is conducted every 2 years among selected high school students throughout the United States. Box 29-2 lists the purposes of the YRBSS. Reports from the survey provide valuable information that can help improve health education programs in schools. See eResource Tool 29A on the book's website, at http://evolve.elsevier.com/Nies/, for a summary of selected YRBSS data; YRBS is also discussed later in the chapter, in relation to sex education.

Injury Prevention

Injury prevention should be taught early in schools, and the information should be age appropriate. For example, bicycle safety, including the importance of wearing a helmet and the proper use of backpacks, must be stressed beginning in elementary schools. Safety on the schoolyard and playground is important for this age group because approximately 220,000 children per year are injured on playgrounds in the United States. Motor vehicle safety should be included in programs for adolescents who are beginning to drive.

Sports safety is particularly important among adolescents as participation in sports continues to grow, especially among girls. More than 3.5 million children younger than 14 years receive medical treatment each year for sports-related injuries (Safe Kids USA, 2011). Injuries occur most commonly on playgrounds, on athletic fields, and in gymnasiums. Orthopedic injuries (e.g., strains, sprains, fractures, and dislocations), dental injuries, neurological problems (e.g., head injury), ophthalmic injuries, cuts, abrasions, and bruises are frequently seen.

Use of proper equipment should be mandatory for children and adolescents. Fitted mouth guards, shin guards, pads, helmets, and other protective gear should be required to prevent injury. Regular hydration and frequent rest periods should be required to prevent heat-related illnesses, especially during hot weather. Effective warm-up and cool-down exercises should be encouraged to prevent muscle strain. Schools that participate in aquatic sports should include pool safety. The nurse has a unique opportunity to work with the athletic staff to promote these kinds of policies.

The sports physical is a good time for the school nurse to talk with and counsel the student about the risk for development of health problems related to physical activity. This is a perfect setting for the nurse to question girls about menstrual irregularities and to ask all students about their eating behaviors, feelings about their weight, and history of musculoskeletal injuries. The nurse can use this setting to teach the importance of stretching exercises to help prevent injuries. Many school districts have school safety committees that make recommendations for sports-related safety. These committees collect data on injuries, develop safety inspection policies, and plan staff training and student education related to school environmental factors. Such committees should include school nurses.

BOX 29-2 PURPOSES OF THE YOUTH RISK BEHAVIOR SURVEY SYSTEM

- Determine the prevalence of health risk behaviors.
- Assess whether health risk behaviors increase, decrease, or remain the same over time.
- Examine the co-occurrence of health risk behaviors.
- Provide comparable data among subpopulations of youth.
- Provide comparable national, state, territorial, tribal, and local data.
- Monitor progress toward achieving the *Healthy People 2020* objectives and other program indicators.

From Eaton DK, Kann L, Kinchen S, et al: Youth Risk Behavior Surveillance System—United States, 2007. *MMWR Surveillance Summaries* 57(SS04):1-131, 2008. Available from <www.cdc.gov/mmwr>.

Tobacco Use

For the past several decades, major concerns have been raised about long-term health problems associated with adolescents' use of tobacco, alcohol, and illegal substances. There is an increased likelihood that these youthful abusers will ultimately engage in other high-risk behaviors. Adolescent smoking has been closely correlated with alcohol use and other drugs. Smoking by young people can cause serious health problems, such as heart disease, chronic lung disease, and cancers of the lung, pharynx, esophagus, and bladder. Factors that have been associated with youth tobacco use include low economic status, peer pressure, smoking by parents, a perception that tobacco use is the norm, low levels of academic achievement, and history of aggressive behavior such as membership in gangs (CDC, 2012d).

Smoking is a major problem in this country and is the single leading preventable cause of death in the United States. Prevention should be emphasized in young people because 80% of adults who use tobacco began before age 18 years. Although the overall percentage of high school students who report smoking has declined in recent years, rates remain high, at about 20%. An estimated 3800 youth under the age of 18 try their first cigarette each day. Of those, approximately 1000 become lifetime smokers. White high school students have the highest rate of current cigarette use at 23%, followed by Hispanics at 18%, and blacks at 9.5%. Percentage rates are about equal when divided among male and female cigarette users (CDC, 2012d).

Approximately 9% of youth report using smokeless tobacco, and these students are more likely to become cigarette smokers (CDC, 2012d). The use of smokeless tobacco can cause cancers of the mouth, esophagus, and pharynx and can increase the risk of development of heart disease and stroke. Of note, 23% of students surveyed report having smoked cigars, cigarillos, or little cigars within the past month (CDC, 2012n).

Risk factors for development of oral cancer include all forms of tobacco; the risk is even higher when tobacco use is combined with alcohol use (CDC, Division of Oral Health, 2006). Therefore, all adolescents should be queried as to their use of both tobacco and alcohol. Education and counseling should be offered to students who use tobacco products. Limiting adolescents' exposure to tobacco advertising and teaching them the negative consequences associated with tobacco are essential in preventing its use.

Substance Abuse

The use of alcohol and other drugs is associated with problems in school, injuries, violence, and motor vehicle deaths. All 50 states and the District of Columbia have outlawed the sale of alcohol to anyone under the age of 21, yet it is still the most commonly used and abused drug among children and adolescents. In 2011, statistics show that 33% of eighth graders and 70% of twelfth graders had tried alcohol with increasing frequency as they progressed in school (CDC, 2012a). Approximately 22% of high school students reported they had five or more drinks of alcohol in a row within a couple of hours at least 1 day within the last 30 days. Additionally, almost 39% reported having had at least one drink of alcohol during the last 30 days. Alcohol use is more prevalent among Hispanics (42.3%) and whites (40.3%) than blacks (30.5%). The reported use of alcohol on school property remains relatively unchanged at 5.1% (CDC, 2012g). Research shows a direct correlation between alcohol use and liver disease, cancer, cardiovascular disease, and neurological and psychiatric problems.

The most commonly used illicit drug in the United States is marijuana. In 2011, 40% of young people reported using marijuana one or more times in their lives. The percentage of students who reported the use of marijuana on high school property was 5.9%, and 25.6% of students say they were offered, sold, or given marijuana (CDC, 2012i). Marijuana use has been linked to the same health problems as tobacco.

The use of other illegal drugs in high school students include cocaine (6.8%), inhalants (11.4%), heroin (2.9%), methamphetamine (3.8%), and steroids (3.6%). Use of an inhalant, the most widely abused substance, involves breathing the contents of an aerosol spray can, sniffing glue, or inhaling paint or spray in order to achieve a high. Even though the use of anabolic steroids has decreased in high school students from 6.1% in 2003 to 3.6% in 2011, the issue should remain a concern to school health nurses because of the number of athletes who abuse the drugs (CDC, 2012i). Many athletes believe that anabolic steroids will produce an increase in strength and muscle mass and enhance their performance. Part of the problem is that students are trying to emulate professional sports figures, such as renowned Tour de France bicyclist Lance Armstrong, who have used these drugs to enhance their performances. There are more than 100 different types of anabolic steroids, and each one requires a prescription. Abuse or improper use of anabolic steroids can result in severe problems, including renal impairment or failure, liver cancer, cardiovascular problems such as high blood pressure and elevated cholesterol levels, and sexual changes such as testicular shrinkage, clitoral enlargement, and accelerated puberty (National Institute on Drug Abuse, 2012).

BOX 29-3   TEEN PREGNANCY

- The U.S. teen birth rate is one of the highest among developed countries.
- 329,797 babies were born to teenagers aged 15 to 19 in 2011.
- Black and Hispanic youth have a disproportionately high rate of teen pregnancy.
- Teen mothers are less likely to complete high school.
- Teen mothers are more likely to be single parents and to live in poverty.
- Birth rates among teenagers vary substantially from state to state.

Data from Centers for Disease Control and Prevention: *About teen pregnancy,* 2012. Available from <http://www.cdc.gov/TeenPregnancy/AboutTeenPreg. htm>.

Sex Education

A number of objectives of *Healthy People 2020* address issues of human sexuality and prevention of pregnancy, STDs, and HIV. These issues are important for the nurse working with older children and adolescents.

Teens are becoming sexually active at earlier ages, and, despite recent declines, pregnancy rates continue to be high (Box 29-3). Data obtained from the YRBSS reveal a decrease from 48.4% in 1997 to 47.4% in 2011 of adolescents in grades 9 through 12 who have had sexual intercourse. Even though 84% of students have been given HIV/acquired immunodeficiency syndrome (AIDS) education in school, HIV transmission remains high among adolescents and young adults (CDC, 2012l). Because HIV transmission is higher in the presence of coexisting STDs, it is imperative that older children and adolescents have age-appropriate information on sexuality issues, including prevention of pregnancy and STDs.

According to the CDC (2012b), there were 1,148,200 people living with HIV in the United States in 2009. The cumulative estimated number of AIDS diagnoses in the United States is 1,129,127. Of these, 9475 occurred in children younger than 13 years. Through 2009 the cumulative number of estimated deaths in the United States of persons with AIDS diagnoses was 641,976; this number includes 4986 children less than 13 years of age at death (CDC, 2012c). It is important to note that HIV reporting is not mandatory in all states and so these data may underestimate the devastation of this illness among school-age children.

Sex education in the school setting is a controversial topic. Opponents of sex education believe that parents have the responsibility for teaching this content to their children. Laws in certain states prohibit or dramatically limit sex education in public schools. However, 21 states and the District of Columbia mandate that public schools teach sex education (National Conference of State Legislatures, 2012). Proponents argue that for many children sex education will not be addressed in the home. If this information is not taught in schools, children may receive inadequate or incorrect information from peers, media, or other sources. There is no research that concludes that sex education in the schools increases sexual activity. According to the Future of Sex Education Initiative (2012), the following seven topics are considered fundamental to a comprehensive sex education curriculum: anatomy and physiology, puberty and adolescent development, identity (sexual orientation), pregnancy and reproduction, sexually transmitted diseases and HIV, healthy relationships, and personal safety. School nurses have been caught in the center of this controversy but historically have advocated for education on normal human sexuality that encourages discussion in an objective, nonjudgmental manner and in which students are free to ask questions and receive correct answers.

Tattoos and Body Piercings

Tattoos and body piercings are a form of self-expression and attention-seeking behavior. Their popularity has risen dramatically in the last several years. The procedures are often done at home, on the streets, or in parlors where sterile technique and safety precautions are not practiced. Both hepatitis C and methicillin-resistant *Staphylococcus aureus* have been linked to tattoos and body piercings. This fact presents an opportunity for the school nurse to teach students the importance of making healthy decisions on whether to have such procedures done and, if so, under what conditions they will be performed.

Dental Health

One of the most common complaints of school-age children is dental caries. There are numerous contributing factors, including poor oral hygiene, lack of fluoridated water, and lack of funds or insurance for dental care. Half of children aged 12 to 15 years have dental caries. This disease is more common in lower-income children, and approximately 66% of those between the ages of 12 and 19 have had tooth decay. Untreated cavities can greatly affect a child's quality of life and cause pain, absence from school, and decreased self-worth (CDC, 2011b). Proper brushing of teeth should be taught along with good nutritional habits and the importance of regular dental checkups. Children should also be taught the relationship between high-sugar foods and dental caries.

Physical Education

One of the major objectives of *Healthy People 2020* is improvement of health and fitness through regular physical activity. Children today are less active than children in the past. Daily enrollment in physical education classes among high school students dropped from 42% in 1991 to 32% in 2011. Children are becoming more sedentary as a result of increased use of computers and television and decreasing requirements for physical education. It was reported in 2011 that 31% of high school children used a computer 3 or more hours a day and 32% watch television 3 or more hours a day (CDC, 2012f).

A sedentary lifestyle is associated with obesity, hypertension, heart disease, and diabetes. Studies show that people who are active have a better quality of life and outlive those who are inactive. Habits in childhood are likely to continue into adulthood, making it imperative that children are taught the importance of being physically active at a young age. Studies also show that children and adolescents who are physically active have increased self-confidence and self-esteem and

decreased anxiety, stress, and depression. Regular physical activity helps build and maintain healthy bones and muscles.

Physical education should focus on activities that children can continue into their adult years, such as walking, swimming, biking, and jogging. The educational content should change as the child ages. For example, what may appeal to a young child, such as playing on the playground with friends, is different from what motivates an adolescent, such as competitive sports and aerobic exercise. The CDC has made ten recommendations for the promotion of lifelong physical activity (Box 29-4).

Health Services

Health care provided in schools includes preventive services such as immunizations and health screenings. This component of a comprehensive school health program may also involve emergency care, management of acute and chronic health conditions, appropriate referrals, health counseling, education about healthy lifestyles, and medication administration.

Immunizations

Immunizations are a vital component of routine health care, providing long-lasting protection against many diseases. Vaccine-preventable deaths (VPDs) are at record-low levels. Many communicable diseases have been reduced by more than 99% as a result of immunizations. Under-vaccination of

---

BOX 29-4   GUIDELINES FOR SCHOOL PROGRAMS: PROMOTING HEALTHY EATING AND PHYSICAL ACTIVITY

1. Use a coordinated approach to develop, implement, and evaluate healthy eating and physical activity policies and practices.
2. Establish school environments that support healthy eating and physical activity.
3. Provide a quality school meal program and ensure that students are offered only appealing, healthy food and beverage choices outside the school meal program.
4. Implement a comprehensive physical activity program with quality physical education as the cornerstone.
5. Implement health education that provides students with the knowledge, attitudes, skills, and experiences needed for healthy eating and physical activity.
6. Provide students with health, mental health, and social services to address healthy eating, physical activity, and related chronic disease prevention.
7. Partner with families and community members in the development and implementation of healthy eating and physical activity policies, practices, and programs.
8. Provide a school employee wellness program that includes healthy eating and physical activity services for all school staff members.
9. Employ qualified persons and provide professional development opportunities for physical education, health education, nutrition services, and health, mental health, and social services staff members as well staff members who supervise recess, cafeteria time, and out-of-school-time programs.

From Centers for Disease Control and Prevention: School health guidelines to promote healthy eating and physical activity. *MMWR Recomm Rep* 60(RR-5):1-76, 2011. Available from <www.cdc.gov/mmwr/pdf/rr/rr6005.pdf>.

children, especially those in large urban areas, is a concern because of the potential for disease outbreaks.

All states now require proof of immunization status or evidence of immunity before a child can enter school. Certain exceptions based on religious and philosophical beliefs or medical contraindications may apply. The school nurse plays an important role in verifying compliance with immunization requirements and in educating children and parents about the benefits of immunization. See the CDC website (http://www.cdc.gov) for current immunization schedules.

Health Screenings

Many children in the United States are not appropriately screened for certain treatable conditions. Impaired vision and hearing can result in poor academic performance, slowed emotional development, and stress-related disorders. Early identification and treatment of these problems is highly effective and less costly. Vision and hearing screenings are provided at most schools according to a schedule set by the state or school district. These screenings usually occur upon a child's initial entry to school and at least once during elementary, middle, and high school. Children and adolescents may need to be screened more often on the basis of family history, developmental delays, recurrent ear infections, or exposure to loud noise.

Vision screening is required in most states, with referrals as needed. The standard Snellen vision chart is the usual screening tool. Screening for strabismus is a nursing responsibility, and this condition must be identified and treated early to prevent amblyopia. If left untreated, amblyopia may result in loss of vision. Referral to an eye specialist is a critical component of all abnormal eye examination results.

Scoliosis or postural screening should be done to identify spinal deviations in an effort to prevent secondary problems. Spinal problems may lead to cosmetic, functional, or emotional problems. Scoliosis screening in the school consists primarily of a visual inspection of the back. The American Academy of Pediatrics and the American Academy of Orthopedic Surgeons recommend screening of all girls at 10 and 12 years and boys once at either 13 or 14 years (Richards and Vitale, 2007).

The assessment of high blood pressure during childhood is important in identifying children who have hypertension and who will benefit from early intervention and follow-up. Vascular and end-organ damage from hypertension can begin in early childhood. Periodic blood pressure measurements are inexpensive and should be performed routinely for all children.

The Children's Health Insurance Program (CHIP) is a national program designed for children of families who earn too much money to qualify for Medicaid but cannot afford the high cost of health insurance. Medicaid-eligible children are guaranteed access to comprehensive health care services and routine dental examinations. Medicaid created the Early and Periodic Screening, Diagnostic, and Treatment (EPSDT) service because of the large number of uninsured children. EPSDT, a comprehensive child health program for the uninsured under the age of 21, includes health education and periodic screening. Services provided under the EPSDT program are often performed through the public health offices in each state but may occur in community health clinics and schools. Screening services must include a comprehensive health and developmental history, an unclothed physical examination, immunizations and laboratory testing that are age appropriate, as well as lead toxicity screenings (Centers for Medicare & Medicaid Services, 2012).

Emergency Care

Schools are a common site of injuries ranging from minor scrapes, and bruises, to fractures, seizures, head injuries, and severe asthma attacks. Injuries may occur in school buildings or classrooms or during physical education classes or athletic events. Emergencies can include natural events such as hurricanes, tornadoes, and earthquakes, or man-made disasters, such as hazardous material spills, fires, and civil disobedience. Basic first aid equipment should be available in all schools. The school nurse must be knowledgeable about standard first aid and certified in cardiopulmonary resuscitation. The school nurse must also be responsible for the development of an Emergency Care Plan (ECP) that provides school staff with a guide to facilitate quick response in case of a student emergency.

Care of the Ill Child

The school nurse is responsible for monitoring the health of all students. For students with acute or chronic illnesses, administration of medications or treatments may be necessary. The nurse is often required to assess an ill child to determine the type of illness or health problem and develop a management plan.

In 2011, 9.6% of U.S. children younger than 18 years had asthma, which was most prevalent among poor children (13.5%) and non-Hispanic black children (17%). Asthma is one of the most common chronic childhood conditions, causing more than 4.6 million people to miss more than 1 day of school or work (CDC, 2011d). Because asthma is so prevalent, it is recommended that school-based support exists for children who have it. Actions undertaken by some schools across the country include immediate access to asthma medications, development and implementation of asthma action plans, and student and staff education on asthma. An assessment tool has been developed to determine how well schools assist children with asthma (Box 29-5). Answers to all the questions in the assessment tool should be "yes." "No" answers indicate that students may not be in an environment conducive to asthma control.

According to the American Diabetes Association (ADA, 2011), diabetes is prevalent in school-age children, affecting 215,000 people younger than 20 years. Type 2 diabetes is now being diagnosed in children, a condition that has historically been diagnosed only in adults. Type 2 diabetes in youth is projected to increase by 49% in the next 40 years while the number of children diagnosed with type 1 diabetes is expected to increase 23%. The figures are disproportionately larger in

---

BOX 29-5 **HOW ASTHMA-FRIENDLY IS YOUR SCHOOL? CHECKLIST**

Children with asthma need proper support at school to keep their asthma under control and be fully active. Use the questions below to find out how well your school assists children with asthma:

☐ Yes ☐ No   1. Is your school free of tobacco smoke at all times, including during school-sponsored events and on school buses?

☐ Yes ☐ No   2. Does the school maintain good indoor air quality? Does it reduce or eliminate allergens and irritants that can make asthma worse? Check if any of the following are present:
     ☐ Cockroaches
     ☐ Dust mites (commonly found in humid climates in pillows, carpets, upholstery, and stuffed toys)
     ☐ Mold
     ☐ Pets with fur or feathers
     ☐ Strong odors or fumes from art and craft supplies, pesticides, paint, perfumes, air fresheners, and cleaning chemicals

☐ Yes ☐ No   3. Is there a school nurse in your school all day, every day? If not, is a nurse regularly available to help the school write plans and give the school guidance on medicines, physical education, and field trips for students with asthma?

☐ Yes ☐ No   4. Can children take medicines at school as recommended by their doctor and parents? May children carry their own asthma medicines?

☐ Yes ☐ No   5. Does your school have a written, individualized emergency plan for teachers and staff in case of a severe asthma episode (attack)? Does the plan make clear what action to take under different emergency situations such as fire, weather, or lock-down? Whom to call? When to call?

☐ Yes ☐ No   6. Does someone teach school staff about asthma, asthma action plans, and asthma medicines? Does someone teach all students about asthma and how to help a classmate who has it?

☐ Yes ☐ No   7. Can students actively participate in physical education class and recess? (For example, do students have access to their medicine before exercise? Can they choose modified or alternative activities when medically necessary?)

If the answer to any question is "no," students in your school may be facing obstacles to asthma control. Uncontrolled asthma can hinder a student's attendance, participation, and progress in school. School staff, health professionals, and parents can work together to remove obstacles and promote students' health and education.

From National Heart, Lung, and Blood Institute, National Asthma Education and Prevention Program, NAEPP School Asthma Education Subcommittee: *How asthma friendly is your school?* 2008. Available from <www.nhlbi.nih.gov/health/public/lung/asthma/friendly.pdf>.

---

minority populations. Childhood obesity and the decline in physical activity are considered major factors in this development (ADA, 2012b). In general, teachers are inadequately prepared to care for children with diabetes and must rely on the school nurse. Children should be able to participate in their care to the extent that they are able (ADA, 2012a). The ADA has specific recommendations based on age, as shown in Box 29-6.

Medication Administration

Administration of medications is a service provided almost universally by school districts across the country. The use of medications by school-age children has increased over the last several years, allowing many children to attend school despite serious health problems.

Medication administration in the schools is a serious undertaking. Issues facing the school nurse include safety, monitoring of both therapeutic and side effects, proper documentation, confidentiality, and ongoing communication with the student and family. Only those medications considered necessary are administered at school.

The following guidelines from NASN (2013a) should be adhered to by the school nurse:

- Properly received, stored, and labeled over-the-counter and prescription medications
- Parental consent for the nurse to communicate with the primary care provider
- Administration of medication without violating standing orders, school district policies, nursing standards of practice, or state nurse practice acts

---

BOX 29-6 **EXPECTATIONS OF THE CHILD WITH DIABETES**

Toddler and Preschool Age
- The child should be able to determine which finger to prick.
- The child can usually choose an injection site.
- The child is generally cooperative.

Elementary School Age
- The child should be able to assist in all diabetes tasks at school.
- The child is usually able to perform his or her own finger-stick glucose monitoring.
- The child can administer his or her own insulin with supervision.
- The child is usually able to let an adult know when he or she is experiencing a hypoglycemic episode.

Middle School and High School Age
- The child should be able to perform self-monitoring of blood glucose.
- Most children should be able to administer their own insulin with supervision; adolescents should be able to administer insulin without supervision.
- All children may need assistance with blood glucose testing when the glucose level is low.

Data from American Diabetes Association: Diabetes care in the school and day care setting, *Diabetes Care* 35:S76-S80, 2012.

- Maintenance of student confidentiality
- Supervision of unlicensed personnel

School nurses must be aware of medications that are being self-administered on school grounds and must provide education as needed to both children and parents. Rescue

TABLE 29-2 OVERVIEW OF INCREASE IN NUMBER OF STUDENTS WITH DISABILITIES*

TYPE OF DISABILITY	1976-1977	1990-1991	2000-2001	2009-2010
All disabilities	8.3	11.4	13.3	13.1
Specific learning disabilities	1.8	5.2	6.1	4.9
Speech or language impairments	2.9	2.4	3.0	2.9
Developmental delays	—	—	0.4	0.7
Serious emotional disturbance	0.6	0.9	1.0	0.8
Hearing impairment	0.2	0.1	0.2	0.2
Orthopedic impairments	0.2	0.1	0.2	0.1
Other health impairments	0.3	0.1	0.6	1.4
Visual impairments	0.1	0.1	0.1	0.1
Multiple disabilities	—	0.2	0.3	0.3
Autism and related disorders	—	—	0.2	0.8

*Children age 3 to 21 years served in federally supported programs for the disabled, by type of disability: Selected years, 1976-1977 through 2009-2010. From National Center for Education Statistics: *NCES fast facts: students with disabilities,* 2012. Available from <www.nces.ed.gov/fastfacts/display_asp?id=64>.

medications such as albuterol must be administered quickly to affect asthma symptoms, and the nurse must be familiar with its expected effects to properly assist the child who needs it. It is now legal in all 50 states for students to carry and self-administer asthma medications (NASN, 2013b). With the growing number of children who have diabetes, it is imperative that the nurse recognize the signs and symptoms of hypoglycemia and hyperglycemia in order to assist children in the monitoring of glucose levels and the administration of insulin or glucagon.

Medications commonly given in schools include analgesics and antipyretics (e.g., acetaminophen [Tylenol] or ibuprofen [Advil]), antacids, antitussives, anticonvulsants, antiemetics and antidiarrheals, antifungals, antihistamines, and antibiotics. Medications used to treat attention deficit hyperactivity disorder (ADHD) are the one of the most commonly administered. In 2007, 5.4 million U.S. children between 4 and 17 years were diagnosed with ADHD, and this number appears to be increasing (Schwarz, 2012).

Alternative and complementary medicine includes practices and products outside the realm of conventional medicine. Medication administration policies should exist that reflect local and state laws that address these products. The request for the administration of any of these medications provides the nurse with an excellent health teaching opportunity.

Children With Special Health Needs

In 1976, Public Law 99-142 was enacted, giving all students, including those who are severely handicapped, the right to public education in the least restrictive environment possible, regardless of mental or physical disabilities. The Education for All Handicapped Children Act of 1973 and the subsequent Individuals With Disabilities Education Act (IDEA) of 1990 enhanced the opportunities for children previously served in acute care and long-term care settings to have access to public education. President George W. Bush signed the reauthorized IDEA into law on December 3, 2004, to support children with disabilities in the U.S. school systems. Children affected by these laws include those who are hearing impaired, mentally challenged, multi-handicapped, orthopedically impaired, "other" health impaired (e.g., chronic or acute health problems such as a heart condition or epilepsy), seriously emotionally disturbed, speech impaired, or visually handicapped, or who have a specific learning disability.

The rapid development of medical technology has enabled students to attend public school whose conditions may have prevented them in the past from leaving an institution or controlled environment. These children need nursing services of varied types to continue their progression in school. Public Law 94-142 requires school nurses to screen or identify children in need of special education and related services and to participate in development of an interdisciplinary Individualized Education Program that includes educational goals and specific services to be provided. The nurse is also responsible for the development of an Individualized Health Care Plan (IHP) for all students requiring continuous nursing management while at school. Table 29-2 gives an overview of the increase in the number of students with disabilities.

Student Records

Health records are maintained for all students according to individual school district policy. At a minimum, student health records should include immunization status, pertinent history, results of screenings and examinations, and IHPs. The Family Educational Rights and Privacy Act (FERPA), a strong privacy protection act, protects student education and health records. Student health records should be afforded the same level of confidentiality as that given to clients and patients in other settings (i.e., sharing confidential information with others without approval is considered unethical and improper except in emergency situations).

The Health Insurance Portability and Accountability Act of 1996 (HIPAA) was published in 2002 and instituted nationwide in 2003. A major component of HIPAA is ensuring confidentiality of personal health information. Public schools that provide health care services fall under HIPAA regulations. Private schools that do not receive federal funding but engage in HIPAA-related activities are also governed by this act.

Delegation of Tasks

Not every school has a full-time nurse available on site. A nurse may be assigned to three or four schools, resulting in delegation of certain tasks to unlicensed personnel. Each state's nurse practice act stipulates which procedures may be delegated. The responsibility for assessment, diagnosis, goal setting, and evaluation may never be delegated. When tasks are delegated, the nurse must provide appropriate education, written procedures, and ongoing supervision and evaluation of the caregivers.

Nutrition

School-age children are undergoing periods of rapid growth and development and have high nutritional needs. They must eat a variety of foods to meet their daily requirements. Diets should include a proper balance of carbohydrates, protein, and fat, with sufficient intake of vitamins and minerals. Children and adolescents share a well-known preference for junk food, and their diet is often high in fat and sugar and frequently consists of fast-food items, such as hamburgers and French fries, instead of fruits and vegetables. Skipping meals, especially breakfast, and eating unhealthy snacks contribute to poor childhood nutrition. Identifying nutritional problems, counseling, and making appropriate referrals are important in the school setting. The school nurse should consider cultural influences on diet when teaching students and assessing their nutritional status.

Poor nutritional status is closely associated with poverty. Federally funded programs such as the School Breakfast Program and National School Lunch Program were initiated to ensure that all children have access to these meals during the school day.

VENDING MACHINE FOOD CHOICES

In 2004, the National Association of School Nurses addressed the issue of unhealthy foods found in school vending machines and sold in school fund-raising projects. The organization specifically resolved that schools should provide healthy food choices in school vending machines and for sale in fund-raising projects.

Data from National Association of School Nurses: *Resolution: vending machines and healthy food choices in schools*, 2004. Available from <www.nasn.org>.

Eating Disorders

It is imperative that the school nurse recognize the association between feelings of inadequacy and unhealthy eating practices in adolescents and young people. These self-perceptions begin early in life; therefore education and counseling must begin in elementary school. Prevention should concentrate on eliminating misconceptions surrounding nutrition, dieting, and body composition and should stress optimal health and personal performance. Outside influences such as commercials and advertisements make this a serious problem; adolescents and young children are bombarded with messages such as "You can never be too thin" and "Life will be wonderful if you look and dress like a model." According to the National Association of Anorexia Nervosa and Associated Disorders (NAANAD, n.d.), only 5% of American females naturally have the body type portrayed in advertising.

Nurses must also be aware of eating disorders. Anorexia, bulimia, and binge eating are the three most common eating disorders, and anorexia is ranked number three in terms of chronic disorders in adolescents (NAANAD, n.d.). *Binge eating* is defined as recurrent, out-of-control eating of large amounts of food whether a person is hungry or not. *Anorexia* is a severely restricted intake of food based on an extreme fear of weight gain. Literature has shown that anorexia is multifactorial, seen primarily in females, and often correlated with family dysfunction or a history of sexual abuse. *Bulimia* is a form of anorexia characterized by a chaotic eating pattern with recurrent episodes of binge eating followed by purging. Health consequences of eating disorders may include reduction of bone density, severe dehydration, tooth decay, and potentially fatal electrolyte imbalances.

FEMALE ATHLETE TRIAD

The "female athlete triad" is a syndrome consisting of eating disorders, amenorrhea, and osteoporosis. Pressure to attain a particular body shape or weight considered desirable in a selected sport may put the female athlete at risk for development of this disorder. The triad is a complex problem with psychological and physiological factors. It can result in menstrual irregularities, premature osteoporosis, and decreased bone mineral density; if taken to the extreme, it can become life threatening.

Data from Nemours Foundation: *Female athlete triad*, 2010. Available from <www.KidsHealth.org/teen/food_fitness/sports/triad.html>.

Obesity

Statistics show that few adolescents feel good about their bodies. Of those surveyed, 15.2% are overweight, 13% are obese, and 4.3% of high school students report taking laxatives or inducing vomiting to lose weight (CDC, 2012j). These kinds of harmful practices have been reported in girls as young as 11.

Obesity is the fastest-rising public health concern in the nation and may overtake tobacco use as the single leading preventable cause of death. The obesity rate has more than doubled in children and tripled in adolescents over the past three decades. More than a third of children and adolescents are considered overweight or obese. Statistics show that obese children and adolescents are more likely to become obese adults. Obesity and its prevention or treatment must be of concern to the school nurse (CDC, 2013).

Although many of the underlying causes of obesity are not well understood, several contributing factors have been identified; they include reduced access to and affordability of nutritious foods, decreased physical activity, and cultural and genetic influences. Obesity is associated with development of diabetes, dyslipidemia, hypertension, and other disorders, such as osteoarthritis, sleep apnea, different cancers, and cholelithiasis. In addition, obesity may result in social and quality-of-life impairment, and obese children are often labeled by their peers and ridiculed (CDC, 2013). The school nurse should determine the body mass index (BMI) for all adolescents. A BMI greater than the 85th percentile for age and gender indicates the need for further assessment and referral. To be successful, the treatment of obesity must begin early and must be multifaceted. Some of the solutions include improved health education related to nutrition and dietary behavior, increased physical activity and physical education programs, healthier school environments, and better nutrition services.

Nutritional Education Programs

Nutritional education is essential and must include parents, teachers, and the child. Children need to know and understand the food pyramid, how to make healthy snack choices, and the importance of balancing physical activity with food intake. Obesity, dental caries, anemia, and heart disease can be reduced or prevented with proper education and lifestyle changes. In addition, all adolescents and school-age children should receive counseling regarding intake of saturated fat.

Congress enacted the Nutritional Education and Training (NET) Program in 1977. NET focuses on healthy nutritional choices and health promotion and disease prevention topics in school and child care settings. Comprehensive school-based nutrition programs and services should be provided to all students. The ultimate goal of these efforts is that children will make healthy nutritional choices both in and outside the school setting.

Counseling, Psychological, and Social Services

The mental health of a child or adolescent is affected by physical, economic, social, psychological, and environmental factors. Children, like adults, often hide problems from themselves and from others. They may see problems as a sign of weakness or as a lack of control. Children may also be trying to protect themselves or someone they love and so do not seek help, with tragic results. Promotion of mental health and reduction or removal of threats to mental health are important to children and adolescents. Mental health is often difficult, yet essential, to assess.

Children and teens often struggle with depression, substance abuse, conduct disorders, self-esteem issues, suicidal ideation, eating disorders, and under- or over-achievement. They may also have to cope with physical or mental abuse, pregnancy, and STDs. Common warning signs of stress in children are presented in Box 29-7. Drugs and alcohol can enter a child's life as early as elementary school. Many children live in single-parent households with little social or economic support. They may not have enough to eat or a safe, warm place to sleep, yet are expected to come to school each day ready to learn. Services aimed at helping children cope with these problems are often lacking or too costly for many families.

The nurse or teacher may be the only stable adult in a child's life who will listen without being judgmental. Therefore, one of the most important roles of the school nurse is to act as counselor and confidante. Children may come to the school nurse with various vague complaints, such as recurrent stomach aches, headaches, and history of sexually promiscuous behavior, and the nurse must look beyond the initial complaint to identify underlying problems.

Major depressive disorders often have their onset in adolescence and are associated with an increased risk of suicide. In 2010 suicide was the fourteenth leading cause of death among children 5 to 9 years old, and the third leading cause in both the 10- to 14-year and 15- to 19-year age-groups. Homicide was the second leading cause of death in children 15 to 19 years old and the fourth leading cause in those 10 to 14 years old (CDC/NCHS, 2012). Suicide attempts are more common than completed suicides. A 2011 survey of students in grades 9 through 12 showed that 8% attempted suicide in the preceding year and 16% seriously considered suicide (CDC, 2012m). The nurse and other school personnel must be on the alert for suicide clusters that are often known to follow a successful suicide. Adolescents may approach school nurses and other school professionals for help before a suicide attempt. The call for help may be subtle and not recognized as such. Therefore, it is important for the school nurse to be cognizant of the warning signs associated with suicide and to recognize and refer at-risk adolescents to appropriate mental health professionals (Box 29-8).

A large number of children are abused daily in this country. Physical and psychological abuse and neglect are usually a result

---

BOX 29-7 WARNING SIGNS OF STRESS

- Problems eating or sleeping
- Use of alcohol or other substances (e.g., sedatives, sleep enhancers)
- Problems making decisions
- Persistent anger or hostile feelings
- Inability to concentrate
- Increased boredom
- Frequent headaches and ailments
- Inconsistent school attendance

BOX 29-8 TRUTHS ABOUT ADOLESCENT SUICIDES

1. Most adolescents who attempt suicide are ambivalent and torn between wanting to die and wanting to live.
2. Any threat of suicide should be taken seriously.
3. Warning signs usually precede a suicide attempt; they may include depression, substance abuse, decreased activity, isolation, and appetite and sleep changes.
4. Suicide is more common in adolescents who are dealing with bisexuality or homosexuality without support or in a hostile school environment.
5. Education concerning suicide does not lead to an increased number of attempts.
6. Females are more likely to consider or attempt suicide, and males are more likely to complete a suicide attempt.
7. One suicide attempt is more likely to result in a subsequent attempt.
8. Sixty percent of completed suicides in children and adolescents are committed with guns.
9. Most adolescents who have attempted or completed suicide have not been diagnosed as having a mental disorder.
10. Suicide affects all socioeconomic groups.

of many interacting factors, such as poverty, social isolation, and drug and alcohol abuse. School nurses and other school personnel are mandated to report cases of child maltreatment and neglect. The nurse must be alert to subtle changes in behavior or physical appearance that may point to abuse. Box 29-9 outlines some of the signs and symptoms of child maltreatment.

The school nurse may help the child learn problem solving, coping mechanisms, and steps to build self-esteem. The role of the nurse may extend outside the school campus. The nurse may need to work closely with families to develop an appropriate health plan for a particular child.

Healthy School Environment

A healthy school environment is one in which distractions are minimized and that is free of physical hazards and psychological health risks. NASN believes that all students and staff have an inherent right to learn and work in a healthy school environment and that the school nurse can "assess the school environment for risk factors, advocate for the school community to address environmental pollution issues, and educate the community to the impacts of environmental issues and exposures." (NASN, 2012).

Violence

Violence is a major public health problem because it threatens the health and well-being, both physical and psychological, of many children and adolescents. According to

the U.S. Department of Justice Bureau of Justice Statistics (2012), during the 2010 school year students were victims of 828,000 crimes, including 470,000 thefts and 359,000 violent crimes. Thirty-one percent of students reported they had been in a physical fight in the last year, and 11% stated that they had been in a fight on school property.

In recent years there have been a number of shootings and other acts of serious violence in schools. The CDC (2012h) reported that 17% of children admitted to having carried a weapon at least 1 day out of the last 30 and that 7% had been threatened or injured with a weapon on school property within the last year. The school shooting at Columbine High School in Littleton, Colorado, in 1999 was probably the first time that people in this country realized how unsafe schools could be. The most recent mass shooting, in Newtown, Connecticut, killed 20 children and 6 adults, making it the nation's worst K through 12 school shooting.

School nurses and other school personnel should be aware of risk factors and signs that could indicate a tendency to violence. Factors common in those who commit violent acts in school include being male and having a history of being ostracized or bullied in school. Media influences that desensitize the impact of violence are being studied more closely as a possible cause of increased violence among children and adolescents. Children involved in school shootings often have a need for instant gratification, have easy access to guns, and may have a history of discipline problems.

Although the number of students who commit violent acts is small, these random acts are frightening, and school officials are struggling with ways to prevent their occurrence and to recognize the signs of troubled youth. Violence prevention programs should begin in elementary schools. Children who exhibit aggressive behavior in elementary school are more likely to exhibit antisocial and violent behavior as adolescents and adults. Programs should target stress management, conflict and anger resolution, and personal and self-esteem development. Nurses should use data collected through the YRBSS and other local data as a means of assessment when developing violence policies and prevention programs in the school and community. Additionally, nurses should initiate and participate in research that examines the complex developmental, social, and psychological factors surrounding violence.

BOX 29-9 POSSIBLE SIGNS OF ABUSE AND NEGLECT

Physical Abuse
- Has unexplained burns, bites, bruises, black eyes, or broken bones
- Is wary of adult contact
- Appears frightened of parents or other relatives and cries when it is time to go home

Neglect
- Is frequently absent from school
- Steals food or money
- Lacks adequate medical or dental care
- Appears dirty or disheveled or is underweight
- Does not have proper seasonal clothing

Sexual Abuse
- Has difficulty walking or sitting
- Reports new onset of nightmares or bedwetting
- Refuses to change into gym attire or participate in physical activities
- Runs away from home
- Becomes pregnant or has a sexually transmitted disease

Emotional Abuse
- Exhibits changes in behavior, such as acting out or extreme passivity
- Exhibits delay in either physical or emotional development
- Has attempted suicide
- Exhibits inappropriate adult or infantile behavior

Data from Child Information Gateway: *What is child abuse and neglect? Recognizing the signs and symptoms*, 2013. Available from <https://www.childwelfare.gov/pubs/factsheets/whatiscan.cfm>.

Terrorism

Schools may not be the primary target in an act of terrorism but they will be affected. Events following the September 11, 2001, terrorist attack illustrate potential problems facing schools, which may include fear and panic among students, teachers, and parents, and anxiety among those directly affected.

Every school is expected to have an emergency management plan. In fact, many states mandate that schools develop plans to address the potential threat of another terrorist attack or natural or man-made disaster. School nurses must be prepared to act after any form of terrorism has occurred. The school nurse has an important role as a potential first responder in any emergency situation and should be an active participant in planning and policy development.

Health Promotion for School Staff

Although specific numbers vary, it is estimated that schools in the United States employ more than 5.5 million teachers and other employees. Health promotion programs at the work site have beneficial results, including positive effects on blood pressure control, daily physical activity, smoking cessation, and weight control. Staff who participate in health promotion programs increase their knowledge and positively change their attitudes and behaviors relative to smoking practices, nutrition, physical activity, stress, and emotional health. Health promotion programs improve morale, reduce job stress and absenteeism, and heighten interest in teaching health-related topics to students. School nurses play an important role in all levels of prevention through assessment, planning, intervention, and evaluation. The school nurse can assist the faculty and staff by giving workshops on exercise and nutrition, screening for increased blood pressure, and establishing weight management programs.

Family and Community Involvement

School nurses are often asked to provide health content to family, parents, and the community on a variety of topics, such as sexuality, STDs, HIV, communicable diseases, and substance abuse. Health education in the community consists of programs that are designed to positively influence parents, staff, and others in matters related to health. School nurses are a resource in the community and can take a leadership role in developing programs that positively affect the community, such as a program for smoking cessation. School nurses may also serve as consultants and advocates for other community health programs.

FAMILY RISK INDEX

Children living in families with four or more of the following characteristics are considered "high risk":

- Child is not living with two parents
- Household head is a high school dropout
- Family income is below the poverty line
- Child is living with parent(s) who does not have steady, full-time employment
- Family is receiving welfare benefits
- Child does not have health insurance

The percentage of children living in "high-risk" families, based on the preceding definition, is 10%.

Data from Annie E. Casey Foundation: *Children at risk: state trends 1990–2000*, 2002. Available from <www.aecf.org/ KnowledgeCenter/Publications. aspx?pubguid={A58448A9-05B2-45EA-A31f-98D7BECCE445}>.

Programs that engage the parents in school activities should be based on community needs and resources. Studies show that students who have parental support are more successful, experience less emotional distress, eat healthier, and are more actively engaged in learning. School nurses can improve parental involvement through the establishment of clear communication, involving parents as volunteers and including them in the planning of health-related events at schools. The nurse must also recognize that an increasing number of children are being raised in nontraditional families—single parents, grandparents, gay or lesbian couples, and interracial couples. When addressing issues with families, the nurse cannot let personal or religious bias alter the plan of care and must be aware that what worked with one family situation will not necessarily work for another.

Nurses should become adept at working in the public sphere by increasing their visibility and becoming skilled in working with the media and legislators. The media can be a useful tool in assisting school nurses with health education advocacy.

SCHOOL NURSING PRACTICE

School nursing is a specialty unto itself. School nurses need education in specific areas, such as growth and development, public health, mental health nursing, case management, program management, family theory, leadership, and cultural sensitivity, to effectively perform their roles. They must be prepared to work with children of all ages and cultures and under variable circumstances. The nurse must also keep abreast of issues affecting children and must participate in research that explores and expands the role. The school nurse's practice is relatively independent and autonomous, even though the school nurse functions as a member of an interdisciplinary team. For entry into school nursing, it is recommended that nurses hold a minimum of a bachelor's degree. Some universities are now preparing school nurses at the master's level. The school nurse must be able to identify and access professional development in order to maintain competency in the care of children and adolescents.

DEFINITION OF SCHOOL NURSING

School nursing is a specialized practice of professional nursing that advances the well-being, academic success, and lifelong achievement and health of students. To that end, school nurses facilitate positive student responses to normal development; promote health and safety, including a healthy environment; intervene with actual and potential health problems; provide case management services; and actively collaborate with others to build student and family capacity for adaptation, self-management, self-advocacy, and learning (NASN, 2011).

School nurses function in many roles. Among these are care provider, student advocate, educator, community liaison, and case manager. Additional skills needed by school nurses include the ability to supervise others, to practice relatively independently, and to delegate care. The American Nurses Association developed competencies relevant to school nurses and updated them in 2011. *School Nursing: Scope & Standards of Practice*, 2nd edition, can be downloaded at http://www.nursesbooks.org/Main-Menu/eBooks/eStandards/eBook-School-Nursing.aspx.

The school setting is a perfect place to conduct research on how children adapt to life transitions such as divorce; illness or death of a loved one; illness of either themselves or a peer; and domestic violence. The health-related behaviors of the young are a rich source of research opportunities. The school nurse must be aware of and interested in participating in different research studies.

RESEARCH HIGHLIGHTS

Research Priorities in School Nursing

Gordon and Barry (2006) surveyed 263 school nurses to identify what the nurses believed to be the top research priorities for the specialty. Ten areas were identified as being priority research topics. These priority areas, and examples for each, are presented here.

- *Obesity/nutrition*—nutrition and weight-loss counseling programs, eating disorders, obesity in children and teens, importance of exercise
- *Role of the school nurse*—presence of the school nurse and better academic outcomes, case management, role of the school nurse as health consultant, delegation to non-nursing personnel, mental health support
- *Legal/ethical issues*—legal liability when delegating to non-medical personnel, ethical issues related to children with Do Not Resuscitate orders, confidentiality, Health Insurance Portability and Accountability Act (HIPAA) mandates
- *Emergencies*—emergency preparedness, administering epinephrine autoinjectors (EpiPens) in school, standing orders for emergencies
- *Health education*—effective curricula for health promotion on hot topics (drugs, sexual activity, nutrition, exercise)
- *Absenteeism/attendance*—the school nurse's impact on student attendance, impact of absenteeism on educational success, strategies to decrease absenteeism
- *Diabetes/insulin*—diabetes management and safe delegation to nonlicensed personnel, managing insulin pumps at school
- *Injuries*—playground safety, sports injuries
- *Health services*—funding of school health services by using matching reimbursement (Medicaid), access to health services for students and their families, benefits and cost-effectiveness of school health services
- *Asthma*—environmentally unsafe schools, asthma education, asthma prevalence, use of peak flow meters

Data from Gordon SC, Barry CD: Development of a school nursing research agenda in Florida: a Delphi study, *J Sch Nurs* 22(2):114-119, 2006.

SCHOOL-BASED HEALTH CENTERS

School-based health centers are one of the best ways to offer comprehensive health care services to school-age children and adolescents. The center or clinic works in collaboration with, but does not take the place of, the school nurse. The collaboration between the school nurse and the school-based health center staff prevents fragmented care and duplication of services. School-based health centers provide an interdisciplinary team approach with personnel such as nurse practitioners, social workers, psychologists, and physicians who provide services. Services provided in these centers include nutrition education, injury treatment, general and sports physicals, prescriptions, pregnancy testing, laboratory services, immunizations, gynecological examinations, medication dispensing, social work services, and management of chronic illnesses. Close collaboration must exist within and among the community, the educational board, and the families for such a center to develop and flourish. The National Assembly on School-Based Health Care (2009) outlined the core values for school-based health care programs. This organization believes that all children should have access to high-quality health care; that the school setting is the appropriate place to deliver health care; that all services should be provided directly; that health care inequities can be reduced; and that fair reimbursement should be provided.

FUTURE ISSUES AFFECTING THE SCHOOL NURSE

Our nation's youth are our greatest asset and our hope for the future. The school nurse's role must constantly evolve to meet the demands of this future hope. Issues that will face the school nurse of tomorrow include ethical dilemmas, use of telehealth, continued threat of school violence, threat of bioterrorism, new and emerging infectious diseases, and increase in antibiotic-resistant diseases. The school nurse will need to understand and appreciate the multicultural community in which he or she will practice.

CASE STUDY   APPLICATION OF THE NURSING PROCESS

The nursing process is a systematic, organized approach to problem solving that nurses use when working with clients. It is neither fixed nor stagnant. It is a flexible process that allows for ongoing changes. This case study illustrates the use of the nursing process in a school setting.

Sandra Baker is a nurse at an elementary school in a small town. A second-grade teacher brought Carrie Broussard to the clinic and told Sandra that Carrie had been scratching her head all day and she was worried that Carrie might have an infection.

Assessment

Carrie was 7 years old. Her shoulder-length blond hair appeared neat and clean. When questioned by Sandra, Carrie replied that her head had been itching for 2 or 3 days, but she denied any pain or trauma. Sandra noted that Carrie did not have a fever or swollen lymph nodes, but examination of her scalp revealed multiple excoriated areas. Carrie's hair was examined with a Wood's light, and Sandra saw adult lice at the base of the hair follicles on the back of her head, near the nape of the neck. She also saw multiple nits. Sandra learned that Carrie had

two brothers in the school and one sister who was a toddler at home.

On Carrie's initial visit to the clinic, Sandra assessed the following:
- Temperature
- Lymph nodes
- Scalp for any abnormal findings

Diagnosis
Individual
- Head lice

Family and Community (School)
- Potential for spread of infestation in both family and school
- Educational opportunity to prevent the spread of lice by teachers and family members

Planning
Sandra was familiar with the school district's policy that covers head lice in schoolchildren. According to the policy, the nurse must do the following:

CASE STUDY APPLICATION OF THE NURSING PROCESS—cont'd

Individual
Long-Term Goal
- Carrie's return to school after successful treatment

Short-Term Goals
- Contact Carrie's parents to tell them about the lice.
- Inform Carrie's parents that she must be picked up from school.
- Recommend treatment based on school protocol.
- Provide guidelines for returning to school.

Family and Community
Long-Term Goal
- Ensure that the teachers, staff, and family members have the necessary education relative to prevention and treatment of head lice.

Short-Term Goals
- Examine the hair of all other children in Carrie's class for lice, and treat each according to the school protocol.
- Check the hair of all siblings who attend the school for lice.
- Check the hair of all students in the siblings' classes if lice are identified.

Intervention
Family
Carrie's brothers, David and Paul, were brought to the clinic for examination. Both brothers had lice. Sandra contacted Mrs. Broussard, explained the situation to her, and requested that she come to the school to pick up her children. When Mrs. Broussard arrived at the school, Sandra gave her written information on treatment and prevention of lice and showed her what nits and lice look like. Mrs. Broussard was also instructed to check other members of the family not attending this school, especially those who share hairbrushes, pillowcases, and towels, because all family members with lice must be treated or the lice would continue to be passed from member to member. Sandra also explained procedures for cleaning combs, brushes, bedding, and potentially contaminated clothing and toys. Finally, Mrs. Broussard was informed that the children could return to school the day after treatment.

It was obvious to Sandra that Mrs. Broussard was embarrassed. To ease her mind, Sandra carefully explained that head lice are highly contagious, are easily passed from child to child, and are not an indication of poor hygiene. Mrs. Broussard repeated the instructions and left with her three children.

Community
Sandra examined all of the students from each of the Broussard children's classes for head lice. From the three classes, she identified five more children with head lice and notified their parents. Those children had siblings in three additional classrooms and she repeated the procedure for each of them. At the end of the day, she had identified a total of 15 children with head lice, and contacted all parents.

Sandra investigated whether the teachers and staff desired an information session on the transmission and spread of head lice because so many students had lice. She discovered that it had been 2 years since this was done, and so she arranged a class for the coming week for the teachers and teachers' aides to learn how to identify and treat head lice.

Evaluation
Individual and Family
Mrs. Broussard brought Carrie, David, and Paul to school the following day and on examination Sandra found their hair to be free of lice and nits. Mrs. Broussard expressed her appreciation for the nurse's help and nonjudgmental approach to the problem.

Community
Over the next two days, Sandra reexamined all of the children in the affected classrooms and found that the infected children had been successfully treated and that there were no new cases. New cases were not identified during the remainder of the semester. The teachers and staff gave her positive feedback about the head lice education class and asked for it to be repeated at the beginning of each school year.

Levels of Prevention and School Health
School nursing encompasses all three levels of prevention (i.e., primary, secondary, and tertiary), and all three may be practiced individually or concurrently. Table 29-3 lists examples of school nursing interventions for each of the three levels of prevention.

TABLE 29-3	EXAMPLES OF PREVENTION AND THE ROLE OF THE NURSE IN THE SCHOOL SETTING
EXAMPLE	**NURSE'S ROLE**
Primary Prevention	
Nutrition education	Provide education to children and parent(s); consult with dietary staff
Immunizations	Provide for or refer to source(s) for immunizations; offer consultation for immunization in special circumstances
Safety	Provide safety education; inspect playgrounds and buildings for safety hazards
Health education	Teach healthy lifestyle education; develop health education curriculum for appropriate grade levels; provide health education to parents, faculty, and staff; develop suicide prevention and sex education programs
Secondary Prevention	
Screenings	Schedule routine screenings for scoliosis, vision and hearing problems, eating disorders, obesity, depression, anger, dental problems, and abuse
Case finding	Identify at-risk students
Treatment	Administer medications; develop individualized health plan; implement procedures and tasks necessary for students with special health needs; administer first aid
Home visits	Assist with family counseling and assess special and at-risk students
Tertiary Prevention	
Referral of student for substance abuse or behavior problems	Serve as an advocate; assist with resource referrals; assist parents, faculty, and staff; consult with neighborhood and law enforcement officials; initiate outreach programs
Prevention of complications and adverse effects	Follow-up and referral for students with eating disorders and obesity; participate with faculty and staff to reduce recurrence and risk factors; serve as a case manager
Faculty and staff monitoring	Follow-up for faculty and staff experiencing chronic or serious illness; follow-up of work-related injuries and accidents

SUMMARY

Components of a comprehensive school health program have been clearly identified and discussed. Many of the *Healthy People 2020* objectives specifically relate to issues that can be addressed in the school setting. The role of the school nurse has changed dramatically since its inception and continues to evolve to meet the demands of school-age children, their parents, and the communities in which they live. School nurses continue to reduce the number of days and the frequency with which students miss school related to illness. They have become child advocates, counselors, health promoters and collaborators, educators, researchers, and resources in both the school and the community.

⚖ ETHICAL INSIGHTS

An Ethical Dilemma: What Would You Do?

You are working as the school nurse in a rural high school when Grace, a 15-year-old female student, enters the clinic. Grace appears very worried, and, after several hesitant starts, she begins to cry and tells you that she is sexually active with a 17-year-old senior. She goes on to tell you that she has missed her last period and that her home pregnancy test result was positive. She states that she is afraid to tell her parents because she feels that they will be very disappointed in her and because she is afraid of what her father will do. She asks you where she can go to get an abortion. You speak with Grace for quite a while and encourage her to speak with her parents. She leaves the clinic a little more composed and promises you that she will think about what you have said. The next day Jenny, Grace's mother, comes into the clinic and asks to speak with you. She confides that she is worried about Grace and asks whether you know what is going on with her child. What would you do in this situation?

Although maintaining confidentiality and a professional relationship respectful of the student's wishes is vital, state laws and school district policies determine what a school nurse may do, and in some cases is required to do, when providing care to minor children. In order to deal with personal and sensitive information such as described here, the school nurse should be well-versed in relevant laws and policies and should follow them. When in doubt, contact a supervisor.

LEARNING ACTIVITIES

1. Explain how the *Healthy People 2020* objectives can be used to shape school-based health care.
2. Attend a meeting of the school nurse association in your area. Identify the major pros and cons of being a school nurse. Look at factors such as working conditions, number of children assigned to each nurse, job functions, and job satisfaction.
3. Visit a comprehensive school-based clinic in your area. Discuss how the care given in this type of clinic differs from the care that a school nurse can provide. Review the protocols of both settings and see how they differ.
4. Log on to one of the websites for school nurses such as http://www.schoolnurse.com/ or https://www.nasn.org/ and review the many sign resources available.
5. Interview a member of the local school board about controversial subjects in health education (e.g., sex education).
6. Review the most common diseases and reported injuries in school-age children in your area. Develop a plan for how the school and the community can work together to decrease their incidence.
7. Interview the parents of several school-age children. Ask what health services they would like to see provided in the school setting.
8. Arrange with the principal of a local school to have a discussion session with children in a particular grade level. Ascertain what their eating habits are and then develop a class that can enhance healthy eating.
9. What is the cultural make-up of your local area? How should this knowledge influence the school nurses' practice?

ⓔ EVOLVE WEBSITE

http://evolve.elsevier.com/Nies

- NCLEX Review Questions
- Case Studies
- Glossary
- Resource Tool 29A: 2012 United States Youth Risk Behavior Survey Data

REFERENCES

Allensworth D, Lawson E, Nicholson L, Wyche J, editors: *Schools and health: our nation's investment*, Washington, DC, 1997, National Academies Press.

American Diabetes Association: *Diabetes statistics*, 2011. Available from <www.diabetes.org/diabetes-basics/diabetes-statistics/?loc=DropDownDB-stats>.

American Diabetes Association: Diabetes care in the school and day care setting, *Diabetes care* 35:S76–S80, 2012a.

American Diabetes Association: *Number of youth with diabetes projected to rise substantially by 2050*, 2012b. Available from <www.diabetes.org/for-media/2012/number-of-youth-with-diabetes-projected-to-rise-by-2050.html>.

Annie E, Casey Foundation: *Children at risk: state trends 1990–2000*, 2002. Available from <www.aecf.org/ KnowledgeCenter/Publications.aspx?pubguid={A58448A9–05B2-45EA-A31f-98D7BECCE445}>.

Centers for Medicare and Medicaid Services: *Early and periodic screening, diagnostic, and treatment*, 2012. Available from <http://www.CMS.gov>.

Centers for Disease Control and Prevention: *National health education standards*, 2011a. Available from <www.cdc.gov/healthyyouth/SHER/standards/index.htm>.

Centers for Disease Control and Prevention: *Oral health: preventing cavities, gum disease, tooth loss, and oral cancers at a glance*, 2011b. Available from <www.cdc.gov/chronicdisease/resources/publications/AAG/doh.htm>.

Centers for Disease Control and Prevention: *The case for coordinated school health*, 2011c. Available from <www.cdc.gov/healthyyouth/cshp/case.htm>.

Centers for Disease Control and Prevention: Vital signs: Asthma prevalence, disease characteristics, and self-management education—United States, 2001-2009, *MMWR Morb Mortal Wkly Rep* 60(17):547–552, 2011d. Available from <www.cdc.gov/mmwr/preview/mmwrhtml/mm6017a4.htm?s_cid=mm6017a4_w>.

Centers for Disease Control and Prevention: *Fact sheets: underage drinking*, 2012a. Available from <www.cdc.gov/alcohol/fact-sheets/underage-drinking.htm>.

Centers for Disease Control and Prevention: *Healthy people 2020 Leading health indicators: Objective HIV-13: Proportion of persons living with HIV who know their serostatus*, 2012b. Available from <http.//healthypeople.gov/2020/topicsobjectives2020/pdfs/HIV.pdf>.

Centers for Disease Control and Prevention: *HIV/AIDS: basic statistics*, 2012c. Available from <www.cdc.gov/hiv/topics/surveillance/basic.htm29-aidsage>.

Centers for Disease Control and Prevention: *Youth and tobacco use*, 2012d. Available from <www.cdc.gov/tobacco/data_statistics/fact_sheets/youth_data/tobacco_use/index.htm29-background>.

Centers for Disease Control and Prevention: Youth risk behavior surveillance—United States, 2011, *MMWR Morb Mortal Wkly Rep* 61(4), 2012e. Available from <www.cdc.gov/mmwr/pdf/ss/ss6104.pdf>.

Centers for Disease Control and Prevention: *YRBSS in brief*, 2012f. Available from <www.cdc.gov/healthyyouth/yrbs/brief.htm>.

Centers for Disease Control and Prevention: *YRBSS: Trends in the prevalence of alcohol use, national YRBS:1991-2011*, 2012g. Available from <www.cdc.gov/yrbss>.

Centers for Disease Control and Prevention: *YRBSS: Trends in the prevalence of behaviors that contribute to violence, national YRBS:1991-2011*, 2012h. Available from <www.cdc.gov/yrbss>.

Centers for Disease Control and Prevention: *YRBSS: Trends in the prevalence of marijuana, cocaine, and other illegal drug use, national YRBS:1991-2011*, 2012i. Available from <www.cdc.gov/yrbss>.

Centers for Disease Control and Prevention: *YRBSS: Trends in the prevalence of obesity, dietary behaviors, and weight control practice, national YRBS:1991-2011*, 2012j. Available from <www.cdc.gov/yrbss>.

Centers for Disease Control and Prevention: *YRBSS: Trends in the prevalence of sexual behaviors and HIV testing, national YRBS:1991-2011*, 2012l. Available from <www.cdc.gov/yrbss>.

Centers for Disease Control and Prevention: *YRBSS: Trends in the prevalence of suicide-related behaviors, national YRBS:1991-2011*, 2012m. Available from <www.cdc.gov/yrbss>.

Centers for Disease Control and Prevention: *YRBSS: Trends in the prevalence of tobacco use, national YRBS:1991-2011*, 2012n. Available from www.cdc.gov/yrbss.

Centers for Disease Control and Prevention: *Childhood obesity facts*, 2013. Available from <www.cdc.gov/healthyyouth/obesity/facts.htm>.

Centers for Disease Control and Prevention, Division of Oral Health: *Oral health for adults*, 2006. Available from <http://www.cdc.gov/OralHealth/publications/factsheets/adult.htm>.

Centers for Disease Control and Prevention, National Centers for health Statistics: *LCWK1*, 2012. Available from <www.cdc.gov/nchs/data/dvs/LCWK1_2010.pdf>.

Children's Defense Fund: *Child poverty in America: 2011*, 2012a. Available from <www.childrensdefense.org>.

Children's Defense Fund: *Policy priorities: Racial and ethnic disparities*, 2012b. Available from <www.childrensdefense.org/policy-priorities/childrens-health/racial-ethnic-disparities/>.

Children's Defense Fund: *Who are the uninsured children, 2010: Profile of America's uninsured children*, 2011. Available from <www.childrensdefense.org>.

Future of Sex Education Initiative: *National sexuality education standards: Core content and skills, K-12*, 2012. Available from <www.futureofsexeducation.org/documents/josh-fose-standards-web.pdf>.

National Assembly on School-Based Health Care: *Core values*, 2009. Available from <www.nasbhc.org/site/ c.jsJPKWPFJrH/b.2663979/k.7566/Vision_Mission_Core_Value>.

National Assembly on School-Based Health Care: *School-based health centers: National census school year 2007-2008*, 2010. Available from <www.nasbhc.org>.

National Association of Anorexia Nervosa and Associated Disorders: *Eating disorders statistics*, n.d. Available from <www.anad.org/get-information/about-eating-disorders/eating-disorders-statistics/>.

National Association of School Nurses: *Resolution: Vending machines and healthy food choices in schools*, 2004. Available from <www.nasn.org>.

National Association of School Nurses: *Caseload assignments*, 2010. Available from <www.nasn.org/PolicyAdvocacy/PositionPapersandReports/NASNPositionStatementsFullView/tabid/462/smid/824/ArticleID/7/Default.aspx>.

National Association of School Nurses: *Role of the school nurse*, 2011. Available from <www.nasn.org/PolicyAdvocacy/PositionPapersandReports/NASNPositionStatementsFullView/tabid/462/smid/824/ArticleID/87/Default.aspx>.

National Association of School Nurses: *Environmental health concerns in the school setting*, 2012. Available from <https://www.nasn.org/PolicyAdvocacy/PositionPapersandReports/NASNIssueBriefsFullView/tabid/445/smid/853/ArticleID/73/Default.aspx>.

National Association of School Nurses: *Medication administration in the school setting*, 2013a. Available from <https://www.nasn.org/PolicyAdvocacy/PositionPapersandReports/NASNPostionStatementsFullView/tabid/462/smid/824/ArticleID/86/Default.aspx>.

National Association of School Nurses: *Self-administration of rescue inhalers for asthma in the school setting*, 2013b. Available from https://www.nasn.org/PolicyAdvocacy/PositionPapersandReports/NASNIssueBriefsFullView/tabid/445/smid/853/ArticleID/122/Default.aspx.

National Conference of State Legislatures: *State policies on sex education in schools*, 2012. Available from <www.ncsl.org/issues-research/health/state-policies-on-sex-education-in-schools.aspx>.

National Institute on Drug Abuse: *Drugfacts: anabolic steroids*, 2012. Available from <www.drugabuse.gov/publications/drugfacts/anabolic-steroids>.

Richards BS, Vitale M: *AAOS-SRS-POSNA-AAP information statement: Screening for idiopathic scoliosis in adolescents*, 2007. Available from <www.aaos.org/about/papers/position/1122.asp>.

Safe Kids USA: *Preventing injuries: At home, at play, and on the way, sport and recreation safety fact sheet*, 2011. Available from <www.safekids.org/our-work/research/fact-sheets/sport-and-recreation-safety-fact-sheet.html>.

Schwarz A: Attention disorder or not, pills to help in school, *The New York Times*, October 9, 2012. Available from <www.nytimes.com/2012/10-/09/health/attention-disorder-or-not-children-prescribed-pills-to-help-in-school.html?pagewanted=all&;_or=0>.

U.S. Department of Health and Human Services: *The Affordable Care Act and the school-based health center capital program*, 2011. Available from http://www.hhs.gov/healthcare/facts/factsheets/2011/12/sbhc.html.

U.S. Department of Health and Human Services, Health Resources and Services Administration: *The registered nurse population: Initial findings from the 2008 national sample survey of registered nurses*, 2010. Available from <http://bhpr.hrsa.gov/healthworkforce/rnsurveys/rnsurveyinital2008.pdf>.

U.S. Department of Justice, Bureau of Justice Statistics: *Indicators of school crime and safety, 2011*, 2012. Available from <www.bjs.ojp.usdoj.gov/index.cfm?ty=pbdetail&;lid=2295>.

30

Occupational Health

Bonnie Rogers

OBJECTIVES

Upon completion of this chapter, the reader will be able to do the following:

1. Describe the historical perspective of occupational health nursing.
2. Discuss emerging demographic trends that will influence occupational health nursing practice.
3. Identify the skills and competencies germane to occupational health nursing.
4. Apply the nursing process and public health principles to worker and workplace health issues.
5. Discuss federal and state regulations that affect occupational health.
6. Describe a multidisciplinary approach for resolution of occupational health issues.

KEY TERMS

Ada Mayo Stewart
Americans With Disabilities Act
disability syndrome
ergonomics
industrial hygiene
National Institute for Occupational Safety and Health
occupational health nursing
Occupational Safety and Health Administration
safety
toxicology
Workers' Compensation Acts

OUTLINE

Evolution of Occupational Health Nursing
Demographic Trends and Access Issues Related to Occupational Health Care
Occupational Health Nursing Practice and Professionalism
Occupational Health and Prevention Strategies
  Healthy People 2020 and Occupational Health
  Prevention of Exposure to Potential Hazards
  Levels of Prevention and Occupational Health Nursing
Skills and Competencies of the Occupational Health Nurse
  Competent
  Proficient
Expert
Examples of Skills and Competencies for Occupational Health Nursing
Impact of Federal Legislation on Occupational Health
  Occupational Safety and Health Act
  Workers' Compensation Acts
  Americans With Disabilities Act
Legal Issues in Occupational Health
Multidisciplinary Teamwork

Occupational health nursing, a subspecialty of public health nursing, is defined by the American Association of Occupational Health Nurses (AAOHN) as the following:

> The specialty practice that focuses on the promotion, prevention, and restoration of health within the context of a safe and healthy environment. It includes the prevention of adverse health effects from occupational and environmental hazards.

> It provides for and delivers occupational and environmental health and safety programs and services to clients. Occupational and environmental health nursing is an autonomous specialty and nurses make independent nursing judgments in providing health care services. (AAOHN, 2012, p. 2)

As depicted in Figure 30-1, occupational health nursing derives its theoretical, conceptual, and factual framework

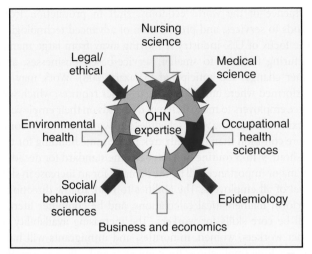

FIGURE 30-1 Occupational health nursing knowledge domains. (From Rogers B: Occupational health nursing expertise, *AAOHN J* 46:477-483, 1998. Copyright Bonnie Rogers, 1998.)

from a multidisciplinary base. Elements of this multidisciplinary base include the following (Rogers, 1998, 2003b):

Nursing science, which provides the context for health care delivery and recognizes the needs of individuals, groups, and populations within the framework of prevention, health promotion, and illness and injury care management, including risk assessment, risk management, and risk communication

Medical science specific to treatment and management of occupational health illness and injury, integrated with nursing health surveillance activities

Occupational health sciences, including toxicology, to recognize routes of exposure, examine relationships between chemical exposures in the workplace and acute and latent health effects such as burns or cancer, and understand dose-response relationships; industrial hygiene, to identify and evaluate workplace hazards so control mechanisms can be implemented for exposure reduction; safety, to identify and control workplace injuries through active safeguards and worker training and education programs about job safety; and ergonomics, to match the job to the worker, emphasizing capabilities and minimizing limitations

Epidemiology, to study health and illness trends and characteristics of the worker population, investigate work-related illness and injury episodes, and apply epidemiological methods to analyze and interpret risk data to determine causal relationships and to participate in epidemiological research

Business and economic theories, concepts, and principles for strategic and operational planning, for valuing quality and cost-effective services, and for management of occupational health and safety programs

Social and behavioral sciences, to explore influences of various environments (e.g., work and home), relationships, and lifestyle factors on worker health and determine the interactions affecting worker health

Environmental health, to systematically examine interrelationships between the worker and the extended environment as a basis for the development of prevention and control strategies

Legal and ethical issues, to ensure compliance with regulatory mandates and contend with ethical concerns that may arise in competitive environments

EVOLUTION OF OCCUPATIONAL HEALTH NURSING

The evolution of occupational health nursing in the United States has mirrored the societal changes in moving from an agrarian-based to an industrial-based economy and then, as we entered the twenty-first century, to a service-based economy. Occupational health nursing dates to the late 1800s with the employment of Betty Moulder and Ada Mayo Stewart (Parker-Conrad, 2002; Rogers, 2003b).

A group of coal-mining companies hired Betty Moulder in 1888 to care for coal miners and their families (American Association of Industrial Nurses [AAIN], 1976). Seven years later, the Vermont Marble Company hired Ada Mayo Stewart to care for workers and their families. Stewart is often referred to as the first "industrial nurse," and her activities are well documented (Parker-Conrad, 1988). In 1897, Anna B. Duncan was employed by the John Wanamaker Company to visit sick employees at home; then, in 1899, a nursing service was established for employees of the Frederick Loeser department store in Brooklyn, New York (AAIN, 1976).

At the turn of the twentieth century, the industrial revolution was well under way, and the concept of health care for employees spread rapidly. Companies hiring industrial nurses in the early 1900s included the Emporium in San Francisco; Plymouth Cordage Company in Massachusetts; Anaconda Mining Company in Montana; Broadway Store in Los Angeles; Chase Metal Works in Connecticut; Hale Brothers in San Francisco; Filene's in Boston; Carson, Pirie, Scott in Chicago; Fulton Cotton Mills in Georgia; and Bullock's in Los Angeles (McGrath, 1946; Parker-Conrad, 1988). The cost-effectiveness of providing health care to employees was achieving greater recognition, and by 1912, after workers' compensation legislation had been instituted, 38 nurses were employed by business firms (McGrath, 1946; Parker-Conrad, 1988). The following year, a registry of industrial nurses was initiated, and in 1915, the Boston Industrial Nurses Club was formed, later evolving into the Massachusetts Industrial Nurses Organization.

In 1916, the Factory Nurses Conference was organized. This group was open only to graduate, state-registered nurses affiliated with the American Nurses Association (ANA), and their efforts identified the industrial nurses' need to explore the uniqueness of this evolving specialty area (AAIN, 1976). More importantly, industrial nurses were practicing in single-nurse settings and recognized the benefit of uniting as a group for the purpose of sharing ideas with peers practicing in the same nursing arena. In 1917, the first educational course for industrial nurses was offered at Boston University's College of Business Administration.

During and after the Great Depression, many nurses lost jobs because employers and business managers viewed industrial nursing as a nonessential aspect of business (Felton, 1985, 1986). The focus of health care for employees again changed as a result of many factors, including the impact of the two world wars. During World War I, the government demanded health services for workers at factories and shipyards holding defense contracts. Demographics in the workplace were also dramatically different during World War II because higher numbers of women entered the workforce. In 1942, the U.S. Surgeon General told an audience of nurses that the health conservation of the "industrial army" was the most urgent civilian need during the war (Felton, 1985).

From 1938 to 1943, the number of occupational health nurses increased by more than 10,000. In 1942, some 300 nurses from 16 states voted to create a national association for the specialty. Catherine R. Dempsey, a nurse at Simplex Wire and Cable Company in Cambridge, Massachusetts, was elected president of the national association. By 1943, approximately 11,000 nurses were employed in industry (AAIN, 1976).

Nine years later, members of AAIN voted to remain an independent, autonomous association rather than merge with the National League for Nursing or the ANA. In 1953, another important step was taken toward formalizing this specialty area of nursing practice when the *Industrial Nurses Journal* (now the *AAOHN Journal*) began publishing. In 1977, the organization changed its name to the AAOHN, reflecting a broader, more diverse scope of practice.

In the 1980s and 1990s, occupational health nursing rapidly increased its role in health promotion, policy development, management, and research while maintaining traditional occupational health nursing practice. In 1989, AAOHN developed its first research agenda, and in 1993, the **Occupational Safety and Health Administration** (OSHA) established the Office of Occupational Health Nursing, reenergizing the concept of occupational health into practice. In 1999, the AAOHN Foundation was established, and competencies in the specialty were delineated. In 2003, the 60-year-old Annual Joint Conference, the American Occupational Health Conference, was abolished by the physicians and nurses even though there was lack of consensus on this decision among the membership at large. Consequently, AAOHN held its first separate occupational health nursing conference in 2005. In the twenty-first century, the AAOHN continues to expand specialty borders, emphasizing the importance of occupational health concepts and population-based practice.

DEMOGRAPHIC TRENDS AND ACCESS ISSUES RELATED TO OCCUPATIONAL HEALTH CARE

At the beginning of the twenty-first century, sweeping transformations in industry are influencing the direction of occupational health nursing. These transformations include changing workforce demographics, rising health care costs, diversity of health care systems with the integration of managed care, influence of the world economy, shift in production from goods to services, and proliferation of advanced technologies. The focus of U.S. industry is moving away from large manufacturing facilities to smaller, service-based businesses, and other changes are anticipated (Salazar, 2006). Work may be performed where and when the customer requires, which will force employers to make different demands on their employees. Flexible and varying work schedules and worksites have become more common than the daily trek to the same building for the 40-hour, 9-to-5 routine that has been the standard for decades. Of major importance will be the demand for an increase in skill level of all employees. The abilities to read, follow directions, perform mathematical calculations, and be computer literate will be core skills for workers. The increasing availability of older workers, women, minorities, and immigrants will have far-reaching implications for employers and will pose specific challenges for occupational health professionals.

According to the U.S. Bureau of Labor Statistics, total employment is expected to increase by 20.5 million jobs from 2010 to 2020. Industries and occupations related to health care, personal care and social assistance, and construction are expected to have the fastest job growth. Service-producing industries are anticipated to produce nearly 18 million jobs; employment in health care–related occupations is expected to grow rapidly (nearly 30%) followed by personal care and service (24%), largely because an aging population will require more medical care. Furthermore, patients increasingly are seeking home care as an alternative to costly hospital or residential care stays (U.S. Bureau of Labor Statistics, 2012). These trends are important to understand because they have a direct impact on the national rate of economic growth, especially in the area of population-sensitive products such as food, automobiles, housing units, household goods, and services such as health care, education, and transportation. With expansion of each of these sectors, there are concomitant hazards.

Within the context of these evolving organizational trends, key characteristics include a focus on a shared vision, strategy, and long-term objectives in an environment composed of individuals working in teams. In contrast to the past, occupational health nurses have opportunities to work on cross-functional teams to shape decisions in areas such as benefits, research, safety, and legal matters. Specifically, occupational health nurses have opportunities to positively affect the transformation of the health care delivery system, establish policies within the managed care environment and within corporations, and assume leadership positions on legislative staffs and in governmental agencies.

Corporations have become driving forces in shaping the development of alternative approaches to health care. Rapidly rising health care costs have spawned a number of alternative approaches to providing health care, such as preferred provider organizations.

It is important that the occupational health nurse remains informed about the various health care options available to the workforce as rapid changes occur regarding corporate benefits. This issue is of particular importance when the nurse is considering the referral of an employee to a health resource.

Participation in one of the managed care plans requires that treatment take place according to the organization's guidelines and within its health service delivery system. Managed care plans have nearly replaced traditional indemnity plans. Access to care is closely managed and often limited. As this trend continues, the role of the occupational health nurse will take on added importance. The nurse must be prepared to accept increasing responsibilities as a primary care provider as well as a tertiary care coordinator/case manager.

As businesses seek ways to maximize the value of the dollars they spend on health care services, occupational health nurses and other health professionals face both an opportunity and a threat. The opportunity comes from being able to demonstrate that cost-effective, quality health programs do improve the health of employees and their dependents, positively influencing their companies' attempts to control rising health care costs. The threat is that if health professionals cannot prove cost-effectiveness and value to companies, their functions may be eliminated or replaced by contract services (Intili and Laws, 2003).

OCCUPATIONAL HEALTH NURSING PRACTICE AND PROFESSIONALISM

As workplaces have continued to change over the past few decades, the role of the occupational health nurse has become even more diversified and complex (Rogers, 2012). Often working as the only on-site health care professional, the occupational health nurse collaborates with workers, employers, and other professionals to identify health problems or needs, prioritize interventions, develop and implement programs, and evaluate services delivered. The occupational health nurse is in a unique and critical position to coordinate a holistic approach to the delivery of quality, comprehensive occupational health services. The Standards of Occupational and Environmental Health Nursing, the Code of Ethics, and AAOHN practice competencies guide the nurse.

AAOHN's Standards of Occupational and Environmental Health Nursing Practice form the basis of the profession's responsibilities and accountabilities (AAOHN, 2012). The 11 standard statements are listed in Table 30-1. For each standard, identifiable criteria are detailed that can be used to evaluate practice relative to the standard. Refer to the complete standards document from the AAOHN for this information.

Guided by an ethical framework made explicit in the AAOHN Code of Ethics, occupational health nurses encourage and enable individuals to make informed decisions about health care concerns (AAOHN, 2009) (Box 30-1). The occupational health nurse is a worker advocate and has the responsibility to uphold professional standards and codes. The occupational health nurse is also responsible to management, is usually compensated by management, and must practice within a framework of company policies and guidelines (Rogers, 2003a). Ethical dilemmas arise because the nurse is loyal to both workers and management. Issues such as screening, drug testing, informing employees about hazardous exposures, and confidentiality of health information, which is integral and central to the practice base, often create ethical debates. As advocates for workers, occupational health nurses foster equitable and quality health care services and safe and healthy work environments.

Occupational health nurses make up the largest professional group providing health care services to employees in highly complex work environments. The roles of occupational health nurses are changing as a result of many factors, including rising health care costs, increased recognition of health

TABLE 30-1	STANDARDS OF OCCUPATIONAL AND ENVIRONMENTAL HEALTH NURSING
Standard I: Assessment	The occupational and environmental health nurse systematically assesses the health status of the client(s).
Standard II: Diagnosis	The occupational and environmental health nurse analyzes assessment data to formulate diagnoses.
Standard III: Outcome identification	The occupational and environmental health nurse identifies outcomes specific to the client(s)
Standard IV: Planning	The occupational and environmental health nurse develops a goal-directed plan that is comprehensive and formulates interventions to attain expected outcomes.
Standard V: Implementation	The occupational and environmental health nurse implements interventions to attain desired outcomes identified in the plan.
Standard VI: Evaluation	The occupational and environmental health nurse systematically and continuously evaluates responses to interventions and progress toward the achievement of desired outcomes.
Standard VII: Resource	The occupational and environmental health nurse secures and manages the resources that support occupational health and safety programs and services.
Standard VIII: Professional	The occupational and environmental health nurse assumes accountability for professional development to enhance professional growth and maintain competency.
Standard IX: Collaboration	The occupational and environmental health nurse collaborates with the client(s) for the promotion, prevention, and restoration of health within the conduct of a safe and healthy environment.
Standard X: Research	The occupational and environmental health nurse uses research findings in practice and contributes to the scientific base in occupational and environmental health nursing to improve practice and advance the profession.
Standard XI: Ethics	The occupational and environmental health nurse uses an ethical framework for decision making in practice.

Data from American Association of Occupational Health Nurses: Standards of occupational and environmental health nursing, *AAOHN J* 60: 151-157, 2012. Copyright American Association of Occupational Health Nurses. Retrieved from <http://www.aaohn.org>.

effects associated with various exposures, emphasis on health promotion and wellness, health surveillance, women's issues, ergonomics, reproductive issues, downsizing, trends in managed care, and multicultural workforces. Box 30-2 reflects this growth in scope of practice and outlines the occupational health nursing services currently mandated by state and federal regulations and those generally mandated by company policies.

⚖ ETHICAL INSIGHTS

Confidentiality of Employee Health Information

The occupational health nurse sometimes experiences ethical dilemmas because of dual responsibility to both the employer and the employees. In dealing with health information, the employee has a right to privacy and should "be protected from unauthorized and inappropriate disclosure of personal information" (AAOHN, 2004, p. 1). Exceptions can, and in some situations must, be made, however. These include (1) life-threatening emergencies, (2) authorization by the employee to release information to others (e.g., insurance company, health care provider), (3) workers' compensation information, and (4) compliance with government laws and regulations.

The AAOHN identifies three "levels of confidentiality" of health information. Level I relates to information required by law (e.g., data on occupational illness and injuries, exposure data, and information derived from special examinations [i.e., tests given to food handlers]). Level II covers information that will assist in management of human resources (e.g., information obtained from job placement and other health examinations to determine "workability status" of the employee). Finally, Level III focuses on "personal health information." This includes non–job-related health problems and health counseling.

Disclosure of Level I and II information to management should be allowed only on a "need-to-know" basis, generally with reference to workability status and regulatory compliance. Disclosure of level III information to management and regulatory agencies should be allowed only as required by law. Finally, disclosure of level III information health insurance providers should be made only with appropriate written authorization of the employee.

Data from American Association of Occupational Health Nurses: *Position statement: confidentiality of employee health information*, 2004. Available from <www.aaohn.org/practice/positions/upload/Confidentiality_of_Emp_Health_Info.pdf>.

According to the most recent National Sample Survey of Registered Nurses, approximately 19,000 nurses, or about 1% of the total nursing population, are practicing in the occupational health field in the United States (Health Resources and Services Administration, Office of Information Technology, 2011). Approximately 60% of these occupational health nurses work alone, making decisions about health and safety issues, influencing policy in health and safety, and planning and implementing myriad health programs. More than 65% of nurses practicing in occupational health are prepared at the baccalaureate level or higher and have been practicing in the field of occupational health for at least 10 years (AAOHN, 2006).

Meeting the needs of employees in smaller businesses is another important practice priority. The integration of occupational health and safety principles into the curricula of schools of nursing, engineering, and management is critical.

BOX 30-1 AMERICAN ASSOCIATION OF OCCUPATIONAL HEALTH NURSES CODE OF ETHICS

- Occupational and environmental health nurses provide health, wellness, safety, and other related services to clients with regard for human dignity and rights, unrestricted by consideration of social or economic status, personal attributes or the nature of the health status.
- Occupational and environmental health nurses, as licensed health care professionals, accept obligations to society as professional and responsible members of the community.
- Occupational and environmental health nurses strive to safeguard clients' rights to privacy by protecting confidential information and releasing information only as required or permitted by law.
- Occupational and environmental health nurses promote collaboration with other professionals, community agencies, and stakeholders in order to meet the health, wellness, safety, and other related needs of the client.
- Occupational and environmental health nurses maintain individual competence in nursing practice, based on scientific knowledge, and recognize and accept responsibility for individual judgments and actions, while complying with appropriate laws and regulations.

From American Association of Occupational Health Nurses: *AAOHN Code of Ethics and Interpretive Statements*, 2009. Available from <www.aaohn.org>.

Community health nurses may assume occupational health nursing roles; therefore community health nurses must be knowledgeable about the specialty area of occupational health nursing. Municipalities, smaller companies, visiting nurse associations, and home care agencies may provide opportunities for community health nurses to be involved in screening programs, health education activities, workplace hazard evaluations, and other occupational health–related activities.

The occupational health nurse's strengths are embedded in assessing, planning, implementing, and evaluating health programs for populations, care plans for individuals, and health education activities for worker aggregates. Often, lack of understanding or misconceptions about the occupational health nurse's role have fostered the invisibility of the nurse, both within the nursing profession itself and within the business environment, thereby exacerbating the difficulties the nurses face in being the sole guardians of health for workers in many companies. Empowered, well-trained, educated occupational and environmental health nurses can help bring about crucial changes in the areas of primary, secondary, and tertiary prevention in occupational health.

In response to societal changes and historical events, the practice of occupational health nursing has changed dramatically, demanding a sophisticated knowledge base and problem-solving skills that are empirically grounded and multidisciplinary in nature (Rogers, 2003b). For example, demographic changes with an aging population requires more knowledge and skills about managing an aged workforce (Rogers et al, 2009b). The roles and responsibilities of the occupational health nurse must be clearly articulated to lay people, managers, workers; union representatives, and colleagues in occupational health, nursing, and medicine

BOX 30-2 OCCUPATIONAL HEALTH NURSING SERVICES

Services Mandated by Federal and State Regulations

- Safe and healthful workplace
- Emergency medical response
- First aid responder selection and training
- First aid space, supplies, protocols, and records
- Designated medical resources for incident response
- Workers' compensation
- Confidentiality of medical records
- Compliance with medical record retention requirements
- Occupational Safety and Health Administration (OSHA) compliance
- Medical personnel requirement (29 *CFR* 1910.15)
- Injury and illness reporting and recording
- Accident and injury investigation
- Cumulative trauma disorder prevention
- Employee access to medical and exposure records
- Medical surveillance and hazardous work qualification
- Personal protective equipment evaluation and training
- Infection control
- Employee Right-to-Know Act notification and training
- Community Right-to-Know Act compliance
- Americans With Disabilities Act (ADA) compliance
- Rehabilitation Act: handicap, preplacement, fitness for duty evaluations, accommodations
- Department of Defense, Department of Transportation, Nuclear Regulatory Commission, and Drug-Free Workplace Act compliance
- Policy development
- Drug awareness education
- Drug testing and technical support
- Employee Assistance Program services
- Threat of violence and duty to warn
- Video display terminal (VDT) local regulations
- State and local public health regulations
- Nursing practice acts
- Board of Pharmacy and Drug Enforcement Agency regulations
- Continuing professional education required for licensure

Services Often Mandated by Company Policy

- Clinical supervision of on-site health services
- Health strategy development
- Health services standards
- Space, staffing, and operational standards
- Occupational illness and injury assessment, diagnosis, treatment, and referral
- Nonoccupational illness and injury assessment, diagnosis, treatment, and referral
- Disability and return-to-work evaluations and accommodations
- Impaired employee fitness for duty evaluation
- Preplacement evaluation and medical accommodation
- Handicap evaluation, placement, and accommodation
- Employee Assistance Program standards
- International health: travel, medical advisory, and immunizations
- Data collection and analysis
- Medical consultation
- Pregnancy placement in hazardous environments
- Professional education and development
- Audit and quality assurance

Optional Services

- Health education and health promotion
- Medical screening for early detection and disease prevention
- Physical fitness programs
- Allergy injection programs

BOX 30-3 RESEARCH PRIORITIES IN OCCUPATIONAL HEALTH NURSING

- Effectiveness of primary health care delivery at the worksite
- Effectiveness of health promotion nursing intervention strategies
- Nature and effects of stress and workplace stressors on worker health
- Strategies that minimize work-related adverse health outcomes (e.g., respiratory disease)
- Health effects resulting from chemical exposures in the workplace
- Occupational hazards of health care workers (e.g., latex allergy and blood-borne pathogens)
- Factors that influence workers' rehabilitation and return to work
- Effectiveness of ergonomic strategies to reduce worker injury and illness
- Health effects resulting from the interaction between aging and workplace hazards
- Evaluation of critical pathways to effectively improve worker health and safety and enhance maximum recovery and safe return to work
- Evaluation of intervention strategies to improve worker health and safety
- Strategies for increasing compliance with or motivating workers to use personal protective equipment
- Emergency/pandemic preparedness in the workplace
- Impact of occupational health nursing interventions on worker's compensation claims

From American Association of Occupational Health Nurses: *Research priorities in occupational and environmental health nursing,* 2012. Retrieved from <www.aaohn.org/practice/priorities.cfm>.

to ensure that occupational health nursing can continue to positively affect workers' health, contribute to reducing health care costs, and foster reduction in health risks. Occupational health nurses must seize opportunities in areas such as program planning, research, and policy making during this era fraught with a health care system in crisis. Issues to be addressed and managed include nursing shortages in many areas of the country, dramatic changes in the business environment, employees' increasing awareness of workplace hazards, and the ever-increasing need to demonstrate the cost-effectiveness of occupational health nursing care and services (Towers Watson/National Business Group in Health, 2011; Ward et al, 2011).

Research is an integral component of occupational and environmental health nursing practice because it provides the basis for scientific discovery that improves practice. That National Occupational Research Agenda (**National Institute for Occupational Safety and Health**) first set the priorities for research in the occupational health field in 1996. Prior to that in 1989, research priorities in occupational health nursing were first identified and published, and were used as a model for the Agenda (Rogers, 1989). They have been updated periodically to serve as the scientific basis to continue to build the body of knowledge in occupational and environmental health nursing for practice improvement and expansion (Box 30-3) (Rogers, 2013).

OCCUPATIONAL HEALTH AND PREVENTION STRATEGIES

Like the practice of all community health professionals, the occupational health nurse's practice is based on the concept of prevention. Promotion, protection, maintenance, and restoration of worker health are priority goals set forth in the definition of occupational health nursing. Prevention of exposure to occupational and environmental safety hazards and specific strategies for each level of prevention are described along with objectives from the *Healthy People 2020* program.

Healthy People 2020 and Occupational Health

Healthy People 2020 is the federal government initiative that focuses on health promotion and illness prevention. One topic area of *Healthy People 2020* concentrates on Occupational Safety and Health (U.S. Department of Health and Human Services [USDHHS], 2014). Objectives from this priority area cover work-related injuries and deaths, repetitive motion injuries, homicide, assault, lead exposure, skin disorders, stress, and hearing loss. In addition, objectives from other topic areas also address issues related to occupational health and safety. The *Healthy People 2020* box lists objectives that deal with occupational health.

 HEALTHY PEOPLE 2020

Objectives for Some Areas of Occupational Health

ECBP-8: Increase the proportion of worksites that offer health promotion programs to employees
ENT-VSL-6: Increase the use of hearing protection devices
NWSS-7: Increase the proportion of worksites that offer nutrition or weight management classes or counseling
OSH-1: Reduce deaths from work-related injuries
OSH-2: Reduce nonfatal work-related injuries
OSH-5: Reduce deaths from work-related homicides
OSH-8: Reduce occupational skin diseases or disorders among full-time workers
OSH-9: Increase the proportion of employees who have access to workplace programs to prevent or reduce employee stress
OSH-10: Reduce new cases of work-related noise-induced hearing loss
PAF-12: Increase the proportion of employed adults who have access to and participate in employer-based exercise facilities and exercise programs
TU-13: Establish laws on smoke-free indoor air that prohibit smoking in public places and worksites
V-3: Reduce occupational eye injuries

From HealthyPeople.gov: *Healthy People 2020: Topics & objectives*, 2013. Retrieved from <http://healthypeople.gov/2020/topicsobjectives2020/>.

Prevention of Exposure to Potential Hazards

To prevent occupational and environmental safety hazards in the work environment, it is important to identify work-related agents and exposures that are potentially hazardous. These can be categorized as follows:

Biological-infectious hazards: Agents such as bacteria, viruses, fungi, and parasites that may be transmitted via contact with infected clients or contaminated objects or substances
Chemical hazards: Various forms of chemical agents, including medications, solutions, and gases, that interact with body tissues and cells and are potentially toxic or irritating to body systems
Enviromechanical hazards: Factors encountered in work environments that cause accidents, injuries, strain, or discomfort (e.g., poor equipment or lifting devices and slippery floors)
Physical hazards: Agents within work environments, such as radiation, electricity, extreme temperatures, and noise, that can cause tissue trauma through transfer of energy from these sources
Psychosocial hazards: Factors and situations encountered or associated with the job or work environment that create stress, emotional strain, or interpersonal problems

Table 30-2 provides examples of work-related exposures in each of these areas. Having a good understanding of the nature of these hazards allows for the development of health promotion and prevention strategies to mitigate exposure risk.

Levels of Prevention and Occupational Health Nursing

Because occupational health nurses usually practice autonomously in their role as health care providers (Thompson, 2012), their activities in primary, secondary, and tertiary prevention strategies are expected to assume an even more important role in the prevention and treatment of illness, injury, and chronic disease in the future. For example, Griffith and Strasser (2010) describe the integration of a pilot full-service primary care, health promotion, and disease prevention program, including screening, early diagnosis, and uncomplicated treatment, into a large U.S. manufacturing company's occupational health services. Results showed significant employee satisfaction with the services as well as cost savings. The results of this initiative validate the expanded functioning in scope of occupational health nursing practice related to surveillance, screening, and prevention activities while recognizing the contributions all providers make to a healthy workforce.

Primary Prevention

In the area of primary prevention, the occupational health nurse is involved in both health promotion and disease prevention. O'Donnell (2009) describes health promotion as follows:

> *The art and science of helping people discover the synergies between their core passions and optimal health, enhancing their motivation to strive for optimal health, and supporting them in changing lifestyle to move toward a state of optimal health. Optimal health is a dynamic balance of physical, emotional, social, spiritual and intellectual health. Lifestyle change can be facilitated through a combination of learning experiences that enhance awareness, increase motivation, and build skills and most importantly, through creating opportunities that open access to environments that make positive health practices the easiest choice (p. iv).*

TABLE 30-2	TYPES OF OCCUPATIONAL HAZARDS AND ASSOCIATED HEALTH EFFECTS	

CATEGORY	EXPOSURES	HEALTH EFFECTS
Biological	Blood or body fluids	Bacterial, fungal, and viral infections (e.g., hepatitis B)
Chemical	Solvents	Headache and central nervous system dysfunction
	Lead	Central nervous system disturbances
	Asbestos	Asbestosis
	Acids	Burns
	Glycol ethers	Reproductive problems
	Mercury	Ataxia
	Arsenic	Peripheral neuropathy
Enviromechanical	Static or nonneutral postures	Musculoskeletal disorders
	Repetitive or forceful exertions	Back injuries
	Lighting	Headache and eye strain
	Shift work	Sleep disorders
	Electrical	Electrocution
	Slips and falls	Musculoskeletal conditions
	Struck by or against object	Injury
Physical	Noise	Hearing loss
	Radiation	Reproductive effects and cancer
	Vibration	Raynaud's disease
	Heat	Heat exhaustion and heat stroke
Psychosocial	Stress	Anxiety reactions and a variety of physical symptoms
	Work-home balance	

Disease prevention, then, begins with recognition of a health risk, a disease, or an environmental hazard. This recognition is followed by measures to protect as many people as possible from harmful consequences of that risk.

The occupational health nurse uses a variety of primary prevention methods, with one-on-one interaction as an important strategy for evaluating risk reduction behavior for individuals. The occupational health nurse has daily contact with numerous employees for many reasons (e.g., assessment and treatment of episodic illness or injury, health surveillance); therefore this contact is an important method of promoting health. The phrase "seize the moment" aptly describes the opportunity that exists with every employee encounter.

Occupational health nurses plan, develop, implement, and evaluate aggregate-focused intervention strategies. The occupational health nurse plans and implements programs such as weight and cholesterol reduction, acquired immunodeficiency syndrome (AIDS) awareness, ergonomics training, and smoking cessation. Performing "walk-throughs" in the workplace on a regular basis, recognizing potential and existing hazards, and maintaining communications with safety and industrial hygiene resources to prevent illness and injury from occurring will continue to be critical work for the occupational health nurse (Levy et al, 2005).

For overall *health promotion*, the nurse may plan, implement, and evaluate a health fair, a multifaceted health promotion strategy that usually includes a number of community health resources to provide expertise on a wide range of health issues and community services. As part of an overall health and wellness strategy, the occupational health nurse may negotiate with the employer for an on-site fitness center or area with fitness equipment; if cost or space is prohibitive, the employer may choose to partially subsidize membership at a local fitness center (Rogers, Randolph, and Mastrianno, 2009b).

Types of *nonoccupational programs* included in the area of primary prevention are cardiovascular health, cancer awareness, personal safety, immunization, prenatal and postpartum health, accident prevention, retirement health, stress management, and relaxation techniques. Occupational health programs could include topics such as emergency response, first aid and cardiopulmonary resuscitation training, right-to-know training, immunization programs for international business travelers, prevention of back injury through knowledge of proper lifting techniques, ergonomics, and other programs targeted to the specific hazards identified in the workplace (Burgel and Childre, 2012; Rogers et al, 2009b).

Women's health and safety issues such as maternal-child health, reproductive health, breast cancer education and early detection, stress management, and work-home balance issues will achieve heightened significance as more women enter the workforce. Thirty percent of women currently in the workforce are between ages 16 and 44 years, and each year approximately 1 million infants are born to these women. Interest in workplace safety and the relationship to reproductive outcomes continues to grow as women of childbearing age enter the workplace in greater proportions than ever before.

The occupational health nurse can play a key role in the development and delivery of prenatal, postpartum, and childhood programs in the workplace. Of primary importance will be the ability to serve as a change agent to initiate needed programs in the work environment. Employers must be educated regarding strategies not only to reduce health care costs for women and infants but also to improve the work environment for mothers (Stewart-Glenn, 2008). Women who believe their employers are interested in the well-being of themselves and their families are more apt to be productive and satisfied employees. The occupational health nurse can play a critical role in the shaping of supportive policies and practices to accommodate the needs of families, including flexible working hours, parental leave, and on-site child care (Rogers et al, 2009a).

Members of *racial and ethnic minority* groups make up a large share of the labor force, and as the number of minority and ethnic workers in the workforce increases, so will the illnesses traditionally associated with these groups of workers (e.g., heart

TABLE 30-3	**WORK-RELATED DISEASES AND INJURIES**
WORK-RELATED DISEASE(S) OR INJURY	**EXAMPLE(S)**
Occupational lung disease	Cancer and asthma
Musculoskeletal injuries	Back, upper extremity, and musculoskeletal disorders
Occupational cancers	Leukemia, bladder, and skin
Trauma	Death, amputation, and fracture
Cardiovascular diseases	Hypertension and heart disease
Reproductive disorders	Infertility and miscarriage
Neurotoxic disorders	Neuropathy and toxic psychosis
Noise-induced hearing loss	Loss of hearing
Dermatological conditions	Chemical burns and allergies
Psychological disorders	Neurosis; alcohol or substance abuse

disease and stroke, hypertension, cancer, cirrhosis, and diabetes). In addition to basic health concerns for this population, available statistics indicate that minority workers have been disproportionately concentrated in some of the most dangerous work, and they are at greater risk for experiencing many of the leading occupation-related diseases and injuries. Table 30-3 illustrates examples of common occupational diseases and injuries.

The occupational health nurse may face challenges in developing programs that are culturally and linguistically appropriate. The occupational health nurse may be in an advocacy role to negotiate with the employer for changes in the work environment that will reduce or eliminate existing or potential occupational exposure to risk factors.

Finally, veterans of our uniformed services are being employed at noteworthy numbers as they return to civilian life. Occupational health nurses should be aware of health problems—both physical and mental—that are sometimes encountered among this aggregate. Nurses should ensure that information for education for potential and anticipated problems is readily available. Furthermore, they can collect and maintain resources for referral to help assist with the most serious issues (see Veterans' Health box).

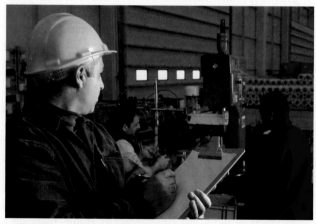

Occupational Health Nurses often perform "walk throughs" in the work place to look for potential hazards and maintain communication with workers to prevent illness and injury. (Copyright © 2013 Thinkstock. All rights reserved. Image # 53446261).

VETERANS' HEALTH

The wars in Afghanistan and Iraq are winding down, and most of our veterans have returned home. Consequently, many have left active duty to return to civilian employment. Occupational health nurses (OHNs) will increasingly have contact with former U.S. soldiers as they transition into civilian life, and it is important that the OHNs understand the potential physical and/or mental health problems some veterans experience following deployment. With this knowledge, the OHN can help facilitate a soldier's reintegration into society and the new worksite.

Brown (2008) presented an overview of some of the more common problems (e.g., blast injuries, posttraumatic stress disorder, traumatic brain injury) associated with military service and summarized some of the resources available for returning soldiers. This information can be used to help identify and address symptoms of overt or delayed responses to the war experience. It will also aid the OHN in assisting the veteran to locate resources for diagnostic and therapeutic interventions when needed.

Data from Brown ND: Transition from the Afghanistan and Iraqi battlefields to home: An overview of selected war wounds and the Federal agencies assisting soldiers regain their health. *AAOHN J* 56: 343-348, 2008.

Secondary Prevention

Secondary prevention strategies are aimed at early diagnosis, early treatment interventions, and attempts to limit disability. The focus at this level of prevention is on identification of health needs, health problems, and employees at risk.

As with primary prevention, the occupational health nurse uses a number of different secondary prevention strategies (Rogers, 2003b). By providing direct care for episodic illness and injury, the occupational health nurse is afforded the opportunity to conduct assessments and provide treatment and referrals for a variety of physical and psychological conditions. The occupational health nurse can offer health screenings, which are designed for early detection of disease, at the worksite with relative ease and at minimal cost. Screenings may focus on vision, cancer, cholesterol, hypertension, diabetes, tuberculosis, and pulmonary function. Other types of screening, such as mammography, may be contracted with a vendor who uses mobile equipment.

Secondary prevention efforts provided by the occupational health nurse include *preplacement, periodic,* and *job transfer evaluations* to ensure that a worker is being placed or is continuing to work in a job that is safe for him or her (Rogers, 2003b). The preplacement evaluation is performed before the worker begins employment in a new company or is placed in a different job. The evaluation is a baseline examination that consists of a medical history, an occupational health history, and a physical assessment that should target the type of work that the employee will be performing. For example, if the employee is going to be lifting materials in a warehouse, special attention should be paid to any history of musculoskeletal problems. Strength testing and range of motion should be performed for all muscle groups. (See ⓔ **Resource Tool 30A: Preplacement Health Evaluation,** and **Resource Tool 30B: Occupational Health History,** on the book's website at http://evolve.elsevier.com/Nies/).

The preplacement examination may also include medical tests to determine specific organ functions that may be affected by exposure to existing agents in the employee's workplace. For example, if the employee is working with a chemical that is a known liver toxin, baseline liver function tests may be appropriate to determine the current health status of the liver and its ability to handle this specific chemical exposure. However, the preplacement examination must be carefully evaluated to ensure compliance with the Americans with Disabilities Act (ADA), which is discussed later in the chapter.

Periodic assessments usually occur at regular intervals (e.g., annual and biannual) and are based on specific protocols for those exposed to substances or irritants such as lead, asbestos, noise, and various chemicals. Examinations of individuals transferring to other jobs are critical to document any changes in health that may have occurred while the employee was working in a specific area or with a specific process. Such examinations are usually done to comply with OSHA regulations or National Institute for Occupational Safety and Health (NIOSH) recommendations. (See ⊖ **Resource Tool 30C** for an example of an OSHA screening and surveillance guide.) For full details of compliance requirements, OSHA standards must be consulted.

Activities must continue to focus on prevention and early detection by increasing awareness of the incidence of commonly occurring health conditions such as breast cancer and providing accessible and affordable screening programs. For example, it is estimated that in 2013 invasive breast cancer will be diagnosed in more than 232,000 women and that about 40,000 women will die of the disease each year, making breast cancer one of the most commonly diagnosed malignancies among women in the United States and the second leading cause of cancer death (after lung cancer) (American Cancer Society, 2013). By detecting early malignancies, breast cancer screening reduces the mortality rate in women between ages 50 and 69 years. Mammography is the most effective method for detecting these early malignancies. The occupational health nurse is in an excellent position to play a key role in reducing morbidity and mortality associated with breast cancer. Increasingly, the occupational health nurse will be expected to document the return on investment for these and other related activities in the workplace.

Tertiary Prevention

On a tertiary level, the occupational health nurse plays a key role in the rehabilitation and restoration of the worker to an optimal level of functioning. Strategies include case management, negotiation of workplace accommodations, and counseling and support for workers who will continue to be affected by chronic disease and disability (Rogers, 2003b; Rogers et al, 2009b).

In the United States, it is estimated that more than 500,000 workers take an estimated 5 months of leave from work each year because of a physical disability; only 48% return to work (Fletcher, 2003). Research findings indicate the importance of developing strategies to reinforce the behavioral change of the individual to avoid what is often referred to as the **disability syndrome**, a state in which an individual chooses not to work when medical clearance has been granted (Curtis and Scott, 2004).

Knowledge of the workplace, the ability to negotiate with the employer for appropriate accommodations, early intervention, and comprehensive case management skills have been and will continue to be essential to the disabled employee's successful return to work. The process of returning an individual to work begins with the onset of injury or illness (Rogers, 2003b; Rogers et al, 2009b). Regardless whether an occupational or a nonoccupational condition is involved, the occupational health nurse is the center of case management (Kalina, Haag, and Tourigan, 2004). The nurse works closely with the primary care provider to monitor the progress of the ill or injured worker and to identify and eliminate potential barriers in the return-to-work process. The nurse has a comprehensive understanding of the workplace and of the physical requirements necessary for the employee to work. The physical demands analysis (Randolph and Dalton, 1989) is a useful tool for objectively assessing the physical demands of any job. (See ⊖ **Resource Tool 30D**, Physical Demands Analysis.) Once the assessment is completed, the occupational health nurse can relay this information to community health professionals caring for the employee.

For workers needing special accommodations, the occupational health nurse can negotiate and facilitate those appropriate to the employee's health limitations (Kalina et al, 2004). The nurse is often the driving force behind the employer's creation of a transitional duty pool. The goal of this type of program is to provide temporary work that is less physically demanding in nature than the employee's regular work. It facilitates the employee's return to the workplace earlier than if he or she required to wait until after regaining full strength.

The occupational health nurse can monitor and support the health of employees returning to work who continue to experience adverse health effects of chronic disease. For example, the employee who is returning to work after sustaining a myocardial infarction may undergo blood pressure monitoring on a routine basis. Counseling regarding adjustment to normal work life and support for behavior modification (e.g., smoking cessation) also may be provided (Byczek et al, 2004).

In addition, because the workforce is aging and because older workers are more prone to chronic disease, the occupational health nurse can implement and monitor treatment protocols and help workers live and work at their optimum comfort level while managing their diseases. Responsibilities for the care of elderly parents or significant others will influence the balance of work and home for older workers. The occupational health nurse's role as counselor, referral resource for workers, and consultant to management can influence future beneficial changes.

SKILLS AND COMPETENCIES OF THE OCCUPATIONAL HEALTH NURSE

Although clinical and emergency care remains an important tenet of occupational health nursing, the current and future practice must focus on a proactive approach with the goal of preventing illness and injury and promoting health. Therefore the occupational health nurse must possess competencies necessary to recognize and evaluate potential and existing health hazards in the workplace. Management and budgeting skills and knowledge of legal and regulatory requirements, toxicology, ergonomics, epidemiology, environmental health, safety, counseling, and health promotion and education are essential to meet the present and future demands of occupational health nursing practice.

Competencies in occupational and environmental health nursing have been delineated in nine categories by AAOHN (2007) (Box 30-4). Each competency delineates comprehensive performance criteria at the competent, proficient, and expert levels. Each level is described here, followed by a description of occupational health nursing practice at that level.

Competent

At the "competent" level of practice, the nurse has gained confidence and his or her perception of the role is one of mastery and an ability to cope with specific situations. There is less of a need to rely on the judgments of peers and other professionals. Work habits tend to stress consistency rather than routine tailoring of care to encompass individual differences (Benner, 1984).

The competent occupational and environmental health nurse has sufficient experience to recognize a range of practice issues and to function comfortably in such roles as clinician, occupational health services coordinator, and case manager. This nurse follows company procedures and relies on assessment checklists and clinical protocols to provide treatment.

Proficient

The "proficient" nurse has an increased ability to perceive client situations as a whole on the basis of past experiences, focusing on the relevant aspects of the situation. The nurse is able to predict the events to expect in a particular situation and can recognize that protocols sometimes must be altered to meet the needs of the client (Benner, 1984).

Occupational and environmental health nursing example: A proficient occupational and environmental health nurse is able to quickly obtain the information needed for accurate assessment and move rapidly to the critical aspects of the problem. Structured goals are replaced by priority setting in response to the situation. The proficient nurse usually possesses sophisticated clinical or managerial skills in the occupational health setting.

Expert

The "expert" nurse has extensive experience and a broad knowledge base and is able to grasp a situation quickly and initiate appropriate action. The nurse has a sense of salience grounded in practice guiding actions and priorities (Benner, 1984).

Occupational and environmental health nursing example: Occupational and environmental health nurses at the expert level include those providing leadership in developing occupational and environmental health policy within an organization, those functioning in upper executive or management roles, those serving as consultants to business and government, and those designing and conducting significant research in the field.

Examples of Skills and Competencies for Occupational Health Nursing

As described, numerous skills and competencies are necessary for occupational health nursing practice. Examples of some of these are outlined here, according to the nine defined areas of competence.

Clinical and Primary Care

- Applying the nursing process in delivery of care
- Providing first aid and primary care according to treatment protocols
- Conducting a physical assessment
- Taking an occupational and environmental health history
- Diagnosing and treating
- Being knowledgeable about immunization protocols
- Identifying employees' emotional needs and providing support and counseling
- Using a multidisciplinary problem-solving approach to occupational health illness and injury
- Maintaining records
- Clinical testing and monitoring
- Responding to medical emergencies
- Being knowledgeable about trends in health-related issues

Case Management

- Identifying the need for case management services
- Conducting case management assessments using a multidisciplinary framework
- Developing case management care plans
- Evaluating resources and vendors for case management
- Implementing early return-to-work programs

- Monitoring and evaluating outcomes
- Developing policies and programs for case management
- Analyzing trends for case management services
- Designing disability management systems
- Conducting case management outcomes-based research

Workforce, Workplace, and Environmental Issues

- Having knowledge of worksite operations, manufacturing processes, and job tasks
- Identifying and monitoring potential and existing workplace exposures
- Influencing appropriate and targeted recommendations for control of workplace hazards
- Having knowledge of toxicological, epidemiological, and ergonomic principles
- Understanding appropriate engineering and administrative controls and personal protective equipment specific to preventing workplace health hazard exposures
- Understanding roles and collaboration with other cross-functional groups as an integral part of a core multidisciplinary team
- Performing risk assessments
- Managing health surveillance programs

Legal and Ethical Responsibilities

- Being knowledgeable of state nursing practice acts and ability to practice occupational health nursing within state guidelines
- Being knowledgeable of federal, state, and municipal regulations pertaining to occupational and environmental health
- Being knowledgeable of the ADA, associated guidelines, and other relevant occupational and environmental health laws
- Being knowledgeable of all aspects of medical record-keeping practices in compliance with nursing practice, state law, and standards of practice
- Being knowledgeable of current legal trends related to negligence and malpractice cases in professional nursing and in the occupational health setting
- Being knowledgeable of confidentiality parameters
- Influencing regulatory and legal processes related to occupational and environmental health

Management and Administration

- Managing budgets
- Hiring staff and management of staff performance
- Fostering professional development plans
- Developing program goals and objectives
- Developing business plans through knowledge of internal and external resources
- Providing comprehensive on-site services and programs
- Knowing needs of business and employees
- Writing reports
- Performing audits and quality assurance
- Handling workers' compensation and disability

- Performing cost-benefit analyses, cost-effectiveness analyses, and outcomes monitoring
- Allocating appropriate staff resources
- Providing leadership in health-related issues
- Negotiating
- Facilitating work accommodations and return-to-work processes
- Coordinating medical response activities and site disaster planning
- Being a resource expert on health issues for employees and management
- Participating in strategic operations planning

Health Promotion and Disease Prevention

- Conducting needs assessments
- Recognizing cultural differences and their relationship to health issues
- Using effective communication styles to match diverse employee and management audiences
- Making effective presentations
- Planning, developing, implementing, and evaluating health programs designed to meet the needs of specific employee groups or organizations
- Evaluating health promotion outcomes
- Applying adult learning theory and principles to health education programs
- Integrating all levels of prevention into company culture

Occupational and Environmental Health and Safety Education

- Creating effective professional and technical support networks both functionally and cross-functionally
- Developing and implementing training programs for workers and professionals

Research

- Identifying researchable problems
- Systematically collecting, analyzing, and interpreting data from different sources
- Recognizing trends in health outcomes by department, work area, or work process
- Planning, developing, and conducting research
- Developing and testing models and theories relative to occupational and environmental health nursing practice

Professionalism

- Engaging in a lifelong learning plan
- Being knowledgeable of AAOHN Standards of Occupational and Environmental Health

Nursing and Code of Ethics

- Maintaining currency in practice
- Acting as a professional role model for students and colleagues
- Advancing the specialty through knowledge and science

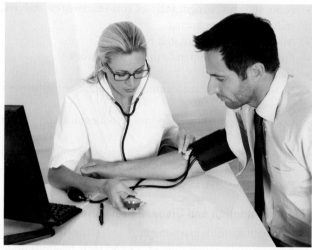

Occupational health nurses may provide pre-employment physical examinations or monitor health problems. (Copyright © 2013 Thinkstock. All rights reserved. Image #167397756).

IMPACT OF FEDERAL LEGISLATION ON OCCUPATIONAL HEALTH

Legislation and associated activities have influenced the practice of occupational health in the United States. Table 30-4 presents a historical perspective of some of the major pieces of legislation that have had, and will continue to have, a direct impact on the general practice of occupational and environmental health nursing. The Occupational Safety and Health Act, Workers' Compensation Acts, and the ADA are highlighted here.

Occupational Safety and Health Act

The Occupational Safety and Health Act of 1970 was enacted 2 years after a major coal-mining disaster in West Virginia. The passage of this legislation came about because of concerns about workers' health, a burgeoning environmental awareness, union activities, and a greater knowledge about workplace hazards. The general duty clause of the act states that employers must "furnish a place of employment free from recognized hazards that are causing or likely to cause death or serious physical harm to employees" (OSHA, 1970). The act also identifies the roles of the various governmental agencies, provides for the establishment of federal occupational safety and health standards, and identifies a structure of penalties, fines, and sentences for violations of regulations. Under the act, any state has the right to implement its own occupational safety and health administration. The only requirement is that the state standards meet or exceed federal standards. Currently, 25 states and the Virgin Islands operate state occupational safety and health administrations. The following organizations were formed under the provisions of the Act:

- Under the jurisdiction of the Department of Labor, the Occupational Health and Safety Administration (OSHA) is responsible for promulgating and enforcing occupational safety and health standards.

TABLE 30-4	HISTORICAL PERSPECTIVE OF LEGISLATION AFFECTING OCCUPATIONAL HEALTH IN THE UNITED STATES
YEAR	**LEGISLATION**
1836	First restrictive child labor law enacted (Massachusetts)
1877	State legislation passed requiring factory safeguards (Massachusetts)
1879	State legislation passed requiring factory inspections (Massachusetts)
1886	State legislation passed requiring reporting of industrial accidents (Massachusetts)
1910	State legislation passed requiring formation of an Occupational Disease Commission (Illinois)
1911	Workmen's Compensation Act passed (New Jersey)
1935	Social Security Act passed (state and federal unemployment insurance program)
1936	Walsh-Healey Act (federal legislation setting occupational safety and health standards for certain government contract workers)
1938	Fair Labor Standards Act (setting minimum age for child labor)
1948	All states now have workers' compensation acts
1964	Civil Rights Act
1965	McNamara-O'Hara Act (extends protection of the Walsh-Healey Act to include suppliers of government services)
1966	Mine Safety Act (mandatory inspections and health and safety standards in mining industry)
1969	Coal Mine Health and Safety Act (mandatory health and safety standards for underground mines)
1970	Occupational Safety and Health Act
1970	Environmental Protection Agency established
1970	Consumer Protection Agency established
1972	Equal Employment Opportunity Act
1972	Noise Control Act
1972	Clean Water Act
1973	HMO Act
1973	Rehabilitation Act
1976	Toxic Substances Control Act
1976	Resources Conservation and Recovery Act
1977	Federal Mine Safety and Health Act
1990	Americans With Disabilities Act
1991	Bloodborne Pathogens Standard
1993	Family Medical Leave Act
1996	National Occupational Research Agenda (NIOSH) established
2000	Needlestick Safety and Prevention Act
2002	Recordkeeping Rule amended
2008	Genetic Information Nondiscrimination Act

- Under the jurisdiction of the USDHHS, NIOSH is responsible for funding and conducting research, making recommendations for occupational safety and health standards to OSHA, and for funding Occupational Safety and Health Education and Research Centers for the training of occupational health professionals.

- The Occupational Safety and Health Review Commission, which is appointed by the President, is responsible for advising OSHA and NIOSH regarding the legal implications of decisions or actions in the course of performing their duties.
- The National Advisory Committee on Occupational Safety and Health, which is also appointed by the President, is a group of consumers and professionals who are responsible for making recommendations to OSHA and NIOSH regarding occupational health and safety.
- The National Commission on State Workers' Compensation Laws, appointed by the President as well, were tasked with studying the adequacy of state workers' compensation laws and making recommendations to the President on its findings. This commission's work ended as of October 30, 1972.

Since it was instituted, OSHA has promulgated occupational health and safety standards. These are published in the *Code of Federal Regulations* (CFR) and updated on a regular basis. Having access to the most recent publication of these standards is a crucial responsibility of the occupational health nurse.

The occupational health nurse must be knowledgeable of Title 29 of the *Code*, part 1910 (29 CFR 1910) (OSHA, 2014a), and other sections that apply to specific hazards in the workplace. For example, 29 CFR 1904 (OSHA, 2014b) pertains to OSHA's record-keeping requirements and mandates the employer's responsibility to keep records of work-related injuries, illnesses, and deaths. These records must be posted in the workplace for 1 month per year and made available for review by OSHA at any time. In many cases, the occupational health nurse has full responsibility for compliance with this standard.

OSHA has ten regional offices throughout the United States. Inspectors are assigned to each region to enforce the standards and to provide consultation to industries. An OSHA inspection can be initiated in one of several ways. Each office plans a schedule of routine visits to the industries in their respective regions. In the past, funding has been an issue, and inspections have not taken place in the number or frequency originally intended. An inspection will occur if a major health or safety problem, such as a death, occurs at the worksite, or if three or more workers are sent to the hospital as a result of the same incident. Inspection also may occur by employer request. A request is not usually made unless the employer has an exemplary occupational health and safety program and wishes to participate in OSHA's voluntary inspection program. Inspection also may be initiated by an employee request if there is concern about a suspected hazardous condition. In this case, OSHA is mandated to respond, and it must keep the employee's name confidential at the employee's request. In the past, penalties for violations have been inconsequential, and sentences have rarely been served. However, events now indicate that fines have increased, and OSHA has made public its intention to criminally prosecute company executives for serious and willful violations.

In many organizations, the occupational health nurse is the interface with the OSHA inspector. This position requires the nurse to be knowledgeable about the potential hazards in the workplace and about the appropriate control measures designed to eliminate or minimize exposure. The nurse should know that employees or their union representatives have the right to accompany the OSHA investigators.

Workers' Compensation Acts

Workers' Compensation Acts are state mandated and state funded. Workers' compensation programs provide income replacement and pay for health care services for workers who sustain a work-related injury, temporary or permanent disability, or death. Workers' Compensation Acts also protect the employer if the compensation received by the employee precludes legal suits against the employer. Each state regulates its own workers' compensation program that is unique to that state. The employer can self-insure, contract with commercial insurance carriers, or purchase a policy with the state-operated insurance fund. Workers receive an average of 66% of their take-home pay before taxes as compensation. Some disabled workers and their families are eligible for other benefit programs, including old age, survivors, disability, and health insurance, supplemental security income (SSI), and any other disability arrangement that they may have purchased through the company or on an individual basis.

In an era of high health care costs and a propensity for injured workers to engage the services of lawyers to represent them in negotiating financial settlements, many employers are claiming that workers' compensation costs are crippling their ability to compete in an international marketplace. The occupational health nurse has a unique opportunity to support both the employee and employer in this arena. For the employee, the nurse may be the initial person to whom the work-related injury or illness is reported. Accurate assessment of the injury or illness and appropriate treatment are essential. Community resources must be identified to ensure that the injured worker is provided with high-quality health care and appropriate medical follow-up.

The occupational health nurse educates the employee regarding benefits under the Workers' Compensation Act and is often the one who files the claim. If the employee is disabled from work for a period, the nurse provides case management support and remains in contact with the employee until the return to work. If the employer uses an insurance carrier, the nurse works closely with the claims adjuster to manage the case. The need for light duty or other workplace accommodations is determined before the employee's return. In most cases, the nurse facilitates this process with the employer.

For the employer, the occupational health nurse provides the expertise in early intervention and case management. The goal is to limit the worker's disability and provide an opportunity for early return to work through appropriate workplace accommodations. The desired outcome is a productive employee with optimum health and productivity, with reduced health care and workers' compensation costs.

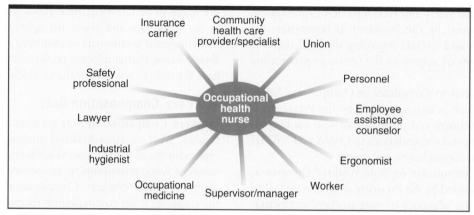

FIGURE 30-2 The occupational health nurse's professional links in the workplace and community.

Americans With Disabilities Act

The Americans With Disabilities Act, enacted by Congress in July 1990, is a comprehensive act that prohibits discrimination on the basis of disability. The core of this law requires employers to adjust facilities and practices for the purpose of making "reasonable accommodations" to enhance opportunities for individuals with disabilities. Employment provisions of this act began on July 26, 1992, for employers with 25 or more employees and were revised in July 1994 to include employers with 15 or more employees. Provisions regarding access to public transportation and accommodations became effective in January 1993.

The ADA defines disability as "physical or mental impairment that substantially limits one or more major life activities; having record of such an impairment; or being regarded as having such an impairment" (Kaminshine, 1991, p. 249). Physical or mental impairment guidelines are the same as those described in the Federal Rehabilitation Act and include "any physiologic disorder or condition, cosmetic disfigurement, anatomical loss affecting any of the major body systems, or any mental or psychological disorder" (Kaminshine, 1991, p. 249). Major life activities include caring for self, walking, seeing, hearing, and speaking. The ADA excludes conditions relating to sexual preference and gender identity, compulsive gambling, kleptomania, and pyromania. The ADA also denies protection for individuals who are currently involved in illegal drug use.

With regard to the ADA, the occupational health nurse has particular responsibility in two areas. The first involves the duty to provide or facilitate reasonable accommodations. This duty is facilitated by the nurse's familiarity with the physical requirements of jobs in the workplace. The second involves preplacement inquiries and health examinations. Preplacement health examinations will be permitted only if phrased in terms of the applicant's general ability to perform job-related functions rather than in terms of a disability and after a job offer has been made. The examination must be job related and consistently conducted for all applicants performing similar work.

As illustrated in this discussion of specific laws pertinent to occupational health, the legal context for occupational health nursing practice is broad and involves many arenas. The occupational health nurse must be knowledgeable about all laws and regulations that govern any industry in which the nurse provides health care to employees (e.g., laboratories, transportation, and utilities).

LEGAL ISSUES IN OCCUPATIONAL HEALTH

In recognition of the dynamic nature of occupational health nursing practice, coupled with the influences and impact of larger policy issues, the occupational health nurse must know the legal parameters of practice and must respond to legislative mandates that govern worker health and safety. Professionally, the occupational health nurse is primarily accountable to workers and worker populations and to the employer, the profession, and self (AAOHN, 2012). In particular, the occupational health nurse must be aware of liability and legal issues related to the following:
- The employee-nurse relationship
- The employment capacity of the occupational health nurse
- Any acts of negligence

The employee-nurse relationship can be confusing when the employer hires the nurse to provide services to the employee. The concern is whether a professional relationship exists under the law or the relationship is based on a co-worker status.

MULTIDISCIPLINARY TEAMWORK

As workplaces have become more complex, a diverse array of expertise has emerged in many functional and technical areas. To be successful, the occupational health nurse must recognize the need to work as part of an interdisciplinary team. The nurse may interact with occupational medicine professionals, industrial hygienists, safety and ergonomic professionals, employee assistance counselors, personnel professionals, and union representatives (Figure 30-2). Community health professionals, insurance carriers, and other support agencies in the community are also critical links.

CASE STUDY APPLICATION OF THE NURSING PROCESS

Leslie Johnston is a 23-year-old woman who was transferred by her employer into a job that required her to work with chemicals used in photolithography. Leslie became concerned when she noticed that the label on one of the pieces of equipment warned of possible adverse effects on reproduction. Because of her concern and related issues, she went to the on-site health clinic to talk with Peter Mitchell, the occupational health nurse.

Peter invited Leslie into his office to ask her questions and do a brief health history. Leslie reported that her health had been "excellent" until recently but that she had not felt well since transferring to her new position. She explained that she was newly married and thought she may be pregnant, but this was unconfirmed. She questioned whether her vague physical complaints (fatigue, headaches, occasional queasiness) might be related to working with chemicals, a pregnancy, or another reason.

Peter reassured Leslie that he had been employed at the company for 8 years, and he was aware that there were no restrictions in Leslie's work area for pregnant women. He pulled up her health file from his computerized database and gave her a set of health history forms to complete. He also had her read and sign several forms related to confidentiality and assured her that none of her health information would be shared with their employer without her consent.

Assessment

To obtain needed information, Peter:
- Completed general health and occupational health histories.
- Performed a modified physical assessment and discussed the symptoms Leslie was experiencing.
- Referred Leslie to her personal health care provider for further evaluation and to obtain a pregnancy test. (NOTE: In some cases, on-site clinics will be equipped for basic procedures such as this. If this is not a service provided by the occupational health nurse, referral must be made to the employee's health care provider. If the employee does not have one, referral must be made to an appropriate community health resource). Peter encouraged Leslie to inform her supervisor and himself if the pregnancy test result was positive so they could adapt her assignments to her condition.
- Assessed Leslie's work area with an industrial hygienist to determine whether there might be problems, such as leaking equipment or problems with ventilation.
- Reviewed the most current industrial hygiene data appropriate to the area.

Diagnosis
Individual
- At risk for chemical exposure
- Vague physical complaints of unknown etiology
- Possible pregnancy
- At risk for possible adverse pregnancy outcomes
- Stress related to concern regarding possible exposure to harmful chemicals

Community
- Potential for exposure of employees to unsafe chemicals and/or working conditions

Planning
- Peter developed a plan of care based on Leslie's health history and concerns. Together they set the following goals:

Individual
Short-Term Goals
- Determine pregnancy status.
- Determine potential exposure levels and review side effects of chemicals.
- Determine reason for her vague physical complaints.
- Reduce stress experiences.

Long-Term Goals
- Ensure that the work environment is safe for future pregnancies (if Leslie is not pregnant at present).
- Collaborate with Leslie and her supervisor on possible work restrictions.

Community (Workplace)
Short-Term Goals
- Company personnel (e.g., the occupational health nurse, the industrial hygienist, and all others who are directly affected) will be knowledgeable in safe handling of all hazardous chemicals.
- All company policies regarding safety and exposure will be followed.

Long-Term Goals
- Policies on handling of chemicals and related information will be reviewed periodically as required by law.
- All employees who work with and around potentially hazardous chemicals will undergo periodic instruction and instruction in and confirmation of knowledge about proper procedures.
- Work areas will be monitored per policy for compliance with safe practices.
- There will be no incidents involving worker exposure to chemicals.

Intervention
Individual

Peter conducted a brief physical examination and did not identify any obvious physical abnormalities. Because Leslie's chief complaints were fatigue, occasional headaches, and queasiness, he encouraged her to make an appointment with her primary care provider or gynecologist for a more extensive workup and to assess for pregnancy.

With her permission, he called the industrial hygienist to counsel Leslie regarding the policies of the company, to explain what chemicals might potentially be hazardous, and to review procedures and restrictions. The hygienist also stated that he would send a team to Leslie's work area to take air samples, check lighting, and perform other tests to ensure there were no problems.

Community (Workplace)

The assigned industrial hygiene team sampled the environment for chemical exposure per established procedure. They also set up a plan to have the area more frequently observed pending the results of the tests. The hygienist assured Peter and Leslie that he would communicate any work restrictions or changes to the personnel department and Leslie's supervisor if needed.

Evaluation
Individual

Following the meeting with Peter and the industrial hygienist, Leslie stated that she felt reassured. She agreed to make an appointment as soon as possible with her doctor for an evaluation and pregnancy test. She also agreed to inform Peter and her direct supervisor if she learned that she was pregnant.

Continued

CASE STUDY　APPLICATION OF THE NURSING PROCESS—cont'd

Community (Workplace)

The industrial hygienist and his assistants performed several tests in close proximity to Leslie's work station; they found no abnormal readings, and all equipment was in good working order. Per agency policy and following OHSA regulations, they charted all findings and submitted reports.

Levels of Prevention

Primary
- Teach about chemicals, exposures, etc.

- Instruct about chemical avoidance.
- Remove employee from environment through work restrictions.

Secondary
- Assess employee for signs and symptoms.
- Assess work environment for exposure.
- Refer for evaluation of possible health problems as needed.

Tertiary
- Provide reproductive counseling.

SUMMARY

This chapter describes the evolution of occupational health nursing during its first century of practice. It also highlighted current and future demographics and business trends as they relate to this nursing specialty area. Aging workers, escalating health care costs, increasing numbers of women and minorities in the workforce, and the competitive international marketplace are key factors shaping occupational health nursing practice.

The occupational health nursing role is challenging and can have a tremendous impact on the quality and delivery of health care to workers and their families. Nurses working in occupational settings should have an excellent understanding of all levels of prevention and possess the skills and competencies outlined here.

For the community health nurse who works in other settings, such as home health, clinics, and schools, knowledge of occupational health nursing practice is also important. Many companies do not have on-site occupational health nurses and therefore must rely on community health nurses to support their occupational health and safety needs.

LEARNING ACTIVITIES

1. A large automobile manufacturer needs a program designed to control respiratory disease among foundry workers. Workers in different areas of ferrous foundries are exposed to different respiratory hazards. The main problems are exposures to silica and formaldehyde. The corporation would like to develop a pilot program for one of its foundries that will then be applied to its other foundries. Health and industrial hygiene data will be collected. Both the corporation and the workers support the project, and both see the project as having the following three purposes:
   - Detecting health effects in individuals who may benefit from intervention
   - Determining the relationship of health effects with environmental exposures
   - Identifying control strategies as appropriate

   Outline a pilot program. Discuss the implications of discovering adverse health effects among current workers. Describe the roles of the occupational health nurse, physician, industrial hygienist, safety professional, manager, and employee.

2. A weight-loss program was conducted during August. Ten people participated in the 6-week program. The total weight loss for the group was 185 pounds. The following chart indicates the weight loss for the individuals:

Weight before program (lb)	Weight after program (lb)
215	190
175	160
139	129
275	245
145	120
198	183
120	115
243	233
185	145
210	200

   Is there a more effective way to show the results of the program? Assume a peer distributed this report for critique. Be creative, filling in any data, facts, figures, or other information that may be missing. Redesign a report to send to management.

3. Take an occupational history on five currently employed workers. Identify the occupation, associated job tasks, and potential health hazards. Describe control strategies that could minimize or eliminate the risk of adverse health effects.

4. Conduct a literature review to identify critical concepts in occupational health nursing, epidemiology, ergonomics, safety, industrial hygiene, and medicine, and describe how these disciplines work together to achieve optimal ends.

ⓔ EVOLVE WEBSITE

http://evolve.elsevier.com/Nies
- NCLEX Review Questions
- Case Studies
- Glossary
- Resource Tools
- – 30A: Preplacement Health Evaluation
- – 30B: Occupational Health History
- – 30C: Example of Screening and Surveillance: Guide to OSHA Standard for Benzene
- – 30D: Physical Demands Analysis

REFERENCES

American Association of Industrial Nurses: *The nurse in industry*, New York, 1976, Author.

American Association of Occupational Health Nurses: *Compensation and benefits study*, Atlanta, 2006, Author.

American Association of Occupational Health Nurses: Competencies in occupational and environmental health nursing, *AAOHN Journal* 55:442–447, 2007. Available from <http://www.aaohn.org>.

American Association of Occupational Health Nurses: *AAOHN Code of ethics and interpretive statements*, 2009. Available from <www.aaohn.org>.

American Association of Occupational Health Nurses: Standards of occupational and environmental health nursing, *AAOHN J* 60:97–103, 2012.

American Cancer Society: *Cancer statistics*, 2013. Available from <http://www.cancer.org/cancer/breastcancer/detailedguide/breast-cancer-key-statistics>.

Benner P: *From novice to expert: excellence and power in clinical nursing practice*, Menlo Park, CA, 1984, Addison-Wesley.

Burgel B, Childre F: The occupational health nurse as the trusted physician in the 21st century, *AAOHN J* 60:143–150, 2012.

Byczek L, Walton SM, Conrad KM, et al.: Cardiovascular risks in firefighters: implications for occupational health nurse practice, *AAOHN J* 52:66–76, 2004.

Curtis J, Scott LR: Integrating disability management into strategic plans, *AAOHN J* 52:298–301, 2004.

Felton JS: The genesis of occupational health nursing: Part I, *Occup Health Nurse* 30:45–49, 1985.

Felton JS: The genesis of occupational health nursing: Part II, *AAOHN J* 34:210–215, 1986.

Fletcher M: Careful integration, management of disabilities helps hospitals trim millions from its corporate costs, *Bus Insur* 37:26–30, 2003.

Griffith K, Strasser PB: Integrating primary care with occupational health services: A success story, *AAOHN J* 58:519–523, 2010.

Health Resources and Services Administration, Office of Information Technology, HSRA Geospatial Data Warehouse: National Sample Survey of Registered Nurses (NSSRN) public use files 2008 country, 2011. http://datawarehouse.hrsa.gov/nssrn.aspx.

Intili H, Laws C: Delivering health care in a large urban hotel: cost-effective, quality care for an underserved and uninsured population, *AAOHN J* 51:306–309, 2003.

Kalina CM, Haag A, Tourigan R: Challenges and solutions in case management, *AAOHN J* 52:143–145, 2004.

Kaminshine S: New rights for the disabled: The Americans With Disabilities Act of 1990, *AAOHN J* 39:249–251, 1991.

Levy BS, Wedman DH, Baron SL, et al., editors: *Occupational and environmental health*, ed 5, Philadelphia, 2005, Lippincott Williams & Wilkins.

McGrath BJ: *Nursing in commerce and industry*, New York, 1946, The Commonwealth Fund.

Occupational Health and Safety Administration (OSHA). Occupational Safety Act, 1970 (P.L. 91–596). https://www.osha.gov/pls/oshaweb/owadisp.show_document?p_table=OSHACT&p_id=3359.

Occupational Health and Safety Administration (OSHSA): Regulations (Standards – 29): 1910. 2014a. Available from: https://www.osha.gov/pls/oshaweb/owasrch.search_form?p_doc_type=STANDARDS&p_toc_level=1&p_key value=1910.

Occupational Health and Safety Administration (OSHSA): Regulations (Standards – 29): 1904. 2014b. Available from: https://www.osha.gov/pls/oshaweb/owasrch.search_form?p_doc_type=STANDARDS&p_toc_level=1&p_key value=1904.

O'Donnell M: Editor's notes: Definition of health promotion 2.0: Embracing passion, enhancing motivation, recognizing dynamic balance, and creating opportunities, *Am J Health Promot* 24, 2009. iv.

Parker-Conrad JE: A century of practice: occupational health nursing, *AAOHN J* 36:156–161, 1988.

Parker-Conrad JE: Celebrating our past, *AAOHN J* 50:537–541, 2002.

Randolph SA, Dalton PC: Limited duty work: an innovative approach to early return to work, *AAOHN J* 37:446–452, 1989.

Rogers B: Establishing research priorities in occupational health nursing, *AAOHN J* 37:493–500, 1989.

Rogers B: Occupational health nursing expertise, *AAOHN J* 46:477–483, 1998.

Rogers B: Nursing: an ethic of caring, *AAOHN J* 51:155–157, 2003a.

Rogers B: *Occupational health nursing: concepts and practice*, ed 2, Philadelphia, 2003b, Saunders.

Rogers B: Occupational and environmental health nursing: Ethics and Professionalism, *AAOHN J* 60:177–182, 2012.

Rogers B: Research priorities in occupational and environmental health nursing, *AAOHN J*, 2013. In press.

Rogers B, Franke J, Jeras J, et al.: The Family Medical Leave Act: implications for occupational health nursing, *AAOHN J* 57(6):239–250, 2009a.

Rogers B, Randolph S, Mastrianno K: *Occupational health nursing guidelines for primary clinical conditions*, ed 4, Beverly, MA, 2009b, OEM Press.

Salazar MK, editor: *Core curriculum for occupational and environmental health nursing*, ed 3, Philadelphia, 2006, Saunders.

Stewart-Glen J: Knowledge, perceptions, and attitudes of managers, coworkers, and employed breastfeeding mothers, *AAOHN J* 56:423–432, 2008.

Thompson M: Professional autonomy of occupational health nurses un the United States, *AAOHN J* 60:159–166, 2012.

Towers Watson/National Business Group on Health: *The road ahead: Shaping health care strategy in a post-reform environment: 16th Annual Employer Survey on Purchasing Value in Health Care*, (www.towerswatson.com) 2011.

U.S. Bureau of Labor Statistics: *Occupational outlook handbook*, 2012. Available from <www.BLS.org>.

U.S. Department of Health and Human Services: Healthy People 2020. www.healthypeople.gov 2014.

Ward JA, Beaton RD, Bruck AM, et al.: Promoting occupational health nursing training: An educational outreach with blended model of distance and traditional learning approaches, *AAOHN J* 59:401–406, 2011.

31

Forensic and Correctional Nursing

Angela Jarrell and Stacy Drake

OBJECTIVES

Upon completion of this chapter, the reader will be able to do the following:

1. Define forensic nursing.
2. Describe the specialties of forensic nurses.
3. Explain issues important to each of the subspecialty areas of forensic nursing.
4. Describe interventions and services forensic nurses perform.
5. Discuss factors affecting health and wellness in a correctional setting.

KEY TERMS

child abuse
coroner
correctional nursing
elder abuse
forensic

forensic nurse death investigator
forensic nurse examiners
forensic nursing
forensic psychiatric nurse
legal nurse consultants

living forensics
medical examiners
nurse attorneys
nurse coroners
sexual assault nurse examiner

OUTLINE

Subspecialties of Forensic Nursing
    Sexual Assault Nurse Examiner
    Medicolegal Death Investigation
    Legal Nurse Consultants and Nurse Attorneys
    Clinical Forensic Nurse Examiner
    Forensic Psychiatric Nurse
Correctional Nursing
    Maintenance of a Safe Environment

Health Issues in Prison Populations
    Chronic and Communicable Diseases
    Women in Prison
    Adolescents in Prison
Mental Health Issues in Correctional Settings
Education and Forensic Nursing

According to the Bureau of Justice Statistics National Crime Victimization Survey, in 2011 approximately 5,805,430 violent crimes were reported (U.S. Department of Justice/Bureau of Justice Statistics [USDOJ/BJS], 2012). These crimes ranged from vandalism and theft, to rape and sexual assault, to aggravated assault and murder. The estimated medical and productivity economic burdens of interpersonal and self-directed violence (suicide, homicide, child maltreatment, youth violence, intimate partner violence, and other assaults) are staggering. Because of the prevalence of violence and violent crimes in society, health care professionals are required to identify and assess victims of trauma, abuse, and/or neglect and provide proper care and referrals as needed. Indeed, screening for violence is now considered to be a minimum standard of care for all women, as is vigilance in looking for indications on when/where to screen for abuse among elders and vulnerable adults (U.S. Preventive Services Task Force [USPSTF], 2013).

The term **forensic** means "pertaining to the law; legal" (Lynch, 2013, p. 3). It refers to instances, activities, or information used in or suitable to courts of law. Health care providers, especially nurses, frequently care for both victims and perpetrators of crime, and they should be prepared to assess for indications of violence and abuse and to intervene as needed.

Forensic nursing is defined as "application of the nursing process to public or legal proceedings, and the application of forensic health care in the scientific investigation of trauma and/or death related to abuse, violence, criminal activity, liability and accidents" (Lynch, 2013, p. 3). Forensic nursing combines the disciplines of nursing science, forensic science, medical science, sociology, and psychology with law enforcement and the criminal justice system. One of the newest specialty areas recognized by the American Nurses Association (ANA), forensic nursing is growing nationally and internationally. It was officially recognized by the ANA in 1995, and the *Scope and Standards of Forensic Nursing Practice* was published in 1997 (Lynch, 2011) and revised in 2009 (ANA, 2009).

The International Association of Forensic Nurses (IAFN) explains that forensic nursing is the practice of nursing where the health and legal systems intersect (ANA, 2009). Thus the forensic nurse's role provides a vital link between the health care system, the investigative process, and courts of law (Lynch, 2011).

Forensic nurses practice in multiple areas and settings of the public health system. Their responsibilities may include screening and the assessment and collection of evidence, and may also include the documentation and expert witness testimony for victims and perpetrators in settings such as hospitals, community clinics, and death scenes. In addition to working with victims and perpetrators, forensic nurses may be involved in paternity disputes and cases involving workplace injuries, malpractice, vehicle accidents, food or drug tampering, and medical equipment defects (Lynch, 2011). The Advanced Practice Forensic Nurse may assist in developing and implementing protocols and systems to help victims or perpetrators of violent occurrences, aid in research and policy changes, develop and supervise systems of care for complex health issues, and provide essential education to others (IAFN, 2004). The *Healthy People 2020* box lists some objectives related to this highly specialized practice area.

♥ HEALTHY PEOPLE 2020

Objectives Related to Forensic Nursing

IVP HP2020-33: Reduce physical assaults.

IVP HP2020-38: Reduce nonfatal child maltreatment.

IVP HP2020-40: Reduce sexual violence.

IVP 2020-43: Increase the number of states that link data on violent deaths from death certificates, law enforcement, and coroner and medical examiner reports to inform prevention efforts at the state and local levels.

MHMD-HP2020-7: Increase the proportion of juvenile residential facilities that screen admissions for mental health problems.

SA HP2020-5: Increase the number of drug, driving while impaired (DWI) and other specialty courts in the United States.

SA HP2020-10: Increase the number of Level I and Level II trauma centers that implement evidence-based alcohol screening and brief intervention.

From HealthyPeople.gov: *Healthy People 2020: Topics & objectives,* 2013. Available from<http://www.healthypeople.gov/2020/topicsobjectives2020/objectiveslist.aspx?topicId=24>.

SUBSPECIALTIES OF FORENSIC NURSING

The IAFN recognizes core specialties within forensic nursing (Box 31-1). Each of the subspecialties will be briefly discussed.

Sexual Assault Nurse Examiner

The **sexual assault nurse examiner** (SANE) is the most widely recognized subspecialty in forensic nursing. In the 1970s, emergency department (ED) registered nurses identified a special client population—sexual assault or rape victims—who were not receiving the appropriate, compassionate care after a terrifying traumatic event (Ledray and Arndt, 1994). They observed that in many cases the staff did not know how to compassionately approach the sexual assault victim entering the ED, to properly assess and collect evidence, or to testify in court; therefore the SANE role was developed.

A SANE is a specially trained registered nurse who applies the nursing process during forensic examinations to victims or perpetrators of sexual assault. The SANE collects forensic evidence related to a reported crime and frequently testifies as an expert witness at subsequent trials (Ledray, 2011). SANEs are usually employed in EDs and community clinics dedicated to victims of interpersonal violence. SANEs may also be employed to complete forensic examinations on deceased individuals for whom sexual assault is presumed.

If the client is medically stable, the SANE is responsible for conducting a thorough examination, including obtaining a history, performing the physical assessment, and collecting forensic evidence (Box 31-2). If the client is medically unstable, he or she will be assessed and stabilized by a physician prior to the forensic examination. Other responsibilities of the SANE are crisis intervention referral, pregnancy risk

---

BOX 31-1   SPECIALTIES OF FORENSIC NURSES

- Sexual assault nurse examiner
- Nurse coroner and death investigator
- Legal nurse consultant and nurse attorney
- Forensic nursing educator and consultant
- Forensic psychiatric nurse
- Forensic nurse examiner
- Correctional nurse

BOX 31-2   TYPE OF EVIDENCE COLLECTED FROM A VICTIM OF SEXUAL ASSAULT

- Documentation of history of the event
- Documentation of injuries (photographic and written)
- All clothing worn at the time of incident
- Trace evidence (fiber, glass, soil, particulate matter)
- Biological evidence for DNA comparison (victim's blood or hair)
- Fingernail swabbing
- Swabs and smears (from the victim's mouth, vagina/penis, and anus)
- Pubic hair combings
- Evidence disbursement sheet
- Any additional evidence, as noted during examination (example: body piercings)

Data from Ferrell J, Caruso C: Sexual assault evidence recovery. In Lynch VA, Duval JB, editors: *Forensic nursing science,* ed 2, St Louis, 2011, Mosby.

assessment and interception as needed, and client referral for additional support (Ledray, 2011).

A registered nurse caring for sexual assault victims may receive SANE certification offered through the IAFN. Both adult and pediatric certifications are available. The requirements for a registered nurse to be eligible for the SANE certification examination are that the nurse must: (1) be in practice for a minimum of 2 years, (2) have successfully completed 40 hours of didactic instruction or 64 hours of course work from an accredited nursing program, (3) demonstrate competency in sexual assault examinations and (4) provide nursing continuing education contact hours (IAFN, 2014).

Medicolegal Death Investigation

According to Hanzlick (2007), there are four different types of death investigation: medicolegal, institution-based, private, and public health. Medicolegal death investigations are usually conducted to clarify the unnatural circumstances in which death occurred. Institution-based death investigations are usually those that occur in the hospital or nursing home setting. Private death investigations are family initiated and are focused on answering questions the family may have surrounding the death. Public health investigations are frequently conducted in cooperation with the medicolegal and/or are retrospective studies. An example of public health death investigation would be elderly mistreatment–related deaths. Typically the forensic nurse is employed in the medicolegal death investigation or public health setting. The medicolegal death investigation system falls within the purview of the public health system as defined by the Centers for Disease Control and Prevention. One of the outputs of death investigation is death certificates. In the United States, medicolegal death investigation systems are characterized as either medical examiner, coroner/justices of the peace, or mixed (Hanzlick, 2007; Lynch, 2011).

Typically, **medical examiners** are licensed physicians who are board certified in anatomic and forensic pathology (Hanzlick, 2007). Usually a medical examiner is appointed for an unspecified term and serves a county, district, region, or state as determined by law. The **coroners**/justices of the peace are usually elected laypersons; that is, persons who have little or no training in medicine or science who conduct medicolegal investigations and certify cause and manner of death. A mixed medicolegal system is a combination of medical examiner and coroners/justices of the peace systems, depending on state law (Hanzlick, 2007).

Most medicolegal death investigation agencies are responsible for issuing death certificates that state the cause and manner of death. These data are collected at city, county, state, and national levels and used to determine the health of the nation and how best to allocate financial resources. The *cause of death* is the event that initiated the progression of events that ended in death (Lynch, 2011). The *manner of death* is categorization that relates to the conditions in which the cause of death occurred (Hanzlick, 2007). The National Association of Medical Examiners (NAME) identifies five acceptable options for recording manner of death: natural, accident, suicide, homicide, and "undetermined" (Hanzlick, Hunsaker, and Davis, 2002).

Role of a Forensic Nurse Death Investigator

Forensic nurses enter the death investigation arena possessing knowledge of anatomy, physiology, pharmacology, growth and development, physical examination, and health history interviewing techniques, all of which are needed to conduct a comprehensive death investigation (Lynch and Koehler, 2011; McDonough, 2013). In most cases related to a death scene investigation, investigators are police officers or homicide detectives—members of professions without medical or science knowledge. The **forensic nurse death investigator** (FNDI) evaluates the death scene from a holistic nursing perspective and might interpret the scene differently (Figure 31-1). The requirements for being a forensic nurse death investigator vary; however, most employers ask for a minimum of 2 years of experience, preferably in the setting of critical care or emergency.

Clinical Example

A police officer entering a house observes several pools of blood located throughout the residence and discovers a deceased male, nude and lying in bed; the police officer suspects murder. The FNDI entering the same death scene notices the same findings as the initial police officer, but also notes bloody emesis in the toilet, blood-soaked towels in the washing machine, and empty alcohol bottles in the trash. A preliminary examination of the decedent by the FNDI reveals ascites, jaundice, and multiple contusions on the body. Communication with family members, the FNDI discovers the decedent was an alcoholic with many health problems; the FNDI suspects that he had ruptured esophageal varices. This suspicion was confirmed by an autopsy, and the manner of death was determined to be from natural causes rather than homicide as initially believed.

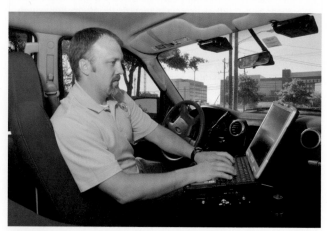

FIGURE 31-1 A forensic nurse death investigator working at the scene. (Used with permission from Harris County Institute of Forensic Sciences.)

Role of Nurse Coroner

In coroner systems in which the chief medicolegal death investigator is elected and state laws do not have specific requirements of the office, nurses may decide to run for the position of coroner or nurse coroner. The nurse coroner is responsible for ensuring that appropriate measures are taken to perform death investigations and to certify death certificates. A nurse coroner's educational background and knowledge enables him or her to identify disease processes that the lay coroner may not recognize or may misinterpret as foul play, as in the preceding clinical example.

Forensic nurse death investigators and nurse coroners exhibit communication skills when dealing with grieving families. Nurses are given education in therapeutic communication and are able to practice those skills in any setting. They are acutely aware of the importance of using open-ended questions, listening attentively, and being fully present with family and friends. The use of these techniques allows family and friends to openly share the feelings and thoughts experienced with the death of a loved one (Potter and Perry, 2009).

Nurse coroners and FNDIs may apply to become board certified in death investigation through the American Board of Medicolegal Death Investigators (ABMDI). ABMDI requires applicants to (1) be certified at the Registry Level and in good standing for a minimum of 6 months, (2) have at least an associate's degree from a postsecondary institution recognized by a national educational accrediting agency, (3) be currently employed at an agency with the job responsibility to conduct scene investigations, and (4) have a minimum of 4000 hours of experience in the last 6 years (ABMDI, 2013). Once an investigator satisfies these requirements, he or she may take a standardized examination and become board certified as a Fellow of the ABMDI.

Legal Nurse Consultants and Nurse Attorneys

Legal nurse consultants (LNCs) and nurse attorneys are nurses who provide assistance within the legal system using specialized nursing knowledge and expertise when interaction between law and health issues arises (Geissler-Murr and Moorhouse, 2006; Pagliaro and Cewe, 2013). Among many activities, LNCs evaluate, analyze, and render informed opinions on the delivery of health care and its outcomes (American Association of Legal Nurse Consultants [AALNC], 2013). LNCs are hired by attorneys and insurers to review and interpret medical records and charts, provide objective opinions based on standards of care, and possibly to testify in court as expert witnesses. A forensic nurse practicing as a LNC may apply for certification through the American Legal Nurse Consultant Certification Board (ALNCCB). The candidate must have: (1) a current nursing license full and unrestricted, (2) a minimum of 5 years' experience as a registered nurse, and (3) evidence of 2000 hours of legal nurse consulting experience within the last 5 years (ALNCCB, 2013). Once the candidate meets these requirements he or she may sit for a standardized examination, and once having passed the examination, he or she earns the Legal Nurse Consultant Certified (LNCC) credential.

Nurse attorneys are educated in both law and nursing. They may practice in health care, public health, or criminal or civil law, which would include malpractice cases. Malpractice cases may require participation of a nurse attorney on either the plaintiff's or the defendant's side, and may involve licensure disciplinary action or agency oversight (Collins and Halpern, 2005). Some practitioners have differing opinions regarding LNCs and nurse attorneys. They may be perceived as either defending the profession or prosecuting peers by testifying against professional colleagues. By providing services as experts and by testifying, nurses serving as legal consultants help hold accountable practitioners who are dangerous to clients. In contrast, meticulous practitioners who are wrongfully accused of negligence are defended by these nurses' actions.

According to the AALNC (2013), an LNC performs many different services and activities, as follows:

- Identify organize and analyze medical records and related materials
- Prepare chronologies or timelines of health care events
- Identify applicable standards of care
- Evaluate causation and damage issues
- Conduct literature research and summarize medical literature
- Evaluate case strengths and weaknesses
- Serve as an expert witness
- Identify plaintiff's future medical needs and associated costs

LNCs read reports and records and determine whether the standards of care were met or breached. In general, if working for a plaintiff in a malpractice case, the LNC will look for breaches in the standards of care; if working for the defense, the LNC will look for nursing care that is given within the standards of care related to the complaint. It is essential that the attorneys be kept informed of all findings—even those that might negatively affect their case (Robson, 2009).

When providing services, the LNC may submit an *affidavit*, a written statement explaining the expert's credentials, background, and licensing or certification(s). It also provides a list of the materials read and considered in the case, and the findings of the review are summarized into a case analysis. Following the submission of an affidavit, the LNC may be asked to provide a deposition. The *deposition* is a pretrial discovery process that allows the attorneys on both sides to learn more about what the courtroom testimony will be. It is given to a court reporter, and the respondent is under oath.

During the deposition, the LNC presents the facts of the case and is questioned by attorneys from both sides. This process may be quite lengthy and stressful. It is essential that the LNC be prepared, having reviewed everything thoroughly. Following this process, the LNC is given a written transcript of the deposition, which needs to be carefully reviewed for accuracy. If the case goes to trial, the LNC will then testify in court (Robson, 2009; Ruiz-Contreras, 2005).

In some cases, the forensic nurse is called on to testify in court, not as an expert witness as described previously, but as a factual witness—one who has firsthand knowledge of the case in question. In these cases, the forensic nurse provides factual statements about the evidence collected and what was observed (Pagliaro and Cewe, 2013). Box 31-3 lists tips that will be helpful for nurses to review prior to testifying in court.

Clinical Forensic Nurse Examiner
Emergency and Critical Care

Registered nurses may be employed in EDs and critical care units as **forensic nurse examiners**. In this role they deliver care to both living and deceased clients who are somehow involved with the legal system, and their services may include several subspecialties. The term **living forensics** refers to individuals who are subject to forensic investigations, including but not limited to survivors of rape, drug and alcohol addiction, domestic violence, nonfatal assaults, motor vehicle and pedestrian accidents, and police detention (Lynch, 2011).

The ED is frequently the initial location of the medicolegal investigation involving these individuals, both living and deceased (Doughtery, 2011). It is imperative that ED registered nurses identify forensic cases, initiate the proper collection, preservation, and chain of custody of all evidence, then provide accurate documentation for this unique population. This collection of evidence plays an important role in the investigation of crimes and can have a major impact on legal decisions. Box 31-4 lists types of evidence.

Clinical Example

A 27-year-old woman arrived at the emergency department (ED) with a circular defect on the head suggestive of a gunshot wound. Emergency medical technicians reported to the ED nurse and doctor that the client was found by her boyfriend barely breathing. The boyfriend called 911, and the client was transported to the hospital. The client arrived at the hospital in asystole and was pronounced dead within 10 minutes of arrival. The ED nurse applied her forensic knowledge and placed brown paper bags on the client's hands, securing them with tape. This procedure is performed to preserve gunpowder or primer residue. Gunpowder or primer residue aids in the identification of the shooter and distance of the gun. When a gun is fired, residue is released and lands on the items close to the gun, specifically the hands and clothing of the person firing it.

The police agency investigated the death. The nurse's intervention, placing paper bags over the client's hands, preserved the presence or absence of gunshot or primer residue. The police agency performed a scanning electron microscope examination for gunpowder residue and did not find any on the client's hands. This finding led police to further investigate the incident and discover that the boyfriend had shot the client, rather than the first presumption, that the gunshot wound was self-inflicted.

Organ and Tissue Donation and Transplantation

Forensic nurses also have a role in providing a detailed physical examination of patients who may be organ and tissue donors. This area of care is complex and requires detailed understanding of related legal and ethical issues. When a patient is declared brain dead, federal law states that the legal next of kin shall be approached for organ and tissue donation. A forensic nurse is able to conduct and provide a detailed physical examination and to collect any evidence that may be required. A thorough death investigation at the hospital may be required for sudden, unexpected, and nonnatural deaths. This involves reviewing medical records and documenting injuries which is essential for the medicolegal investigation agency to identify acceptable candidates and potential organs and tissues for harvest. The nurse involved in this process must be knowledgeable about legal specifications related to organ donation and familiar with agency policies and procedures for determining brain death. The nurse must also have excellent communication skills as well as the ability to relate empathetically to grieving families. In this capacity, the forensic nurse working harmoniously with organ and tissue procurement agencies can obtain release authorization for lifesaving organs (Shafer, 2011).

Care of Vulnerable Populations

The youngest, oldest, and disabled populations are the most vulnerable to abuse and neglect. Nurses dedicating their practice to these vulnerable populations have an essential role in advocacy for individuals who cannot protect themselves.

Child Abuse and Neglect. Child abuse and neglect are major concerns for society; therefore the role of a forensic nurse examiner is especially imperative. The Federal Child Abuse Prevention and Treatment Act defines child abuse and neglect as:

> Any recent act or failure to act on the part of a parent or caretaker which results in death, serious physical or emotional harm, sexual abuse or exploitation; or an act or failure to act which presents an imminent risk of serious harm. (U.S. Department of Health and Human Services, Administration for Children and Families, 2011)

In 2011, approximately 676,569 children were victims of child abuse and neglect, and nearly 87.6% of the perpetrators were the parents. Furthermore, reported cases of child abuse or neglect resulting in death in were estimated to be 1530 children. (U.S. Department of Health and Human Services [USDHHS], Administration for Children and Families [ACF], 2011).

States have varying definitions of what constitutes or determines child abuse and neglect. If a forensic nurse suspects that a child is being abused or neglected, the nurse should refer to the state's legislation surrounding the reporting of these suspicions. The following definitions are provided by the USDHHS, ACF (2011):

Neglect: Failure of a parent, guardian or caregiver to provide basic needs. Neglect may be physical (deprivation of adequate food, clothing, shelter, or supervision); medical (failure to provide necessary medical treatment); educational (failure to educate a child or attend to special education needs); or emotional (failure to attend to emotional needs or provide psychological care or allowing the usage of alcohol or other drugs).

Sexual abuse: Range of activities from noncontact indecent exposure to production of pornographic materials, to incest, rape, fondling, and genital contact to actual adult-child sexual intercourse.

Physical abuse: Intentional physical injury, including striking, kicking, burning, and biting.

Emotional abuse (or psychological abuse): A pattern of behavior that impairs the child's emotional development or sense of self-worth, including constant criticism, threats, and rejection.

For the well-being and safety of the child, a forensic nurse examiner ensures that abuse and neglect are swiftly identified and reported to proper authorities (Finn, 2011). The nurse obtains a thorough history and assessment, focusing on several facets of abuse and neglect. These include child-parent interaction, the child's appearance and behavior, child-child interaction, and the environment.

A forensic nurse may be employed in a variety of clinical settings that assess, diagnose, and treat children. These settings may include pediatric or general EDs, hospitals, physician offices, schools, home health, hospice, and child advocacy agencies.

Elder Mistreatment. Forensic nurse examiners caring for the geriatric population play an important role similar to that of pediatric forensic nurses. Elder mistreatment is thought to be one of the most underdiagnosed and underreported crimes in the United States (Pearsall, 2011). Unfortunately, there is no exact accounting of elder mistreatment cases, for several reasons: an absence of standardized reporting systems, no consistency in state definition of elder mistreatment, and lack of national data collection (Hammer and Hammer, 2013).

There are several forms of elder abuse: physical, psychological or emotional, financial, neglect, and sexual abuse (Pearsall, 2011). Physical abuse is the intentional harm or injury of another person resulting in bruises, abrasions, lacerations, fractures, or all of these (Pearsall, 2011). In a study by Acierno and colleagues (2009), 1.6% of subjects reported physical mistreatment, and family members accounted for 76% of the mistreatment; specifically, in 57% of cases the abuser was a partner and/or spouse.

Psychological or emotional abuse occurs when there is mental or emotional anguish (e.g., humiliating, intimidating, or threatening comments directed toward the elder) (Hammer and Hammer, 2013). Acierno and colleagues (2009) reported that 4.6% of elders experienced emotional abuse, and for 25% of them, the abuse came from the partner and/or spouse. Financial exploitation occurs when the elder person's financial resources are utilized for another person's benefit without the elder's consent. In the study by Acierno and colleagues (2009), more than 5% of subjects reported being a victim of financial exploitation.

Sexual abuse is the nonconsensual intimate contact between two people. The elder population is at risk for sexual abuse because of inability to resist pursuit or inability to recognize the abuse owing to mental illness or other advanced disease process. Less than 1% of respondents in the study by Acierno and colleagues (2009) reported sexual abuse, and for 40% of those who did report the abuse, the partner and or spouse was responsible.

Lastly, neglect is the most common form of elder abuse, whether it is caregiver neglect or self-neglect. Caregiver neglect occurs when the caregiver does not provide appropriate clothing, food, or health services or in the case of abandonment of the elder client. Self-neglect occurs when the elder discounts personal well-being—this could be the result of medical or mental illnesses. Acierno and colleagues (2009) report that 5.1% of elders experienced caregiver neglect.

The elderly client may be hesitant to report abuse, ask for assistance, or acknowledge the maltreatment because the abuser might be a spouse and/or partner, child, or close relative, or because the disclosure would possibly result in litigation and institutionalization (Pearsall, 2011). Forensic nurses may be employed in any setting, treating or seeing elder clients. Some settings are EDs, hospitals, physician offices, nursing homes, home health agencies, and geriatric day care centers.

Clinical Example

A home health care nurse has received a referral from the hospital for a 80-year-old female residing at her home with her son. The patient had been discharged from the hospital with the diagnosis of urinary tract infection and pneumonia. Her son reports she was confused and coughing for 2 months before he took her to the hospital. Her past medical history includes dementia, impaired mobility, and dysphasia from a prior stroke. Upon arrival at the residence, the nurse greets the patient, who is lying in bed. The home is cluttered and dirty, with visible roaches, and the refrigerator/freezer is filled with meat, cheese, milk, and beer. The nurse's assessment findings include the following: clothing is loose fitting and adult brief is soiled, strong body and urine odor present, body is emaciated with upper and lower extremity contractures, contusions of various coloring are located on the upper thighs and posterior torso, stage II decubitus ulcers are present on the right hip and sacral areas (both are covered with soiled dressing), and dentition is poor. The son explains that the patient obtained the contusions because at times she becomes confused and strikes out hitting things. Furthermore, this happens during times that he attempts to bathe and turn the patient.

Upon leaving the residence, the nurse contacts her supervisor to discuss the findings and her concerns about physical and sexual abuse and neglect. The supervisor agrees and a call is placed to Adult Protective Services (APS) for further evaluation and investigation. The hospital is also contacted to discuss why the patient was discharged back into this environment.

Disabled Population. It is well documented that children and elderly with disabilities are more likely to be mistreated. Mandatory laws addressing the reporting of abuse or neglect of a disabled person aged 18 to 64 years varies within states. Throughout their life span, the risk for one or more forms of mistreatment of individuals with disabilities is three times higher than that for individuals without disabilities (Harrell, 2012).

Forensic Psychiatric Nurse

The **forensic psychiatric nurse** bridges the gap between the criminal justice, legal, and mental health systems. Forensic psychiatric nurses apply the nursing process to clients who await a criminal hearing or trial while maintaining a neutral, objective, and detached position (Mason, 2011). Forensic psychiatric nurses collect evidence by determining intent or diminished capacity in the client's thinking at the time of the incident. To do so, they often spend several hours interviewing and observing the client, carefully documenting conversations and observations.

The forensic psychiatric nurse may be called to court to testify as an expert witness in a mental health issue; therefore it is imperative that the nurse have an understanding of mental illnesses and personality disorders. Roles filled by or activities performed by psychiatric forensic nurses include the following (Mason, 2011):

- Sanity or competency evaluation (for legal purposes)
- Assessment of violence potential
- Assessment of capacity to formulate intent
- Parole and probation considerations
- Assessment of racial or cultural factors in crime
- Assistance in jury selection
- Sexual predator screening
- Provision of expert witness testimony

CORRECTIONAL NURSING

Correctional nursing is a specialized subset of forensic nursing. It requires a significant amount of knowledge as well as an understanding and awareness of the unique needs and perspective of the clients served. Several issues specific to correctional nursing and related issues are described in this section.

Unlike in any other care setting, clients are inmates, and care is negotiated and provided with recognition of safety and security issues for the nurse and the constitutional right of prisoners to receive adequate and timely health care. The primary goal in correctional facilities is to maintain a safe, secure, and humane environment for inmates. Health care, including nursing care, is a necessary and essential part of that environment.

Maintenance of a Safe Environment

Correctional facilities are violent environments, and nurses practicing in correctional settings must continually negotiate personal safety and nursing care. Nurses in this setting must be aware that medical supplies issued to inmates can be a safety threat to the environment. For example, a simple elastic bandage can be used to improve the grip on a homemade weapon. Virtually any prescribed medication can have value on the prison "black market." Furthermore, nurses are subject to manipulation by inmates, who may seek nursing care for reasons other than health.

As the following clinical example illustrates, the nurse must maintain an escape route to use if a situation of personal violence is imminent. In addition, no nursing care in a correctional environment requires a nurse to be locked in an enclosed environment with an inmate. Although it might appear that providing humane, therapeutic nursing care in an environment of potential violence is contradictory, it is ultimately a prerequisite for nursing practice in correctional settings.

Clinical Example

Safety in Correctional Facilities

In a county jail in Georgia in 1996, two nurses were attacked and beaten by an inmate being held on aggravated assault charges. The deputy on duty responsible for protecting them was also subdued by the inmate. These nurses were locked inside the jail with the inmate with their freedom, mobility, and flight to safety limited. The nurses sued the sheriff and deputy for failing to protect them in their work environment. The lawsuit was dismissed because the court determined that the nurses did not have a constitutional right to protection from harm in the work environment (Cohen, 1999c, p. 34).

RESEARCH HIGHLIGHTS

Hearing-impaired Prisoners

Miller, Vernon, and Capella (2005) compared the incidence and types of violent offenses of a deaf prison population with a hearing prison population in the Texas correctional system. A total of 99 individuals with severe-to-profound hearing loss were included in the study population. Of those offenders, 64.6% had been convicted of violent offenses including robbery, homicide, assault, and sexual assault.

The study found that in comparison with hearing violent offenders, a lower percentage of deaf violent offenders committed robberies. The researchers speculated that this difference might be due to the circumstances involved in a robbery, such as communication issues. The findings also revealed that deaf offenders had a higher percentage of sexual assault convictions compared with hearing offenders. The researchers thought that one reason for this finding might be that offenders were sexually assaulted as children.

Miller and colleagues proposed improving education for the deaf population and developing regional centers for deaf defendants charged with crimes. It is hoped that the regional centers will give the deaf defendant time to understand the linguistics of the criminal system and will allow for due process.

Data from Miller KR, Vernon M, Capella ME: Violent offenders in a deaf prison population, *J Deaf Stud Deaf Educ* 10(4):417-424, 2005.

HEALTH ISSUES IN PRISON POPULATIONS

Today's prison inmate often enters prison with health care issues. Nurses employed in the correctional setting are likely to see health care problems that are similar to those in an acute care setting or a community outpatient clinic. The daily operation of a correctional clinic includes management of acute and chronic illness. Most health care clinics in correctional environments screen each inmate upon entry into the facility. The health care triage process generally includes a physical and a mental health history. Many significant health care issues are recognized during the screening process, often for the first time.

Chronic and Communicable Diseases

The most critical heath care issues among the incarcerated population are chronic and communicable diseases. Of particular concern are human immunodeficiency virus (HIV), hepatitis, and tuberculosis (TB). According to the Bureau of Justice Statistics, the rate of HIV infection decreased from 194 cases per 10,000 inmates in 2001 to 146 per 10,000 at year end in 2010 (Maruschak, 2012). The rate of HIV infection in this population is associated with high-risk behaviors, including current and previous drug use, unprotected sexual intercourse, and tattooing.

Hepatitis is a serious health care issue in correctional facilities. According to the Bureau of Justice Statistics, 5.3% of state inmates and 4.2% of federal inmates reported hepatitis as a medical problem in 2004 (Maruschak, 2008). The National Commission on Correctional Health Care (NCCHC, 2013) recommends that all inmates be screened and, if indicated, treated for hepatitis upon incarceration.

Another serious health care issue in correctional facilities is TB. The 2004 Bureau of Justice Statistics report on the subject indicated that 9.4% of state inmates and 7.1% of federal inmates reported having tuberculosis (Maruschak, 2008). The rate of infection in correctional facilities is related to overcrowding, poor ventilation, and rapid movement of inmates into and out of jail. In 2006, the Centers for Disease Control and Prevention released general recommendations for the prevention and control of TB in correctional facilities, including the following:

- TB screening for all staff members and inmates, identifying persons with active TB disease and latent TB infection
- Containment by preventing transmission and providing adequate treatment to inmates with the disease
- Assessment, ongoing monitoring, and evaluation of screening and containment efforts
- Collaboration between correctional facilities and public health departments

As it is for the general population, TB, especially in its antibiotic-resistant forms, will continue to be a major threat to the health of incarcerated people in the foreseeable future.

Women in Prison

In mid-year 2007, there were 65,500 mothers in jail who reported having 147,400 children under the age of 18 years (Glaze and Maruschak, 2008). More than four in every ten women in prison admit to being abused before the current imprisonment: 34% physically abused and 34% sexually abused (Snell and Morton, 1994). Almost half of the women in prison report being under the influence of drugs or alcohol at the time of the offense and using drugs months prior to the offense.

Drug use and victimization, combined with the stress associated with being separated from their children, put incarcerated women at risk for many mental and physical health problems, including the risk of HIV infection and other sexually transmitted diseases. Unfortunately, health care providers in correctional facilities have limited experience and training to meet the health care needs of women in prison, and quality of care is adversely affected. For example, women who have been sexually assaulted are often reticent about obtaining regular gynecological examinations. The NCCHC confirms that routine gynecological examinations are not consistently a part of health screening for women upon entry into a correctional facility or a routine part of ongoing health care. The NCCHC (2013) offers the following to guide the provision of health care for women:

- Correctional institutions' health care intake procedures should include comprehensive gynecological examinations.
- Comprehensive health care services should be available to incarcerated women that give special consideration to the reproductive health needs of women, the high rate of victimization among incarcerated women, counseling related to parenting issues, and accessibility to drug or alcohol treatment.

⚖ ETHICAL INSIGHTS

Inmates' Refusal of Medications

An inmate's right to refuse treatment is a legal and ethical issue that nurses working in a correctional environment sometimes experience. The right to refuse treatment and the state's power to enforce treatment are both highly charged legal and political issues and have gained attention in state and local courts. The issue of forced medication and competence to stand trial is of particular concern. The legal and ethical principles that guide forced treatment against the will of an inmate have historically been potential for violence toward self or others and the capacity to understand the consequence of refusing medical treatment. A court decision determined that a judicial hearing is required to forcibly treat a nondangerous incompetent offender to render competence to stand trial. The court decision was based on the following three-factor analysis (Cohen, 1999b, p. 17):

1. Individual's interests
2. State's interest
3. Value of the suggested treatment

Unlike in nursing practice with the general population, prison inmates who refuse health care do not leave the facility and return home. Nurses practicing in correctional facilities continue to provide care and address the consequences of an inmate's refusal of treatment. For example, an inmate who refuses to adhere to treatment protocols for HIV infection may experience declining health status. Nurses are obliged to treat any resultant health issues. Individuals who are incarcerated by the state have a constitutional right to refuse and receive health care. Nurses practicing in correctional settings must respect the right to refuse care even if the result is an adverse outcome.

The correctional institute nurse must be mindful of the need to view incarcerated women holistically, realizing that many factors, such as early childhood trauma, violent victimization, gender discrimination, drug use, and a context of economic impoverishment, have often contributed to their current situations.

Adolescents in Prison

Increasing numbers of adolescents are committing violent crimes, and many states have lowered the age limit at which adolescents may be tried and sentenced as adults. Consequently, adolescents who have been convicted of violent crimes are often incarcerated in adult facilities. Incarcerating adolescents in an adult population presents barriers to meeting the distinct developmental needs of adolescents. These developmental needs include rapid physical and emotional growth and nutritional needs, all influenced by environment, genetics, and family experiences. Adult correctional facilities are not generally equipped to deal with the challenges of adolescent development. Adolescents in an adult correctional facility are five times more likely to be sexually assaulted, three times more likely to be beaten by prison guards, and 50% more likely to be assaulted with a weapon than adolescents held in a juvenile center (Coalition for Juvenile Justice, 2005). Juveniles in adult correctional facilities are five times more likely than the adult population and eight times more likely than juveniles in the juvenile center to commit suicide.

To ensure the safety of adolescents in an adult facility, the nurse must be aware of their individual vulnerability. A mechanism for adolescents to access medical and mental health care is essential. Services and interventions should be provided that consider the developmental stage and the experience of adolescence.

MENTAL HEALTH ISSUES IN CORRECTIONAL SETTINGS

Approximately 34% of state inmates, 24% of federal inmates, and 17% of jail inmates received treatment for mental health problems (James and Glaze, 2006). Being in prison with a mental illness such as schizophrenia, bipolar affective disorder, major depressive disorder, or personality disorder makes adjustment to incarceration extremely difficult. The great number of inmates with mental illnesses in today's prisons makes it difficult to meet the needs of this population.

In the late 1950s and early 1960s, deinstitutionalization moved people with mental illness out of state hospitals into communities that were often ill-prepared to care for them. As a result, many people with a mental illness reside in nursing homes, residential homes, prisons, or jails. People with mental illness are often jailed for crimes committed in response to the symptoms of mental illness. With community services declining and increasing numbers of people with mental illness being incarcerated, the "criminalization of the mentally ill" has become a significant political topic (National Alliance for the Mentally Ill [NAMI], 2013).

According to NAMI, most jail inmates with symptoms of mental illness are charged with minor crimes. A far smaller number of inmates with severe mental illness commit more serious crimes, again frequently a consequence of either inadequate or no treatment. NAMI (2013) takes the position that many dangerous or violent acts by people with severe mental illness are a result of inappropriate or inadequate treatment. The following strategies have been suggested to reduce the number of incarcerated people with severe mental illness:

- Train police officers to recognize severe mental illness in the community and to respond appropriately to people who are experiencing psychiatric crises
- Divert non-violent offenders with severe mental illnesses away from incarceration into appropriate treatment

- Establish "mental health courts" to hear all cases involving individuals with severe mental illness charged with misdemeanors or nonviolent felonies in order to divert as many as possible away from incarceration and into treatment and services
- Create specialized units within departments of parole and probation to coordinate services for people with severe mental illness on probation

Mental illness became increasingly understood as a neurobiological illness; therefore the professionals prescribing psychiatric medications have changed their objective from attempting to control behavior to targeting the symptoms of mental illness. Antipsychotic medications, along with psychosocial support, have become the standard of treatment for people with a diagnosis of schizophrenia or other mental illnesses that result in alterations in perception. Access to mental health treatment, including psychiatric medication, is a right for prison inmates. Correctional facilities must supply inmates with psychotropic medication after discharge for a time reasonable to seek community mental health treatment. Consequently, the state's responsibility for providing psychiatric medication extends beyond discharge from a correctional facility into the community (Dole, 2011).

Nurses employed in correctional settings must always be aware of the vulnerabilities of people with mental illness who are incarcerated. Depression, schizophrenia, bipolar disorder, and other neurobiological disorders can be readily treated with newer-generation psychiatric medications that reduce or ameliorate symptoms, but the unique vulnerabilities of incarceration often remain.

EDUCATION AND FORENSIC NURSING

According to Kent-Wilkinson (2011), because of the amount and depth of knowledge and skills needed by forensic nurses, whatever their subspecialty area, simply completing a continuing education course is not adequate for practice. As a result, several colleges and universities offer a variety of programs to educate practitioners. This is the direct result of the identified need and growing knowledge base for practice of this specialty area. Table 31-1 gives an overview of basic curricula for forensic nursing programs. In addition, during the formal programs of study, the student usually completes a minimum specified number of supervised clinical hours; a clinical internship also may be required.

TABLE 31-1	BASIC CURRICULA FOR FORENSIC NURSING PROGRAMS
SUBJECT	**TOPIC(S)**
Fundamentals for forensic nursing	Evidence collection
	Documentation
	Interviewing skills
	Basic criminal, procedural, and constitutional law
	Scope of practice
	Interdisciplinary collaboration
	Testifying in court as an expert witness
Forensic law	Legal concepts (culpability, burden of proof, rationale for punishment, mitigating circumstance)
	Defense issues (justification, insanity, entrapment, duress)
Forensic science	Collection and preservation of evidence
	Interpretation of DNA and laboratory reports
	Forensic chemistry and toxicology
	Cause of death
	Blood spatter interpretation
	Manner and mechanism of injury; wound identification and cause

Data from Burgess AW, Berger AD, Boersma RR: Forensic nursing: investigating the career potential in this emerging graduate specialty, *Am J Nurs* 104(3):58-64, 2004.

For those interested in seeking additional education in the growing and interesting specialty of forensic nursing, Box 31-5 lists nursing colleges and universities that have programs in forensic nursing. It should be noted that some of these programs offer a certificate in forensic nursing, whereas others provide a minor or concentration, and still others grant a graduate degree (typically a master of science in nursing degree).

The American Nurses Credentialing Center offers an Advanced Forensic Nursing certification (AFN-BC). To become eligible to obtain an AFN-BC, a nurse must (1) hold an active RN license, (2) have practiced at least 2 years as a full-time registered nurse, (3) have obtained a graduate degree in nursing, (4) have practiced a minimum of 2000 hours within a specialty area of forensic nursing with the last 3 years, and (5) have completed a minimum of 30 continuing education hours within the specialty forensic nursing area (ANCC, 2012).

BOX 31-5 SCHOOLS OFFERING PROGRAMS IN FORENSIC NURSING (GRADUATE AND CERTIFICATE PROGRAMS)*

California
University of California at Riverside, Riverside, California—*online*

Colorado
University of Colorado at Colorado Springs, Beth-El College of Nursing, Colorado Springs, Colorado

Florida
University of Florida, Gainesville, Florida—*online*

Illinois
University of Illinois at Chicago, College of Nursing, Chicago, Illinois—*online*

Louisiana
Bossier Parish Community College, Bossier City, Louisiana

Maryland
Johns Hopkins University, Baltimore, Maryland—*online*

Massachusetts
Boston College, Chestnut Hill, Massachusetts
Fitchburg State College, Fitchburg, Massachusetts—*online*

Nebraska
Bryan LGH College of Health Sciences, Lincoln, Nebraska

New Jersey
Fairleigh Dickinson University, Teaneck, New Jersey

Monmouth University, West Long Branch, New Jersey—*online*

New York
Binghamton University, Binghamton, New York—*online*
Kaplan College, New York, New York—*online*

North Carolina
Charlotte Mecklenburg Forensic Medicine Program, Charlotte, North Carolina

Ohio
Cleveland State University, Cleveland, Ohio—*online*
Xavier University, Cincinnati, Ohio

Oklahoma
University of Central Oklahoma, Edmond, Oklahoma—*online*

Pennsylvania
Duquesne University, Pittsburgh, Pennsylvania—*online*
University of Pennsylvania, Philadelphia, Pennsylvania
University of Pittsburgh, Pittsburgh, Pennsylvania

Virginia
George Mason University, Fairfax, Virginia—*online*

Washington
University of Washington, Seattle, Washington

*As of 2013.

CASE STUDY 31-1 APPLICATION OF THE NURSING PROCESS: CORRECTIONAL NURSING

Mr. Smith is a 65-year-old African-American male serving a sentence for aggravated assault. Mr. Smith has a medical history of diabetes mellitus, hypertension, coronary artery disease, and peripheral vascular disease. Three weeks ago, his right foot was amputated because of gangrene. Mr. Smith has been admitted to the infirmary six times since the procedure, stating, "I'm not feeling well; can you double-check my sugar?"

The incision site is healing well, and his diabetes mellitus is under control with medication. Mr. Smith takes his medications as prescribed, and his doctor believes he is doing well and continues with his current medication regimen.

Mr. Smith's daughter visits him only once every 6 months because she lives out of state. His son is also in prison but at another location. Mr. Smith's wife recently died from a motor vehicle accident, and he was unable to attend the funeral.

Assessment

Mr. Smith has a flat affect and does not make eye contact. He constantly looks at the ground and does not speak clearly when asked questions. Many times the nurse must ask him to repeat himself. According to medical records, he has lost approximately 18 pounds since surgery and he says, "I'm not hungry, that's why I don't eat." When asked about his sleeping habits, Mr. Smith states he sleeps all day except when the guards make him get up. He says he has not played cards with his buddies in more than a week. He also reports that he has been buying soma "from them" and has not taken a bath in 3 days.

Diagnosis

Individual
- Despair, gloom, hopelessness
- Inability to overcome mental and emotional difficulties
- Powerlessness

Family
- Situational crises

Community
- Lack of mental health services

Planning

Mr. Smith will set goals with the health care provider and will ask for assistance with communication with his daughter and son.

Individual
Long-Term Goal
- Client will reestablish positive relationships with fellow inmates within 2 weeks.

Short-Term Goal
- Client will verbalize and recognize his feelings.
- Client will participate in diversion activities of his choice (e.g., playing cards).

CASE STUDY 31-1 APPLICATION OF THE NURSING PROCESS—cont'd

Family
Long-Term Goal
- Family will demonstrate coping skills appropriate to the situation.

Short-Term Goal
- Family will verbalize and recognize feelings.

Community
Long-Term Goal
- Program will be available for all individuals.

Short-Term Goal
- Begin mental health programs for individuals in need, utilizing forensic nurses.

Intervention
Individual
- Mr. Smith will be encouraged to express his feelings in an open and nonjudgmental environment, allowing for the development of a therapeutic relationship.
- The forensic nurse will schedule several visits to the clinic and encourage Mr. Smith to participate in activities, such as card playing, with his friends.

Family
- Mr. Smith's daughter will be included in the plan of care and encouraged to express her thoughts and feelings relating to her father's imprisonment.

Community
- The forensic nurse will arrange several activities for inmates suffering from mental illnesses, including group activities and group talk.

Evaluation
Individual

Mr. Smith slowly engaged the forensic nurse individually and in group therapy. He gained 5 pounds over 2 weeks and was able to make eye contact. Mr. Smith expressed his grief for the death of his wife. He gradually stopped buying soma and spent more time with his friends.

Family

Mr. Smith's daughter continued to visit only once every 6 months but was able to fully explain her thoughts and feelings about her father's incarceration. The time the daughter spent with her father increased and was more meaningful.

Community

A forensic nurse was on constant duty to assist inmates with mental health illnesses.

Levels of Prevention
Primary
- Encourage interaction with colleagues and family.
- Promote participation in prison activities.

Secondary
- Screen for depression.
- Provide outreach services to inmates with mental illness.

Tertiary
- Encourage therapy to reduce symptoms of mental illness.

CASE STUDY 31-2 APPLICATION OF THE NURSING PROCESS: FORENSIC NURSING

Transcript of a 911 telephone call:
- *Emergency operator:* "This is 911, what is your emergency?"
- *Caller:* "My son isn't breathing, he's not moving, I need help!"
- *Emergency operator:* "We will send an ambulance and police to assist you."
- *Caller:* "Thank you, please hurry!"

Emergency medical personnel arrived at the house to discover James Oats, a 14-year-old white male, lying face-up on his bed. The young man was unresponsive and not breathing. Emergency medical personnel immediately began lifesaving interventions, but, despite all efforts, they were unsuccessful. James Oats was pronounced dead at his house.

Police officers arrived at the residence during the rescue attempt and secured the scene. They then notified homicide detectives and the medical examiner's office. Teresa Fernandez, a forensic nurse death investigator (FNDI), was dispatched to the residence to work in collaboration with the homicide detective, Pete Smith, to investigate the death.

The police determined that there was no indication of foul play. The house was in order, there was no evidence of a robbery, and all the doors and windows were locked. A PlayStation was attached to the television, various clothes were strewn about the room, and schoolbooks were on the desk.

The decedent's mother, Jane Oats, informed the FNDI that James was in fine health. She explained that he had undergone a physical examination last week for athletics and that the findings were unremarkable. James had an older brother and younger sister, both in excellent health. James's father has hypertension and a history of heart disease, and diabetes and cancer were present in grandparents.

Teresa (the FNDI) tried to comfort Mrs. Oats, who was extremely upset; she was crying and hyperventilating. Teresa turned to Mr. Oats, who was also present. In answer to Teresa's questioning, Mr. Oats reported that other parents and teachers had been concerned about rumors of the increasing use of "bars" in area schools. Teresa was alarmed by this information and questioned him further about what he meant; he confirmed that the school kids were reportedly using the antianxiety medication Xanax.

Assessment

Teresa performed an assessment of the decedent. James was wearing blue jeans, a yellow shirt, and socks. Her findings: "Livor mortis is consistent with body position and blanchable; rigor mortis is breakable in the jaw, arms, and legs. Frothy white foam cone was present at mouth and within bilateral nares. There are no visible signs of trauma."

The decedent was removed from the residence by the medical examiner's office, and an autopsy was performed the following day. The pathologist reported that the physical findings from the autopsy were unremarkable. During the autopsy, toxicology samples were collected from the heart, liver, and stomach.

Toxicology results were returned and were positive for an extremely large amount of alprazolam (Xanax). The final, official cause of death for James Oats was alprazolam toxicity; the manner of death was accident.

Continued

CASE STUDY 31-2 APPLICATION OF THE NURSING PROCESS—cont'd

Along with James's parents and Detective Smith, Teresa was informed of the cause and manner of death. Mr. and Mrs. Oats were devastated by the news and, upon questioning, stated that they did not understand how James had obtained the Xanax pills. They assured the detective and the FNDI that the only prescription medications in the residence were locked in the master bedroom cabinet and that James had no access to them.

Mr. Oats reported that Mrs. Oats has not been eating and had lost 25 pounds in 3 weeks. She had not been able to return to work, cried continuously, and did not care for their other children. Mr. Oats reported that the entire family was withdrawn; the younger child was misbehaving in school and received detention several times. Mr. Oats expressed exasperation with the need to provide all child care, perform routine chores, and go to work; he admitted that he did not know how much more he could handle.

Mr. Oats told the investigators that community and church members were extremely helpful and sensitive to the family. The school officials and area churches agreed to support and offer programs to encourage children to say no to drugs; these programs were to focus more attention on prescription medications. Furthermore, the school James attended was investigating drug and alcohol abuse. The school social worker told Mr. Oats that a support group was being formed to assist students with James's death.

Detective Smith interviewed several of James's classmates and discovered that Xanax was used by many of them. From the information that he was able to gather, it appeared that this was the first time James had tried the drug. Detective Smith discovered that some of the students were obtaining Xanax from their parents and selling it to their peers. Furthermore, he learned that students are trying the "bars" because "it's cool."

Diagnosis
Family
- Mental and emotional distress
- Grief
- Lack of family support
- Excessive stress

Community
- Readiness for healing

Planning
Family
- The Oats family will initiate counseling to assist with acceptance of and coping with James's death.

Long-Term Goal
- Family will identify need for outside support and seek such support.

Short-Term Goals
- Family will verbalize and recognize feelings surrounding the death.
- Family will express feelings honestly.

Community
Long-Term Goal
- Members of the community will establish a plan to deal with problems and stressors, including premature deaths.

Short-Term Goal
- Members of the community, including school personnel and students, will identify positive and negative factors affecting management of current and future problems and stressors.

Intervention
Family
Teresa Fernandez:
- Listened to the family's comments, remarks, and expression of concerns, noting nonverbal behaviors and responses
- Encouraged family members to verbalize feelings openly and clearly
- Referred family to appropriate resources for assistance as indicated (e.g., counseling, psychotherapy, spiritual guidance)

Community
With police, school personnel, and community leaders, Ms. Fernandez:
- Reviewed the community plan for dealing with substance abuse problems among schoolchildren and assessed the related stressors
- Determined the community's strengths and weaknesses
- Identified available resources
- Established a mechanism for self-monitoring of community needs and evaluation of efforts

Evaluation
Family
- The Oats family began family counseling and slowly accepted James's death.
- James's siblings began educating fellow classmates about the ill effects of abusing prescription medications.

Community
- The community implemented quarterly meetings for grieving families that included licensed counselors.
- The community members employed "just say no" rallies focusing on school-aged children.

Levels of Prevention
Primary
- Initiate drug teaching in middle and high schools, focusing on drug resistance training, social skills, and personal management.
- Support programs that encourage students to role play and apply life skills to deal with peer pressure.
- Provide life skills training (e.g., skills to cope with peer pressure, improve self-esteem/confidence).

Secondary
- Organize group sessions in school to discuss illegal prescription medication abuse.
- Provide information to school personnel and parents on how to identify or screen for evidence of use of drugs and alcohol among school-aged children.
- Provide information on area groups that provide support for students who want to avoid using drugs or want to stop using drugs.
- Reduce or stop harm that is done to individuals or groups while they are using drugs.

Tertiary
- Reduce risk that additional students will abuse prescription medication.
- Provide support to those who are abusing such substances.
- Refer to support systems (e.g., Narcotic Anonymous).

SUMMARY

Forensic nursing is an innovative, stimulating specialty that combines multiple aspects of nursing science into the care of patients and families with forensic or legal concerns. Most often, the forensic nurse is employed in a hospital, clinic, correctional facility, or medicolegal death investigation office. Specialized skills and knowledge are essential to the practice and require advanced education and training.

As mentioned previously, assessing for evidence of violence and intervening as needed are fundamental requirements of care that all health professionals must perform. Therefore, every nurse has the potential to be a forensic nurse, regardless of the client population or setting of care. With the increase in violence in society, forensic nurses are faced with the challenge of advocating for victims of violence, living or deceased, and the need for practitioners in this specialty area is expected to grow.

LEARNING ACTIVITIES

1. Spend a few hours working with a forensic nurse in an ED. Observe the nurse's interventions and processes related to evidence collection and preservation and to collaboration with, for example, police officers. Take note of the techniques used for interviewing and counseling.
2. Attend a session of local or state mental health court (court proceedings to determine the status of an individual's mental status and disposition—e.g., confinement to a mental institution or release in the care of a guardian or family member). Report on the experience to classmates.
3. Spend a day in a jail or correctional facility working with a correctional forensic nurse. Pay particular attention to differences in care delivery related to legal and ethical issues unique to this subspecialty. Develop impressions into a paper.

ⓔ EVOLVE WEBSITE

http://evolve.elsevier.com/Nies
- NCLEX Review Questions
- Case Studies
- Glossary

REFERENCES

Acierno R, Hernandez-Tejada M, Muzzy W, et al.: *National Elder Mistreatment Study*, 2009. Available from <https://www.ncjrs.gov/pdffiles1/nij/grants/226456.pdf>.

American Association of Legal Nurse Consultants: *What is an LNC?*, 2013. Available from <http://www.aalnc.org/>.

American Board of Medicolegal Death Investigators: *Board certification (advanced)*, 2013. Available from <http://abmdi.org/index.php?page=board-certification-advanced>.

American Legal Nurse Consultant Certification Board: *Eligibility criteria*, . Available from <http://www.aalnc.org/page/EligibilityCriteria/?>, 2013.

American Nurses Association: *Scope and standards of forensic nursing practice*, Washington, DC, 2009, American Nurses Publishing.

American Nurses Credentialing Center: *Advanced forensic nursing certification eligibility criteria*, 2012. Available from <http://www.nursecredentialing.org/AdvForensicNursing-Eligibility.aspx>.

Burgess AW, Berger AD, Boersma RR: Forensic nursing: Investigating the career potential in this emerging graduate specialty, *Am J Nurs* 104(3):58–64, 2004.

Coalition for Juvenile Justice: *Childhood on trial: The failure of trying and sentencing youth in adult criminal court*, 2005. Available from <http://www.juvjustice.org/media/resources/public/resource_115.pdf>.

Cohen F: Judicial hearing and strict scrutiny required to forcibly medicate incompetent detainees, *Corrections Mental Health Rep* 1(2):17, 1999b.

Cohen F: Prisons' duty to provide psychotropic medication includes post-release supply, *Corrections Mental Health Rep* 1(4):49, 1999c.

Collins SE, Halpern KJ: Forensic nursing: a collaborative practice paradigm, *J Nurs Law* 10(1):11–19, 2005.

Dole PJ: Forensic nursing in correctional care. In Lynch V, Duval JB, editors: *Forensic nursing science*, ed 2, St. Louis, 2011, Mosby.

Doughtery CM: Evidence collection in the emergency department. In Lynch V, Duval JB, editors: *Forensic nursing science*, ed 2, St. Louis, 2011, Mosby.

Ferrell J, Caruso C: Sexual assault evidence recovery. In Lynch V, Duval JB, editors: *Forensic nursing science*, ed 2, St. Louis, 2011, Mosby.

Finn O: Child maltreatment: Forensic biomarkers. In Lynch V, Duval JB, editors: *Forensic nursing science*, ed 2, St. Louis, 2011, Mosby.

Finn O: Relationship crimes. In Lynch V, Duval JB, editors: *Forensic nursing science*, ed 2, St. Louis, 2011, Mosby.

Geissler-Murr A, Moorhouse MF: Legal nurse consulting. In Lynch V, editor: *Forensic nursing*, St. Louis, 2006, Mosby.

Glaze LE, Maruschak LM: *Parents in prison and their minor children* (Bureau of Justice Statistics Rep No NCJ 222984), 2008. Available from <www.ojp.usdoj.gov/bjs/pub/pdf/pptmc.pdf>.

Hammer TC, Hammer RM: Crimes against the elderly. In Hammer RM, Moynihan B, Pagliaro EM, editors: *Forensic nursing: A handbook for practice*, ed 2, Burlington, MA, 2013, Jones and Bartlett.

Hanzlick R: *Death investigation systems and procedures*, Boca Raton, FL, 2007, CRC Press. Taylor Francis Group.

Hanzlick R, Hunsaker III JC, Davis GJ: *National Association of Medical Examiners: A guide for manner of death classification*, 2002. Available from <https://netforum.avectra.com/Public/DocumentGenerate.aspx?wbn_key=38c0f1d2-11ec-45c7-80ca-ff872d0b22bc&SITE=NAME>.

Harrell E: *Crime against persons with disabilities: 2009-2011 statistical tables* (Bureau of Justice Statistics Rep No NCJ240299), 2012. Available from <http://bjs.ojp.usdoj.gov/content/pub/pdf/capd0911st.pdf>.

International Association of Forensic Nurses: *Core competencies for advanced practice forensic nursing*, Pitman, NJ, 2004, Author.

International Association of Forensic nurses: 2014 SANE Certification Handbook. 2014. Available from: http://c.ymcdn.com/sites/www.forensic-nurses.org/resource/resmgr/Certification/2014_SANE_CERTIFICATION_EXAM.pdf

James DJ, Glaze LE: *Mental health problems of prison and jail inmates* (Bureau of Justice Statistics Rep No NCJ 213600), 2006. Available from <www.ojp.gov/bjs/pub/pdf/mhppji.pdf>.

Kent-Wilkinson A: Forensic nursing educational development: an integrated review of the literature, *J of Psychiatric & Mental Health Nursing* 18(3):236–246, 2011.

Ledray LE: Sexual violence. In Lynch V, Duval JB, editors: *Forensic nursing science*, ed 2, St. Louis, 2011, Mosby.

Ledray LE, Arndt S: Examining the sexual assault victim: a new model for nursing care, *J Psychosoc Nurs* 32(2):7–12, 1994.

Lynch V: Evolution of forensic nursing science. In Lynch V, Duval JB, editors: *Forensic nursing science*, ed 2, St. Louis, 2011, Mosby.

Lynch V: Forensic nursing science. In Hammer RM, Moynihan B, Pagliaro EM, editors: *Forensic nursing: A handbook for practice*, ed 2, Burlington, MA, 2013, Jones and Bartlett.

Lynch V, Koehler SA: Forensic investigation of death. In Lynch V, Duval JB, editors: *Forensic nursing science*, ed 2, St. Louis, 2011, Mosby.

Maruschak, LM: *HIV in Prisons, 2001-2010* (Bureau of Justice Statistics Rep No NCJ238877), 2012. Available from<http://bjs.ojp.usdoj.gov/content/pub/pdf/hivp10.pdf>.

Maruschak LA: *Medical problems of prisoners* (Bureau of Justice Statistics Rep No NCJ 221740), April 2008. Available from<http://www.bjs.gov/content/pub/pdf/mpp.pdf>.

Mason T: Psychiatric forensic nursing. In Lynch V, Duval JB, editors: *Forensic nursing*, ed 2, St. Louis, 2011, Mosby.

McDonough ET: Death investigation. In Hammer RM, Moynihan B, Pagliaro EM, editors: *Forensic nursing: A handbook for practice*, ed 2, Burlington, MA, 2013, Jones and Bartlett.

Miller KR, Vernon M, Capella ME: Violent offenders in a deaf prison population, *J Deaf Stud Deaf Educ* 10(4):417–424, 2005.

National Commission on Correctional Health Care: *Women's health care in correctional settings*, 2013. Available from <http://www.ncchc.org/women-s-health-care-in-correctional-settings>.

National Alliance for the Mentally Ill [NAMI]: The criminalization of people with mental illness. 2013. Available from: http://www.nami.org/Content/ContentGroups/Policy/WhereWeStand/The_Criminalization_of_People_with_Mental_Illness___WHERE_WE_STAND.htm

Pagliaro EM, Cewe BRB: The forensic nurse witness in the American justice system. In Hammer RM, Moynihan B, Pagliaro EM, editors: *Forensic nursing: A handbook for practice*, ed 2, Burlington, MA, 2013, Jones and Bartlett.

Pearsall C: Elder maltreatment: Forensic biomarkers. In Lynch V, Duval JB, editors: *Forensic nursing science*, ed 2, St. Louis, 2011, Mosby.

Potter PA, Perry AG: *Fundamentals of nursing*, St. Louis, 2009, Mosby.

Robson B: From emergency nurse to legal nurse consultant and independent practitioner: legal nurse consulting? What is that? *NENA Outlook* 32(2):24–26, 2009.

Ruiz-Contreras A: The nurse as an expert witness, *Top Emerg Med* 27(1):27–35, 2005.

Shafer TJ: Organ donation. In Lynch V, Duval JB, editors: *Forensic nursing science*, ed 2, St. Louis, 2011, Mosby.

Snell TL, Morton D: *Women in prison: survey of state inmates, 1991*, (Bureau of Justice Statistics Special Rep No NCJ 145321), 1994. Available from<www.ojp.gov/bjs/pub/pdf/wopris.pdf>.

U.S. Department of Justice/Bureau of Justice Statistics [USDOJ/BJS]: Criminal victimization. 2012.

U.S. Department of Health and Human Services, Administration for Children and Families, Administration on Children, Youth and Families Children's Bureau: *Definitions of child abuse and neglect 2011*, Washington, DC, 2011, Author. Also available from <https://www.childwelfare.gov/systemwide/laws_policies/statutes/define.pdf.>.

U.S. Department of Health and Human Services, Administration for Children and Families, Administration on Children, Youth and Families Children's Bureau: *Child maltreatment 2011*, Washington, DC, 2011, Author. Also available from <http://www.acf.hhs.gov/sites/default/files/cb/cm11.pdf>.

U.S. Preventive Services Task Force: *Screening for intimate partner violence and abuse of elderly and vulnerable adults: Clinical summary of U.S. Preventive Services Task Force recommendation*, 2013. Available from <http://www.uspreventiveservicestaskforce.org/uspstf/uspsipv.htm>.

Faith Community Nursing

Beverly Cook Siegrist

OUTLINE

Faith Communities: Role in Health and Wellness
Foundations of Faith Community Nursing
Roles or Functions of the Faith Community Nurse
Education of the Faith Community Nurse
The Faith Community Nurse and Spirituality
Issues in Faith Community Nurse Practice

Providing Care to Vulnerable Populations
End-of-Life Issues: Grief and Loss
Family Violence Prevention
Confidentiality
Accountability

Nurses seem to have one foot in the sciences and one in the humanities; one foot in the spiritual world and one in the physical one…they [nurses] have insight into the human condition. (Maginnis and Associates, 1993, p. 1)

The purpose of this chapter is to present an overview of faith community nursing and to explore the challenges of providing nursing care to faith communities. On the basis of centuries-old philosophies from churches and religious groups, nurses are applying the science of nursing and caring to address the biopsychosocial health needs of individuals and groups in church congregations and faith communities across the country. The following scenarios illustrate models of faith community nursing

found in the United States and suggest the unique ways that faith community nurses (FCNs) provide nursing care.

Clinical Example

Faith Community Nursing Model 1

Sandra Mills began her FCN practice as a volunteer when her parish priest recruited her to help establish a cancer support group and coordinate classes for caregivers. Within 6 months, her church's social concerns committee established a paid position on their ministry team and employed her as a full-time, paid staff member. After completing a faith community nursing program through a local university, she began to develop a health ministry in her church. She describes her days as full and rewarding. Each day, she visits ill or homebound parish members and provides support through prayer, education, and listening. She is challenged to locate and refer community resources, provide health education to church groups (e.g., mother's day out and the over-55 group), and coordinate the efforts of other volunteers in the church. She is practicing holistic nursing for the first time in her 15 years of practice. She has found that the church, as a healing community, allows her to focus on the body-mind-spirit connection she believes is necessary to improve the health of congregation members.

Clinical Example

Faith Community Nursing Model 2

Marilyn Michaels is a former home care and hospice nurse who works as an FCN coordinator for St. Luke's Hospital, which is a 400-bed medical center serving a Midwestern rural population. Her position was created to assist community churches in developing and maintaining parish nurse programs. She supervises 12 registered nurses employed by the hospital, who provide nursing through a contract to area congregations until the churches' budgets can support a nurse's salary. She also works with churches that have a volunteer model of health care ministry. She coordinates educational programs, including a 34-hour preparation program for beginning FCNs, an advanced program for FCN coordinators in individual churches, and monthly educational programs offered through an FCN support group. Marilyn developed the support group and facilitates communication among the 200 nurses and 100 church communities that St. Luke's Hospital serves. She also assists the many faith community programs by connecting them with other services that the hospital and community agencies provide (e.g., screening, support groups, and speakers). The program at St. Luke's Hospital is self-supporting through grants and educational programs.

The preceding clinical examples illustrate how faith community nursing is evolving in the United States and worldwide, from its beginning with fewer than a dozen nurses in Chicago. The practice now involves in excess of 15,000 nurses in more than 23 countries (International Parish Nurse Resource Center [IPNRC], 2013a). The growing number of registered nurses (RNs) in faith community nursing documents this practice as a significant role for the community health nurse. FCNs are now recognized as leaders with the ability to positively impact the health and wellness faith communities. In Figure 32-1, the Reverend Dr. Deborah Patterson, former Director of the IPNRC while in St. Louis, is being greeted by President Obama. Rev. Patterson is currently the Executive Director for the Northwest Parish Nurse Ministries (NPNM) in Portland, Oregon. She was at the White House in Washington, DC, on March 7, 2013, with FCNs from NPNM to be recognized by First Lady Michelle Obama and the President as one of 60 faith-based and community organizations providing national leadership in the Let's Move Faith & Communities initiative. This initiative

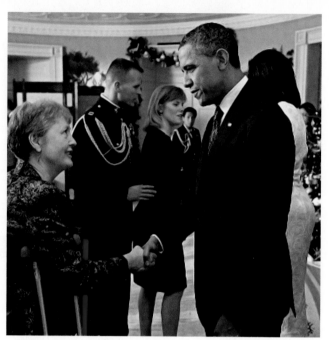

FIGURE 32-1 The Rev. Dr. Deborah Patterson, Executive Director of Northwest Parish Nurse Ministry, receives congratulations from President Obama on March 7, 2013, for faith community nursing work in First Lady Michelle Obama's Let's Move Faith and Communities initiative. (Courtesy of the White House Press.)

identified best practices in promoting healthy lifestyles for children and adults in the United States. Mrs. Obama's presentation can be viewed through a video-streamed White House press conference (http://www.whitehouse.gov/photos-and-video/video/2013/03/07/lets-move-faith-and-community-challenge-winners).

Community health nursing has evolved from early church efforts to provide care for the sick and disenfranchised. Modern parish nursing focuses on the global health and wellness issues of all people and has its roots in more recent efforts to encourage the reemergence and blending of health care roles into the healing ministry of faith communities (Hickman, 2007, Patterson, 2004; Solari-Twadell and McDermott, 1999).

FAITH COMMUNITIES: ROLE IN HEALTH AND WELLNESS

Former President Jimmy Carter, faculty and founding member of Strong Partners Interfaith Health Program at Emory University in Atlanta, Georgia, understands the importance of faith communities for Americans. President Carter is quoted as follows on the Interfaith Health Program website (http://www.interfaith.emory.edu):

> What if churches, mosques, and temples worked together to improve the health of their communities? If faith groups adopted one small area and made sure that every single child was immunized…that every person had a basic medical exam…that every woman who became pregnant would get prenatal care? Are these possible? We believe the answer is yes. (Interfaith Health Program, 2005)

Throughout history, church communities have provided care for the indigent and disenfranchised, meeting basic human needs for food, clothing, and basic health care. The majority of the world's populations belong to organized faith communities. Approximately one third of the people in the world identify themselves as Christians (2.1 billion), followed by Islam (1.5 billion), Hindus (900 million), and Buddhists (380 million) (Jacobsen and Hustedt Jacobsen, 2012; IPNRC, 2013). All of these religions have traditions and rituals related to health and healing, including specific prayers and practices. Some of the religions give specific guidelines for ministering to the ill, homebound, or dying members. All of the major religions describe the relationship among health, healing, and wholeness. The Old Testament discusses Shalom, or God's desire for health and wholeness for the earth and its people. The New Testament documents the healing activities of Jesus, restoring health to people. The Talmud describes the importance of maintaining physical health and vigor so that Jewish people will understand God's will in their lives. Followers of Buddhism believe that health and healing are interconnected and that illness occurs when there is an imbalance between life and the environment (IPNRC, 2013).

Koenig, King, and Carson (2012) cite, in the *Handbook of Religion and Faith,* a positive correlation between religion and health that has recently been termed the faith factor. These writers also note that more than 1,800 research studies have been completed since 2000 studying longevity and religiosity. Williams and Sternthal (2007) completed a meta-analysis of studies related to spirituality, religion, and health. In 17 studies, individuals who reported intrinsic religion (internalized or regularly practiced) and regular attendance at a religious service reported decreased stress. In 147 studies, these researchers found that there was an inverse relationship between religiosity and depression. They found evidence in another 49 studies indicating that people who practiced religious coping had lower levels of anxiety, depression, and stress and coped more positively with many chronic diseases, such as human immunodeficiency virus (HIV), hypertension, and cancer. One reason for this variance may be that the people who reported the highest level of religious involvement also reported practicing healthier lifestyles, including exercising more and smoking less (Myers, 2004, 2008; Tsuang, Williams, and Lyons, 2002). Eckersley (2007) suggests that "religion provides things that are good for health and well-being, including social support, existential meaning, a sense of purpose, a coherent belief system and a clear moral code" (p. S54). Myers (2011) and Koenig and George (2004) suggest that faith communities contribute to the well-being of their members through support, prayer, and providing a sense of hope. The importance of stress management in health promotion and disease management is well documented.

Organized religions are attempting to meet the needs of members in many nontraditional ways, such as exploring Internet church services, developing support groups, and including modern music and drama in traditional worship services to improve intergenerational communication. FCNs, because of their educational preparation and goals, are ideal health professionals to ensure that the health information provided in congregations is accurate and accessible. FCNs also understand the importance of spirituality in health and healing. The role of the FCN therefore complements the ministry of health found in faith communities.

FOUNDATIONS OF FAITH COMMUNITY NURSING

The Reverend Granger Westberg, a Lutheran minister, is considered the founder of the modern faith community nursing movement. Educated as a chaplain and minister, he worked with nurses in hospitals, medical schools, and church communities. Westberg was a visionary, with an understanding of the possibilities that church leaders, health care professionals, and congregational members could make in improving whole person health (body-mind-spirit). In one sermon he noted, "the church has not assumed its share of the responsibility for the health of the community" (Solari-Twadell and McDermott, 2006, p. 6). He later proposed to the W.K. Kellogg Foundation and the Department of Preventive Medicine of the University of Chicago College of Medicine the founding of "Wholistic Health Centers" where family physicians provided primary health care in churches with a team of nurses and clergy (Holistic Health Centers, 1976). These projects were implemented with success in various Illinois communities over the next decade. Evaluators later identified that a major reason for the success of the centers was the nurses, who could act as bridges between the ministers and the physicians because they understood both the science of medicine and the importance of religion in health and wellness (Holistic Health Centers, 1976). Impressed with the nurses' ability in viewing the physical, emotional, and spiritual challenges of human illness, Westberg described parish nursing as the culmination of his lifelong work in relating theology and health care. In 1984, he first proposed a parish nurse program to Lutheran General Hospital (LGH) in Chicago. Westberg envisioned a partnership between the hospital and all church congregations in the hospital's community. He proposed that participating churches would make contributions to fund a nurse's salary and identified seven roles the nurse could use to provide services to faith communities (Hickman, 2007; O'Brien, 2003; Patterson, 2004).

In 1985, six FCNs were hired in the Chicago area. Initially, LGH and the participating churches' contributions primarily funded the nurses' salaries. As the program grew and the International Parish Nurse Resource Center (IPNRC) became a reality, oversight was provided by the Lutheran-rooted Advocate Health Care System. Located in Park Ridge, Illinois, the center offered education, development guidance, and contact with parish nurses nationally and internationally. In

2001, ownership of the IPNRC moved from Advocate Health Care System to the Deaconess Foundation of St. Louis, Missouri. The Deaconess ministries in the United States have their roots in the Deaconess service movement founded in Germany in the mid-1800s. Deaconess Foundation has been involved in faith community nursing since the late 1980s and, as the Deaconess Parish Nurse Ministries, is a leader in the specialty in the United States. The Deaconess Parish Nurse Ministries served as the parent organization of the IPNRC until 2011 (IPNRC, 2009; Westberg, 2007).

On October 1, 2011, the IPNRC became the newest section of the community outreach division of the Church Health Center located in Memphis, Tennessee. The Church Health Center was founded in 1987 by Scott Morris, family practice physician and ordained United Methodist minister, to provide quality and affordable health care for working, uninsured people and their families. His vision is to "reclaim the Church's biblical commitment to care for our bodies and spirits" (Church Health Center, n.d.). The organization is now the largest faith-based health care organization of its type in the country. Using a volunteer interprofessional team of physicians, nurse practitioners, dentists, and others, the Church Health Center currently provides care to more than 58,000 patients without government funding. Patients pay an average of $25 per visit on a sliding fee scale. A wellness model of care is the foundation for all programs of the Church Health Center. The philosophy of the IPNRC and the Church Health Center is a complementary one related to a belief in the importance of the role of the church in health and wellness. Figure 32-2 illustrates the wellness model that is the basis for the vision, mission, and programs related to the Church Health Center. Part of the community outreach of the Center is to build congregational relationships and to "encourage, educate and equip" people to live healthier lives. Additionally, Scott has a personal knowledge of Westberg's vision for faith community nursing. He had previously met and discussed faith community nursing with Westberg as he was developing his plan for designing a plan for merging church and health. The Church Health Center has the resources to move faith community nursing to the next level. Susan Jacob, RN, PhD, has retired as Interim Dean of the School of Nursing at the University of Tennessee Health Science Center and has assumed the position as Manager of Faith Community Outreach at the Church Health Center (Church Health Center, 2013).

In 1998, the American Nurses Association (ANA), in collaboration with the newly formed Health Ministries Association, Parish Nurse Division, published the first *Scope and Standards of Parish Nurse Practice*. This was a landmark publication for parish nurses, officially recognizing their practice as a nursing specialty. ANA revised the standards in 2012, providing a clearer definition of the practice, including advanced nursing practice and changing the name of the specialty from parish nurse to faith community nurse. While acknowledging the importance of the

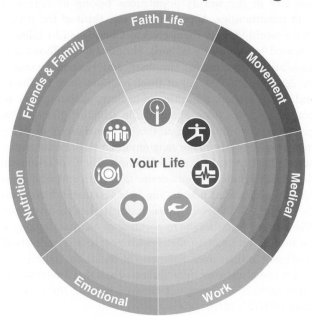

The Church Health Center
Model for Healthy Living

 Faith Life

Building a relationship with God, your neighbors, and yourself.

 Movement

Discovering ways to enjoy physical activity.

 Medical

Partnering with your healthcare provider to manage your medical care.

 Work

Appreciating your skills, talents, and gifts.

 Emotional

Managing stress and understanding your feelings to better care for yourself.

 Nutrition

Making smart food choices and developing healthy eating habits.

 Family & Friends

Giving and receiving support through relationships.

FIGURE 32-2 The Church Health Center Model for Health Living. (From Church Health Center: *Model for healthy living*, n.d. Available from <http://www.chreader.org/contentPage.aspx?resource_id=712&listWebPage_id=1>.)

Judeo-Christian basis of the practice, the authors of *Scope and Standards* believed that the change better reflected the diversity now found in the specialty. The IPNRC (2009) reports that faith community nursing is now practiced in more than 23 countries—Australia, Bahamas, Canada, England, Ghana, Kenya, South Korea, Madagascar, Malawi, Malaysia, New Zealand, Nigeria, Pakistan, Palestine, Scotland, Singapore, South Africa, Swaziland, Ukraine, United States, Wales, Zambia, and Zimbabwe—serving Muslim, Jewish, and Christian faith communities. Many FCNs continue to identify themselves as parish nurses in deference to Westberg and the origins of the practice. For this reason, the terms are used interchangeably in the literature and at conferences. Other FCNs may be known as congregational nurses or church nurses, choosing to identify themselves in the manner most accepted by their individual faith communities.

RESEARCH HIGHLIGHTS

A Community-Based Parish Nurse Intervention Program for Mexican American Women with Gestational Diabetes

The birth rate of Hispanic women has grown more than that of any other ethnic population in the United States. This group generally has a better pregnancy outcome than other groups, possibly owing to social support including family and church. The purpose of a study by Mendelson and associates (2008) was to determine whether the strong traditional ties that Mexican American women have with the church could be used to affect health outcomes of pregnant women, especially in the area of gestational pregnancy. These researchers enrolled 100 Mexican American women who were patients in an outpatient clinic for pregnant women with gestational diabetes in a randomized controlled trial, in which all the women participated in a 1-hour educational program and completed the Health Promoting Lifestyle Profile. Two measures of glycemic control (pre- and post-intervention) were measured, as well as newborn size and days in the hospital. The women were assigned to either a usual follow-up through the clinical or a faith community nurse (FCN) follow-up through their churches. All of the FCNs who provided the follow-up had bachelor's of science degrees in nursing and were fluent in Spanish. Each subject received individual sessions in which they discussed diabetes, risk factors, diet, and activity, explored their individual belief systems, and had prayer. Group sessions were also available. There was a significant statistical difference between the two groups related to the Health Promoting Lifestyle Profile, with the FCN group showing the most improvement but no other difference. There were indications of the benefits of working with the FCN in promoting the health of mothers.

Data from Mendelson SG, McNeese-Smith D, Koniak-Griffin D, et al: A community-based parish nurse intervention program for Mexican-American women with gestational diabetes. *JOGN*, 37(4), 2008, 415-425.

Solari-Twadell and McDermott (1999) and Westberg (1990) described the philosophical basis of parish nursing as encompassing the following five key elements:

1. The spiritual dimension is central to the practice.
2. The role balances nursing science and technology with service and spiritual care.

3. The nurse's clients are members of the **faith community** defined by the church and its public service philosophy.
4. Parish nursing services are built upon principles of self-care and capacity building, with a focus on understanding the connection between health and the individual's relationship with God, faith traditions, nursing, and the broader society.
5. The parish nurse understands that holistic health is a dynamic process that requires connections among the person's spiritual, psychological, physical, and social dimensions.

These beliefs direct the parish nurse in planning nursing care and defining health not only as wellness but also as wholeness of body and spirit. They also emphasize spiritual health as a motivating factor in seeking wellness care, participating in education, and enhancing self-care capabilities (Hickman, 2007; Patterson, 2004; Smith, 2003). The IPNRC (2009) identifies a vision that "every faith community in the future will have access to a FCN."

The defining characteristics and roles of the FCN in any setting arise from these philosophical foundations.

The following current mission statement for parish nurses was developed and approved in 2000 by more than 600 attendees at the Fourteenth Annual Westberg Symposium:

♥ HEALTHY PEOPLE 2020

Faith Community Nursing

Topic Area
Educational and community-based programs

Goal
Increase the quality, availability, and effectiveness of education and community-based programs designed to prevent disease and improve health and quality of life.

Faith community nursing practice may vary depending upon the needs of the faith community served. Programs and services may contribute to many *Healthy People 2020* goals. The Topic Area, Educational and Community-Based Programs—directs public health agencies to form partnerships with many community-based organizations, including faith communities, to improve the quality and effectiveness of health education programs. A free toolkit is available for faith communities to implement some of the ideas from the top 60 faith community nursing programs and community programs in the Let's Move Initiative selected as the best in the U.S. at promoting activity in all ages of Americans. It can be downloaded at http://www.letsmove.gov/faith-communities-toolkit.

From U.S. Department of Health and Human Services: *Healthy People 2020: Educational and community-based programs*, Washington, DC, 2013, U.S. Government Printing Office. Available from <http://www.healthypeople.gov/2020/topicsobjectives2020/overview.aspx?topicid=11>.

Parish nursing (aka faith community nursing) is the intentional integration of the practice of faith with the practice of nursing so that people can achieve wholeness in, with, and through communities of faith in which the parish nurse serves. Parish nurses educate, advocate, and activate people to take positive action regarding wellness, prevention, appropriate treatment of illness, and social and spiritual connections with God, members of their congregations, and their wider community. (Patterson, 2004, p. 32)

ROLES OR FUNCTIONS OF THE FAITH COMMUNITY NURSE

The faith community nursing practice focuses on health promotion and wellness. It is based on a holistic nursing practice that holds the spiritual dimension central to health and healing within the context of the faith community. In the nursing process, the FCN improves the health of a faith community by implementing interrelated roles or functions, including those of health educator, personal health counselor, **referral agent**, health advocate, coordinator of volunteers, developer of support groups, and integrator of health and healing (Hickman, 2007; IPNRC, 2013a).

As a **health educator**, the FCN provides or coordinates educational offerings for people of all ages and developmental stages. The educational efforts may target lifestyles, values, and wellness and may incorporate the spiritual aspects of individual and community well-being. The educator role includes educating the church leaders and members about the roles and purposes of a parish nurse. Educational efforts are based on the church community's priorities and *Healthy People 2020* (DHHS, n.d.). Because the faith community membership includes people of all ages, church-based educational programs can address all ten major health indicators (IPNRC, 2013a; King and Tessaro, 2009). Early in the development of a parish nurse program, and periodically thereafter, the parish nurse should assess the health status and needs of the congregation members to determine educational priorities. ⓔ **Resource Tool 32A** on the book's website, http://evolve. elsevier.com/Nies/, presents an example of an adult congregational health and wellness survey. The FCN should complete an assessment on each population group served by the congregation and should include children grouped by developmental stages. Examples of educational efforts are teaching cardiopulmonary resuscitation to new mothers; teaching signs and symptoms of hypertension and stroke to adults in the congregation; educating lay church ministers visiting homebound individuals on the signs and symptoms of acute illness; and teaching basic health and safety to school-age children. With increasing frequency, FCNs are implementing comprehensive wellness programs. One such program is "Get My People Going," developed by the IPNRC. It provides an 8-week healthy lifestyle program based on the Exodus story that includes exercise, nutrition, and community support (IPNRC, 2009).

As a **personal health counselor**, the FCN discusses health problems with individuals and families within the church community. The nurse may focus on self-care issues such as explaining a prescribed medical regimen; assessing the need for further resources and referrals; or making visits to homes, nursing homes, or hospitals (McGinnis, 2008).

The FCN utilizes referral skills and knowledge of community resources to guide individuals as they access available resources. The nurse may function as a liaison and, with the client's approval, may provide referrals to resources or health care providers. The FCN recognizes the difficulties encountered by vulnerable populations within the faith community and helps them maneuver the health care maze to access needed resources. These vulnerable populations may include non–English-speaking individuals, those who speak English as a second language (ESL), individuals living in poverty, individuals without health care insurance, and individuals living with complicated chronic or catastrophic illness.

In the role of **health advocate**, the FCN "facilitates clients' efforts in obtaining needed health services and appropriate care management plans, promotes community awareness of significant health problems, lobbies for beneficial public policy, and stimulates supportive action for health" (Clemon-Stone, McGuire, and Eigsti, 2002, p. 45). Advocacy can present challenges for the nurse in any setting. The nurse must always remember that the client (individual, family, or group) has the right to self-determination. The FCN's role may be that of educating clients to make the best choices or empowering them to speak for themselves. The nurse also must understand the policies and beliefs of the congregation in relation to specific health issues. Church doctrine may guide members to adopt values and beliefs that are in conflict with current health care recommendations. Individuals may request that the parish nurse provide education and support in making decisions related to issues of infertility, stem cell technology, birth control, and sex education for teens and youth. Although assuming the role of advocate implies a commitment to change, the parish nurse must understand that the politics of working within the faith system require acceptance of individual and system values and beliefs.

The role of **coordinator of volunteers** involves recruiting, training, and directing volunteers to work with the faith community nursing program or health ministry. The nurse may work with other nurses and lay people within the congregation. The faith community nursing program may encompass all programs related to the health of the church community. For example, the community needs assessment may identify the need for development of a transportation committee or respite program. These services affect the ability of church members to access health and related services; these programs may be delegated to the nurse. As a coordinator of volunteers, the nurse would plan, implement, and direct these programs. Many FCNs work through existing health ministry frameworks within their churches, such as health or social welfare committees. The membership of these committees may be interdisciplinary or representative of the entire church congregation. The FCN may be delegated the responsibility for developing specific health-related programs and activities. In the **facilitator** role, the nurse would also connect the church with existing resources and programs to meet identified health and educational needs. For example, the nurse might facilitate available health screenings, flu shots, or immunizations through the local public health department.

The role of **developer of support groups** requires skills in assessment, and the FCN uses community assessment and program evaluation skills. The nurse may practice within a community rich in resources and support groups or one with few health-related resources. Support groups are people who meet for support and sharing of issues related to common problems. Examples are bereavement groups and new mother groups. Support groups are different from self-help groups, which focus on personal growth (e.g., Alcoholics Anonymous). Some individuals prefer support groups to be physically located within their faith community, where they have existing support systems and can network with individuals who have common values and beliefs. The FCN must evaluate the need for a support or self-help group within the faith community. Situations that might indicate the need for support groups include the increased incidence of a sudden and shared experience by members—for example, the death of five or more members from cancer in a short timeframe; several incidences of suicide; or eating disorders within a teen group. A needs assessment of the faith community also might indicate the need for development of a support group. There are many models that the parish nurse may use as guidance in the development of groups. For example, the University of Kansas provides a Community Tool Box to help with creating and facilitating support groups (http://ctb.ku.edu/en/tablecontents/). If acceptable to the client, an individual referral may be made to an existing community group. It is also important to remember that groups usually have an anticipated "life expectancy." After the needs of a particular support group are met through education or support, there may no longer be a need for the group. The FCN should document the history of the group and move forward toward new goals.

As an **integrator of health and healing**, the nurse acknowledges and integrates spirituality as the basis of his or her nursing practice. For example, in teaching a class on healthy aging, the nurse will discuss lifestyle, compliance with prescribed medical treatment, attitudes, and values and their connections to well-being. In a home visit to a terminally ill person, the nurse will explore the meaning of healing versus cure and provide emotional support and encouragement. In certain faith communities, the nurse may lead, or contribute to, healing services as a member of the health ministry team. A basis for successful integration of health and healing in faith community nursing practice is an understanding of spirituality as a foundation for parish nurse practice. The importance of spirituality to faith community nursing practice and health is discussed later in the chapter.

These examples illustrate the diversity and autonomy found in faith community nursing. Depending on the needs of the church community and its members, the roles may be implemented in a variety of ways and through various organizational structures. Some organizational models use volunteer and paid nurses in the role of parish nurse. Hospitals provide parish nurses to community churches through grants, contracts, and public service. Many faith communities have incorporated positions for part-time and full-time nurses within their ministerial teams. Job descriptions and programs vary; examples can be found online at websites for individual parish nurse programs or at the IPNRC website (http://www.churchhealthcenter.org/fcnhome).

EDUCATION OF THE FAITH COMMUNITY NURSE

A baccalaureate-prepared RN with several years of experience in clinical practice is best prepared to implement the roles of the FCN; however, many schools of nursing provide faith community nursing education in baccalaureate prelicensure, RN to BSN (bachelor of science in nursing), and MSN (master of science in nursing) programs. The self-direction and independent decision making required by the autonomous roles of the FCN require a nurse experienced in clinical nursing and community-based nursing practice. The educational preparation of the baccalaureate nurse in community health nursing provides the theoretical basis needed to plan and implement programs for diverse populations in a congregational setting and to function as a beginning member of a pastoral team (Church Health Center, n.d.) All FCNs should complete a formal program of study (Church Health Center, n.d.; IPNRC, 2013b; Smith, 2003; Solari-Twadell and McDermott, 1999; Westberg and McNamara, 1990). Universities, hospitals, and faith community nursing programs now offer hundreds of courses that nurses may take for college credit, continuing education, or postgraduate certification. Courses are offered online, in seminars, and in regular classrooms. More than 136 international educational partners offer parish nurse courses. A list of these educational providers can be found on the IPNRC website.

Many universities are incorporating existing basic preparation programs into advanced nursing degree programs. Programs are generally offered at beginning and advanced levels and consist of approximately 32 to 40 contact hours of planned classroom instruction, self-study, or clinical experiences at each level. Box 32-1 provides an example of the curriculum content for a beginning faith community nursing program as suggested by the IPNRC. The curriculum is currently being revised and is expected to be more flexible. The revised curriculum incorporate other topics needed to provide comprehensive nursing care and health promotion for specific faith communities, such as disaster management, care of families, and special needs of rural congregations. As faith community nursing programs grow in number and in the services they provide to faith communities, continuing education programs will increase in availability and in diversity of content. The IPNRC conference held annually at the Westberg Symposium provides the greatest opportunity for education and networking among FCNs in the world.

Implementation of the FCN's roles requires the use of the nursing process to plan nursing interventions in wellness and physical, emotional, and spiritual health. Other chapters in this text provide useful information concerning health promotion and planning activities to promote physical and mental health. Spirituality, as a major focus of nursing care, presents different challenges for the nurse.

THE FAITH COMMUNITY NURSE AND SPIRITUALITY

Westberg (2007) described the ideal FCN as one who is spiritually mature and able to apply spiritual aspects to the health care of congregation members. Many FCNs find the need for further education to develop spiritual assessment skills, acquire theological knowledge, and learn the nurse's role in healing.

Wright (2005) defines spirituality as "the human desire for a sense of meaning, purpose, connection, and fulfillment through intimate relationships and life experiences" (p. xviii). In nursing, spiritual distress is more often the focus of care. The North American Nursing Diagnosis Association (1992) defines spiritual distress as "a disruption in the life principle that pervades a person's entire being and that integrates and transcends one's biological and psychosocial nature" (p. 46). FCNs understand that Christian-based beliefs consider spiritual distress to be a "metaphor to describe the experience of loneliness and desolation in one's life associated with a crisis in faith or with profound spiritual concerns about the relationship with God" (Dura-Vila and Dein, p. 544) (e.g., loneliness, isolation, and hopelessness). Spirituality is the basis of nursing care in the church setting. The Joint Commission, the International Council of Nursing, and the National Council of State Boards of Nursing and related National Council Licensure Examination for Registered Nurses (NCLEX) include as important "religious and spiritual influences on health" and list spiritual care as a characteristic in indicators of "quality care" (McEwen, 2005).

There are many models available to help nurses assess the spiritual dimensions of care including the HOPE Model and the JAREL Spiritual Well-Being Scale (McEwen, 2005). The FCN should learn to use a tested model that facilitates his or her practice, because knowledge deficiencies are identified as a major barrier to spiritual nursing care (McEwen, 2005). Schnorr (1988, 2003) suggests the CIRCLE Model of Spiritual Care. This model illustrates the following concepts of care that guide nursing practice and interventions:

Caring
Intuition
Respect for religious beliefs and practices
Caution
Listening
Emotional support

Caring includes caring practices and attitudes. Swanson (1991) provided an understanding of the caring processes through her early research, which identified five caring processes: knowing (trying to understanding what events mean to the patient); being with (both emotionally and in person); doing for (as needed); enabling (helping through transitions and life stages); and maintaining belief (helping the person sustain faith or hope). These processes were later further defined and identified as caring behaviors. The top caring behaviors in nursing as derived from the literature are: attentive listening, comforting, honesty, patience, responsibility, providing information so the patient can make an informed decision, touch, sensitivity, respect, and calling the patient by name (Swanson, 1991; Watson, 1998; Wolf, 1986; Wolf, Zuzelo, and Costello, 2004). Nurse theorist Jean Watson described caring as "professional, ethical, scientific, esthetic, personalized giving-receiving behaviors that allow for contact between the nurse and client" (quoted in Dossey, 1999, p. 45). Intuition requires acting on instinct, hunches, or "gut feelings." Benner (1984) described intuitive abilities as responses that expert nurses have after several years of experience; these abilities enable the nurse to "read between the lines." Schnorr (1988) described respect as understanding the importance of religious beliefs and practices. The nurse allows time for prayer and sacrament and supports and encourages religious activities. Caution in spiritual care advises the parish nurse to avoid proselytizing or "preaching" religion to clients. The ANA's (2012) *Code of Ethics for Nurses* also provides the nurse with direction to avoid judgments and respect the client's right to self-determination. Listening is a skill that is highly developed in most experienced nurses. It allows an understanding of spoken and unspoken words and feelings, encourages open communication, and supports and empowers patients to communicate needs and desires. Emotional support is the link between the physical and spiritual. Among the emotional interventions, Schnorr (1988) includes working with feelings, showing love, and using appropriate touch and empathy.

Prayer is a commonly used spiritual intervention that can provide comfort and support. Many nurses are not comfortable with sharing individual or group prayer (see ⓔ **Resource Tool 32B** on the book's website, at http:// evolve.elsevier.com/Nies/, for guidelines to help nurses in the development of group prayer sessions). Clients may ask FCNs to offer prayer for healing or recovery. Many faith traditions, such as Catholic and Jewish, have traditional prayers that the parish nurse can read or memorize. A guideline to follow is to keep the prayer simple and offer the request to the client's higher power. The nurse may have a poem for healing that is meaningful, which may be also be used. Silence may also be used after a simple prayer, or the nurse may request that the client offer his or her own prayer. Hickman (2007) suggests that through prayer, spiritual assessment, and hope and faith, the FCN facilitates important client outcomes for spiritual health and well-being, including self-esteem, self-actualization, hope, trust, and peace.

Clinical Example

During a meeting of the health ministry committee, the FCN nurse learned that Mrs. James, a church member, had been diagnosed with end-stage breast cancer. Mrs. James is a 45-year-old wife and mother of two school-age children. She returned home after surgery and had to decide whether to seek further treatment within the following weeks. Her husband attended church with his family although he was a member of another faith community. A home health nurse was involved with Mrs. James's postoperative care, and it was possible that a referral to hospice would occur following her decisions regarding further treatment. The nurse called Mrs. James and offered to make a home visit to assess how the FCN and church community could support and care for the family's well-being. Mrs. James welcomed the visit. Showing respect for their faith beliefs, the nurse offered prayer and waited for a request from the couple. The nurse's instincts and experience in working with patients with cancer and their families guided her in using listening as a nursing intervention during this initial visit and in using caution when Mrs. James asked for guidance in making treatment decisions. The nurse further explored the home situation, the needed educational support, and the physician's prognosis and treatment options with the patient. Emotional support was important for Mrs. James, and the FCN offered support through touch and words of concern. This model helped develop an initial nurse-client relationship of trust and open communication.

ISSUES IN FAITH COMMUNITY NURSE PRACTICE

The practice of faith community nursing is affected by many issues common to community health practice as well as issues specific to parish nursing. Selected issues discussed in this section include working with vulnerable populations and the legal and ethical issues of confidentiality and accountability. Other issues identified as important by the IPNRC are end-of-life and family violence issues; these are required content in faith community nursing courses.

Providing Care to Vulnerable Populations

The philosophical foundations of faith communities related to caring, outreach, and support of vulnerable populations place the parish nurse in a position to positively influence the health of diverse groups. Historically, churches have been among the first groups to sponsor and support refugees, develop programs for homeless individuals and families, offer assistance and resources to low-income families, and provide resources to entire communities during disasters (e.g., floods and tornadoes). FCNs are able to provide care for diverse populations using skills in assessment, planning, and interventions.

Faith community nurses can be instrumental in helping diverse populations access services; however, nurses should not attempt to meet the population's many needs alone (Boss, 1996, 1999; Hickman, 2007). When one is using available health resources, "more is not necessarily better." The nurse in the educator role can assess the needs of vulnerable populations and teach the faith community about the people and their spiritual, emotional, and physical needs. A community of caring that can collectively meet the many needs of vulnerable populations will emerge from the congregation. Boss (1999) called this the Nehemiah approach, meaning that people collectively share their talents and desire to do the work. The FCN works as a member of a caring church community to meet the health and related needs of vulnerable populations. For example, as Hispanic populations grow in rural populations, the need for churches to meet the needs of this population also grows. Established churches may provide resources for Hispanic populations to form their own churches. The FCN may serve an outreach church in addition to the parent church.

End-of-Life Issues: Grief and Loss

Faith communities have long been the first-line provider of support related to loss, grief, and dying. The aging population, the increased prevalence of chronic diseases such as cardiovascular disease and cancer, and public awareness have contributed to the need for improved end-of-life care. FCNs become partners with hospice and home care nurses in providing palliative care to congregation members. The IPNRC suggests that the FCN needs a theoretical base that includes an understanding of grief and loss from a developmental and social perspective, knowledge of the manifestations of normal and complicated grief, and nursing interventions to facilitate healthy grieving.

FCN activities related to end-of-life care may include educational sessions on drawing up living wills, establishing health care surrogates, and understanding hospice and palliative care; providing home visits to dying congregational members and emotional support to family and survivors; and developing grief support groups.

Family Violence Prevention

Education and prevention of family violence directly relate to *Healthy People 2020* objectives, and all nurses must be informed in this area (IPNRC, 2009; Smith, 2003). The FCN must have an understanding of risk factors for family, child, and elder abuse; knowledge of the cycle of abuse; and assessment skills to identify individuals and families at risk for violence. Family violence affects all racial, ethnic, religious, and socioeconomic classes in the United States.

In intimate partner violence (IPV) (also known as domestic abuse, spouse abuse, domestic violence, courtship violence, battering, marital rape, or date rape), it is important to understand that the main issue is an imbalance of power. There are no standard reporting laws (across the United States) related to IPV; however, it is essential that the FCN recognize signs and symptoms of IPV and have an intervention plan that includes providing support, establishing a trusting relationship, discussing safety issues, making appropriate referrals for shelter and counseling, and documenting the abuse according to the organizations policy (IPNRC, 2013a).

Child abuse and neglect are reportable in all 50 states:

All 50 States, the District of Columbia, and the U.S. territories have enacted statutes specifying procedures that a mandatory reporter must follow when making a report of child abuse and neglect. Mandatory reporters are individuals who are required by law to report cases of suspected child abuse or neglect. In most States, the statutes require mandatory reporters to make a report immediately upon gaining their knowledge or suspicion of abusive or neglectful situations. In all jurisdictions, the initial report may be made orally to either the child protection services agency or to a law enforcement agency. (U.S. Department of Health and Human Services [DHHS], n.d.)

Nursing interventions for suspected or actual child abuse include the following:

1. Report to the appropriate authority.
2. Provide resources and referrals.
3. Establish a trusting relationship with the child or adolescent.
4. Provide presence.
5. Listen.
6. Document according to policy, law, or both.

The National Center on Elder Abuse (2013) reported that 13% of the U.S. population, or 40.3 million people, were aged 65 years or older (based on the 2010 U.S. Census) and possibly as many as 10% experienced some type of abuse in 2010. Women were more likely to be exploited than men, and major financial exploitation may occur at the rate of 41 per 1000 individuals. Elder abuse includes not only physical abuse but also psychological neglect, with or without verbal threats; violation of personal choice or rights; financial theft or misuse of the elder's money; and failing to provide basic needs (food, shelter, clothing, and medical care). The parish nurse or another church volunteer may be the first individual to identify signs and symptoms of elder abuse. The nurse's role may also include educating church volunteers on identifying abuse and making reports and referrals. The nurse must have skill in recognizing symptoms of abuse and must possess assessment or screening questions to identify specific problems. Specific nursing interventions include the following:

⚖️ **ETHICAL INSIGHTS**

Principles of Applied Ethics in a Faith Community

Applied ethics refers to the utilization of ethical principles in real-life situations. The values and beliefs of faith communities raise additional ethical considerations for the parish nurse. Actions of the parish nurse may result in a conflict between established nursing interventions and beliefs of the faith community. The IPNRC (2009) identifies these potential areas of ethical conflict:

- Infertility treatment
- Organ donations
- Blood transfusions
- Proper dress or behavior
- Withdrawal of and withholding nutrition
- DNR (do not resuscitate) orders
- Pro-life versus pro-choice
- Use of advance directives
- Distribution of scarce resources
- Competency for decision making
- Clergy sexual conduct

The FCN's roles include understanding the scope of practice for parish nurses related to ethical practice and the values and beliefs of the community served. The nurse must understand his or her own beliefs and values that are in conflict with the faith community's beliefs. It is necessary that the parish nurse know when to seek help, when to refer, and when to remove himself or herself from the ethical decision-making process (O'Brien, 2003).

---

1. Recognizing that all states have laws against elder abuse but that reporting varies from state to state so it is important to know state laws
2. Establishing a trusting relationship with the elder and being a presence (being with the elder as needed)
3. Providing appropriate referral and resources
4. Documenting the abuse, according to policy, law, or both

Confidentiality

The *Code of Ethics for Nurses* (ANA, 2008) and the *Scope and Standards of Faith Community Nursing Practice* (Health Ministries Association and ANA, 2012) provide ethical guidance to parish nurses. FCNs are accountable to state boards of nursing, employing agencies (i.e., including churches), and the faith communities they serve. Many ethical and legal issues are generic to clinical practice settings; however, confidentiality issues have the potential to be problematic in a church community. Nurses who volunteer in faith communities, as in any other community organization in which they use the title nurse or employ nursing skills, must maintain active licenses as required by the state in which they reside. Many state boards of nursing provide practice guidelines related to the accountability and responsibility of the registered nurse as a volunteer. Basically the nurse should assume he or she is accountable and responsible for knowing and following established policies and procedures.

Concerned church members may identify individuals in need and refer them to the parish nurse. In the role of health minister, the parish nurse may receive private and sensitive information. The nurse does not act in the role of minister or priest. Congregation members should not relate information in the form of confession or repentance; however, the connection with the church ministry team may put the nurse in a position to hear this type of sensitive information.

The nurse should protect clients' rights to confidentiality in relation to information concerning their health or health-related condition. Although the nurse must share information with the church minister in certain instances, the nurse should share confidential information with other church ministry leaders (or prayer groups) only when given permission by the client. Exceptions are found in religious sects or congregations that require the public confession of members' behaviors or conditions so that members may benefit from divine intervention and forgiveness. As a care provider, the FCN should be aware of these rituals and practices before counseling members of the faith community (Fowler, 1999). General guidelines for medical record management should be followed by the FCN. Policies and procedures for managing and storing records and sharing and requesting medical information must be established. Faith community nursing programs within faith communities generally are not required to follow Health Insurance Portability and Accountability Act (HIPAA) guidelines related to medical records and confidentiality, because churches are not in the category of identified health care providers. An exception is parish nurse services provided by a licensed health care provider such as a hospital; in this instance, HIPAA regulations do apply (IPNRC, 2009).

Accountability

Sister Mary Angela Shaughnessy (1998) provides direction for the FCN by listing the following information related to church law:

- Volunteers in a church are held to the same degree of accountability as are paid employees.

- The doctrine of separation of church and state does not exempt churches from discrimination laws.
- Ministers, both ordained and nonordained, may be required to disclose confidential information in court.

As volunteers or paid employees, nurses are accountable to the nursing standards and civil laws designed to protect individuals from abuse, neglect, and discrimination. FCNs, as nonordained ministers, do not have client-professional privileges and should be aware of appropriate standards in documenting provided services. In documenting parish nurse services, "less is better." Many churches may not have the facilities to store medical records in a secure locked area. In this instance, the nurse should have a file storage system that locks and can be kept in a secure location. Simple records of blood pressure screenings or health education programs could include only numbers of attendees or blood pressure results categorized by American Heart Association standards as hypertensive, borderline, or normal. Also included in the documentation could be numbers of individuals referred for services. Faith community governing boards or committees need not have the names of individual clients but will be interested in the types of services and numbers of clients served. Individual client services require a nurse's note or assessment and development of a nursing care plan. Prior to beginning a faith community nursing program, the nurse should develop and follow general policies and guidelines for record keeping and storage. Shaughnessy (1998) provides further information related to contract law. The handbooks, brochures, or programs that church-related institutions offer are contracts. The FCN should ensure that health information is current and based on accepted practices and standards. These suggestions are not intended to limit the parish nurse's creativity or scope; rather, they emphasize that the professional nurse is accountable for his or her practice in any role.

CASE STUDY APPLICATION OF THE NURSING PROCESS

Nancy Elliot, an FCN at Living Hope Baptist Church, just completed a needs assessment of her faith community of 200 families. Nancy is new to the faith community nursing role, having recently been hired. Living Hope, considered a moderate-sized church, is located in a rural community of 40,000. Nancy decided to perform the needs assessment of the congregation and community prior to planning programs and services for the faith community.

Assessment

The community has one hospital and a variety of voluntary and official community agencies. Many private practitioners are available, either in the town or within a 1-hour drive in a larger city. Recently the town was awarded a grant to develop community parks and recreational facilities. Nancy is surprised by the demographic picture she finds after completing of assessment. Young families with toddlers to young school-age children comprise more than 70% of the congregation. She notes that these families are in the childbearing developmental stage of family growth and development. The remaining 30% of the members are elders, more than half of whom are 80 years or older. The survey indicates that the

members are most interested in health screening and educational opportunities presented at the church. Only 3% of the members reported having no health insurance.

A discussion with the minister provides additional information. Two new industries have recently relocated to the area. The parent home of both of these industries was formerly located in distant states. Many new members have relocated to the area. Nancy understands that these young families may have decreased family and social support and little knowledge of existing community resources. The minister also informs her that the current church ministries focus on the elderly members and that new services are needed. Nancy schedules a meeting with the young parents following a church social gathering. Fifty mothers and fathers attend the session to discuss the health-related needs of the families. They identify that a "mother's-day-out" program is a priority and also request information on community resources, parenting classes, and health and wellness programs for the children and parents. On the basis of the needs assessment and sessions with the parents, the FCN determines the following goals, nursing diagnoses, and population-focused nursing interventions.

Continued

CASE STUDY   APPLICATION OF THE NURSING PROCESS—cont'd

Diagnosis
Individual

- Readiness for health promotion, as evidenced by requests for health information related to parenting, health, and wellness
- Potential for parent support, as evidenced by developmental stage of families, requests for education, and presence of new community members with limited knowledge of community resources
- Potential for community building, as evidenced by individual concerns related to limited social support and lack of social networks

Family

- Potential need for family support, related to recent relocation to new community and lack of social network

Community (Faith Community)

- At risk for community (congregation) disorganization, related to recent change in membership demographics, lack of developed resources, and new or developing faith community nursing role

Planning

A plan of care is developed to address the needs of the individuals, families, and the Living Hope faith community. Goals suggested by the FCN are mutually agreed upon by the ministerial team and congregational members.

Individual
Long-Term Goals

- Monthly educational programs will be offered addressing current issues in parenting and health and wellness of young families.
- Congregation will establish a social network for young parents.
- Ministerial leaders will dedicate funds to increase resources for children and young adults.

Short-Term Goals

- Establish parent steering committee for educational program ideas, identification of parent talents (assist with education programs).
- Explore development of mother's-day-out program.

Family
Long-Term Goals

- Parent members will report increased social networks.
- Parent members will identify adequate resources to support growing family.

Short-Term Goal

- Identify community and congregation support for new and growing families.

Community (Faith Community)
Long-Term Goal

- Programs will be established to support growing families.

Short-Term Goal

- Implement one new program (educational, social) or resource for families each quarter of the church year.

Interventions

Nancy utilized diverse interventions to meet the goals established for families of Living Hope.

Individual

Nancy asked the parents (men and women) to complete a talent survey to identify the resources available within the families of Living Hope. From this survey, Nancy identified two RNs willing to help provide educational programs and three previously certified early childhood teachers. The teachers were willing to develop a committee to explore the development of a mother's-day-out program, a playgroup, and a new parent support group. Additional members were willing to begin a ministry to provide meals to new parents. Community resources were identified at the local health department to help teach parenting classes and provide immunizations. A plan was established to begin the mother's-day-out program part-time within 2 months. The playgroup and educational programs were implemented immediately.

Family

The ministerial team and a parent advisory group were formed to identify family needs. Family social events were planned, including a church picnic. Planning was made for age-appropriate activities, such as the development of a soccer team for the youth, a softball team for the young adults, and a literary club for those interested. The advisory committee developed a budget to submit to the ministerial team, requesting financial support to develop a playground for the children attending the mother's-day-out program and the hiring of a part-time employee to supervise the related activities. The families reported greater feelings of support from the faith community, increased social support and networks, and a feeling of belonging to the greater community.

Community (Faith Community)

The faith community developed a budget to support individual and family requests. Monthly health education programs became the standard, with topics noted on the monthly calendar. Members reported increased feelings of "community" not only among the young families but also across generational lines, as new members increasingly participated in leadership roles within the congregation. The minister documented an increase in weekly attendance, which had a positive impact on the long-range goals identified by the congregational members.

Evaluation
Individual and Family

Attendance at the health and wellness and parenting sessions increased with each educational session offered. Initial attendance was 5 to 7 people for each session, and after 6 months, the average attendance was 15 to 20 people for each session. The request from attendees changed from offering additional educational sessions to planning intervention programs such as a yoga class and a weight reduction program. The playground was completed in less than the planned time because of the increased budget. The mother's-day-out program, which began as a part-time, 3-day-per-week program, grew to a Monday-through-Friday program within 12 months. The program became self-sufficient by the end of the year because of established fees, parent volunteers, and donations. Men and women verbalized an increased satisfaction with their spiritual growth and support from the faith community. Nancy developed a health ministry committee of volunteers from within the church and was able to increase the number and variety of related parish nurse activities.

Community (Faith Community)

The health and wellness activities attracted the attention of sister churches, and a grant was offered to increase the number of family support services and wellness programs offered within the church. Health and wellness programs were expanded to include additional methods for reaching congregational members, such as through a website. The greater attendance and participation of congregational members positively affected all members, who benefited from the leadership and positive environment. The educational offerings and intervention programs were developed on the basis of *Healthy People 2020* goals, in particular increasing activity and exercise, healthy eating, and obesity prevention (DHHS, 2010).

CASE STUDY APPLICATION OF THE NURSING PROCESS—cont'd

Levels of Prevention
The roles of the FCN direct the interventions and programs planned for faith communities. The following are examples of all three levels of prevention applied to this case study.

Primary
- Assessment and teaching about parenting, health, and wellness
- Development of programs and social support systems to prevent social isolation and increase resources for successful parenting and healthy behaviors

Secondary
- FCN assessment and screening to identify individuals and families at risk
- Congregational resources and educational programs developed to meet individual and family needs

Tertiary
- FCN provides, or refers to, resources for rehabilitation, for families coping with children with disabilities or chronic health problems (parents and children).

SUMMARY

This chapter provided an overview of the FCN's role in providing nursing care for faith communities, and it explored the historical and philosophical foundations of the modern faith community nursing practice. Traditional roles of the nurse are used in unique ways to allow the FCN to provide nursing care to church communities. The FCN's role in the development of spiritual health and well-being becomes significant and requires the nurse to focus on the spiritual needs of congregation members. The CIRCLE model for planning spiritual nursing may be used to guide nursing interventions. Faith community nursing offers new opportunities for increasing the health and wellness of clients and requires the nurse to refocus skills and knowledge.

Many educational programs are available throughout the United States to provide faith community nursing education after basic nursing education. These programs are offered as continuing education and through formal university courses as part of degree programs. Church law, nursing ethics, and standards are the basis for the legal and ethical faith community nursing practice. As a relatively new area of community health nurse practice, FCN offers the RN many opportunities to improve the health of faith communities through a holistic nursing practice that connects the body, mind, and spirit in the celebration of health and healing.

LEARNING ACTIVITIES

1. Speak with an FCN in the community. Ask the nurse about congregational health needs and discuss how the roles of the faith community nurse are implemented through the faith community nursing programs and ministry. Observe the nurse in his or her daily activities and identify how spirituality is a basis for congregational nursing care.
2. Speak with a minister, priest, rabbi, or church leader in the community from a faith belief system different from your own. Explore the philosophical basis for the church's role in health and healing.
3. Visit websites devoted to faith community nursing and identify the models of faith community nursing programs or read the descriptions of their practice. Share these with the clinical group.

ⓔ EVOLVE WEBSITE
http://evolve.elsevier.com/Nies
- NCLEX Review Questions
- Case Studies
- Glossary
- Resource Tool 32A: Parish health assessment form
- Resource Tool 32B: Guidelines for Simple Prayer Services

REFERENCES

American Nurses Association: *Faith community nursing: Scope and standards*, ed 2, Silver Springs, MD, 2012, Author.

Benner P: *From novice to expert*, Menlo Park, CA, 1984, Addison-Wesley.

Boss J: Lesson learned over time: great teachers—St. Francis, St. Clare, and Eleanor, *Health Dev* 2:7–19, 1996.

Boss J: Parish nursing with under organized, underserved, and marginalized clients. In Solari-Twadell PA, McDermott MA, editors: *Parish nursing: promoting whole persons health within faith communities*, Thousand Oaks, CA, 1999, Sage.

Church Health Center: *About us: Our mission*, 2013. Available from <http://www.churchhealthcenter.org/>.

Clemon-Stone S, McGuire S, Eigsti D: *Comprehensive community health nursing*, ed 6, St. Louis, 2002, Mosby.

Dossey MD: Dynamics of healing and the transpersonal self. In Dossey MD, Keegan L, editors: *Holistic nursing: a handbook for practice*, Gaithersburg, MD, 1999, Aspen.

Eckersley RM: Culture, spirituality, religion and health: looking at the big picture, *Med J Aust* 186(Suppl 10):S54–S56, 2007.

Fowler M: Ethics as a context for the practice. In Solari-Twadell PA, McDermott MA, editors: *Parish nursing: promoting whole persons health within faith communities*, Thousand Oaks, CA, 1999, Sage.

Health Ministries Association and American Nurses Association: *Faith community nursing: scope & standards*, Washington, DC, 2012, American Nurses Association.

Hickman JS: *Faith community nursing*, Philadelphia, 2007, Lippincott Williams & Wilkins.

Holistic Health Centers: *Survey research report*, Hinsdale, IL, 1976, Society for Holistic Medicine.

Interfaith Health Program: *Strong partners: interfaith health program*, Atlanta, GA, 2005, Emory University.

International Parish Nurse Resource Center: *Basic parish nurse preparation curriculum*, St. Louis, 2009, Deaconess Parish Nurse Ministries.

International Parish Nurse Resource Center: *Role of parish nurse, mission and resources*, Memphis, TN, 2013a, Church Health Center.

International Parish Nurse Resource Center: *International parish nursing*, Memphis, TN, 2013b, Church Health Center.

Jacobsen D, Hustedt Jacobsen R: How religion is making a comeback on college campuses, Daily Beast, December 23, 2012. Available from <http://www.thedailybeast.com/articles/2012/12/23/how-religion-is-making-a-comeback-on-college-campuses.html>.

King MA, Tessaro I: Parish nursing: promoting health lifestyles in the church, *J Christ Nurs* 26(1):22–24, 2009.

Koenig HG, George L: Religion, spirituality, and health in hospitalized older patients, *J Am Geriatr Soc* 52A:532–541, 2004.

Koenig HG, King D, Carson VB: *The handbook of religion and health*, ed 2, New York, 2012, Oxford.

Maginnis and Associates: *Combining health care and theology: the parish nurse (Maginnis Communique)*, Louisville, KY, 1993, Author.

McEwen M: Spiritual nursing care, *Holistic Nursing Practice* 19:161–168, 2005.

McGinnis DL: The emerging role of faith community nurses in prevention & management of chronic disease, *Policy Polit Nurs Pract* 9(3):173–180, 2008.

Mendelson SG, McNeese-Smith D, Koniak-Griffin D, et al.: A community-based parish nurse intervention program for Mexican-American women with gestational diabetes, *JOGN* 37(4):415–425, 2008.

Myers DG: Stress and health: spirituality and faith communities. In Myers DG, editor: *Psychology*, ed 7, New York, 2004, Worth Publishers.

Myers DG: Religion and human flourishing. In Eid M, Larsen R, editors: *The science of subjective well-being*, New York, 2008, Guilford.

National Center on Elder Abuse: 2013. Available from <www.ncea.aoa.gov/ncearoot/Main_Site/pdf/publication/FinalStatistics050331.pdf>.

North American Nursing Diagnosis Association: *NANDA nursing diagnosis: definitions and defining characteristics*, Philadelphia, 1992, Author.

O'Brien ME: *Parish nursing: Healthcare ministry within the church*, Sudbury, MA, 2003, Jones and Bartlett.

Patterson D: Parish nursing: a beneficial partner for clergy, *The Clergy Journal* 53:32–33, 2004.

Schnorr MA: *Spiritual nursing care: theory and curriculum development*, Doctoral dissertation. DeKalb, IL, 1988, Northern Illinois University (Dissert Abstr Int 50:601-A, DA8912525).

Schnorr MA: Parish nurse pedagogy or andragogy. In *Proceedings of the 17th Annual Westberg Parish Nurse Symposium*, St. Louis, MO, 2003, International Parish Nurse Resource Center.

Shaughnessy MA: *Ministry and the law: what you need to know*, New York, 1998, Paulist Press.

Smith SD: *Parish nursing: a handbook for the new millennium*, New York, 2003, Haworth Pastoral Press.

Solari-Twadell PA, McDermott MA: *Parish nursing: Promoting whole person health within faith communities*, Thousand Oaks, CA, 1999, Sage.

Solari-Twadell PA, McDermott MA: *Parish nursing: Development, education, and administration*, Thousand Oaks, CA, 2006, Sage.

Swanson KM: Empirical development of a middle range theory of caring, *Nursing Research* 40(3):161–166, 1991.

Tsuang MT, Williams WM, Lyons MJ: Pilot study of spiritual and mental health in twins, *Am J Psychiatry* 159:486–488, 2002.

U.S. Department of Health and Human Services: *Healthy people 2010*, Washington, DC, 2010, Government Printing Office. Also available at <www.healthypeople.gov>.

U.S. Department of Health and Human Services (DHHS), National Center on Elder Abuse, Administration on Aging: *Statistics and data*, n.d. Available from <www.ncea.aoa.gov/library/Data.index.aspx#problem>.

Watson MF: New dimensions in human caring theory, *Nursing Science Quarterly* 1(4):175–181, 1998.

Westberg G: *The parish nurse: Providing a minister of health for your congregation*, Minneapolis, 1990, Augsburg.

Westberg G: A personal historical perspective of whole person health and the congregation. In Williams DR, Sternthal MJ, editors: *Spirituality, religion and health: evidence and research directions, Med J Aust* 186(10 Suppl):S47–S50, 2007.

Williams DR, Sternthal MJ: Spirituality, religion and health: evidence and research directions, *Med J Aust* 186(10 Suppl):S47–S50, 2007.

Wolf ZR: The caring concept and nurse identified caring behaviors, *Topics in Clinical Nursing* 8(2):84–93, 1986.

Wolf ZR, Zuzelo PR, Costello R, et al.: Development and testing of the caring behaviors: Inventory for elders, *International Journal of Holistic Care* 8(1):48–54, 2004.

Wright LM: *Spirituality, suffering and illness*, Philadelphia, 2005, FA Davis.

Home Health and Hospice

Carrie L. Buch and Mary A. Nies

KEY TERMS

advance directive
durable power of attorney
home health care
living will

OUTLINE

Home Health Care
  Purpose of Home Health Services
Types of Home Health Agencies
  Official Agencies
  Nonprofit Agencies
  Proprietary Agencies
  Hospital-Based Agencies
Certified and Noncertified Agencies
Special Home Health Programs
Reimbursement for Home Care
OASIS
Nursing Standards and Educational Preparation of Home Health Nurses
Conducting a Home Visit
  Visit Preparation
  The Referral

  Initial Telephone Contact
  Environment
  Improving Communication
  Building Trust
Documentation of Home Care
Application of the Nursing Process
  Assessment
  Diagnosis and Planning
  Intervention
  Evaluation
Formal and Informal Caregivers
Hospice Home Care
  Caring for the Caregiver
  Pain Control and Symptom Management
  Cultural Differences Related to Death and Dying

♥ **HEALTHY PEOPLE 2020**

2020 Objectives for Home Health and Hospice Care

> *MICH HP2020-14:* Increase the proportion of children with special health care needs who receive their care in family-centered, comprehensive, coordinated systems.
> *MICH HP2020-24:* Increase the percentage of women giving birth who attend a postpartum care visit with a health worker.
> *OA-HP2020-2:* Reduce the proportion of unpaid caregivers of older adults who report an unmet need for caregiver support services.
> *OA-HP2020-4:* Reduce the proportion of non-institutionalized older adults with disabilities who have an unmet need for long-term services and supports.

From HealthyPeople.gov: *Healthy People 2020: Topics & objectives, 2013.* Retrieved from <http://www.healthypeople.gov/2020/topicsobjectives2020/default.aspx>.

The purpose of home health services is to provide nursing care to individuals and their families in their homes. The specific objectives and services nurses offer vary according to the type of agency providing services and the population served. Nurses who work for public health departments, visiting nurse associations, home health agencies, hospice agencies, or school districts usually provide home visits.

Nurses from clinics or health departments often conduct home visits as part of patient follow-up. These public health nurses make visits to follow patients with communicable diseases and to provide health education and community referrals to patients with identified health problems. Home health nurses who work for home health agencies that are affiliated with hospitals or nursing registries often make home visits to assist patients in their transition from the hospital to home. In addition, health care providers in private practice may order these visits when patients experience exacerbation of chronic conditions.

The focus of all home visits is on the individual for whom the referral is received. In addition, the nurse assesses the individual-family interaction and provides education and interventions for the family and the client. The nurse evaluates how the individual and family interact as part of an aggregate group in the community. The nurse identifies the need for referrals to community services and performs the referrals as necessary.

Nurses who make home visits receive referrals from a variety of sources, including the patient's physician, nurse practitioner or nurse midwife, hospital discharge planner or case manager, schoolteacher, and clinic health care provider. The patient or the patient's family can also originate requests for nursing visits to assess and assist in the client's health care.

Home visits have been an integral part of nursing for more than a century, originating with Florence Nightingale's "health nurses" in England. In the United States in 1877, the Women's Branch of the New York City Mission sent the first trained nurses into the homes of the poor to provide nursing care. Under the direction of Lillian Wald, pioneering efforts were initiated to provide services to the poor in their homes in the late nineteenth century (Kelly and Joel, 1995).

HOME HEALTH CARE

The term **home health care** describes a system in which health care and social services are provided to homebound or disabled people in their homes rather than in medical facilities (U.S. Department of Commerce and International Trade Administration, 1990). The U.S. Department of Health and Human Services (USDHHS) set forth a definition of home health care that an interdepartmental work group developed, which follows:

> *Home health care is that component of a continuum of comprehensive health care whereby health services are provided to individuals and families in their places of residence for the purpose of promoting, maintaining or restoring health, or maximizing the level of independence, while minimizing the effects of disability and illness, including terminal illness. Services appropriate to the needs of the individual patient and family are planned, coordinated, and made available by providers organized for the delivery of home care through the use of employed staff, contractual arrangements, or combination of the two patterns. (Warhola, 1980)*

Purpose of Home Health Services

The primary purpose of home health services is to allow individuals to remain at home and receive health care services that would otherwise be offered in a health care institution, such as a hospital or nursing home setting. The home health industry grew tremendously in the 1980s but began to decline in the 1990s in relation to changes in Medicare home health reimbursement. However, with the development of the home health prospective payment system (PPS), the number of home care agencies has increased since 2001 (National Association for Home Care and Hospice [NAHC], 2010). Numerous factors generated the growth of home health services, including the rising costs of hospital care and the subsequent introduction of the PPS by P.L. 98-21 of the Social Security Amendments in 1983. Under the PPS, hospitals receive a fixed amount of money based on the relative cost of resources used to treat Medicare patients within each type of diagnosis-related group (Guterman and Dobson, 1986). Moreover, many other third-party payers negotiate preferred provider programs or managed care systems. In a managed care arrangement, the health care provider is paid a set fee for providing care to clients enrolled in the program. Providing home care services contributes to cost containment in a managed care environment. This cost containment is accomplished through timely hospital discharges and by providing nursing services in the home setting and supporting clients at home rather than in skilled facilities. Home care is also popular with consumers, who prefer to receive care in their own homes rather than in an institution.

Home health care services have changed to address the needs of the population. Home health nurses visit acutely ill clients, patients with acquired immunodeficiency syndrome, the elderly, terminally ill clients, high-risk pregnant women, and ill infants and children (Feldman, 1993). Home health care continues to focus on the care of sick patients and could expand to include health promotion and disease prevention interventions. Currently, most reimbursement for nursing services is based on the patient's need for skilled nursing. On each patient visit, the nurse must document that the care provided is of a skilled nature that requires the knowledge and assessment skills of a nurse and must verify that the patient or a family member could not provide the same level of care.

Services coordinated in the home include not only skilled nursing care provided by registered nurses (RNs) but also the services of physical, occupational, and speech therapists; social workers; and home health aides. The broader home care industry definition of *home health care* includes supportive social services, respite care, community nursing centers, group boarding homes, homeless shelters, adult day care, intermediate-skilled extended care facilities, and assisted living facilities (American Nurses Association [ANA], 2008).

TYPES OF HOME HEALTH AGENCIES

Home health agencies differ in financial structure, organizational structure, governing board, and population served. The most common types of home health agencies are official (i.e., public), nonprofit, proprietary, chains, and hospital-based agencies. The number of freestanding proprietary agencies has grown faster than that of any other type of Medicare-certified home health agency. Freestanding proprietary agencies now account for 62% of all home health agencies, and hospital-based agencies for 12% of all certified home health agencies (NAHC, 2010).

There continues to be an increase in the number of managed care agencies, which may have any type of financial structure. Managed care agencies contract with payers, such as insurance companies, to provide specified services to the enrolled clients at predetermined prices. Managed care agencies receive payment before offering services and are responsible for taking the financial risk of providing care to patients within the budgeted allotment. This arrangement works well with large numbers of enrolled clients, because the financial risk is spread across a larger number of people, many of whom are healthy and will not require skilled services.

Official Agencies

Local or state governments organize, operate, and fund official (i.e., public) home health agencies. These agencies may be part of a county public health nursing service or a home health agency that operates separately from the public health nursing service but is located within the county public health system. Taxpayers fund official home health agencies, but the agencies also receive reimbursement from third-party payers such as Medicare, Medicaid, and private insurance companies.

Nonprofit Agencies

Nonprofit home health agencies include all home health agencies that are not required to pay federal taxes because of their exempt tax status. Nonprofit groups reinvest any profits into the agencies. Nonprofit home health agencies include independent home health agencies and hospital-based home health agencies. Not all hospital-based home health agencies are nonprofit, even if the hospital is nonprofit. The home health agency can be established as a profit-generating service and serve as a source of revenue for the hospital or medical center. In this situation, the home health agency is categorized organizationally as for-profit and it pays federal taxes on the profits.

Proprietary Agencies

Proprietary home health agencies are classified for-profit and pay federal taxes on the profits generated. Proprietary agencies can be individually owned agencies, profit partnerships, or profit corporations. Provided that the agencies make profits, investors in corporate proprietary partnerships receive financial returns on their investments in the agencies. A percentage of the profits generated are also reinvested into the agencies. Agencies within chains have a financial advantage over single agencies. The chains have lower administrative costs because a larger single corporate structure provides many services. For example, a multiagency corporation has greater purchasing power for supplies and equipment because it purchases a larger volume. A single corporate office can provide administrative services such as payroll and employee benefits for all chain employees, thereby avoiding duplication of these services at each location. Criticism of proprietary and chain agencies includes concerns over the quality of services provided by agencies that are profit driven.

Hospital-Based Agencies

Since the implementation of the home health PPS, the number of hospital-based home health agencies has significantly increased (NAHC, 2010). This trend is not surprising in light of the fixed reimbursement under PPS and the hospitals' incentive to decrease patients' length of stay. By establishing home health agencies, hospitals are able to discharge patients who have skilled health care needs, provide the necessary services to the patients, and receive reimbursement through third-party payers such as Medicare, Medicaid, and private insurance companies. The rising number of home health agencies affiliated with hospitals indicates that these agencies are profitable endeavors that provide hospitals with an additional revenue source.

CERTIFIED AND NONCERTIFIED AGENCIES

Certified home health agencies meet federal standards; therefore they are able to receive Medicare payments for services provided to eligible individuals. Not all home health agencies are certified. The number of Medicare-certified home health agencies increased to approximately 10,444 in 1997, decreased to 6861 in 2001, and increased to 10,581 in 2009 (NAHC, 2010).

The noncertified home care agencies, home care aide organizations, and hospices remain outside the Medicare system. Some operate outside the system because they provide non–Medicare-covered services. For example, they do not provide skilled nursing care and are not eligible to receive Medicare reimbursement.

SPECIAL HOME HEALTH PROGRAMS

Many home health agencies offer special, high-technology home care services. Offering high tech services at home is both beneficial to the patient's health and financially advantageous. Through the implementation of these special programs, patients who require continuous skilled care in an acute or skilled nursing institution are able to return to receive care in their homes. From the financial perspective, skilled services provided at home are less costly than hospitalization.

Examples of special services are home intravenous therapy programs for patients who require daily infusions of total parenteral nutrition or antibiotic therapy, pediatric services for children with chronic health problems, follow-up for premature infants who are at risk for complications, ventilator therapy, and home dialysis programs. The key to the success of all these programs is the patient's, family's, or caregiver's ability to learn the care necessary for a successful home program and the motivation of these individuals to provide the care. If family or caregiver support is not available in the home, the patient cannot be a candidate for any of these programs, and other arrangements for care must be found.

Home dialysis programs are a growing trend. Through such programs, patients learn how to do dialysis at home with a helper who is often a family member or friend. Patients and their helpers receive 3 to 8 weeks of training from the dialysis clinic to learn how to use the equipment, monitor their vital signs, and keep good records of their treatment. The clinic provides the machine and all of the supplies and furnishes 24-hour telephone support. The patient follows up at the clinic monthly to ensure that treatments are working and to discuss any issues or concerns (National Kidney and Urologic Diseases Information Clearinghouse [NKUDIC], 2010).

REIMBURSEMENT FOR HOME CARE

Before the establishment of Medicare in 1965, individuals who required home health services paid cash for the services; donations to the service agency providers helped subsidize care services for patients who were unable to pay (Kent and Hanley, 1990). Since 1965, individuals who are eligible for Medicare benefits under Title XVIII of the Social Security Act or for Medicaid benefits under Title XIX and people with private health insurance have been reimbursed by the federal government through the Medicare program to receive short-term, skilled health care services in their homes. Provided services include nursing care, social service, physical therapy, occupational therapy, and speech therapy, and the program is individualized to meet each patient's needs.

Any individual older than 65 years who is homebound, under the care of a physician, and requires medically necessary skilled nursing care or therapy services may be eligible for home care through a Medicare-certified home health agency. These services must be intermittent or part-time and require physician authorization and periodic review of the plan of care. The only exception is hospice care. Any individual older than 65 years who is certified by a physician or a nurse practitioner (NP) to be terminally ill with a life expectancy of 6 months is eligible to receive the Medicare Hospice Benefit (DHHS, 2013). There is no requirement for the individual to be homebound or in need of skilled care or for the services to be intermittent or part-time. The hospice physician or hospice NP must recertify the patient after the first 90 days and then every 60 days to determine whether he or she is still eligible for hospice care (DHHS, 2013).

The rapid growth of the home health market is reflective of the following:

- Increasing proportion of people aged 65 years and older
- Lower average cost of home health care compared with institutional costs
- Active insurer support for home care
- Medicare promotion of home health care as an alternative to institutionalization

Patient or family payments comprise 46% of the private financing (12% of total spending) for home health services. Private health insurance and nonpatient revenue pay the remaining private financing. Private health insurance includes managed care plans that often involve pre-approval of services and referrals from primary care providers. Private insurance companies require pre-certification to verify patient eligibility for services. The home care RN speaks to the RN at the insurance company, who determines the number of visits that the insurance company covers. In contrast, for Medicare patients, the home care RN determines the schedule and number of visits without calling Medicare to get pre-approval. Medicare pays the home care agency a predetermined amount based on the health condition and needs of the patient. Medicare pays for home care services based on 60-day episodes. If a patient is still eligible for home care services after the first episode, a second episode can begin. There are no limits to the number of episodes for each patient. However, if the patient receives four visits or fewer per episode, the home health care agency is paid a standardized per visit amount instead of an episode payment. These payment adjustments are called Low Utilization Payment Adjustments (Centers for Medicare and Medicaid Services [CMS], 2013).

Between 1967 and 1985, the number of home health agencies certified to provide care to Medicare recipients tripled, from 1,753 to 5,983. In the mid-1980s, this number leveled off at 5900 as a result of an increase in the volume of paperwork required and unreliable payment policies. This led to a lawsuit against the Health Care Financing Administration (HCFA) charged by Representatives Harley Staggers (D-WV) and Claude Pepper (D-FL), and a coalition of members of the U.S. Congress, consumer groups, and the NAHC. The successful conclusion of the lawsuit gave NAHC the opportunity to participate in rewriting the Medicare home care payment policies. New payment policies brought an increase in the home health benefit and increased the number of Medicare-certified home health agencies to more than 10,000. The number is now declining as a direct result of the changes in Medicare home health reimbursement enacted as part of the Balanced Budget Act of 1997. However, because of this decline, the CMS enacted a new payment system whereby home care agencies are reimbursed on a prospective payment system based on the patient's diagnosis. The amount provided to home health agencies is determined on the basis of the average national cost of treating a home health client for 60 days. The goal of this system is to encourage efficient use of home health services without sacrificing quality (NAHC, 2010).

OASIS

The Outcome and Assessment Information Set (OASIS) is a data set that determines Medicare pay rate and measures outcomes for adult home care patients to monitor outcome-based quality improvement. The data set includes sociodemographic, environmental, support system, health status, and functional status attributes of adult patients as well as information about service utilization. These items are used to monitor outcomes, plan patient care, provide reports on patient characteristics for each agency, and evaluate and improve clinical performance. Nurses must use OASIS for all patients receiving skilled care that is reimbursed by Medicare and Medicaid (CMS, 2008).

NURSING STANDARDS AND EDUCATIONAL PREPARATION OF HOME HEALTH NURSES

The ANA (2008) has revised its standards for home health nursing practice. According to the ANA, the generalist home care nurse should be educated at the baccalaureate level because of the autonomy and critical thinking skills that are necessary in home care. The generalist home health nurse must have community health assessment skills to assess client and caregiver needs, provide client and caregiver education, perform nursing actions following the client's plan of care, manage resources to facilitate the best possible outcomes, provide and monitor care, collaborate with other disciplines and providers to coordinate client care, and supervise ancillary staff and caregivers. In home care, the nurse has a primary function of managing an interdisciplinary team that includes physical therapists, occupational therapists, social workers, nurse assistants, chaplains, and so on. In addition, the responsibilities of the generalist home health nurse include, but are not limited to, performing holistic, periodic assessments of client and family/caregiver resources; participating in performance improvement activities; collecting and using research findings to evaluate the plan of care; educating clients and families on health promotion and self-care activities; being a client advocate; promoting continuity of care; using the *Scope and Standards of Home Health Nursing Practice* to guide clinical practice; and identifying ethical issues and exploring options with the necessary individuals and staff members to achieve resolution (ANA, 2008).

In addition to the ANA standards, home health nurses should use the competencies developed by the QSEN (Quality and Safety Education for Nurses) Institute as a guide for best practices in home care (QSEN Institute, n.d.). The QSEN competencies were developed by a national advisory board that included distinguished faculty to establish effective teaching approaches to ensure that nurses graduate with essential competencies in: (1) patient-centered care, (2) teamwork and collaboration, (3) evidence-based practice, (4) quality improvement, (5) safety, and (6) informatics. These six competencies in QSEN are being used by several health care institutions to monitor and ensure that their nurses are providing safe, high-quality patient care.

The advanced practice home health nurse has a master's or doctoral degree in nursing and can perform all of the duties of the generalist home health nurse. In addition, the advanced practice nurse contributes significant clinical expertise to home health patients and their families, demonstrates proficiency in care management and consultation, and is an expert in implementing and evaluating health programs, resources, services, and research for clients with complex conditions. The duties of the advanced practice home health nurse include, but are not limited to, prescribing pharmacological and nonpharmacological treatment to manage chronic illnesses, providing consultation and serving as a resource to the generalist home health nurse, participating at all levels of quality improvement and research, educating all members of the health care team about emerging trends in home health care, performing direct care of the client and family, managing and evaluating the care the client is receiving from caregivers, monitoring trends in reimbursement for home health services, consulting with staff about any ethical issues that may arise, managing an interdisciplinary team, and disseminating practice and research findings to colleagues (ANA, 2008).

Albrecht's conceptual model (1990) for home care clearly identifies educational content areas for students in undergraduate and graduate nursing programs that have specialties in home health care. An underlying premise of the model is that professional satisfaction and effective patient outcomes depend on the education and experience of the home health nurse. Implications that are apparent in the model include the following (Albrecht, 1990, p. 125):

- Nursing programs at the undergraduate and graduate levels must prepare competent providers of home health care.
- Curricula must include concepts related to the suprasystem, health service delivery system, and home subsystem, which includes structural, process, and outcome elements.
- Students at the undergraduate level need at least one clinical observation or experience in a home care agency.
- Graduate-level students need specific courses that cover concepts present in the model, including knowledge of education; preventive, supportive, therapeutic, and high-tech nursing interventions for home health care; a multidisciplinary approach to home health care; health law and ethics; systems theory; economics covering supply, demand, and productivity; and case management and coordination.

The home health nurse serves as a case manager for patients who receive care either from the staff of the home health agency or through contract services. The success of the case management plan is contingent upon the nurse's ability to use the nursing process to develop a plan of treatment that best fits the individual needs of the patient and the patient's family or caregiver. Patient and family assessment is the first step in developing the treatment plan and nursing care plan.

The Albrecht nursing model for home health care provides a framework for nurses, patients, and their families to interact and identify mutual goals of interventions and promote the patient's self-care capability at home (Figure 33-1) (Albrecht, 1990). Three major elements for measuring the quality of home health care patient outcomes are structural, process, and outcome elements.

Structural elements include the client, family, provider agency, health team, and professional nurse. The process elements include the type of care, coordination of care, and intervention. Outcome elements consist of patient and family satisfaction with care, quality of care, cost-effectiveness of care, health status, and self-care capability.

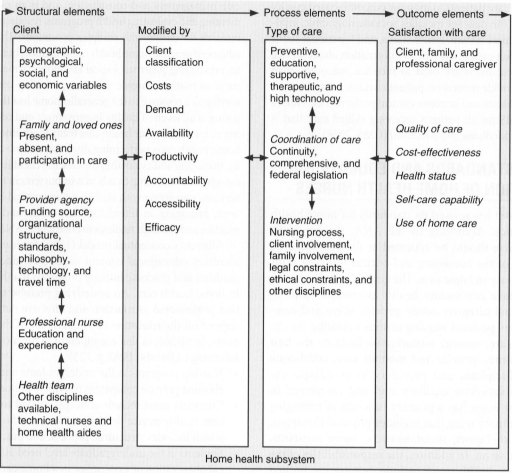

Structural elements →		Process elements →	Outcome elements →
Client	**Modified by**	**Type of care**	**Satisfaction with care**
Demographic, psychological, social, and economic variables	Client classification	Preventive, education, supportive, therapeutic, and high technology	Client, family, and professional caregiver
	Costs		
	Demand		
Family and loved ones Present, absent, and participation in care	Availability	*Coordination of care* Continuity, comprehensive, and federal legislation	*Quality of care*
	Productivity		*Cost-effectiveness*
	Accountability		*Health status*
Provider agency Funding source, organizational structure, standards, philosophy, technology, and travel time	Accessibility	*Intervention* Nursing process, client involvement, family involvement, legal constraints, ethical constraints, and other disciplines	*Self-care capability*
	Efficacy		*Use of home care*
Professional nurse Education and experience			
Health team Other disciplines available, technical nurses and home health aides			

Home health subsystem

FIGURE 33-1 Albrecht nursing model for home health care. (Based on Albrecht MN: The Albrecht model for home health care: implications for research, practice, and education, *Public Health Nurs* 7:118-126, 1990. Reprinted by permission of Blackwell Scientific Publications, Inc.).

In the Albrecht model for home care, the relationship between the structural elements and the process elements directs the interventions. The nurse executes the nursing process, including assessment, nursing diagnosis, planning, intervention, and evaluation, and then the nurse coordinates patient care (Albrecht, 1990).

CONDUCTING A HOME VISIT

Visit Preparation

It is important that the nurse prepare for the home visit by reviewing the referral form, which should furnish the purpose of the visit, the geographic residence of the family, and any other pertinent information. The first home visit gives the nurse the opportunity to establish a trust relationship with the client and family to establish credibility as a resource for health information and community referrals in a nonthreatening environment.

The Referral

The referral is a formal request for a home visit. Referrals come from a variety of sources, including hospitals, clinics, health care providers, individuals, and families. The type of

agency that receives the referral varies, depending on the necessary client services. Public health referrals are made for clients who are in need of health education (e.g., infant care education and resource allocation) or for follow-up of clients with communicable diseases.

Home health referrals are requested to provide clients with short-term, intermittent, skilled services and rehabilitation. Visits can last from 30 to 90 minutes and are scheduled on an intermittent basis according to the specific needs of the client. For example, a client who had a stroke requires skilled nursing assessments, physical therapy visits for gait training, speech therapy for speech deficit improvement, and occupational therapy for retraining in activities of daily living (ADLs) such as bathing and cooking.

By reviewing the referral form before the first visit, the community health nurse (CHN) obtains basic information about the client, such as name, age, diagnosis or health status, address, telephone number, insurance coverage, and reason for the referral. The form also specifies the source of the referral—clinician, health care provider, communicable disease service, hospital, client, or client's family.

Public health referrals usually provide information on the client's condition that necessitates public health nurse (PHN) visits. For example, for a client who is positive for tuberculosis (TB), the PHN is notified of the client's place of residence, type and location of employment, and any known contacts, including family and friends. Another example of a public health referral is one to a 16-year-old girl for antepartum visits because she is 7 months' pregnant and has just initiated prenatal care.

Additional information provided in the home health referral includes current client medications, prescribed diet, physician's orders, care plan goals, and other disciplines involved in the client's care. This information is important because it helps the nurse become familiar with the client's condition.

Initial Telephone Contact

The nurse contacts the client and informs him or her about the service referral. The first telephone contact with the client or family consists of an exchange of essential information, including an introduction by the nurse, identification of the agency that received the referral, and the purpose of the visit. After the initial exchange of information, the nurse informs the client of his or her desire to make the home visit, the client gives permission, and the group sets a mutually acceptable time for the visit. The nurse is a guest in the client's home; therefore, it is important that the client agrees to the visit. The nurse then verifies the client's address and asks for specific directions to the client's home.

During a home health visit, the nurse requests proof of insurance, such as a Medicare, Medicaid, health maintenance organization membership identification, or insurance card. The nurse should forewarn the client so the client or family can locate the information before the visit. If the client is unable to provide this verification, the nurse assists with locating the information during the visit. Clients who receive a public health home visit do not require evidence of insurance coverage because these services are not billed directly. County public health budgets or state or federally funded programs generally cover these visits.

Not all clients have telephones. For a client without one, the nurse should check the referral for a telephone number where messages can be left. It is also worthwhile to contact the health care provider who made the referral to see whether the telephone number was omitted unintentionally. If the client does not have a telephone, the nurse may choose to make a drop-in visit. This type of visit consists of an unannounced visit to the client's home, during which the nurse explains the purpose of the referral, receives the client's permission for the visit, and appoints a time for a future visit with the client. The client may agree to have the first visit while the nurse is there.

If the client is not at home for the drop-in visit, the nurse should leave an official agency card and a brief message asking the client to contact the agency to schedule a nursing visit. The nurse informs the referring agency that the visit was attempted but that the client was not available for contact. A formal agency letter, identifying the agency and the reason for the referral, is often sent to clients who are difficult to contact. The nurse's primary responsibility, when he or she has been unsuccessful in locating the client, is to keep the clinic, physician, or referring agency informed of efforts to establish contact with the client.

Environment

An environmental assessment begins as the nurse leaves the agency en route to the client's home. The nurse should make specific observations, which follow (Keating and Kelman, 1998):

- How does the client's neighborhood compare with other neighborhoods in the area?
- Are there adequate shopping facilities, such as grocery stores, close to the client's home?

The nurse should also note the client's dwelling; for example, whether the client lives in a single-family home, in a single room in a home or hotel, in an apartment, or in a shared apartment or house. Specific assessments include the following:

- Is the client's residence easily accessible by the client given the client's age and functional ability? For example, if the client has limited endurance, can he or she negotiate several flights of stairs when entering or leaving the dwelling?
- Are handicapped facilities available as necessary? Is the dwelling in an area with high rates of drug abuse or crime?
- Is the building or home secure? Does the client live alone? If so, how does the client get to the physician or clinic? How does the client purchase groceries?
- Does the client have food in the home? If so, who prepares the client's meals? Are the meals nutritious?
- Are there rodents, cockroaches, or other potential vectors of disease present in the client's home?
- Does the client's home have hot running water, heat, sanitation facilities, and adequate ventilation?
- Is the client's residence safe relative to the client's physical status, or is the home cluttered with debris and furniture?

Improving Communication

When the nurse meets with the client, whether in the home or at another mutually agreeable location, the initial conversation revolves around social topics. The nurse assumes a friendly manner and asks general questions about the client, the client's family, and health care services that will benefit the client. These questions help the nurse assess the client's needs and create a comfortable atmosphere for communication.

Building Trust

Many clients in need of nursing visits do not trust the health care system and are uncomfortable with the representative from an agency visiting their home. For example, a client who is pregnant and does not have legal status in the United States will be hesitant to allow a nurse to visit; the client will be afraid of being reported to immigration authorities. The nurse's role in visiting this client is to focus on the health and safety of the client and her fetus. The nurse must build a trust relationship early in the visit or the client will not allow additional visits. If a trust relationship is not established and the client believes that the nurse will report her to immigration authorities, it is highly probable that the client will move to another location to avoid future contact.

DOCUMENTATION OF HOME CARE

The nurse documents assessment data and interventions for all home visits. The patient record also contains a copy of the nursing care plan. The patient must be homebound in order to receive home health care benefits. It is critical that the nurse document the homebound status of the patient at each visit.

Many home health nurses would probably identify documentation issues as the most frustrating part of providing home health care. Medicare holds a prominent position as a home health care payer; therefore the HCFA's regulations determine the home health industry's documentation. Correct and accurate completion of required Medicare forms is the key to reimbursement. For more information, the reader should visit http://www.cms.gov/Medicare/CMS-Forms/CMS-Forms/CMS-Forms-List.html. Payment or denial of payment for visits is based on the information presented on the forms. If the nurse does not clearly document the provided skilled care in the electronic nursing notes, the fiscal intermediaries will argue that the care was either unnecessary or not performed and will deny reimbursement. The home health nurse must have an excellent clinical foundation and the ability to identify and document actual and potential patient problems that require skilled nursing interventions (Morrissey-Ross, 1988).

Documenting the care provided to record the patient's quality of care is just as important as documenting for reimbursement purposes. The documentation of home visits records the nurse's observations, assessments of the patient's condition, provided interventions, and the patient's and family's ability to manage the care at home. In addition, documentation of patient visits serves as a formal communication system among other home health professionals who also interact with the patient and family.

APPLICATION OF THE NURSING PROCESS

Assessment

During the first home visit, the type of client assessment will vary depending on the purpose of the home visit. The home health nurse assesses the client's knowledge of his or her health status. The nurse identifies knowledge deficits and uses this information to develop a care plan.

Subjective information is obtained from the client and the client's family and includes the client's perception of the situation and what the client identifies as problems. The nurse assesses whether the client is isolated from others physically or socially and whether the client is a member of a close-knit, nurturing, supportive family or kinship network. The amount of support the client perceives as available may or may not be accurate; therefore the nurse asks several questions about the client's family, friends, and daily routine to assess the client's level of social support.

During the first home visit, the home health nurse assesses the client's health knowledge; his or her physical, functional, and psychosocial status; physical environment; and social support. The nurse collects information through observations, and questions the patient and family or caregivers in the home environment. It is not unusual to find inconsistencies between information the patient provides during hospitalization about the amount of physical and emotional support available to the patient in the home and the amount of help actually available to the patient in the home. The nurse validates or modifies the referral information to reflect the actual home situation. Home health nurses often use contracts that the nurse, patient, and family jointly develop to delineate the responsibilities of the patient in the home.

The client's physical assessment is generally performed in the home health visit and includes a review of all systems, with an emphasis on the systems affected by the client's present condition. The nurse obtains objective data through the use of essential physical assessment skills, such as observation, palpation, auscultation, and percussion. The physical assessment also includes information regarding the client's functional status. Assessment of the functional status is important for Medicare reimbursement and for the development of an individualized plan of care. This assessment includes information regarding the client's ability to ambulate, to perform ADLs independently, and to use an assist device such as a cane or wheelchair. Specific functional limitations, such as shortness of breath and muscle weakness, are assessed at this time.

Information obtained during the assessment phase is used to identify nursing diagnoses and develop a plan of care. Data collection continues while the patient receives home health services. Changes in the patient's condition, environment, or social structure necessitate modifications in the treatment plan and the nursing care plan.

There are differences between the treatment plan and the nursing care plan. The plan of treatment includes the type of home health services received, the projected frequency of visits by each discipline (Albrecht, 1991), and the necessary interventions. The nursing care plan addresses specific nursing interventions designed to treat the patient's actual or potential problems and includes identified goals with measurable outcomes.

Diagnosis and Planning
Develop a Plan for the Client and Family

After the assessment phase of the home visit, the nurse identifies the nursing diagnoses that address the patient's problems and identifies actual or potential problems. The identification of nursing diagnoses serves as the basis for the nursing care plan. This plan is developed in consultation with the client and the family. The plan identifies short-term and long-term goals and measurable outcomes for the patient. The plan identifies nursing interventions that are necessary and additional home health services that are appropriate to help the patient achieve the identified goals. To maximize the plan's success, it is important that the patient and family are involved in the planning process and that they access community resources. Planning is a dynamic process that continues while the patient receives nursing services. The plan is modified as needed, depending on the patient's condition, until the identified goals are met.

Often the nurse develops a contract with the client that delineates the role and responsibilities of the nurse regarding the client's health and the role of the client and family (Spradley, 1990). If the client expresses a disinterest in contracting to improve health during the planning phase, the nurse will be limited in possible interventions. Goals are identified that the client is willing to work toward with the nurse's assistance.

The goal of home visits for both public health and home health nursing is to involve the client and family in taking an active role in health promotion. The nurse is careful not to allow the client to become dependent on the nurse's interventions, because the nurse's involvement is short term.

Outline the Client and Family Roles

Written contracts are helpful for both the nurse and the client because the client's role and the nurse's role in implementing the plan are clearly delineated (Spradley, 1990). If either the client or the nurse forgets his or her role in the plan, the written contract becomes a reference. The client and the nurse can modify the contract by mutual agreement.

Intervention

Implementation of the care plan begins during the first home visit. The nurse begins to provide the client and family with health information concerning the client's health status and informs them about the availability of and access to community resources. In the case of the home health visit, the nurse provides skilled nursing care. At the end of the initial home visit, the nurse discusses the need for another home visit. The nurse and client discuss the goal of the next visit; specifically, they discuss what the client should do before the visit. The nurse informs the client and family about any information or skills he or she will provide during the next visit, and the nurse and client agree on a day for the next visit.

Referral for Community Services

During the first visit, the nurse provides the client and family with information regarding community resources, including the purpose of the resources, their eligibility for the services provided, any involved expense, and agency telephone numbers. Referrals depend on the availability of community resources, the client's eligibility for the services, the client's and the family's willingness to use the services, and the resources' suitability for the client and family. Examples of such services are immunization clinics for children in the family; adult day care or senior centers for elderly clients who could benefit from socialization; adult education classes or continuation of high school for pregnant teen clients who have dropped out of high school; Meals on Wheels (MOW) services for clients who are not able to prepare meals; homeless shelters for men, women, and families; soup kitchens; resources for clothing and housing; mental health clinics; resources for battered spouses; and primary care clinics for low-income clients with and without insurance.

If necessary, the client or client's family may request the nurse's assistance in contacting the community resources. The client and family are encouraged to make the contacts, but if the client and family are unable to make the calls or do not speak English, the nurse needs to intervene on behalf of the client. By providing referral information during the first home visit, the nurse can follow up on the client's or the family's success in contacting and using community services.

Terminating the Visit

The nurse terminates the first visit when the assessment is completed and a care plan has been established with the client. The average visit should not exceed 1 hour. The client receives a great deal of information during that hour, and the nurse collects a great deal of information. Most clients are tired at the end of a 1-hour visit and often cannot retain additional information. It is preferable to set a date for another home visit to reinforce the information provided and to work progressively toward achieving goals.

Evaluation
Evaluation of Progress toward Goals

The evaluation phase occurs when the nurse can determine whether the mutually established goals are realistic and achievable for the patient and the patient's family. The evaluation process is continuous and allows the nurse to determine the success or progress toward the patient's identified goals. The nurse can identify the need for revisions in the nursing care plan and treatment plan through the collection of additional data during the evaluation phase. The nurse can intervene to make necessary changes. An example is an elderly wife who, during the initial home visit, stated that she preferred to provide the physical care for her frail, nonambulatory husband. On a subsequent visit, the nurse assessed that the patient was not receiving the care required for the patient's personal care, specifically bathing. The nurse discussed the problem with the wife and presented her with available options. These included the services of a home health aide to provide personal care and bathing three times a week. A new plan was developed, and it included the home health aide. The plan was implemented and evaluated during future visits. Input from the client is critical to determine whether the goals established are realistic and achievable for the client.

Modification of the Plan as Needed

The evaluation process also allows the nurse and client or family to discuss what is working well and where modifications are necessary in the plan. Evaluation occurs through open communication between the nurse and client, and the nurse asks questions about specific parts of the care plan. If a trust relationship exists, the client feels comfortable telling the nurse about problems in the care plan.

When Goals Are Achieved

The overall purpose of home visits is to assist the client with necessary information and nursing care to enable the client to function successfully without nursing interventions. When the care plan goals are achieved, the client does not need the nurse any longer. The client knows what community resources are available and how to access health care services for primary, secondary, and tertiary interventions.

FORMAL AND INFORMAL CAREGIVERS

Formal caregivers include professionals and paraprofessionals who provide in-home health care and personal services. They are compensated for the services they provide. The largest number of employees consists of home care aides and RNs. Informal caregivers are family members who are caring for the client. The presence or absence of an involved family member can make the difference between the successful completion of the plan of treatment, with the patient remaining in the home, and the need to transfer the patient to an extended-care facility or board-and-care facility. When a capable family member or caregiver is available to assist the patient, the home health nurse spends much of the visit assessing the skills of the caregiver. The home health nurse instructs the caregiver in the correct procedures for providing care and in recognizing the signs and symptoms of problems that must be reported to the health care provider. The goal of the home health nurse's instruction is to provide the caregiver with the skills necessary to care for the patient successfully in the home without intervention of the nurse or other members of the home health team.

The home health nurse faces a special challenge with patients who lack a family member or caregiver capable of learning and providing necessary care. When the patient lives alone and does not have caregivers, the nurse explores other resources available to supplement the patient's self-care activities in the home. For example, if the patient has extensive physical care needs and sufficient financial resources, the nurse may suggest hiring an attendant. Medicare and private insurance companies do not pay for attendant care. If the patient's income is low enough, in-home county support services may be an option. The nurse may consider other services for the patient, such as Meals on Wheels for nutritious meals delivered to the patient's home. Friendly Visitors, a volunteer service, sends a volunteer to the patient's home once a week or more to provide socialization for the patient. Other options that are available in some communities are adult day health centers and senior service centers. Both of these options require arranged patient transportation to and from the centers. A variety of transportation methods are available in different communities; volunteers may transport patients to the centers, or public transportation systems may be available, such as minivans, that provide door-to-door service. Selected services and referrals are based on the patient's individual needs and on the patient's level of functional ability.

⚖ ETHICAL INSIGHTS

Ethics: Home Health and Hospice Care

- Most legal and ethical issues in home health care involve the care of terminally ill patients.
- Early education about these issues is essential to the prevention of problems.
- Early education also gives patients the opportunity to make decisions for themselves and to communicate those decisions to family members and health care providers.
- All competent adults have the right to make decisions that will direct health care providers in the type of care they administer.
- This communication can occur through the completion of advance directives, durable power of attorney for health care, and living wills.

Advance Directive

An **advance directive** is a written document in which a competent person gives instructions about future health care in the event that the individual is unable to make decisions. These directives are completed on a voluntary basis. Medicare-certified health care agencies must ask patients about advance directives and must provide the patient with the advance directive form if the patient is interested in completing it.

Durable Power of Attorney for Health Care

A **durable power of attorney** for health care is one type of advance directive. Also called a health care proxy, the durable power of attorney for health care gives another person the power to make medical decisions related to care of the patient. This person, as identified by the patient, acts as the patient's agent in all decisions regarding health care, personal care, and custody in the event that the patient becomes incompetent or disabled and is unable to make decisions.

Living Will

A **living will** is a written document in which a patient voluntarily informs doctors and family members about the type of medical care desired should the patient become terminally ill or permanently unconscious and unable to communicate. In the living will, the patient can describe the type of care desired, depending on the clinical situation. For example, if the patient is terminally ill and unconscious, the patient can direct the health care team to perform only those measures that will provide comfort and nothing further. The patient can specifically indicate his or her opposition to lifesaving measures; for example, the patient may request the denial of cardiopulmonary life support in the event of a cardiac arrest. Other examples are indicating the exclusion of chemotherapy, blood transfusions, and respirator use in an attempt to prolong life.

HOSPICE HOME CARE

Hospice and palliative nursing care is becoming increasingly important as there is a tremendous need to improve end-of-life care for the terminally ill. Nurses who work with the terminally ill seek to enhance the patient's quality of life by focusing on relieving suffering throughout the illness, supporting the patient and family through the dying process, and providing grief support to the family after the patient has died (ANA, 2007). Hospice and palliative care nurses have a holistic approach to their patients and are responsible for taking a comprehensive health history and physical examination, including an evaluation of mental status; evaluating functional abilities; performing appropriate laboratory and diagnostic studies; determining effective pharmacological and nonpharmacological therapies to manage symptoms; identifying patient and/or family/caregiver goals; providing culturally competent care that is consistent with the patient's health beliefs, values, and practices; evaluating the patient's emotional state and the response to his or her illness and impending death; identifying coping strategies and support systems; evaluating financial resources; and conducting a spiritual assessment (ANA, 2007).

The advanced practice hospice and palliative nurse is an important role for nurses with a master's degree or higher in nursing. The advanced practice hospice and palliative nurse functions as an expert clinician who performs the duties of the generalist hospice nurse in addition to assuming the responsibilities of advanced-level care, which may include prescribing pharmacological treatment to manage symptoms. It is recommended that all advanced practice hospice and palliative nurses obtain certification in advanced practice hospice and palliative nursing (ANA, 2007).

Patients are admitted into hospice care when they have a life expectancy of 6 months or less, and the focus of care shifts from curative to comfort care. However, many patients with terminal illnesses want to continue curative treatments and are not ready to be admitted into a hospice program. Those patients who do not have a life expectancy of 6 months or less and/or want to continue curative treatment can receive the benefits of palliative care. Palliative care focuses on symptom management while the patient is still receiving other treatments, such as chemotherapy. It is important to note that Medicare fully covers all hospice-related expenses. Medicare covers all expenses, including medications, related to the terminal diagnosis. However, Medicare does not cover any expenses, including medications, related to other diagnoses.

Hospice and palliative nursing care is provided in a variety of settings, including hospitals, nursing homes, residential homes, and palliative care clinics. For the patient receiving hospice services in the home, the goal is to keep the client as comfortable at home as long as possible and to provide support and instruction to caregivers. Some patients insist on staying home until they die, and others allow their caregivers to decide whether they should remain at home or be admitted to an extended-care facility or a hospital. Each family unit has different needs, and each must be supported in its decisions. Home death should not be the standard that determines excellence in any case, nor should home death be the ultimate measure of "successful" home care. It is vital to realize that caring for a terminally ill person also includes caring for the family or caregivers. Not all caregivers want their loved one to die at home, and not all caregivers are capable of allowing that to happen. The goal of having a home death must be the goal of the patient and family, regardless of the nurse's personal preference.

When caring for a terminally ill person at home, the hospice nurse must be skilled in physical and psychosocial care for both the patient and the caregiver. The patient is viewed as a whole person, not as an isolated disease. Caring for a terminally ill person at home demands that the nurse view the family system as a unit. In addition, it is important to note that hospice care is a team approach. Each patient has a physician, a nurse, a social worker, a nurse assistant, and a spiritual counselor to provide a multidisciplinary, holistic approach to caring for that patient and his or her family. The team coordinates care with each other and additional resources, such as pain management, as necessary. Furthermore, many hospice agencies have weekly interdisciplinary meetings in which the various members of the hospice team meet to discuss the patients and work together to resolve issues and make sure the patients are receiving the best possible care.

Caring for the Caregiver

Although the dying patient is the focus of all skilled nursing care, the experienced home care nurse knows that a careful assessment of the caregiver's mental and physical health is important. The spouse, lover, children, friends, and neighbors who have made the commitment to stay until the end need the nurse's time and attention as much as, if not more than, the patient. Although the patient's wishes are important, all decisions regarding care are made considering the health of the caregivers. Gaynor (1990) found that women with more caregiving experience had more physical health problems than those with less caregiving experience and that younger women found caregiving more psychologically burdensome than older women. Nursing interventions must be directed toward preventing a decline in the caregiver's health.

Caregivers need reassurance that their judgment is sound, and they need reminders that they cannot do anything "wrong" if it is done for the patient's comfort. The caregivers must understand that they will not mistakenly overdose the patient, and they must be reminded repeatedly that the patient will not die from something they did or did not do. Caring for the terminally ill requires that the home care nurse is willing to nurse the entire family. In addition, the nurse must involve all members of the hospice team to ensure that the caregivers receive the care they need.

Pain Control and Symptom Management

Pain control is an important goal for hospice nurses and their patients. Hospice nurses perform regular pain assessments that involve asking patients the following questions about their pain: (1) history, (2) character (such as sharp, dull, aching), (3) severity or intensity, which is most commonly rated on a pain intensity scale from 0 to 10 with 0 being no pain and 10 being the worst pain imaginable, (4) location, (5) effects on quality of life, (6) precipitating factors, and (7) relieving factors (Norlander, 2008). It is vital that the hospice nurse not only performs regular pain assessments but also remembers that pain is highly subjective and every person experiences pain differently and uniquely; therefore, the patient's pain is whatever he or she says it is regardless of the nurse's objective evaluation of the situation.

Pain medication is administered in doses sufficient to keep the patient free of pain and is administered on a regular schedule to prevent pain from recurring before the next dose. Hospice methods of pain control are particularly well suited to home care. The vast majority of patients can be pain free until their deaths. The key to successful pain control for the terminally ill is to persuade patients to take their medications on a regular basis, not just when they "can't stand it any longer." Generally, these medications are long acting and are administered every 8 to 12 hours. In addition, patients have fast-acting pain medications to take for "breakthrough pain," which happens when the patient experiences an increase in pain before it is time for the next dose of scheduled pain medication. The fast-acting medications are generally administered every 1 to 2 hours as needed.

Many patients, especially the elderly, are afraid of becoming "junkies" or "druggies" and want to delay using pain medication until they "get really bad." Many people believe that using these medications signals "the end of the line," and they are amazed to learn that patients do well while receiving such agents for months, even years, before death occurs. Almost every family must learn that addiction is not the same as tolerance and that their physicians will not "cut off the supply" if they "take too much."

In addition to pain control, hospice nurses help in managing other symptoms such as nausea and vomiting, constipation, diarrhea, fatigue, and decreased appetite. Nurses assist patients in management of these symptoms through medications and/or strategies to help cope with the symptoms. Strategies include such things as increasing fluids to prevent constipation, frequent rest periods to minimize fatigue, and eating small amounts as desired to cope with the decrease in appetite. In addition, the nurse educates the patient and family that some of these symptoms, such as fatigue and decreased appetite, are related to the dying process and are signs that the patient is declining.

Furthermore, the nurse, along with other members of the hospice team, provides emotional support to patients and families as they adjust to the patient's impending death. The nurse educates the patient and family about what physical symptoms the patient will most likely experience as he or she approaches death. In addition, the nurse, along with the social worker and spiritual counselor, provides emotional support and helps the patient and family work through any anxiety or fears they have about dying. Finally, the nurse is there to support the family immediately after the patient dies,

and hospice provides bereavement support to families up to a year after the patient's death.

Cultural Differences Related to Death and Dying

When caring for patients and their families in hospice, the nurse must remember that beliefs, attitudes, and values about death, dying, grief, and loss are influenced by society and culture (TNEEL, 2003). However, these societal and cultural influences are often difficult to recognize. Furthermore, many individual differences within a cultural group, such as spirituality, age, and gender, affect a person's interpretation about the meaning of death. Although there are these individual differences, some general characteristics regarding death and dying are common to people of a certain cultural group. It is important to understand some of these differences to provide culturally sensitive care and ensure a peaceful and dignified death.

For example, among African Americans, health status should be reported to the eldest family member, spouse, or parents, and there is often open and public displays of emotion; although this possibility varies from person to person. African Americans generally care for dying elders at home until death is imminent and then they bring their loved one to the hospital, because some believe that death in the house brings bad luck. Among Mexican Americans, the extended family takes care of the sick and dying person, and there are often several family members present at the same time. In general, Mexican Americans prefer to die at home because the hospital environment may be too restrictive in meeting the needs of the extended family and because some believe that their spirit may get "lost" if they die at the hospital. In comparison, among American Indians some tribes prefer to remain close to the dying person, but other tribes avoid contact with the dying. Similarly, those tribes that prefer to avoid contact may prefer that their loved one dies in the hospital; whereas those tribes that prefer to remain close may prefer to have the person die at home.

These are just some examples of cultural characteristics that influence death and dying beliefs and practices. It is important to understand and respect the differing values and beliefs of patients and their families. Furthermore, it is essential to ask patients and/or families about their beliefs and practices to avoid overgeneralizations and to ensure that nursing care is patient-centered and culturally sensitive.

CASE STUDY 33-1   PUBLIC HEALTH VISIT: COMMUNICABLE DISEASE FOLLOW-UP

The public health nurse received a referral from the county hospital to see Ray, a 57-year-old white man with newly diagnosed TB. The first purpose of the referral was for the public health nurse to meet with the client to ensure that he received the appropriate information about TB and received follow-up medical care on a regular basis. The second purpose of the referral was for the public health nurse to meet with Ray and identify the people with whom he had been in close contact. The nurse then established contact with these people, notified them that they had been exposed to TB, and encouraged them to have follow-up tests for TB.

The nurse contacted Ray and established a time for the home visit. The nurse noted that he resided in a residential hotel in a lower-middle-class neighborhood of a large urban area. During the initial visit, the nurse discovered that the client was an unemployed construction worker. He did not know where he might have contracted TB. Ray assured the nurse that he was taking his medication as directed. He gave the nurse the names of the friends he played poker with every week at a hotel and told the nurse that he advised his friends to be tested for TB. The nurse made a note of the names and later talked with them individually by telephone. During these subsequent conversations, the nurse was very careful to maintain the client's confidentiality. The nurse informed these individuals that they could have been exposed to TB and that they should seek testing through their health care providers or through their local health department.

Ray indicated that he did not have family and he had minimal contact with other people besides his friends at the hotel. The nurse recorded this information on the communicable disease form and returned the information to the public health department's communicable disease division.

Assessment

The public health nurse's assessment of the client with a communicable disease involved the individual, family, and community. The public health nurse assessed whether the client received appropriate information and regular medical care for TB and whether the client followed the prescribed treatment regimen.

Although Ray stated that he did not have family, his friends in the hotel constituted a working support network. The public health nurse was familiar with kinship networks and their importance as alternative family systems (Stack, 1974). Nursing assessment of Ray's kinship network involved determining whether the members were tested for TB. In addition, the public health nurse assessed the client's network for the following:

- Network composition
- Network's knowledge of TB
- Functional capacity
- Network stressors
- Network strengths and weaknesses
- Network's ability to provide support for Ray
- Health beliefs and practices
- Use of health services

The public health nurse was aware that the number of new cases of TB in the community had increased over the past 12 months. The public health nurse further noted that there was an increase in the number of area residents immigrating from various developing countries, and that this population might be at increased risk for development of TB (Dowling, 1991).

Diagnosis

Individual

- Lack of awareness regarding the disease process and transmission of TB

Family

- Lack of awareness regarding the disease process and transmission of TB, location of communicable disease clinics, and the importance of screening those exposed to TB

Community

- Potential for development of TB among community residents, indicated by an increased incidence of new cases of TB over the past 12 months

Planning

A plan of care is established with mutually agreed-upon goals based on the nurse's assessment of the individual, family, and community.

Individual

Long-Term Goal

- Client will perform self-care activities related to treatment of TB and follow up as necessary with appropriate health care professionals.

Short-Term Goal

- Client will verbalize knowledge of transmission of TB; signs and symptoms of complications of TB; purpose, administration schedule, and side effects of medications.

Family

Long-Term Goal

- Support network members with positive test results will receive appropriate treatment.

Short-Term Goal

- Support network members will demonstrate basic knowledge of cause and transmission of TB and will agree to be tested for TB.

Community

Long-Term Goal

- Incidence of TB in the community will decrease over the next 3 years.

Short-Term Goal

- Community members will demonstrate knowledge of increased incidence of TB in their community and of available community resources for treatment and prevention of TB.

Intervention

Implementation of the plan of care for the client with TB occurs at the individual, family, and community levels.

Individual

The public health nurse referred Ray to the communicable disease clinic at the local health department. TB is a reportable communicable disease; therefore the public health nurse obtained information from the client regarding people with whom he had been in close contact.

Family

The public health nurse contacted members of Ray's support network and referred them to the communicable disease clinic as appropriate. The nurse provided these people with information concerning TB transmission and the importance of early treatment and follow-up.

Community

The public health nurse met with professionals from the communicable disease clinic and the health department and with members of the community to establish a program to raise public awareness about the increased incidence of TB in the community. The public was informed about the importance of preventive measures, the availability of community screening services for TB, and the existing health care resources in the community.

Evaluation

Individual

The client's knowledge of the disease process, transmission, treatment, and signs and symptoms of TB is an indicator in evaluating the care plan. Confirmation of the client's follow-up with the communicable disease clinic can also be used for evaluation.

Family

The support network's knowledge of the disease process, transmission, treatment, and signs and symptoms of TB is an indicator in evaluating the care plan. Confirmation of the support network's follow-up with the communicable disease clinic can also be used for evaluation.

Community

The incidence rate of TB in the community and the rate at which TB clinics and related resources are used are measures that can be used to evaluate the effectiveness of interventions at the aggregate level.

Levels of Prevention

The public health nurse is actively involved in all three levels of prevention through education programs, early detection programs,

Continued

CASE STUDY 33-1 PUBLIC HEALTH VISIT: COMMUNICABLE DISEASE FOLLOW-UP—cont'd

and appropriate referrals for patients with TB. Examples of each of these levels of prevention are as follows:

Primary

Goal: Prevention of specific disease occurrence such as TB.
* Development of programs that increase public awareness of the disease process and of the transmission, diagnosis, and treatment of TB.

Secondary

Goal: Early detection of existing conditions.
* Tuberculin skin testing and subsequent follow-up of positive test results.

Tertiary

Goal: To reduce the effects and spread of TB.
* Referral for early, effective treatment and education of clients for self-care.

CASE STUDY 33-2 PUBLIC HEALTH HOME VISIT: ANTEPARTUM CLIENT

The public health nurse received a referral to see a 17-year-old African-American woman named Ali, who was referred by the county prenatal clinic. Ali was 5 months pregnant with her third pregnancy within the past year. Ali miscarried the previous two pregnancies during the first trimester.

When the nurse made the home visit, she noted that Ali was 5 feet 9 inches tall and weighed 120 lb. She resided in a two-room apartment with her boyfriend, who was the father of the baby. The nurse began the first visit with social talk, asking Ali general questions about her employment, education, and the duration of her residence in the area. Ali appeared to be pleased that the nurse was interested in her. Once a trusting relationship was initiated, the nurse asked Ali how she felt about the pregnancy. Ali revealed that she was happy about the pregnancy but was worried that there would be problems because she had had two previous miscarriages. She had not planned any of the pregnancies, but she did not use contraceptives to prevent the pregnancies either. Ali's boyfriend worked and was able to pay the rent and buy food for her. Ali dropped out of high school during her junior year, but she wanted to complete her high school education. She had Medicaid coverage for her health care.

During the initial home visit, the nurse assessed that Ali was underweight and had several knowledge deficits in the areas of prenatal nutrition, infant care, breastfeeding, and contraception. The nurse also identified the need for a referral to the public school for the continuation of Ali's high school education. The nurse briefly discussed her assessment with Ali in a nonthreatening, nonjudgmental manner. The nurse informed Ali that, if she was interested, she could schedule future home visits to provide Ali with more information and answer her questions. Ali agreed to receive future visits to discuss the topics the nurse identified during the assessment phase. They mutually agreed upon the plan for future visits. As the visits progressed, the nurse and Ali modified the plan on the basis of progress evaluation.

The nurse terminated home visits with Ali when the mutually established goals were achieved. The nurse scheduled a postpartum visit with Ali after the baby was born to assess infant care and answer any questions Ali had concerning infant care.

Assessment

Although it was important to perform an individual assessment of Ali, the public health nurse assessed Ali as a member of a family and as a member of the community. *Community* in this case referred to the aggregate of publicly insured adolescent pregnant women. Assessment of Ali revealed an underweight 17-year-old pregnant woman who was unable to demonstrate knowledge of nutrition in pregnancy, infant care, breastfeeding, contraception, or educational options for pregnant teenagers.

An individual assessment of Ali mandated the need for an assessment of the composition and function of Ali's family. The public health nurse assessed the following factors with regard to Ali's family (Logan, 1986):
* Family composition
* General support network

* Family and network patterns related to Ali's psychosocial and economic support
* Family and network attitude toward health
* Family and network beliefs regarding use of health-related services
* Beliefs and attitudes of family and network regarding infant care, breastfeeding, and nutrition
* Attitude of infant's father regarding involvement with Ali and their baby, health beliefs, ability to assume the role of parent, and knowledge of pregnancy and birth

The public health nurse was aware of the need to see the larger, aggregate picture. Identifying the aggregate as the pregnant adolescent community, the public health nurse used the following techniques in an ongoing assessment (Bayne, 1985):
* Observations
* Resource analysis
* Key informant interviews
* Environmental indexes

Using these techniques, the public health nurse gathered information regarding the following:
* Educational and employment options for pregnant teens and teens with infants
* Availability of health services targeting low-birth-weight infants
* Availability of support groups for this aggregate
* Availability of teen parenting classes

Diagnosis

The public health nurse formulated nursing diagnoses based on thorough individual, family, and community assessments.

Individual
* Lack of awareness regarding nutrition in pregnancy, infant care and feeding, contraception, availability of community resources, and educational options for pregnant teenagers
* Inadequate nutritional support related to low-income status and inadequate knowledge of nutritional requirement for pregnancy

Family
* Lack of family support related to Ali's living away from home
* Altered family communication patterns related to role confusion among family members

Community
* Minimal availability of health care services, parenting classes, contraception counseling, and educational opportunities for pregnant teenagers
* Lack of coordination of existing services

Planning

Planning health services and interventions for pregnant teenagers involves formulation of mutually agreed-upon short-term and long-term goals for the individual, family, and community.

Individual
Long-Term Goal
- Ali will carry her infant to term without evidence of maternal or fetal complications.

Short-Term Goals
- Ali will gain at least 3 lbs. per month.
- Ali will demonstrate knowledge of community resources for pregnant adolescents by the next nursing visit.

Family
Long-Term Goal
- Ali, her partner, and other family members will be able to perform mutually determined role responsibilities.

Short-Term Goal
- Ali and her partner will attend teen parenting classes.

Community
Long-Term Goals
- Establishment of effective, comprehensive prenatal health, contraception, and education services for pregnant teenagers
- Decline in rate of teen pregnancies and birth of compromised neonates over the next 24 months

Short-Term Goals
- Increased community awareness of resources for pregnant teenagers
- Increased awareness of contraception counseling services for adolescents

Intervention
Individual
Implementation of Ali's individual care plan involved visits by the public health nurse with a referral to existing prenatal services for pregnant teenagers.

Family
Family intervention was composed of Ali's and the father's referral to a support group for pregnant teenagers and partners.

Community
Implementation of the care plan for the aggregate of adolescent pregnant women included the following:
- Meeting with community leaders
- Meeting with local school administrators and faculty to disseminate information for pregnant teenagers
- Formation of community organizing groups (Bayne, 1985)

Evaluation
Individual
Evaluation included measures of the client's nutritional status and her use of support groups and educational and nutritional services.

Family
Evaluation included measures of the family's use of support groups and educational and services.

Community
Evaluation of the effectiveness of interventions at the aggregate level focused on measurement of available options for pregnant teenagers, measures of teen awareness and use of services, and determination of changes in incidence rates of teen pregnancy and compromised neonates.

Levels of Prevention
The public health nurse not only works with the patient and the patient's support network but also provides care to the entire community through education and intervention programs. The public health nurse is actively involved in working with individual teenagers, their friends and families, and the community in reducing the incidence of teenage pregnancy and assisting pregnant teenagers with prenatal care and available resources. Examples of providing care at the three levels of prevention are listed here.

Primary
- Activities that prevent teen pregnancy from occurring, such as individual and family counseling and school and community education programs

Secondary
- Interventions for early detection of teen pregnancy and early intervention, such as counseling for prenatal care

Tertiary
Goal: To reduce the effects of adolescent pregnancy
- Provision of prenatal education in areas such as nutrition, parenting, and infant care

CASE STUDY 33-3 HOSPICE HOME VISIT

Anne McMillan is 80 years old and is terminally ill with metastatic breast cancer. She has been a widow for 5 years and has three daughters and two sons. All of her children are married with kids of their own, except one son who is handicapped and lives with Anne. Anne is too weak to care for herself and is moving in with her youngest daughter. Her daughter's house is a colonial with all bedrooms upstairs. There is a first floor bathroom. During her first visit, the hospice nurse talks with Anne and her daughter and explains what hospice is all about. The nurse then admits Anne into the hospice program and begins her initial assessment. Anne's primary physical complaints are back pain and constipation. She is still eating and drinking regularly. The nurse immediately recognizes that Anne will need a hospital bed. Anne already has a walker, but the nurse informed Anne and her daughter that they could have a bedside commode if needed in the future as Anne becomes weaker. Anne's biggest concern is her handicapped son,

saying, "He can't be by himself for long and I don't know where he can go now that I can't take care of him." Except for the handicapped son, all of her children and many of her grandchildren are active in her care.

Assessment
On her initial visit, the hospice nurse collects the following data about Anne, her family, and her community. In this case, the community consists of Anne's social support outside of her family, such as her neighborhood and church.
- Pain assessment, including history, character, severity, location, effects on quality of life, precipitating factors, and relieving factors
- Other physical symptoms, such as fatigue, nausea, vomiting, constipation, diarrhea, decreased appetite, and decreased mobility
- Client and family fears, anxiety about dying and the dying process

Continued

- Support network and family dynamics
- Client's anxiety about situation concerning handicapped son
- Additional support network outside of family
- Effect of diagnosis and prognosis on Anne's social support, including her neighbors and her church community

Diagnosis
Individual
- Pain related to disease process
- Potential for constipation and discomfort related to decreased mobility
- Apprehension related to concerns about safety and well-being of handicapped son

Family
- Strong support system indicated by active family participation in Anne's care

Community
- Anticipatory grieving related to social isolation after leaving neighborhood and moving in with daughter

Planning
Individual
Long-Term Goals
- Pain will remain controlled until client expires.
- Client will have regular bowel movements for the next 2 months.
- Client will verbalize satisfaction about resolution of situation concerning handicapped son.

Short-Term Goals
- Pain will be well controlled within 24 to 48 hours.
- Client will have a bowel movement within 24 to 48 hours.
- Client will have decreased anxiety about handicapped son within 24 to 48 hours because the social worker will have found a place for the son to live.

Family
Long-Term Goals
- Family will remain active in Anne's care until she is buried.
- Family will provide a support network for each other and use hospice services for continued support through Anne's death and burial and for months afterward.

Short-Term Goal
- Family will actively participate in Anne's care.

Community
Long-Term Goal
- Client will continue to receive support from friends.

Short-Term Goal
- Client will verbalize feelings about moving in with daughter and leaving friends behind.

Intervention
Individual
After talking with the doctor, the hospice nurse starts Anne on methadone 20 mg daily and Roxanol 5 mg as needed for breakthrough pain. The nurse explains to Anne and her daughter that she is constipated because of her decrease in mobility. The nurse obtains an order for a stool softener and instructs Anne to take it twice daily. The nurse also explains to Anne and her daughter that, as Anne declines, her appetite will decrease and she will eat less and less and may not have bowel movements very frequently. Anne should let the nurse know if she ever feels uncomfortable because she has not had a bowel movement in a few days. The nurse talks to the social worker, who finds a group home for Anne's handicapped son.

Family
The nurse and social worker talk with the family and help them develop a system so that Anne always has someone with her and to help ensure that all of the responsibility for Anne's care does not fall on one person. They also inform the family about resources to support the family.

Community
Anne has a nurse, social worker, spiritual counselor, and nurse assistant assigned to her care. Each of these hospice workers helps Anne discuss her feelings about her situation and works with her to continue to receive support from her friends and neighbors.

Evaluation
Individual
All of Anne's goals are met, because she has good pain control until she dies, she no longer experiences discomfort and problems with constipation, and she expresses less anxiety and worry about her handicapped son. Although she still has some concerns, she feels much better about the situation.

Family
The family's goals are met, because they remain active in Anne's care until she dies. In addition, they use hospice resources appropriately and as necessary, and they support one another through the entire process.

Community
The goals are met, because Anne expresses her feelings about her situation, and her closest friends remain supportive to Anne through visits and phone calls.

Levels of Prevention
In this case, the three levels of prevention focus on helping the client and family through all phases of hospice care from admission until death. Some examples are as follows.

Primary
- Anticipating needs and intervening early on to prevent problems such as skin breakdown and lack of pain control
- Educating the client and family about hospice and the dying process

Secondary
- Responding quickly to needs as they arise
- Continued education about the hospice and dying experience

Tertiary
- Assisting the client and family through the active phase of dying
- Providing follow-up bereavement support to the family

SUMMARY

This chapter presents information on performing public health, home health, and hospice nursing visits to clients in their homes. A general overview of the nursing process for clients in the home setting is presented and expanded to include the individual, family, and community. Case studies involving communicable disease, teen pregnancy, traumatic injury, and terminal cancer are described. The home visit is the foundation of community health nursing and provides a forum for important interventions with individuals, families, and communities. The CHN is responsible for bringing the concerns of individuals and families into the community.

LEARNING ACTIVITIES

1. Make arrangements to accompany a public health nurse, a home health nurse, and a hospice nurse on home visits.
2. Interview a public health nurse about the types of client referrals received, and ask what interventions are usually performed. Repeat this activity with a home health nurse and a hospice nurse. Ask the nurses what they like best about their jobs.
3. Contact a local home health agency and interview the agency director. Ask what type of agency it is, the profit status, and whether it is Medicare certified. Report findings to classmates.
4. Attend a team meeting in a home health agency or a hospice program to see how the roles of the various team members blend together to provide family-centered care.
5. Interview a public health nurse and a home health nurse, and ask how the community affects the care they provide.

EVOLVE WEBSITE

http://evolve.elsevier.com/Nies
- NCLEX Review Questions
- Case Studies
- Glossary

REFERENCES

Albrecht MN: The Albrecht nursing model for home health care: implications for research, practice, and education, *Public Health Nurs* 7:118–126, 1990.

Albrecht MN: Home health care: reliability and validity testing of a patient-classification instrument, *Public Health Nurs* 8:124–131, 1991.

American Nurses Association: *Scope and standards of hospice and palliative nursing practice*, Washington, DC, 2007, Author.

American Nurses Association: *Scope and standards of home health nursing practice*, Washington, DC, 2008, Author.

Bayne T: The pregnant school-age community. In Higgs AR, Gustafson DD, editors: *Community as client: assessment and diagnosis*, Philadelphia, 1985, FA Davis.

Centers for Medicare and Medicaid Services: *Home health compare*, 2008. Available from <http://www.medicare. gov/HHCompare/Home.asp?dest=NAV|Home|Search#TabTop>.

Centers for Medicare and Medicaid Services: *Home health PPS*, 2013. Available from <http://www.cms.gov/Medicare/Medicare-Fee-for-Service-Payment/HomeHealthPPS/index.html?redirect=/homehealthpps/>.

Department of Health and Human Services (DHHS): *Centers for Medicare and Medicaid services: Payment system fact sheet series*, 2013. Available from <http://www.cms.gov/Outreach-and-Education/Medicare-Learning-Network-MLN/MLNProducts/downloads/hospice_pay_sys_fs.pdf>.

Dowling PT: Return of TB: screening and preventive therapy, *Am Fam Physician* 43:457–476, 1991.

Feldman R: Meeting the educational needs of home health care nurses, *J Home Health Care Pract* 5:12–19, 1993.

Gaynor SE: The long haul: the effects of home care on caregivers, *Image J Nurs Sch* 22:208–212, 1990.

Guterman S, Dobson A: Impact of the Medicare prospective payment system for hospitals, *Health Care Financing Rev* 7:97–114, 1986.

Keating SB, Kelman GB: *Home health care nursing: concepts and practice*, Philadelphia, 1998, JB Lippincott.

Kelly L, Joel L: *Dimensions of professional nursing*, ed 8, New York, 1995, McGraw-Hill.

Kent V, Hanley B: Home health care, *Nurs Health Care* 11:234–240, 1990.

Logan BB: Adolescent pregnancy. In Logan BB, Dawkins CE, editors: *Family-centered nursing in the community*, Menlo Park, CA, 1986, Addison-Wesley.

Morrissey-Ross M: Documentation: If you haven't written it, you haven't done it, *Nurs Clin North Am* 23(2):363–371, 1988.

National Association for Home Care and Hospice: *HomeCare online: Basic statistics about home care*, 2010. Available from <http://www.nahc.org/assets/1/7/10HC_Stats.pdf>.

National Kidney and Urologic Diseases Information Clearinghouse [NKUDIC]: *Home hemodialysis*, 2010. Available from <http://www.kidney.niddk.nih.gov/kudiseases/pubs/homehemodialysis/>.

Norlander L: *To comfort always: a nurse's guide to end of life care*, Indianapolis, IN, 2008, Sigma Theta Tau International.

QSEN Institute: QSEN competencies, n.d. Available from <http://qsen.org/competencies/>.

Spradley BW: *Community health nursing: concepts and practice*, ed 3, Glenview, IL, 1990, Scott, Foresman and Little, Brown.

Stack C: *All our kin*, New York, 1974, Harper & Row.

TNEEL Investigators: *8-hour grief: sociocultural aspects, part 1: The influence of culture on attitudes toward dying, death and grieving*, 2003. Available from <http://www.tneel.uic.edu/tneel-ss/demo/grief/frame1.asp>.

U.S. Department of Commerce and International Trade Administration: *U.S. industrial outlook*, Washington, DC, 1990, Government Printing Office.

HealthyPeople.gov: *Healthy People 2020: Topics & objectives*, 2013. Available from <http://www.healthypeople.gov/2020/topicsobjectives2020/default.aspx>.

Warhola C: *Planning for home health services: a resource handbook (USDHHS Pub No HRA 80–14017)*, Washington, D.C, 1980, Public Health Service, U.S. Department of Health and Human Services.

INDEX

Page numbers followed by "f" indicate figures, "t" indicate tables, and "b" indicate boxes.

A

ABC strategy, 274
Abortion, 319
Abstinence, substance abuse and, 527
Abuse, stage of addiction, 524–525, 525t
Abusive head trauma, 547
ACA. *see* Affordable Care Act (ACA)
Acceptability
  health care and, 438–439
  learner verification and, 144t
Access
  definition of, 204b
  of health care, 438–439
  see also Health care, access to
Access limitation, 214
Accidental injuries, 293–296
Accreditation, 197
Achieving Health for All, 278
Acquired immunity, 494–495
  types of, 495t
Acquired immunodeficiency syndrome (AIDS)
  ABC strategy, 274
  in children, 585
  death from, 274
  demographics of, 274
  eradication of, 510
  Healthy People 2020 and, 507–510
  homeless population and, 437
  prevalence of, 274, 509f
  transmission and control of, 511t
  treatment of, 510
  in women, 328
Active immunity, 494–495, 495t
Activities of daily living (ADL)
  assistance with, 412
  and disability, 409
Activity orientation, 227
Activity theory, 356
Actuarial classification
  definition of, 204b
  insurance premiums and, 211–212
Addiction, 522
  assessment process for, 524
  behavior and cognition changes with, 524–525
  during pregnancy, 525, 525b
  stages of, 525t
Administration for Children and Families, 190b
Administration on Aging, 190b
Administrative agencies, 167, 170b
Administrative costs, 204b
Adolescent
  body mass index (BMI) of, 590–591
  dental health of, 586
  health care coverage programs for, 304–305, 304f
  illicit drug use by, 519
  immunization for, 296–297
  mental health of, 591

Adolescent *(Continued)*
  methamphetamine use in, 520–521
  poverty in, 301
  in prison, 624
  public health programs for, 304–306
  self-perceptions of, 590
  sexual risk behavior in, 298–300
  smoking in, 584
  substance abuse in, 533–534
  suicide in, 591b
  tobacco, alcohol and drug use in, 300
  traumatic brain injury, 293
  violence in, 300, 550
  see also Child health
Adolescent health, 286–313, 312b
  factors affecting, 301–302
  Healthy People 2020, 303, 303b
  legal and ethical issues in, 308–311, 308b
  sexual activity in, 298–299
  sharing responsibility for improving, 306–308
    community health nurse's role, 307–308
    community's role, 307
    employer's role, 307
    government's role, 307
    parents' role, 306
  strategies to improve, 302–304
    monitoring and tracking, 302b, 303
Adolescent pregnancy, 299, 299b
  consequences of, 299
  nursing process, application of, 309b–311b
  prevention models for, 299
Adult learner
  characteristics of, 127t
  community support group and, 125b–126b
  Knowles's assumption about, 126
Adults, health status of, 436–437
Advance directives, 374
Advanced nurse practitioner (ANP), 193
Advanced practice home health nurse, 649
Advanced practice hospice/palliative nurse, 655
Adverse selection, 204b
Advisory Commission on Consumer Protection and Quality in the Health Care Industry, 194
Advocacy, 198
  public health intervention, 15t
Advocate, community health nurse as, 218
Affordability, of health care, 435
Affordable Care Act (ACA), 9, 217, 217b, 304, 469
Africa
  AIDS in, 274
  malaria in, 274
  TB and HIV in, 274
  Team Reach Out in, 283b

African American
  child population, 287f
  culture-bound syndrome in, 237t
  death, leading cause of, 341t
  disabilities and death due to fetal alcohol exposure, 301
  HIV, in men, 341
  homeless population and, 433
  life expectancy for, 340
  nurses as, 222
  population of, 222
  poverty in, 229
  as single-parent family, 384t
  teen birth rate in, 384t
  treating substance abuse and addiction problems in, 535b
Age-adjustment, of rates, 76
  advantages/disadvantages, 77t
Age-specific rates, 76
  advantages/disadvantages, 77t
Agency for Healthcare Quality and Research, 190b
Agency for Toxic Substances and Disease Registry, 190b
Aggregate, 4
  assessment of, 109–111
  community as, 93
  family health intervention extending to, 394–397
  government grants for, 209
  health of, impact on, 19–20
  intervention by, 112t
  prevention levels for, 115t
  vulnerable, protection of, 264b
Aggregate-focused nursing, 95
Aging
  concept of, 356
  culture and, 231–232
  disability prevalence/severity with, 412
  incontinence and, 366
  normal physiological changes associated with, 361t–362t
  psychosocial issues in, 359, 360f
  theories of, 356–357
    biological, 356, 356b
  workforce and, occupational health nurse and, 607
Aging families, 392b
Agoraphobia, effects of, 476
Agrichemicals, food safety and, 259
Agricultural workers
  accidents/injuries in, 455
  acute/chronic illnesses, 455–456
  health disparities in, 455
Air pollutants, major, 256t
Air pollution
  carbon monoxide and, 273
  environmental health issues and, 255b
  environmental stressors and, 273
  from industry, 257
Air quality, outdoor, environmental health and, 256–258, 257b
  definition of, 252t
  problems relating to, 252t
Air quality index (AQI), 257, 257f
Airborne transmission, 494

Albrecht nursing model, for home health care, 649, 650f
Alcohol
  in adolescents, 300
  dating violence and, 545
  death from, 61
  driving under the influence of, 525
  economic value of, 524
  excessive use of, 61
  health and, 60–62
  historical overview of, 517
  homelessness and, 435
  incidence and trends in, 518
  liver disease and, 61
  pharmacotherapy and, 529
  during pregnancy, 291–292
  slavery and, 535
  underage drinking of
    clinical implications of, 61
    prevalence of, 61
    prevention of, 61
  USDA recommendations for, 63
Alcohol consumption, actual causes of death, 4–5
Alcoholics Anonymous (AA), 371–372
  as 12-step programs, 530
Alcoholism
  CAGE test and, 526
  harm reduction and, 531
  pregnancy and, 525
  prevalence of, 517–521
Alliances, within family, 391
Allocation of resources, ethical issues in, 133b
Alma-Ata, Declaration of, 275, 276b
Alprazolam (Xanax), 545
Alternative housing options, for older adults, 358
Alzheimer's disease, 372–373
  behavioral and physical changes due to, 373
  diagnosis of, 372
  strategies for caring for, 373
Ambulatory care, 204b
  use by gender, 342
Ambulatory care centers, 212
Ambulatory care setting, nurses in, 19
American Academy of Family Physicians (AAFP), 448
American Association of Colleges of Nursing, 278
American Association of Occupational Health Nurses (AAOHN), code of ethics, 602b
American Board of Medicolegal Death Investigators (ABMDI), 619
American Cancer Society, older adults, recommendations for, 362–363
American Diabetes Association (ADA), 14
  diabetes in children, 587–588

American Healthcare Commission, 197
American Heart Association, 362–363
American Hospital Association, 31
  on medical waste management, 266
American Indian
  death, leading causes of, in older adult, 365t
  population of, 222
  as single-parent family, 384t
  teen birth rate in, 384t
American Medical Association, vital statistics collection and, 23
American Nurses Association (ANA)
  case management, definition of, 155
  code of ethics, self-determination, 638
  Code of Ethics of, 2
  Scope and Standards of Parish Nurse Practice, 634–635
American Nurses Credentialing Center, case management, 159
American Red Cross
  disaster management and, 568–569
  shelter-in-place, 568, 568t
  type of assistance from, 569t
  volunteers, 569f
American Statistical Association, 24
Americans with Disabilities Act (ADA), 413, 612
  disability, definition of, 612
  purpose of, 612
Americans with Disabilities Act (ADA) Amendments Act of 2008, 413
Amyotrophic lateral sclerosis (ALS), support group for, 125b–126b
ANA. see American Nurses Association (ANA)
Analytic epidemiology, 83–90
Androgen, 343
Annual Homeless Assessment Report (AHAR), 431
Anorexia, in adolescents, 590
Anorexia nervosa, 477
Antabuse (Disulfiram), 529
Antepartum client, home visiting and, 658b–659b
Anthrax, as bioterrorism agent/disease, 561b
Anthropology, nursing and, 223
Anxiety disorder
  in older adult, 370
  types of
    generalized, 475
    obsessive-compulsive disorder, 476
    phobias, 476
    post traumatic stress disorder, 476
Arthritis, in women, 323–324
Asian culture
  culture-bound syndrome in, 237t
  sibling relationship, 228
  sick role behavior and, 232–233
  silence and, 233
  yin-yang theory, 235–236

Asian population, 222
  children as, 287f
  death, leading causes of, 341t
    in older adult, 365t
  nurses as, 222
  poverty in, 229
  sibling relationship of, 228
  as single-parent family, 384t
  teen birth rate in, 384t
Assertive Community Treatment (ACT) program, 482–483
  key features of, 483b
Assessment
  of aggregate, 109–111
  core public health functions, 6b
  as health planning model/objective, 108f, 109b
  see also Community assessment; Needs assessment
Assessment Protocol for Excellence in Public Health (APEX-PH), 115
Association, strength of, cause-and-effect relationship, 79
Assurance, core public health functions, 6b
Asthma
  in children, 587
  schools assisting children with, 588b
At-risk families, home visitation program for, 396
Attack rates, 75
Attention deficit/hyperactivity disorder (ADHD), 477
  cause of, 477
  symptoms of, 477
Attraction, learner verification and, 144t
Attributable risk, 78
Authority, in disaster management, 570

B

Baby boomers, 357
"Back to Sleep" campaign, SIDS and, 293b
Barriers, communication and, 232–233
Barton, Clara, 166
Behavior
  definition of, 51–53
  gender-linked, 345–346
  gender-role, 343b
  good health and, 205–206
  health-protective, 344
  high-risk, in children, 583
  sexual risk, in adolescent, 298–300
  spiritual needs assessment and, 231b
Behavioral intentions, 55
Behavioral responses, to traumatic event, 578t
Behavioral Risk Factor Surveillance System, 99
Behavioral science, 599
Behavioral therapy, 480
Being, 227
Belief, family and, 391
Benzodiazepines, 529–530

Bill and Melinda Gates Foundation, 277
Bill of rights, 170
Binge drinking, 61
Binge eating, in adolescents, 590
Biochemical incidents, 565
  detection of, 565b
Biocultural variations, of culturally diverse people, 244
Biological attack, 567b
Biological factors
  influencing mental health, 471
  influencing sex differences, 343
Biological-infectious hazard
  exposures and health effects of, 605t
  in workplace, 604
Biological plausibility, cause-and-effect relationship, 79
Biological theories, of aging, 356, 356b
Biological weapons, of mass destruction, 560, 562t
Biomedical perspective, illness causation, 235–236
Biosolids, 261
Bioterrorism agents/diseases, 490b, 561b
Bioterrorist attacks, imminence of, 562
Bipolar disorder, 475
  management of, 475
Birth rate
  male and female births, 343
  in teenagers, by ethnic group, 384t
  for unmarried women, 383–384
Black Death, 21
Bladder control. see Incontinence
Blended family, 227
"Block grants," 209
Blue Cross, 31
Board of Health
  for England, 22
  for New York Metropolitan, 27
Body mass index (BMI), 62, 590–591
Body piercings, 586
Body weight, 62
Botulism, 493
  as bioterrorism agent/disease, 561b
Boundary, 389t
Breast cancer
  education, launching and outreach screening program, 134b
  incidence of, 324
  resource materials for, 325b
  in women, 324–325, 325b
Breastfeeding, 292, 306b
Brewster, Mary, 28
  case management programs and, 156
Brucellosis, as bioterrorism agent/disease, 561b
Buddhism
  "Golden Rule" and, 231b
  healing and recovery, 633
Built environment, environmental health and, 253–254, 254b
  conceptual model of, 253f

Built environment, environmental health and (Continued)
  definition of, 252t
  problems relating to, 252t
Bulimia nervosa, 476
  in adolescents, 590
Bullying, 546, 546b
Buprenorphine, 529
Bush, George, National Incident Management System, 559
Business theories/concepts/principles, occupational health, 599

C

Cafeteria plans, 210
CAGE alcohol screening instrument, 372b
CAGE test, 526
Caloric balance equation, 62f
Calorie, restaurant eating and, 64
Campaigning, nurses and, 181
Canada, Achieving Health for All, 278
Cancer
  African American mortality from, 223
  death rates from, 317
  five-year survival rate for, 318
  reducing risk of, 318
  survival of, 318
  in women, 317–318
  see also specific types of cancer
Cannabis, 523t
Capital cost, 204b
Capitated reimbursement, 213–214
Capitation, 204b
Carbon dioxide, breakdown of, 257
Carbon monoxide (CO)
  air pollution and, 258, 273
  sources and effects of, 256t
Cardiovascular disease (CVD)
  in men, 348–349
  in women, 316–317
Cardiovascular system, of older adult, 361t–362t
Care coordination
  and access to, 198
  example of, 159
  of health care services, 156
Care management, 155–156
  definition of, 204b
  framework for, 155
  people served by, 155
Caregiver
  caring for, 655
  formal and informal, 654
Carnegie Foundation, 27
Carrier, 204b
Carter Center, 275
Carve-out service, 204b
Case-control study. see Retrospective studies
Case finding, public health intervention, 15t
Case management, 154–164, 164b
  aim of, 155
  as client-centered and system-centered, 157
  clients with chronic diseases, 161
  in community health
    high-risk clinic settings, 161

Case management *(Continued)*
　occupational health settings, 161
　public health clinic settings, 161
　definition of
　　by American Nurses Association, 155
　　by Case Management Society of America, 155
　disease-specific, 157
　elderly and, 156–157
　ethical issues in, 157b
　function of, 155b
　goal of, 155
　for HIV and AIDS clients, 160
　in home health and hospice settings, 161
　in home health care, 159
　identification of clients, 160
　international, 162–163
　in mental health, 156
　origins of, 156–157
　overview of, 154–156
　programs in, 155
　public health intervention, 15t
　purpose of, 157
　referral process in, 160
　research in, 161–162
　screening in patient, 160
　trends influencing, 158
　utilization review and managed care, 157
Case management models, community, 161
Case Management Society of America (CMSA)
　case management
　　definition of, 155
　　philosophy of, 155
　　standards of, 160b
　case manager
　　certification by, 159
　　role of, 159
Case managers
　certification options for, 159
　　by ANCC, 159
　　by CMSA, 159
　characteristics of, 159–160
　education and preparation for, 158–159
　flexibility of, 160
　length of services, 159
　nurse as, 158–159
　services provided by, 159
　social workers as, 158
Casualty
　classification of, 559
　scope and number of, 562
Cataract, in older adults, 365
Catholic religion
　dietary practice of, 230
　population of, 230
Causality, establishing, 79
Cause-and-effect relationship, 79
Census
　data, 97
　data collection on, 23
　"hidden pockets" of need and, 99b
　metropolitan statistical areas and, 97
　see also U.S. Census Bureau

Census tracts, 93
Center for Mental Health Services (CMHS), 482, 483t
Centers for Disease Control and Prevention (CDC), 168, 190b, 277
　AIDS in children, 585
　bioterrorism agents/diseases, 490b
　disaster management and, 567
　health planning and, 115
　high-risk youth behaviors, 583
　notifiable infectious diseases, 496
　shifts in philosophy at, 168b
Centers for Medicare and Medicaid Services, 190b
Central nervous system depressants, 523t
Central nervous system stimulants, 523t
Certificate of need (CON), 116–117
Certified home health agency, 647
Cervical cancer, 317–318
Cesarean section, 320
Chadwick, Edwin, 22
Change
　stages of, 56t
　transtheoretical model and, 54
Channels, health communication and, 135
　and methods, selection of, 138b
Charges, 204b
Check/balances, 171
Chemical attack, 567b
Chemical hazard
　exposures and health effects of, 605t
　in workplace, 604
Chemical weapons, of mass destruction, 560, 562t
Chickenpox, 500t–501t
Child abuse
　definition of, 297
　definition of, by Federal Child Abuse Prevention and Treatment Act, 621
　forensic nurse examiner in, 621
　long-term effects of, 297
　perpetrators of, 297–298
　physical and behavioral indicators of, 548t
　reporting, 298
Child care, power/empowerment and, 43
Child health, 286–313, 312b
　factors affecting, 301–302
　Healthy People 2020, 303, 303b
　legal and ethical issues in, 308–311, 308b
　sharing responsibility for improving, 306–308
　　community health nurse's role, 307–308
　　community's role, 307
　　employer's role, 307
　　government's role, 307
　　parents' role, 306
　strategies to improve, 302–304
　　monitoring and tracking, 302b, 303
Child labor, 22
Child maltreatment, 546–549

Childhood obesity, goals/objectives for reduction of, 112b
Children
　accidental injuries in, 293–296
　AIDS in, 585
　asthma in, 587
　　school assistance of, 588b
　culturally diverse background of, 228
　death in, 288
　dental health of, 586
　depression in, 475
　diabetes in, 296, 587–588
　　expectations, 588b
　disability in, 418b
　　prevalence of, 410–411
　disability in, types of, 589t
　environmental history assessment for, 251, 251f
　exposure to pesticides, research on, 112b
　of gay or lesbian families, 384
　health care coverage programs for, 304–305, 304f
　health of, long-term implications of, 287
　health promotion and disease prevention for, 303–304
　as homeless, 431
　　health status of, 437–438
　as insured, 581
　　by ethnicity, 581t
　lead poisoning in, 297
　mental health of, 591
　mortality and morbidity rates of, 287
　obesity
　　factors influencing, 296
　　prevalence of, 296
　　prevention of, 296
　　rate of, 296
　obesity in
　　causes of, 590–591
　　diabetes and, 587–588
　population of, 287
　poverty in, 228–229, 228t, 301
　preventive health care in, 301–302
　primary caregiver for, 228
　public health programs for, 304–306
　by race and ethnicity, 287, 287f
　special health care needs of, 298
　with special health needs, 589
　spirituality and, 231
　of substance abusers, 532
　toy-related injuries to, 296b
　traumatic brain injury in, 293
　as uninsured, reasons for, 305
　vaccine-preventable diseases in, 500t–501t
　violence in, 300
　vital statistics for, 288b
Children's Bureau Act of 1912, 173
Children's Health Insurance Program (CHIP), 304–305, 587
Chiropractor, 193
Chlamydia trachomatis, transmission and control of, 508t–509t
Chlorine (pulmonary agent), 562t
Cholera, 23

Christianity, "Golden Rule" and, 231b
Chronic conditions, in men, 341–342
Chronic diseases, in prison, 623
Chronic illness
　in families, nurse working with, 386–387
　in older adult, 364
　in women, 323–327
Chronically homeless, 438
Church-based educational programs, 636
Church Health Center, 634
　model for health living, 634f
Circadian rhythm, 66
CIRCLE Model of Spiritual Care, 638
Circular communication, 390
Civil Rights Act, women's health and, 330
Civilization, disease history, stages and, 19
Classical times, public health in, 21
Clean Air Act, 257
Client-centered health care, 198
Client rights, 198
Clinical nurse leader (CNL), 193
Clinical nurse specialist (CNS), 193
Clinical research, in United States, 206
Clinton, Bill, and health care reform, 216
Clonazepam (Klonopin), 545
Closed system, 389t
Co-payment, 204b
Coal worker's pneumoconiosis, 343
Coalition
　within family, 391
　forming, critical environmental health nursing practice and, 265–266
　nurses and, 179–180
Coalition building, public health intervention, 15t
Codependency, substance abuse and, 531
Cognitive-behavioral therapy, 480
Cognitive change, in older adult, 361t–362t
Cognitive responses, to traumatic event, 578t
Cognitive theory, 125
Cohabitation, 227
　definition of, 383
Cohort study, 85–86, 86b
Coinsurance, 204b
Cold chain, 498
Cold stress disorder, in older adult, 368
Collaborating centers, 279
Collaboration, public health intervention, 15t
Collateral relationships, 227
Collective strategy, for community health, 266
Colorectal cancer, 317
Combined statistical areas (CSAs), 97
Common law, 167t
Communal family, 227

Communicable diseases, 21, 488–514, 512b–514b
defining and reporting of, 496
definition of, 491–492
Healthy People 2020 and, 490–491, 491b
home health visit follow-up for, 656b–658b
nurse's responsibility with, 491b
prevention of, 510
primary, 510
secondary, 510
tertiary, 510
in prison, 623
Communicable period, of infection, 492, 492f
Communication
as community assessment parameter, 100t–101t
with culturally diverse client, 242
during disasters, 570
enhancing, 132–133
home health nurse and client, 651
overcoming barriers to, 232–233
prostate cancer and treatment options for, 144b
social media and, 148
see also Health communication; Nonverbal communication; Verbal communication
Community, 3–4
case management and, 161
disaster response by
disillusionment phase, 573–576
heroic phase, 573
honeymoon phase, 573
environmental health issues affecting, 255b
family as component of, 387
family health and, 387
features of, 93b
functions of, 94
geographic, 94
health promotion in, 50b–51b
healthy, 94–95
determinants of, 97f
"hidden pockets" of need in, 99b
human factors and, 93
improving child health, 307
literacy and health program planning, 140
nature of, 93–94
aggregate as, 93
location defining, 93–94
social system and, 94
of solution, 4
substance abuse intervention and, 537–538
Community as client, 107, 107f
Community assessment, 92–105, 95f, 105b
for disasters, 576b–578b
parameters for, 100t–101t, 107f
sources of data, 95–99
statistical methods in, 26b
Community-based care, 458–460
faith communities/parish nursing, 459
home health/hospice care, 458–459
informal care systems, 459

Community-based living, disability and, 420
Community-based mental health care, 481–484, 482b
Community-based nursing, 11
Community-based participatory method, 123–124
Community-based practice, social injustice and, 45b
Community-based problems, attacking at their roots, 457
Community care, new concepts of, 350–353
Community caregiver, 27–28
Community competence, 95
Community development/ planning, 100t–101t
Community diagnosis
components of, 101–102
format for, 102f
Community empowerment, 130–132
Community forum, 99–101
Community health
definition/focus of, 6
interaction and integration in rural areas, 464
interventions, 13–14
planning, implementation, and evaluation of, 106–121, 107b, 120b
Community health center, development of, 187
Community Health Centers (CHC) program, 460–461
Community health education, 122–153, 149b
basis of, 123–124
concepts for, 130
connecting with everyday realities, 122–123
ethical issues related to, 133b
nurse role in, 123–124
teaching-learning format for, 135t
Community health nurse, 5
community functions and, 95
cost containment and, 385
cultural competence in, 244, 301
cultural knowledge of, 244
cultural self-assessment, 244
culturally based health practices, recognition of, 244–245
data collection by, 99
environmental health and, 252
families and
assessment tools for, 392–393
interacting with, 383
working with, 384
families and, models of care for, 396–397
health care economics, role in, 217–218
health planning, role in, 107
home visiting by, 397, 399b–400b
improving child health, 307–308
in improving health for culturally diverse people, 241–245
biocultural variations, 244

Community health nurse (Continued)
communication, 242
cultural sanctions/restrictions, 242
developmental considerations, 244
disease incidence, 244
educational background, 243
ethnic/racial origins of, 242
health-related beliefs and practices, 242–243
nutrition, 243
organizations providing cultural support, 243
religious affiliation, 243
socioeconomic considerations, 243
values orientation, 242
international health care and, 279
political issues, recognition, 244
population-focused, 11
role of, women's health and, 334
counselor, 334
direct care, 334
educator, 334
safety issues for, 553b
strategies of, in caring for people with disabilities, 419
substance abuse intervention and, 537
Community health nursing, 2, 10
cultural diversity and, 220–248, 248b
faith community nursing and, 632
health promotion and, 49–51, 50b
historical factors for, 18–35
images of, 33b–34b
levels of, 108t
managed care and health reform, 15–16
organizations for, 39
policy, politics, legislation and, 165–185
practice, 11
services for men, 348b
theoretical scope in, 39
transcultural perspectives in, 221
Community health services, 191
Community health visit, 294b–295b
Community mental health
brain neuroimaging, genetics, and hope for new treatments, 470–471
deinstitutionalization, 470
gender, racial, and sexual orientation disparities, 472
medicalization of mental illness, 470
mental health reform, 470
overview and history of, 469–471, 470t
Community Mental Health Centers Act (CMHCA), 469
Community mental health nurse, role of, 484–486
Community of solution, 93

Community organization, 130
Community organizing, public health intervention, 15t
Community participatory research, to assess substance use in rural community, 94b
Community public health nursing, 438–440
framework for, 438–440
models of justice, 438–439
public health intervention wheel, 439–440
social determinants of health, 431b, 439, 439t
thinking upstream, 439
Community resource map, for disasters, 561, 564f
Community risk map
for disasters, 561, 563f
Community support group, adult learner and, 125b–126b
Community violence, 549–551
gangs as, 551
hate crimes as, 551
human trafficking as, 551
prison violence as, 551
terrorism as, 551
in workplace, 549–550
youth-related, 550
Complex community system
functions of, 94
health care system as, 94
Comprehension, learner verification and, 144t
Comprehensive Health Planning, 116
Comprehensive Health Reform, 117–118
Confidentiality, of health information, 602b
Confucianism, "Golden Rule" and, 231b
Conservative scope of practice, 39
Consistency, with other studies, cause-and-effect relationship, 79
Consolidated Omnibus Budget Reconciliation Act of 1985, 175
Constitution, of the government, 170, 170b
Consultation, public health intervention, 15t
Consumer Assessment of Healthcare Providers and Systems (CAHPS), 197
Consumerism, 198
Contagious fever, 23
Continuation stage of addiction, 524, 525t
Continuity of care, 240
Continuity theory, 356
Continuum of care (CoC), 156
homeless, reducing of, 431
Control, of communicable disease, 496
Coordinator, of volunteers, faith community nurse as, 636–637
Coronary vascular disease (CVD), in women, 323
Coroners, 618
Correctional facilities, safe environment in, 622, 623b

Correctional nursing, 622–623, 629b
    maintenance of a safe environment and, 622–623
    nursing process, application of, 626b–628b
Correctional settings, mental health issues in, 624–625
Cost-based reimbursement, 211
Cost containment
    community health nurse and, 385
    current trends in, 213–214
    definition of, 204b
    ethical insights, 213b
    through access limitation, 214
    through rationing, 214, 214b
Cost contract, 204b
Cost sharing, 214–215
Cost shifting
    definition of, 204b
    by hospitals, 211
Counseling
    for children, 591
    public health intervention, 15t
Couple therapy, 480
Coxcomb charts, 25f
Crime, against older adult, 369–370
Crimean War
    disease during, 23
    mortality statistics for, 24, 26t
Crime prevention, 369
Crime watch
    as health planning project, 113, 113b
    intervention by aggregate/system level, 112t
    prevention for, 114t
Crisis Intervention Team (CIT), 483
    core elements of, 483b
Critical care, forensic nurse examiner in, 620
Critical consciousness, 129
    creation of, 131t
Critical interactionism, 44, 45t
Critical question(s), about environmental health problems, 264, 265b
Critical social theory, 44
Critical theoretical perspective, 43–45
    application of, 43–44
    values/assumptions for, 43–45
Critical theory
    definition of, 250
    environmental health, approach to, 250–252
Cross-addiction, 532–533
Cross-cultural communication, 232–235
Cross-cultural nursing, 223
Cross-linkage theory, 356b
Cross-sectional studies, 84, 84f
Crossing the Quality Chasm, 195
Crude rates, 75
    advantages/disadvantages, 77t
Cuba, "health for all," 278
Cue to action, 40, 55t, 127t
Cultural belief, affecting existing illnesses, 273

Cultural care diversity and universality, Leininger's theory of, 223, 224f
Cultural competence, in community health nurse, 221, 301
Cultural diversity
    community health nursing and, 220–248, 248b
    concept of, 221
    health problem management and, 239–241
    nutritional assessment and, 229–230
    in population trends, 221–222
    spiritual needs assessment and, 231b
Cultural effectiveness, ethical issues in, 133b
Cultural expression
    of illness, 236–237
    of pain, 237
Cultural health, *Healthy People 2020* and, 222b
Cultural identity, food and, 229
Cultural imposition, 223–224
Cultural negotiation
    definition of, 238–239, 238b
    goal and use of, 238
Cultural sanctions and restrictions, 242
Cultural self-assessment, 244
Cultural stereotyping, 230
Cultural values, of clients *versus* nurse, 223–224
Culturally and linguistically appropriate services (CLASs), nurse role in, 133
Culturally effective care, 133
Culture
    aging and, 231–232
    characteristics of, 224
    definition of, 224–228
    dietary practices in, 230
    family and, 227–228
    health-related beliefs/practices, 235–237
    nurse knowledge of, 221
    nutrition and, 229–230
    religion and, 230–231
    socioeconomic status and, 228–229
    values formation and, 225–227
    veterans and, 225b
Culture-bound syndrome, 237, 237t
Culture shock, 232
Culture specific, 223
Culture universal, 223
Culturological assessment, 241–244
Current procedural terminology (CPT) codes, 204b, 211
Customary charge, 204b
Customer-centered health care, 198

D

Dark age, 24
Data collection
    on census, 23
    by community health nurse, 99
    sources of, 342b

Data interpretation, theories of men's health, 344
Data retrieval, 102b
Dating violence, 545
    date rape drugs, 545
    physical, from middle to high school, 544b
Day care centers, shelter-in-place instructions at, 568t
Death
    actual causes of, 4–5
    alcohol consumption and, 61
    causes of, 58, 59f
        in men, 341t
        in older adult, 365t
    cultural differences related to, 656–661
    in developing country, 273
    from homicide, 544
    precursors of, 347b
    risk factors for, 59t
Death investigator
    forensic nurse, role of, 618–619, 618f
    medicolegal, 618–619
Declaration of Alma-Ata, 275, 276b
Deductible
    definition of, 204b
    for Medicare, 207–208
Deinstitutionalization, 470
Delegated functions, public health intervention, 15t
Demographics, of health belief model, 127t
Dental concerns, of older adult, 366
Dental health, of school-age children, 586
Department of Health, Education, and Welfare, 188
Dependence
    conceptualizations of, 522
    diagnosis of, 522
    from initiation to, 524, 525t
    stage of addiction, 525t
Depressants, 523t
Depression
    in children and adolescents, 475
    geriatric, scale-short form, 371b
    in older adult, 370–371
    prevalence of, 474
    suicide and, 372
    symptoms of, 475b
    treatment for, 475
    in women, 326–327
Descriptive epidemiology, 70, 83, 83b
Destiny, 226
Determinants of health
    Healthy People 2020, 51
    relationship among, 53f
    types of, 51–53, 52t
Detoxification, 527
    pharmacotherapy and, 529
    withdrawals and, 527
Developed country, mortality in, 274
Developing country
    infectious disease in, 274
    malnutrition, disease, or death in, 273
    mortality in, 274
    sanitation facilities in, 273

Developmental theory, 391–392
Diabetes
    in children, 296, 587–588
        expectations, 588b
    health promotion plan for, 386
    in women, 318, 323
Diagnosis-related group (DRG)
    definition of, 204b
    Medicare and, 211
Diet
    health and, 62–65
    and religion, 230
    for special populations, 63
    USDA recommendations for, 63–64
Dietary practices, in culture, 230
Differentiation, 389f
Diphtheria, 500t–501t
Direct health care delivery programs, for children and adolescents, 305–306
Direct transmission, 493
Direct victim, of disaster, 559
Disability
    aging and, 412
    attitudes toward people with early, 407
        eighteenth and nineteenth centuries, 407–408
        twentieth century, 408
    characteristics of, 409–412
    in children, 418b
        family and caregiver responses to, 417–418
        family research outcomes, 417–418
    in children, types of, 589t
    community health nurse in caring for, strategies of, 419
    contemporary conceptualizations of people with, 408–409
    costs associated with, 414–415
    culture and, 411–412
    definition of, 404–407
        Social Security Administration, 414b
    differentiating illness from, 407
    dos and don'ts for interacting with, 410t
    economic well-being and employment for, 414–415, 415t
    experience of, 416–419, 417t
    health status and causes of, 411
    Healthy People 2020 and, 415–416
    historical perspective for, 407–409
    intellectual, 415–416
    knowledgeable client/nurse, 418–419
    language usage surrounding, 409t
    "living" with, 421b–423b
    measurement of, 409
    measures of, 410
    misconceptions surrounding, 409b
    models for, 404–407
        disability model, 406
        example of, 405f

Disability (Continued)
  medical model, 406
  moral model, 406
  rehabilitation model, 406
  Nagi model and, 404–405
  needs of people with, 415–416
  nurse with, 423–426
  nursing process, application of, 424b–426b
  paradigm influences policy and actions, 418t
  people with disabilities (PWD), 404
  personal assistance for, 412
  populations affected by, 403–428, 406b, 414b, 421b, 426b
    ethical issues for, 419–426
  prevalence of, 409–411
    by race and sex, 410
  public assistance programs for, 414
  and public policy, 412–414, 412b
    Individuals with Disabilities Education Act (IDEA), 412–413
    legislation affecting, 412–413
  reasonable accommodations for, 413
  self-assessment of, 404
  as socially constructed issue, 407
  spiritual issues and, 420b
  systems of support for, 416f
  terminology for, 405t
Disability model, 406
Disability syndrome, 607
Disabled population, forensic nurse examiner and, 622
Disadvantaged Minority Health Improvement Act of 1990, 245
Disaster
  characteristics of, 560–563, 562b
  community assessment process for, 576b–578b
  community resource map for, 561, 564f
  community response to
    disillusionment phase, 573–576
    heroic phase, 573
    honeymoon phase, 573
  community risk map for, 561, 563f
  consequences of, 558–559
  counseling support for victims of, 576
  definition of, 559
  frequency of, 560
  imminence of, 562
  intensity of, 562–563
  mitigation of, 561
  natural and man-made, 558–579
  nurse's role in, 559
  posttraumatic stress disorder and, 576–578, 578t
  predictability of, 561
  preparation for, 559
  preventability of, 561
    primary, 561
    secondary, 561
    tertiary, 561
  reactions to, 576–578, 578t

Disaster (Continued)
  scope of, 562
  types of, 560, 560b
    Natech (natural-technological), 560
    terrorism, 560
Disaster management, 563–569
  American Red Cross and, 568–569
  areas of operation in, 571f
  Centers for Disease Control and Prevention and, 567
  Department of Health and Human Services and, 567
  evacuation routes as, 571
  public health system and, 567–568
  reconstruction phase of, 576
  responsibilities during
    of federal government, 565–567
    of local government, 564–565
    of nurse, 564, 564b
    of state government, 565
  search and rescue, 571
  shelter-in-place, 568t, 571
  stages of
    preparedness and planning, 570
    prevention, 569–570
    recovery, 578
    response, 571–578
    staging area, 571–572
Disaster plan, 561
  effectivity of, 570
  expectations in, 570
  initiation of, 570
  logistical section of, 570
  principles of, 570b
Disaster programs, as community assessment parameter, 100t–101t
Disaster triage
  focus of, 572
  "hot zone" of, 572–573
  steps in, 572
Disaster triage tag
  color coding for, 572
  example of, 572f
  hazmat as, 572
Discharge planner, 158
Discharge planning, case management model and, 161
Disclosure of HIV/AIDS status, 242b
Discrimination, in health care, 447b
Disease
  conditions affecting, 22
  definition of, 20t
  determinants of, 4–5
  in developing country, 273
  drug-resistant, 490b
  history, stages in, 19, 19f
  natural history of, 78
  and other health event investigation, 15t
  patterns of, 273–275
  racial and ethnic disparities and, 223
  spontaneous generation theory of, 24
  vaccine-preventable, 498b
  work-related, 606t
Disease avoidance, 40

Disease causation
  spontaneous generation theory of, 24
  theories of, 31
Disease eradication, criteria for, 496b
Disease prevention
  for children, 303–304
  examinations for, 363b
  impact on health care costs, 215
  Metropolitan Life Insurance Company and, 156
Disengagement theory, 356
Disillusionment phase, of community response to disaster, 573–576
Displaced persons, 559
Distance zone
  as culturally appropriate, 232
  functional use of, 232t
District nursing, 28
District nursing, Florence Nightingale and, 382
Disulfiram (Antabuse), 529
Divorce, 392
Do-not-resuscitate (DNR), 374
Dock, Lavinia, 166
Doctor of nursing practice (DNP), 278
Documentation, of home health care, 652
Doing, 227
Domestic abuse
  nursing process, application of, 555b–556b
  power and control wheel, 547f
Domestic Abuse Intervention Project, 546
Domestic violence, 544
  in women, 329, 329b
Dominant value orientation, 226
Dose-response relationship, cause-and-effect relationship, 79
Downstream health care, 37
Driver safety, older adult and, 367–368, 367b
Drug-resistant pathogens/diseases, 490b
Drug trafficking, 525
Drugs
  economic value of, 524
  legalization or decriminalization, 526
  war on, 526
Drunk driving, 531b
Dual diagnosis, substance abuse and, 535–536
Dysmenorrhea, in women, 327

E

Early and Periodic Screening, Diagnosis, and Treatment (EPSDT), 304–305, 587
Earthquakes, 560
  injury and death from, 562
Eating disorders, 476–477
  in adolescents, 590
  risk factors for, 477
  treatment for, 477
  types of
    anorexia nervosa, 477
    bulimia nervosa, 476

Ecological balance, stressors interfering with, 273
Ecological framework, 395
Ecomap
  example of, 393f
    of Garcia family, 394f
  as family assessment tool, 385, 393
Economic theories/concepts/principles, occupational health, 599
Economics
  affecting existing illnesses, 273
  of health care, 202–219, 218b
  resource allocation and, 203
Ecosocial epidemiology, 72–74
Ectopic pregnancy, 319
Education
  about illicit drug use, 525
  as community assessment parameter, 100t–101t
  of culturally diverse client, 239–240
  of faith community nurse, 637–638, 638b
  and forensic nursing, 625–629
    school programs in, 626b
  foundation of, 132–133
  health, focus of, 111
  for home health nurse, 649–650
  of older adults, 357
  of parent, 301
  problem-solving, 129
  socioeconomic status and, 229
Education for Homeless Children and Youth (EHCY), 431–432
Educator, community health nurse as, 217
Effectiveness, 204b
Egalitarianism, disability and, 412b
Eighteenth century, public health in, 22
Elder abuse, 368–369, 549
  forensic nurse examiner in, 621
  indicators of, 550t
Elder mistreatment. see Elder abuse
Elder safety and security needs, 366–370
  falls, 366–367
Elderly
  needs of, recognizing, 359b
  substance abuse in, 534
Electoral information, 179t
Electronic medical records (EMRs), health care system and, 198
Eligibility, for Medicare, 207
Elimination, of communicable disease, 496
Elizabethan Poor Law, 22
Emergency care
  forensic nurse examiner in, 620
  as health services, 587
Emergency Care Plan (ECP), 587
Emergency preparedness, in rural communities, 460
Emergency response, in rural areas, 460
Emotional abuse, 548, 548t
  definition of, 621
  signs of, 592b
Emotional communication, 390

Emotional neglect, 548t
Emotional response, to traumatic event, 578t
Employer, improving child health, 307
Employment
  diseases and injuries during, 606t
  employee health information, 602b
Empowerment
  child care, quality of, 43
  community, 130–132
  of community members, 111
  health communication and, 134
  health education, model of, 128–130
  health education and, 131t
  history/concept of, 129
  spheres of, 111
Empowerment education, 130
  examples of, 129–130
Enabling, substance abuse and, 531
End-of-life issues
  advance directives as, 374, 374b
  nurse's role in, 374–377
Endemic disease, 492
  definition of, 20t
Energy
  definition of, 389t
  and fat, 63
England
  General Board of Health for, 22
  public health nursing in, 28
English clients, silence and, 233
Enrollees, in health care insurance plans, 209
Enviromechanical hazard
  exposures and health effects of, 605t
  in workplace, 604
Environment
  as community assessment parameter, 100t–101t
  damaging effects of, 250
  as determinant of health, 278
  health and, 263
  healthy school, 592
  infectious disease and, 491
  spiritual needs assessment and, 231b
Environmental assessment, home visit and, 651
Environmental factors, disease in human populations, 72t
Environmental hazards, 266
  effects of, 261–262, 261f
Environmental health, 249–271, 269b
  approaching, at population level, 263–264, 264b
  areas of, 252–261, 252t
  core, competencies, 265b
  critical, nursing practice, 264–268
    advocating for change, 264
    facilitating community involvement, 265
    forming coalitions for, 265–266
    questions for, 264

Environmental health (Continued)
  using collective strategies, 266–268
  critical theory approach to, 250–252
  definition of, 250, 599
  emerging issues, 263
  global, 263
  Healthy People 2020
    elements of, 250f
    objectives for, 264b
  nurses work in, 46, 46f
  problems
    efforts to control, 262–263, 262b
    example of, 252t
  World Health Organization (WHO) and, 250
Environmental health history
  for adults, 251
  assessment, 251f
  benefit of, 250–251
  for children, 251
  occupational exposure, 250–251
Environmental health issues, affecting communities, 255b
Environmental health nursing, standards of, 601t
Environmental health problems, critical questions about, 265b
Environmental health services, 191
Environmental justice, 254
Environmental legislation, landmark federal, 254b
Environmental Protection Agency (EPA), 253
  air quality index, 257f
Environmental Response Compensation and Liability Act, 261
Environmental stewardship, 266
Environmental stressor
  consequences of, 273
  types of, 273
Epidemic
  definition of, 492
  effects of, 489
Epidemic disease
  definition of, 20t
  theory of, 22
Epidemiological approach, 71b
Epidemiological triangle, 70, 70f
Epidemiology, 69–91, 90b
  analytic, 83–90
  data analysis and, 95
  definition of, 599
  descriptive, 70, 83, 83b
  in disease control/prevention, 70–74, 72t, 78–82
  ecosocial, 72–74
  in health services, 82–83, 83b, 88b–89b
  methods of, 83–90
  social, 347b
Equal protection, disability and, 412b
Equilibrium, definition of, 389t
Equity, ethical issues in, 133b
Eradication, of communicable disease
  criteria for, 496b
  definition of, 496

Ergonomics, and occupational health science, 599
Error theory, 356b
Escherichia coli, 259
Ethical issues, in children and adolescents, 308–311
Ethnic disparities
  in health care, 223
  Healthy People 2020 and, 222
Ethnic disparity
  child and adolescent health and, 301
  infant mortality and, 288, 290f
Ethnic disparity, in health care, 447b
Ethnic group
  single parent families and, 384t
  teen birth rate by, 384t
Ethnicity, of children, 287, 287f
Ethnicity, substance abuse and, 535, 536b
Ethnocentrism, 223–224
Ethnocultural considerations, substance abuse and, 535, 536b
Etiological factors, disease in human populations, 72t
Evacuation, during disaster, 571
Evaluation
  as health planning model/objective, 108f, 109b
  types of, 112
Evidence
  in sexual assault, 617b
  types of, 620b
Executive branch, of the government, 170t
Exercise
  health and, 65
  walking as, 65
Experience, adult learner, 127t
Experimental studies, 87–90, 88f
Explosions, 567b
Exposure variables, 83–84
Expressed need, 110
Expressive functioning, 390
Extended family, 227
External structure, of family, 390

F

Facilitator, faith community nurse as, 636–637
Factory Nurses Conference, 599
Faith communities, in rural areas, 459
Faith community nurse
  CIRCLE Model of Spiritual Care and, 638
  as coordinator of volunteers, 636–637
  as developer of support groups, 637
  education of, 637–638, 638b
  as facilitator, 636–637
  as health advocate, 636
  as health educator, 636
  as integrator of health/healing, 637
  interventions by, 637–638
  as personal health counselor, 636
  as referral agent, 636
  roles/functions of, 636–637
  spirituality of, 638–639, 639b

Faith community nursing, 631–644
  accountability, 641–643
  confidentiality, 640–641
  family violence prevention, 639–640
  foundations of, 633–636, 635b
  Healthy People 2020, 635b
  issues in, 639–643
    end-to-life issues, 639
    providing care to vulnerable populations, 639
  models of, 631b–632b
  nursing process, application of, 641b–643b
  principles of applied ethics in, 640b
  role in health/wellness, 632–633
Faith factor, 633
Falling, improving balance, 367b
Family, 381b–382b
  with adolescents, 392b
  assessment tools for, 392–393
  characteristics of, 383–384
  chronic illness in, nurse working with, 386–387
  as component of community, 387
  culture and, 227–228
  definition of, 383
  divorce and remarriages in, 392
  functional diversity of, 227
  health care, access to, 387b
  health promotion for, 593
  healthy, characteristics of, 389–390
  as homeless, 433, 437
  instrumental functioning of, 390
  Japanese-American, 228
  as launching centers, 392b
  Mexican-American, 228
  models of care for, 396–397
    Health Access Nurturing Development Services Program, 396–397
    Kentucky Partnership for Farm Family Health and Safety, 396
  moving to community, 387–388
  newborn assessment, involving in, 386
  occupational health nurse and, 386
  risk index, 593b
  school nurses and, 386
  social system and
    ecological framework, 395
    network framework, 395
    transactional model, 395–396
  structural-functional conceptual framework, 390–391
  structure of
    external, 390
    internal, 390
  substance abuse and
    effect on, 532
    as social network for, 531–532
  types of, 384t
Family and Medical Leave Act, women's health and, 330–331

Family Educational Rights and Privacy Act (FERPA), 589
Family functional assessment, 391b
 expressive functioning as, 390
 instrumental functioning as, 390
 purpose of, 394
Family health, 380–402, 381f, 382b, 391b
 approaches to, 388–392
 community and, 387
 HANDS program and, 396–397
 needs of, 388
Family health assessment, 398b
 form for, 394
 guidelines for, 394
 social and structural constraints, 394
 tools for
  development of, 394
  ecomap, 393
  family health tree, 392
  genogram, 392–393, 393f
Family health intervention, extending, to larger aggregates and social action, 394–397
Family health tree, 392
 information on, 392
 purpose of, 392
Family interviewing
 components of, 385
  genogram and ecomap, 385
  manners, 385
  strengths of family or individual, commending, 386
  therapeutic conversations, 385
  therapeutic questions, 385
 issues in, 386
Family life cycle, 391b
 of middle-class North American, 392b
Family nursing, 382–383
Family Support Act of 1988, 175
Family theory, 388
Family therapy, 479
Family violence prevention, 639–640
Farm family, health and safety of, 396
Fasting, 230
Fats, role of, 63
Fecal incontinence, 366
Fecal-oral transmission, 494
Federal Child Abuse Prevention and Treatment Act, 621
Federal Emergency Management Agency (FEMA), 559, 566f
 mission of, 566
Federal government, 170
 different types of emergencies, 567b
 disaster responsibilities of, 565–567
 disaster supply kit, 566b
Federal health centers, 435
Federal legislation, occupational health, impact of, 610–612, 610t
Federal-level subsystem, 189–190
 activities of, 189
 health services of, 189–190

Federal poverty guidelines, 174t
Federalism, 170
Fee schedule, 204b
Feedback, 389t
Female athlete triad, 590b
Fertilizer
 food quality in, 260
 land pollution and, 273
Fetal alcohol spectrum disorders (FASDs), 291
Fetal development, 287–288
 smoking and, 291
Fire-related injuries, in older adult, 368
Firearm, in violence, as a factor of, 552
First responders, to disasters, 564–565
Flexible spending account (FSA), 204b, 215
Flexner Report, 27
Floods
 picture of, 573b–574b
 predictability of, 561
Flow and transportation, 389t
Flunitrazepam (Rohypnol), 545
Focus groups, 99–101
Folk healers, 27, 236
Fomites, 493
Food
 cultural identity and, 229
 social contact during, 229–230
Food and Drug Administration, 190b
Food safety
 agrichemicals, 259
 environmental health and, 259–261, 260b
 definition, 252t
 problems, 252t
 Escherichia coli, 259
 genetically modified, 260
 handling of, 259
 steps to, 259f
Food safety meat inspection, environmental health issues, 255b
Food systems, healthy and sustainable, 260b
For-profit health care, shift to, 207
For-profit hospitals, 203
Forensic, definition of, 616
Forensic nurse death investigator, role of, 618–619, 618f
Forensic nurse examiner
 clinical, 620–622, 620b
 in emergency and critical care, 620
 in organ and tissue donation and transplantation, 620–621
 in vulnerable populations care, 621–622, 622b
  child abuse and neglect, 621
  elder abuse, 621
Forensic nursing, 616–617, 629, 629b
 education for, 625–629
 Healthy People 2020 and, 617b
 programs, basic curricula for, 625t
 responsibilities of, 617

Forensic nursing (Continued)
 schools offering programs in, 626b
 subspecialties of, 617–622, 617b
  coroner, 619
  death investigator, 618–619, 618b
  legal consultants and attorneys, 619–620
  nurse examiner, clinical, 620–622
  sexual assault nurse examiner (SANE), 617–618
Forensic psychiatric nurse, 622
Formal caregivers, 654
Format, 135
Formative evaluation, 112
Framingham Heart Study, 87
Free radical theory, 356b
Freire, Paulo, 129
Frequency, of disasters, 560
Friends, as substance abuser social network, 531–532
Frontier, 445
Fruits, USDA recommendations for, 63
Fujita Tornado Intensity Scale, 563
Full capitation, 204b
Functional activities, 409
Functional diversity, of family, 227
FURCO Service Learning Model, 281f

G

Gamma-hydroxybutyrate (GHB), 545
Gangs, as community violence, 551
Garcia family
 ecomap for, 394f
 family health assessment of, 398b
 genogram for, 393f
Gastrointestinal system, of older adult, 361t–362t
Gatekeeper, 204b, 205
 physicians as, 214
Gatesville Medical Center, 283b
Gay, 227
Gay/lesbian family, 384
Gender, 234
 life expectancy by, 340t
 medical care use by, 342
  ambulatory care, 342
  health services, 342
  hospital care, 342
  preventive care, 342
 of older adults, 357
Gender-linked behavior, 345–346
Gender-role behavior, stereotyped, 343b
General Board of Health for England, 22
General health services, in rural areas, 448
General systems theory, 388–389
Generalized anxiety disorder, 475
Genetic disorder, screening of newborns for, 293b
Genetic factors, 471
Genetically engineered foods, 260
Genetically modified (GM) foods, 260

Genital herpes, 508t–509t
Genitourinary system, of older adult, 361t–362t
Genogram
 example of, of Garcia family, 393f
 as family assessment tool, 385, 392
 symbols for, 393f
Geographic community, 94
Geography, as community assessment parameter, 100t–101t
Geopolitical communities, 3
Geriatric care management for low-income seniors, 162b
Glaucoma, 365–366
Global environmental health, 263
Global warming, 262
 as environmental stressor, 273
Globalization
 definition of, 272
 international health and, 199
"Golden Rule," 231b
Gonorrhea, 508t–509t
Government, 169
 branches, 170t
 improving child health, 307
Great Britain, 22
Greeks, culture-bound syndrome in, 237t
Grief, faith community nursing and, 639
Group home, for developmentally delayed
 as health planning project, 113, 113b
 prevention for, 114t
 problematic step for, 113t
Group therapy, 480
Growing, 227
Guardianship, 374

H

Haemophilus influenzae, 500t–501t
Hallucinogens
 effect and withdrawal symptoms of, 523t
 illicit use of, 517–519
Handicap, 404–407
 terminology for, 405t
Harm reduction, 531
Harmony, 226
Hate crimes, as community violence, 551
Hazmat tag, 572
Head injury, 293
Healing services, faith community nurse integrating, 637
Health, 3
 affecting existing illnesses, 273
 of aggregate
  consequences for, 30–31
  impact on, 19–20
 alcohol consumption and, 60–62
 child and adolescent, 286–313
 of children, long-term implications as, 287
 community view, 1–17
 conditions affecting, 22
 culture and, 235
 definition of, 50

Health *(Continued)*
determinants of, 4–5
diet and, 62–65
emphasizing the "doing" aspects of, 457
evolution of, 19–23
faith community role in, 632–633
in global community, 272–285
and homeless populations, 435
indicators of, 5
literacy and, 140–144, 140b
patterns of, 273–275
perceptions of, 454–455
gender, race, and ethnicity, 454–455
physical activity and, 65
poverty influencing, 228–229
during pregnancy, 287–288
preventive approach to, 7–10
promotion, 7–8
risk to, relationship of, 57–66
sleep and, 65–66
Health, United States, 342b
Health Access Nurturing Development Services Program, 396–397, 397t
Health advocate, faith community nurse as, 636
Health Amendments Act of 1956, 174
Health behaviors
intervention foci and, 44f
reporting, 344
Health belief model (HBM), 40–41, 53–54
application of, 40–41
basis/purpose of, 126
components/example and explanation of, 127t
concepts/definitions of, 55t
constructs of, 54
example of, 56f
limitations of, 41, 127
Milio's framework *versus*, 42
personal behavior pattern and, 44
purpose of, 42
variables/relationships in, 40f
Health care
access to, 53, 158
coordination and access to, 198
delivery system, 166
economics of, 202–219, 218b
expenditures for, 278
family access to, 387b
fraud and abuse in, 207, 207b
governmental grants for, 209
Hispanics and, 223
homeless population and, market and social justice approaches to, 438–439
industry, restructuring of the, 182–183
insurance plans, 209–212
historical perspective, 209–210
reasons for lack of, 209–210
legislation, 172–173, 172b
federal, 173–176, 173t
limited, 199b
mission-oriented, 346

Health care *(Continued)*
modern, advent of, 23–30
philanthropic foundations influencing, 27
policy, nurses' historical/current activity in, 166
public financing of, 207–209
racial/ethnic disparities in, 223, 447b
reform, 182–183
reimbursement, changes in, 158
system, major legislative actions and the, 173–176
technological advances in, 206
use of, 205
Health care alliances, 215
Health care cost
containment, 212
factors influencing, 203–207
historical perspective of, 203–205
Health care cost, upward spiral in, 157
Health care coverage programs, for children and adolescents, 304–305
Affordable Care Act, 304
Children's Health Insurance Program, 304–305
direct health care delivery programs, 305–306
Maternal and Child Health Block Grant, 305
Medicaid, 304–305
school-based health centers, 305–306
Special Supplemental Nutrition Program for Women, Infants, and Children, 306
Health care delivery
critical issues in, 197–199
managed care, 197
quality care, 197
disparity in, 199
in rural areas, 448, 457–458, 464
Health care dollar, spending of, 211f
Health care expenditure
increasing with age, 206
projection for, 278
Health care financing
philanthropy and, 209
reform, 215–217
trends in, 214–215
Health care professionals, 192–194
substance abuse among, 532
Health care providers, 192–194
accreditation and, 197
definition of, 204b
fee for services by, 203
nontraditional, 194
organizations, 192
changes in, 192
in rural areas, 445, 457–458
telemedicine, 458
types of, 192
Health care reform, 117, 199, 217
Bill Clinton and, 216
Health care services
coordination of, 159
school-based health centers, 305–306

Health care system, 186–201, 201b
components of, 187–194
cost-effectiveness and cost containment, 187
distribution of resources, 229
federal legislation in
Medicaid, 191
Medicare, 191–192
future of, 199–200
learning activities of, 200–201
market-based, 278
population-based *versus*, 278
men as consumers in, 348
overview of, 187
private *versus* public, 187, 187f
subsystems as, 94
Health Care without Harm, 266
Health center, school-based, 594
Health communication
framework for developing, 133–140, 139f
assessing effectiveness and making refinements, 138–140, 139b
developing and pretesting concepts/messages/materials, 135–138, 138b
feedback, 139b
implementing program, 138, 138b
planning and strategy development, 134–135
Health data. *see* Census
Health delivery systems, Milio's framework for, 42–43
Health determinants
Healthy People 2020, 51
relationship among, 53f
types of, 51–53, 52t
Health disparities, 133
Healthy People 2020, 223
in quality and access, 415
Health education, 583–586
definition of, 124
effective teaching tips for, 143–144
focus of, 111
goal of, 124
learner verification, components of, 144t
minority population and, 239–240
nurse role in, 132, 132b
nursing process, application of, 145b–146b
for older adults, 359
during pregnancy, 291
resources of, 140–147
teaching-learning format for, 135t
see also Community health education
Health education empowerment, model of, 128–130
Health education material
assessment of, 144–145
aesthetic quality and appeal, 147
format/layout, 146
learner verification, 147
reading level, 147
relevancy, 145–147

Health education material *(Continued)*
type, 146
verbal content, 146–147
visual content, 147
pamphlets as, 144
Health education model, 126
Health educator, faith community nurse as, 636
"Health field concept," 278
"Health for all," 278
social justice *versus* market justice ethics, 347b
Health Impact Assessments (HIAs), 95
Health indicator, focus areas for, 52t
Health information campaigns, planning, 239
Health initiatives, throughout the world, 280–284, 280f
Health insurance
changes in, 31
for children and adolescents, 304–305, 304f
Children's Health Insurance Plan, 203
covered services by, 212
development of, 203
Medicare as, 358
national, 216
reform in, 118
reimbursement mechanisms of, 210–211
in rural areas, 448–449
types of, 210
Health Insurance Portability and Accountability Act of 1996 (HIPAA), 175
component of, 589
Health insurance-purchasing cooperative, multistate networks/alliance as, 210
Health issue, description of, 135b–136b
Health literacy, 128–129
definition of, 141
ethical issues related to, 133b
intervention for, 141
nurse role in, 141
screening for, 142
Health maintenance organization (HMO), 187, 204b, 210
advantages and disadvantages of, 212t
Health Maintenance Organization (HMO) Act of 1973, 174–175
Health manpower, as community assessment parameter, 100t–101t
Health Objectives Planning Act of 1990, 175
Health plan, 204b
Health Plan Effectiveness Data and Information Set (HEDIS), 197
Health planning
changing focus of, 117–120
community involvement in, 111
concept of, 109–111
focus of, 107
nurse role in, 107
overview of, 107, 107f

Health planning (Continued)
  prioritizing problems in, 110
  project objectives of, 109b
  in public health, 115–116
Health planning federal legislation, 116–120
  influences on, 116
  student nurse involvement in, 118b–119b
Health planning model, 108–112, 108f
Health planning project
  childhood obesity reduction as, 112b
  evaluation during, 112
  goals and objectives of, 111
  intervention for, 111–112
  nursing process importance in, 114
  as successful
    crime watch as, 113, 113b
    rehabilitation group as, 113, 113b
    in textile industry, 113, 113b
  as unsuccessful, 113, 113t
Health policy, 167, 171–173, 177
  and the private sector, 171
Health problem management, in culturally diverse populations, 239–241
Health problems, diagnosing, 101–105
Health professional organizations community services, as community assessment parameter, 100t–101t
Health Professions Education, 196
Health promotion, 78
  for children, 303–304
  in community, 50b–51b, 593
  community health nursing and, 49–51, 50b
  definition of, 49–50
  diabetes and, 386
  examinations for, 363b
  to family and community, 593
  and financial resources, 347
  impact on health care costs, 215
  lack of, men's health, 346–347
  Metropolitan Life Insurance Company and, 156
  models of, 240
  occupational health nursing and, 605
  in older adults, 360–364
  population-based approaches to, 278
  risk reduction and, 49–68, 67b
  risk to health and, 57–66
  for school staff, 593
  theories in, 53–56
Health Promotion Model (HPM), 53, 55t, 55f
  application of, 128
  components/definitions of, 128t
Health protection, 50
Health-protective behavior, 344
Health records, for students, 589
Health reform, 15–16
Health-related beliefs/practices, 235–237

Health-related quality of life (HRQOL), 9
Health Resources and Services Administration (HRSA), 178
Health risk, tobacco and, 58–60
Health screening, as health services, 587
Health services
  delivering and financing, 240
  use by gender, 342
Health statistics, as community assessment parameter, 100t–101t
Health status, in United States, rank of, 206
Health teaching, public health intervention, 15t
Health visiting, 28
Healthy communities, 94–95
  determinants of, 97f
Healthy family, characteristics of, 389–390
Healthy home, environmental health and, 258, 258b
  definition, 252t
  problems, 252t
Healthy People 2020, 9–10, 168, 277, 520, 520b
  communicable disease and, 490–491, 491b
  content related to public health infrastructure, 169b
  cultural health and, 222b
  cultural perspectives and, 222–223
  environmental health and elements of, 250f
  objectives for, 264b
  faith community nursing and, 635b
  focus areas for, 45–47
  forensic nursing objectives, 617b
  goals of, 51, 277
  health disparities and, 223
  and health needs of people with disabilities, 415–416
  health planning and, 118
  HIV/AIDS, 507–510
  home health and hospice care objectives, 646b
  immunization and infectious diseases, 499
  leading health indicator topics, 5b
  mental health and, 471, 471b
  minority health and, 446
  model, 4f
  objectives for child and adolescent health, 303, 303b
  objectives for data collection and reporting, 81b
  objectives for school health, 583b
  objectives of, 222
  and occupational health, 604
    objectives for, 604b
  for older adults, 360–362, 360b
  selected objectives for women's health, 315b
  sexually transmitted diseases and, 506–507
  substance abuse and, 520, 520b
  surveillance, 81

Healthy People 2020 (Continued)
  in thinking upstream, 45–47
  topic areas, 9b–10b
  violence and, 552
    objectives related to injury, 552b
Hearing, loss of, in older adults, 366, 366b
Hearing-impaired prisoners, 623b
Heart disease, 341
Heat stress disorder, in older adult, 368
Heavy metal, in water treatment, 258–259
Hebrews, hygiene code by, 21
Hepatitis
  in prisons, 623
  transmission and control of, 504t–505t
Herd immunity, 495
  example of, 495f
Heroic phase, of community response to disaster, 573
Heroin, 517, 519
Herpes, 508t–509t
Hierarchy of system, 389t
High-risk clinic setting, case management in, 161
Hill-Burton Act, 116, 174
Hinduism
  dietary practice of, 230t
  "Golden Rule" and, 231b
Hispanic culture
  adolescent pregnancy and, 299, 302f
  child population of, 287, 287f
  culture-bound syndrome in, 237t
  health and, 223
  health care and, 223
  nurses as, 222
  population of, 222
  poverty in, 229
Hispanic population
  death, leading cause of, 341t
  life expectancy for, 340
  of older adults, 357
  as single-parent family, 384t
  substance abuse and, 535
  teen birth rate in, 384t
Historiography, 27b
Holistic care, 32
Home, shelter-in-place instructions at, 568t
Home health agencies
  certified and noncertified, 647
  types of, 647
    hospital-based, 647
    nonprofit, 647
    official, 647
    proprietary, 647
Home health care, 646–647, 654b
  Albrecht nursing model for, 649, 650f
  for communicable disease, 656b–658b
  documentation of, 652
  formal and informal caregivers and, 654
  Healthy People 2020, 646b
  hospital readmission and PPS, 213b

Home health care (Continued)
  managed care and, 646
  models of, 279
  nursing process, application of, 652–654
    assessment, 652
    client and family roles, outlining, 653
    community service referral, 653
    diagnosis and planning, 652–653
    evaluation, 653–654
    intervention, 653
  OASIS and, 648–649
  pain control and symptom management in, 655–656
  purpose of, 646–647
  reimbursement for, 648
  in rural areas, 458–459
  service provided by, 647
  special programs for, 647–648
Home health nurse
  family members/caregivers and, 654
  standards and education for, 649–650
Home health services
  purpose of, 646–647
  types of, 647
Home visiting, 658b–659b
  antepartum client, 658b–659b
  conducting a, 650–651
    building trust, 651
    environment, 651
    improving communication, 651
    initial telephone contact, 651
    preparation, 650
    referral, 650–651
  cultural differences related to death and dying, 656–661
  environmental assessment and, 651
  evaluation phase of, 653–654
    goal achievement, 654
    goal progress, 653
    plan modification, 653
  Florence Nightingale and, 646
  focus of, 646
  HANDS program and, 396–397
  hospice, 659b–660b
  initial telephone contact for, 651
  preparation for, 650–651
  proof of insurance, 651
  referral for, 650–651
  terminating, 653
Homeless
  definition of, 429–430
  prevalence of, 431–433
Homeless Information Management System (HMIS), 431
Homelessness
  definitions of, 429–431
    conceptual approaches to, 430
    legal approaches to, 430–431
  factors contributing to, 433–435
    affordable housing, shortage of, 433–434

Homelessness *(Continued)*
  income insufficiency, 434
  supportive services, scarcity,
    434–435
  prevalence estimates, 432
Homeless population, 429–442,
    440b
  children as, 431
    health status of, 437
  counting of
    early efforts of, 431
    recent efforts of, 431
  demographic characteristics
    of, 433
  families as, 437
  health and, 435
  health care, access to, 435
  health experiences of, 47b
  health status of, 436–438
    women, 436–437
  number of, 432
  in shelters, 432
Homicide, 544
Homosexual family. *see* Gay/
    lesbian family
Homosexuality, 345b
Honeymoon phase, of community
    response to disaster, 573
Hookworm, 27
Hospice, 645–661, 661b
Hospice care, in rural areas,
    458–459
Hospice home care, 654–661, 654b
Hospice nurse, pain control and
    symptom management, 655
Hospice setting
  case management for, 161
  in rural areas, 458–459
Hospital
  cost shifting, 211
  nurses and, 2
  types of, 203
  use by gender, 342
Hospital-based care, alternatives
    to, 278
Hospital-based home health
    agencies, 647
Hospital care, gender differences
    in, 342
Hospital readmission, prospective
    payment system and, 213b
Hospital statistics
  classification of, 24
  lack of, 24
Host factors, disease in human
    populations, 72t
Host of disease, 491
  resistance/immunity of, 494–495
Host susceptibility
  definition/factors of, 493t
  to infectious disease, 494
House on Henry Street, 28, 29b
"Household science," 382
Housing
  as affordable, shortage of,
    433–434
  for older adults, 357–358
Human factors, 93
Human host
  of infectious disease, 491
  resistance/immunity of, 494–495

Human immunodeficiency virus
    (HIV), 274
  acquired immunodeficiency
    syndrome (AIDS) and, 489
  course of infection, 510f
  eradication of, 510
  exposure to, 510
  Healthy People 2020 and, 491b,
    507–510
  homeless population and, 437
  intervention for, 124b–125b
  prevalence of, 509f
  in prisons, 623
  transmission and control of,
    511t
  treatment of, 510
  in women, 328
Human-made disasters, mental
    illness and, 472–473
Human nature orientation, 226
Human papillomavirus (HPV)
  immunization, 507b
  transmission and control of,
    508t–509t
Human Rights Campaign, 382
Human rights violations, 168
Human trafficking, as community
    violence, 551
Humankind, disease history, stages
    and, 19, 19f
Hunting/gathering stage in disease
    history, 19, 19f
Hurricane
  categories of, 563
  death from, 562
  frequency of, 559–560
  injury from, 558–559
  predictability of, 561
  Saffir-Simpson Hurricane Scale,
    563, 564b
Hurricane Katrina, 558–559
  disaster relief during, 574b–575b
  scope of, 562
Hurricane Rita, scope of, 562
Hurricane Scale, 563, 564b
Hydrogen cyanide, 562t
Hygeia, *versus* Panacea, 30
Hygiene code, 21
  in Middle Ages, 21–22
Hypersensitivity, to vaccine,
    498–499
Hypertension, in women, 323
Hysterectomy, in women, 320

I

Iatrogenic disease, 24
Illicit drug use
  in adolescent, 300, 519, 585
  anxiety disorders, 370
  demographics for, 520
  educating about, 525
  by gender differences, 519–520
  historical overview of, 517
  incidence and trends in, 518–519
  during pregnancy, 291–292
  prescription-type psychothera-
    peutics, 519
  treatment for
    guidelines for, 528b
    harm reduction as, 531
    pharmacotherapy and, 529

Illness
  "as a river" metaphor, 439
  biomedical perspective on,
    235–236
  cross-cultural perspectives on
    causes of, 235
  cultural expressions of, 236–237
  differentiating disability from,
    407
  folk healers and, 236
  indicators of, 5
  magicoreligious perspective
    on, 236
  manufacturers of, 37
  naturalistic perspective on,
    235–236
Illness orientation, 344
Immigrants
  depression in, 232
  nutritional patterns of, 241b
  older adult as, 232
  values of children of, 228
Immigration, population and, 222
Imminence, 562
Immunity
  types of, 494–495
  vaccines providing, 495
Immunization
  for children, 296–297
  as health services, 586–587
  Healthy People 2020 and, 491b,
    499
  and infectious disease, 274
  for older adult, 363b
  precautions for, 497
  recommendation for, 297
  types of, 497–498
Immunological theory, 356b
Impairment, 404
  terminology for, 405t
Inactivated vaccines, 498, 499t
Incest, 548
Incidence rate
  example of, 75t
  of infectious disease, 492
  for morbidity, 74–75
Incineration, of waste, 261
Inclusion and trust
  establishment of, 132
  nurse enhancing, 132–133
Income
  insufficiency of, homeless and,
    434
  in rural areas, 449–451
  sources for older adults,
    358–359
Incontinence, in older adult, 366
Incubation period, of infection,
    492, 492f
Indemnity fee for service,
    advantages and disadvantages
    of, 212t
Indemnity health care insurance,
    205
Indemnity plan, 204b
Indian Health Service (IHS), 190b,
    245–247
Indirect transmission, 493
Indirect victim, 559
Individual behavior, models of,
    126–128

Individual is focus of change,
    40–41, 43t
Individual relationships, 227
Individual therapy, 479
Individualized education plan
    (IEP), 411
Individualized Health Care Plan
    (IHP), 589
Individuals, as homeless, 433
Individuals with Disabilities
    Education Act (IDEA), 412–413,
    589
Industrial cities stage in disease
    history, 19f, 20
Industrial engineering, 278
Industrial hygiene, and
    occupational health science,
    599
Industry, as community assessment
    parameter, 100t–101t
Infant
  accidental injuries in, 293–296
  health and safety of, 288
  preconception health of mother,
    290–291
  primary caregiver of, 228
Infant death
  definition of, 288b
  leading causes of, 288
Infant mortality rate, 288, 289f
  definition of, 288b
  demographic characteristics
    of, 445
  factors influencing, 288
  male and female, 343
  mother's ethnicity and race and,
    290f
  race and ethnicity and, 288
  smoking and, 291
  United States *versus* other
    nations, 288, 289t
Infection
  definition of, 491–492
  multicausation of, 491
  occurrence, principles of,
    491–492
  spectrum, 491–492
  stages of, 492, 492f
Infectious agent, 491
  definition/factors of, 493t
  transmission of, 492–493
Infectious diseases
  definition of, 491–492
  in developing countries, 274
  Healthy People 2020 and, 491b,
    499
  multicausation of, 491
  prevention of, 512t
  public health control of,
    495–496
Inflicted traumatic head injury, 547
Influence, behavior and, 391
Influenza, 500t–501t
Informal care systems, in rural
    areas, 459
Informal networks, maximizing the
    use of, 457
Information technology, 197–198
  in rural communities, 462–463
Infrastructure, affecting existing
    illnesses, 273

Inhalant
  effect and withdrawal symptoms of, 523t
  illicit use of, 519
Initiation stage of addiction, 524, 525t
Injury
  accidental, 293–296
  from disasters, 558–559
  fire-related, in older adult, 368
  intentional, 543
  in men, 341
  motor vehicle-related
    in children, 293
    in men, 343
  objectives related to, and violence, in *Healthy People 2020*, 552
  work-related, 606t
Injury prevention, as school health program, 584
Inpatient drug treatment programs, 528
Input, 389t
Institute of Medicine (IOM), 6
  Best Care at Lower Cost, as report, 218
  health care quality monitoring, 194–197
Institutional policies, 167
Instrumental activities of daily living (IADL), disability and, 409
Instrumental functioning, 390
Insurance reimbursement plans, 212t
Integrated health maintenance model, 187
Integrator, of health/healing, faith community nurse as, 637
Intellectual disabilities, 415
Intended audience, description of, 135b–136b
Intensity
  of disasters, 562–563
  Fujita Tornado Intensity Scale, 563
Intentional injuries, 543
Intercultural communication, 232
Intercultural nursing, 223
Internal structure, of family, 390
International Association of Forensic Nurses (IAFN), 617
International Community Assessment, application of, 281b–282b, 281f
International Council of Nurses (ICN), 277
International health, research in, 279
International health care, community health nurse and, 279
International Health Care Delivery Systems, 277–279
International nursing research, focus of, 279
International Parish Nurse Resource Center (IPNRC), 633–634
Interpersonal relationship, spiritual needs assessment and, 231b

Interpersonal violence, power and control wheel, 547f
Intervention, 111–112
  by aggregate/system level, 112t
  follow up to, 112
  health, effect on, 53
  as health planning model/objective, 108f, 109b
  home health care and, 653
  planning of, 111
  at prevention levels, 114
  STI/HIV risk reduction, 124b–125b
  for substance abuse, 525–531, 530t
  at community level, 537–538
Intervention foci, health behaviors, continuum of, 44f
Intervention Wheel. *see* Public Health Intervention Wheel
Intimacy, nurse-client, 232
Intimate partner violence, 640
  signs of, 329b
Intimate partner violence (IPV), 544–546
  myths associated with, 546b
  during pregnancy, 545
Intimate zone, 232t
IOM. *see* Institute of Medicine (IOM)
IPNRC. *see* International Parish Nurse Resource Center (IPNRC)
Islam
  dietary practice of, 230t
  "Golden Rule" and, 231b
Isolation, 494
Issue selection, health education and, 131t
Italian culture
  health and, 235
  sick-role behavior of, 232–233

J

Jamaican culture, health and, 235
Japanese-American families, 228
Jenner, Edward, 22
Jesus, 633
Jewish clients, eye contact and, 233
Job transfer, and community health nurse, 607
Johns Hopkins School of Hygiene and Public Health, 27
Johns Hopkins University Medical School, 27
Joint Commission, 197
Judaism
  dietary practice of, 230t
  "Golden Rule" and, 231b
Judicial branch, of the government, 170t

K

Keeping Patients Safe: Transforming the Work Environment of Nurses, 196–197
Kentucky Cabinet for Health and Family Services, 396
Kentucky Partnership for Farm Family Health and Safety, 396
Ketamine (ketamine hydrochloride), 546

Key informants, 99–101, 110
Koch, Robert, 25

L

Laboratory research, in United States, 206
Lalonde Report, 278
Land pollution
  causes of, 273
  as environmental stressor, 273
Language, 233–234
Language barriers, overcoming, 234b
Late preterm birth
  definition of, 288b
  prevalence of, 290
Latency period, of infection, 492, 492f
Latinas Unidas por un Nuevo Amanecer, Inc. (LUNA)
  community empowerment-collaboration-participation, 131b–132b
  development of, 131
Launching centers, family as, 392b
Launching stage, of family life cycle, 392b
Laws, 167
Lead, sources and effects of, 256t
Lead poisoning, 297
  as environmental stressor, 273
Leadership by Example, 195
Learner verification
  components of, 144t
  of health education material, 147
Learning, 124
Learning theory, 124–126
Legal issues, in children and adolescents, 308–311
Legal nurse consultants, 619–620
Legislation, 166
  health care, 172b
  process of, 171–173, 172f
Legislative branch, of the government, 170t, 171
Legislative information, sources for, 179t
Leininger, Madeleine, 223
Leininger's Sunrise Model, 223, 224f
Licensed practical nurse (LPN), 193
Life expectancy, 356–357
  for men, 340t
  by sex and race, 340t
  in women, 316
Lifestyle, 43
  affecting existing illnesses, 273
  barriers and facilitators to changes in, 215
  as determinant of health, 278
  good health and, 205–206
  sedentary, 586
Lineal relationships, 227
Lister, Joseph, 25
Literacy
  definition of, 141
  health and, 140–144, 140b
  health care services and, 141
  history/concept of, 129
Live attenuated vaccines, 499t

Liver disease, 61
Living arrangements, of older adults, 357–358
Living forensics, 620
Lobby, 180, 181b
Lobbyist, 180
Local government
  disaster management and, 564–565
  home healthcare and, 647
Local health department
  subsystems, 191
  activities of, 191
  categories of, 191
Location, defining community, 93–94
Longevity, in men, 340, 340t–341t
Loss, faith community nursing and, 639
"Love drug," 545
Low birth weight, 290
  infant mortality and, 290
  prevention of, 290
Lubic, Dr. Ruth Watson, 166
Lung cancer
  death rates from, 317
  in men, 340t, 341
  in women, 317, 325–326

M

Macroscopic approaches
  concept of, 39
  microscopic *versus*, 38–39, 38t
Macroscopic focus, 38–39
Macular degeneration, in older adults, 365
Magicoreligious perspective, illness causation, 236
Major depressive disorder, panic disorder, 475–476
Malaria, 274
Male-female relationship, 234–235
Malnutrition, in developing countries, 273
Man-made disaster, 558–579, 560b
  examples of, 573b–574b
Managed care, 15–16
  case management and, 157
  home healthcare and, 647
  in rural areas, 458
    interaction and integration, 464
Managed care group, 211–212
Managed care organizations (MCOs), 9
  accreditation of, 197
Managed care plan, 204b
Mandate, 204b
Mania, 475
Manners, 385
Manufacturing plant
  as health planning project, 114, 114b
  prevention for, 114t
  problematic step for, 113t
Marijuana, adolescent use of, 521, 521b
Marital status, of older adults, 357
Market-based health care system, 278

Market justice
 models of, 438–439
 versus social justice, 347b
 social justice and, 45b
 social justice *versus*, health care
  for homeless, 438–439
Marriage, family life cycle and,
 392b
Mass casualty event, 559
Materials and media, 135
 types of, 136t–137t
Maternal and Child Health Block
 Grant, 305
Maternal mortality, 318–319, 319t
Maximum allowable costs, 204b
McCarren-Ferguson Act of 1945,
 174
MCOs. *see* Managed care
 organizations (MCOs)
Measles
 blindness from, 489
 transmission and control of,
  500t–501t
Measurable objectives, 111
Media, in violence, as a factor of,
 552
Medicaid, 330
 case management and, 158
 for children and adolescents,
  304–305
 creation of, 205
 definition of, 204b
 federal legislation in health care
  system and, 191–192
 health care economics and,
  208–209
 homeless access to, 435
 for older adults, 358–359
 Title XIX Social Security
  Amendment, 174
Medical care
 men's health and patterns of, 346
 use by gender, 342
  ambulatory care, 342
  hospital care, 342
  other health services, 342
  preventive care, 342
Medical examiner, 618
Medical model, for disability, 406
Medical science, 599
Medical treatment, types of, 24
Medical waste management, 266
Medicalization, 43
 of mental illness, 470
Medicare, 330
 case management and, 158
 creation of, 205
 deductible for, 207–208
 definition of, 204b
 in diagnosis-related group, 211
 eligibility for, 207
 federal legislation in health care
  system and, 191–192
 fraud, 207b
 health care economics and,
  207–208, 208f
 OASIS and, 648–649
 pharmaceutical benefit for, 207
 Rural Hospital Flexibility, 461
 Title XVIII Social Security
  Amendment, 173–174

Medicare Advantage Plan, 204b,
 208, 358
Medicare-certified home health
 agency, 647
 number of, 648
Medicare home health expenditure,
 controlling, 213b
Medicare Modernization Act, 175,
 207
Medicare Part A, 207–208
Medicare Part B, 208, 358
Medicare Part C, 208
Medicare Part D, 208
Medicare Prescription Drug, 207
Medications
 administration of, by school
  districts, 588
 economic value of, 524
 inmates' refusal of, 624b
Medigap insurance, 204b, 358
Men
 addressing health concerns in,
  350b
 chronic conditions in, 341–342
 community health nursing
  services for, 348b
 death in, leading causes of, 341t
 health services for, 349
 heart disease in, 341
 as homeless, 433
 interest groups for, 348
 longevity in, 340
 lung cancer in, 341
 morbidity rate in, 341–342
 mortality in, 340–341, 344
 as older adult, physiological
  changes, 361t–362t
 reproductive health needs of,
  345b
 screening services for, 349
 testicular cancer in, 345b
Meningitis, type B, 500t–501t
Menopause, 327
Men's health, 339–354, 340b, 353b
 factors impeding, 346–347
  access to care, 346
  health promotion, lack of,
   346–347
  medical care patterns, 346
  mission orientation, 346
  time factors, 346
 life expectancy for, 340t
 needs of, 347–348
  skills for addressing, 348b
 nursing process, application of,
  351b–353b
 policies related to, 349
 status, longevity and mortality
  of, 340–342
 theories explaining, 342–346
  biological factors, 343
  socialization, 343–344
Mental disorders
 depression, 474–478
 encountered in community
  settings, 474–478, 474b
 evidence-based practice
  management of, 479
 identification, 479–481, 480f
  and management of, 478–481
 mental health and, 471

Mental disorders *(Continued)*
 overview of selected, 474
 psychotherapy for, 479–481
 in women, 326–327
Mental health
 of child or adolescent, 591
 factors influencing, 471–474
  biological, 471
  brain structure and
   functioning, abnormalities,
   471
  genetic factors, 471
  political, 473–474
 Healthy People 2020, 471
 of homeless population, 434–435
 nursing process, application of,
  485b–486b
 organizations that promote
  education and advocate for,
  484t
Mental health care
 community-based, 481–484
 in rural areas, 460
Mental Health Parity and
 Addiction Equity Act of 2008,
 175, 469
Mental health reform, 470
Mental health services, 191
Mental illness
 definition of, 469, 475b
 medicalization of, 470
 natural and human-made
  disasters and, 472–473
 nursing process, application of,
  485b–486b
 populations affected by, 468–487,
  486b
 in violence, as a factor of, 552
Mesothelioma, 343
Metabolic syndrome, in women,
 323
Methadone, 529
Methamphetamine
 administration of, 520–521
 effects of, 521
 prevalence of, 521
 treatment for, 527
Methane gas, 261
Methylenedioxymethamphetamine,
 519
Metropolitan area, 445
Metropolitan statistical areas
 (MSAs), 97, 445
Mexican-American families, 228
Micropolitan area, 445
Microscopic approach
 concept of, 39
 macroscopic *versus*, 38–39, 38t
Microscopic focus, 38–39
Middle Ages, public health in,
 21–22
Middle-class North American
 family life cycle, stages and tasks
 of, 392b
Midwifery, 27
Migrant farmworkers, 456–457
 enumeration of, 456
 hearing, 456–457
 preventive care for, 456
Migrant health, 443–467
Migrant Health Clinic (MHC), 461

Migrant Health Program (MHP),
 461
Milio's framework for prevention,
 41–43, 42t
 HBM *versus*, 42
 personal behavior patterns and,
  43
Military sexual trauma (MST),
 437
Millennium Development Goals,
 275
Mini-Cog, 373b
Minority Health, Office of (OMH),
 245, 245t
Minority health issues, research
 agenda on, 241
Minority population
 health professionals from,
  240–241
 substance abuse prevention and,
  526
Mission-oriented health care, 346
Mitigation, of disasters, 561
Mobilizing for Action Through
 Planning and Partnerships
 (MAPP) model, 116
Modern nursing, evolution of,
 23–24
Modifiable risk factor, 57–58
Monitoring, child and adolescent
 well-being, 302b, 303
Mood, exercise and, 65
Moral model, for disability, 406
Morbidity rate, 74–75
 of children, 287
 example of, 75t
 in men, 341–342
Mormonism
 dietary practice of, 230t
 population of, 230
Mortality
 during Crimean War, 24, 26t
 in twenty-first century, 30
Mortality rate, 75
 of children, 287
 comparison of, 76t
 example of, 75t
 in men, 340–341, 344
Mothers Against Drunk Driving
 (MADD), 525
Motivation, adult learner, 127t
Motor vehicle emissions,
 environmental health issues,
 255b
Motor vehicle-related injury, 293
Moulder, Betty, 599
Multicausation
 of infectious disease, 491
 principle of, 491
Multicultural nursing, 223
Multiple casualty event, 559
Multiple family configuration,
 women and, 322
Multispecialty group, 187
Multistate networks/alliance, as
 health insurance-purchasing
 cooperative, 210
Mumps, 500t–501t
Murder, 544
Musculoskeletal system, of older
 adult, 361t–362t

Muslim religion
   dietary practice of, 230
   eye contact and, 233
   modesty in women, 233
Mutual help groups
   12-step programs as, 530, 530t
   for substance abuse, 530
My Plate, 63–64, 64f
Myomectomy, in women, 320
MyPyramid
   for older adults, 363
   see also My Plate

N

Nagi model, 404–405
Naltrexone, 529
Narcotics, 523t
Natech (natural-technological)
   disaster, 560, 560b
National Agenda for Prevention
   of Disabilities Model (NAPD),
   405–406
   disabling process, 405–406
   quality of life issues, 406
National Alliance on Mental Illness
   (NAMI), 470
National Association of School
   Nurses, 412–413
National Center for Health
   Statistics (NCHS)
   data collection by, 342b
   National Health Interview
      Survey data, 99
National Center on Minority
   Health and Health Disparities
   (NCMHD), 241
National Committee for Quality
   Assurance (NCQA), 197
National Council on Elder Abuse,
   640
National Health and Nutrition
   Examination Survey (NHANES),
   84
National health insurance, 216
National Health Interview Survey
   (NHIS), 341, 342b
National Health Planning and
   Resources Act of 1974, 175
National Health Planning and
   Resources Development Act,
   117
National Healthcare Disparities
   Report, 415
National Incident Management
   System (NIMS), 559
National Institute for Occupational
   Safety and Health, 603
   occupational injuries, 343
National Institute on Alcohol
   Abuse (NIAA), 530t
National Institute on Drug Abuse
   (NIDA), 517
National League for Nursing
   (NLN), family nursing and, 382
National Organization for Public
   Health Nursing, 29–30
National Response Framework,
   565
National Response Plan, 565
National Women's Health Network
   (NWHN), 331

Native American
   alcohol and, 535
   culture-bound syndrome in, 237t
   eye contact and, 233
   health in rural areas, 451
   nurses as, 222
   population of, 222
   sick-role behavior of, 232–233
Natural disaster, 558–579
   effects of, 273
   examples of, 573b–574b
   types of, 560b
Natural history of disease, 78
Natural immunity, 494–495
Naturalistic perspective, illness
   causation, 235–236
Need, types of, 110
Need to know, adult learner, 127t
Needs assessment
   steps in, 102b
   strategies for, 99–101
Neglect, 547
   in children, physical and
      behavioral indicators, 548t
   definition of, 621
   forensic nurse examiner in, 621
   in older adults, 549
      indicators of, 550t
   signs of, 592b
   see also Emotional neglect;
      Physical neglect
Networking, 332
Network therapy, 395
Neural tube defects, 82b
Neuroendocrine control theory,
   356b
New Freedom Commission on
   Mental Health (NFCMH), 481
   goals and recommendations of,
   482t
New York Metropolitan Board of
   Health, 27
Newborn assessment
   genetic disorder screening in,
   293, 293b
   involving family in, 386
Newest Vital Sign (NVS), 143
NHANES. see National Health and
   Nutrition Examination Survey
   (NHANES)
Nicotine addiction, 58
   during pregnancy, 291
   see also Smoking
Nightingale, Florence, 166
   Coxcomb charts by, 25f
   district nursing and, 382
   health teaching by, 123
   home visiting, 646
   international health care and,
   279
   legislation and politics, influence
      on, 166
   modern nursing and, 23
   nursing practice, foundation
      for, 37
   statistical methods and, 24, 26b
Nineteenth century
   health care in, 23
   public health in, 22–23
Nitrogen oxides, sources and effects
   of, 256t

Noise, as environmental stressor,
   273
Noncertified home health agency,
   647
Non-English-speaking clients
   interpreter for, 233
   language barrier, overcoming,
   234b
Nonfederal sector, cooperative
   efforts with, 241
Nongovernmental environmental
   organizations, 263b
Nongovernmental organizations
   (NGOs), 275
Non-Hispanic white population
   as single-parent family, 384t
   teen birth rate in, 384t
Nonmodifiable risk factor, 57–58
Nonprofit home health agency,
   647
Nonstochastic theories, 356b
Nontraditional health care
   providers, 194
Nonverbal communication, 233
   eye contact as, 233
   handshaking as, 233
   nurse understanding, 233
   silence as, 233
   touching as, 234
   types of, 390
Norm
   definition of, 225–226
   questions related to, 226
Normalization, disability and,
   412b, 417
Normative belief, 55–56
Normative need, 110
North American family,
   middle-class, life cycle of, 392b
North American Nursing
   Diagnosis Association, spiritual
   distress and, 638
Notifiable infectious diseases, 496
   types of, 497b
Nuclear blast, 567b
Nuclear dyad family, 227
Nuclear family, 227, 383
   in varying cultures, 383
Nuclear Regulatory Commission,
   262
Nurse attorneys, 619–620
   testifying in court, 620b
Nurse case managers, 158–159
   elderly and, 161
   in pediatric settings, 161
Nurse-client relationship, 232
Nurse coroner, role of, 619
Nurse-family partnership program,
   88
Nurse-midwife (NM), 193
Nurse practitioner (NP), in rural
   areas, 448
Nurse Reinvestment Act of 2003,
   175
Nurses, 2, 580–581
   and campaigning, 181
   as change agents, 179
   and coalitions, 179–180
   communicable diseases and,
   491b
   in community/public health, 16

Nurses (Continued)
   cross-cultural communication,
   232–235
   disaster responsibilities of, 564,
   564b
   effective use of, 178
   as health educator, 123–124, 123b
   health literacy, role in, 142
   and leadership in health policy
      development, 183–184
   as lobbyist, 180
   national sample of registered,
   183b
   and political action committees,
   180
   in public office, 181–182
   religion and, 230
   role of, improving child health,
   307–308
   roles in political activities,
   178–182, 178b
   spirituality and, 230
   transcultural perspectives of, 221
   and voting strength, 181
Nurses' Health Study, 87
Nursing, anthropology and, 223
Nursing actions, 263
Nursing decisions and actions,
   models of, 223
Nursing policy, 167
Nursing practice, critical
   environmental health, 264–268
   advocating for change, 264
   facilitating community
      involvement, 265
   forming coalitions for, 265–266
   questions for, 264
   using collective strategies,
   266–268
Nursing process
   application of, 266b–268b
   adolescent pregnancy,
      309b–311b
   assessment and diagnosis,
      103b–104b
   case management and,
      162b–163b
   in community health,
      119b–120b
   community health nursing,
      246b–247b
   correctional nursing,
      626b–628b
   disability and, 424b–426b
   domestic abuse and,
      555b–556b
   in environmental health,
      266b–268b
   health education and,
      145b–146b
   home health care, 652–654
   home visiting and, 397,
      399b–400b
   men's health and, 351b–353b
   mental illness, 485b–486b
   occupational health and,
      613b–614b
   older adult, 375b–377b
   in school health, 594b–595b
   in health planning, 114
   substance abuse, 538b–539b

Nursing research, historical methodology for, 27b, 30b, 32b
Nursing science, 599
Nursing theory
  approaches to, 39–45
  development of, 38
  direction to, 38
  goal of, 38
  historical perspectives on, 37–38
  theory definitions and, 38b
Nutrient, fat as, 63
Nutrition
  culture and, 229–230, 243
  see also Diet
  educational programs for, 591
  for older adult, 363–364
  for school-age children, 590, 590b
Nutrition checklist, for older adults, 364t
Nutritional Education and Training (NET) program, 591
Nutritional education programs, 591
Nutritional patterns, of immigrants, 241b

O

OASIS. *see* Outcome and Assessment Information Set (OASIS)
Obesity
  causes of, 590–591
  in children
    diabetes and, 587–588
    factors influencing, 296
    prevalence of, 296
    prevention of, 296
    rate of, 296, 590
  contributing factors of, 62
  prevalence of, 62, 63f
  reduction of, goals/objectives for, 112b
Object, assuming role of, 129
Observational studies, 83–87
Obsessive-compulsive disorder, 476
Occupational exposure, 250–251
Occupational hazards, types of, and associated health effects, 605t
Occupational health, 598–615, 614b
  federal legislation on, impact of, 610–612, 610t
  and *Healthy People 2020*, 604
    objectives for, 604b
  legal issues in, 612
  levels of prevention for system levels in, 115t
  nursing process, application of, 613b–614b
  prevention strategies for, 604–607
    exposure to potential hazards, 604, 606f
Occupational health care, demographic trends/access issues related to, 600–601
Occupational health nurse, 13–14
  ADA and, 612
  families, working with, 386
  multidisciplinary teamwork and, 612–614
  OSHA and, 611

Occupational health nurse (*Continued*)
  pre-employment physical examinations, 610f
  professional links in workplace and community, 612f
  role of, 600–601
  skills and competencies of, 607–610, 608b
    in case management, 608–609
    in clinical and primary care, 608
    competent nurse, 608
    expert nurse, 608
    in health promotion and disease prevention, 609
    legal and ethical responsibilities, 609
    in management and administration, 609
    in nursing and code of ethics, 609–610
    in occupational/environmental health/safety education, 609
    professionalism of, 609
    proficient nurse, 608
    in research, 609
    in workforce/workplace/environmental issues, 609
  Workers' Compensation Act and, 611
Occupational health nursing, 598, 602b
  definition of, 598
  elements of, 598–599
  evolution of, 599–600
  knowledge domains, 599f
  levels of prevention and, 604–607
    primary, 604–606
    secondary, 606–607
    tertiary, 607
  nonoccupational programs in, 605
  practice and professionalism of, 601–603
  racial and ethnic minority groups and, 605–606
  research priorities in, 603b
  services, 603b
  standards of, 601t
  women's health and safety issues and, 605
Occupational health risks, 454
  for agricultural workers, 455–456
Occupational health sciences, 599
Occupational Safety and Health Act women's health and, 330, 331t
Occupational Safety and Health Act of 1970, 174
Occupational Safety and Health Administration (OSHA), 600, 610–611
  environmental conditions regulation of, 254
  establishment of, 610
  inspection program for, 611
  occupational health nurse and, 611
  record-keeping requirements for, 611

Occupational therapist (OT), 193
Office of Emergency Management, 565
Older adult
  Alzheimer's disease in, 372–373
  cataract in, 365
  chronic illness in, 364
  common health concerns for, 364–365
  crime against, 369–370
  culture shock of, 232
  death, leading cause of, 365t
  demographic characteristics of, 357–359
    education, 357
    geographic location, 357
    living arrangements, 357–358
    marital status, 357
    population, 357
    poverty and health education, 359
    racial and ethnic composition, 357
    sources of income, 358–359
  depression in, 370–371
  driver safety and, 367–368, 367b
  end-of-life issues for, advance directives, 374, 374b
  examinations for, 362–363
  health care screenings for, 362–363
  health concerns for
    additional, 365–366
    common, 364–365
  health promotion and, 360–364
    Healthy People 2020, 360–362
  hearing loss in, 366, 366b
  incontinence in, 366
  macular degeneration in, 365
  Medicaid for, 358–359
  medication use by, 364–365
  needs of, recognizing, 359b
  nursing process, application of, 375b–377b
  nutrition for, 363–364
    checklist, 364t
  physical activity and fitness for, 363, 363f
  physiological changes in, 360
  psychosocial disorders in, 370–373
  psychosocial issues in, 359–360, 360b
  sensory impairment in, 365–366
  spirituality of, 373–374
  substance abuse in, 371–372
  suicide in, 372
  traumatic brain injury in, 367
  widowhood and, 357
Omnibus Budget Reconciliation Acts, 175
Open mine waste, nurses and, 46
Open system, 389t
Opioids, 523t
Oral cancer, risk factors for, 584–585
Orem, Dorothea, 40
Organ/tissue donation/transplantation, 620–621
Organization, providing cultural support, 243

Organizational policies, 167
Organizations, 167
Orientation to learning, adult learner, 127t
Osteoarthritis (OA), in women, 323
Osteoporosis, in women, 324
Ostrich phase, and disability, 417
Out-of-pocket expenses, 204b
Outcome, 204b
Outcome and Assessment Information Set (OASIS), 648–649
Outcome evaluation, 103b
Outpatient drug treatment programs, 528
Output, 389t
Ovarian cancer, in women, 326
Overweight
  contributing factors of, 62
  prevalence of, 62
  restaurant eating and, 64
Ozone, 257
  sources and effects of, 256t

P

Pacemaker theory, 356b
Pacific Islander
  death, leading causes of, 341t
    in older adult, 365t
  nurses as, 222
  as single-parent family, 384t
  teen birth rate in, 384t
Pain
  cultural expressions of, 237
  nurse attitudes toward, 237
Pain control, hospice nurse and, 655–656
Palliative nursing care, 654–655
Pamphlet, patient value of, 144
Pan American Health Organization (PAHO), 275
Panacea, Hygeia *versus*, 30
Pandemic, 492
Pandemic disease, definition of, 20t
Panic disorder, 475–476
Paramedical technologists, 194
Parenting
  educational status and, 301
  improving child health, 306
  values and practices of, 228
Parish nursing
  mission statement for, 635
  philosophy of, 633
  in rural areas, 459
Participation, principle, 131t
Participatory action research (PAR), 129, 266, 266b
Participatory method, 129–130
Particle matter, sources and effects of, 256t
Partnership for Health Program (PHP), 116
Passive immunity, 494–495, 495t
Pasteur, Louis, 25
Pathogens, as drug-resistant, 490b
Patient-centered medical home, 157, 298b
  principles of, 157b
Patient protection, 217b

Patient Protection and Affordable Care Act (PPACA), 15–16, 118–120, 175–176
Pediatrician, in rural areas, 448
Pelvic inflammatory disease (PID)
ectopic pregnancy and, 319
effects of, 507
Pender's Health Promotion Model. see Health Promotion Model
"People factors," 93
People with disabilities (PWD), 404
nursing process, application of, 424b–426b
Perceived barriers, 55t, 127t
Perceived benefits, 55t, 126, 127t
Perceived need, 110
Perceived seriousness, 40
Perceived severity, 55t, 127t
Perceived susceptibility, 40, 55t, 127t
Perinatal Periods of Risk (PPOR) model, reducing infant mortality rates using the, 82b
Periodic assessment, and community health nurse, 607
Person-nature orientation, 226
Person-place-time model, 70, 70b
Personal behavior patterns
HBM/Milio's prevention model focus on, 44
lifestyles and, 43
Personal distance, 232t
Personal health care, 187
Personal health counselor, faith community nurse as, 636
Personal health services, 6, 191
Persuasion, learner verification and, 144t
Pertussis, 500t–501t
Pesticide poisoning, in agricultural workers, 455
Pesticides, food safety and, 259
Pew Health Professions Commission, 188
Pharmaceuticals, 206–207
Pharmacist, 193
Pharmacotherapies, 529–530
Phenomenological communities, 3
Phobia, 476
Physical abuse, 547, 548t
definition of, 621
signs of, 592b
Physical activity
guidelines for school programs in promoting, 586, 586b
and health, 65
for older adults, 363
walking as, 65
Physical environment, 53
Physical fitness, and lifestyle, for men's health, 348–349
Physical hazard
exposures and health effects of, 605t
in workplace, 604
Physical inactivity, actual causes of death, 4–5
Physical neglect, 548t
Physical responses, to traumatic event, 578t
Physical therapist (PT), 193

Physician
current procedural terminology (CPT) codes, 204b
as gatekeepers, 214
in rural areas, 448
Physician assistant (PA), 193
Physician (MD or DO), 193
Physiological changes, in older adult, 360, 361t–362t
Plague, 21
as bioterrorism agent/disease, 561b
documented cases of, 22b
Planned behavior, theory of, 57f
Planning
as health planning model/objective, 108f, 109b
of interventions, 111
Planning Approach to Community Health (PATCH) model, 115
Plausibility, biological, cause-and-effect relationship, 79
Play therapy, 480
PMR. see Proportionate mortality ratio (PMR)
Pneumococcal disease, 500t–501t
Point-in-time (PIT) count, 431, 432t
Point-of-service (POS) plan, 204b, 210
advantages and disadvantages of, 212t
Point prevalence study, of homeless population, 431–433
Point prevalences, 75
Policy, 166–167
formulation
the ideal, 177
the reality, 177
steps in, 177–178
health, effect on, 53
Regulatory, and Organizational Constructs in Educational and Environmental Development (PROCEED), 115
Policy analysis, 177
Policy development/enforcement, public health intervention, 15t
Polio, 500t–501t
Polio vaccine, 40, 296–297
Political action committees (PACs), 180
Political organization, as community assessment parameter, 100t–101t
Politics, 166
affecting existing illness, 273
Pollutant, 273
Pollution, 21
as environmental stressor, 273
Polypharmacy, 364
Poor
communicable disease in, 23
federal/state health insurance for, 31
Poor diet, actual causes of death, 4–5
Population, 4
based care, 16
characteristics of, 273
of children, 287
as community assessment parameter, 100t–101t

Population (Continued)
cultural diversity in, 221–222
in developing countries, 273
disability and, 403–428, 406b, 414b, 421b, 426b
distribution of, 273
growth, effects of, 273
"hidden pockets" of need, 99b
immigration and, 222
in rural areas, declining, 448
in workforce, 600
Population-based approach, to health promotion, 278
Population-based health care system, 278
Population-based statistics, 24
Population-focused nursing, 11, 13t
Portability, 204b
Portal of entry
controlling, 494
definition/factors of, 493t
types of, 493
Portal of exit
controlling, 494
definition/factors of, 493t
types of, 493
Portion
definition of, 62
restaurant eating and, 64
Portion distortion, 64
Positive predictive value, 80–81
Post-traumatic stress disorder (PTSD), 476
raising awareness of, 473b
Posttraumatic stress disorder (PTSD)
disaster and, 573, 576–578, 578t
risks for, 573
Poverty
in children, 301
definition of, 581
family and children in, 228–229, 228t
influences on health and well-being, 228–229
in older adult, 359
in rural areas, 449–451, 449f, 450t
Power
child care, quality of, 43
distribution of, 229
PPACA. see Patient Protection and Affordable Care Act (PPACA)
Practice guidelines, 204b
Prayer, 638–639
Preadolescents, substance abuse in, 533–534
PRECEDE-PROCEDE model, 115, 115f
Preconception health, 290–291
Predictability, of disasters, 561
Predisposing, Reinforcing, and Enabling Constructs in Educational Diagnosis and Evaluation (PRECEDE), 115
Preferred provider organization (PPO)
advantages and disadvantages of, 212t
definition of, 204b
overview of, 210

Pregnancy
addiction during, 525b
in adolescents, 299, 299b
alcohol and illicit drug use during, 291–292
intimate partner violence (IPV) during, 545
mother's health during, 287–288
nutrition and, 328
preconception health, 290–291
substance abuse during, 534
substance use during, 291–292
smoking and, 291
Preindustrial cities stage in disease history, 19f, 20
Premature deaths, from air pollution, 256–257
Premium, definition of, 204b
Prenatal care, 288
infant death and, 291
model of, 319b
types of, 291
Prenatally and Postnatally Diagnosed Awareness Act of 2008, 420
Prepaid health provision contract, 203
Preparedness and planning stage, of disaster management, 570
Preplacement evaluation, and occupational health nurse, 606
Prescription drug
expenditure of, 206–207
Medicare and, 207
Prescription-type psychotherapeutics, 519
Present stage in disease history, 19f, 20
Preterm birth
definition of, 288b
factors associated with, 290
infant health and, 290
prevention of, 290
smoking and, 291
Prevalence rate, 75, 76f
Preventability, of disasters, 561
Prevention
of communicable diseases, 510
concepts of, 8b
versus cure, 8–9
for health planning project, 114t
of infectious diseases, 512t
levels of, 7–8, 7f, 7t
Milio's framework for, 41–43
and occupational health nursing, 604–607
primary, 604–606
secondary, 606–607
tertiary, 607
school nurse role in, 595t
substance abuse and, 526
minority population and, 526
of violence, 552–554, 553b, 554t
Prevention stage, of disaster management, 569–570
Preventive behavior determinant, model for, 126
Preventive care
gender differences in, 342, 344
lack of, 205
for migrant/seasonal farmworkers, 456

Preventive health care, 278
   in children, 301–302
Primary care
   definition of, 279
   health care system and, 223
   in rural areas, 448
Primary care provider, 204b
   for managed care organization,
      214
Primary health care
   definition of, 279
   purpose of, 275
Primary prevention, 7, 7t, 78, 111
   case management for, 161
   of communicable diseases, 510
   for disasters, 561
   for health planning project, 114t
   of infectious disease, 512t
   for men's health, 348–349
      health education, 348
      interest groups for, 348
      physical fitness and lifestyle,
         348–349
      policy related, 349
   school nurse role in, 595t
   strategies for occupational health
      nurse, 604–606
   substance abuse and, 526
   for system levels, 115t
   for textile industry, 114t
   of violence, 553, 554t
   women's health and, 332
Primary vaccine failure, 495
Principle of participation, health
   education and, 131t
Principle of relevancy, health
   education and, 131t
Priority Areas for National Action:
   Transforming Health Care
   Quality, 196
Prison populations, 623–624
   adolescents in, 624
   health issues in, 623
      chronic and communicable
         diseases, 623–624
   women in, 623–624
Prison violence, as community
   violence, 551
Prisoners, as hearing-impaired, 623b
Private health care subsystem,
   187–188, 187f
   voluntary agencies and, 188
Private health insurance, 31
Private hospitals, 203
Private insurance, 210
Problem solving, 391
Problem-solving education, 129
Process evaluation, 112
Product evaluation, 112
Professional association, 167
Professional enablers, 532–533
Programmed theory, 356b
Promotion, health, 78
Proportionate mortality ratio
   (PMR), 76
Proportions, 74
Proprietary home health agency, 647
Prospective payment system (PPS),
   158
   hospital readmission after home
      health care, 213b

Prospective reimbursement,
   211–212
Prospective studies, 85–87, 86b, 86f
Prostate cancer, treatment options
   for, patient communication, 144b
Protestants, 226
   population of, 230
Provider of care, community health
   nurse as, 217–218
Providers, terms pertaining to, 204b
Psychological abuse, 621
   see also Emotional abuse
Psychological services, for children,
   591–592
Psychological triage, 573
Psychology, learning theories and,
   124
Psychosocial disorders, 370–373
   anxiety, 370
Psychosocial hazard
   exposures and health effects of,
      605t
   in workplace, 604
Psychosocial issues, in older adult,
   359–360, 360b, 360f
Psychosocial theories, 356
Psychotherapeutic medications,
   479
   nonmedical use, 519
Psychotherapy, 479–481
Psychotropic medications, 479
Public development, core public
   health functions, 6b
Public distance, 232t
Public financing, of health care,
   207–209
Public health, 188–189
   achievements, 31b–32b
   case management and, 156
   in classical times, 21
   core, functions, 6b
   definition/focus of, 6
   early efforts, evolution of, 20–23
   in eighteenth century, 22
   future of, 199–200
   health planning in, 115–116
   infectious diseases control by,
      495–496
   interventions, 15t
   in middle ages, 21–22
   mission of, 2
   in nineteenth century, 22–23
   objectives of, 22–23
   prerecorded historic times in,
      20–21
   purpose of, 16
   in the Renaissance, 22
   in rural areas, 459–460
      interaction and integration,
         464
   three levels of, 191–192
   in United States, 28–30
Public Health Act of 1944, 174
Public health care subsystem, 187f,
   188–192, 189f
   concerns of, 189
   at federal level, 188
   federal policies and practices
      under, 188
   at local health, 191
   at state-level, 190–191

Public health clinic setting, case
   management in, 161
Public health infrastructure, 169b
Public Health Intervention Wheel,
   14–15, 14f
Public health law, 22–23
   definition of, 167
   example of, 167t
Public health nursing, 2, 6, 10
   challenges for, 32–34
   competencies, 12t–13t
   in England, 28
   establishment of, 28–30
   Milio's framework in, 42t
   organizations for, 39
   practice, 11
   research agenda, 10b
   scope/standards of practice for,
      11b
   in United States, 28–30
Public health policy, 171
Public health programs, for children
   and adolescents, 304–306
Public health rates, major, 77t
Public Health Service Act, women's
   health and, 330
Public health services, 6b
   Romans provided, 21b
Public Health Services
   Amendments of 1966, 116
Public health system, disaster
   management and, 567–568
Public hospitals, 203
Public Law 99-142, 589
Public office, nurses in, 181–182
Public policy, 171
   blueprint for governance,
      176–178
   definition of, 167
   disability and, 412–414, 412b
      Individuals with Disabilities
         Education Act (IDEA),
         412–413
      legislation affecting, 412–413
   example of, 167t
Public services, as community
   assessment parameter, 100t–101t
Puerperal fever, 26
Pure Food and Drugs Act of 1906,
   173

Q

Quad Council of Public Health
   Nursing, 39
Quality care, 194–197
   accreditation and, 197
   concern of, 194
Quality care monitoring, 197
Quarantine, 494

R

Rabies vaccine, 26
Race
   of children, 287, 287f
   disability prevalence by, 410
   infant mortality and, 290f
   life expectancy by, 340t
   poverty and, 451
      children and, 451
   substance abuse and, 535
   suicide rates by, 451–452

Racial disparities
   child/adolescent health and, 301
   diseases and, 223
   in health care, 223, 447b
   Healthy People 2020 and, 222
   infant mortality and, 288
Radiation dispersion device event
   outdoors, 567b
Radon, 258
Randomized clinical trial, 87–88,
   88f
Rapid Estimate of Adult Literacy in
   Medicine (REALM), 142
Rates, 74, 74b
   advantages/disadvantages of, 77t
   age-adjustment of, 76
   age-specific, 76
   attack, 75
   calculation of, 74–77, 75t
   crude, 75
   incidence, 74–75
   morbidity, 74–75
   mortality, 75, 76t
   public health, 77t
   raw counts conversion to, 74
   standardization of, 76
Ratio, for disease prevalence, 74
Raw counts, 74
Readiness to learn, adult learner,
   127t
Reasonable accommodations, 413
Reasoned Action, theory of, 55–56
   example of, 57f
Recovery stage, of disaster
   management, 578
Recreation, as community
   assessment parameter, 100t–101t
Recycling
   Hollie Shaner and, 266
   in waste management, 261
Referral
   for community service, 653
   for home health care nursing,
      650–651
Referral agent, faith community
   nurse as, 636
Referral/follow-up, public health
   intervention, 15t
Refugees, 559
Regional Medical Programs
   (RMP), 116
Registered dietitian (RD), 193
Registered nurse (RN)
   education of, 193
   employment of, 2
   national sample of, 183b
Registered Nurse Safe Staffing Act
   of 2013, 182–183, 183b
Regulation, 167t
Rehabilitation group
   as health planning project, 113,
      113b
   intervention by aggregate/system
      level, 112t
   prevention for, 114t
Rehabilitation model, for disability,
   406
Reimbursement
   capitated, 213–214
   for home health care, 648
   prospective, 211–212

Relationships
 categories of, 227
 collateral, 227
 individual, 227
 interpersonal, 231b
 lineal, 227
 male-female, 234–235
 nurse-client, 232
Relative need, 110
Relative risk ratio, 78
Relevancy, principle of, 131t
Religion
 as community assessment
  parameter, 100t–101t
 culture and, 230–231
 diet and, 230
 fasting and, 230
 "Golden Rule" and, 231b
 healing and health, 633
 illness and, 243
 life and death, influence on, 231
 medical care, influence on, 231
 nurses and, 230
 spirituality and, 230–231
 stress and, 633
Religious affiliation, 243
Relocation, as psychosocial issue,
  359
Remarriage, 392
Renaissance, 22
Renal system, of older adult,
  361t–362t
Reproductive health, of men, 345b
Reproductive system, of older
  adult, 361t–362t
Research
 in case management, 161–162
 on gender differences, 344
 on health education and health
  screening in older men, 345b
 in international health, 279
 on medicalization of disability,
  407b
 occupational health nursing and,
  603b
 on physical dating violence, 544b
 for rural health, 462–464
 in school setting, 593
 in women's health, 334–335
Researcher, community health
  nurse as, 217
Reservoir
 controlling, 494
 definition/factors of, 493t
 eradicating, 494
 types of, 493
Residential services, for older
  adults, 357–358
Resistance, of host, 494–495
Resource map, for disasters, 561, 564f
Resources
 distribution of, 8b, 229
 for vaccine schedules, 498b
Respiratory system, of older adult,
  361t–362t
Respiratory therapist (RT), 193
Response stage, of disaster
  management, 571–578
Restaurant
 overweight and, 64
 portions in, 64

Retirement
 culturally defined, 231
 social status change with, 359
Retrospective reimbursement,
  210–211
Retrospective studies, 84–85, 85f,
  86b
Rheumatoid arthritis (RA), in
  women, 323–324
Risk, 77–78
 attributable, 78
 definition of, 56–57
 and health, relationship of,
  57–66
 types of, 57–58
Risk assessment, 57, 204b
Risk communication, 58
Risk factors, 71–72, 77–78
 alcohol as, 60
 coronary heart disease, 73b
 criteria for, 56
 for death, 59t
 diet as, 62
 insufficient sleep as, 65–66
 smoking as, 58
Risk map, for disasters, 561, 563f
Risk reduction
 definition of, 58
 health promotion and, 49–68,
  67b
Robert Wood Johnson Health
  Policy Fellowship, 183
Rockefeller Foundation, 27
Rockefeller Sanitary Commission
  for the Eradication of
  Hookworm, 27
Rogers, Linda, 29
Roles, within family, 390b, 391
Rome
 decline of, 21
 public health services in, 21b
Roosevelt, Franklin, 216
Roosevelt, Theodore, 216
Rubella, 500t–501t
Rural, 445
Rural aggregate
 agricultural workers as, 455–456
 migrant/seasonal farmworkers
  as, 456–457
Rural community
 classification of, 463b
 community participatory
  research in, 94b
 emergency preparedness of,
  460
 information technology in,
  462–463
Rural community health nursing,
  461–462
 characteristics of, 461–462
Rural health, 445–446
 leadership/workforce capacity
  for, 463–464
 legislation/programs affecting,
  460–461
 performance standards in, 463
 priorities, 462b
 theories/thinking upstream
  concepts to, application of,
  457
 upstream interventions for, 457

Rural health care delivery system,
  457–458
 community-based care, 458–460
 emergency services, 460
 faith communities/parish
  nursing, 459
 health care provider shortages,
  457–458
 informal care systems, 459
 managed care and, 458
 mental health care, 460
 new models of, 464
 public health department,
  459–460
Rural health disparities
 composition, 446–455, 447b
  related to persons, 449–454
 context, 446–455
  access to care, 447–449
  related to place, 446–449
Rural health research, 462–464
Rural Hospital Flexibility (RHF),
  461
Rural mental health care, 460
Rural nursing
 characteristics of, 461–462
 concept of, 461
Rural population
 defining, 445
 education/employment of,
  452–453, 453f
 emergency preparedness in, 460
 health care delivery system in,
  448, 457–458, 464
 health needs of, 446
 health risk, injury, and death,
  451–452
 income/poverty in, 449–451
 managed care for, 458
 suicide in, 454
 as uninsured, 449
 vulnerable groups in, 452
Rural poverty, 449–451, 449f, 450t
 children, 451
 family composition, 451
 racial/ethnic minorities, 451
 regional differences, 451
Rural public health departments,
  459–460
Rural United States, 444–446
 health of, 446
 population in, 444–445
 poverty in, 444
Rural-urban continuum, 445

S

Safe rides program
 as health planning project, 113,
  113b–114b
 prevention for, 114t
 problematic step for, 113t
Safety, and occupational health
  science, 599
Saffir-Simpson Hurricane Scale,
  563, 564b
Sandwich generation, 381, 381f
Sanitary Revolution, 22
Sanitation facilities, in developing
  countries, 273
Sarin (nerve agent), 562t
Schizophrenia, 474

School
 healthy environment in, 592
 registered nurses working in,
  580–581
 shelter-in-place instructions at,
  568t
 student health records in,
  582–583, 589
 terrorism and, 592
 violence in, 592
School-based health centers,
  305–306, 594
School health, 580–597
 history of, 581–582
 nursing process in, application
  of, 594b–595b
 selected objectives for, 583b
School Health Policies and
  Programs Study (SHPPS), school
  health services and, 582
School health programs
 components of, 583f
 family and community
  involvement in, 593
 for injury prevention, 584
 nutrition and, 590–591, 590b
  eating disorders and, 590
  education programs for, 591
  obesity and, 590–591
 for physical education, 586, 586b
 for sex education, 585–586
 staff involvement in, 593
 for substance abuse, 585
 for tobacco use, 584–585
School health services
 care of ill child in, 587–588
 for children with special health
  needs, 589, 589t
 definition of, 582
 emergency care as, 587
 health screenings as, 587
 immunizations as, 586–587
 medication administration as,
  588–589
School nurses, 580–581, 596b
 delegation of tasks by, 590
 emergency preparedness and,
  569b
 families, working with, 386, 388b
 function of, 593
 future issues affecting, 594–596
 role in prevention, 595t
 in twentieth century, 29
School nursing
 definition of, 593b
 research priorities in, 594b
Scientific theory, 27b
Screening
 public health intervention, 15t
 purpose of, 79–81
Screening program, 80
 guidelines for, 80b
 outreach, launching, 134b
Search and rescue, 571
Seasonal farmworkers, 456–457
 enumeration of, 456
 hearing, 456–457
 preventive care for, 456
Secondary prevention, 7–8, 7t,
  78, 111
 case management for, 161

Secondary prevention (Continued)
of communicable diseases, 510
for disasters, 561
for health planning project, 114t
of infectious disease, 512t
for men's health, 349
health services for, 349
screening services for, 349
school nurse role in, 595t
strategies for occupational health
nurse, 606–607
substance abuse and, 526
for system levels, 115t
of violence, 553–554, 554t
women's health and, 332–334
Secondary vaccine failure, 495
Seeds of disease, 22
Self-actualization, and disability,
417
Self-care deficit theory, 40
application of, 40
Self-concept, adult learners and,
127t
Self-efficacy, 55t, 127t
definition of, 126
learner verification and, 144t
Self-esteem, exercise and, 65
Self-insurance, 215
Senior health, 355–379, 377b
Sensitivity, screening program,
80, 81t
Sensory impairment, in older adult,
365–366
Service learning, 283b
definition of, student responses
for, 284b
Service Learning Questionnaire,
student and provider responses
to, 284t
Serving, 62
Settled village stage in disease
history, 19f, 20
Seventh-Day Adventism, dietary
practice of, 230t
Severe mental illness (SMI), 469
Sex, disability prevalence by, 410
Sex education, as school health
program, 585–586
Sexual abuse, 548
definition of, 621
indicators of, 548t
signs of, 592b
Sexual Assault Nurse Examiner
(SANE), 617–618
evidence collected by, 617b
requirements for, 618
Sexual harassment, in women, 330
Sexually transmitted diseases
(STDs)
as epidemic, 345b
Healthy People 2020 and, 491b,
506–507
substance abuse and, 536
transmission and control of,
508t–509t
in women, 328
Sexually transmitted infections
(STIs)
in adolescents, 299
intervention for, 124b–125b
types of, 299

Shaken baby syndrome, 547
Shaner, Hollie, 266
Shattuck, Lemuel, 23
Shelter-in-place
American Red Cross and, 568
disaster management and, 571
instructions, 568t
"Shoe leather epidemiology," 95
Short Assessment of Health
Literacy for Spanish-speaking
Adults (SAHLSA), 143
Sibling relationship, 228
Sick building syndrome, 258
Sidewalks in disrepair,
environmental health issues,
255b
Silence, as nonverbal
communication, 233
Simple phobia, 476
Single agent theory, 27b
Single Item Literacy Screener
(SILS), 143
Single parent family, 227, 301
increase in, 383–384
percentage by ethnic group of,
384t
risks associated with, 383–384
Single specialty group, 187
Sixteenth century, life in English
household in, 21b
Slavery, alcohol during, 535
Sleep
drowsy driving and, 66
health and, 65–66
interruptions of, 66
older adult and, 361t–362t
requirements for, 65f
Sleep assessment, 66
Sleep hygiene, 66
Smallpox
as bioterrorism agent, 561b
eradication of, 496
Smokeless tobacco, 60
youth using, 584
Smoking
in adolescents, 584
health risk and, 58
during pregnancy, 291
prevalence of, 58
school health program for, 584
Smoking cessation, 205
steps to, 58
withdrawals and, 58
Snow, John, 23
Social, 3
Social action, 22
family health intervention
extending to, 394–397
Social capital
environmental health and,
253
health education and, 131t
Social changes, community health
nursing and, 31–32
Social classes, 229
Social consequences, of substance
abuse, 516
Social demography, 347b
Social distance, 232t
Social environment, 53
Social epidemiology, 347b

Social factors
influencing mental health,
471–472
for substance abuse, 535
Social institution, 53
Social justice
community-based practice and,
45b
ethical issues in, 133b
versus market justice, 347b
market justice versus, health care
for homeless, 438–439
model for, 438–439
Social learning theory, 125
Social marketing, public health
intervention, 15t
Social media, 148
and cancer care, 148
Social network framework, 395
Social orientation, 227
Social phobia, 476
Social policy, 167
Social problems, as community
assessment parameter,
100t–101t
Social readjustment rating scale,
481f
Social science, 599
Social Security, as older adult
income source, 358
Social Security Act, 173, 216
women's health and, 330
Social Security Amendments
PL 98-21, 158
prospective payment system
(PPS), 158
Social Security Disability Insurance
(SSDI), 414b
Social services, for children,
591–592
Social status, of older adult, 359
Social system, 94
Social worker (SW), 193
Socialization, explaining sex
differences in health, 343–344
Societal beliefs, 206
Societal perceptions, in health
care, 216
Society, aging of, in economics and
health care, 206
Society is focus of change, 41–45,
43t
Socioeconomic class, 229
Socioeconomic conditions
child and adolescent health and,
301
infant death and, 288
Socioeconomic status (SES)
calculation of, 229
culture and, 228
education and, 229
health status and, 229
Solo practice, of a physician, 187
Solution, community of, 93
Somatic mutation theory, 356b
South Africa, Team Reach Out in,
283b
Sovereign power, 169–170
Space
as culturally appropriate, 232
functional use of, 232t

Special designation, and disability,
417
Special health needs, children with,
589, 589t
Special Supplemental Nutrition
Program for Women, Infants,
and Children, 306
Specific protection, 78
Specificity
cause-and-effect relationship, 79
screening program, 80, 81t
Speech-language pathologist, 193
Spiritual distress, 638
Spiritual needs assessment, 231b
Spirituality
childhood and, 231
faith community nurse and, 633
nurses and, 230
in older adults, 373–374
religion and, 230–231
Spit tobacco, 60
Spontaneous generation theory, of
disease causation, 24
Sports safety, 584
Stabilization, pharmacotherapy
and, 529
Stalking, 546
Standardization, of rates, 76
"Standards of Practice for
Culturally Competent Nursing
Care," 221
Staphylococcus aureus, tattoos and
body piercings linked to, 586
START triage system, 572
State Child Health Improvement
Act (SCHIP) of 1997, 175
State government
disaster responsibilities of, 565
home health care and, 647
State legislatures, role of, 176
State-level subsystem, 190–191
activities of, 191
Statistical data, collection of, 97
Statistical methods, 24
Florence Nightingale and, 26b
Status, distribution of, 229
Statutes, 167
Steroids use, 521, 534b
Stewart, Ada Mayo, 599
Stimulants, 523t
Stimulus-response (S-R)
conditioning, 124
Strengths of family or individual,
commending, 386
Streptococcus, 26
Stress
as gender-linked behavior, 345
and religion, 633
warning signs of, 591b
in women, 326–327
Structural-Functional Conceptual
Framework, 390–391
Student learning activity, 411b,
415b
Student records, 589
Subclinical infection, 491–492
Subcultural group
definition of, 224–225
types of, 225
Subculture, 225
Subject, assuming role of, 129

Substance abuse, 515–541, 540b
abstinence and, 527
in adolescent, 519, 533–534
conceptualizations of, 522
definition of, 522
denial, 537
diagnosis of, 522
dual diagnosis and, 535–536
in elderly, 534
ethnocultural considerations for, 535, 536b
etiology of, 516–517
as gender-linked behavior, 345
health care professionals and, 532
homeless population and, 434–435
from initiation to dependency, 524
legal and ethical concerns with, 525
modes of intervention, 525–531, 530t
nursing perspective on, 536–540
nursing process, application of, 538b–539b
in older adult, 371–372
during pregnancy, 534
prevalence of, 517–521
prevention of, 526
professional enablers of, 532–533
school health program for, 585
sexually transmitted diseases (STDs), 536
social consequences of, 516
social network involvement for family and friends, 531–532
sociocultural and political aspects of, 522–524
stage of, 524
substance dependence versus, 522
treatment for, 526–529
detoxification, 527
guidelines for, 528b
harm reduction as, 531
inpatient and outpatient programs for, 527
measuring effectiveness of, 529b
mutual help groups, 530
pharmacotherapies and, 529–530
trends in, 520–521
vulnerable aggregates, 533–536
in women, 534–535
Substance Abuse and Mental Health Services Administration, 190b
Substance dependence
diagnostic criteria for, 522
substance abuse versus, 522
Subsystem
definition of, 389t
health care system as, 94
prevention levels for, 115t
Sudden infant death syndrome (SIDS)
"Back to Sleep" campaign for, 293b
infant death and, 292
smoking and, 291

Sudden unexplained infant death (SUID), 292
Suicide, 477–478, 544
in adolescent, 591b
in older adult, 372
prevention of
and referral resources, 479t
strategy for, 473b
protective factors and risk factors for, 477, 478b
risk factors of, 544
warning signs for, 477, 478b, 478t
Sulfur dioxide, sources and effects of, 256t
Summative evaluation, 112
Supplemental Security Income (SSI), 414b
eligibility, 414b
Suprachiasmatic nucleus (SCN), 66
Suprasystem
definition of, 389t
prevention levels for, 115t
Surveillance, 81–82, 82b
public health intervention, 15t
Survey of Income and Program Participation (SIPP), 409
Symbolic interactionism, 44
Syndrome, sick building, 258
Syphilis, transmission and control of, 508t–509t
System
definition of, 389t
hierarchy of, 389t
Systems framework premises, 109b
Systems interrelationships, example of, 94b
Systems theory, 388–390
definitions from, 389t

T

Tabun (nerve agent), 562t
Tafelsig Community Health Center, 283b
Taoism, "Golden Rule" and, 231b
Tattoos, 586
Tax Equity and Fiscal Responsibility Act of 1982, 175
Teaching-learning format, for health education, 135t
Team Reach Out
in South Africa, 283b
student reflections on, 284t
Technology literacy, 177–178
Teen dating violence, 300
Teen parenting, 227–228
Teen pregnancy
birth rate by ethnicity, 384t
rate of, 585b
rise in, 383–384
Telehealth, 197–198, 206, 458, 463
Telemedicine, 458
Temporally correct relationship, cause-and-effect relationship, 79
Term birth, 288b
Terminally ill, hospice home care for, 655
Terrorism
as community violence, 551
as disaster, 560
effects of, 273

Terrorism (Continued)
events of, 560
and schools, 592
weapons of mass destruction as, 560
Tertiary prevention, 7t, 8, 78, 111
case management for, 161
of communicable diseases, 510
for disasters, 561
for health planning project, 114t
of infectious disease, 512t
for men's health, 349–353
community care, new concepts of, 350–353
sex-role and lifestyle rehabilitation, 349–350
school nurse role in, 595t
strategies for occupational health nurse, 607
for system levels, 115t
of violence, 554, 554t
women's health and, 332–334
Test of Functional Health Literacy in Adults (TOFHLA), 142–143
Testicular cancer, 345b
Tetanus, 500t–501t
Textile industry
as health planning project, 113, 113b
intervention by aggregate/system level, 112t
prevention for, 114t
The Substance Abuse and Mental Health Services Administration (SAMHSA), 517
Themba Care Orphanage, 283b
Theoretical scope, 39
Theory
definition of, 38, 38b
goal of, 38
of men's health, 342–346
biological factors, 343
data interpretation, 344
socialization, 343–344
Theory-based practice, 38
Theory of planned behavior, 57f
Theory of Reasoned Action (TRA), 55–56
example of, 57f
Therapeutic conversation, 385
Therapeutic questions, 385
Therapeutic relationship, 385
Thinking upstream, 36–48
focus of, 37
poor health, causes of, 37
society is focus of change, 41–45
theory of, 36–48, 47b
Ticket to Work and Work Incentives Improvement Act (TWWIIA), 413, 414b
Time orientation, 226–227
Tissue/organ donation/transplantation, 620–621
To Err Is Human: Building a Safer Health System, 194
Tobacco
actual causes of death, 4–5
in adolescents, 300
clinical implications of, 60
death from, 274
economic value of, 524

Tobacco (Continued)
as gender-linked behavior, 345
and health risk, 58–60, 60b
school health program for, 584–585
see also Smoking
Tobacco control, 274
Tobacco Free Initiative, 274
Tobacco-free policy, 274
Tobacco Laboratory Network, 274
Tornado, 573b–574b
Tornado scale, 563
Touch, as cross-cultural communication, 234
Toxic chemical, in water treatment, 258–259
Toxicology, and occupational health science, 599
Toy-related injuries, 296b
Tracking, child and adolescent well-being, 303
Traditional healer, 27
Transactional model, 395–396
Transcultural nursing, 223–224
definition of, 223
Transition stage of addiction, 524, 525t
Transmission
breaking chain of, 494–495
controlling agent, 494
reservoir, eradicating, 494
chain of, 492–494
for infectious agents, 492–493
links of, 492f, 493t
mode of
definition/factors of, 493t
direct transmission, 493
indirect transmission, 493
Transportation, as community assessment parameter, 100t–101t
Transtheoretical model (TTM), 54
change and, 54
constructs and descriptions of, 56t
example of, 57f
Trash production/disposal, 261
Traumatic brain injury (TBI)
in adolescents, 293
in older adult, 367
Traumatic event, responses to, 578t
Treaty, 167t
Treaty of Geneva, 166
Trust, building of, in home care visits, 651
Truth, Sojourner, 166
Tsunami
death from, 562
example of, 573b–574b
Tubercle bacillus (TB), 26
Tuberculosis (TB)
incidence of, 489
prevalence of, 274
in prisons, 623
transmission of, 494, 506t
Tularemia, as bioterrorism agent, 561b
Tuskegee Syphilis Study, 86b–87b
Twelve-step programs
Alcoholics Anonymous (AA) as, 530
tenets of, 530b

Twentieth century
  attitudes toward people with disabilities, 408
  community health nursing and, 31b–32b
  school nurses in, 29
Twenty-first century, mortality in, 30
"Two diseases, one patient" strategy, 274

U

Underage drinking
  clinical implications of, 61
  prevalence of, 61
  prevention of, 61
Uninsured children, 581, 581t
Uninsured population
  children as, 304
  increase in, 432–433
  in rural areas, 449
United Nations (UN), 275
United Nations International Children's Emergency Fund (UNICEF), 277
United States
  drug prohibition and, 525
  epidemic disease in, 23
  health status in, 206
  infant mortality in, 288, 289t
  laboratory and clinical research in, 206
  plague in, 22b
  rural areas in, 444–446
  status, power and wealth in, 229
  structure of the government of the, 169–171
Universal coverage, societal perceptions, 216
Universal health care, 192b
Unlicensed assistive personnel (UAP), 194
Upstream thinking. see Thinking upstream
Urban sprawl, 253
Urbanization, world population growth and, 273
Urinary incontinence, 366
U.S. Census Bureau
  homeless population and
    early efforts of, 431
    recent efforts of, 431
  household income, 434
  purpose of, 97
  see also Census
U.S. Department of Agriculture (USDA), 63
  My Plate by, 63–64, 64f
U.S. Department of Health and Human Services (USDHHS), 277
  governmental grants by, 209
  homeless and, definition of, 431
  poverty guidelines of, 444b
  structure of, 190b
U.S. Department of Homeland Security
  disaster management and, 565–566
  FEMA and, 566
  mission of, 565
  security advisory system, 566

U.S. Department of Housing and Urban Development
  homeless and, definition of, 430
Utilization review
  case management and, 157
  definition of, 204b

V

Vaccination
  definition of, 497
  development of, 296–297
  discovery of, 22
  failure of, 495
  immunity from, 495
  schedules for, 498b
  for travelers, 499
Vaccines
  administration of, 498
  documentation of, 499
  hypersensitivity and contraindications of, 498–499
  and infectious disease prevention, 497–499
  needs for special groups, 499
  preparation of, 498
  related injuries and, 499
  spacing of, 498
  storage, transport, and handling of, 498
  types of, 498, 499t
Vaccine Adverse Event Reporting System (VAERS), 499
Vaccine-preventable diseases, 297, 489
  transmission and control of, 500t–501t
  types of, 498b
Value
  culture and, 225–226
  imposing on others, 223–224
  norms and, 225–226
Value orientation, 226
  perspectives of, 227
Vector-borne diseases, 262
Vectors, 493–494
Vegetables, USDA recommendations for, 63
Vehicle, shelter-in-place instructions at, 568t
Verbal communication
  focus of, 390
  importance of, 232
Verbalization, spiritual needs assessment and, 231b
Very preterm birth, 288b
Veterans
  epidemiological examination of suicide among, 90b
  as homeless, 433, 434b
Veteran's health, 606b
Violence, 542–557, 556b
  in children and adolescents, 300
  drug, 545
  factors influencing, 551–552
    firearms, 552
    media, 552
    mental illness, 552
  Healthy People 2020 and, 552
  objectives related to injury, 552b
  history of, 543–544

Violence (Continued)
  interpersonal, 544–549
    versus community violence, 549
    homicide and suicide, 544
    intimate partner violence, 544–546
  in nursery rhymes, 543
  overview of, 543
  power and control wheel, 547f
  prevention of, 552–554, 553b, 554t
    primary, 553
    secondary, 553–554
    tertiary, 554
  in prisons, 551
  from public health perspective, 552
  in schools, 592
  victims of, considerations for working with, 545b
  wife beating, 543–544
  see also Community violence; Dating violence; Domestic abuse
Virchow, Rudolf, 22
Vision
  cataract and, 365
  glaucoma and, 365–366
  macular degeneration and, 365
Visiting Nurse Association, 28
Vital statistics
  data in, 98–99
  "hidden pockets" of need, 99b
Vital statistics, collection of, 23
Voluntary agencies
  classification of, 188
  future of, 188
  private health care subsystem and, 188
  services provided by, 188
Vulnerable populations, care of, 621–622, 622b
VX nerve agent, 562t

W

Wakefield, Mary, 181–182
Wald, Lillian, 166
  case management programs and, 156
  "community as client," 107, 107f
  home visiting, 646
  House on Henry Street and, 28, 29b
  National Organization for Public Health Nursing and, 29–30
Walking, 65
War, effects of, 273
"War on Drugs," 526
Warts, 508t–509t
Waste incineration, 261
Waste management
  environmental health and, 261, 261b
  definition, 252t
  problems, 252t
  medical, 266
  recycling as, 261
  trash production/disposal and, 261

Water pollution, 273
  environmental health issues, 255b
Water quality
  environmental health and, 258–259, 259b
  definition, 252t
  problems, 252t
  water treatment technologies in, 258
Water treatment technologies, 258
Wealth, distribution of, 229
Weapons of mass destruction, types of, 560
  biological organisms as, 562t
  chemical warfare agents as, 562t
Wear-and-tear theory, 356b
Weather patterns, 263
Web of causation, 71–72, 73f
Welfare Reform Act of 1996, 175
Well-being
  poverty influencing, 228–229
  and religion, 633
West Nile virus, 262
Westberg, Reverend Granger, 633
Wheel model, of human-environment interaction, 70–71, 73f
White Anglo-Saxon Protestant (WASP), 226
White population
  children as, 287, 287f
  countries of origin for, 226
  culture-bound syndrome in, 237t
Who Will Keep the Public Healthy?, 195–196
Wide Range Achievement Test, Level IV, 142
Widowhood, 359
Wife beating, 543–544
Wildfire, 573b–574b
Windshield survey
  example of, 96b
  purpose of, 95
  questions for, 98b
Withdrawal syndromes, 516
  detoxification and, 527
Women
  breast cancer, 324–325, 325b
  cancer in, 317–318
  cardiovascular disease in, 316–317
  chronic conditions/limitations of, 320
  chronic illness in, 323–327
    arthritis, 323–324
    coronary vascular disease/metabolic syndrome, 323
    diabetes, 318, 323
    hypertension, 323
  death, cause of, 317t
  disability and, 329
  education/work for, 321, 321t
  employment/wages of, 321, 321t
  family configuration/marital status of, 322
  gynecological cancers, 326
  health and safety issues, 605
  health care access for, 321
  health promotion strategies for, 322–329

Women (*Continued*)
  as homeless, 433
    with children, 437
    factors contributing to,
      436–437
    health status of, 436–437
  hospitalization of, 320
  human immunodeficiency virus
    and acquired immunodefi-
    ciency syndrome in, 328
  lung cancer, 325–326
  maternal mortality in, 318–319,
    319b, 319t
  mental disorders/stress in,
    326–327
  mental health of, 320
  nutrition of, 328
  as older adult, physiological
    changes, 361t–362t
  osteoporosis, 324
  in prison, 623–624
  reproductive health of, 327–328
  sexually transmitted diseases
    in, 328
  substance abuse in, 534–535
  surgery for, 320
  working, and home life of,
    321–322, 322t
Women, Infants, and Children
  (WIC), 161, 306
Women for Sobriety, 530

Women's health, 314–338
  community health nurse, roles
    of, in, 334
    counselor, 334
    direct care, 334
    educator, 334
  community voluntary services
    for, 332
  health/social services to
    promote, 331–332, 331b
  legislation affecting, 329–331
    Civil Rights Act, 330
    Family and Medical Leave Act,
      330–331
    Occupational Safety and
      Health Act, 330, 331t
    Public Health Service Act, 330
    Social Security Act, 330
  levels of prevention and,
    332–334
    primary prevention, 332
    secondary prevention,
      332–334
    tertiary prevention, 332–334
  major indicators of, 315–320
    life expectancy, 316
    mortality rate, 316–319, 316b
  in the military, 316b
  nursing process, application of,
    332b–334b
  objectives for, 315b

Women's health (*Continued*)
  research in, 334–335
  social factors affecting, 321–322
  unintentional injury/accidents
    and domestic violence, 329,
    329b
  working with, 327b
Women's health services, 331
Work, shelter-in-place instructions
  at, 568t
Work Incentives Improvement Act,
  Ticket to Work and (TWWIIA),
  413, 414b
Work-related diseases/injuries,
  606t
Work-related exposure,
  environmental health and,
  254–256, 256b
  definition, 252t
  problems, 252t
Workers' Compensation Act, 611
Workplace violence, 549–550
World Bank, 277
World Framework Convention on
  Tobacco Control, 274
World Health Organization
  (WHO), 168
  3 by 5 Initiative, 274
  collaborating centers in nursing,
    279
  Declaration of Alma-Ata, 275

World Health Organization
  (*Continued*)
  disability and, 404
  in environmental health,
    266–268
  goal of, 275
  health, definition of, 50
  primary care *vs.* primary
    prevention, 192b
  "two diseases, one patient"
    strategy, 274
  violence, definition of, 543
World population
  distribution of, 273
  growth and urbanization, 273
World Trade Center, bombings
  of, 559
  picture of, 573b–574b

Y

Yin-yang theory, 235–236
Youth
  health status of, 437–438
  at risk, 581b
Youth-related violence, 550
  risk factors for, 551t
Youth Risk Behavior Surveillance
  System, 298
Youth Risk Behavior Survey
  System, 584
  purposes of, 584b

SPECIAL FEATURES

CASE STUDY APPLICATION OF THE NURSING PROCESS

Using an Epidemiological and Public Health Approach to Managing a Food-Borne Outbreak (Chapter 5), pp. 88-89

Assessment and Diagnosis (Chapter 6), pp. 103-104

School Bilingual Program (Chapter 7), pp. 119-120

Selected Teaching Approaches and Learning Needs (Chapter 8), pp. 145-146

Comprehensive Case Management Program (Chapter 9), pp. 162-163

Asian Family and Cultural Practices (Chapter 13), pp. 246-247

Air Pollution (Chapter 14), pp. 266-268

International Community Assessment Model (ICAM): A Collaborative Model for Community Assessment, Education, and Health Care Delivery (Chapter 15), pp. 281-282

Team Reach Out South Africa (Chapter 15), pp. 283

Pregnant Teenager (Chapter 16), pp. 309-311

Pregnant Inmate in a Correctional Facility (Chapter 17), pp. 332-334

Gender-Appropriate Care for Men (Chapter 18), pp. 351-353

75-Year-Old Widow (Chapter 19), pp. 375-377

Student Absenteeism (Chapter 20), pp. 399-400

Client with Progressive Swallowing Difficulties (Chapter 21), pp. 424-426

Client with Mental Illness (Chapter 24), pp. 485-486

Employee with a Communicable Disease (Chapter 25), pp. 512-514

Client with an Alcohol Abuse Problem and Hepatitis C (Chapter 26), pp. 538-539

Domestic Violence (Chapter 27), pp. 555-556

Coastal City: Preparedness for a Disaster (Chapter 28), pp. 576-578

Student with Lice (Chapter 29), pp. 594-595

Employee Exposure to Chemicals (Chapter 30), pp. 613-614

Correctional Nursing (Chapter 31), pp. 626-627

Forensic Nursing (Chapter 31), pp. 627-628

Needs Assessment of a Faith Community (Chapter 32), pp. 641-643

Public Health Visit: Communicable Disease Follow-Up (Chapter 33), pp. 656-658

Public Health Home Visit: Antepartum Client (Chapter 33), pp. 658-659

Hospice Home Visit (Chapter 33), pp. 659-660

HEALTHY PEOPLE 2020 *Objectives Related to*

Data Collection and Reporting (Chapter 5), p. 81

Public Policy (Chapter 10), p. 169

Cultural Health (Chapter 13), p. 222

Environmental Health (Chapter 14), p. 264

Child and Adolescent Health (Chapter 16), pp. 303

Women's Health (Chapter 17), p. 315

Family Planning (Chapter 17), p. 327

Older Adults (Chapter 19), p. 360

Access to Health Care (Chapter 20), p. 387

Social Determinants of Health (Chapter 22), p. 431

Rural Health Priorities (Chapter 23), p. 462

Mental Illness and Health (Chapter 24), p. 471

Communicable Disease (Chapter 25), p. 491

Substance Abuse (Chapter 26), p. 520

Violence (Chapter 27), p. 552

School Health (Chapter 29), p. 583

Occupational Health (Chapter 30), p. 604

Forensic Nursing (Chapter 31), p. 617

Faith Community Nursing (Chapter 32), p. 635

Home Health and Hospice Care (Chapter 33), p. 646

RESEARCH HIGHLIGHTS

Public Health Nursing Research Agenda (Chapter 1), p. 10

Understanding the Health Experiences of Homeless Populations (Chapter 3), p. 47

Reducing Infant Mortality Rates Using the Perinatal Periods of Risk Model (Chapter 5), p. 82

Using Community Participatory Research to Assess a Substance Use in a Rural Community (Chapter 6), p. 94

What about the Children Playing Sports? Pesticide Use on Athletic Fields (Chapter 7), p. 112

Linking Theory to Practice: An Example of a Sexually Transmitted Infection/Human Immunodeficiency Virus Risk Reduction Intervention in a Primary Care Setting (Chapter 8), p. 124

Geriatric Care Management for Low-Income Seniors: A Randomized Controlled Trial (Chapter 9), p. 162

National Sample of Registered Nurses (Chapter 10), p. 183

Hospital Readmissions from Home Health Care Before and After Prospective Payment (Chapter 12), p. 213

Nutritional Patterns of Recent Immigrants (Chapter 13), p. 241

I PREPARE: Development and Clinical Utility of an Environmental Exposure History Mnemonic (Chapter 14), p. 262